Game/Set/Match

A Tennis Guide 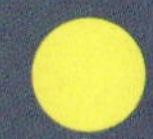 Fifth Edition

James E. Bryant, Ed.D.
San Jose State University

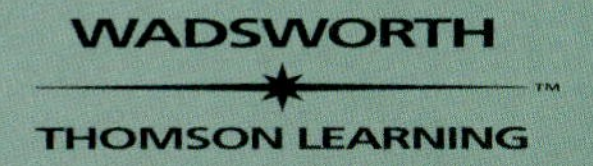

Australia • Canada • Mexico • Singapore • Spain • United Kingdom • United States

WADSWORTH
THOMSON LEARNING™

Publisher: Peter Marshall
Associate Editor: April Lemons
Assistant Editor: John Boyd
Editorial Assistant: Andrea Kesterke
Marketing Manager: Joanne Terhaar
Project Editor: Sandra Craig
Print Buyer: Mary Noel
Permissions Editor: Stephanie Keough
Production and Composition: Ash Street Typecrafters, Inc.
Text and Cover Designer: Harry Voigt
Copy Editor: Kristi McRae
Cover Image: Joe McBride/© Tony Stone Images
Printer: Transcontinental Printing

Printed in Canada
2 3 4 5 6 7 04 03 02 01

Library of Congress Cataloging-in-Publication Data

Bryant, James E.
Game, set, match: a tennis guide / James E. Bryant.—5th ed.
p. cm.
Includes index.
ISBN 0-534-57146-8
1. Tennis—Handbooks, manuals, etc. I. Title.

GV995 .B77 2001
796.342—dc21

00-43974

Wadsworth/Thomson Learning
10 Davis Drive
Belmont, CA 94002-3098
USA

For more information about our products, contact us:
Thomson Learning Academic Resource Center
1-800-423-0563
http://www.wadsworth.com

International Headquarters
Thomson Learning
International Division
290 Harbor Drive, 2nd Floor
Stamford, CT 06902-7477
USA

UK/Europe/Middle East/South Africa
Thomson Learning
Berkshire House
168-173 High Holborn
London WC1V 7AA
United Kingdom

Asia
Thomson Learning
60 Albert Street, # 15-0 1
Albert Complex
Singapore 189969

Canada
Nelson Thomson Learning
1120 Birchmount Road
Toronto, Ontario M1K 5G4
Canada

Contents

Preface

This fifth edition of *Game, Set, Match . . . A Tennis Guide,* is written primarily for the beginning or novice tennis player, but it is also appropriate for the intermediate player. It is for students who are actively receiving instruction and who plan on continuing to play tennis as a lifelong activity.

New features will enhance the learning experience of players. There is an extensive revision of the Physical Aspects of Playing Tennis chapter, a more detailed explanation regarding the two-hand backhand groundstroke, and a reorganization of several chapters to provide a better continuity of reading. Photographs and diagrams have been updated, adding improved clarity and perception for the reader. The USTA Tennis Rules have been replaced with USTA's The Code. The Player's Guide for Unofficial Matches. The *Instructor's Guide* has been revised to assist the instructor in coordinating use of the book with the practical experience of learning to play the game on the tennis court.

Tennis is a highly popular sport played at all levels of skill and by people of all ages. It requires a strong foundation of skill, an in-depth comprehension of the intricacy of the flow of the game, and an insight into the rules of play. It is a game played at an intense level of competition by some and in a spirit of enjoyment by all who understand that tennis is a game. Tennis, as played today, is a never-ending learning experience for the player. It is a complex game that, when played and practiced over the years, becomes surprisingly simple and yet always remains challenging.

Game, Set, Match provides players with a visual and written analysis of tennis. Students will profit from reading the descriptions of the skills and reviewing the photographs to gain a mental image of execution of the skill. They also will gain from reading and understanding how physical fitness and mental preparation are critical to their improvement and development as a player.

The two strategies chapters provide a base for development of thinking on the court, and the tennis court behavior and interpretation of rules section will enable the student to make sense of the intangibles of tennis. And, a chapter combining the tennis court, equipment, and tournament play and resources will aid students in understanding the fringe parts of the game.

This material is a guide for the tennis player who is receiving instruction through a course or private lessons, or who is simply attempting to learn to play the game. I hope everyone who reads and studies this book will continue to grow with the game and reap its rewards through the years.

James E. Bryant, Ed. D.

Acknowledgments

Since 1986 individuals have contributed to the continual development of *Game, Set, Match* as reviewers, models, illustrators, and as sources to provide as complete and accurate of a book as possible. I want to extend a personal thank you to all those who have in some way permitted me to gain from their knowledge and talents in order to write a book for the beginning tennis player that allows for skill development and growth. In particular, I want to convey a thank you to my former students who have given feedback and served as a true test for the practicality and applicability for the book.

Specifically, I want to thank those who have been instrumental in the development of this fifth edition. Photographers Kevin Sam and Eric Risberg, who created the quality photographs that show tennis skill at its best. Mark Newton and Fred Safpoir who assisted in finding facilities and models. In addition, I extend a thank you to the Walnut Creek Tennis Club, Walnut Creek, California and Cupertino Tennis Center, Cupertino, California, who provided facilities for the photographs. And finally, a major thank you goes to Heidi Kromschroder and Shane Velez, college tennis players, Anh-Dao Nguyen, San Jose State University Women's Tennis Coach, and John Hubbell, Northern California USTA Coordinator who not only performed the proper skills as models but also asked questions and made suggestions that truly enhanced the overall development of the book.

James E. Bryant, Ed. D.

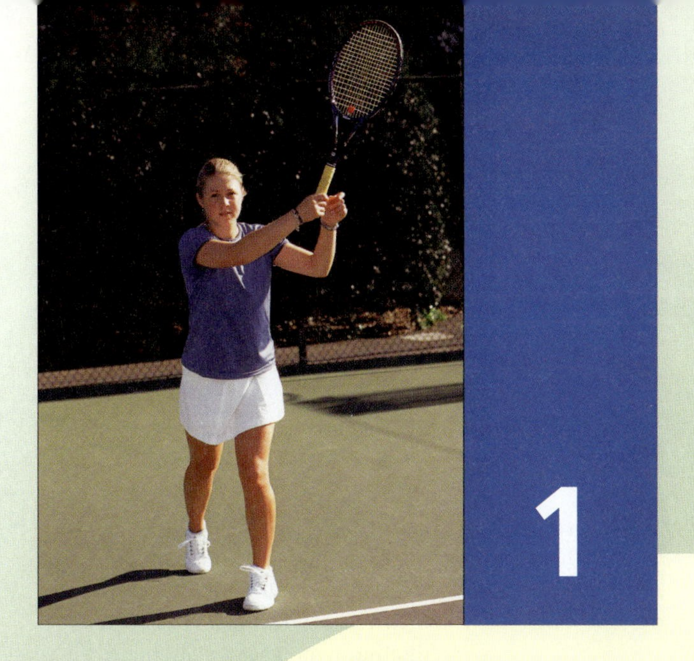

1

The Preliminaries to the Strokes in Tennis

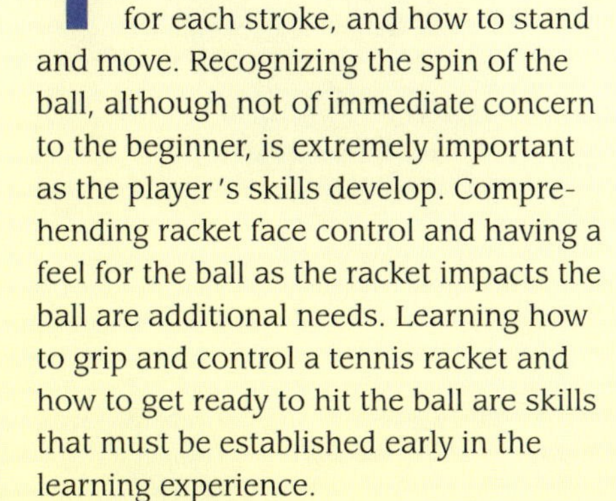

To play tennis, a person has to know how to hold a tennis racket for each stroke, and how to stand and move. Recognizing the spin of the ball, although not of immediate concern to the beginner, is extremely important as the player's skills develop. Comprehending racket face control and having a feel for the ball as the racket impacts the ball are additional needs. Learning how to grip and control a tennis racket and how to get ready to hit the ball are skills that must be established early in the learning experience.

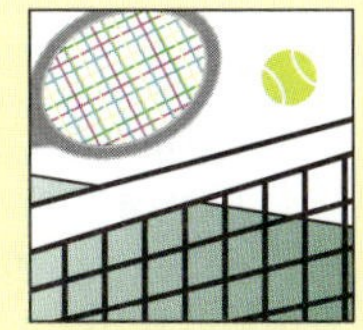

Basic Tennis Grips

The tennis grip used when hitting a particular stroke is directly related to execution of that stroke. Selecting a tennis grip that fits the stroke is necessary to complete the stroke with acceptable form.

The *eastern forehand grip*, a universally used grip designed for executing the forehand groundstroke, is also called the "shake hands" grip (Figures 1.1–1.3). Place your racket hand on the strings of the racket, and bring your hand straight down to the grip. As your hand grasps the racket grip, your fingers will be spread along the length of the racket grip with the index finger spread the farthest in a "trigger finger" style, providing control. The thumb will be situated on the back side of the racket, and the thumb and four fingers will form a "V" on the racket grip. The "V" points to the racket shoulder when the player holds the racket in front at a right angle to the body.

The *eastern backhand grip* is a conventional backhand grip used extensively in tennis (Figures 1.4–1.5). From the eastern forehand grip, roll your hand over the top of the racket grip and place your thumb diagonally across the rear plane of the racket grip. You should be able to see all four knuckles of the racket hand from this position when holding the racket perpendicular to the body. The "V" formed by the thumb and fingers will point to the non-racket shoulder when the racket is held in front of the body.

The *continental forehand grip* and *continental backhand grip* are essentially the same (Figures

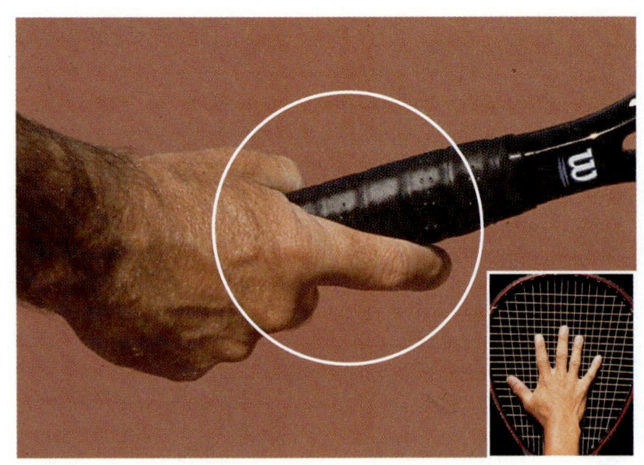

Figure 1.1 "Trigger-finger" position.

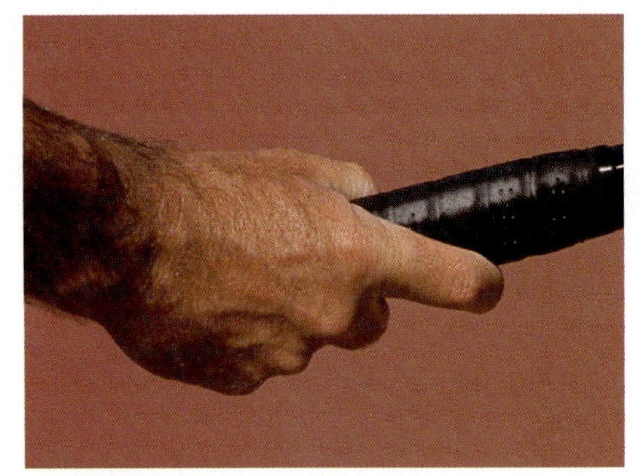

Figure 1.2 Eastern forehand grip (back view).

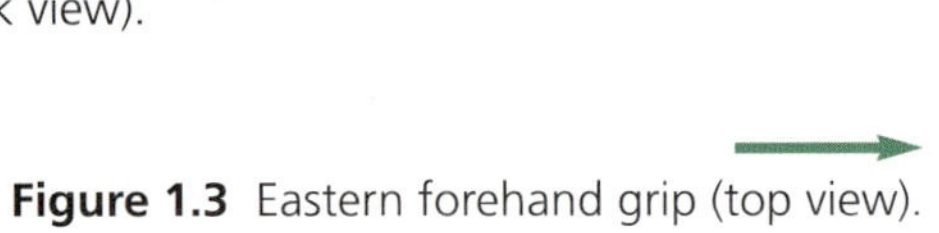

Figure 1.3 Eastern forehand grip (top view).

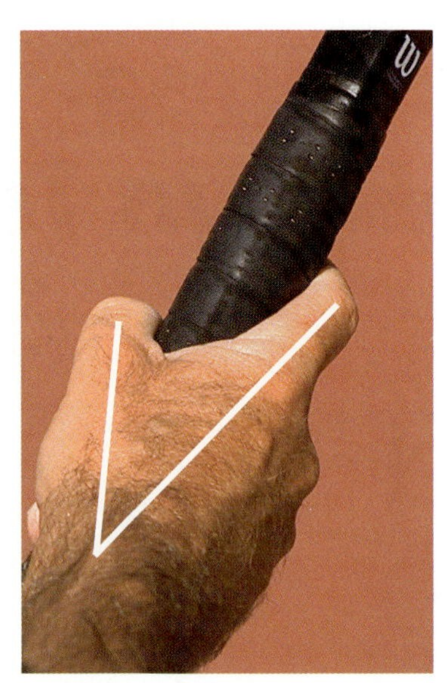

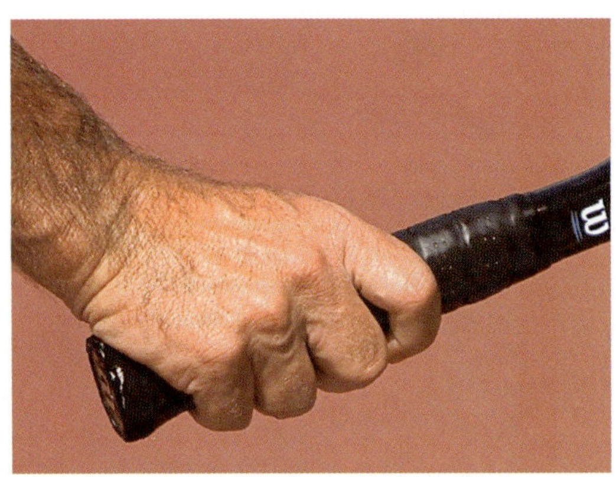

Figure 1.4 Eastern backhand grip (front view).

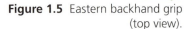

Figure 1.5 Eastern backhand grip (top view).

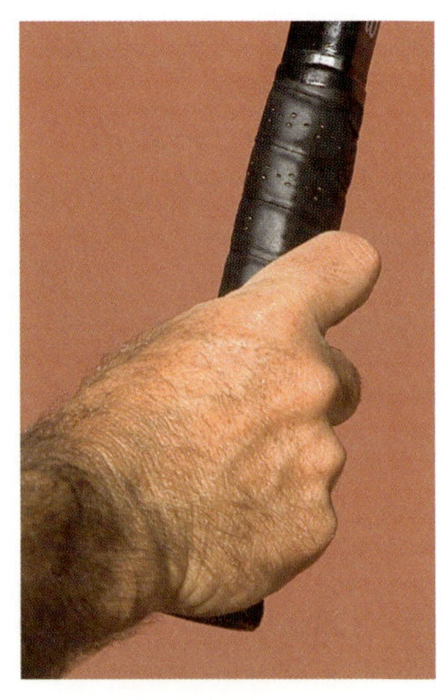

1.6–1.7). They differ from the eastern forehand and backhand grips in that the hand is placed midway between the positioning of the two eastern grips. The "V" formed by the thumb and fingers points to the middle or center of the body halfway between the racket and non-racket sides of the body when the racket is held in front of the body. The subtle difference between the forehand and backhand placement of the hands for the continental grip is that, in the forehand grip, the thumb grasps the racket grip, whereas in the backhand, the thumb is placed diagonally across the rear of the racket grip.

The *western forehand grip* (Figures 1.8–1.9) is often the forehand groundstroke grip of choice used by highly skilled players, and by young developing players who are taught to impart exaggerated topspin when hitting forehand groundstrokes. It is also a grip used by those who pick up a tennis racket for the first time and start to play. The grip is best achieved by laying the racket on the court and picking it up naturally. The palm of the hand faces flat against and under the back side of the racket grip. The "V" formed by the thumb and fingers, when the racket is held in front of the body, points beyond the racket shoulder.

The two-hand grip in tennis has become quite popular. The *two-hand backhand grip* (Figures 1.10–1.11) is achieved when the dominant hand grasps the racket grip in a continental grip with the non-dominant hand butted above that grasp in an eastern forehand grip. The two-hand backhand grip must be a snug fit of two hands working together to execute the stroke. A few players use a two-hand forehand grip, but the grip is not popular, thus not considered necessary as a choice of grips for the beginning player.

Selection of a grip is based on the stroke used. Eastern forehand grips are used for the forehand groundstroke. The eastern backhand grip is used for the backhand groundstroke and for special serves.

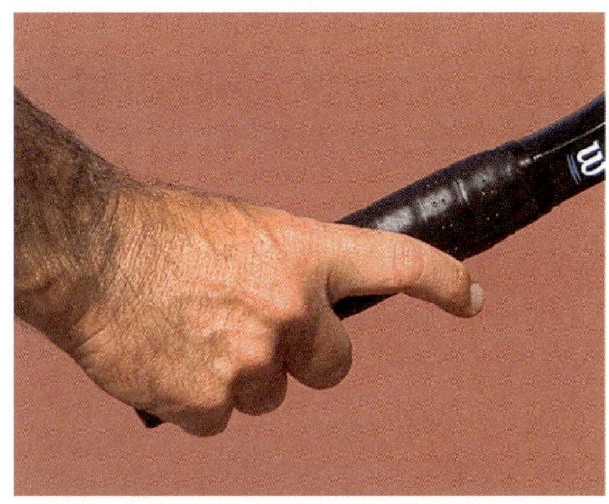

Figure 1.6 Forehand-backhand continental grip (back view).

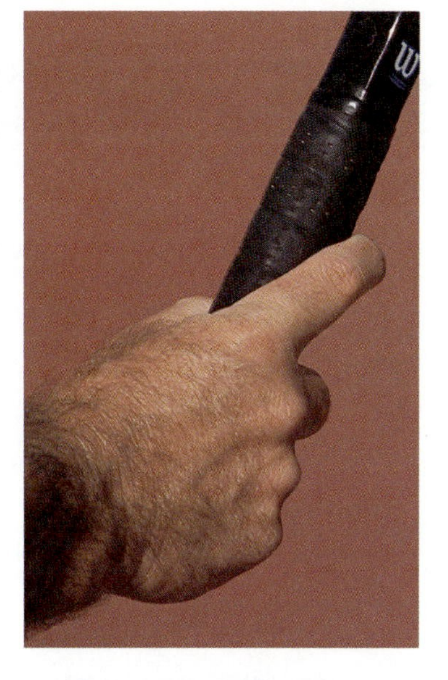

Figure 1.7 Forehand-backhand continental grip (top view).

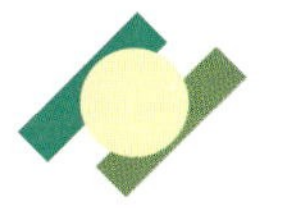

Trigger Finger

Remember: All grips require that the index finger serve as a trigger finger to provide control of the racket along with a relaxed and flexible grip.

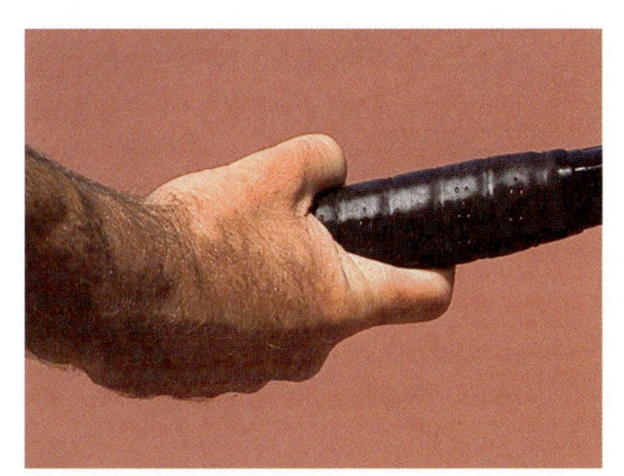

Figure 1.8 Western forehand grip (back view).

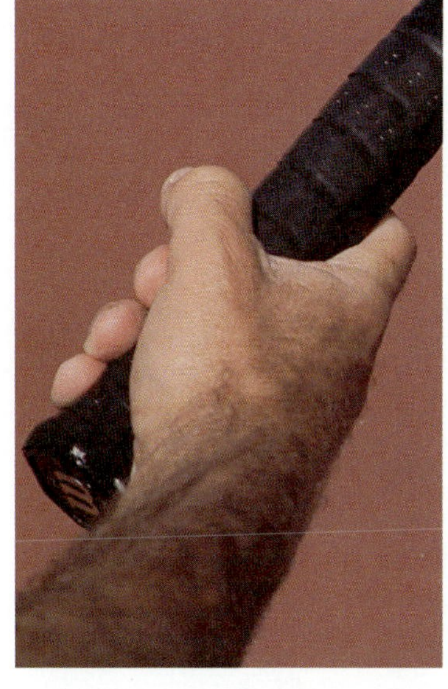

Figure 1.9 Western forehand grip (top view).

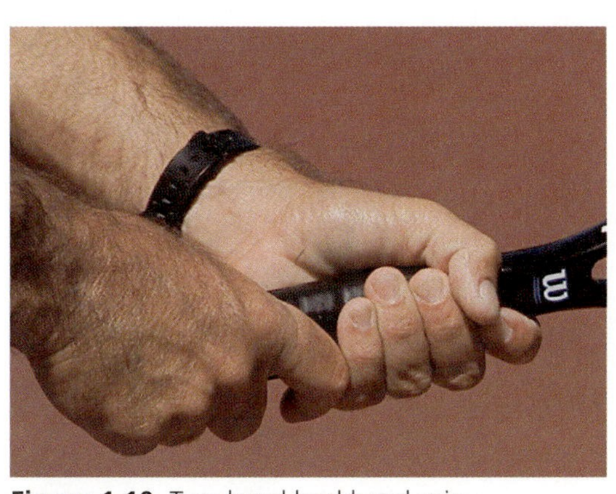

Figure 1.10 Two-hand backhand grip (front view).

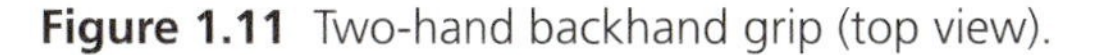

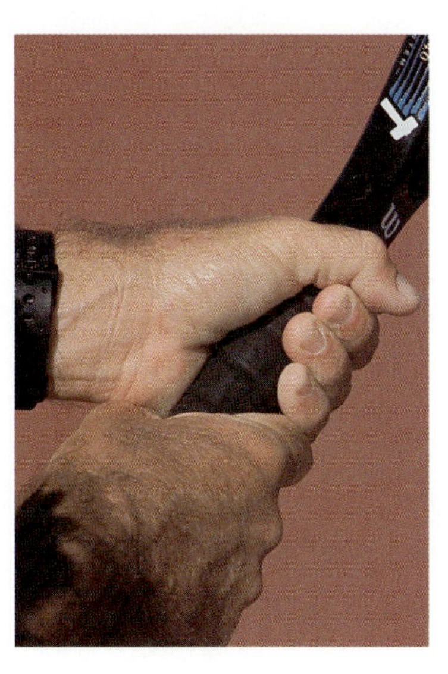

Figure 1.11 Two-hand backhand grip (top view).

The continental grips are used for groundstrokes, net play, and serving. The continental grip has the added advantage of requiring little in the way of grip adjustment for different strokes; consequently, strokes are disguised when using this grip. The western forehand is used with success when hitting topspin forehand groundstrokes. The two-hand backhand grip is used by players who seek both power and control for their backhand groundstroke. Selection of a two-hand backhand grip requires the player to cover more distance on a court in order to reach shots hit wide.

From the perspective of *what grip to use for what stroke situation*, it is suggested that the eastern grip be used by a player who intends to stay at the baseline and hit groundstrokes. An alternative to using the eastern grip when hitting from the baseline is to use a two-hand backhand grip for backhand groundstrokes. When serving, the continental grip will provide control, accuracy, and power for an effective service. As a beginner, you may want to start by using the eastern forehand grip for the serve; however, you should switch to the continental grip as soon as possible. Going to the net to play a volley shot requires reaction and timing, which means that the grip should not be changed much for a forehand or backhand volley. It is recommended that the player maintain a continental grip for play at the net to avoid mis-hitting the ball and being confused at the net.

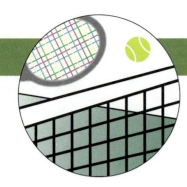

Learning Experience Reminders

Grip

1. Keep the fingers spread down the racket grip with the index finger serving as a "trigger finger."
2. Be aware of the location of the "V" in relation to the racket and non-racket shoulders.
3. Grasp the racket firmly when assuming a grip.
4. Understand the subtle differences between each grip and the purpose for each grip.

Elimination of Errors (Grip)

The Error	What Causes the Error	Correction of the Error
Lack of control of the racket.	Grasping the racket in a fist-like position.	Make sure the fingers are spread along the racket grip with a trigger finger.
Mis-hitting a ball or poor execution.	Grip is too tight.	Relax the grip. Grasp the racket firmly, not tightly.
	Grip is too loose.	Tighten the grip. Grasp the racket firmly, not tightly. Check grip size. If the grip is too small the racket will turn in the hand when a return shot has high velocity.
	Wrong grip for the stroke.	Check purpose for each grip.

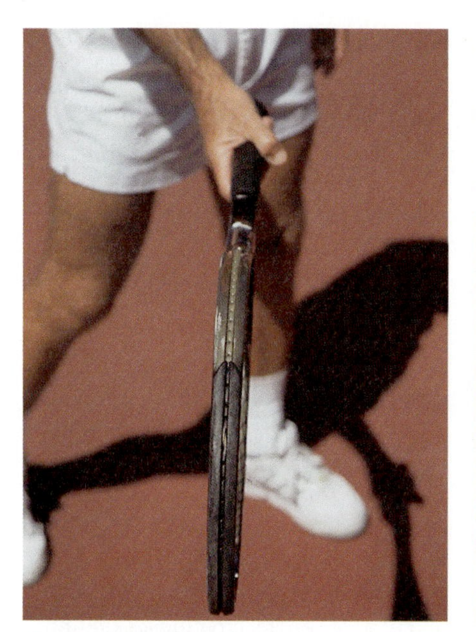

Figure 1.12 Flat racket face.

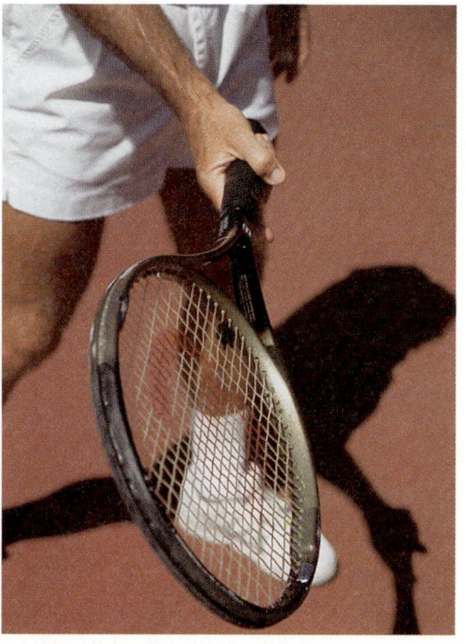

Figure 1.13 Open racket face.

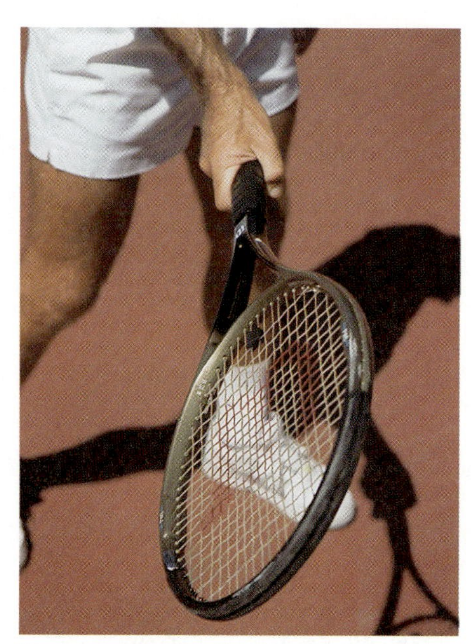

Figure 1.14 Closed racket face.

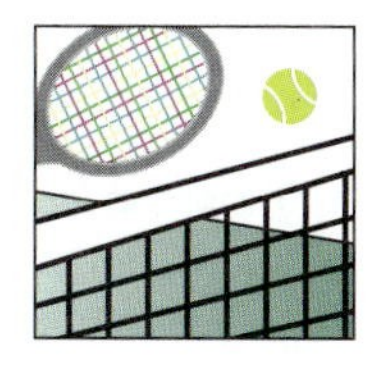

Controlling the Racket and Getting Ready to Hit

Racket control is essential to good strokes, and thus to successful play. Three basic actions when swinging a racket will provide racket head control and consequently will accomplish a stroke. The basic *swing action* is reflected in the forehand and backhand groundstrokes and the various lobs. The serve and overhead smashes are described through the *action of throwing*. The *punch action* is used with forehand and backhand volleys. By executing each of these actions or patterns, you will eliminate all extraneous motion, which will help you to simplify the action of each stroke.

Also, three basic *racket face* positions will affect the control and flight pattern of the ball and the bounce of the ball on the surface of the court. The effect of these three positions on the resultant action of the ball depends on the speed of the racket head hitting through the ball and on the angle of the racket face when it contacts the ball. If contact is made with the *racket face flat* to the ball (Figure 1.12), the flight of the ball will be straight, and the ball will fall to the court surface due to gravity. An *open racket face* (Figure 1.13) will cause the ball to have a floating action in its flight, spinning in a backward motion. A *closed racket face* (Figure 1.14) will force the flight pattern of the ball downward because the ball has a forward spin.

Each racket face position is important to all skill levels of players. Understanding what causes the drop or rise of the ball gives the beginning player greater insight into the total concept of hitting the ball and reacting to the bounce.

Comprehending spins is a direct carryover from understanding racket head and racket face control. A tennis shot that is hit without spin is affected by three aspects of the overall stroke. First, as the ball strikes the racket face, a direct force is applied to the ball that provides velocity and determines the ball's flight pattern. Second, that velocity is countered by air resistance and gravity; the former impedes the velocity of the tennis ball and the latter

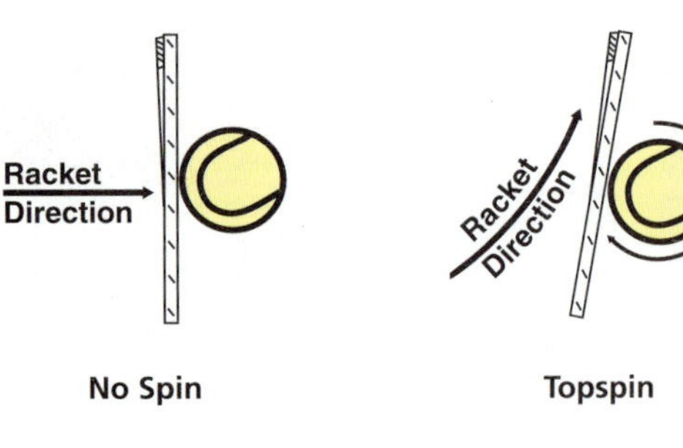

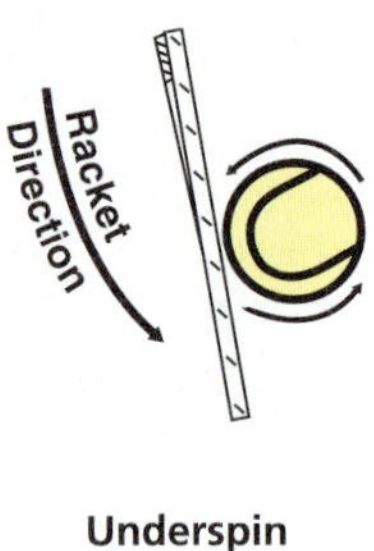

Racket Direction

Sidespin

Figure 1.15 Basic actions for balls in flight.

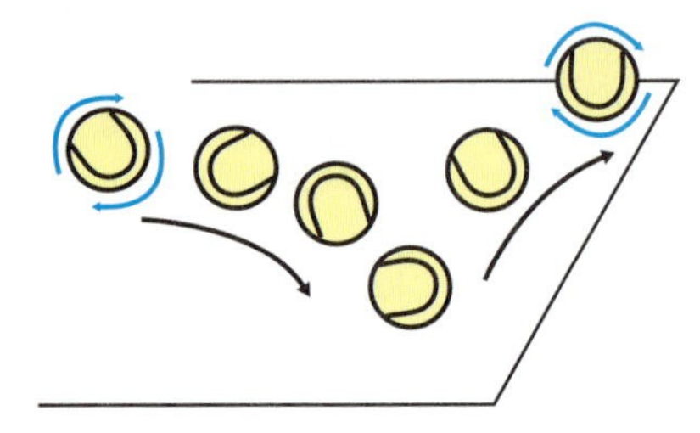

Action of ball striking court—topspin

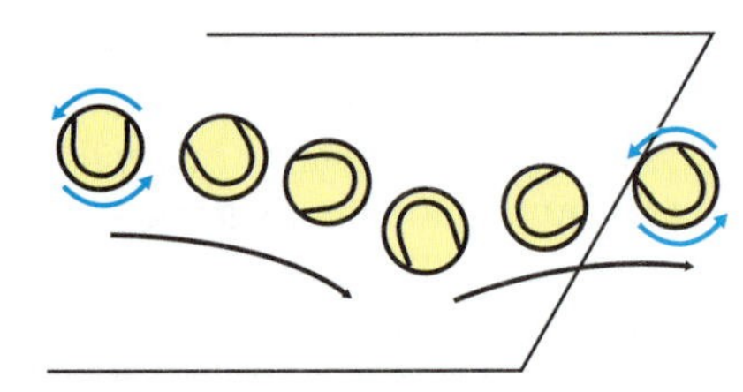

Action of ball striking court—underspin

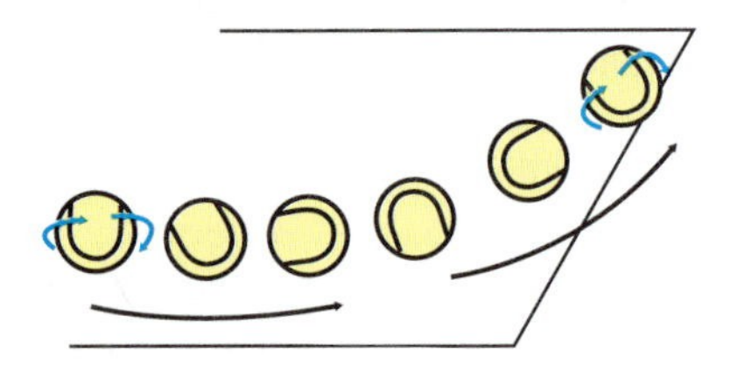

Action of ball striking court—sidespin

Figure 1.16 Basic actions for ball striking the court.

pulls the ball down toward the court. Finally, the ball will strike the tennis court surface at an angle equal to the rebound of the ball off the court surface.

When a ball spins in its flight pattern, the tennis player also must cope with the behavior of the ball as it strikes the court surface. There are three *basic actions for balls in flight* (see Figure 1.15). First, *topspin* is caused by the action of the top surface of the ball rotating against air resistance. This creates friction on the top part of the ball, forcing the ball in a downward path. A second spinning rotation, *underspin*, is caused by the bottom of the ball meeting air resistance and forcing the ball to stay up longer than normally is found with a non-spinning ball. The final spin action of a ball—*sidespin*—is created when the side of the ball meets air resistance and pressure. This causes the ball to veer to the opposite side.

The *action of the ball striking the court surface* is the end result of racket control action on the ball and the spin of the flight of the ball (Figure 1.16). As the tennis ball makes contact with the tennis court, the ball will behave in a highly predictable manner. A *topspin* action will hit the court surface with a high, deep bounce because of the forward rotation of the ball. A ball hit with *underspin* usually is hit with power and at a low angle, creating a skidding action as ball meets surface. The *sidespin* strikes the court with the same action and direction as the sidespin on the ball.

In summary, racket control and spin of the ball have a cause-effect relationship. A flat racket face at contact will cause a flat flight pattern and flat equal angle bounce off the court. An open racket face will result in underspin during the flight of the ball and a skidding action upon contact with the court surface. A closed racket face will provide a topspin ball action with a resulting high and deep bounce off the court surface. The player should understand that these two racket positions for the slice and topspin groundstrokes produce only a subtle change at contact.

A closed racket face striking the ball on the side will create a sidespin action followed by a sideward bounce when the ball strikes the court. The beginning player needs to understand the various spins applied to a ball in order to cope with balls hit with spin and to learn how to supply spin to various strokes.

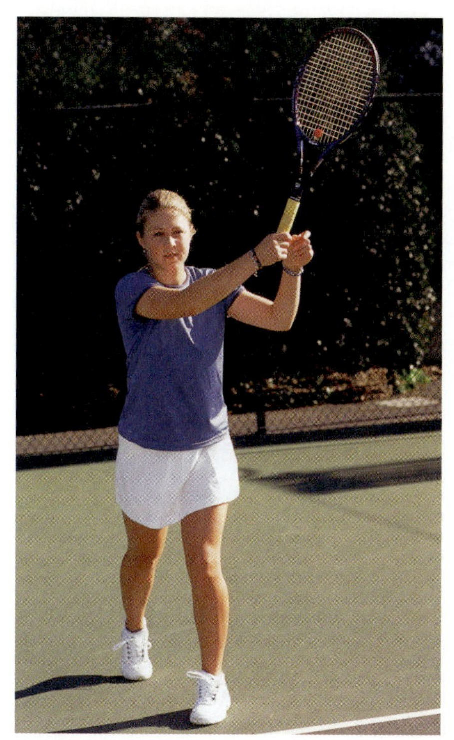

Figure 1.17 Forehand groundstroke follow through.

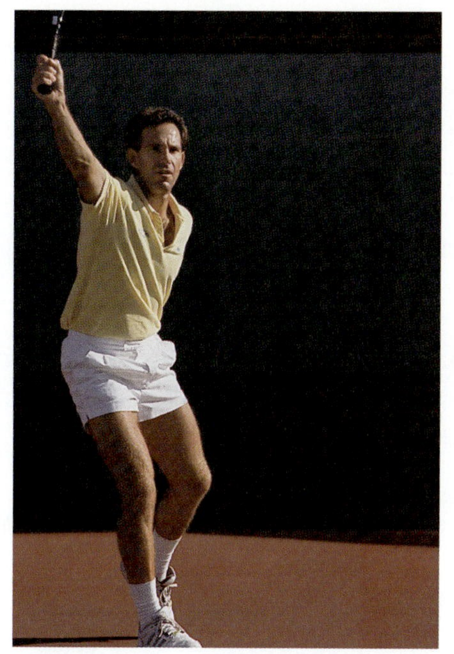

Figure 1.18 Backhand groundstroke.

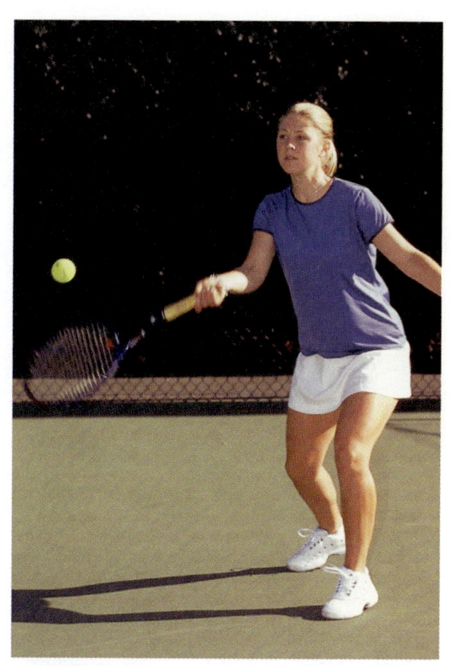

Figure 1.19 Lob.

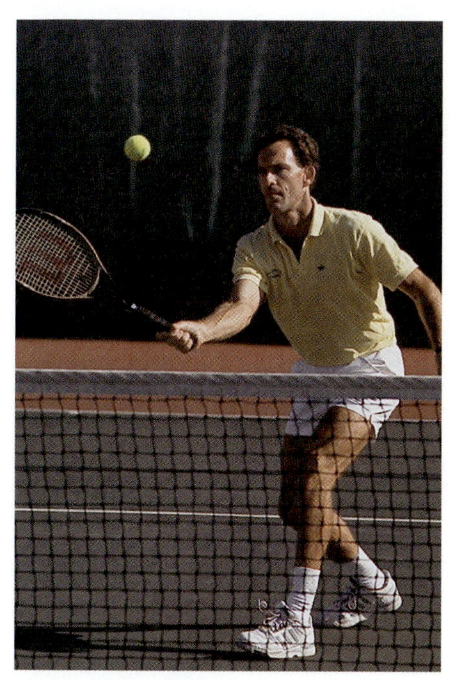

Figure 1.20 Volley.

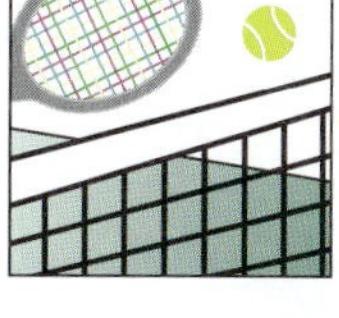

Types of Strokes

As an introduction to strokes in tennis, a definition of the various strokes should enable better understanding of the basic skills of the game.

The basic *forehand groundstroke* (Figure 1.17) is a stroke hit from the baseline following the bounce of the ball. The stroke is executed with a swinging action that produces a flat, no-spin (actually, most flat shots have a small amount of topspin) movement to the ball. The *backhand groundstroke* (Figure 1.18) is played under the same conditions as the forehand groundstroke, with the same ball action. Both are swinging action strokes with the forehand hit on the racket side of the body and the backhand hit on the non-racket side of the body.

Both strokes are foundations for more advanced strokes, including *topspin* and *slice (underspin) groundstrokes. Approach shots*, which are an extension of groundstrokes, are characterized by a player advancing to the middle of the court to hit a ball. All *lobs* (Figure 1.19) are also an extension of groundstrokes in terms of the swinging action except there is a lifting action designed to hit the ball deep to the baseline and with a loft.

The *volley* (Figure 1.20) is a punching action characterized by playing the ball before it contacts the court surface. Both forehand and backhand volleys usually are played at the net. *Half-volleys* are an extension of a volley shot.

The fourth type of stroke is the basic *flat serve* (Figure 1.21), and it is described as a throwing action. Strokes that develop from the flat service are the slice service (sidespin), the topspin service, and an advanced stroke known as the American twist (another sidespin rotation).

The *overhead smash* (Figure 1.22) is a continuation of the basic flat service. The key parts of the serve are reflected in the smash. It differs from the serve in that the ball is hit either on the fly or after a bounce on the court surface when the offensive player is positioned near the net.

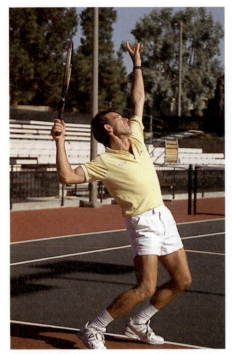

Figure 1.21 Flat Serve.

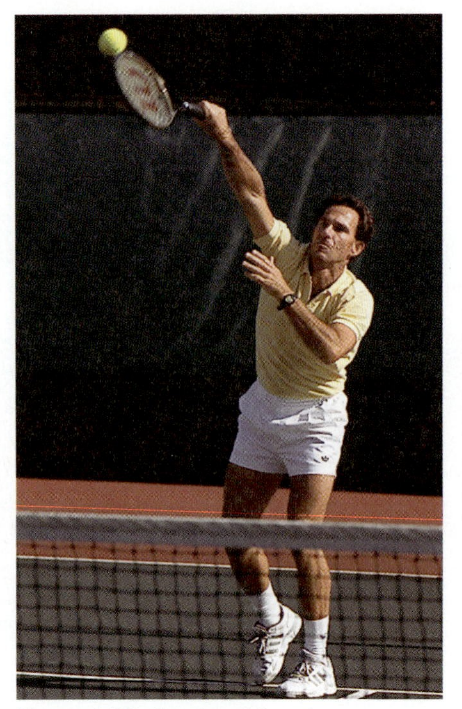

Figure 1.22 Overhead Smash.

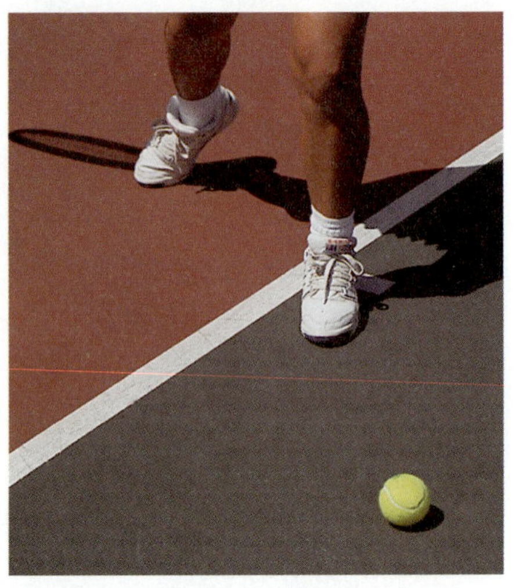

Figure 1.23 Position of ball and feet away and behind the ball.

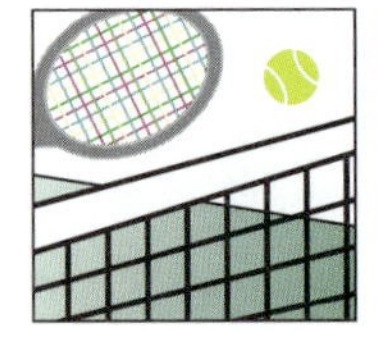

Feel and Timing of the Tennis Ball

The development of *timing and feel for the tennis ball* is a prerequisite for successful tennis play. Regardless of the racket control, the spin of the ball, and various stroke fundamentals, execution of each stroke depends on feeling and timing of the ball through *eye-hand coordination*, *timing*, and *focus*. Eye-hand coordination is based on past experiences of throwing and catching an object similar in size to a tennis ball. The swinging, throwing, and punching actions associated with tennis are fundamental to the ball games of batting, throwing, and catching that most American children play during their childhood. If you have played softball or racquetball, or have engaged in activities like playing catch, the game of tennis will be easy for you compared to individuals who have not had those experiences.

Timing also is related to where the ball eventually will be positioned to be hit rather than where it bounced originally. You must comprehend where the ball will go after it bounces, and set up behind and away from the ball so you can step into the ball to hit it (Figure 1.23). Players tend to get too close to the ball or too far away, which causes them to lurch to hit the ball rather than smoothly step into the ball. If the ball is too far away, the player can adjust (and not lose timing) by stepping toward the ball with a weight transfer (Figure 1.24). If the ball is too close, the player should step away, yet forward, to hit the ball (Figure 1.25). The key factor in stepping away is the opening of the upper body as the racket is brought through the ball at contact.

Part of timing involves controlling the racket head speed. Players under pressure tend to swing too hard or fast, particularly with the return of service. You must remember to play from a relaxed position and control the racket head speed. The same is true with

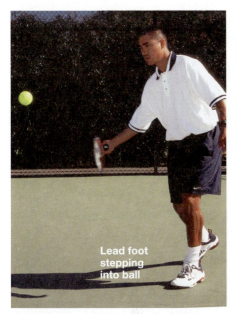

Figure 1.24 Stepping into the ball.

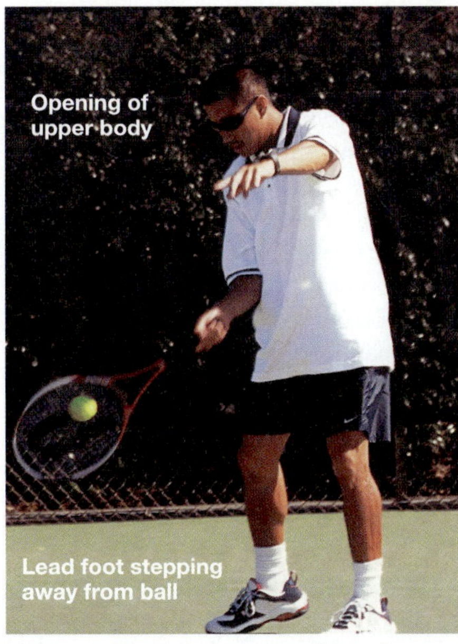

Figure 1.25 Stepping away from the ball.

hitting overhead smashes and groundstrokes when the opposing player is at the net. The added pressure tends to break down timing, forcing the player to rush through the stroke. The focal points have to be relaxation, confidence in hitting the ball, and concentration on the ball. Timing is improved immeasurably by watching the ball as long as possible. This is the part of focus that is most often ignored.

The ability to *focus* is extremely important in tennis. The ability to "see" the ball and perceive the racket striking the ball will help the developing player improve rapidly. Being able to focus on the ball is based on the same past experiences as with eye-hand coordination. Recognizing the bounce of the ball in terms of height, the distance the ball is in relation to the player, and the relationship of the ball to the body are part of the focus. Additional focus points include moving to the ball, transferring weight into the ball at contact, and being in the correct position at the correct time. A final consideration in focusing is the ability to block all outside distractions and keep the tennis ball as the only target.

The foundation for timing and feel of the ball rests with establishing a *ready position* from which to hit groundstrokes and volleys (Figure 1.26). The ready position is the first actual skill presented for the developing player, and it is the foundation for all strokes.

The feet should be spaced slightly wider than shoulder width and should be parallel to each other. The knees are slightly bent, and the weight of the body is centered over the balls of the feet. The buttocks should be "down," with the upper body leaning slightly forward in a straight alignment. The head should be

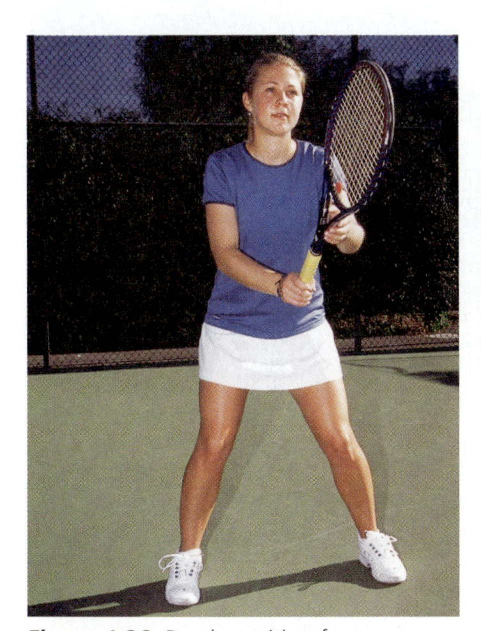

Figure 1.26 Ready position for a groundstroke.

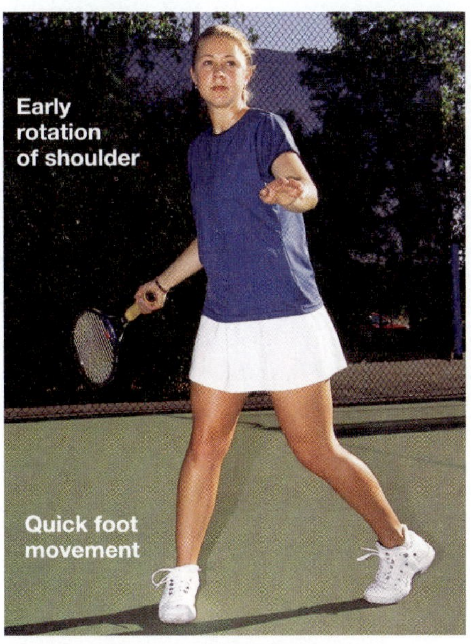

Figure 1.27 Ready position—turn of shoulders (forehand).

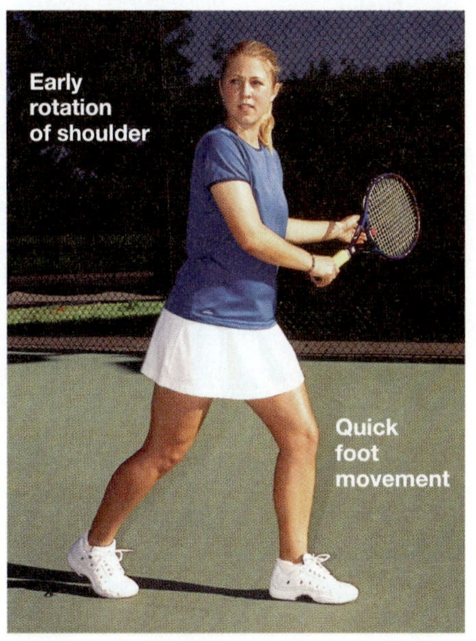

Figure 1.28 Ready position—turn of shoulders (backhand).

"up," looking toward the ball on the opposite side of the net. The racket is held "up" with a forehand grip on the handle, with the non-racket hand lightly touching the throat of the racket. The racket head is above the hands, and the elbows are clear of the body.

The ready position gives the player the opportunity to move equally to the right or left, as well as advance forward or retreat backward. The first response from a player in the ready position is to rotate the shoulders immediately when recognizing the direction of the ball from across the net (Figures 1.27–1.28). A player with good mobility will be able to move the feet quickly from the ready position. If a player can be relaxed in a ready position, keep the weight on the balls of the feet, and then react to the approaching ball with an early turn of the shoulders and quick foot movement, the stroke has been initiated positively.

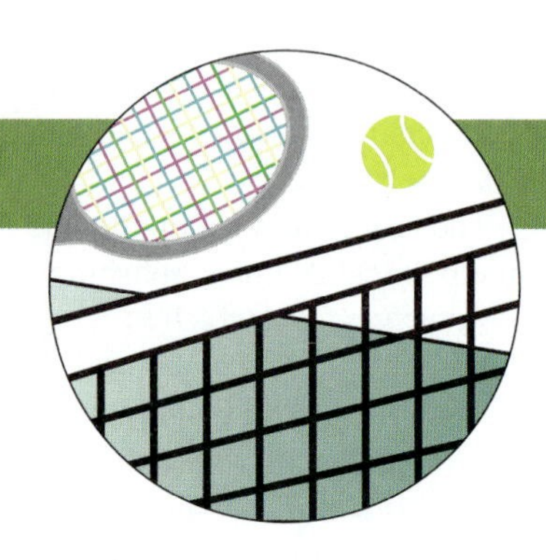

Learning Experience Reminders

Ready Position

1. Maintain a base with the feet shoulder-width apart.
2. Focus on the ball on the other side of the net.
3. Keep the knees bent slightly and the weight on the balls of the feet.
4. Be relaxed and ready to react.
5. As the ball crosses the net, turn the shoulders and move the feet.

Elimination of Errors (Ready Position)

The Error	What Causes the Error	Correction of the Error
Falling off balance.	Feet too close together.	Widen the base.
Mis-timing the ball.	Not focusing on the ball and not getting shoulders rotated early with feet moving.	Watch the seams of the ball and rotate your shoulders early.

Check Points

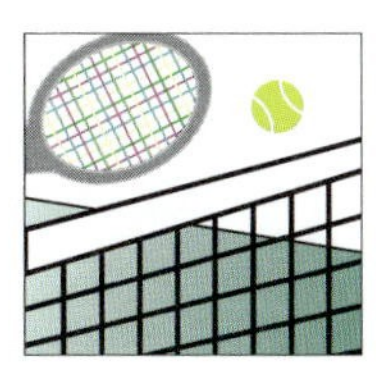

1. The eastern forehand grip is described as
   a. trigger finger, V formed by index finger and thumb with V pointed to racket shoulder.
   b. grasp of racket, V formed by index finger and thumb with V pointed to the racket shoulder.
   c. trigger finger, V formed by index finger and thumb with V pointed to center of chest.
   d. trigger finger, V formed by index finger and thumb with V pointed to non-racket shoulder.

2. The continental grip is described as
   a. similar to a two-hand grip.
   b. halfway between an eastern forehand and western forehand grip.
   c. halfway between an eastern forehand and eastern backhand grip.
   d. halfway between an eastern backhand and western forehand grip.

3. The continental grip is used most effectively for
   a. playing the baseline.
   b. playing the baseline and the net.
   c. playing the baseline and serve.
   d. playing the net and serve.

4. The basic racket control actions are
   a. punch action, swing action, and throw action.
   b. punch action and swing action.
   c. throw action and swing action.
   d. punch action and throw action.

5. The three types of spin imparted on a ball in flight are
   a. topspin, sidespin, underspin.
   b. reverse spin, topspin, backspin.
   c. reverse spin, sidespin, topspin.
   d. sidespin, reverse spin, and slice.

6. Timing and feel for the tennis ball requires
   a. eye-hand coordination, focus, and foot coordination.
   b. eye-hand coordination, timing and focus.
   c. focus, foot coordination and timing.
   d. foot coordination, eye-hand coordination and timing.

7. The first response from a ready position is to
   a. rotate shoulders.
   b. turn the racket-side shoulder.
   c. turn the non-racket-side shoulder.
   d. rotate the shoulders with the direction of the ball seen across the net.

8. The tennis racket should be grasped
   a. tightly.
   b. loosely.
   c. firmly.
   d. in a fist-like grip.

Answers to Check Points can be found on page 145.

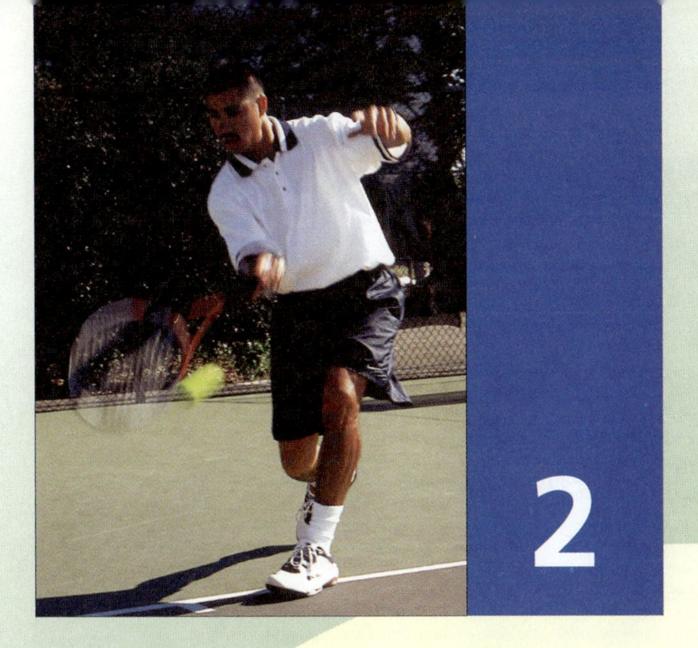

2

Groundstrokes

Groundstrokes are crucial to success in tennis. They are executed by the player hitting the tennis ball from the baseline area following one bounce of the ball on the court. The groundstroke involves a swinging action designed to hit the ball deep to the opponent's baseline. Both forehand and backhand groundstrokes develop from the basic (little spin) flat stroke and evolve into other groundstrokes termed *topspin* and *slice* (underspin) groundstrokes. In order to initiate the groundstroke, get in the ready position and then decide whether to use the forehand or the backhand.

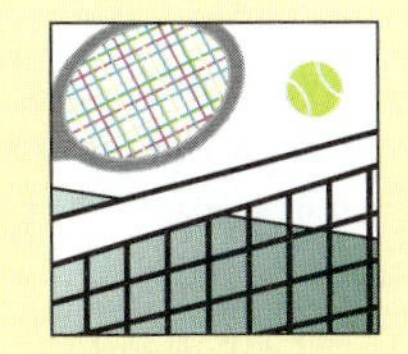

Groundstrokes—Basic Forehand

The *basic forehand groundstroke* is the foundation for all forehands hit with spin. It is the stroke players use most often if they are given the choice between a backhand and a forehand.

The eastern forehand grip—also known as the "shake hands" grip—is used to execute the basic forehand groundstroke. The basic forehand groundstroke has three stages: preparing to hit the ball, contacting the ball, and following through. Each stage must be performed in sequence.

Preparing to hit the ball begins with the player in the ready position. Two reactions follow: (1) rotation of the shoulders, and (2) movement of the feet. The racket is placed in an early backswing position as a result of the shoulder and foot movement. To do this, the player may either bring the racket straight back or loop the racket. Either is acceptable because the goal is to get the racket back in a low position to hit from a semi-low to a high position. The loop will be emphasized in this situation as the best method to get the racket back early and in proper position.

The *loop* is divided into three parts: (1) the shoulders turn allowing the racket to pull back in a line even with the eye (Figure 2.1), (2) the racket moves to a general perpendicular position aligned to the fence located behind the baseline, with the racket positioned slightly higher than the hand and wrist (Figure 2.2), and (3) the racket drops

Figure 2.1 Pull the racket back in a line even with the eye (eastern forehand grip).

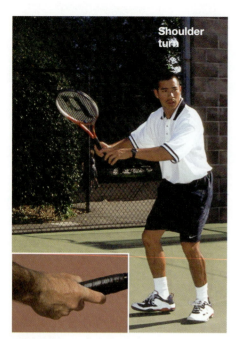

Figure 2.2 Backswing—racket perpendicular and high.

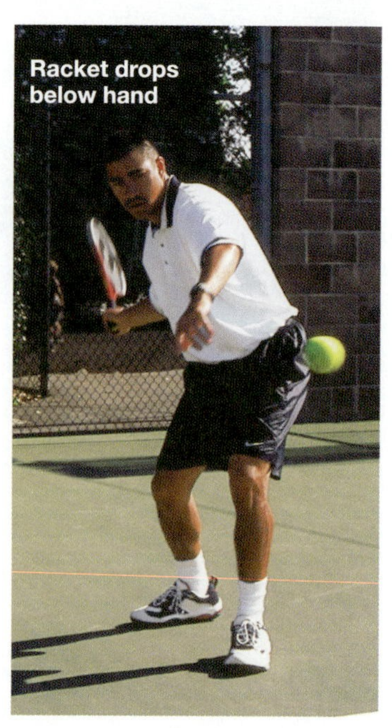

Figure 2.3 Drop the racket below the line of the ball.

below the line of the flight of the ball at about a 12-inch position below and behind the intended contact area to the ball (Figure 2.3). The loop will provide a rhythm to the swing, add extra velocity to the ball following impact, and ensure a grooved swing.

The full pattern for this preparation is to bring the racket back as quickly as possible by reacting early to the ball and turning the shoulders at a 45-degree angle to begin inertia. As the racket starts back in the loop following the shoulder turn, both feet will move and pivot automatically to accommodate the upper body turn. When the racket moves to a perpendicular position to the fence beyond the back court, the wrist and arm should be firm, with the elbow bent slightly and away from the body. The final part of the preparation is bending the legs (Figure 2.3).

Contact with the ball begins when the racket moves from the backswing in a semi-low to a high pattern. The lead leg steps into the ball with a transfer of weight from back foot to lead foot. The lead leg is bent at contact while the back leg is beginning to straighten. The palm of the hand grasping the racket is behind the ball at impact, with a very firm wrist and with the arm extended 8 to 10 inches from the body. The non-racket arm is extended toward the ball, giving direction to the ball and balance to the body. The ball is hit off the lead leg at slightly above mid-thigh to above waist level. The sequence of backswing to contact with the ball requires stepping into the ball, transferring your weight forward, and keeping the ball away from the body at a position toward the net and sideline (Figure 2.4).

The final part of the sequence is the *follow through*. The wrist remains firm and fixed and the arm extends out across the body, with the inside of the upper arm touching the chin. The legs lift throughout the follow through, with the lead leg fully extended and the back leg slightly bent. The purpose of the follow through is to eliminate a premature lifting or pulling of the ball before it leaves the racket strings at contact (Figure 2.5).

The *position of the elbow and wrist* and the *transfer of weight* are crucial to execution of the stroke. It must be emphasized that the wrist and arm remain firm but relaxed throughout the stroke. The tendency is to lay back the wrist and to hyperextend the elbow. The wrist should not rotate, and the elbow can remain straight or slightly bent. Both

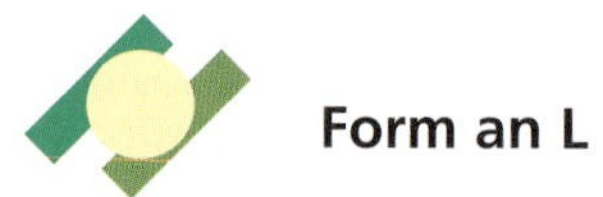

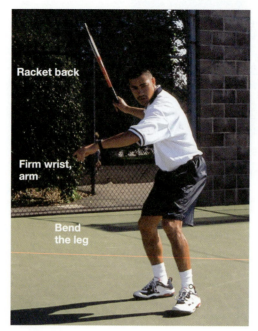

Form an L

When making contact with the ball on a forehand groundstroke, the racket and forearm should form an L.

C. Chappuzeau, Tennis, 6/95, pp. 75

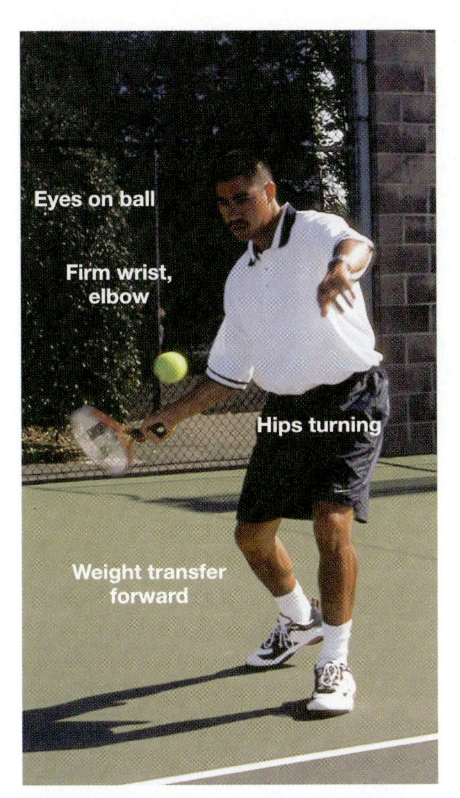

Figure 2.4 Forehand groundstroke contact.

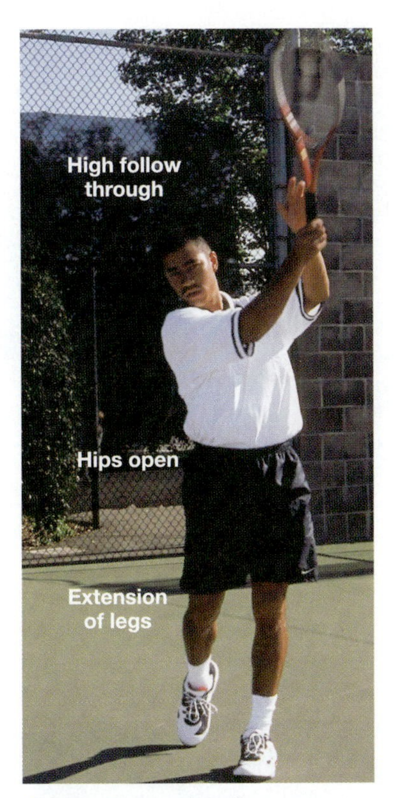

Figure 2.5 Forehand groundstroke follow through.

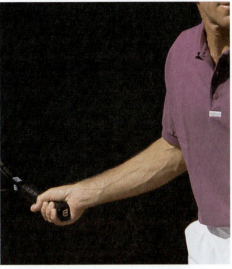

Figure 2.6 Forehand groundstroke closeup of shoulder, elbow, and wrist.

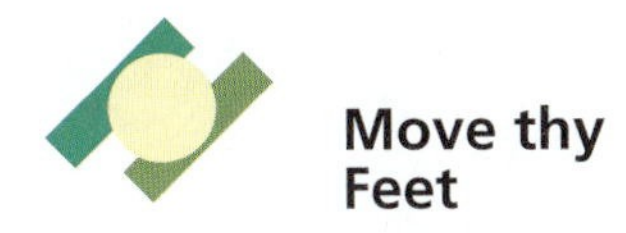

Move thy Feet

Remember, to be ready to hit the next groundstroke you have to keep your feet moving.

should remain firm (Figure 2.6). Weight transfer provides the needed drive behind the ball, with the center of gravity directed forward through the stroke by a stepping motion into the ball. During the weight transfer, the legs must be bent with a change of the degree in bend through the full stroke.

Footwork and *early preparation* are both critical to success with the forehand groundstroke. Footwork supplies the mobility and balance that will provide the base for the stroke, and it sets the stage for weight transfer and leg power. Weight has to be centered over the balls of the feet to effect ease of movement, and the pivoting and lifting actions aid throughout the stroke in placing the body in a position to hit the ball (Figures 2.7 and 2.8). The early preparation includes good shoulder rotation and accompanying foot pivot with a loop backswing. That early response to the opponent's shot is the base for all that follows.

The stroke must be performed in full sequence, with a fluid movement from one part to the next. Any jerky, non-grooved action will detract from the stroke. The acceptable sequence has to include a coordination of feet, legs, shoulder, arm, and wrist. See Figures 2.9–2.11.

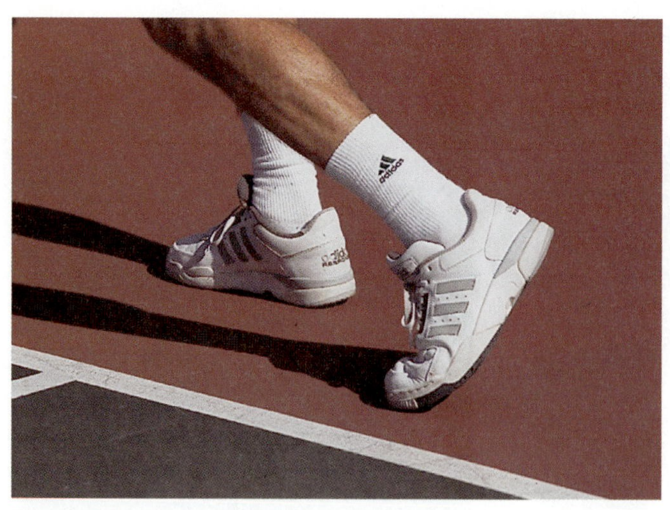

Figure 2.7 Weight centered over balls of the feet.

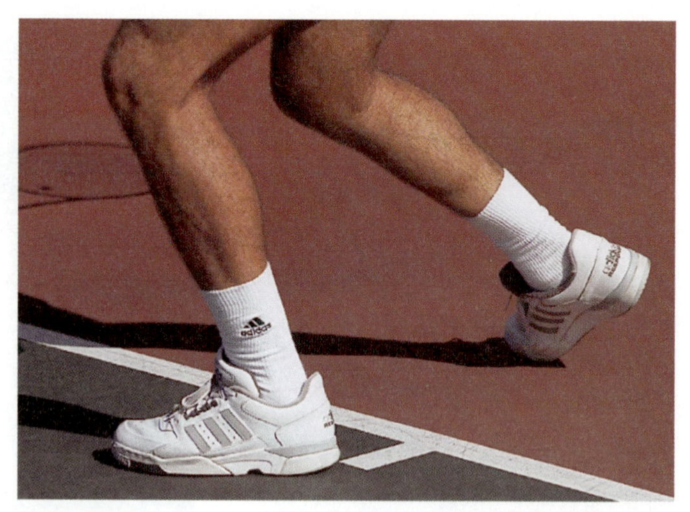

Figure 2.8 Pivoting and lifting actions through the stroke.

Basic Forehand Groundstroke

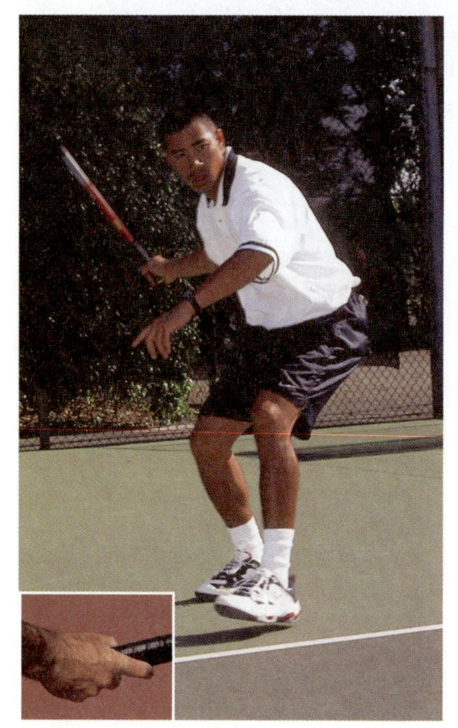

Figure 2.9 Backswing.

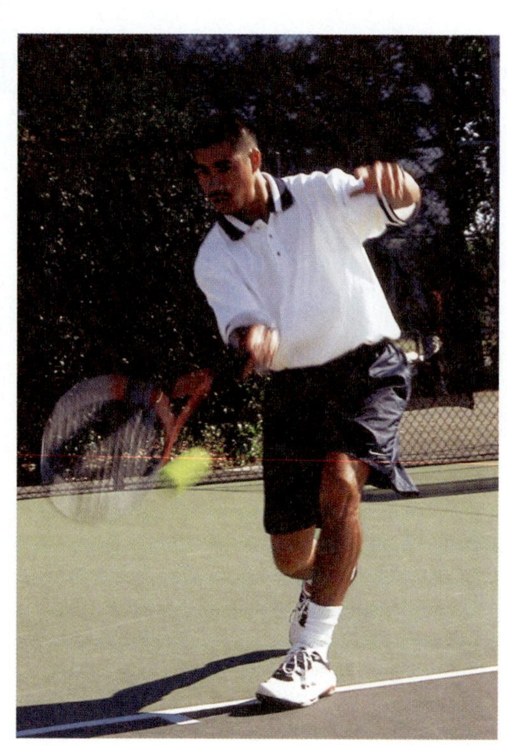

Figure 2.10 Contact.

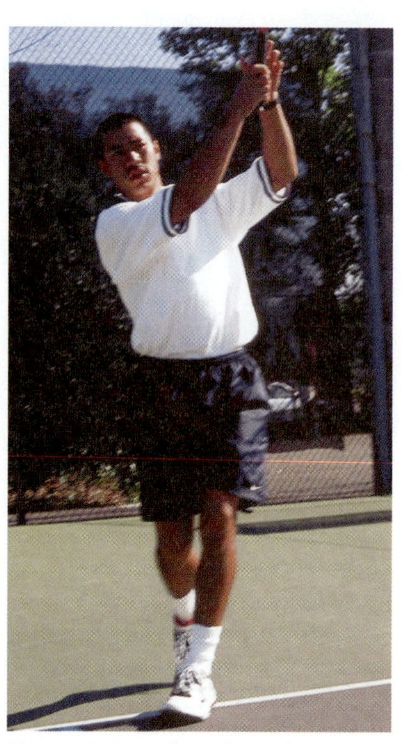

Figure 2.11 Follow through.

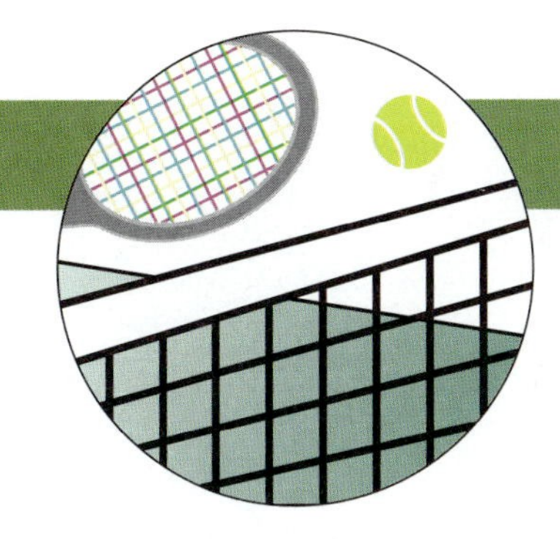

Learning Experience Reminders

Basic Forehand Groundstroke

1. Always start from a ready position.
2. Prepare with an early shoulder rotation and pivot of the feet.
3. Activate the loop or a straight-back backswing.
4. Step into the ball at contact by transferring your weight forward.
5. Contact the ball with the palm-of-the-hand position and firm wrist.
6. Swing from slightly low to high, with the follow through extending high and across the body.
7. Maintain a full synchronized sequence to the timing of the stroke.

Elimination of Errors (Basic Forehand Groundstroke)

The Error	What Causes the Error	Correction of the Error
Ball pulled to the non-racket side of the court.	Hitting too far out in front of the body or turning the racket shoulder too much through the stroke.	Step into the ball, hitting off the lead leg. Keep non-racket shoulder consistent with transfer of weight forward. Keep non-racket hand out in front of your body.
Ball directed to the near racket side of the court.	Being late in the backswing position, backswing beyond the perpendicular position to the fence, or laying the wrist too far back.	React early to the flight of the ball with a 45-degree turn of the shoulders, initiating an early backswing.
Balls hit short with little velocity.	Not stepping into the ball with weight transfer, and poor racket pattern from high to slightly low. Racket may also be too high at the lowest part of the backswing.	Transfer weight into the ball at contact; change the swinging pattern to slightly low to high.
Balls hit long or high against opponent's back fence.	Hitting the ball with poor timing, or too hard with the weight on the back foot, or in a lifting pattern at contact; also "breaking wrist" at contact.	Synchronize the timing of the stroke with the slightly low-to-high racket pattern; use good weight transfer. Keep wrist firm; don't lean back at contact with the ball.

Forehand Slice Groundstroke

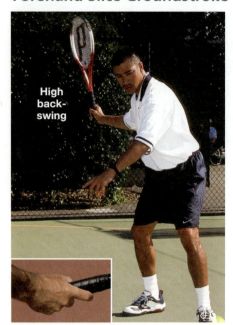

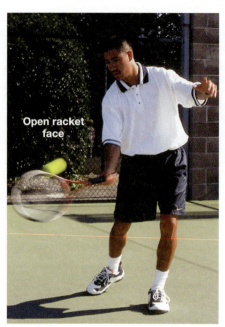

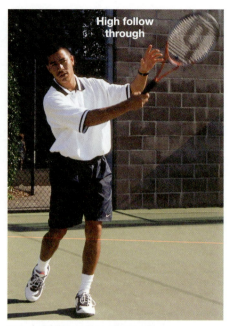

Figure 2.12 Backswing (eastern forehand grip).

Figure 2.13 Contact.

Figure 2.14 Follow through.

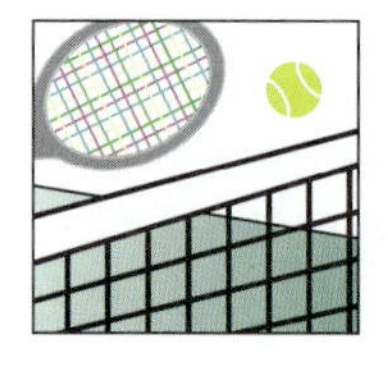

Forehand Groundstroke— Slice and Topspin

The basic forehand groundstroke is the stroke that beginners start with, but they need to identify and eventually hit a *forehand slice groundstroke* and a *forehand topspin groundstroke*. All three strokes are similar, but the slice requires a high backswing and a slightly open face contact point, followed by a high follow through (Figures 2.12–2.14). The spin imparted to the ball is underspin, with the ball staying low to the net, followed by a skidding action, or low bounce, when rebounding off the court.

The topspin stroke begins with a very low backswing, a slightly closed racket face at contact, and a high follow through. At contact the forearm rotates somewhat. In addition, the legs play a part in this stroke with a low bend of the knees during the backswing, followed by an extension of the legs in the follow-through position (Figures 2.15–2.17). The spin of the ball is an overspin, or topspin, and the ball action upon striking the court surface is a high bounce. The grip used for a slice is still the eastern forehand grip, but to gain additional spin, the grip for the topspin changes to a more western grip.

The beginner needs to first develop the basic stroke, then move to the slice and topspin in a progression. For most beginners, the slice is more difficult to develop. In contrast, the forehand topspin groundstroke comes naturally to many players.

Forehand Topspin Groundstroke

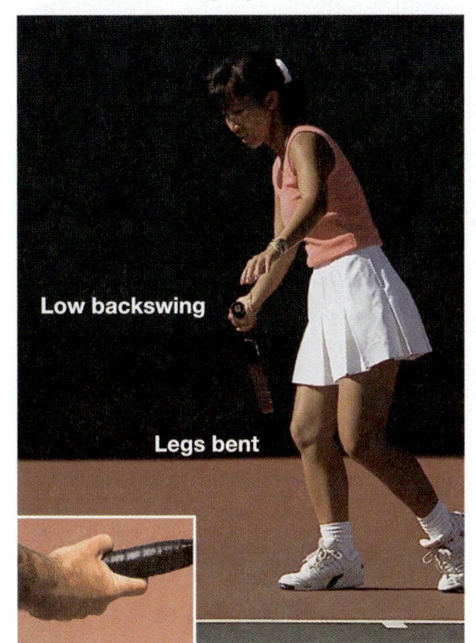

Figure 2.15 Backswing (western forehand grip).

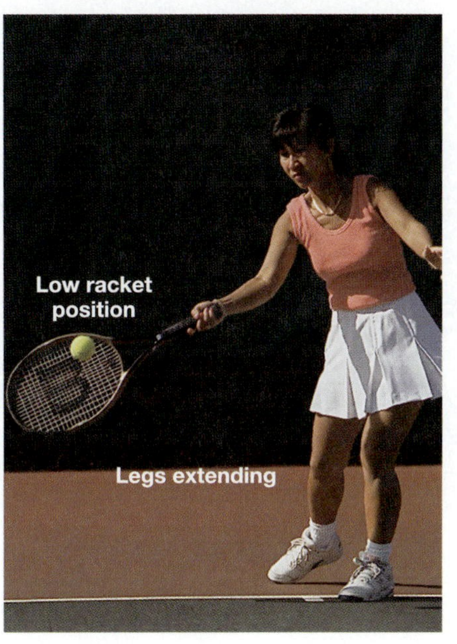

Figure 2.16 Contact.

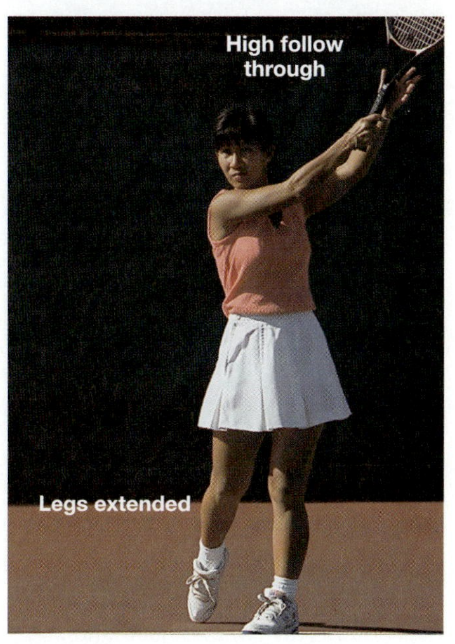

Figure 2.17 Follow through.

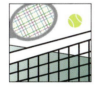

Groundstrokes—Basic Backhand

The basic backhand groundstroke is the easier of the two strokes to hit (i.e., forehand vs. backhand) mechanically, yet it is the stroke that most players fail at in competition. Hitting a backhand is easy and fun, but the player must first develop confidence.

The *grip* used for the basic backhand is the *eastern backhand grip*, with the hand rolled onto the top of the racket grip so that the "V" is pointed to the non-racket shoulder when the racket is held in front of the body. Another guide for the grip is that the knuckles of the racket hand are aligned with the net when the racket makes contact with the ball.

As with all forehand strokes and subsequent backhands, there are three phases to the stroke that all mesh into a consistent, grooved feeling. *Preparation in hitting the ball* is based on an early reaction to the ball with an immediate rotation of both shoulders. The feet pivot during the shoulder rotation, and the racket starts its backswing movement with either the loop or straight back technique. The loop is pulled back at eye level and then dropped about eight inches below the contact point of the ball. The swinging pattern is a low-to-high action that is initiated by the backswing in preparation (Figure 2.18).

A change of grips also occurs in the preparation phase. The player begins the stroke from a ready position with an eastern forehand grip. As the player reacts to the ball and turns the shoulders and pivots the feet, the racket begins its backward journey. As the racket moves back, the player uses the non-racket hand to adjust the grip by turning the racket at the throat until the top of the hand is seen as the racket follows the shoulder to the backswing position (Figure 2.19). The non-racket hand stays in contact with the throat of the racket throughout the backswing and into the movement forward to hit the ball. The racket is perpendicular to the back fence during the final extension backward. The weight of the body is centered over

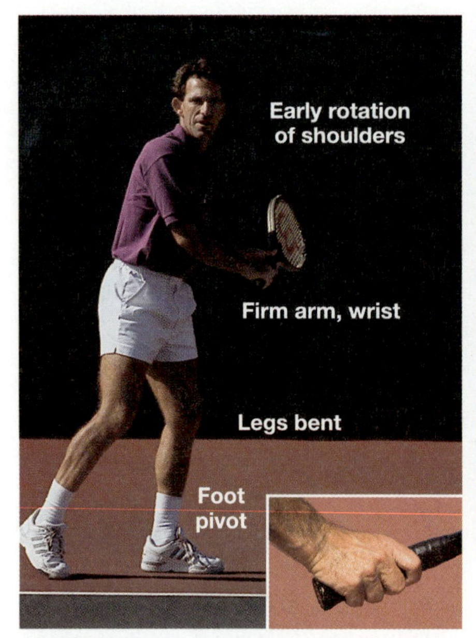

Figure 2.18 Backhand groundstroke preparation (eastern backhand grip).

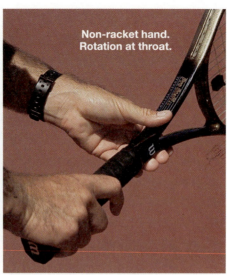

Figure 2.19 Changing grips for the backhand.

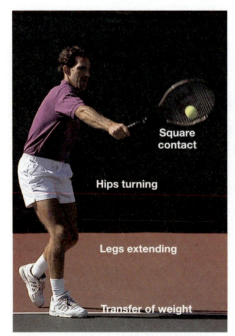

Figure 2.20 Backhand groundstroke contact.

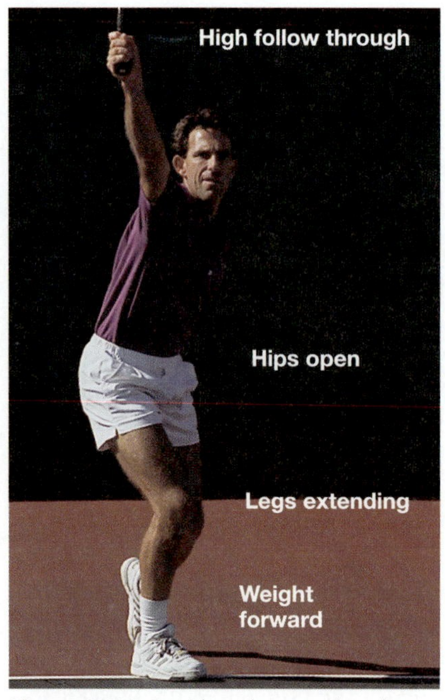

Figure 2.21 Backhand groundstroke follow through.

the back foot and the legs are bent, permitting the body to be coiled for the next phase of the stroke.

Contact with the ball occurs with a semi-low-to-high swinging pattern that will insure direction for the ball. The shoulder leads the elbow into the swing, and the elbow leads the wrist. This provides an accumulating effect so that at contact the racket is nearly square to the ball and the joint alignment from shoulder to wrist is a straight line. That joint alignment provides a firm base of support as the ball strikes the racket face. The weight of the body is transferred to the lead leg just prior to contact with the ball, and the position of the racket to the lead leg at contact is mid-thigh to above waist level (Figure 2.20).

The *follow through* is an extension of the semi-low-to-high swinging action, with the weight continuing forward off the lead leg as the lead leg straightens and the back leg bends slightly (Figure 2.21). This provides a degree of balance to the base of the stroke. The wrist remains firm as the racket finishes high, facing the racket side of the sideline.

The *wrist, elbow,* and *shoulder positions* are key elements in the basic backhand groundstroke. The initial shoulder turn followed by the shoulder leading into the stroke are essential in completing the action. The elbow and the wrist should never physically be ahead of the racket (Figure 2.22). The racket should rotate around the wrist, and the wrist should rotate around the elbow from backswing to contact with the ball. At follow through, the racket should lead the wrist and elbow. If the elbow or wrist leads the racket at contact, a pushing action will result, decreasing the velocity of the ball. The racket arm stays closer to the body than with the forehand at a distance of perhaps six to eight inches.

Racket control, weight transfer, footwork, and *leg power* all contribute to the success or failure of the backhand groundstroke. Racket control is characterized by the loop—pulling the racket back at eye level (Figure 2.23), then dropping the racket below the projected contact point of the ball (Figure 2.24).

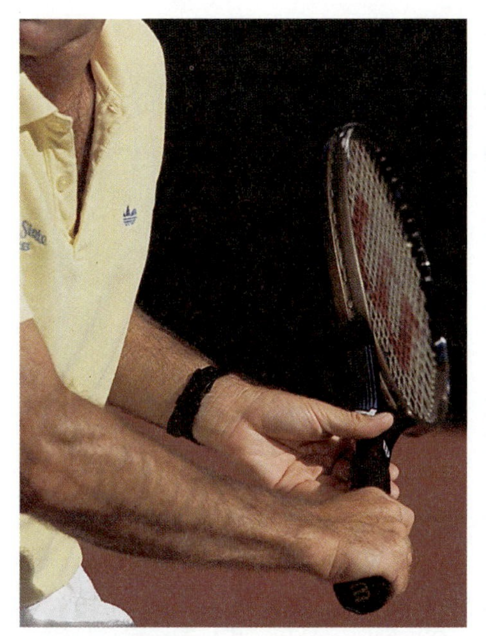

Figure 2.22 Backhand groundstroke closeup of shoulder, elbow and wrist.

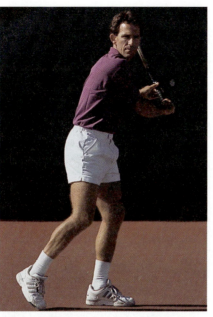

Figure 2.23 Backhand groundstroke loop — pull the racket back at eye level.

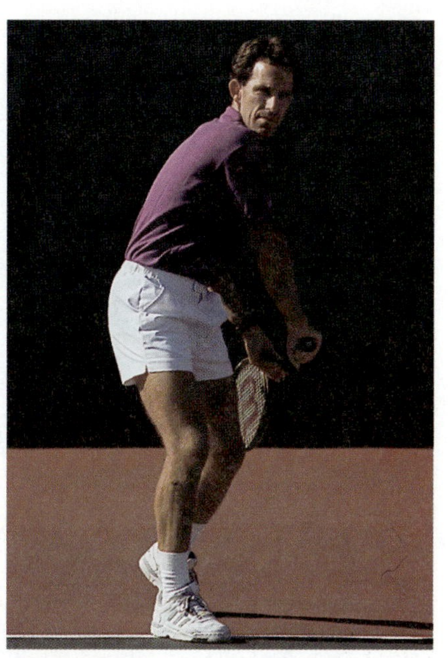

Figure 2.24 Backhand groundstroke loop — drop the racket below the projected contact point of the ball.

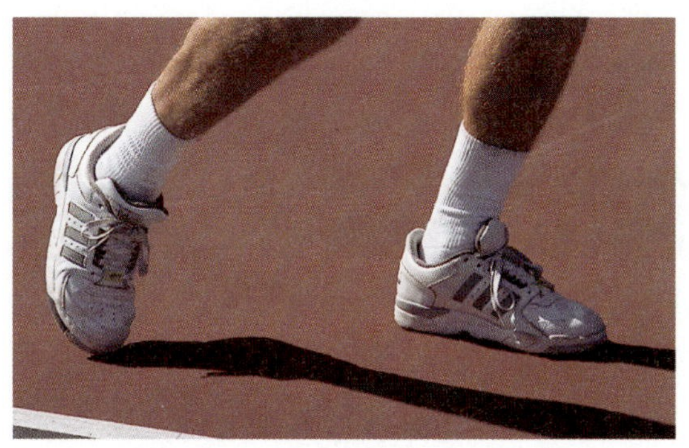

Figure 2.25 Turn the non-racket foot when the shoulder rotates.

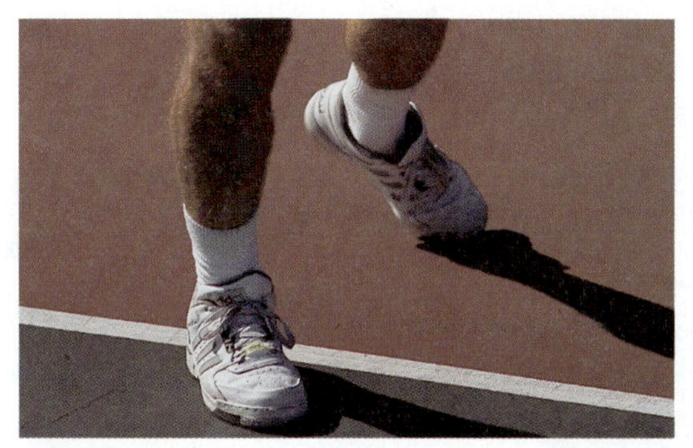

Figure 2.26 Step into the ball with the racket-side foot just prior to contact with the ball.

Balance and weight transfer occur when the player uses proper footwork from the ready position to the final follow through. The critical part of the footwork involves the singular turn of the non-racket foot when the shoulder rotates (Figure 2.25) and the subsequent stepping into the ball with the racket-side foot just prior to contact with the ball (Figure 2.26). The weight transfer is a total exchange from moving weight from the back foot during preparation to the lead leg at contact on through to follow through.

The full sequence of actions involved in the basic backhand groundstroke will determine the outcome of the stroke. There must be a fluid sequence of movement void of all jerky or shaky movement. That sequence should include coordination of shoulders, feet, legs, elbow, and wrist into a mechanically smooth, grooved stroke that causes the racket to make contact with the ball in a nearly square position and that flows to an ultimate follow through (Figures 2.27–2.29). As a final thought, the mechanics of the stroke have to be combined with the belief that the backhand is easier to execute and mechanically more sound than the forehand.

Basic Backhand Groundstroke

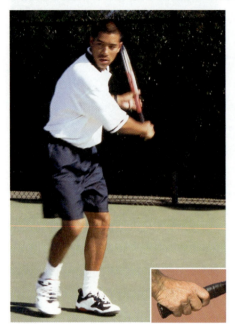
Figure 2.27 Backswing.

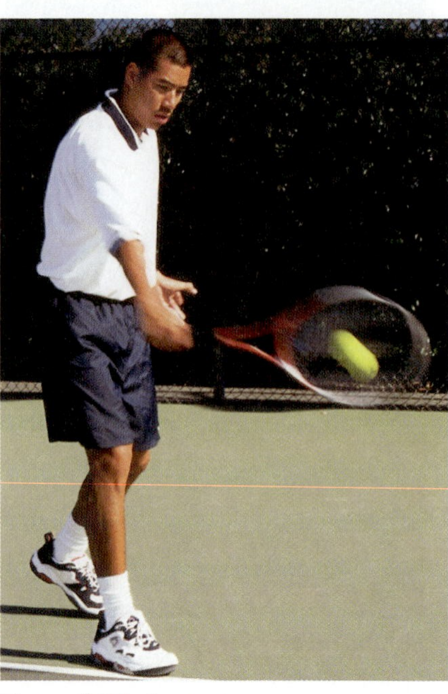
Figure 2.28 Contact.

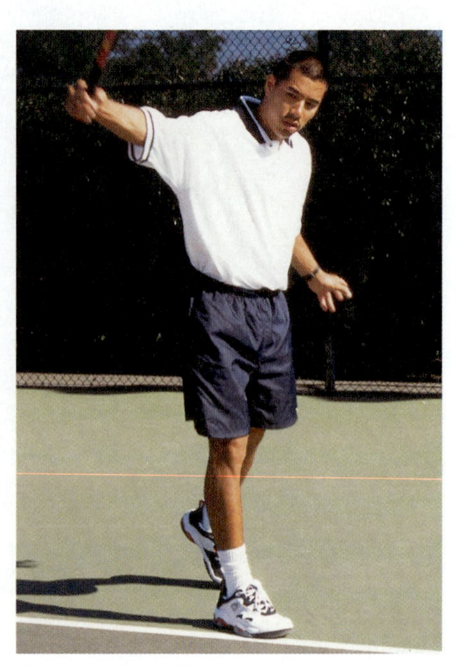
Figure 2.29 Follow through.

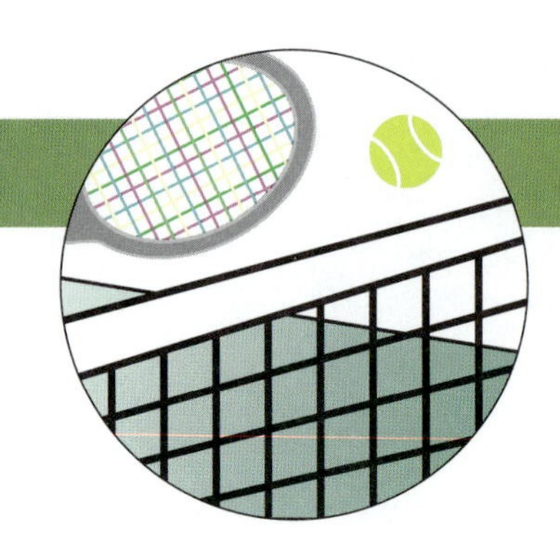

Learning Experience Reminders

Basic Backhand Groundstroke

1. Always start from the ready position.
2. Prepare with an early shoulder rotation and pivot of the feet.
3. Activate the loop or a straight-back motion backswing.
4. Change the grip from eastern forehand to eastern backhand as the racket is brought to the backswing position.
5. Keep a firm wrist, and keep the elbow and wrist behind the racket through contact.
6. Transfer the weight from the back foot to the front as the racket moves from backswing to contact to follow through.
7. Contact the ball slightly in front of the lead leg, with the knuckles facing the net at that contact point.
8. Swing low to high, with the racket finishing high and parallel to the racket-side sideline.
9. Keep a full synchronized sequence to the timing of the stroke.

Elimination of Errors (Basic Backhand Groundstroke)

The Error	What Causes the Error	Correction of the Error
Ball pulled to the non-racket side of the court.	Hitting too far out in front of the body, or turning the racket shoulder too early.	Stay sideways as long as you can during the swing.
Ball directed to the non-racket side of the court.	Too late in shoulder turn to initiate a backswing.	Early anticipation and shoulder turn to set up the backswing.
Ball hit short or into the net with little velocity.	Not stepping into the ball at contact with minimal weight transfer, or not keeping your racket arm or elbow extended or fixed through contact.	Step into the ball and transfer weight forward. Hit with a flat racket face and follow a racket pattern from semi-low to high. Hit with an extended and fixed racket arm.
Ball hit long or high against opponent's fence.	Hitting with poor timing, or weight, on back foot. Also opening racket face too much and not following through, or the racket side elbow may be raised.	Synchronize the timing and transfer weight to lead foot at contact and follow through. Step into the ball at contact. Make sure to follow through. Also check grip and make sure it is an eastern backhand grip.

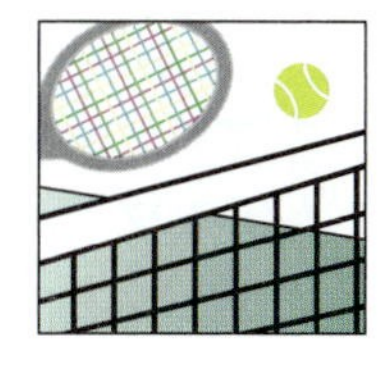

Groundstrokes—Two-hand Backhand

The two-hand backhand is immensely popular today with people who need the added strength for force and velocity, and more control particularly for the beginner who has trouble hitting the sweet spot of the racket face. The player using the two-hand backhand will gain confidence in the backhand and at the same time sacrifice the reach related to a more conventional stroke. With the exception of the lack of reach, the two-hand backhand provides the opportunity to hit both topspin and slice without changing grips; rather, the change occurs in swing action and in the position of the arms in reference to the body.

In the *two-hand backhand*, the dominant hand grips the racket with a continental grip at the butt end of the racket handle. The non-dominant hand rests on top of the racket-side hand in an eastern forehand grip. The heel of the support hand is nestled snugly between the thumb and index finger of the racket-side hand.

Preparation for hitting the ball involves basic rotation of the shoulders, except that the rotation will be limited because of the two-hand position. Rather than a loop backswing, the racket is brought straight back and then dropped low toward the feet. The same foot pivot and weight transfer occur with the two-hand backhand as with conventional eastern forehand and backhand (Figure 2.30). *Contact with the ball* involves continuation of the low- to high-pattern with the arms close to the body and the wrists firm. The weight, as with all strokes, is transferred forward

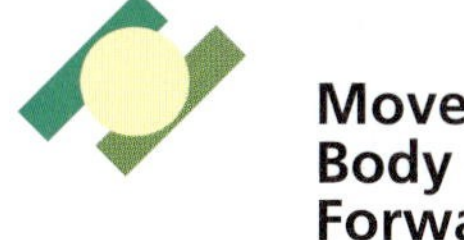

Move that Body Forward

Remember to transfer your weight, at contact, on each groundstroke.

to the lead foot as the player steps into the ball to make contact off that lead foot (Figure 2.31). The *follow through* is a simple continuation of the stroke, with the legs extended, and the hands extended and at eye level, your belly button turned to your target. The full swing comes from your shoulders and requires a solid, compact swing action. The hands work together throughout the swing (Figure 2.32).

Basic Two-Hand Backhand Groundstroke

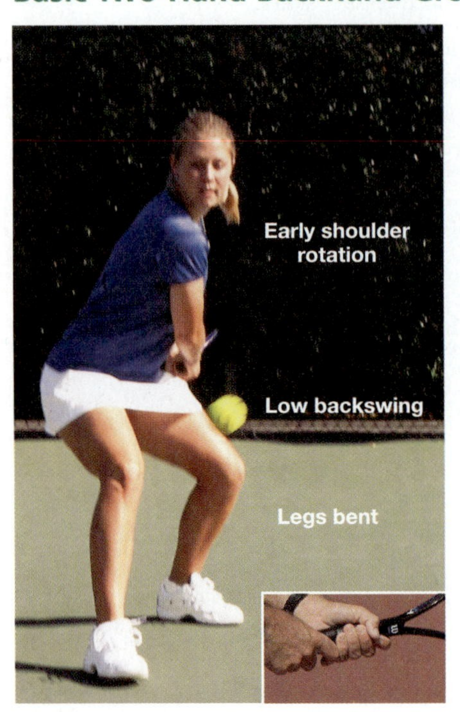

Figure 2.30 Backswing (two-hand backhand grip).

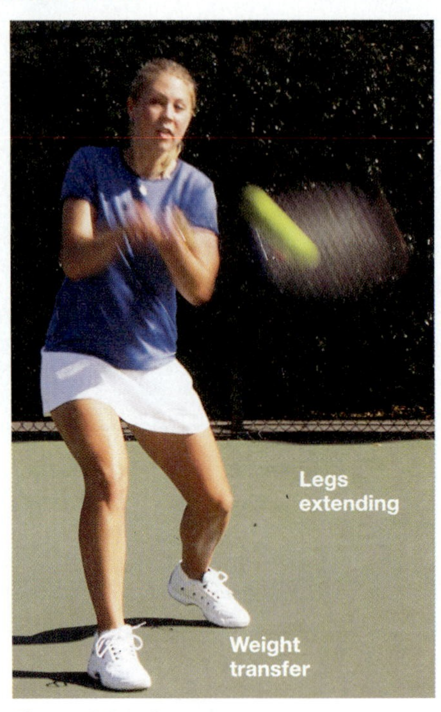

Figure 2.31 Contact.

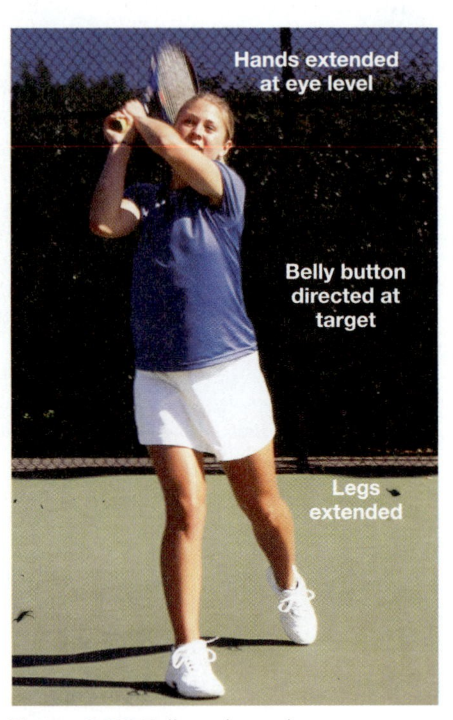

Figure 2.32 Follow through.

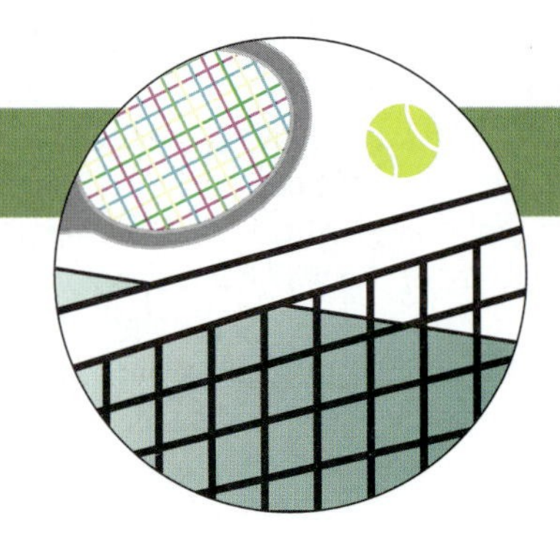

Learning Experience Reminders

Two-Hand Backhand Groundstroke

1. Keep the arms close to the body throughout the stroke, and keep the wrists firm.
2. Make sure that the two hands are snug to each other on the grip.
3. Use a low backswing to a high follow through.
4. Incorporate a compact, full swing.

Elimination of Errors (Two-Hand Backhand Groundstroke)

The Error	What Causes the Error	Correction of the Error
Stroking the ball into the net.	Hitting too far in front of the lead leg or not following the low-to-high pattern.	Hit off the lead leg and follow through to a high position.
Hitting the ball long or high against the fence.	Dropping the racket to a low position and bending the knees in an exaggerated low-to-high follow through and leg extension.	Swing low to high, and use a low leg bend followed by an extension of the legs, but eliminate the exaggerated movement.
Hitting the ball off the end of the racket or not getting to the ball in time.	Poor reaction time and little anticipation of where the ball will be hit.	Concentrate on the ball when it is in on the far side of the net. Remember that the radius of the reach is shorter with a two-hand backhand than with a one-hand backhand.

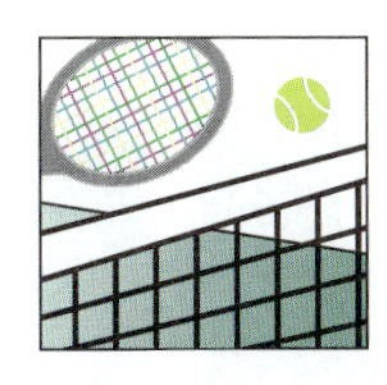

Backhand Groundstroke—Slice and Topspin

As with the forehand slice and topspin groundstroke, it is important to recognize that the basic backhand is the starting point for a beginner, but two additional strokes are available, known as the *backhand slice groundstroke* and the *backhand topspin groundstroke*. The slice is executed with a high backswing, a slightly open racket face at contact, and a high follow through (Figures 2.33–2.36). The ball action is the same underspin with a skidding action as it rebounds from the court. The eastern grip is used with this stroke.

The topspin groundstroke starts with a low backswing, a slightly closed face at contact, and a high follow through (Figures 2.37–2.40). The forearm does rotate slightly from contact to follow through, and the legs bend and extend from backswing to follow through. The eastern backhand grip is used for both the slice and the topspin.

A two-hand slice groundstroke has the same action as an eastern backhand slice stroke. And a two-hand backhand topspin stroke is particularly successful because the stroke is compact and already programmed to begin low in the backswing and continue on through to an extensive high follow through. A two-hand backhand becomes particularly successful when hitting a topspin backhand because the stroke is compact and already programmed to begin low in the backswing and continue on through to an extensive follow through.

Just as with the comments regarding the forehand groundstroke, beginners need to start with the basic backhand and progress to spin strokes as they develop. Often the slice becomes an extremely reliable stroke for the developing player, and the topspin can become quite lethal for a player who develops a two-hand backhand.

Backhand Groundstroke Slice

Figure 2.33 Backswing.

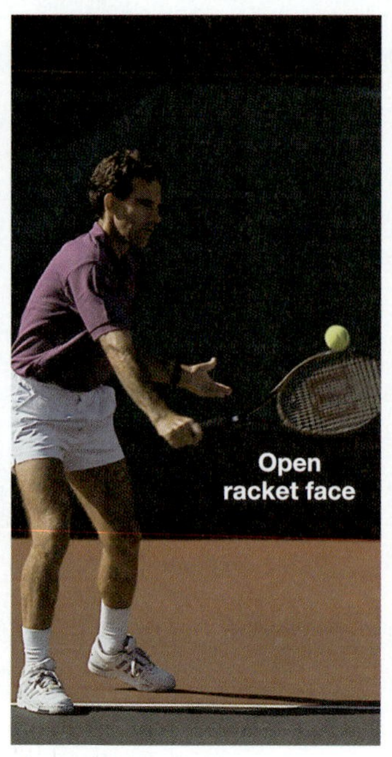

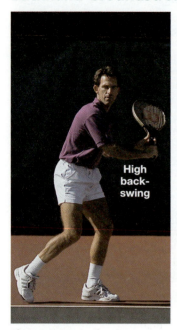

Figure 2.34 Contact.

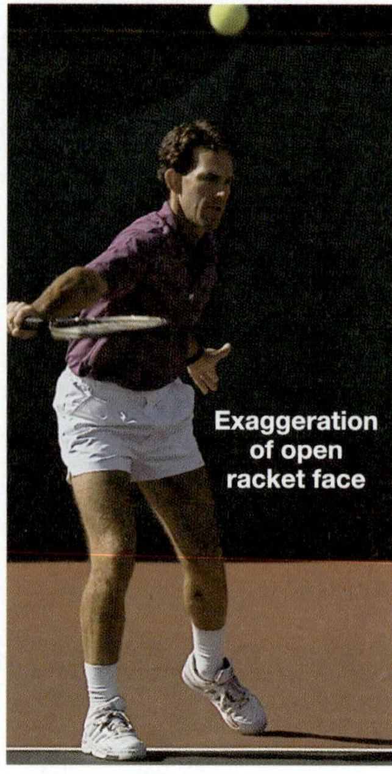

Figure 2.35 Follow through.

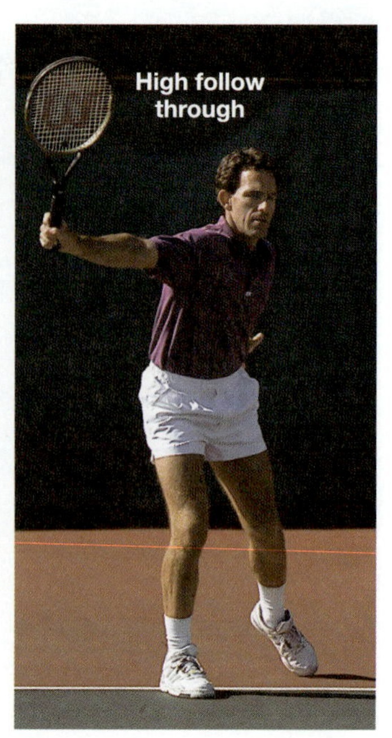

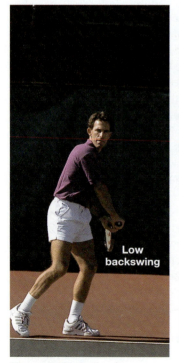

Figure 2.36 Follow through.

Backhand Groundstroke Topspin

Figure 2.37 Backswing.

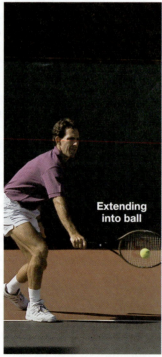

Figure 2.38 Contact.

Figure 2.39 Follow through.

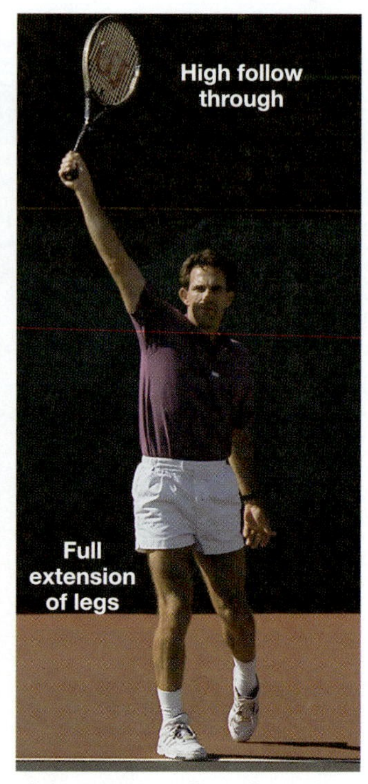

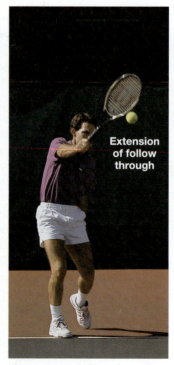

Figure 2.40 Follow through.

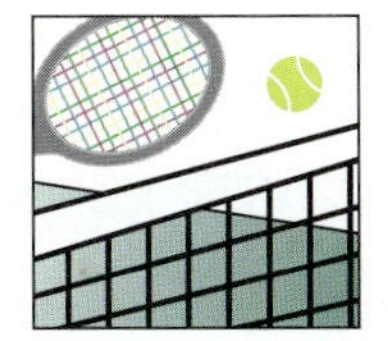

Synopsis of the Groundstroke

Groundstrokes are the basis of all play in tennis. The developing player needs to grow with the game and progress from a stationary position of hitting groundstrokes to a moving situation that will allow setting up to hit a ball. To balance the skill aspect of hitting groundstrokes, the player needs to work on both sides of the body equally to develop both forehand and backhand. The beginning player needs to be skilled at simple tasks ranging from dropping a ball and hitting a groundstroke to knowing where home base is and moving from home base to retrieve and stroke the ball.

Learning how to *drop and hit the ball* to begin a rally is necessary if a player is going to practice, warm up, or actually play the game. In a forehand groundstroke, the drop should be toward the sideline and toward the net so the player has to extend the arm to reach the ball and step, transferring weight to the lead leg to hit the ball. Dropping the ball anywhere else would confuse the player, eliminate the same form development for each stroke, and provide a difficult setup to begin a rally. One of the reasons for a forehand developing more quickly is that the player practices more on the forehand side. This is because it is more convenient to drop the ball on that side to begin a rally (Figures 2.41 and 2.42).

The drop for the backhand should be attempted as often as the forehand drop to encourage development of the backhand stroke. The backhand differs from the forehand drop only in that the drop is completed under the racket on the backhand side, and the racket is not yet in a complete backswing position. The ball is dropped in a palm-up position, and a lifting action allows the ball to bounce and come straight back up off the rebound to mid-thigh level to be hit. During the drop and swing, the body is turned to the side, facing the appropriate sideline (Figures 2.43 and 2.44). The drop for the two-hand backhand is the same as for the basic backhand except you need to re-grasp with your two-hand grip after dropping the ball.

Practice with groundstrokes usually begins from a stationary position. The area behind the baseline is known as *home base* (Figure 2.45). It is a great learning experience for the player just beginning to develop the mechanics of a sound groundstroke to have all balls hit deep to that position. The rationale for having balls thrown to students in the early stages of skill development or having a ball machine toss balls directly to a player is to ensure that home base is identified and that practice is as consistent as possible. There comes a time, however, when the player has to leave home base and move after a ball hit a distance away. The player must leave the home base area, move toward the ball, and hit a groundstroke—then return to home base.

Self-Drop For Forehand

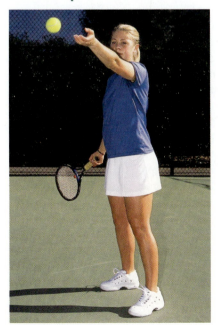

Figure 2.41 Drop the ball toward the sideline and toward the net.

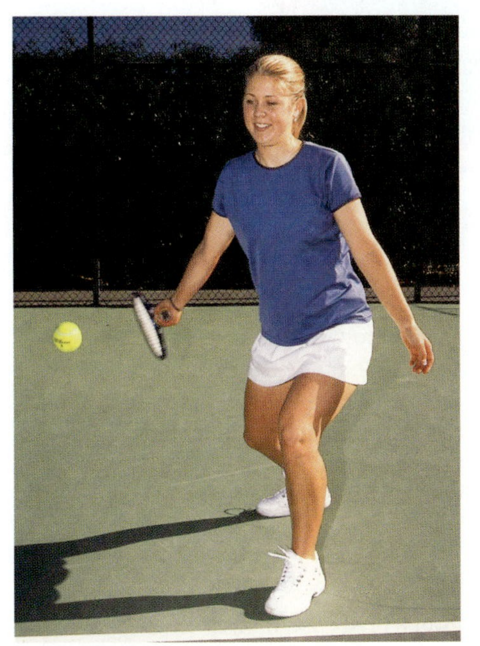

Figure 2.42 Ball should bounce and come straight back up to mid-thigh.

Self-Drop For Backhand

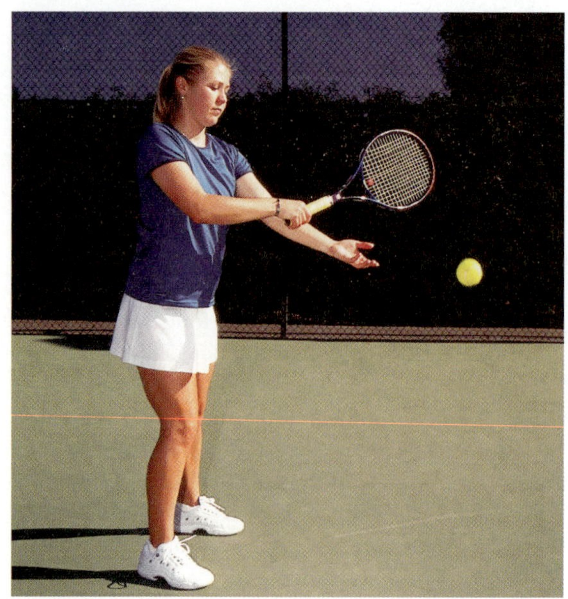

Figure 2.43 Drop the ball toward the sideline and toward the net.

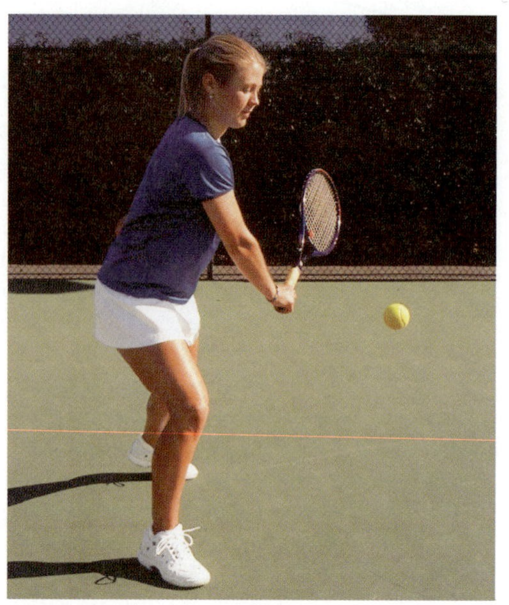

Figure 2.44 Ball should bounce and come straight back up to mid-thigh.

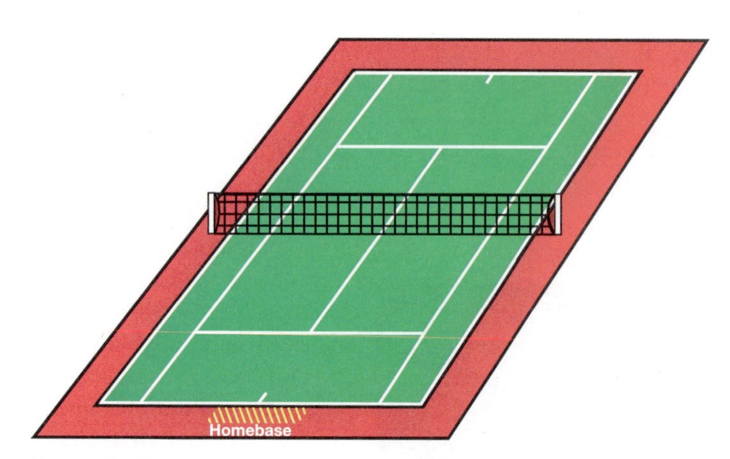

Figure 2.45 Home base.

Moving to the ball, which involves proper footwork, is a major problem for the beginning tennis player. If the ball is hit deep with a high and deep bounce, the player must retreat behind the baseline to get to the ball, set up, then step back into the ball with good weight transfer. To respond to a deeply hit ball, the player first must turn the shoulder (remember—the player always starts from a ready position) and take a sideward step with the foot that is on the same side as the turning shoulder. From that point, the movement is either a sideward response or a total turn and run to at least a step behind and away from the ball. The turning movement must occur as soon as possible, preferably before the ball crosses the net (Figure 2.46).

Moving to the ball when it is in front of the player is a little easier, but it requires the early anticipation of where the ball is going. The player moves in a direct line forward with a timing that will provide opportunity to set up behind the ball and away from the line of the ball's flight. The last part of the movement involves slowing down and gathering the body in a controlled manner, then stepping in a direct line to the ball with the racket-side foot first, thus aligning the body to the path of the ball and establishing the next sequential step.

The next step involves stepping into the ball with the non-racket-side leg in a timed movement to synchronize with the contact part of the full stroke. As the racket-side leg steps first, the racket is in a backswing position, then it comes through into the ball at contact. (See Figure 2.47.) There is no difference

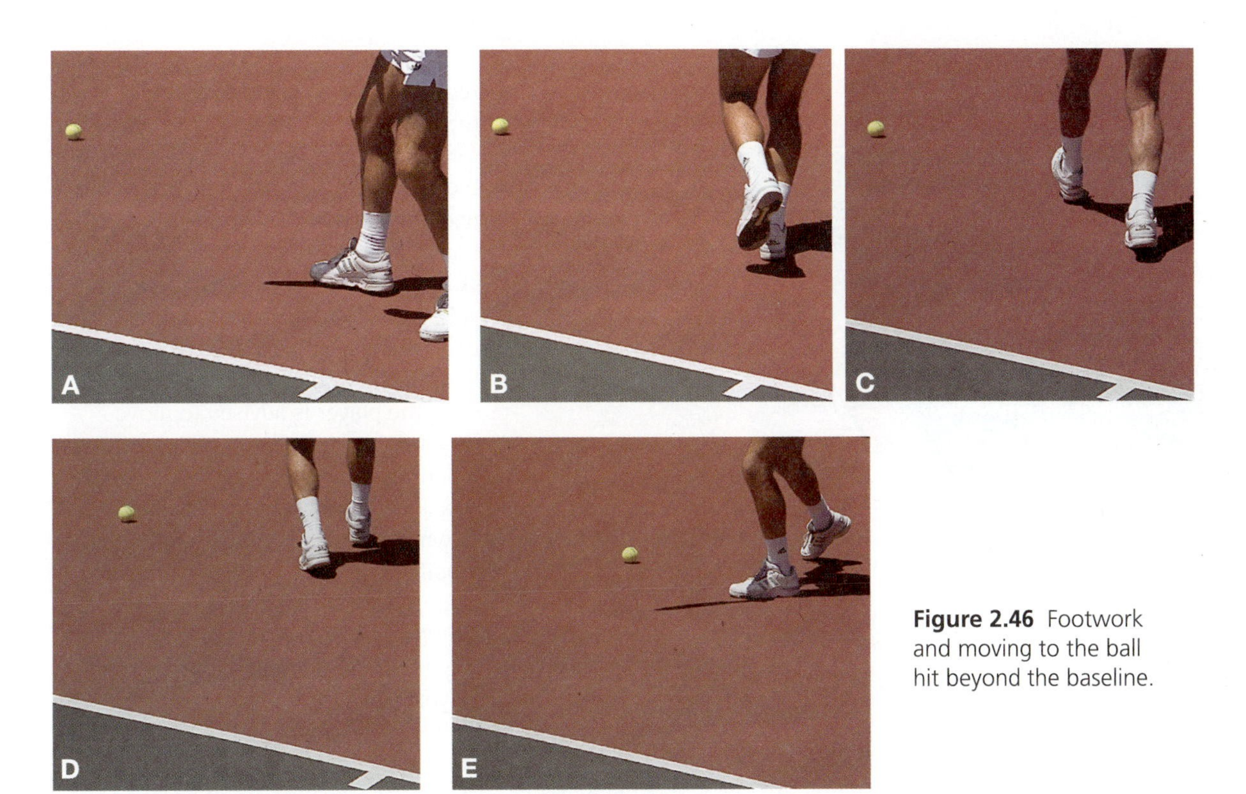

Figure 2.46 Footwork and moving to the ball hit beyond the baseline.

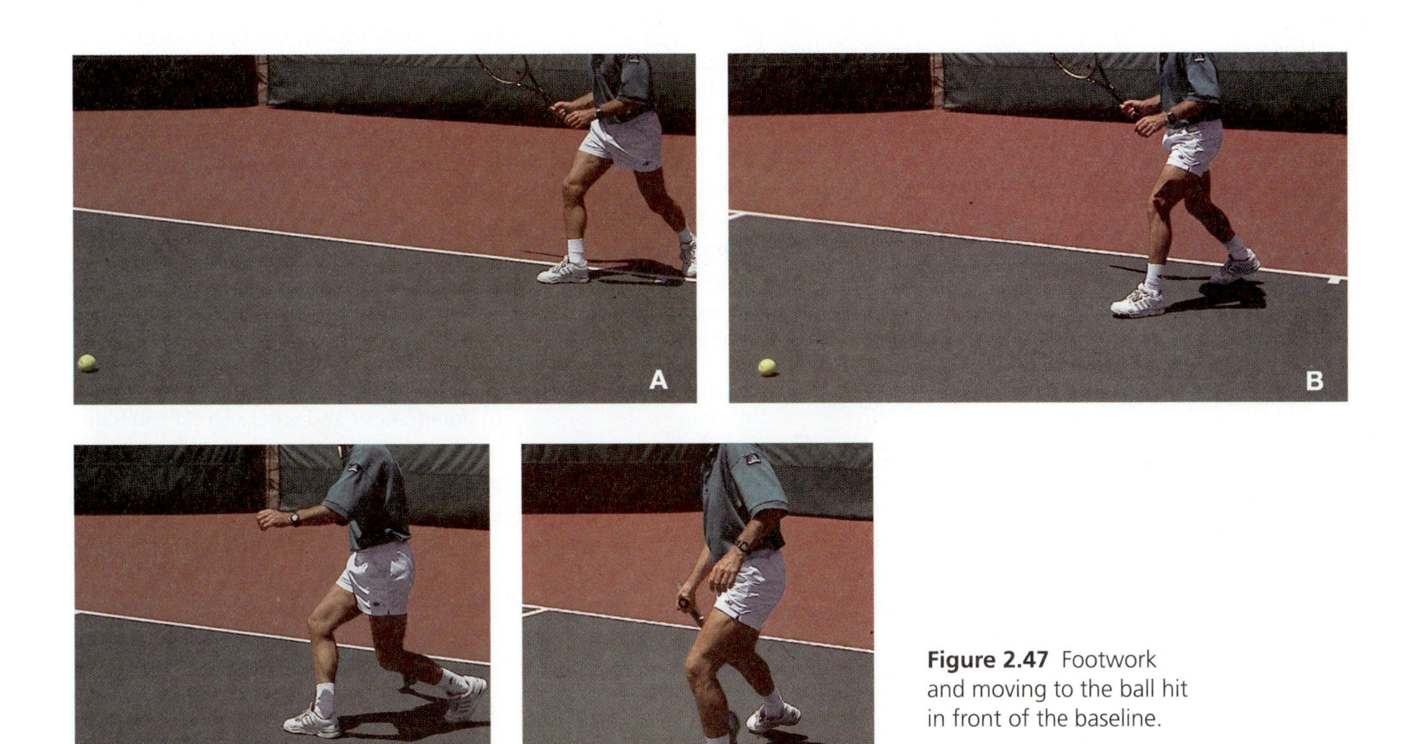

Figure 2.47 Footwork and moving to the ball hit in front of the baseline.

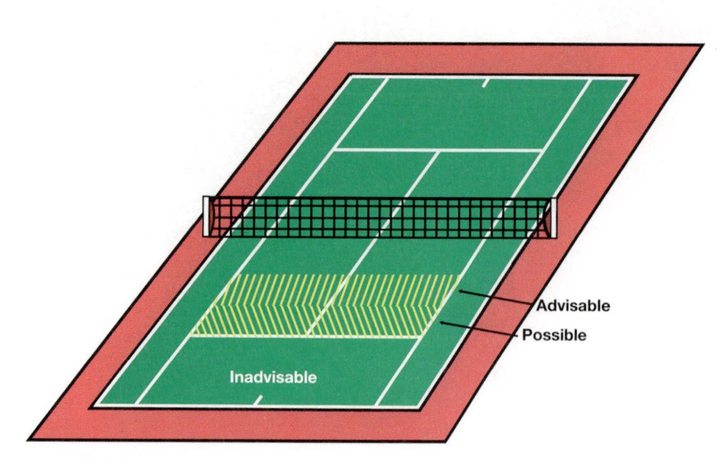

Figure 2.48 Foundation—when to go to the net, when to stay at home base.

between hitting a forehand and a backhand groundstroke. The point is to set up behind and to the side of the ball as described when dropping the ball to start a rally.

Moving to the ball or hitting from the baseline will be enjoyable if a foundation is built from the baseline that is consistent for all groundstrokes. The foundation of hitting with a stepping movement, having good weight transfer, and developing a sound stroke pattern is basic. The foundation must be repeated so often that each stroke is an instinctive reaction that does not require thought.

Using the Groundstroke to Hit an Approach Shot

Moving to hit a ball situated between the baseline and the net is related not only to foot movement but also to decision making. It is now important to recognize which shots require the player to step into the ball, stroke the ball, then return to home base, or to move up to the ball and hit it, then advance to the net. Shots that are hit at the service court line require the decision to continue to advance to the net to play a potential volley, or to retreat back to home base. Balls that are hit between the service court line and the net require no decision: the player is advised to move forward to play at the net (Figure 2.48). When a decision must be made to either attack the net or retreat to the baseline, or when the player must go to the net, a modification of the groundstroke called an *approach shot* is called for.

When it is determined that a player is going to hit an approach shot that player must develop certain perceptions. First, a player must realize that the approach shot is simply a groundstroke they must move toward in order to hit the ball. Second, the approach must be viewed as a gift given as a reward for excellent play on the baseline that forced the opponent to hit the ball short rather than deep. Third, a player must recognize that approach shots often allow for too much time to decide what to do with the ball, resulting in a shabby attempt at hitting an approach shot. Fourth, the approach shot must be considered a modified version of the full groundstroke swing.

The third and fourth concepts have to be discussed in more detail. Being given time to hit a shot allows the player to decide how and where to hit the ball. A problem exists, however, when the player changes the decision once it has been made. The player must make one

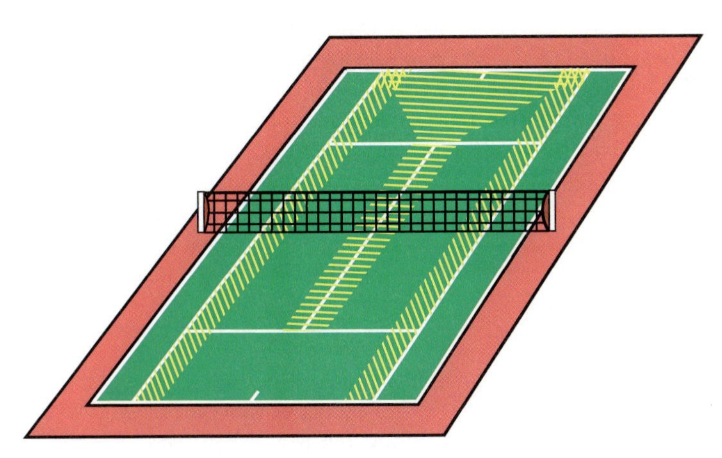

Figure 2.49 Approach shots down the line and in the corners.

decision on *how* to hit the ball, and another on *where* to hit the ball (deep or at an angle). Both judgments are difficult for beginning players, and as a result, they simply bang away at the ball, usually missing everything but the back fence. A player must be aware of the choices and continue to learn from mistakes, gaining confidence from each opportunity to hit an approach shot. The target areas are based on zones. An approach shot positioned on the side zones should be hit down that sideline; a shot positioned in the center zone should be hit down the center of the court or deep to either corner (Figure 2.49).

Modifying the approach shot to cope with the target area is the skill adaptation to the groundstroke. Three adaptations to the approach shot from the groundstroke are: (1) shorten the backswing, (2) visualize the target, and (3) select the appropriate shot sequence.

An approach shot doesn't require extensive force behind it, as does a shot from the baseline. Instead of bringing the racket back in a full backswing motion, it should be brought back perhaps two-thirds of that distance. If, when preparing to hit an approach shot, a player will develop a mental imagery of the target as being located at the opponent's service court line, the ensuing distance the ball travels probably will increase by a third of the distance. As a result, the ball will really travel to the opponent's baseline. The baseline is the spot desired for a deep hit, but the mental imagery has to give a shortened target distance to allow for the shortened distance the ball actually must travel.

Selecting the appropriate shot is based on the position of the ball to be hit. Balls that are returned low are usually hit to the backhand of the opponent, with the player then moving to the net to hit a volley off the opponent's assumed weaker backhand return. Returns that hit the center of the court have a target area of the corners. Hitting a ball cross-court that is positioned down the line opens up too much court for the opposing player to return successfully.

The sequence of moving from the baseline to hitting an approach shot is continued by the player moving on to the net to play a potential volley return of the opponent's reaction to the approach shot. Discussion of the volley sequence is found in the following chapter.

Check Points

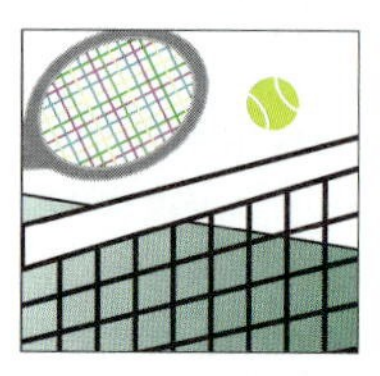

1. The three parts to a basic forehand groundstroke are
   a. preparation, loop backswing, and follow through.
   b. preparation, contact, and follow through.
   c. loop backswing, contact, and follow through.
   d. preparation, loop backswing, and contact.

2. When hitting a forehand groundstroke the
   a. wrist and forearm remain firm but relaxed.
   b. wrist is laid back and the elbow is hyperextended.
   c. wrist remains firm with the elbow hyperextended.
   d. wrist is laid back and the elbow is firm but relaxed.

3. The correction of the error of shots hit short with little velocity requires
   a. changing the swing from slightly low to high.
   b. changing the swing from slightly high to low.
   c. transfer of weight into the ball at contact.
   d. stepping away from the ball at contact.

4. To hit a topspin forehand groundstroke requires an adjustment from the basic stroke that includes
   a. eastern grip, low-to-high swing, and leg flexion and extension.
   b. western grip, low-to-high swing, and leg flexion and extension.
   c. western grip, flat backswing to high follow through, and leg flexion and extension.
   d. eastern grip, low-to-high swing, and leg flexion.

5. A characteristic of hitting a basic backhand groundstroke includes
   a. shoulder leading into contact with racket rotating around the wrist and elbow leading the racket.
   b. shoulder leading into contact with the wrist and elbow leading the racket.
   c. shoulder held back with the wrist and elbow leading the racket.
   d. shoulder leading into contact with the racket rotating around the wrist and elbow.

6. A backhand groundstroke hit long is caused by
   a. hitting with poor timing and/or weight on the back foot.
   b. too much of an open racket face with no follow through.
   c. hitting with an open racket face, poor timing, and not following through.
   d. all three of the above causes.

7. The two-hand backhand groundstroke requires that the follow through is a
   a. racket finish in a wrap-around of shoulders and head, and the belly button turned toward the hitting target.
   b. racket finish high with the belly button turned toward the hitting target.
   c. racket finish in a wrap-around of shoulders and head, and the belly button turned to the racket side of the body.
   d. combination of a, b and c.

8. Hitting the ball off the end of the racket when hitting a two-hand backhand is caused by
   a. not dropping the racket to a low position.
   b. poor reaction timing and limited anticipation.
   c. hitting too far out in front of the lead leg.
   d. not swinging low to high.

9. When attempting to hit a moving ball that is short or deep the player must
   a. set up even with the ball and step up even with the ball to hit it.
   b. set up in front of the ball and step into the ball to hit it.
   c. move at an angle to set up behind the ball and step into the ball to hit it.
   d. move straight to the ball and step into the ball to hit it.

10. Approach shots should be hit
    a. with a visual image target to the opponent's service court line.
    b. with a reduced backswing.
    c. with a target of down-the-line to the corners and to the center.
    d. using b in combination with a and c.

Answers to Check Points can be found on page 145.

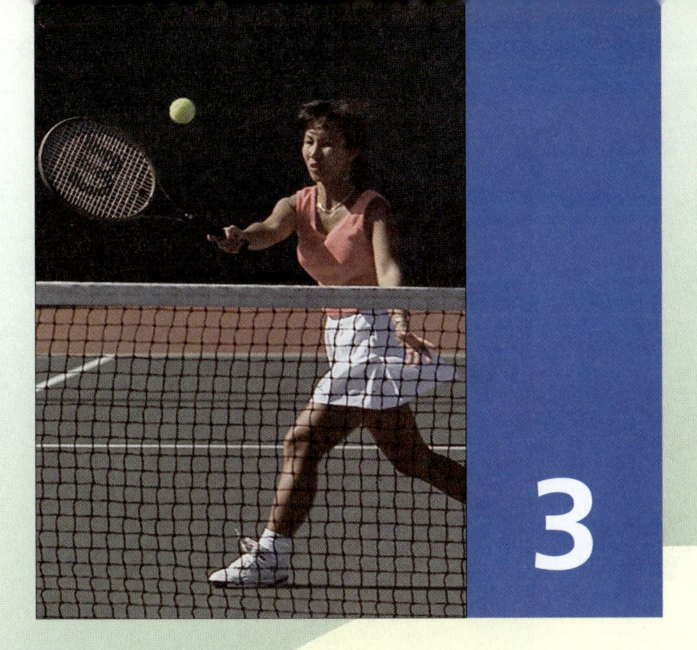

3

Net Play

The volley is one of two strokes hit when the ball is in mid-air prior to striking the court on the bounce. It is an uncomplicated punching action stroke also described as a "blocking-the-ball action." The volley is used in singles play following an approach shot or in a serve-and-volley combination. In doubles, the volley also is used following an approach shot and as a serve-and-volley combination, and it is used with a player positioned at the net during a serve. Early in their development all players must learn the skills involved in the volley. A singles player may avoid most situations involving the volley, but in doubles play there is no choice but to be located at the net on most shots played.

The volley shot begins from the *ready position* as described when preparing to hit a groundstroke, except that the racket is held higher, at chin level (Figure 3.1). From this position the player may respond to either a forehand or a backhand volley while located at the net. Part of the preparation in the ready position is to assume a grip that is both comfortable and functional.

The *continental grip* usually is recommended for the volley, as no adjustment has to be made for a forehand or a backhand volley (Figure 3.1). Often there is not enough time to change grips when at the net because of the high velocity of a ball and the short distance from the opposing player. The strength of the continental grip is that the backhand is firm and solid when punching the volley. The weakness is that the grip for a forehand provides a weaker base, forcing the player to adjust at the net by changing to an eastern forehand when time permits. Most successful players do "cheat" and move the hand on the grip for most volley shots providing that they have the time not only to change but also to change back following the stroke.

Keep your back against the wall.

An attacking volley requires meeting the ball out in front of your body with forward weight transfer. Maintain the image of a wall directly behind you forcing you to move forward and not allowing you to take a long backswing.

L. Naelon, Tennis, 11/95, p. 34

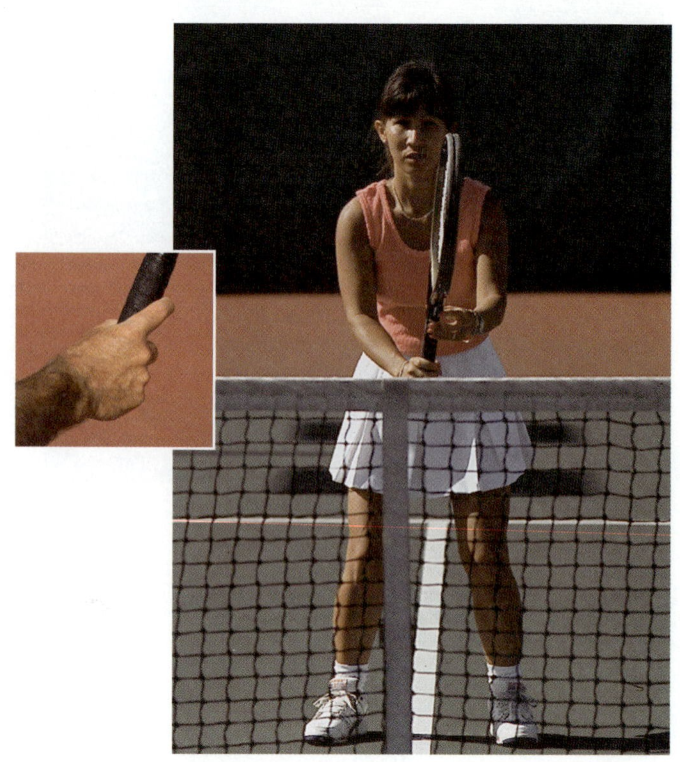

Figure 3.1 Volley ready position (continental grip).

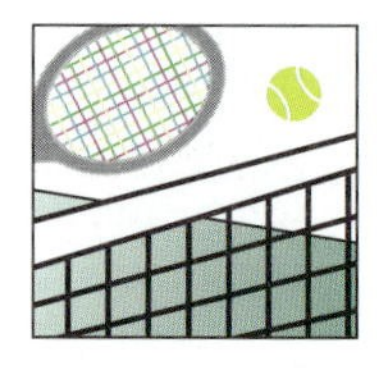

Forehand Volley

The *forehand volley* begins with a "short" backswing created by a shoulder turn. The racket head is located above the hand as the racket is taken back even with the racket shoulder (Figure 3.2). The *preparation* is completed with the weight centered on the racket-side foot. The racket comes forward at *contact* with the ball, with the face of the racket striking the back of the ball squarely at the front of the lead leg (Figure 3.3). A slight downward path of the stroke with a slightly open racket face imparts some underspin to the ball. At contact, the racket head is positioned above the hand, the wrist remains firm, and the grip is also firm in order to prevent the racket from turning in the hand at impact. A step is taken with the opposing leg, and the weight is transferred to that leg. The knees are bent from backswing to contact. It should be repeated that the racket must be in front of the lead leg at contact.

The *follow through* (Figure 3.4) is the final part of the punching action. A short downward motion, with the bottom edge of the racket leading, completes the stroke. The lead leg is still bent during follow through, with the weight centered over that leg. Upon completion of follow through, the player must return to a ready position in preparation for the next volley.

Forehand Volley Sequence

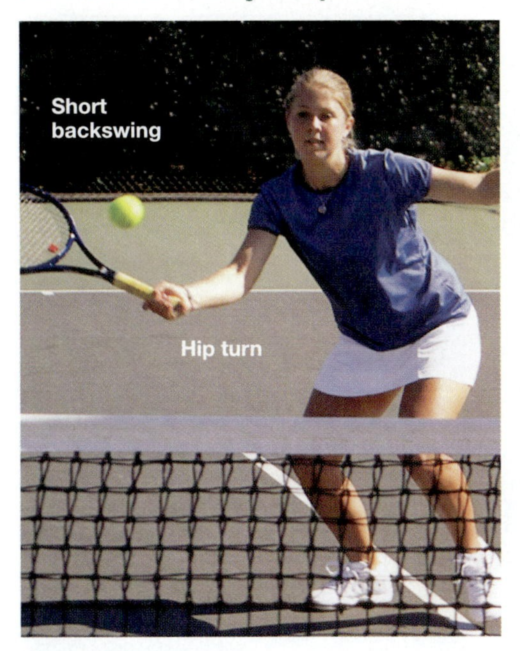

Figure 3.2 Preparation.

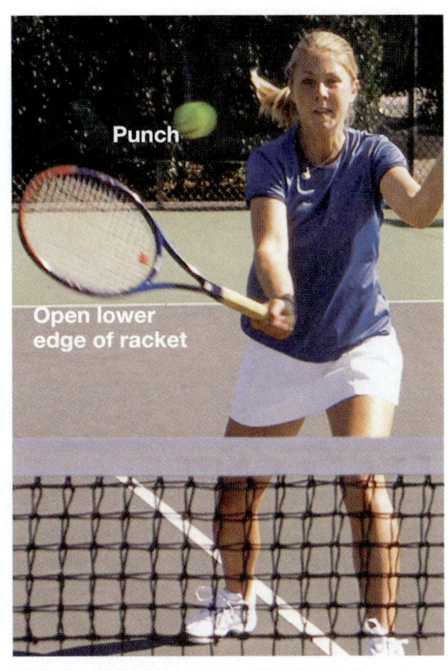

Figure 3.3 Contact with the ball.

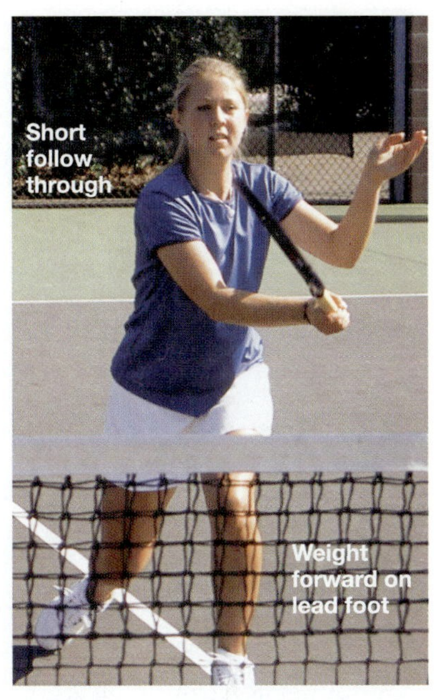

Figure 3.4 Follow through.

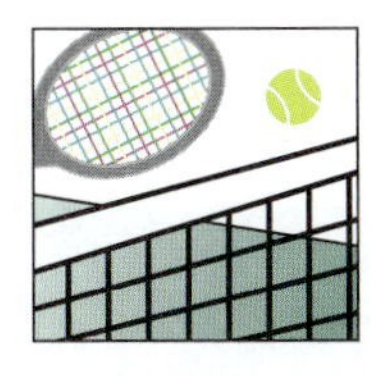

Backhand Volley

The *backhand volley* is executed like the forehand volley, but it is easier to complete mechanically because the shoulder turn is already to the backhand side and the elbow and shoulder work as a firm backboard when striking the ball. In *preparation*, the racket head is brought back to the non-racket side and is positioned above the hand. The weight of the body is centered over the non-racket-side foot, and the backswing is short with a firm wrist.

At *contact*, the weight shifts forward to the racket leg as that leg steps into the ball (Figure 3.5). The racket face strings make full square contact with the back of the ball with a punching action that includes a firm wrist and arm, and a firm grip on the racket. Contact is made slightly in front of the lead leg, with the racket above the hand (Figure 3.6). The knees are bent from preparation through contact and into the follow through.

The *follow through* is a continuation of the punch action, with the bottom edge of the racket leading to apply a slight spin to the ball (Figure 3.7). At the end of the follow through, the weight is centered on the leading leg and the racket is extended a short distance forward. The recovery must be quick as the player returns to the ready position at the net.

Two-hand Backhand Volley

A *two-hand backhand volley* can also be used at the net. The stroke is the same as the *basic backhand volley*, but you are limited in terms of your arm and leg extension. This is a relatively severe limitation, but with good footwork and the reminder to keep your arms into your body, it is an effective volley stroke (Figures 3.8–3.10). As you develop confidence and skill at the net you need to move away from two hands to a more effective one-hand backhand volley stroke.

Backhand Volley Sequence

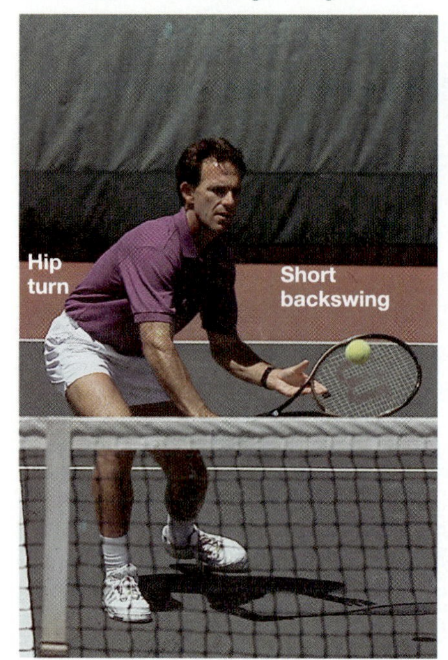

Figure 3.5 Preparation.

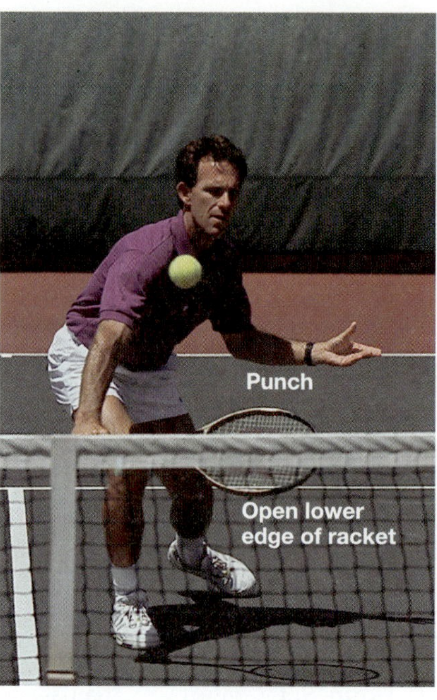

Figure 3.6 Contact with the ball.

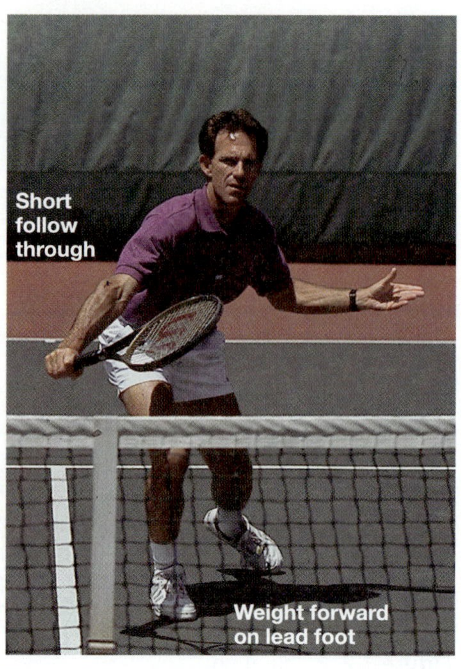

Figure 3.7 Follow through.

Two-hand Backhand Volley Sequence

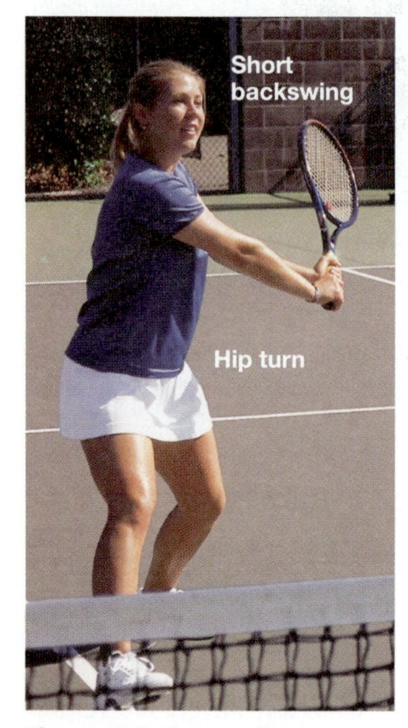

Figure 3.8 Preparation.

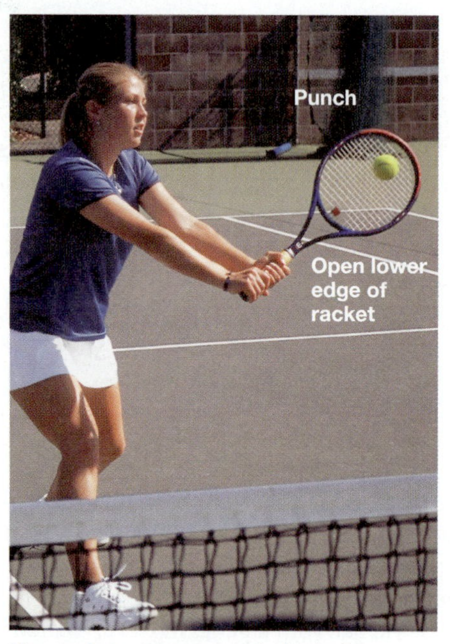

Figure 3.9 Contact with the ball.

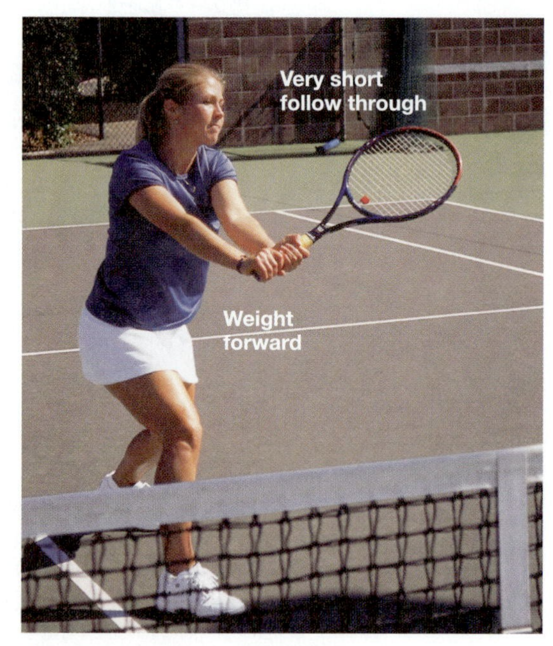

Figure 3.10 Follow through.

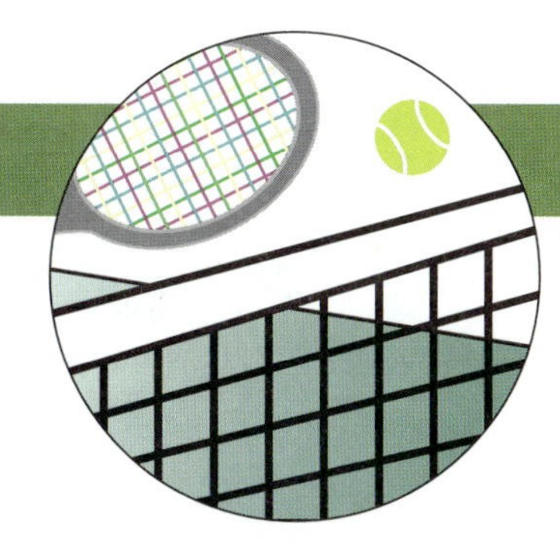

Learning Experience Reminders

Volley

1. Punch the ball—do not swing at it.
2. Keep backswing and follow brief.
3. Keep the racket above the hand throughout the stroke.
4. Step into the ball if time allows.
5. Stay low on the ball.
6. Hit behind the ball, then follow through with the bottom edge of the racket leading.
7. Make contact in front of the lead leg.
8. Begin with the continental grip, but "cheat" when time allows.
9. Maintain control of the racket with a firm grip and firm wrist throughout the stroke.

Elimination of Errors (Volley)

The Error	What Causes the Error	Correction of the Error
Balls that have no pace or just drop off the racket strings.	Not hitting in front of the lead leg; not transferring weight into the ball at contact.	Hit slightly in front of the lead leg between the body and net. Step into and punch through the ball.
Racket turns in the hand, causing lack of control of the ball.	Lack of a firm grip, or grip size is too small.	Tighten the grip or increase the size of the grip for better control.
Ball strikes the net following contact.	Player not getting "down on the ball" and bending the knees when the ball is below the height of the net. Or, racket face is not open enough at contact.	Bend the knees all the way through the shot. If ball is below the net open the racket face and punch through the ball.
Ball is hit long.	Elbow usually not firm.	Keep elbow away from the body through contact.

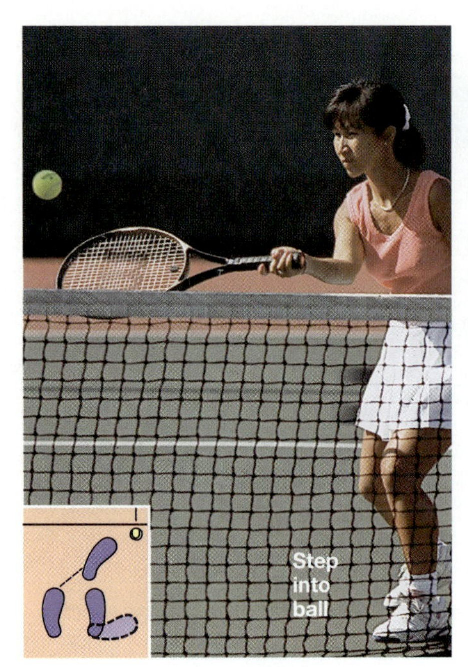

Figure 3.11 Footwork for the setup volley (forehand).

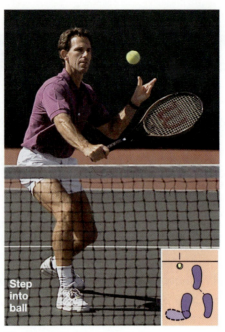

Figure 3.12 Footwork for the setup volley (backhand).

Evade the Ball

On balls hit at you when at the net, evading the ball means getting out of its way by rotating your shoulders and hitting a backhand volley.

D. Van Der Meer, Tennis, 4/92, p. 89

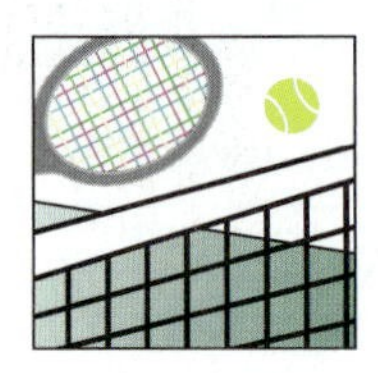

Insight When Hitting a Volley

Anticipation is a key to playing well at the net. If the player at the net is afraid of the ball, there will be no anticipation. If the player "sees" the ball early, reacting as the ball comes off the opposing player's racket rather than waiting until the ball arrives at the net, the volleying player will be effective at the net. Once the reaction has been improved, the next important phase is to attack by stepping into the ball rather than waiting for the ball to arrive at the net. Even guessing, as part of anticipation, is better than standing at the net and waiting.

Footwork for the volley is an important aspect of the stroke so that form can be added to the total maneuver. Footwork enables the player to step into the ball with body weight behind the punch, and to move efficiently to get to the ball. The first part of the footwork involves a shoulder turn and hip pivot. From a ready position, the player should pivot the hips toward the anticipated position of the ball. With the hip turn, the shoulders will turn also, and the racket-side foot will react by pivoting until the body weight centers over that foot.

Three basic ball positions presented to the volleyer are: (1) the setup with the shoulder and hip turn, involving a small cross-step, (2) the wide ball that forces the player to take a lengthened cross-step, and (3) the ball hit at the player that requires a defensive reaction. The *setup* is initiated with the shoulder and hip turn, followed by the turn of the inside of the foot and a step forward and a little across the body with the opposite leg (Figures 3.11 and 3.12). The *wide ball* is reached by the same movement used for the setup, but the step across the body with the opposite leg requires an elongated, direct movement (Figures 3.13 and 3.14).

Figure 3.13 Footwork for the wide-ball volley (forehand).

Figure 3.14 Footwork for the wide-ball volley (backhand).

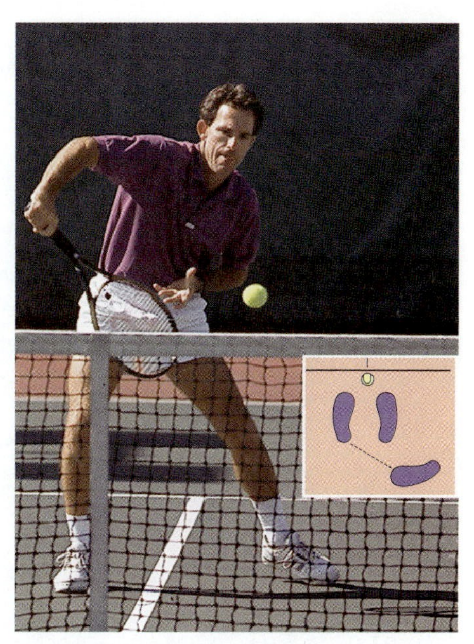

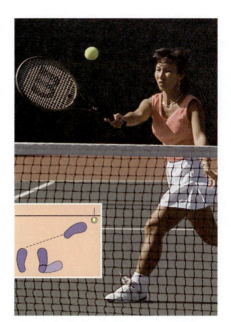

Figure 3.15 Footwork for the ball hit at the net player (backhand).

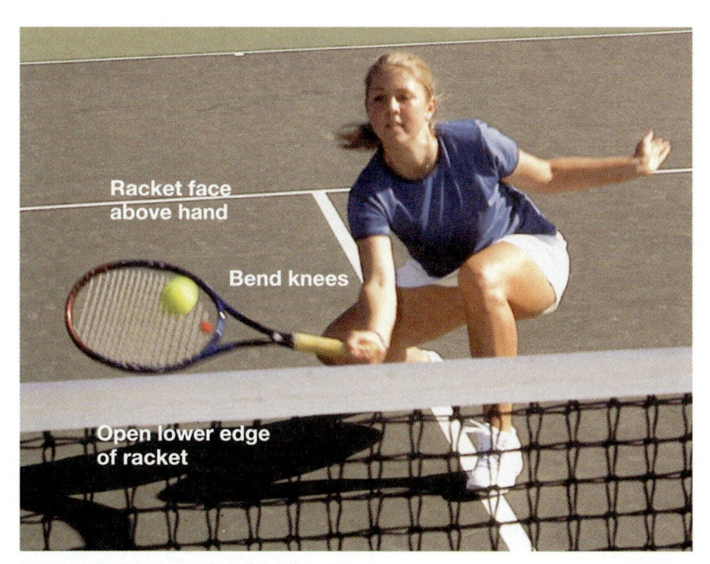

Figure 3.16 Low forehand volley.

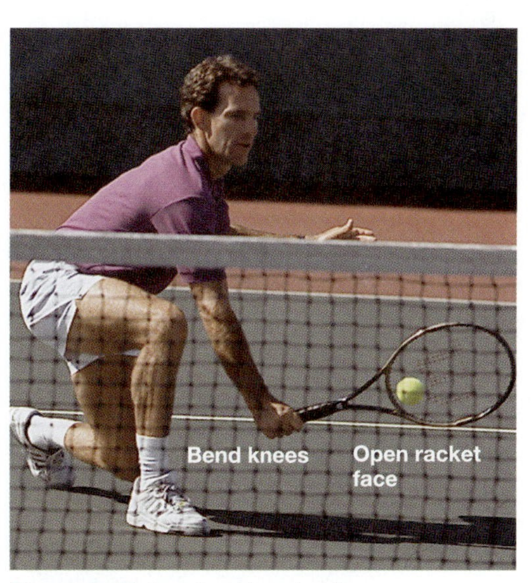

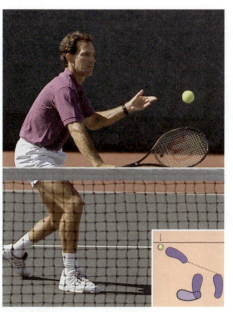

Figure 3.17 Low backhand volley.

The *ball hit at the player* requires that the player hit with a backhand volley, if at all possible. The player must pivot off the racket foot and step with the non-racket foot behind the opposite foot to turn the shoulder sideways to the ball. The player then must lean back into the path of the ball (Figure 3.15).

Body elevation also is important to successful completion of the volley, as balls are not going to be returned at shoulder level in all situations. The legs must be either bent or extended for many of the volley stroke situations.

A *low volley* forces the player to bend the knees and get low to the ball (Figures 3.16 and 3.17). The hip and shoulder turn must occur to position the shoulder to the ball, and the legs must bend as low as possible. The volleyer steps into the ball with the opposite foot and punches under and through the ball, using underspin to lift the ball over the net. The underspin is achieved by

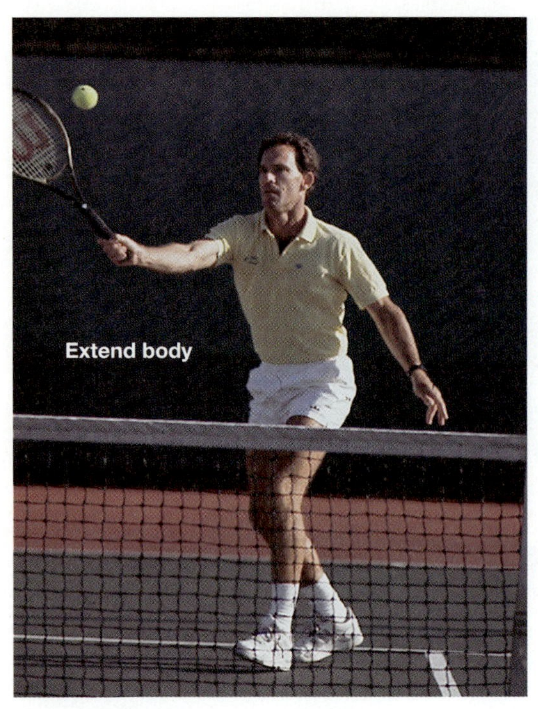

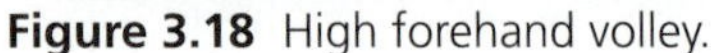
Figure 3.18 High forehand volley.

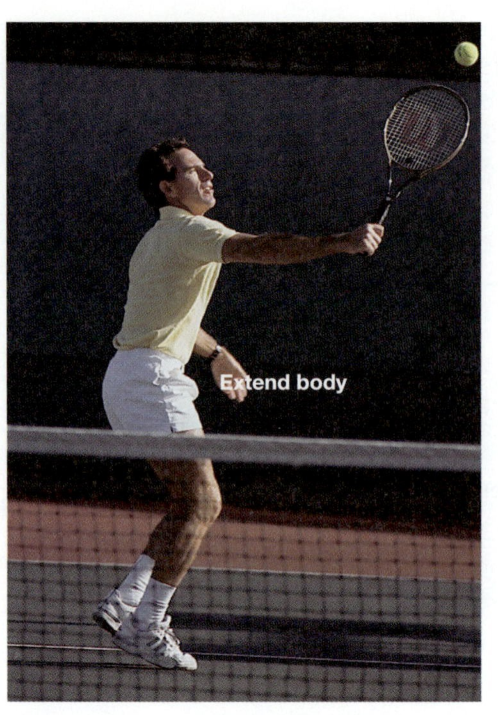

Figure 3.19 High backhand volley.

opening the racket face. The closer the ball is to the court at contact, the more open the racket face should be. The follow through of the low shot continues with an upward, short movement of the racket, with the knees remaining bent. Throughout the stroke, the racket should stay above the hand, if possible, to ensure proper technique and stroking action.

The *high volley* forces the volleyer to extend the body and the legs to reach the ball. The shoulder turn must occur early to permit the racket to be taken back a little farther and higher than for the basic volley. The player then steps into the ball with the opposite leg and punches down and through the ball. The follow through moves in the direction of the ball just hit and ends at waist level. The punching pattern is a high-to-low closing stroke. The wrist is locked, and the stroke is firm. (See Figures 3.18 and 3.19.)

The volley has to be *incorporated into the total game* of the beginning player. At this point, the volley is an extension of the player hitting a groundstroke and advancing to the net, or hitting an approach shot and moving to the net, or hitting at the net in doubles play. The volley is a reward for forcing the opponent into a mistake, and it is executed best between the service court line and the net.

Beginning players will play most volleys off the net at a range of one to one and one-half racket lengths away from the net. More advanced players have a wider range back to the service court line, but the same players have the goal of moving closer to the net to be less vulnerable to a well-placed low shot at the feet.

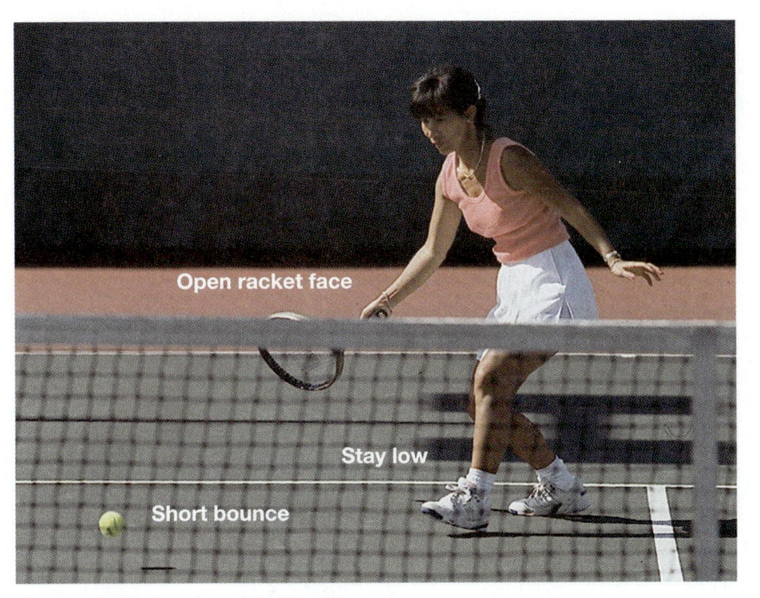

Figure 3.20 Forehand half-volley.

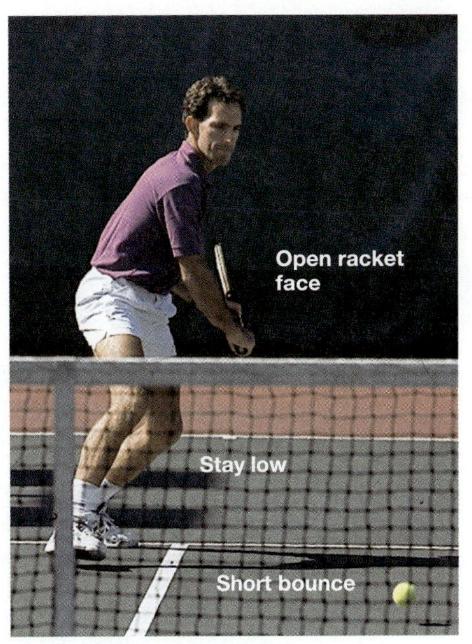

Figure 3.21 Backhand half-volley.

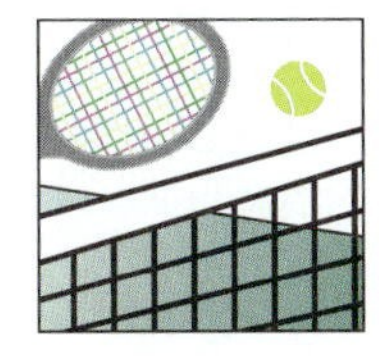

Half Volley

Half volleys are necessary when the player is positioned in the midcourt area and is confronted with a return shot placed just in front of the feet. The player uses an eastern forehand or backhand grip, or a continental grip, and strokes the ball as a combination groundstroke and volley. The player must bend both legs to the extreme, with the lead leg bent at a right angle and the back leg nearly scraping the court surface. The ball must be contacted on the "short" bounce or before it rises. The wrist is firm at contact, and the angle of the racket face is open just enough to permit the ball to clear the net. The backswing is short, as with an approach shot, and the follow through lifts the body up from the low position. Throughout the shot, the head should stay down to ensure that the body does not lift early. The forehand half-volley contact point is at the lead leg, and the backhand point is in front of the lead leg. (See Figures 3.20 and 3.21.)

Check Points

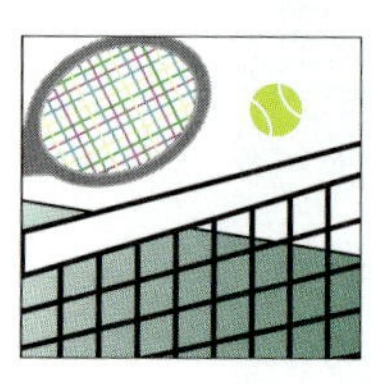

1. The type of grip used for the volley is the
   a. eastern forehand.
   b. eastern backhand.
   c. western forehand.
   d. continental.

2. The backswing for a volley shot is
   a. shortened.
   b. lengthened.
   c. the same as a regular groundstroke.
   d. any of the three depending on the situation.

3. Contact with the ball is made
   a. in front of the lead leg.
   b. behind the lead leg.
   c. even with the lead leg.
   d. with all three depending on the situation.

4. The correction for the shot that hits the net following contact is
   a. tighten the grip.
   b. align the wrist, arms, and shoulders in a firm position.
   c. bend the knees through the shot.
   d. close the racket face.

5. The body position for a ball hit directly at the body of the volleying player is
   a. use a backhand volley.
   b. drop step to hit the ball.
   c. use a forehand stroke.
   d. use a and b in combination with each other.

6. A low volley position requires
   a. opening the racket face at contact.
   b. closing the racket face at contact.
   c. hitting with a square face at contact.
   d. hitting off the back foot.

7. The beginning player has a comfort zone range at the net of
   a. 1 to 1 ½ racket length from the net.
   b. from the service court to the net.
   c. 2 to 2 ½ racket length from the net.
   d. anywhere on the court.

8. A half volley is hit with
   a. an open racket face at the top of the ball bounce.
   b. a closed racket face off a short bounce.
   c. a square face off a short bounce.
   d. an open face off a short bounce.

Answers to Check Points can be found on page 145.

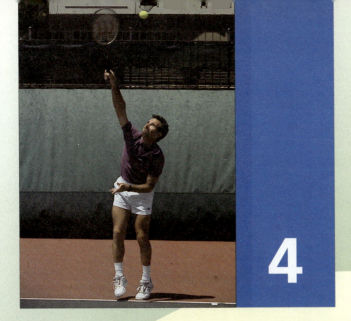

4

The Service and Service Return

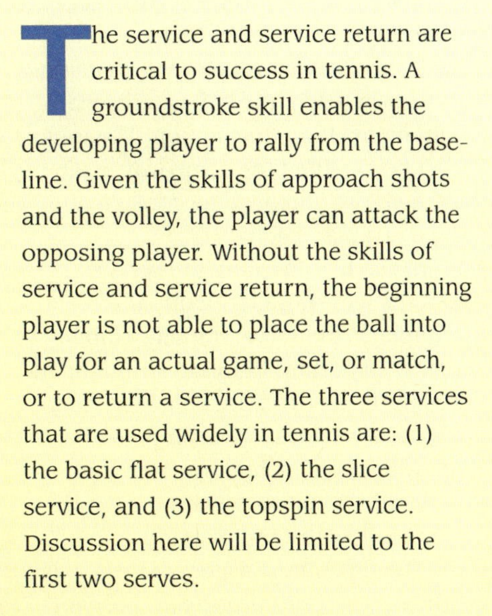

The service and service return are critical to success in tennis. A groundstroke skill enables the developing player to rally from the baseline. Given the skills of approach shots and the volley, the player can attack the opposing player. Without the skills of service and service return, the beginning player is not able to place the ball into play for an actual game, set, or match, or to return a service. The three services that are used widely in tennis are: (1) the basic flat service, (2) the slice service, and (3) the topspin service. Discussion here will be limited to the first two serves.

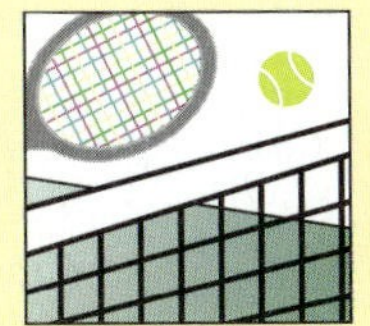

Basic Flat Service

The *basic flat service* is a model for the service. A *service stance* is used in all serves. The feet are approximately shoulder-width apart, with the lead foot positioned approximately the length of a tennis ball from the baseline and the center mark of the baseline. The shoulder is pointed toward the service court target, the knees are slightly flexed, and the body from the waist up is upright (Figure 4.1).

The *grip* for the *flat service* (and for the two other services) is the continental, with some possible slight variations. The continental grip provides a flat surface for a square contact point. When learning to serve, you may begin by using an eastern forehand or a western forehand grip, but you should change to a continental grip as soon as possible.

Skill is involved in *holding the ball for the toss* that initiates the serve action and also *in actually tossing the ball.* To begin any service, you must have two tennis balls in your possession. Keep one ball in the pocket of your tennis shorts so you have to cope with only one ball during any one serve. Grasp the ball to be tossed with the fingertips and the thumb, with the heel of the hand pointing in the direction of the toss (Figure 4.2). From the support base, the ball is placed into a position off the lead shoulder between the player and the sideline, and higher than the reach of the racket. A straight arm lifts the ball from the waist to above the head. The

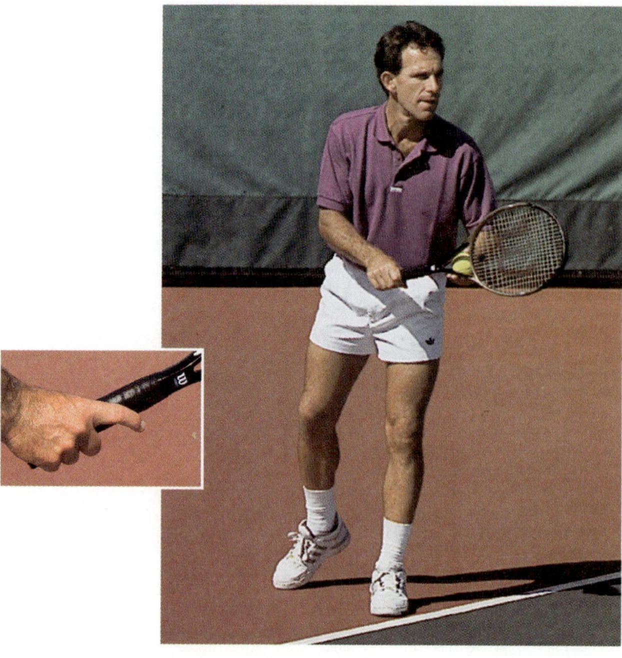

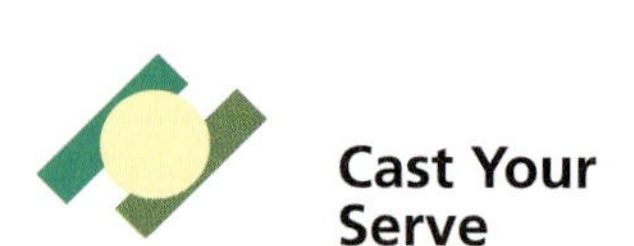

Figure 4.1 Service stance (continental grip).

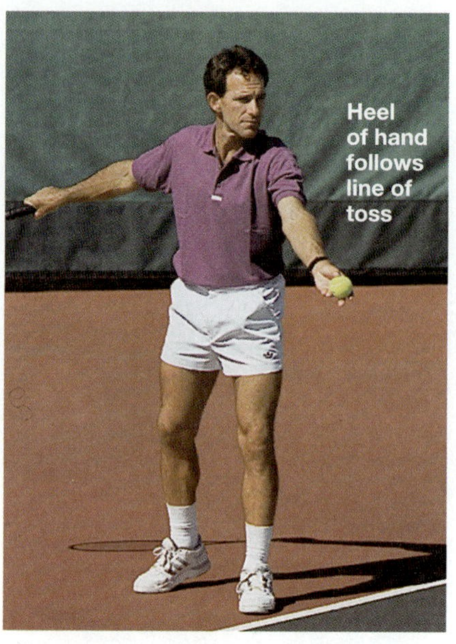

Figure 4.2 Beginning of toss.

Cast Your Serve

Relax your arm and visualize that you are fly fishing.

J. Langolis & J. Langolis, Tennis, 5/93, p. 25

heel of the hand is raised during the full arm movement. As the tossing arm begins the upward movement, the racket arm brings the racket back in synchronization with the toss. At the extension of the arm reach, the ball is released, culminating the lifting action. The toss must be executed the same way again and again so you become consistent (Figures 4.3 and 4.4).

When first learning the service, keep the feet shoulder-width apart throughout the serve. Initially, stability is more important than extra rhythm. Although the feet will not come together in the early stages of learning, the back foot will automatically come forward as the weight transfers toward the target on the follow through (Figures 4.5–4.7).

The first timing aspect of the service is the *toss synchronization as preparation for the service.* As the tossing hand begins the upward lift of the ball, the racket begins a backward movement with the arm straight. The two arms move in opposition. The racket continues back, with the elbow bending as the racket approaches the shoulder-blade area. The back of the elbow is at a right angle, and the arm is in an overhand throwing position. As the ball reaches the top of the placement and begins to fall, the tossing hand will drop away and the hitting elbow will stay in a right-angle position. (See Figures 4.8–4.12.)

Following the backswing, the initiation of contact now occurs. The legs straighten from a bent position in preparation for bringing the racket through in a striking position, with the wrist and forearm breaking, and along with the shoulders, rotating through the contact of the ball. The arm and body are stretched fully. The back and top of the ball is hit with the racket face at about 4 inches down from the height of the toss. The body, led by the shoulder, opens up to the position of the ball at contact (Figure 4.13).

The follow through continues as momentum carries the racket through the ball and on down to the far non-racket-side leg. A definite weight transfer occurs during follow through, with the momentum of the racket side pulling the body down and forward. This forces the back foot at the last moment to step forward for a balanced finish (Figures 4.14–4.16).

The basic flat service is designed mechanically to hit through and down on the ball. The ball cannot be hit directly down in a straight line unless the server is at least 6'7" tall. The racket

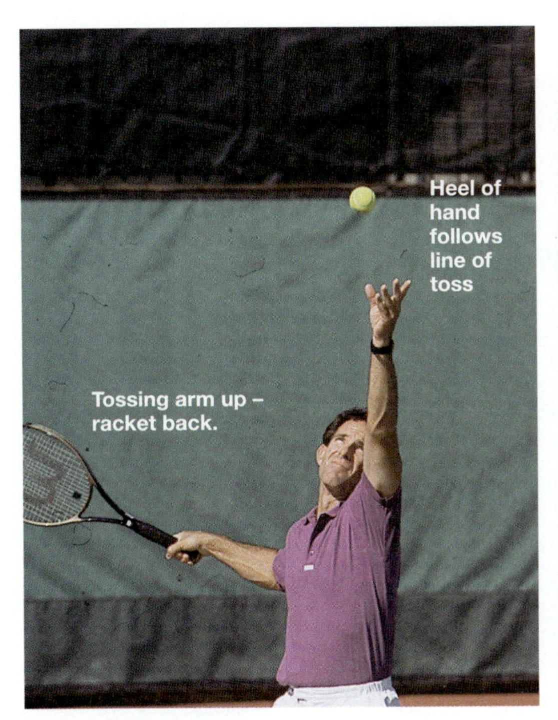
Heel of
hand
follows
line of
toss
Tossing arm up –
racket back.

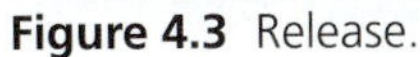
Figure 4.3 Release.

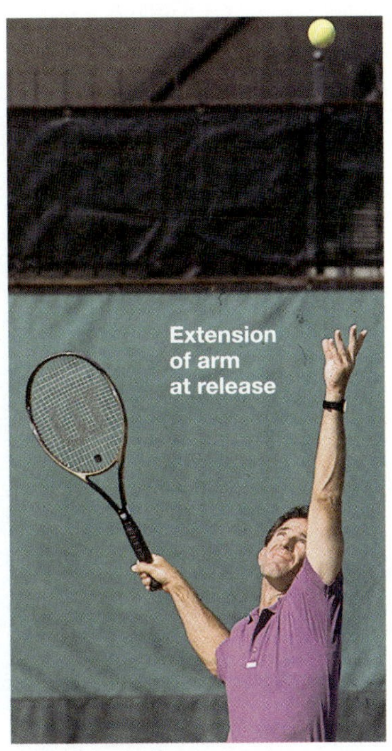
Extension
of arm
at release

Figure 4.4 Height of toss.

makes an upward movement at contact, followed by a breaking of the wrist and forearm through the ball. Most beginning players have a great desire to hit the flat serve as hard as they can, assuming that the idea is to hit the service with blazing speed. The problem with that view is that few balls are placed accurately into the appropriate service court, which, in turn, means that the ball hasn't been placed in play to begin a point. This takes away from the fun of playing the game and minimizes the possibility for success by first serves that miss the target. The idea is to hit a firm, controlled, rhythmical service placed in the service court effectively. Rhythm and ball placement are far more effective than a sometimes accurate, high-velocity serve.

The *execution of a full versus a half-service* requires discussion. Some beginning instruction starts the player with the racket already positioned between the shoulder blades to eliminate the initial take-back portion of the stroke preparation. The purpose is to keep the stroke as simple as possible and not complicate coordination of the stroke. The choice of a full serve versus a half-serve is a simple one of efficiency. Some highly skilled players use a half-service position, and many less skilled players use a full service. Some players are more comfortable initially with a full-service sequence, but all players need to see the half-service position to understand the upward position of the elbow and the location of the racket during the backswing to permit accurate timing of the stroke. Refer to Figures 4.8–4.16.

Footwork for Service

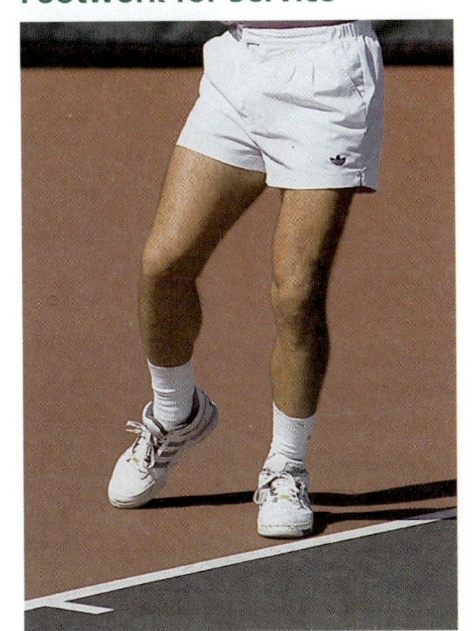
Figure 4.5 Backswing.

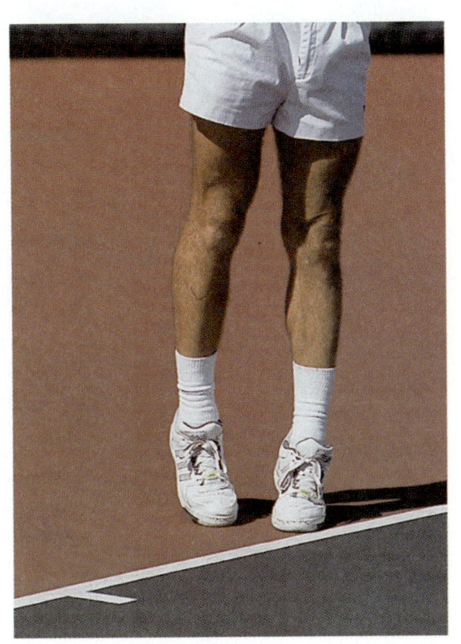
Figure 4.6 Contact.

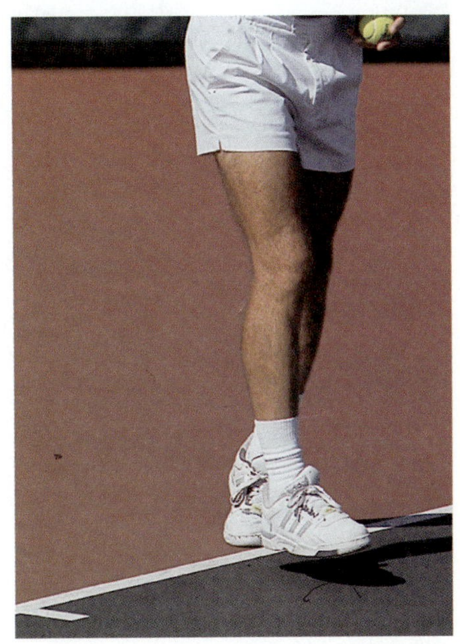
Figure 4.7 Follow through.

Flat Service

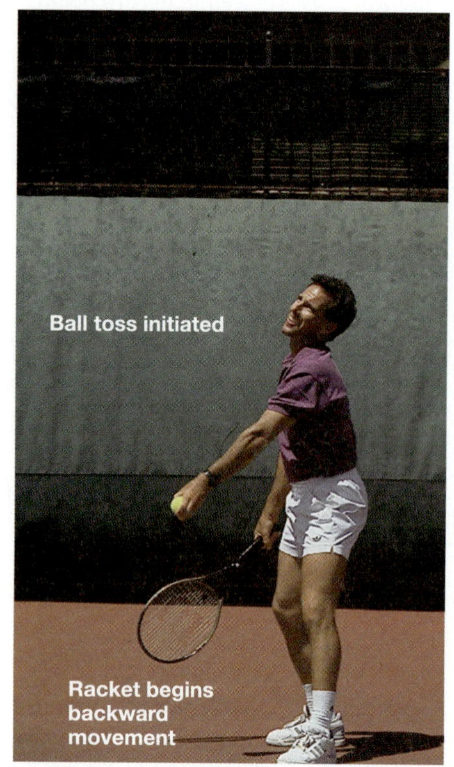

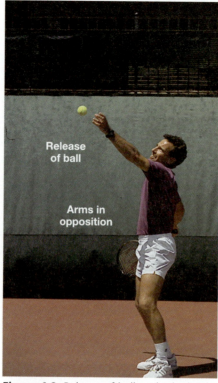

Figure 4.8 Beginning of toss.

Figure 4.9 Release of ball and take back of racket.

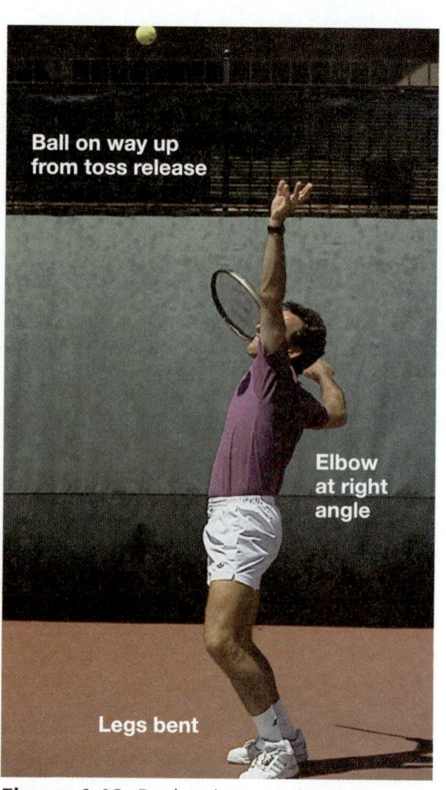

Figure 4.10 Backswing continuation in preparation sequence.

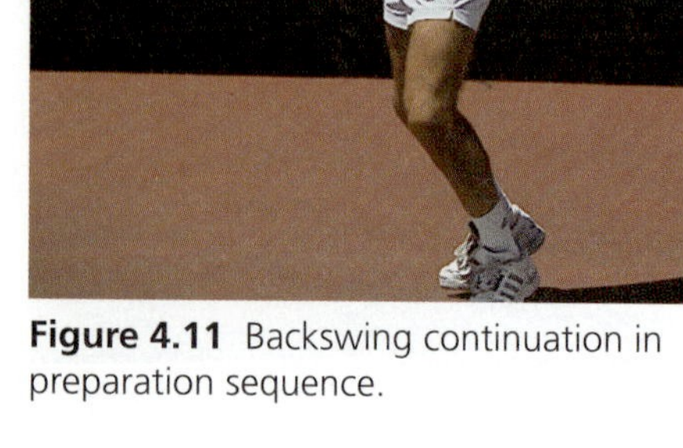

Figure 4.11 Backswing continuation in preparation sequence.

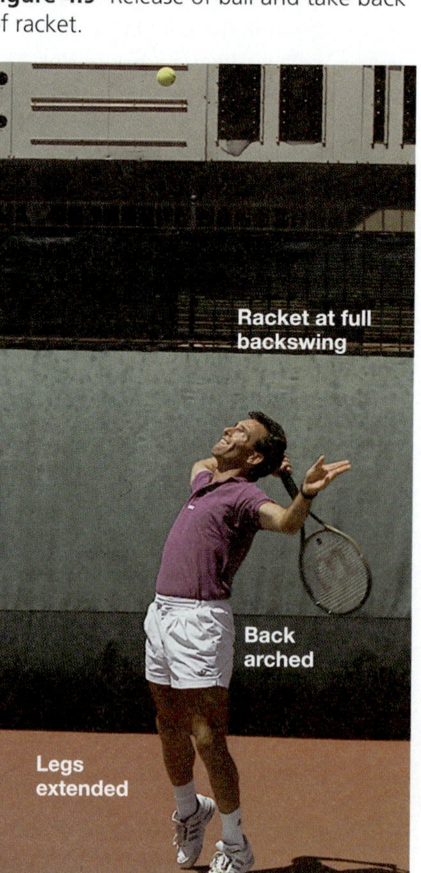
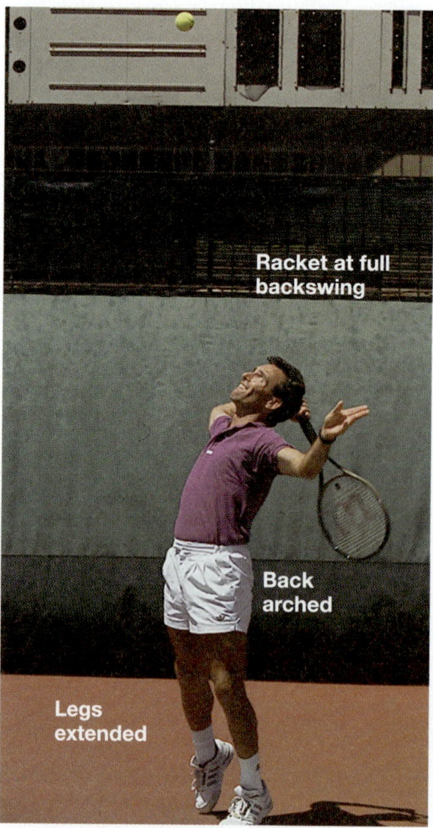

Figure 4.12 Full backswing preparation sequence.

Figure 4.13 At contact.

Flat Service (continued)

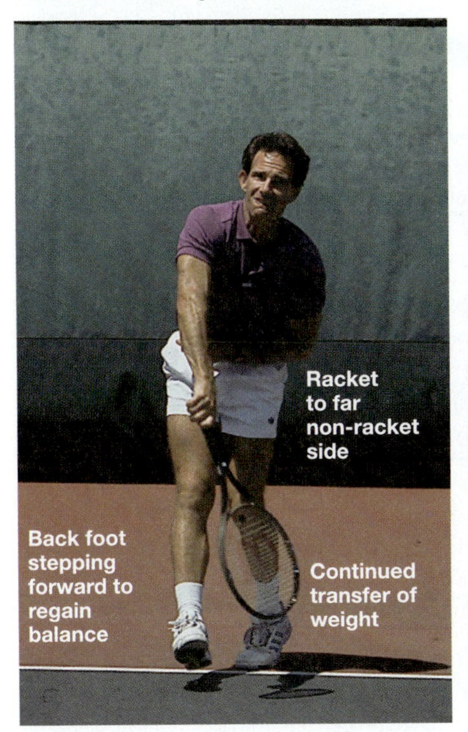

Figure 4.14 Follow through sequence.

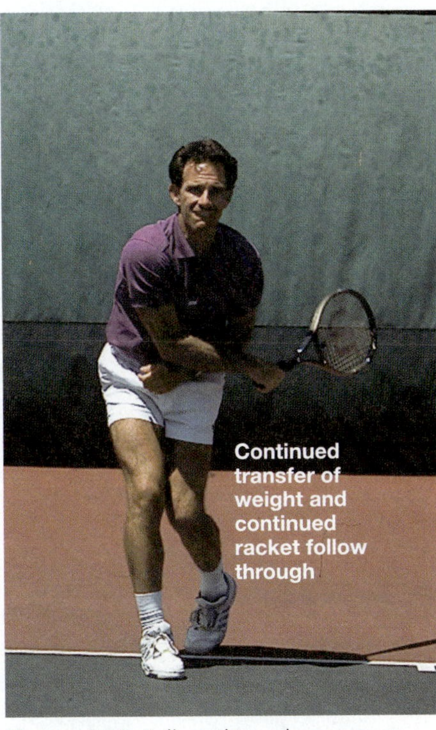

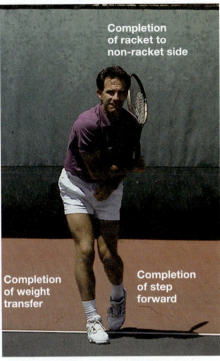

Figure 4.15 Follow through sequence.

Figure 4.16 Completion of follow through sequence.

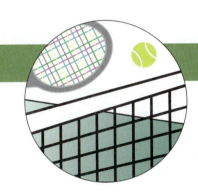

Learning Experience Reminders

Basic Flat Serve

1. Use the continental grip as soon as possible.
2. Time the toss with the take-back of the racket.
3. Keep the tossing arm straight, with the heel of the hand lifting in the direction of the toss.
4. Make the toss higher than the racket can reach.
5. Release the ball at the extension of the arm.
6. Keep the elbow up and at a right angle at the extension of the backswing.
7. Coil the body by arching the back and bending the knees during preparation.
8. Bring the racket through the ball with a slight upward, followed by a downward wrist and forearm break, and shoulder turn.
9. Let the weight transfer carry the body and racket forward in the direction of the ball, with the back foot coming forward to regain balance.
10. Make sure the racket follows on through to the non-racket-side hip.

Elimination of Errors (Basic Flat Serve)

The Error	What Causes the Error	Correction of the Error
Erratic placement of the serve.	Inconsistent toss.	Toss the ball by placing it off the lead shoulder between the shoulder and the sideline at a height above the reach of the racket.
Balls served short.	Ball hit too far out in front of the server toward the net; or server attempting to hit over ball; or ball too low at contact.	Toss the ball off the lead shoulder, at a height above the reach of the racket and between the server and the sideline. Focus on brushing through the back and top of the ball.
Ball toss goes behind the head.	Not lifting in a straight line with the tossing arm.	Use the heel of the hand as the lifting agent, along with a straight arm, thus giving direction to the ball.
Ball served long.	Racket under the ball at contact, pushing the ball up; trying to hit the ball too hard.	Toss the ball off the lead shoulder, at a height above the reach of the racket and between server and sideline. Focus on brushing through the back, top of the ball at contact.
Stepping on the baseline during the serve.	Toss is too far over baseline toward net, or player steps with foot as if throwing a ball.	Toss the ball by laying it off the lead shoulder between the shoulder and the sideline at a height above the reach of the racket. Keep the lead foot firmly on the court.

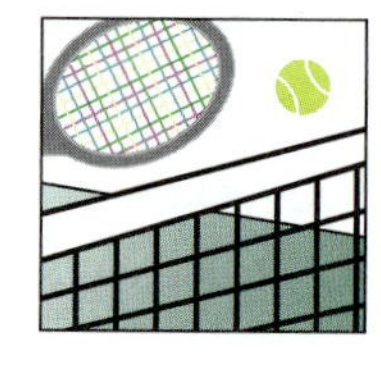

Slice Service

The slice service involves a sidespin action to the ball and it usually is used as a second serve in singles and a first and second serve in doubles. The spin permits the server to hit with greater accuracy and still place the serve deeply. A sidespin is imparted by contacting the back and side of the ball in sequence. The racket grip is a continental grip, and as more spin is needed, the grip can be adjusted to an eastern backhand grip. The result is that the ball lands in the court and kicks away from the position of the server.

The *slice service differs from the flat service* in the toss position and in the movement pattern of the racket. The toss is the same distance from the body, but with less height (one of the advantages in the wind is a lower toss with a slice service). The ball is tossed between the lead shoulder and the middle of the body. More spin and less velocity is achieved the closer the toss is to the back of the racket shoulder. The difference between the slice and flat serve toss is that the flat serve toss is above the reach of the racket as compared to the shorter toss for a slice service, and the toss is off the lead shoulder instead of between the lead shoulder and the middle of the body. See Figures 4.17–4.20 for comparison.

Toss for Flat Serve

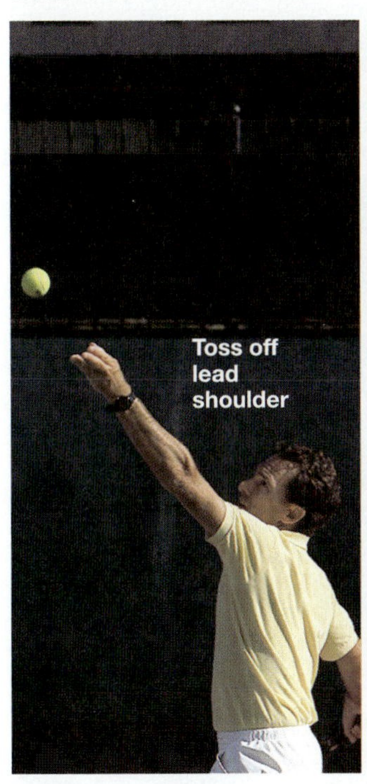

Figure 4.17 Toss off the lead shoulder.

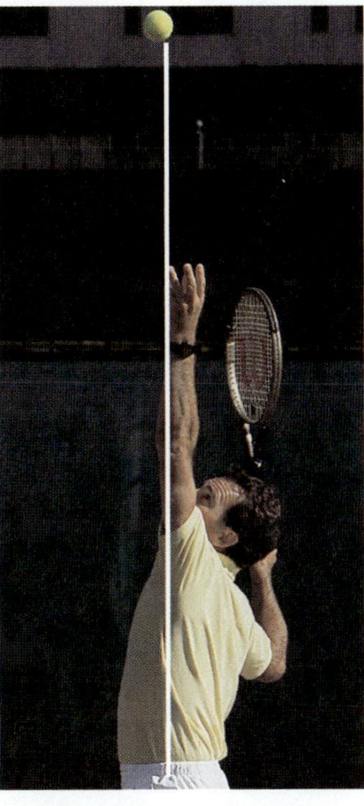

Figure 4.18 Toss above the reach of the racket.

Toss for Slice Serve

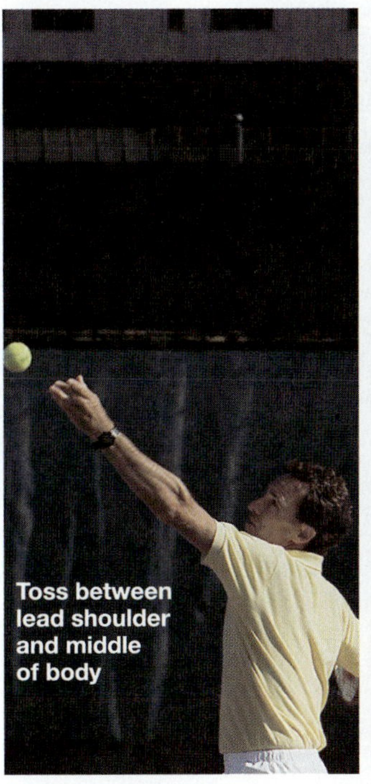

Figure 4.19 Toss between lead shoulder and middle of body.

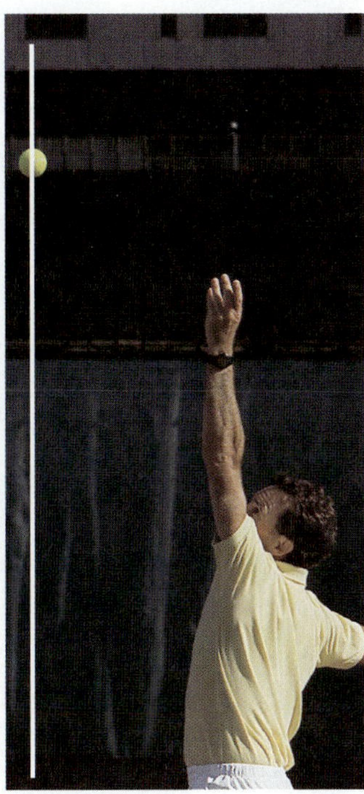

Figure 4.20 Toss short of reach of racket.

During a slice service, contact is made on the side and back of the ball just below center, with the racket moving from high to low. The wrist and forearm move through a controlled movement and forceful action at contact. The shoulders are turned more with a slice service, leaving the body even more open at contact than with the flat service (Figures 4.21–4.22). That openness results from a small change in foot position, with the back foot placed slightly behind the lead foot (Figures 4.23–4.24).

The *full sequence of the slice service,* including the exceptions identified, is a rhythmical one with the take-away, followed by the contact with the ball, and culminating with a follow through down off the hip of the non-racket side. The weight transfer is an aid to that sequence, as is the leg bend followed by extension of the leg at contact (Figures 4.25–4.28).

A *summary of the differences and commonalities* of the two services may be helpful to the developing player. The differences, related to ball toss position, racket pattern movement, and foot position on the baseline, are outlined in Table 4.1. The commonalities involve weight transfer, elbow position on the backswing, and follow through off the non-racket-side hip.

One additional commonality that will enhance the rhythm and timing of the total stroke is a change in foot movement from preparation through contact for the developing player. Instead of maintaining stability with a stationary foot position, the developing player may bring the back foot up even with the lead foot as the racket pattern begins to close on the ball at contact. This small change should be utilized when the player has developed balance and stroke timing from a more stationary position.

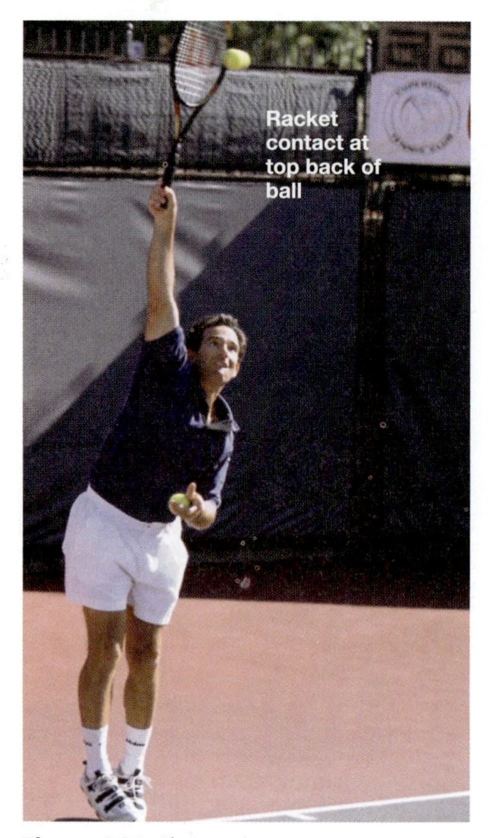

Figure 4.21 Flat service contact.

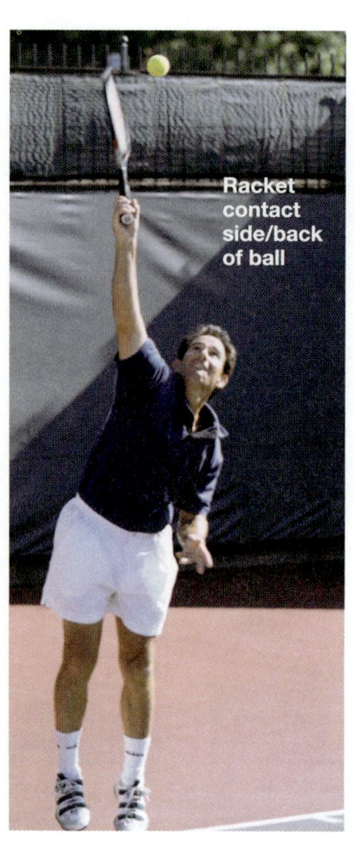

Figure 4.22 Slice service contact.

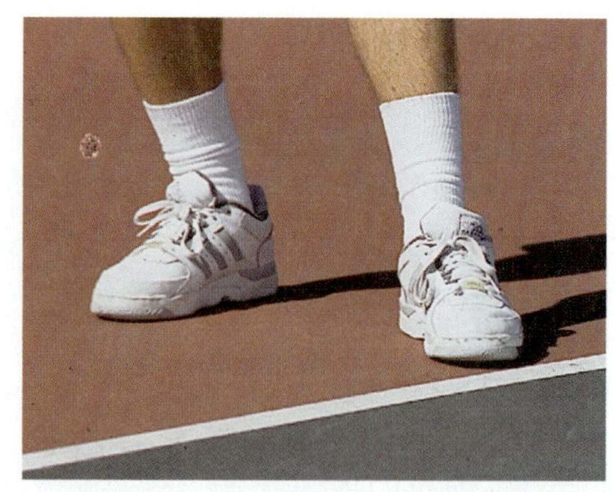

Figure 4.23 Flat-service foot position.

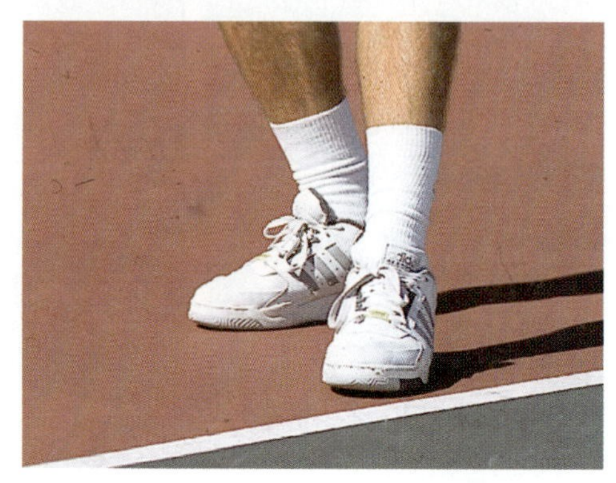

Figure 4.24 Slice service foot position.

Slice Serve

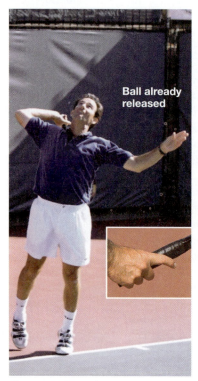

Figure 4.25 Backswing (continental grip).

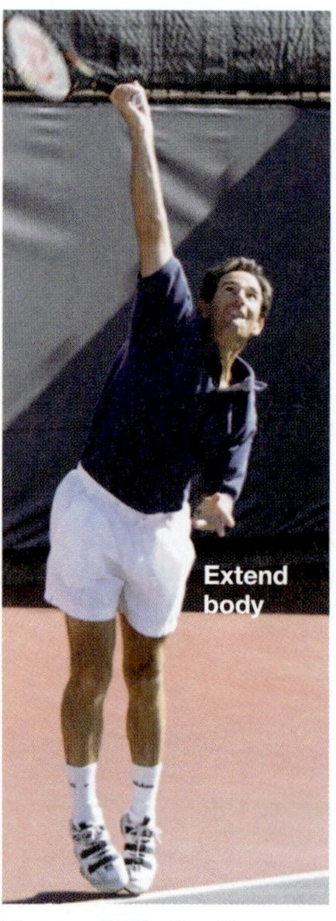

Figure 4.26 Continuation of backswing.

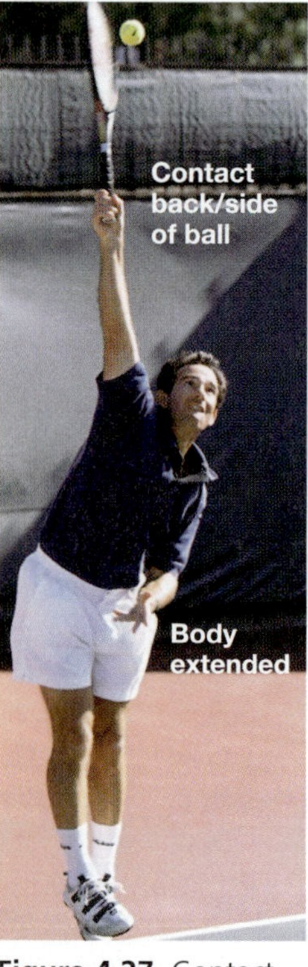

Figure 4.27 Contact.

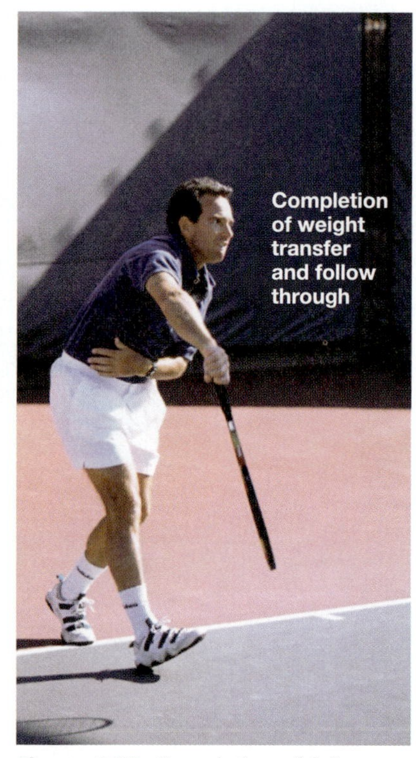

Figure 4.28 Completion of follow through.

Table 4.1 Differences Between the Two Major Services

TYPE OF SERVICE	BALL TOSS PLACEMENT	FOOT POSITION ON BASELINE	RACKET PATTERN MOVEMENT	CONTACT POSITION ON BALL
Flat	off lead shoulder, above racket reach	even	straight through	back-top
Slice	between lead shoulder and racket shoulder, lower than racket reach	back foot slightly back	curving line	back-side just below center

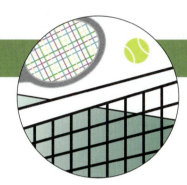

Learning Experience Reminders

Slice Serve

1. Use a continental grip.
2. Open the serving stance more than with the flat service.
3. Toss the ball lower than on the flat service, and toss more toward the back shoulder to obtain more spin.
4. Contact the ball sequentially on the back and side below center.
5. Transfer weight forward through the sequence of the service, allowing the back foot to move forward to regain balance after contact.

Elimination of Errors (Slice Serve)

The Error	What Causes the Error	Correction of the Error
Lack of spin on the ball.	Toss not far enough back to the racket shoulder; no continental grip; body doesn't open to the ball.	Toss between the two shoulders; check to make sure the grip is continental; or turn the lead shoulder more through the stroke.
Pulling the ball out of the serving court.	Turning the non-racket shoulder into the ball too early, and pulling the shoulder too far through the ball.	Point the non-racket shoulder to the service court target area from contact through follow through, thus reducing excessive shoulder turn.
A great amount of spin, but little velocity or distance.	Hitting ball too far back on back shoulder, or racket pattern too far to the outside of the ball at contact.	Move toss toward the lead shoulder and/or control racket pattern through a sequential brushing action of the back and side of the ball.
Hitting the ball off the racket edge.	Too much of an eastern backhand grip.	Use a continental grip.

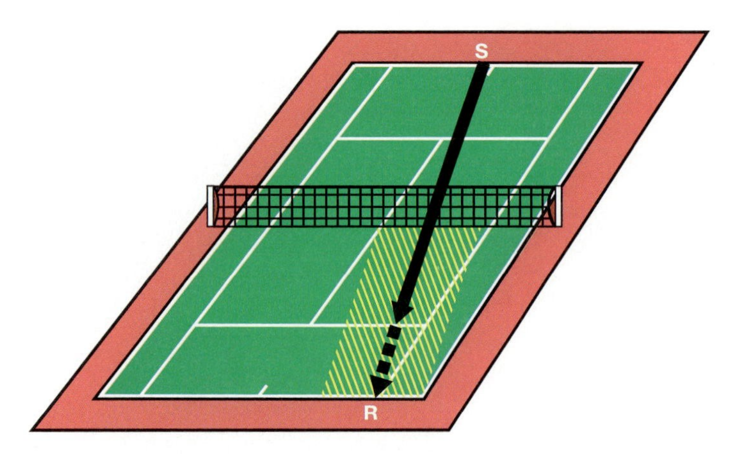

Figure 4.29 Return of serve position.

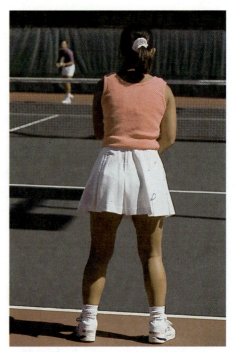

Figure 4.30 Return of serve ready position.

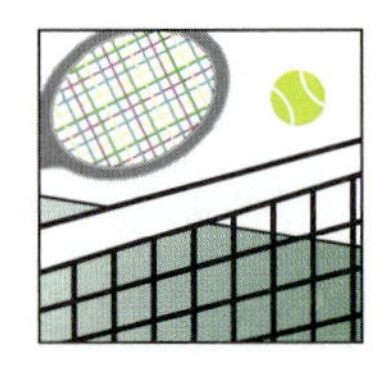

Return of Service

Because the different services have different velocities, trajectories, and spins, the beginning player may be confronted with a series of decisions related to coping with each type of serve.

Return of serve positioning is a matter of mathematics. The receiver must split the court in half in a line from the server to the receiver (Figure 4.29). The receiver cannot overplay to the side, attempting to return all serves with a forehand, since a server with an adequate slice serve can place a ball that will kick off the court and out of the reach of the player favoring the side. It is much better for the receiver to position with the potential to hit either a forehand or backhand equally.

The depth of the receiver's position depends on the strength of the server and the velocity of the ball. If a player pushes the ball when serving and simply gets the ball in play, the receiver can move up and stand inside the baseline about halfway between the baseline and the service court line. If the server has a strong serve with high velocity, the receiver should stand at or slightly behind the baseline.

Returning the served ball effectively requires a special set of skills. First, the receiver should develop a relaxed attitude and physical position. The ready position (Figure 4.30), as a second check, should be high to permit quick lateral movement and enable the receiver to hit through the ball with minimal adjustment. The third reaction is for the receiver to rotate the shoulders to a hitting position at the earliest possible moment. Fourth, the receiver must transfer weight into the stroke by stepping into the ball at contact. A fifth consideration is for the player to adopt a volley concept to the stroke. The backswing and follow through have to be shortened to a movement longer

Return of Serve: Forehand

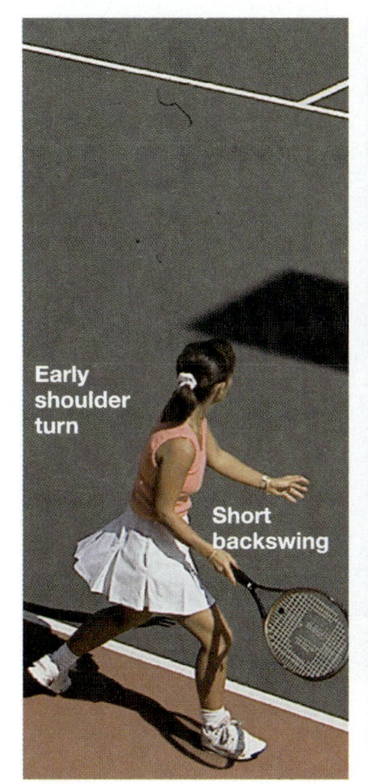

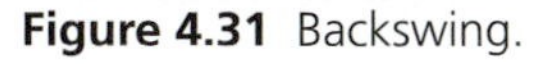
Figure 4.31 Backswing.

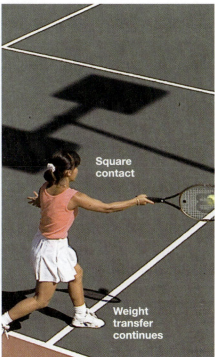

Figure 4.32 Contact.

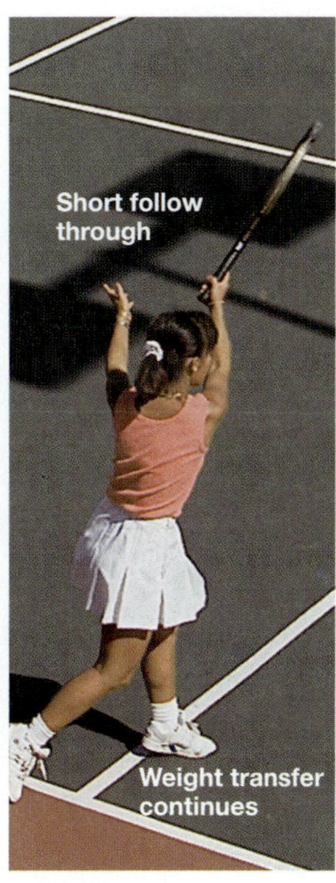

Figure 4.33 Follow through.

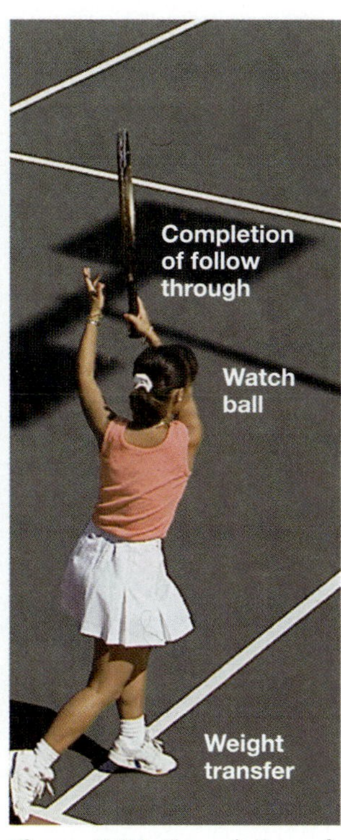

Figure 4.34 Completion of follow through.

than a volley but shorter than a groundstroke. The shortened backswing enables the receiver to control the racket and bring it through in time to contact the ball. The action of the racket is more of a blocking or punching movement that pushes the ball back across the net, reversing the velocity of the serve. The racket should be square to the ball and a little out in front of the lead leg, with a short follow through to add direction to the ball. Sixth, the racket should be held firmly throughout the stroke, and particularly at contact. Finally, the receiver must watch the ball as long as possible up to the point of contact. Return of serve follows the same process and skill pattern whether hitting a forehand (Figures 4.31–4.34) or backhand (Figures 4.35–4.38). The key to selecting the side to hit from depends on the spin and direction of the ball and a responsive early rotation of the shoulders based on anticipating the position of the ball.

Target for return of serve is a moot point if the return player is just trying to get the racket on the ball. But with a degree of skill at returning a serve, the receiver can return the ball to spots on the court. The first consideration is where *not* to place the ball. Balls hit short to the server are a reward to that server, so it is important to eliminate short returns. Serves that pull a return player off the court should be returned down the sideline rather than crosscourt, and most returns hit soft and "up" should be avoided. If the receiver can remember to return deep with pace and velocity on the ball, subsequent play should enable the receiver to gain equal footing in a baseline rally.

Anticipation of the serve is both a physical and mental phase of return of service. The receiver must look at the body language of the server and concentrate on the ball. The body language will provide clues to the spin and velocity of the ball. If the racket-face pattern of the server is to the outside of the ball and the toss is short and back toward the racket shoulder, the serve will be a slice. If the toss is off the lead

Return of Serve: Backhand

Figure 4.35 Backswing.

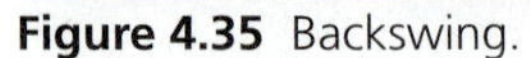

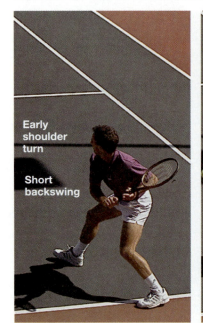

Figure 4.36 Contact.

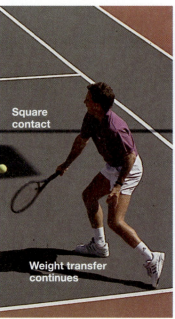

Figure 4.37 Follow through.

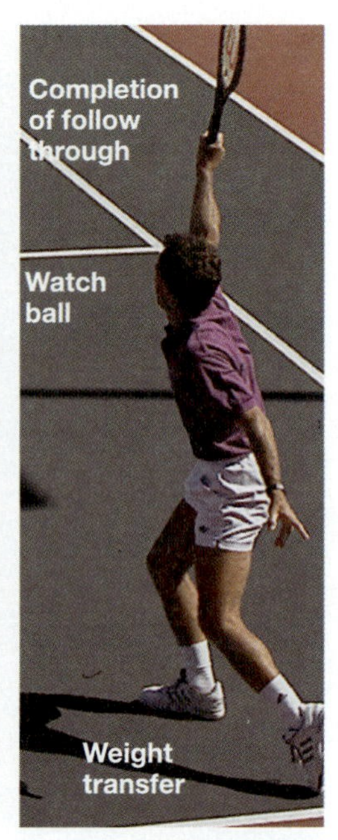

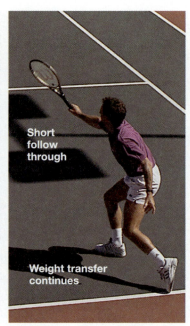

Figure 4.38 Completion of follow through.

shoulder and toward the net, the ball will be a flat serve. A topspin serve will be interpreted by a toss above the head and/or more back arch than usual. Velocity of the ball can be observed to some extent by the server's effort. Concentrating on the seams of the ball will permit the receiver to react physically to the direction of the ball. The mental efforts all combine to allow the receiver to make an early shoulder turn and pivot of the feet, thus placing the racket in a backswing position.

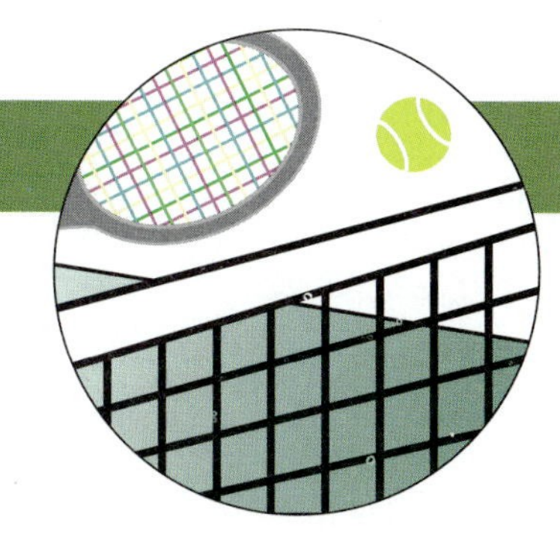

Learning Experience Reminders

Return of Serve

1. Be relaxed when waiting to return a serve.
2. Throughout the serve, concentrate on the server's body language and on the ball.
3. Get the racket back early.
4. Be aggressive and step into the ball at contact.
5. Use a compact swing with a short backswing and follow through.
6. Maintain a firm grip on the racket at contact.
7. Hit deep on all return of serves, and hit with a groundstroke swing on soft serves that are deep to the receiver's service court.
8. Return soft and short serves using an approach-shot concept.
9. Block all high-velocity serves, and block deep and to the baseline.
10. Return every serve by placing the racket on the ball on every service.

Elimination of Errors (Return of Serve)

The Error	What Causes the Error	Correction of the Error
Hitting the ball out beyond the server's baseline.	Swinging with a full groundstroke swing.	Use a compact swing; block high-velocity serves.
Pulling the ball across the court to the sidelines.	Racket contact with the ball too far out in front of projected contact point.	Judge the velocity of the ball, and time the swing.
Ball coming off the racket late with direction toward the near sideline.	Not anticipating early and, as a result, not getting the shoulders turned and the racket back early.	Watch the ball, and communicate mental observation to the physical reaction of turning the shoulders and pivoting the feet.
Cannot control direction of the ball.	Wrist isn't firm and grip isn't tight.	Keep a firm wrist and grip at contact.

Check Points

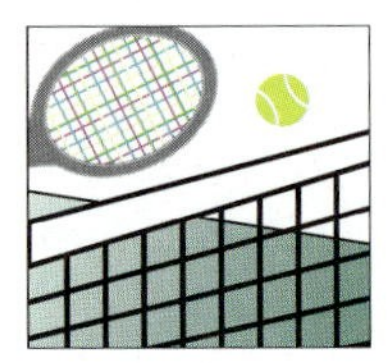

1. The toss for serve is a key to success. It should be executed
   a. by grasping the ball with the finger tips and thumb.
   b. with the heel of the hand pointed in the direction of the toss.
   c. by a straight lifting action of the arm.
   d. by using all three skills above.
2. The toss synchronization requires
   a. the racket beginning a backward movement as the lift of the tossing hand occurs.
   b. the racket placed in the middle of the shoulder blades as the lift of the tossing hand occurs.
   c. the racket beginning backward movement as the toss reaches its top height.
   d. the use of all three techniques listed above.
3. The racket follow through
   a. continues on a downward pattern finishing off the non-racket leg.
   b. continues on a downward pattern finishing off the racket leg.
   c. stops at waist level.
   d. can be any of the three depending on the type of serve used.
4. Weight of the body should
   a. be transferred forward by stepping with the lead foot.
   b. be centered at contact with the ball.
   c. rest on the back foot at contact with the ball.
   d. be transferred forward at contact with the ball.
5. The cause of the ball being consistently served into the net is
   a. that the toss is too high.
   b. that the server is attempting to hit over the ball.
   c. that the ball toss is too far out in front of the server.
   d. any of the three causes listed above.
6. The contact position on the ball for a slice serve is
   a. top-back.
   b. side-back.
   c. top.
   d. side.
7. The position of the ball on the toss for a slice serve is
   a. off the lead shoulder.
   b. off the racket shoulder.
   c. between lead shoulder and racket shoulder.
   d. in any of the three positions.
8. A lack of spin applied to the ball when hitting a slice serve is caused by
   a. the toss being placed not far enough back toward the racket shoulder.
   b. turning the racket shoulder into the ball too soon.
   c. too extreme of a continental grip.
   d. contact on the side of the ball.
9. The return of serve ready positioning should be
   a. with the receiver standing to the forehand side of the line of the serve.
   b. with the receiver standing 2–4 feet inside the baseline.
   c. with the receiver standing 2–4 feet behind the baseline.
   d. with the receiver splitting the court in half in a line from the server to the receiver.
10. The correction for hitting a return of serve long is
    a. to use a compact swing and swing through the ball.
    b. to use a compact swing and block all serves.
    c. to use a compact swing and block all high-velocity serves.
    d. to use a full swing.

Answers to Check Points can be found on page 145.

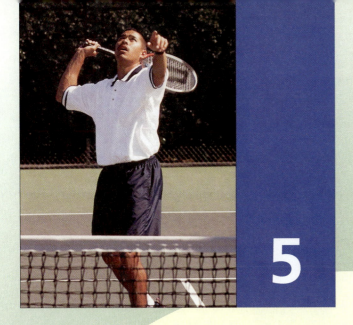

5

The Aerial Game

The lob and overhead smash combinations are basic strokes for the beginning player. Each skill complements the other in tennis. The lob is an extension of the groundstroke, discussed in Chapter 2, and the overhead smash is an elaboration of the service discussed in Chapter 4. Overhead smashes are attacking weapons. Lobs are used to react to an opponent playing at the net.

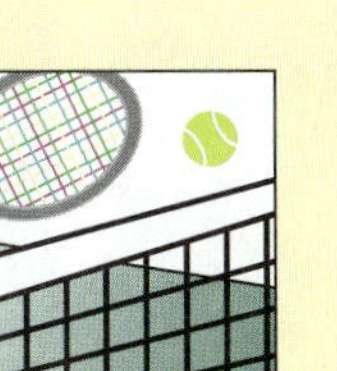

Overhead Smash

The basic forehand overhead smash is executed as a flat serve from the half-swing position. The overhead is hit from either the forehand or the backhand side, but most players run around the backhand to play a forehand overhead. The two overhead smashes in tennis are the simplistic orthodox overhead with little foot movement and a simple swing, and the more complex overhead characterized by additional agility and timing (Figure 5.1). The orthodox overhead smash is the only smash to be discussed here. The eastern forehand or continental grip is used for all forehand overheads.

The *orthodox forehand overhead smash* is a simple transition from the flat service. The player must maneuver underneath the ball that is hit as a lob, and from that position bring the racket back to the middle of the shoulder blades with the racket elbow at a right angle. The position of the racket physically touching between the shoulder blades provides a reference point for the player hitting the overhead. The reaction that occurs simultaneously with the racket moving to a ready position is for the player to point with the non-racket arm and hand to the ball as a second reference point. The line of the flight of the ball is similar to the ball toss, but the ball falls more rapidly and at a slightly different angle. The feet are shoulder-width apart, and the non-racket shoulder has turned to face the net and the intended target area (Figure 5.2).

In executing the overhead, the player's body is coiled and gathered, ready to time the stroke. The ball is hit off the lead shoulder, with the legs

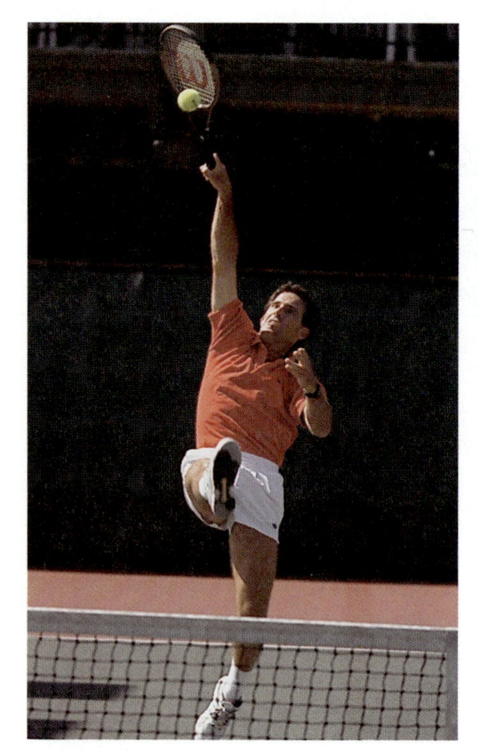

Figure 5.1 Complex overhead smash.

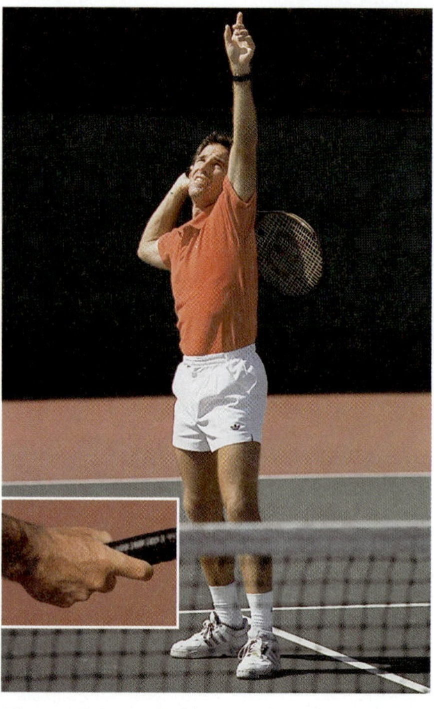

Figure 5.2 Orthodox overhead smash ready position (eastern forehand or continental grip).

extending and the body uncoiling. Contact of racket to ball involves an up-and-over motion, providing a little topspin for greater net clearance and depth. The racket comes through the ball with a wrist break and a follow through to the far hip, but the action is shortened to accommodate the return of a ready position for the next shot (Figures 5.3–5.6).

The full stroke is simplistic, eliminating wasted motion and extraneous actions. The feet remain stable until the follow through pulls the back foot forward to catch the balance of the player at completion of the follow through. The player is encouraged to hit out on the ball with smooth, rhythmical timing and control.

Advancing to more agility with the forehand overhead smash involves adding a few parts to the stroke. First, it is important to set up to hit the overhead. That movement consists of long running strides to get to the general area as fast as possible allowing time to set up the stroke. Once in the general area, the player will be situated behind the anticipated drop of the ball. At this point, the player takes small steps to

Orthodox Forehand Overhead Smash

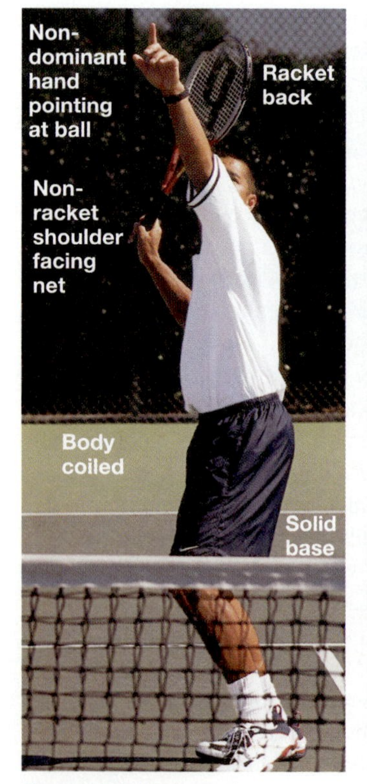

Figure 5.3 Preparation.

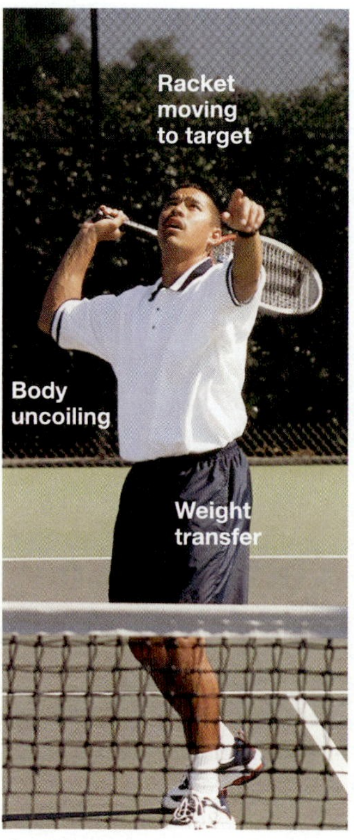

Figure 5.4 Initiation of swing.

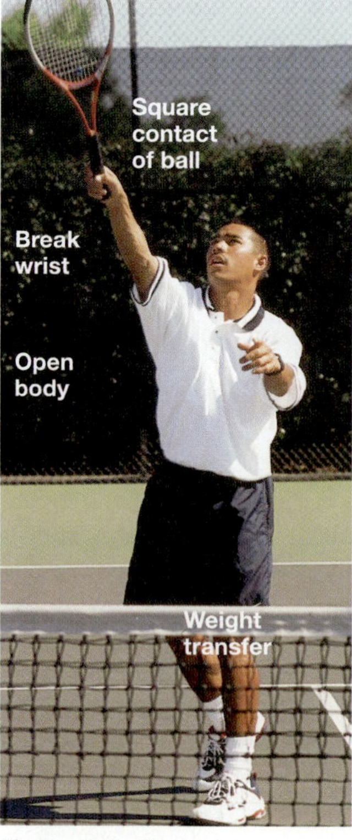

Figure 5.5 Contact.

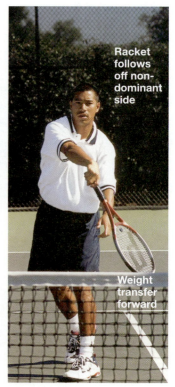

Figure 5.6 Follow through.

Backhand Overhead Smash

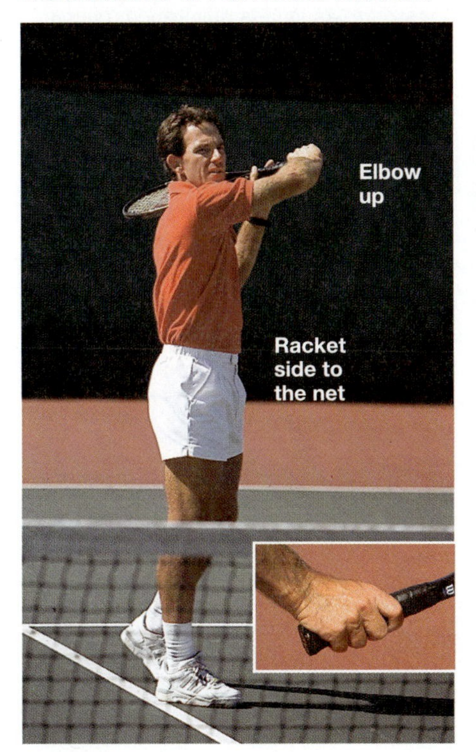

Figure 5.7 Preparation (eastern backhand grip).

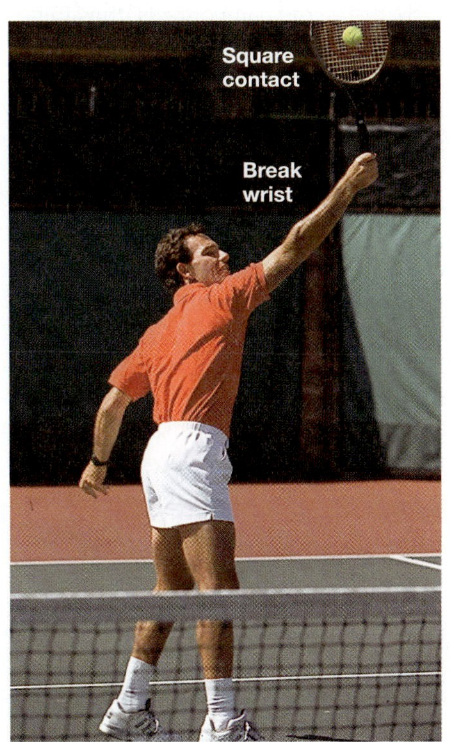

Figure 5.8 Contact.

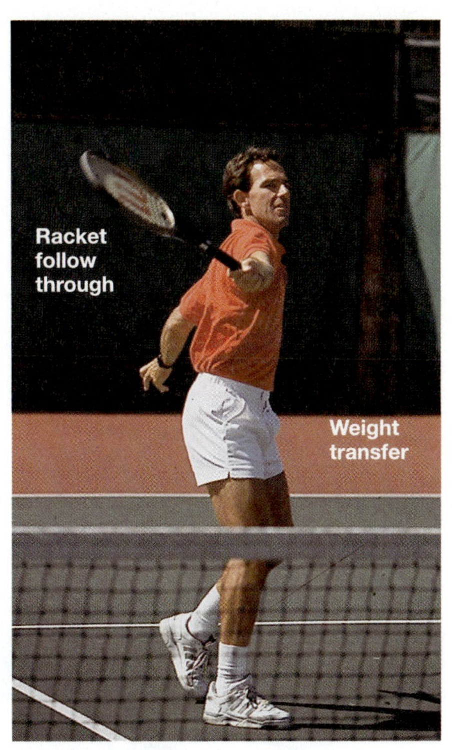

Figure 5.9 Follow through.

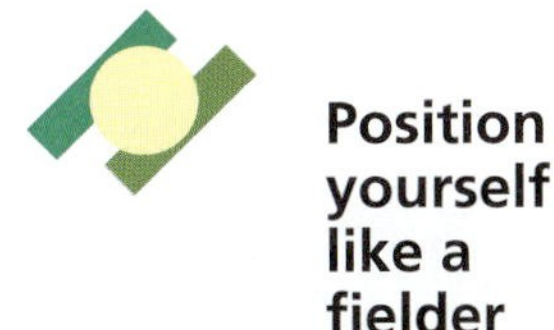

Position yourself like a fielder

Visualize how a softball or baseball player gets in position to catch a fly ball. Like a fielder, you want to keep your feet moving and adjusting to the position of the ball until time to catch —or, in this case, hit the ball.

G. Williams, Tennis, 8/95

adjust to the position of the ball. Balls that are hit over the player's head are handled in the same manner: taking long strides to get behind the ball, then short steps to adjust to the falling pattern of the ball.

Bouncing the overhead means permitting the ball to bounce before executing an overhead smash. There are two situations in which the lob is allowed to bounce prior to being hit as an overhead smash. Lobs that have a very high loft are permitted to bounce for better timing when hitting the overhead. Lobs that are short at the net, eliminating a good set position for the overhead, also are allowed to bounce.

Hitting a high lob following a bounce is similar to hitting the overhead from a mid-air position following a lob. The additional time generated when permitting a bounce gives the opponent an opportunity to reposition in anticipation of returning an overhead return, but it also gives the player hitting the overhead a chance to place the ball more effectively. When hitting a lob that bounces short, you need to stay low enough so the stroke is still angled down and through the ball. The goal for the overhead return of a short ball is a short, hard-hit, high-bouncing ball that carries out beyond the baseline.

The *backhand overhead smash* is used when the player cannot run around the ball to hit a forehand smash. To begin a backhand overhead, the player should use an eastern backhand or continental grip, and turn the shoulder so the racket side actually faces the net. The elbow on the racket side is up and points to the ball, and the racket head is below the hand. The weight is on the player's back foot and the head is up, eyes fixed on the ball. The ball is contacted above the head slightly in front of the racket shoulder, with the racket face moving through the ball with a strong break of the wrist. The weight is transferred forward through the ball, with the follow through carrying the racket head downward and parallel to the court surface (Figures 5.7–5.9).

Incorporating the overhead smash into the total game blends favorably with the player's total game plan. The overhead is the second type of shot that is hit before the ball bounces, thus joining the volley shot as a stroke hit in the air near the net. When a player is at the net, the opponent must either hit a groundstroke that hopefully can be volleyed by the net player, or a lob that the net player can return as an overhead smash. The player, with improving skill and confidence, can hit an overhead from any location on the court, while the beginning player should hit overheads when lobs are short between the service court line and the net. The beginning player would also be wise to let the ball bounce before executing an overhead so that timing can aid in the stroke. As skill is developed, overheads should be hit on the fly, and the scissors kick should be added. Regardless of skill development, the player needs to remember that the overhead smash is an offensive shot that must be hit under control and with confidence. The player should also remember that the overhead is the first in a series of overheads if the opponent returns the first overhead. Returns of overheads tend to be shorter lobs than the first lob hit, consequently setting up the player at the net for an eventually "easy" overhead.

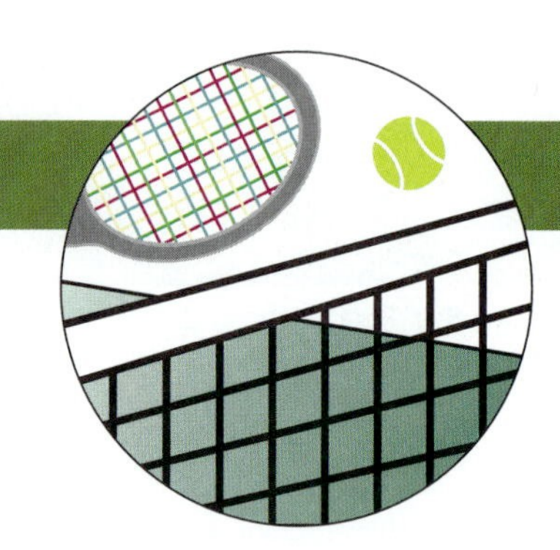

Learning Experience Reminders

Backhand Overhead Smash

1. Point the racket elbow at the ball on the backhand overhead, and turn the racket side to the net during the preparation phase.
2. Bring the wrist through the ball forcefully on the backhand overhead smash.

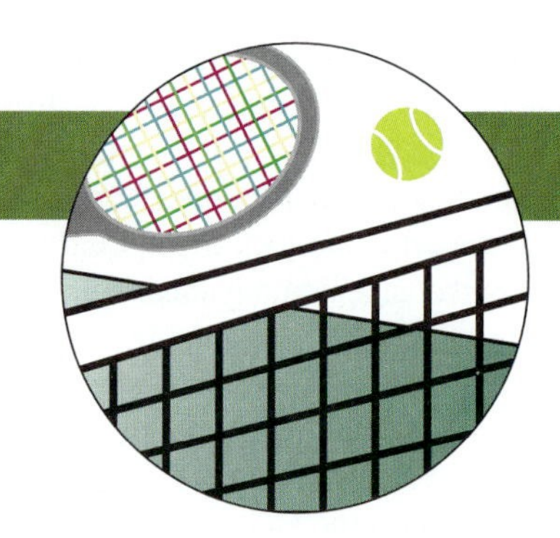

Learning Experience Reminders

Orthodox Forehand Overhead Smash

1. Keep in mind that the forehand overhead smash is a basic throwing action that imitates the flat serve.
2. Place the racket head between the shoulder blades on the backswing.
3. Point the non-racket arm at the ball for a reference point to the ball.
4. Keep the base of the orthodox overhead wide throughout the stroke.
5. Bring the racket through the ball with a wrist snap and a downward follow through.
6. "Bounce" the ball when it is lobbed extremely high or is hit short to the net.

Elimination of Errors
(Forehand Overhead Smash or Backhand Overhead Smash)

The Error	What Causes the Error	Correction of the Error
Hitting into the net.	Ball too far out in front of lead shoulder, or hitting ball downward.	Get directly underneath the ball. Keep chin up.
Hitting out beyond the baseline of the opponent.	Hitting too hard with poor timing, or hitting up into the ball.	Get directly underneath the ball and hit through the ball breaking at the wrist at contact.
Inconsistency in placing the ball.	Racket not placed between the shoulder blades on the back-swing, and player's position under the ball is random.	Get directly underneath the ball and always place the racket between the shoulder blades.
Hitting the ball off the edge of the racket at the top, or off the bottom edge, causing the ball to be hit long or to hit the court surface immediately.	Swinging too early or too late.	Point the non-racket arm to the ball for a reference point, check the position of the racket on the back-swing, and develop a rhythmical timing to the stroke.

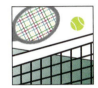

The Lob

The lob is an extension of the ground-stroke incorporating the same grip and basic swinging action. Mechanics of the stroke do require the racket face to open and lift the ball up rather than hit through the ball. Lobs, characterized by a high *flight pattern*, can be both offensive and defensive. The flight patterns are different for each type of lob, and the differences are based on the purpose of the stroke and the amount of spin applied to the ball. The two basic lobs used in tennis are discussed on the following pages and are diagrammed in Figure 5.10.

The *offensive lob* is hit over the outstretched reach of the net player, bouncing near the baseline and kicking on beyond the baseline. The *defensive lob* has a higher flight pattern and is hit off a strong opposing player return, with an underspin rotation.

The *offensive lob* requires use of an eastern forehand or backhand grip. The racket is brought back low with an extensive knee bend. The racket is brought back with the wrist cocked. The racket then moves into the ball with a slightly open face at waist height, meeting the ball from underneath and lifting up. The wrist breaks at contact, imparting topspin to the ball. The follow through continues with the racket finishing at an exaggerated high position off the middle of the body, with a roll of the wrist (Figures 5.11–5.16). The more

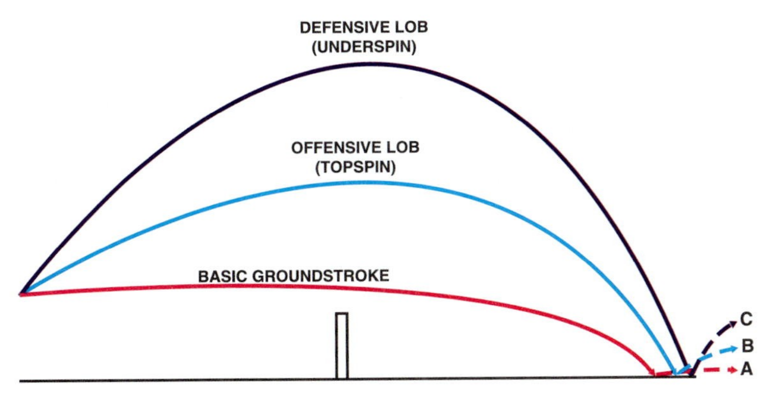

Figure 5.10 Flight patterns of lobs and groundstroke.

Forehand Offensive Lob with Topspin

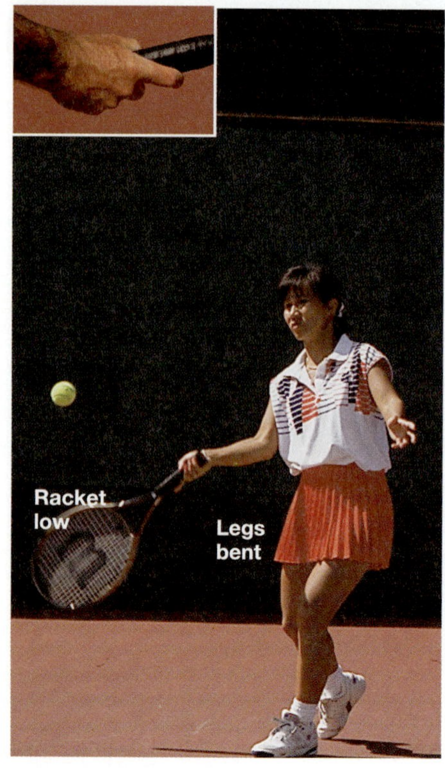

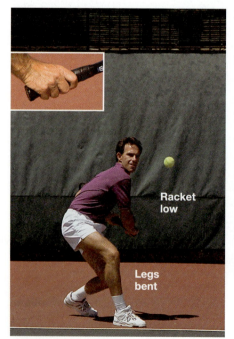

Figure 5.11 Prior to contact (eastern forehand grip).

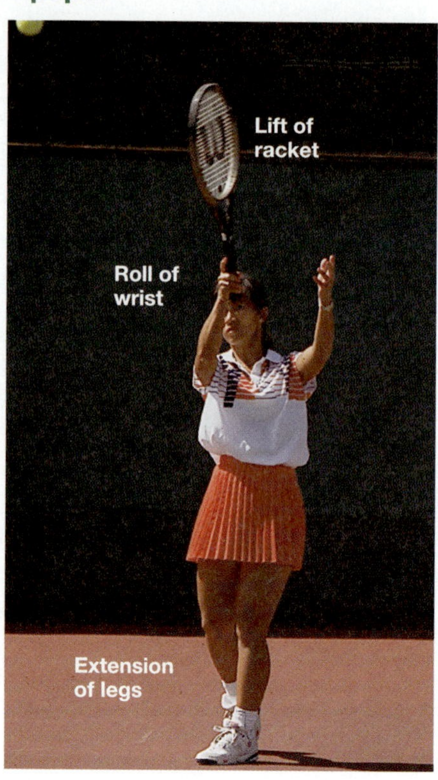

Figure 5.12 Just after contact.

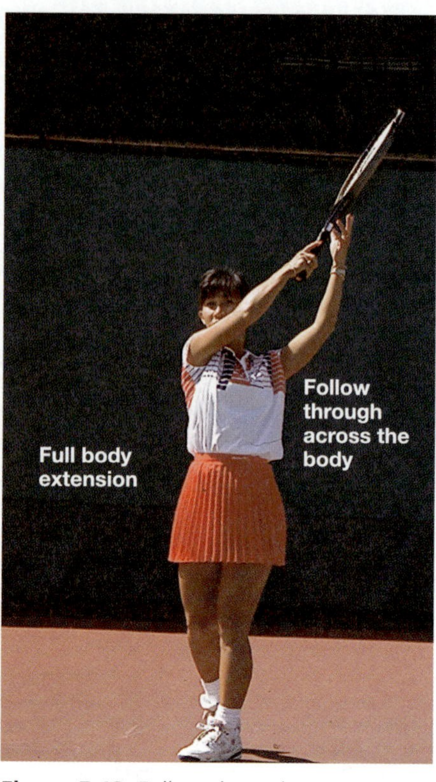

Figure 5.13 Follow through.

Backhand Offensive Lob with Topspin

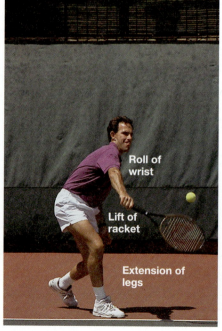

Figure 5.14 Preparation (eastern backhand grip).

Figure 5.15 Contact.

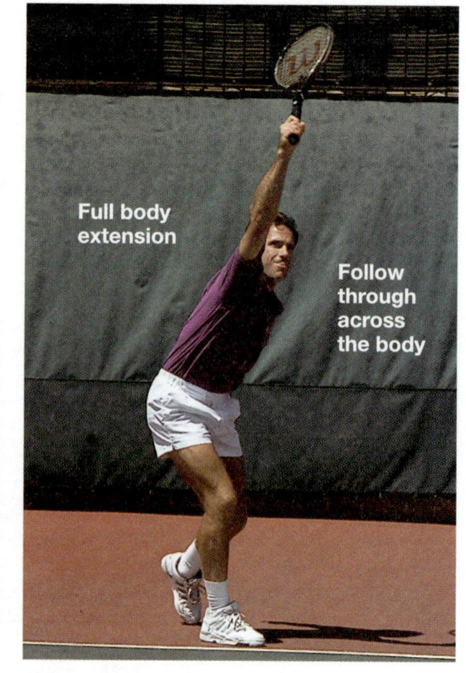

Figure 5.16 Follow through.

Defensive Lob with Forehand Underspin

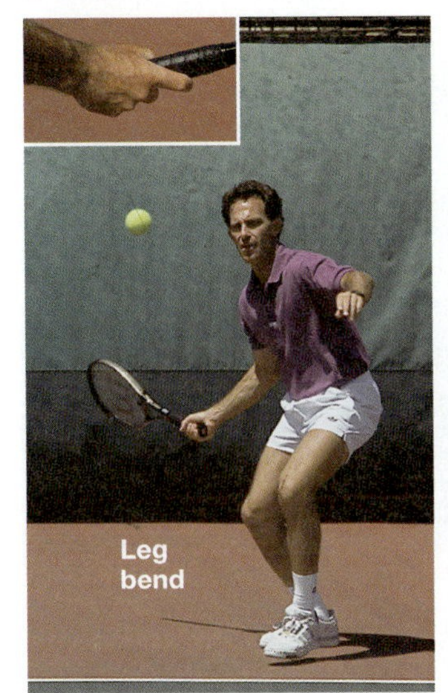

Figure 5.17 Preparation (eastern forehand grip).

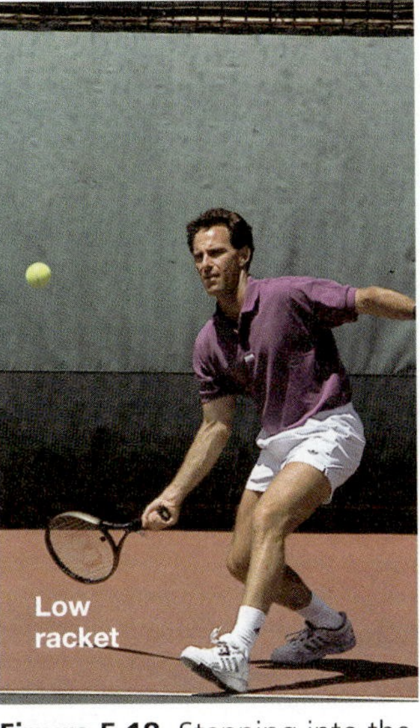

Figure 5.18 Stepping into the ball.

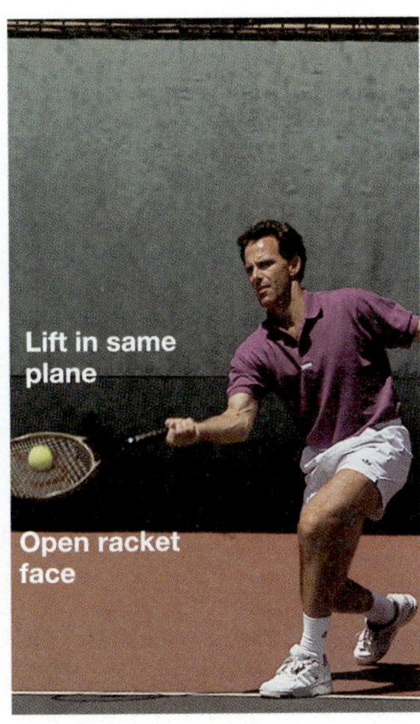

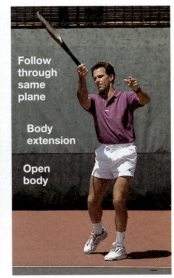

Figure 5.19 Contact.

Figure 5.20 Follow through.

Defensive Lob with Backhand Underspin

Figure 5.21 Preparation (eastern backhand grip).

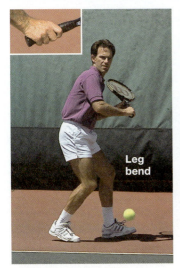

Figure 5.22 Stepping into the ball.

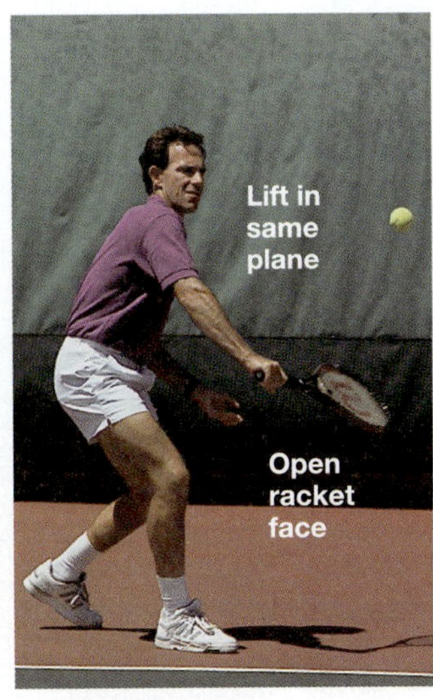

Figure 5.23 Contact.

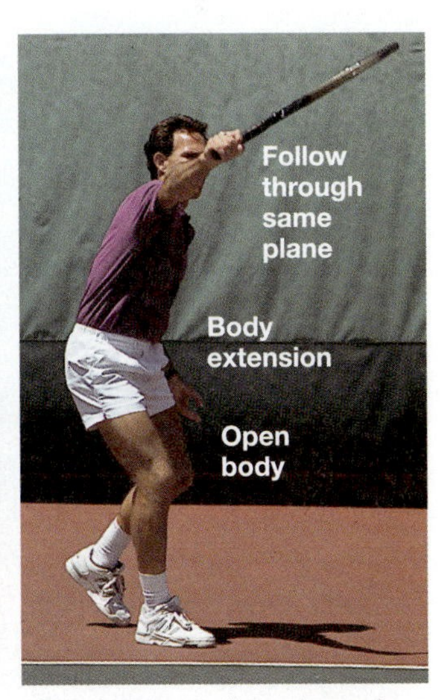

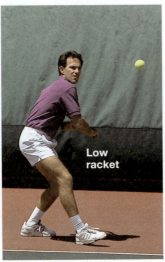

Figure 5.24 Follow through.

speed generated by the racket head, the more topspin generated, and the faster the ball will drop.

The *defensive lob* is a reaction, in many situations, to an opponent's overhead smash. With an eastern forehand or backhand grip, the racket is brought back into a short backswing position with a firm wrist. The racket is brought forward to hit the ball off the lead shoulder. The bottom edge of the racket leads, opening the racket face. The follow through is high, and the racket face remains open. The racket stays in the same plane as during the swing from preparation to contact. The wrist remains firm throughout the stroke, and the weight transfer, although important, is minimal compared with other strokes. The legs are bent and extended through the swing pattern, but only with a minimum amount of change. The lob is a reaction to an aggressively hit ball, and the total stroke has to be in moderation to combat the high velocity of the ball (Figures 5.17–5.24).

Moving Laterally to Hit a Lob Behind the Baseline—Forehand

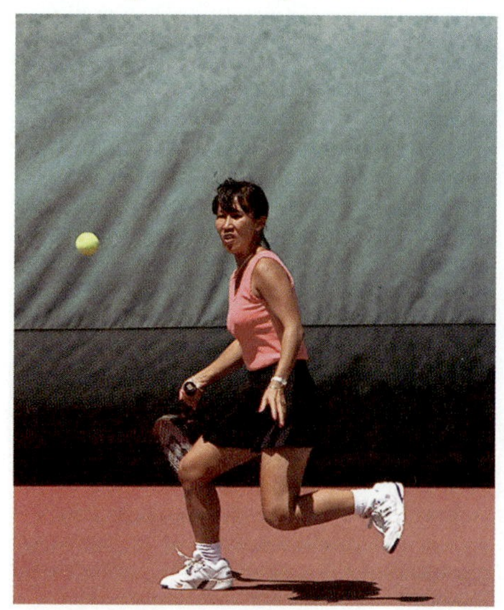

Figure 5.25 Backswing.

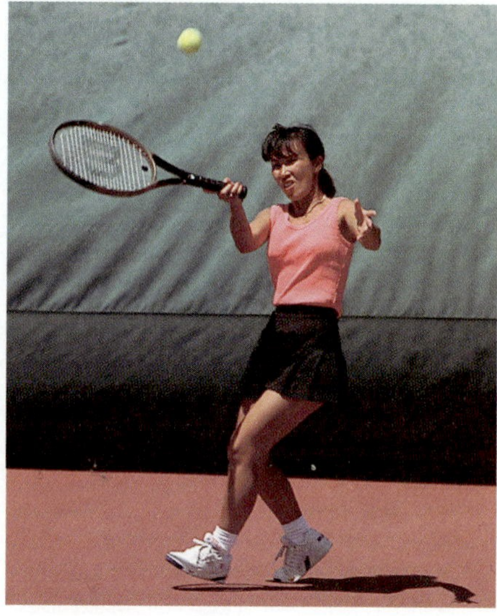

Figure 5.26 Contact.

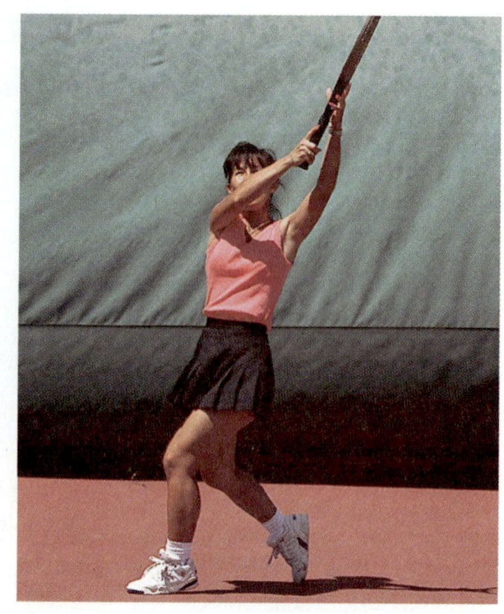

Figure 5.27 Follow through.

Retreating to Hit a Lob Behind the Baseline—Backhand

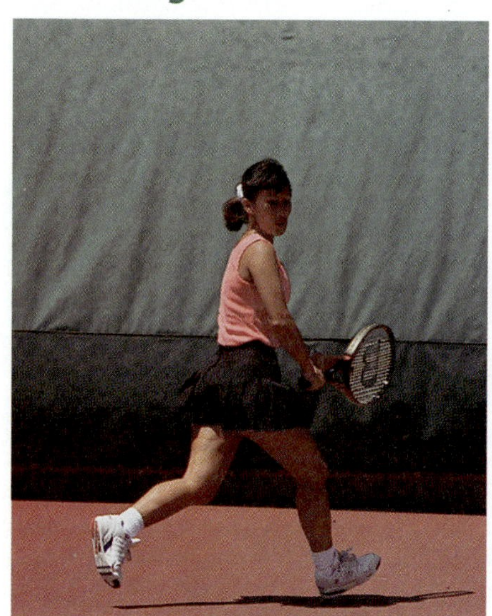

Figure 5.28 Backswing.

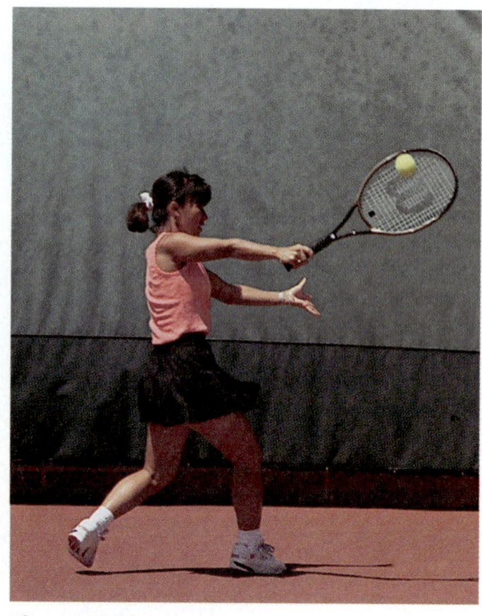

Figure 5.29 Contact.

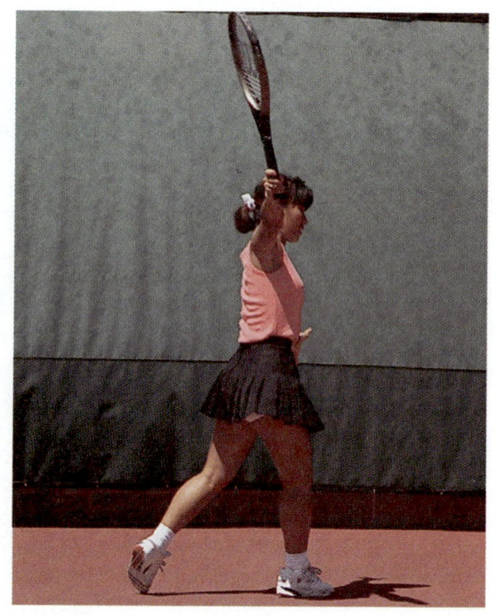

Figure 5.30 Follow through.

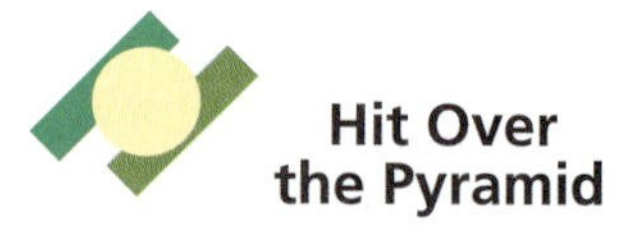

Hit Over the Pyramid

Visualize a pyramid at the apex of the net, and hit your defensive lob over that apex. A defensive lob hit with height at the apex of the net will bounce in-court and deep.

B. Hartwick, Tennis, 11/91, p. 28

Racket control, weight transfer, and movement of the feet are essential to hitting lobs. Racket control is used to apply topspin of varying degrees, underspin, or a simple block of the ball.

Weight transfer, as with all shots, is important with the lob, but the transfer has more to do with the hips and a little step transfer than with a long step into the ball. It is more of a center-of-gravity movement forward. Most lobs are hit on the move rather than from a stationary position. The player either is retreating from the net to hit the ball or is moving laterally along the baseline. As a result of having to hit a lob on the run, the lob isn't always a nice setup from a ready position that permits easy execution of the stroke. Moving the feet to get to the ball, then recovering enough to place the racket on the ball, while attempting to hold form, are all based on the initial foot movement and anticipation as to the location the opponent has intended for a target (Figures 5.25–5.30).

Incorporating the lob into the total game is important to the developing player. Without the lob, there is no response to the overhead smash, and the options for hitting a ball when the opponent is at the net decrease by one. The lob also serves as an occasional change-of-pace stroke, and it can be frustrating for the opponent who likes pace associated with the game or who cannot hit an overhead effectively. The lob is an extension of a groundstroke, and developing the skill is only a transition rather than development of a totally new stroke.

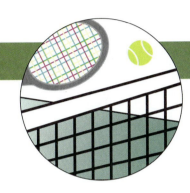

Learning Experience Reminders

Lobs

1. To produce an offensive lob with topspin, roll the forearm from contact through follow through.
2. Strive for all lob follow throughs to finish high.
3. Follow the principle that the more defensive a lob, and the more change from some topspin to an underspin, the more firm the wrist and shorter the backswing.
4. Follow through an underspin to a ball on the defensive lob in the same plane.
5. To regulate topspin in an offensive lob, vary leg bend and extension. The more topspin, the more leg bend and extension.
6. Open the racket face on lobs at contact.
7. Move to the ball as quickly as possible to incorporate form into the stroke.

Elimination of Errors (Lobs)

The Error	What Causes the Error	Correction of the Error
Lobs hit long beyond the opponent's baseline.	Too much velocity and lift applied to the ball.	The lob requires touch and feel. Focus on a shorter target. Adjust the upward angle of the racket.
Balls hit short just over the net.	Usually not enough follow through and backswing.	If stroking the lob, rather than blocking, the backswing and follow through should be equal in distance, and the more distance, the farther the ball will travel.
Lobs that are blocked rebound off at different angles.	Racket face isn't square to the ball.	Provide a firm arm and wrist base with an open racket face.

Check Points

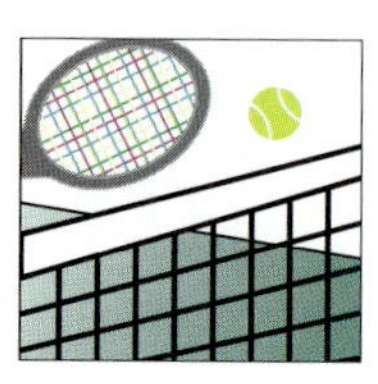

1. Positioning to hit an overhead smash requires the body to
   a. be positioned behind the ball.
   b. be positioned in front of the ball.
   c. be positioned underneath the ball.
   d. adjust depending on the height of the lob.

2. The overhead smash should be hit after allowing the ball to bounce when
   a. a lob is hit short at the net.
   b. a lob has a very high loft.
   c. both situations in a and b exist.
   d. the player is unsure of how to hit the ball.

3. When hitting a backhand overhead smash the position of the elbow is
   a. up, pointed at the ball.
   b. out, pointed in line with where the ball is to be hit.
   c. down, positioned to allow the racket to swing through the ball.
   d. none of the above.

4. Overhead smash shots hit long are caused by
   a. hitting the ball too hard.
   b. hitting the ball with an open racket face.
   c. hitting the ball with the ball positioned behind the head.
   d. all three examples above.

5. The follow-through pattern when hitting an offensive lob requires the racket
   a. to cross the upper body and finish high.
   b. to stay in the same plane as with the backswing and contact positions.
   c. to stop following contact with the ball.
   d. to cross the upper body and stay low.

6. The ball action off a defensive lob is
   a. underspin.
   b. topspin.
   c. slice.
   d. no spin.

7. The flight patterns of a basic groundstroke, offensive lob, and defensive lob are
   a. high, middle, low.
   b. middle, high, low.
   c. low, middle, high.
   d. middle, low, high.

8. The keys to hitting successful lobs include
   a. leg bend and extension, open racket face, and fast racket movement.
   b. leg bend and extension, open racket face, and a high follow through.
   c. leg bend and extension, closed racket face, and a high follow through.
   d. leg bend and extension, closed racket face, and fast racket movement.

Answers to Check Points can be found on page 145.

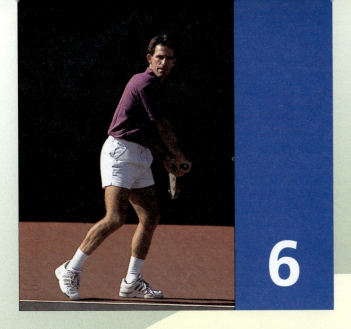

6

Mental Aspects of Tennis Competition

Physical effort and mental planning of strategy are necessary to be successful in tennis. Without the physical skill, an individual would have a difficult time winning. Mental effort is the intangible that accents the physical and gives purpose to playing tennis. The mental aspects of tennis are the true key to success on a tennis court.

A beginning tennis player should ask, "Why participate in a game that requires so much from a player, both physically and mentally?" To play tennis requires a bit of a childlike personality. The player has to want to play for play's sake. Associated with that is the idea of playing for fun and for the sheer joy of physical movement and abandon. The tennis player needs to feel the game, feel the aesthetics, and appreciate the execution of skill.

Playing for fitness or skill development and playing for fun are playing tennis for the right reasons. A player should feel the sun and breeze caressing the body and absorb the sound of balls striking rackets, the chatter of people, and the sounds of effort as a player reaches for an overhead or completes a serve. Tennis is not bigger than life. It isn't life itself, and it never is a life or death situation. Tennis is a life experience that can enhance your self-worth. It is about your inner self (Picture This, by J. Loehr, *World Tennis,* April 1989, p. 22.) If the game is played for the correct reasons, all the other parts, including winning, fall into place.

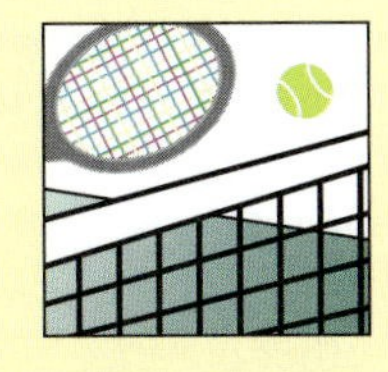

Understanding What Competition Really Means

Competition and winning often are confused as being the same, but they are barely related. In competition, winning is a byproduct for one of the participants. Competition is not opponent against opponent. It is player against barrier. If the tennis player can visualize that the player on the other side of the net is providing barriers, an understanding of competition begins to emerge. The opponent—through a serve, a volley, or a lob—is placing a barrier for the other player to respond to. The barrier is erected for a challenge. It is nothing personal. A tennis player must understand that concept to be really successful in a match and to learn to truly compete.

A player must learn to emphasize *execution over winning*. If execution is the important aspect, the winning will take care of itself. Worrying about winning or losing interferes with both execution and winning. Thinking about appearances or pleasing others interferes with execution and winning. The emphasis is on execution, the concentration is on execution, and the goal is execution.

A clarification is in order when using the term "execution." The emphasis is not on thinking about executing a skill pattern; it is on completing the skill pattern. The mind should be focused on feeling a barrier and responding to it by a reflex action, and that reflex action is execution. If a player begins to analyze movement and strokes, or begins to think of ulterior motives behind execution, skilled play collapses.

The beginning tennis player may never have been exposed to this concept before and so may have difficulty understanding why thinking about winning is not acceptable. If the player will realize that emphasis on winning places pressure to excel and pressure not to fail, the idea of eliminating those pressures might become palatable. If executing by doing provides the realization of the long-term goal of winning, execution begins to make sense.

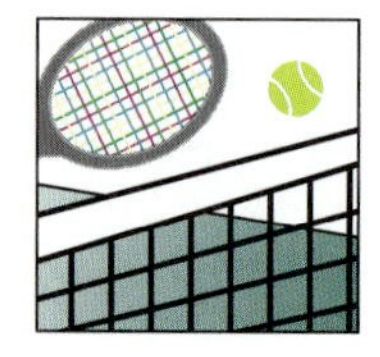

Eliminating Negative Attitudes

When participating in tennis, a *negative attitude or negative feelings* contribute to a negative response. If a player is ready to receive a serve and the thought "please don't make the serve; double fault—please" flashes, a negative attitude has been established. Other thoughts that are apt to enter the mind include, "What if I miss the shot?" or "If I hold my serve, I can win," or "You dummy—why can't you hit the ball?" Each of these plants a negative thought that contributes to a less than successful experience.

Negative attitudes arise when a player gets upset and begins to talk to the other self: "How could you hit such a stupid shot," or "I can't believe you're real—how could you miss such an easy setup?" If a player keeps making derogatory statements about performance, that player will exceed all expectations of failure through negative thought.

Fear of winning and fear of losing both contribute to negative thought. Fear places pressure on the player not to make mistakes, and that negative thought reemphasizes fear of failure. The player becomes anxious to do well, and that anxiousness contributes to tension, which restricts performance (as performance must be accomplished in a relaxed, controlled manner).

Becoming *angry and losing one's temper* is another negative. Anger is a means of releasing energy, and this will take a toll on the player when a demand for extra effort is needed and the body cannot provide it. Losing one's temper also places pressure on that player. A player who gets mad at himself or herself is venting anger internally. That internal anger creates the same anxiety as the fear of winning or losing, with the player trying to please "self." The effect of the cycle of anger-anxiety-pressure is the collapse of the player's performance during competition.

Another negative associated with performance and tennis play is the opponent's behavior. A popular term in sport is *psych out*. Behavior by an opponent can be upsetting if permitted to be upsetting. Body language, verbal comments, gamesmanship, and outbursts by an opponent can create negative reactions that will cause anxiety for the other player.

Negative thoughts can be changed by realizing what is happening and replacing them with positive thoughts. Instead of worrying about a missed shot, concentration should be on remembering a similar shot that was executed well. Instead of hoping that an opponent will miss a serve, a player should hope the serve will be good so that "I can have the opportunity to return a winner."

The fear of winning or losing is eliminated if the player will remember and practice what competition means and shut out the emphasis on winning and losing. Certainly, attacking one's own person verbally and sometimes physically is not being a friend to oneself. The developing player should treat the inner self with respect and dignity, stop arguing with and embarrassing one's other self, and begin to compliment the other self on a good shot or a good point played. Finally, not allowing an opponent to psych you out is extremely helpful in competition.

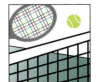

Concentration

Concentration is an important part of tennis. Blocking out all factors other than executing a shot is required for success. A focus on the ball and the task of hitting the ball helps a player to concentrate. When engaged in a rally, the player should look at the seams of the ball all the way to the racket face. Research indicates that a player can see a ball only to within four feet of the racket, but just the effort to look the ball into the racket improves concentration.

Concentration also is enhanced by being in touch with one's own body. The ability to synchronize breathing with each stroke and to sense the heartbeat as a body function permit the player to be in touch and concentrate better.

Another sense that enhances concentration is hearing—as in hearing the tennis ball make contact with the racket strings. And the kinesthetic sense is evoked when feeling the impact of ball and racket and recognizing muscle contraction and tension during the stroke. To really concentrate requires the player to eliminate all extraneous aspects of the environment.

Exchanging sides of the court can be a time for concentration. The concentration should be on the game plan and on thinking positive thoughts. If a player keeps saying "I'm playing well," that thought will become reality. In sum, concentration is focusing on the task at hand.

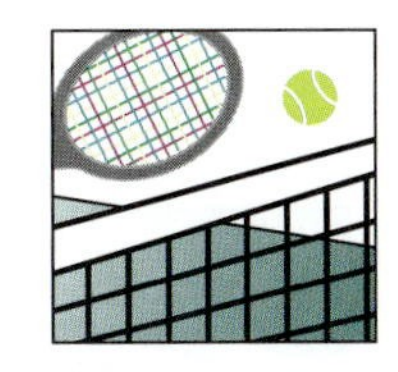

Anxiety and Slumps

There will be times when everything "clicks" during a game—a *flow* to movement and to the play in general. That flow may last for a few points in a match, for a larger portion of a match, for a few days, or for months. Then there will be down times, when nothing seems to work and Murphy's Law is real! The down time is described best as a *slump*. Slumps seem to appear for no reason, but they usually are a result of worrying, tension, or a fear of winning or losing. In short, slumps occur as a result of self-induced pressure, and that pressure causes anxiety. Once a player becomes anxious, the muscles tense, which in turn forces physical errors because there is no relaxation during play. When the errors mount, the tension increases and the slump continues. As long as the player permits the pressure to interfere with performance, the cycle will continue.

The cure to the slump is to eliminate the anxiety by reducing muscle tension. This can be done in two ways: (1) the player begins to think positive, and (2) the player begins to relax and hit out on each ball, eliminating concern for the end result. To reduce muscle tension, the player needs to rebuild confidence. Participating in a match with a player who hits at a consistent pace is a start at redeveloping that confidence. Self-talk ("good shot—way to play") aids in raising self-confidence. Believing that the flow will return and relaxing are keys to coping positively. As a means of relaxing, the player must work at minimizing the number of times the muscle groups will be permitted to tense, which decreases interference with relaxed performance.

During competition, the flow may disappear when the player realizes "I shouldn't be playing this well." A self-fulfilling prophecy begins to make the player anxious, and the whole cycle within the match begins to develop. In the next match a slump may not be evident, but somewhere in the match, if similar circumstances occur, play will deteriorate just as before. Regardless of the length of the slump, the anxiety causes muscle tension, which reduces performance.

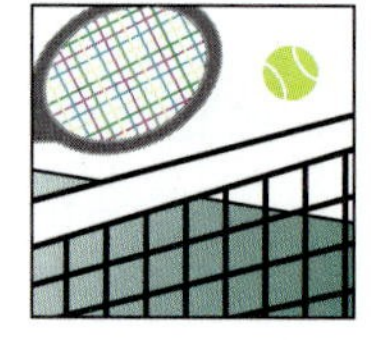

Relaxation

The ability to relax contributes greatly to physical performance. Learning how to relax in a tennis match requires first recognizing muscle tension. If the player grips the racket too tightly (an exception when hitting volley shots), the muscles tense too much. Shoulder and arm muscles that are tight can be recognized with a little practice. A check of the jaw will reveal tenseness in the mouth and jaw areas. The whole body can tense during the pressure of a point or game, and shortness of breath, excessive sweating, and mental confusion are signals that the stress is too great. Relaxation during play can be attained in several ways: (1) by immediately responding to tension on the court, (2) by preparing to play through mental rehearsal and mental imagery, and (3) by relaxing before the match.

The *immediate response to tension on the court* is to learn how to recognize the tension and then relax those muscle groups. If the player feels tension in the shoulders and neck, a clockwise rotation of the head followed by a counterclockwise motion will relax that area. Tension in the arms and legs can be eliminated by running or skipping in place. Another exercise that aids in total body relaxation is to take a deep breath and hold for a count of five, finally expelling the air.

Preparing to play by using *mental rehearsal* or *mental imagery* requires practice, but it can be learned in a short time. The idea is to prepare so well mentally that it enhances confidence, which, in turn, reduces anxiety and tension. Among the several approaches to this way of developing relaxation, one is to correct a skill problem by visualizing the mistake, then repeatedly reviewing the proper skill with the mind.

Sometimes the skill problem is more related to the sequence of shots or a game plan. The corresponding mental practice should be to use imagery emphasizing the acceptable shot or sequence of shots in a game plan. This mental imagery is a foundation for the actual tennis match and will assist the player in recognizing certain situations. Mental rehearsal even helps during a match when a player visualizes a positive picture of the next sequence of serves or a strategy for moving the ball from one side of the court to the other in a baseline rally.

The third form of relaxation is *pre-match relaxation.* The most widely used technique is *progressive relaxation*, which involves developing a habitual 20-minute-per-day relaxation exercise plus a before-a-match session. Skill development centers on recognizing muscle tension followed by relaxing each muscle group. The tension recognition and relaxation response provides a foundation from which to approach life in general, and tennis, in a more relaxed way.

This skill carries over to a tennis match by permitting the player to recognize pressure during play, and immediately relaxing enough to prevent a deterioration of performance.

Other forms of relaxation include meditation and self-hypnosis, which are compatible with tennis players who want to improve their performance. The progressive relaxation technique and additional forms of pre-match relaxation also contribute to the player's using mental rehearsal or imagery after attaining relaxation. The mental aspects of tennis preparation can raise a player's skill level to an optimum not considered possible. The game is more mental than physical. By applying various forms of relaxation, the player will improve rapidly.

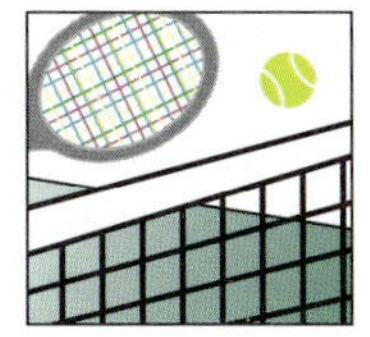

Mental Toughness

Jim Loehr (How to get Mentally Tough/ Part I and II, *Tennis*, July/August 1992, pp. 45–61) provides an excellent view on mental toughness and insight into the positive approach to mentally preparing for a match. He uses terminology analogous to muscular strength—resilience, strength, flexibility, and responsiveness—to define mental toughness.

Resilience is related to any emotional excess baggage you carry into the next point of a match following a mistake. If your skill errors come in bunches, you may struggle with your temper and develop a negative attitude. If a bad call upsets you, you are not a resilient tennis player. To overcome low resilience, focus on the positive. Avoid drooping or whining after you miss a shot. Turn away from the net—and leave the mistake behind you.

Players with *emotional strength* generate positive emotional support for themselves and reject negative emotional distress. Those who lack emotional strength are shy about pumping a fist in the air or showing positive emotion, are fearful of looking an opponent in the eyes, make a line call softly, and rarely question obviously bad calls. Emotional strength is displayed on the court through body language, voice patterns, and general attitude. Opponents sense weak behavior and uncertainty. The key is to assume a court presence: stand up straight, move with a purpose, use a firm voice in your calls, and stop complaining.

The *flexible* player is one who creates a relaxed atmosphere in stressful situations. Laughing at a stupid mistake, ignoring poor court conditions or an obnoxious opponent, eliminating tantrums, and looking and feeling positive under all circumstances are signs of a flexible player. Positive thought and action are critical flexibility.

Finally, a *responsive* player is one who maintains alertness and intensity. Behaviors such as playing in a daze, being too casual, forgetting the score, and not caring contribute to an unresponsive attitude. A responsive player focuses on the event and maintains a standard of expectation for a high performance level.

A great deal of mental effort is involved when playing tennis. Understanding what competition really is, eliminating negative attitudes, and developing relaxation techniques are extremely helpful. Positive mental imagery contributes as well.

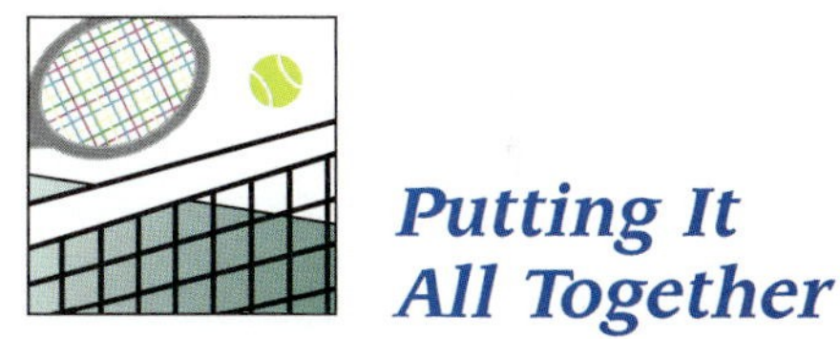

Putting It All Together

Even though you are a beginner, it is important to take the subjects discussed in the previous pages and apply them. It's time to think a little about how you might be most effective against another player in terms of mental outlook.

First, never be intimidated by an opponent. Remember you are playing a barrier, not an opponent. What you need is a level of confidence that you are going to play as well as you are capable of playing. Second, establish a plan of attack. When you read the next two chapters you will have the opportunity to develop a strategy to compete in singles or doubles play. Think through what you are going to do—make it a mental plan. Third, once you have started playing recall what has been going on during the match. What are the strengths of the other player? Just as important, what are the weaknesses? Take advantage of the weaknesses. Within your skill level try to hit shots to the weakness of the other player, and try not to hit the ball to any of the player's strengths (Mind over Matter, by J. F. Murray, *Tennis*, May 1999, p. 20).

Confidence breeds confidence. Believe in yourself and what you have learned as a player up to the point of the most recent match you have played. Focus in on your task. Think about what you have to do. It helps to have a desire to play well, and to be mentally and emotionally ready. You also must focus on the process, not the result. Enjoy the moment. Hit each ball as if it is your best shot. Have fun. And play for the shear joy of playing. Finally, learn to play with low anxiety. Dismiss being nervous, relax your body without becoming a wet noodle, and believe that you can play the game (Even the Odds, by J. Taylor, *Tennis*, November 1999, p. 15).

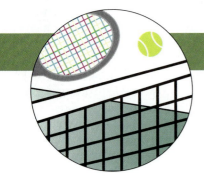

Learning Experience Reminders

The Mental Game

1. Competition is not opponent against opponent. It is player against barrier.
2. Emphasize execution over winning.
3. Eliminate negative attitudes like fear of losing, becoming angry, and self-defeating negative conversation with yourself.
4. Concentrate by blocking our extraneous interference.
5. Eliminate anxiety.
6. Learn to relax on court through relaxation techniques, including mental imagery and progressive relaxation.
7. Develop a mental toughness that includes resilience, emotional strength, flexibility, and responsiveness.
8. Establish a strong mental outlook that includes confidence, match planning, and readiness.

Check Points

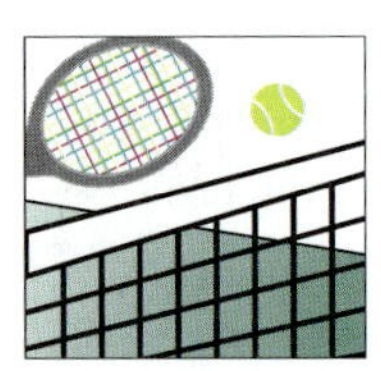

1. Competition associated with tennis is most closely allied with
   a. winning.
   b. execution.
   c. thinking about execution.
   d. opponent against opponent.

2. Negative attitudes associated with tennis include all but one of the following:
   a. Anger
   b. Fear of winning
   c. Psyching out
   d. Shutting out emphasis on winning

3. Concentration associated with tennis includes all but one of the following:
   a. Focus
   b. Synchronized breathing
   c. Competing
   d. Hearing the tennis ball bounce

4. Slumps when playing tennis are caused by all but one of the following:
   a. Anxiety
   b. Flow
   c. Muscle tension
   d. Self-induced pressure

5. Relaxation during play can be attained by
   a. overcoming tenseness with will power.
   b. immediately responding to tension on the court.
   c. preparing to play through mental rehearsal.
   d. relaxing before the match.

6. A mentally tough tennis player is a player who meets all but one of the following profiles:
   a. Resilience
   b. Emotional strength
   c. Anxiousness
   d. Flexibility

Answers to Check Points can be found on page 145.

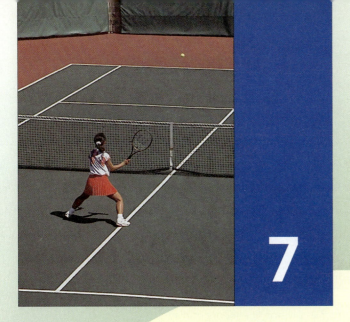

7

Singles Strategy

Strategy in singles is part physical and part mental. The physical provides the mechanics to execute what the mental suggests be done to win a point. The mental is divided into two parts: (1) thinking and broadening thought to plan for the whole match, and (2) using the mind to control the match. This chapter is concerned with the physical or mechanical execution of what the mind suggests and requires in developing a game plan.

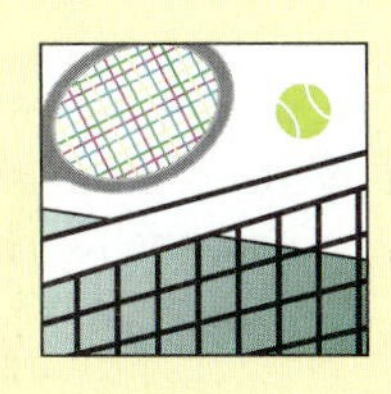

Percentage Tennis

Tennis is a game of mistakes. The player who makes the most mistakes loses. To win at tennis requires *percentage tennis*. Percentage tennis is specific to hitting every ball deep and within the lines of the tennis court. This sounds easy, and actually it is, if the player is devoted to the system of play. The problem with percentage tennis is that players would rather hit the one spectacular shot than play the ball methodically. A percentage player is one who plays within the limits of skill, hitting only the shots that skill development will permit. In addition, the percentage player hits the appropriate stroke for a given shot. A percentage tennis player should grasp two concepts. The first is to comprehend what shot should be hit from what position on the court, and the second is to understand and be able to apply the *division theory of play.*

Court-Division-for-Position-Play Strategy

The tennis court is divided into three parts: backcourt, wasteland, and forecourt (Figure 7.1). The backcourt extends a yard deep behind the baseline, and this is where the percentage player returns all deeply hit shots from the opponent. The percentage concept requires that the player return every shot from the backcourt deep to the opponent's court.

The forecourt is between the service court line and the net. All shots in this area are volleys, overhead smashes, or approach shots. This is the area the

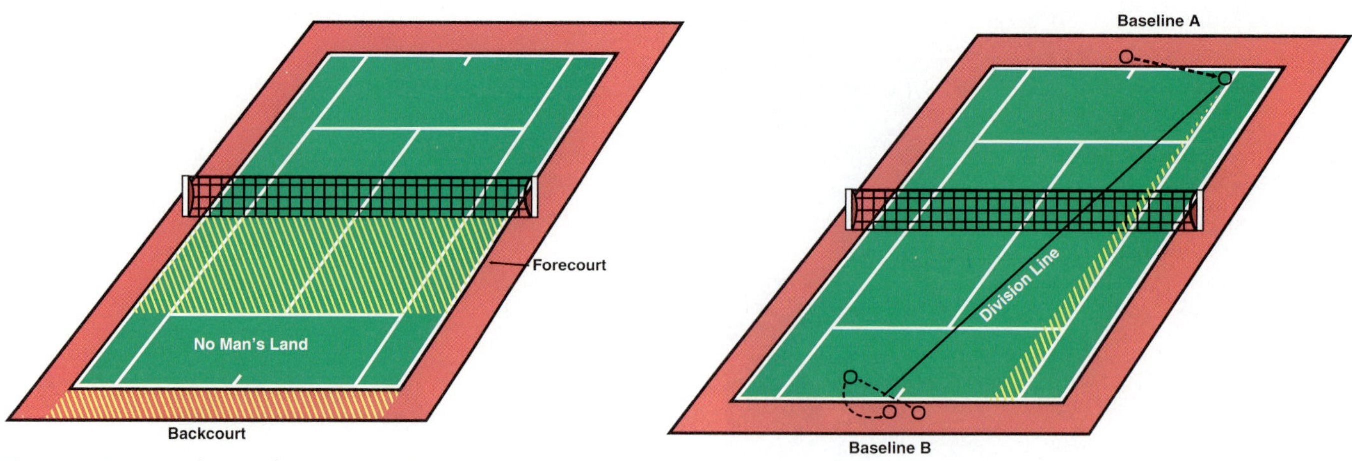

Figure 7.1 Court division for position play.

Figure 7.2 Division line theory of play.

player should enjoy, because a ball hit in the forecourt represents an opponent's error and permits the percentage player to control the net area.

The wasteland is the portion of the court where the percentage player must step to return a shot, then retreat to the baseline to play the next shot. A player never should stand in the wasteland. It is a highly vulnerable area and should be avoided.

Understanding and Applying Division-Line-Theory-of-Play Strategy

A second consideration in percentage tennis is to understand and apply the *division line theory of play.* This involves dividing the court into two equal parts on every stroke. If two players are rallying from the baseline and the ball is coming straight back to each player, the court is divided at the center mark on the baseline (Figure 7.2). If Baseline A player hits a ball angled to the left of Baseline B player, and then the return is a comparable cross-court return, there is a division line that needs to be established. This division line is established for Baseline B player by that player setting up on the baseline a step and a half to the left of the center mark. The intent is to maintain an equal court coverage for a forehand or backhand return. The yellow shaded area in Figure 7.2 helps illustrate this equal court balance.

If the percentage player can stay out of the wasteland except to return a shot, can apply the division line theory, and can hit each return deeply at least three times in a row, the percentage of the opposing player losing the point is quite high. When hitting from the baseline, the percentage player should use the topspin groundstroke when possible because of the high, safe trajectory and the deep, abrupt drop of the ball at the far baseline.

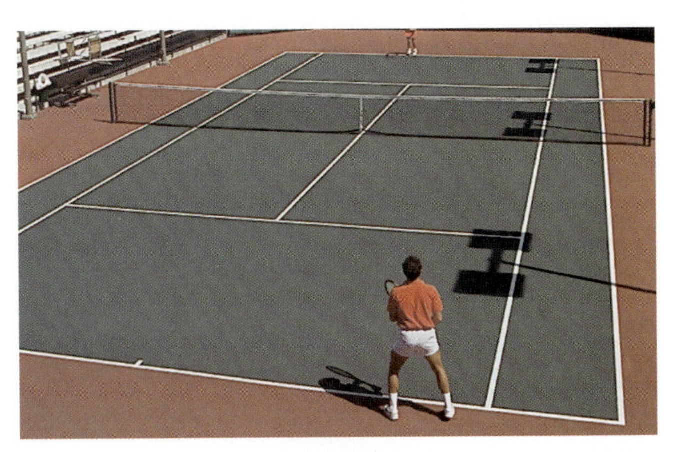

Figure 7.3 Service and service return position.

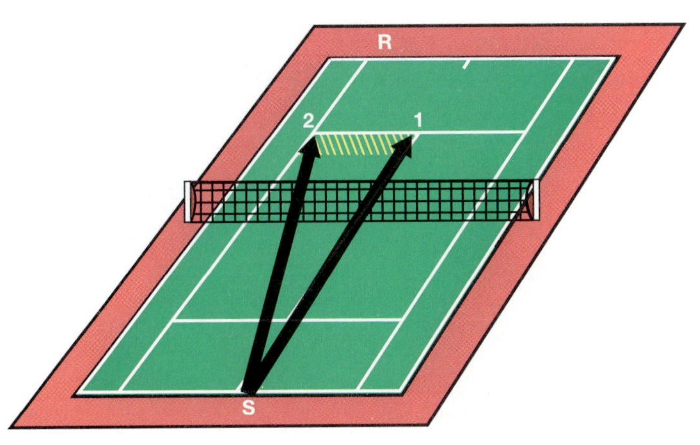

Figure 7.4 Hitting deep serves.

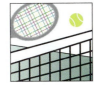

Service and Service-Return Strategy

Using the *service as a part of strategy* is a necessity (Figure 7.3). Most beginners breathe a sigh of relief when their serve strikes the appropriate service court. The strategy comes in when the serve strikes the service court because the server had confidence, hit the ball with velocity, and had a plan as to where to place the ball in the service court. If a server can hit a serve repeatedly with modest speed and place the ball in the corners of the opponent's service court 70 percent of the time, the chances for success are enhanced greatly. If spin can be applied to the ball during service, with accuracy, a variety of serves can be used to confuse the receiver. In addition, the server can capitalize on the receiver's weakness in returning a serve if those weaknesses can be recognized.

Placement-of-Service Strategy

Placement of the service should be deep (Figure 7.4). Then choices can be made as to where to direct the ball to cause the most problems for the receiver. From a position of S1 (Figure 7.5) a serve may be hit down the center of either service court. From a position of S2 a serve is hit wide to either service court. These placements are excellent spots to place a service. In addition, if a server puts reasonable velocity on a flat serve, the receiver will have problems even if the ball is placed directly in front of the body.

A slice serve can be hit wide to the right side of the right service court, pulling the receiver off the court and consequently opening the whole court for the next shot by the server (Figure 7.6). A slice service to the right corner of the left service court pulls the receiver to the middle of the court, causing a down-the-middle return (Figure 7.7).

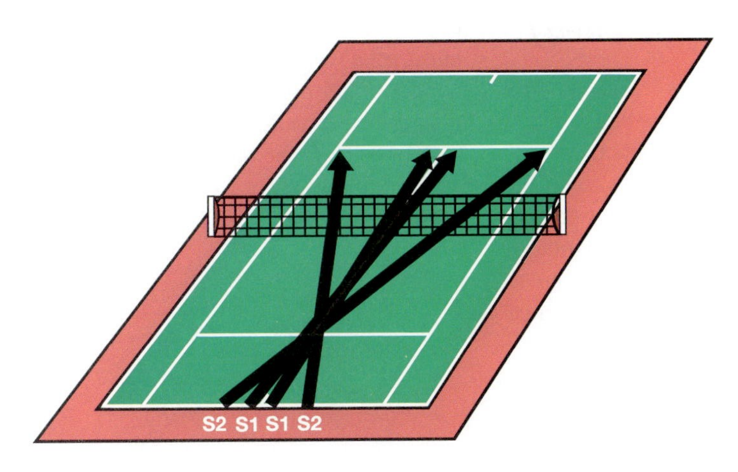

Figure 7.5 Hitting the corners on the serve.

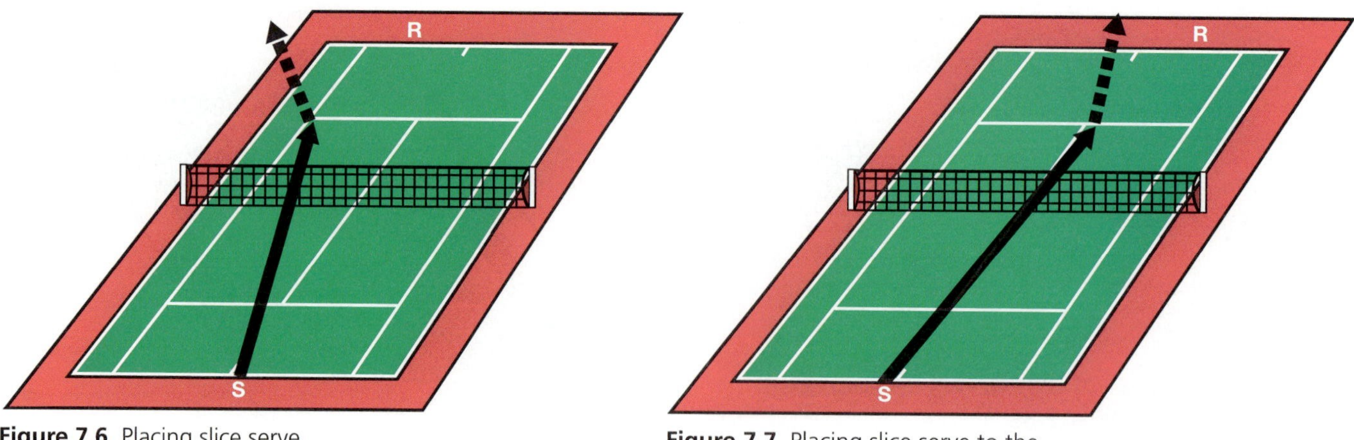

Figure 7.6 Placing slice serve.

Figure 7.7 Placing slice serve to the left service court.

Second-Service Strategy

The second service is even more important in the sense that if it is not placed accurately in the appropriate service court, the point is lost without a response from the receiver. The second serve not only must be reliable and accurate but also should have some pace. Many servers make the mistake of pushing the ball into the service court rather than hitting with good form. The three requirements of a sound second serve are: (1) the serve must have accuracy coupled with pace, (2) the serve must have spin to ensure accuracy, and (3) the serve never is pushed or blooped into the service court. Accuracy is enhanced by a slice or service with some attention to placement of the ball and pace.

Return-of-Service Strategy

Return of service strategy is crucial. The server's role is to place the ball in play, and the return player's role is to keep the ball in play. The strategy is to hit the ball back with pace, and to hit it deep to eliminate the server's initial advantage. The server who relies on the serve to win points will begin to lose confidence if the ball keeps coming back.

A cause-effect relationship indicates that the receiver should respond to the server's pace and depth of serve by standing beyond the baseline to return serve. Such thought must be dispelled. If the server has a strong spin, it is best to step inside the baseline and cut down the sidespin or high bounce before the effect can occur. A serve that is pushed over the net should be returned firmly and deeply, and the receiver should avoid the tendency to "kill" the ball.

When returning the serve, the receiver can use various placements that will enhance the play at that point. Returning *down the line* is usually a mistake when the server has the ability and court position to move easily down the baseline to reach the ball, as it will leave the court open for a cross-court winner by the server (Figure 7.8). Service returns are most effective when hit back along the line of flight of the serve, and at the feet of the server. When serves are hit with little pace, the receiver has more options, including down the line, cross-court, and angled cross-court. The effort off a weak serve should be to hit a winner under control, forcing the opposing server to hit while moving to the ball, or to miss the ball entirely.

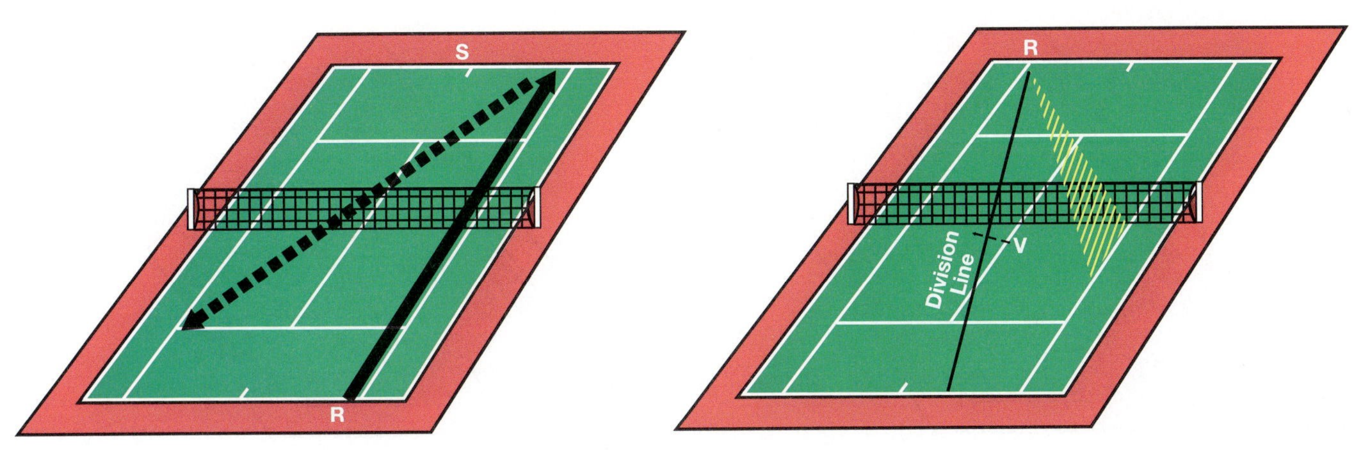

Figure 7.8 Consequences of return of serve down the line.

Figure 7.9 Division line theory.

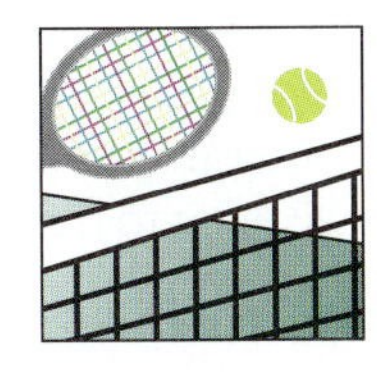

Attacking the Net and Beating the Net Player

Judgments a player must make include when to go to the net and, once there, when to stay and when to leave. A player should go to the net in three situations: (1) off a serve, (2) off an approach shot, and (3) off a firmly hit groundstroke that forces the opponent to move behind the baseline when returning the shot. When at the net, there are two times to stay and continue play at the net: (1) when following one volley with another, and (2) when hitting an overhead smash from between the service court line and the net. The player should retreat in only one situation—when a lob is hit deep to the baseline, compelling the net player to leave the net to return the lob. The player attacking the net should apply the *division line theory* by following the path of the ball to the net, dividing the court in half between the two players. The division line will enable the net player to cover all territory equally between the forehand and the backhand and give the opponent only one possible winning shot. If, as an example, the net player hits to the deep, right baseline corner of the opponent and takes a step and a half to the left of the center of the net, the only possible return for a winning shot is to the far right corner angled at the net (Figure 7.9).

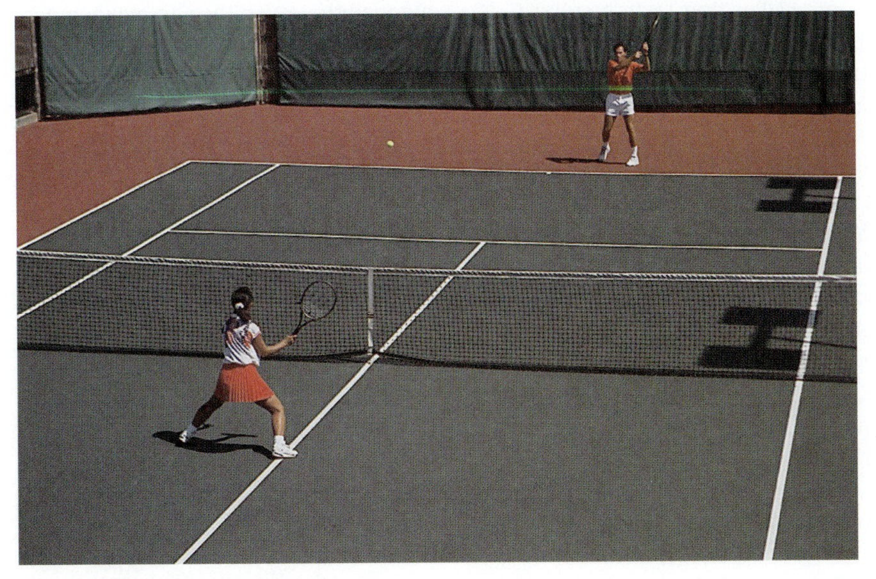

Figure 7.10 Server going to the net.

Going-to-the-Net Strategy

Going to the net following a serve suggests the execution of an accurate serve (Figure 7.10). In fact, an accurate serve with pace provides the opportunity to effectively advance to the net. If the serve is returned with pace, penetration is as close as it is going to be if the

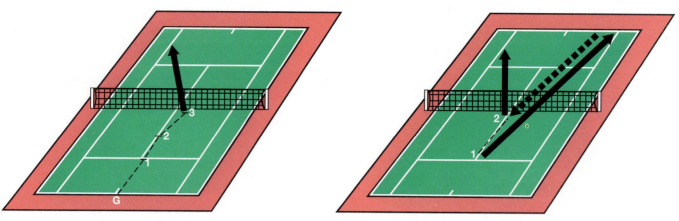

Figure 7.11 Going to the net following a serve.

Figure 7.12 Going to the net following an approach shot from the middle of the court.

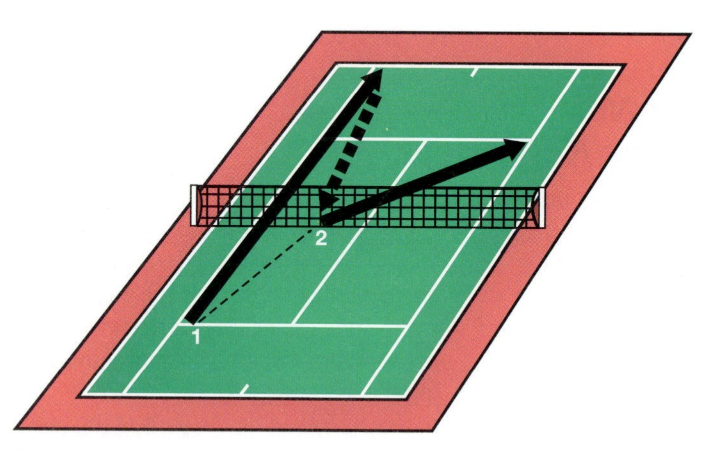

Figure 7.13 Going to the net following an approach shot from the sideline area of the court.

server can get to the service court line (Figure 7.11/Position 1). If the return of the serve is a mis-hit, the server can pounce on the return with an efficient volley from the net position (Figure 7.11/Position 2 or 3). If the return of serve is at the feet of the server, who has advanced on the net, a 20-foot return distance from the net may become a liability. The server now has to be an exceptional volleyer because the ball at the feet creates vulnerability. A slice service permits the server to advance closer to the net before being forced to stop and respond to the opponent's return of serve.

Going to the net following an approach shot is an ideal time to advance on the net (Figure 7.12). If the return from the opponent is short—at the service line in the middle of the court—the approach shot can be played to a corner (Figure 7.12/Position 1). Once the ball is hit to the corner, the player advances to the net, in line with the ball, and volleys cross-court (Figure 7.12/Position 2). If a return shot is hit to the service line, close to and parallel to a sideline, the approach shot should be down the sideline (Figure 7.13/Position 1) followed by a short angled volley cross-court as the player advances on to the net (Figure 7.13/Position 2).

Going to the net off a groundstroke must be done with some prudence. It is inadvisable to go to the net when the groundstroke (1) has not been hit with authority, (2) has not been hit deep to the baseline, and (3) has not forced the opponent to return the shot while moving away from the net. If the player has hit an effective groundstroke, however, that player must learn to *close in on the net.* As the player advances to the net from the baseline, a ready position must be assumed prior to the return shot crossing the net. Once the advancing player has hit a return, that player continues on to the net in a line with the ball, and again stops in a ready position before the return shot crosses the net.

Between two and three stops are required to gain control of the net and be in control of hitting a winning shot if the opponent is able to respond with some degree of authority in returning the shots hit by the advancing player. Three thoughts should be on the mind

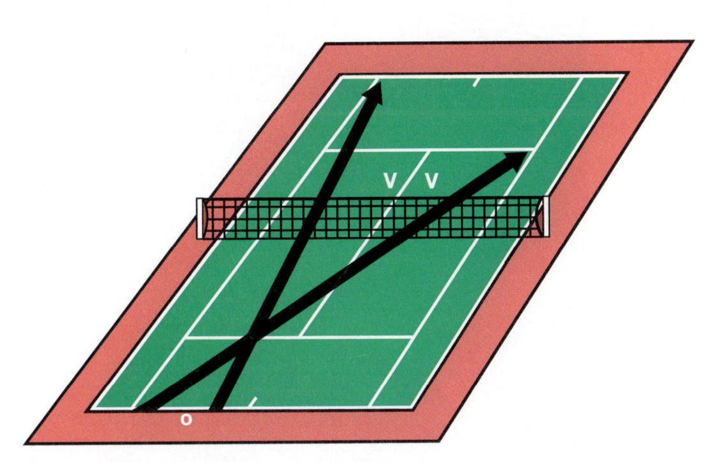

Figure 7.14 Hitting a passing shot to beat a net player.

of the player advancing from the baseline: (1) volley and advance, (2) punch the ball deep to the baseline, and (3) hit at the feet of the opponent so the return is "up."

Advancing to the net is an adventure and a reward if the end result is a winning shot. The choice of going to the net is based on the advantage that it will give the player to advance. Some final thoughts associated with attacking the net are: First, the volleyer always must stop and assume a ready position prior to the return shot crossing the net. Second, when attacking, the player should follow the path of the ball to provide the division line. Third, the player has to get close to the net to hit a volley. A beginning player needs to be a racket-and-a-half length away from the net, whereas a skilled player can volley from the service court line. All players who volley must remember to stay low and punch the ball.

Beating-the-Net-Player Strategy

A *threefold strategy to beat the player who attacks the net* is: (1) hit at the feet of the net player, (2) hit a passing shot, and (3) hit a lob.

Hitting at the feet of the net player forces the player to hit the ball up in the air, providing a setup to hit a winning return. Two shots are most often used to hit at the feet of a player at the net. A topspin stroke usually is hit from the baseline to the feet of a player at the net, and from a return of serve a ball often is blocked back to the feet of an advancing net player.

Hitting a passing shot to beat a net player is a second means of defeating the volleyer at the net. The passing shot may be hit down the line or as a short-angled cross-court shot. As an example, if a player is to the left of the center mark at the baseline, a shot down the net player's right sideline could pass that player. A ball hit farther to the left of the baseline player can be played as a short-angled cross-court passing shot, as the net player has moved to the right of center to establish the division line (Figure 7.14).

The third method of *beating the net player is with a lob.* A net player tends to get too close to the net to avoid hitting balls at the feet. This diminishes the ability to retreat and cover a deep lob, and the player at the baseline has a clear-cut choice of hitting an offensive, topspin lob to the net player's baseline. If the players are beginners, any form of a lob that gets over the head of the net player will be effective. The important point is to drive the opponent back from the net, ensuring a return on the move with the back to the net.

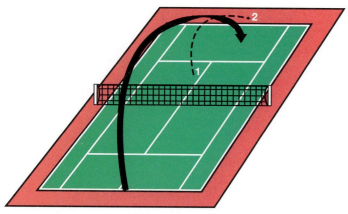

Figure 7.15 Retrieving a lob.

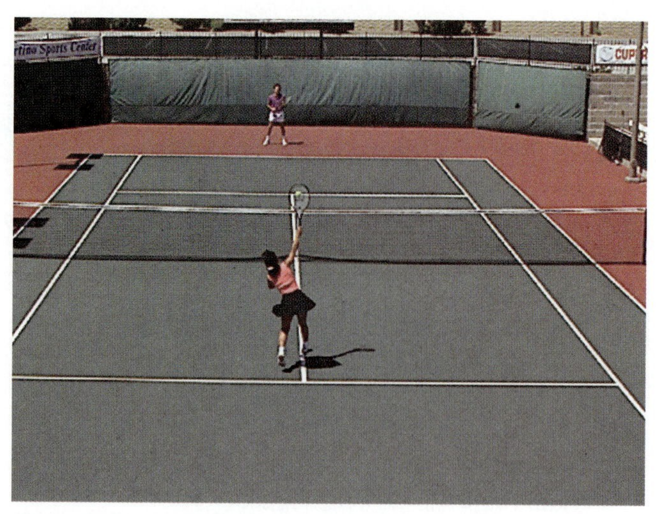

Figure 7.16 Overhead smash set up.

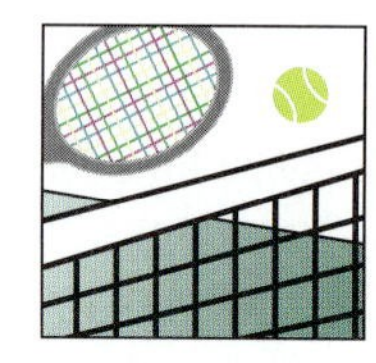

Lob and Overhead-Smash Strategy

Lobs and overhead smashes are an integral part of overall court strategy. The lob can be either a defensive or an offensive shot, and the overhead smash is a reward for effective serve or groundstroke play.

Lob Strategy

The question in singles play is *when to hit a lob, and what kind to hit.* Defensive lobs should be hit whenever the opponent has forced the play, and whenever a player needs to "buy time" to recover from a strong shot. The important part of a defensive lob is to hit to the opponent's backhand, forcing the opponent to run around the ball to hit an overhead smash, or to return the ball going away from the net with a backhand stroke.

When retrieving a lob, the player, instead of running in a straight line, should run to the outside of the ball and come from behind it to hit a return lob, or a forceful groundstroke, or an overhead smash (Figure 7.15/Positions 1–2). A lob that has the effect of an offensive shot should, of course, be hit when the opposing net player is too close to the net.

Overhead-Smash Strategy

Overhead smashes are used in singles strategy to respond to lobs that are hit between the service court and the net (Figure 7.16). Setting up is an important part of that strategy. A crisp volley down the opponent's right sideline forces that player to execute a lob that travels to the middle of the court, which, in turn, can be hit as an overhead smash to the opponent's left corner (Figure 7.17). This example illustrates that a firm offensive shot creates a weak lob return, and for each lob return, there is a wide variety of targets for the overhead smash. Balls hit deep to the opponent's baseline are always acceptable as effective overheads (Figure 7.18).

When the return lob is closer to the net, smashes can be angled and bounced out of the opponent's court. The angle and bounce carry the ball into a nonreturnable location (Figure 7.19). Angled and deeply angled overhead smashes are also effective (Figure 7.20). They ensure that the opponent has to move to retrieve the overhead rather than remain stationary and hit a lob with control. An angled overhead (Figure 7.20/Position 1) is an excellent placement for a backhand overhead

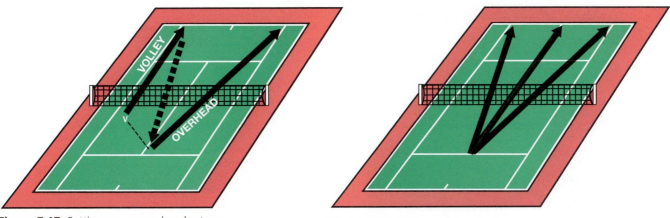

Figure 7.17 Setting up an overhead return with a volley shot.

Figure 7.18 Hitting overheads deep.

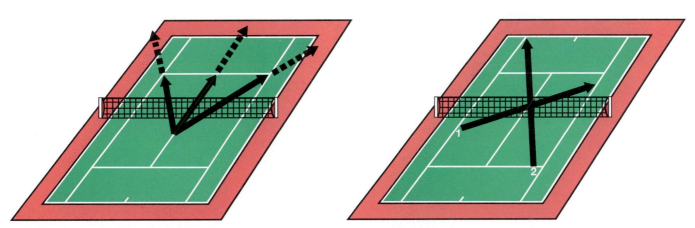

Figure 7.19 Hitting angled overhead smashes.

Figure 7.20 Angled and deeply angled overhead smashes.

because accuracy in placement is more important than speed in completing the shot successfully, while a forehand overhead angled deep is often a winning shot (Figure 7.20/Position 2).

Often the first overhead smash is not a winning shot, nor should it be expected to be. The first overhead "softens up" the opponent, who can return the shot only from a defensive position. Strategically, if the player hitting the lob keeps the overhead consistently deep and angled, the opponent returning lobs eventually wears down or breaks down skillwise and hits a short lob that can be returned as a winning overhead.

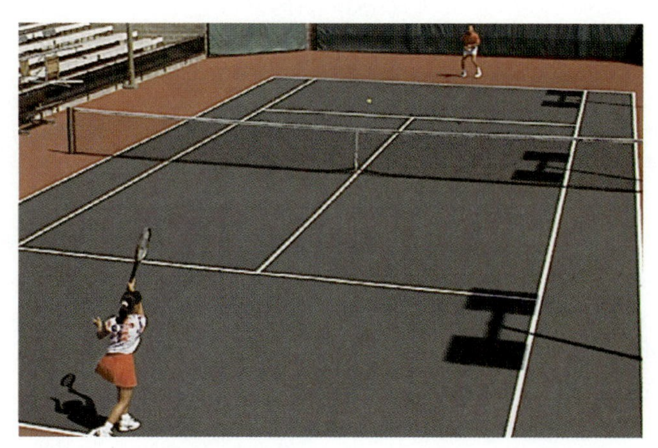

Figure 7.21 Baseline play set up.

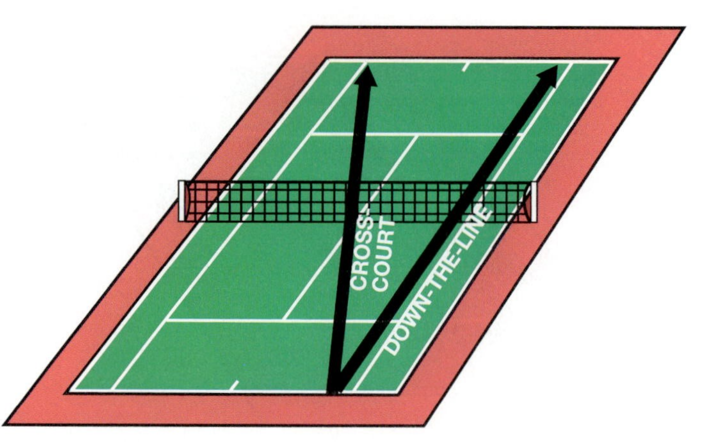

Figure 7.22 Duplication groundstroke returns.

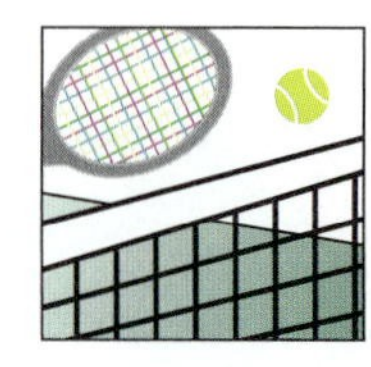

Baseline-Play Strategy

Baseline play involves giving complete, undivided attention to hitting groundstrokes deep and relying on percentage tennis to its fullest. The idea is to force the opponent to make a mistake with a mis-hit shot or poorly hit return. Among the several ways of forcing an error from the opponent are cross-court and down-the-line shots (Figure 7.21).

Duplicating-the-Opponent's-Groundstroke-Return Strategy

Duplicating the opponent's return is good strategy because it puts pressure on the opponent to change the direction of the ball. Singles strategy dictates that if the opponent hits cross-court, the return should be cross-court until the opponent hits down the line. At that point, the player hitting has the option of returning in duplication down the line or coming back cross-court. In either case, the advantage is with the player returning a shot rather than the opponent because the return angle favors the return player's stroke and because there is an element of the unknown in the return direction (Figure 7.22).

Moving-the-Opponent Strategy

Another strategy is to move the opponent back and forth across the baseline, forcing alternate forehand and backhand returns. If the opponent can be driven from one side of the court to the other, reaching for shot returns, the ball eventually will be returned short or "up" so an approach shot, volley, or overhead can be used as a follow-up to good baseline play.

With skill and experience, the baseline player can develop strategy using varied strokes, always coming back to hit with depth and angle that will cause the opponent to make a mistake. Sometimes varying the stroke is disguised by hitting down the sideline with a groundstroke to the opponent's backhand for a succession of shots, then switching to a cross-court shot that pulls the opponent out of a groove and requires a totally new stroke in the rally. Hitting the groundstroke again and again to the same side also will wear down an opponent's confidence, and the skill of the stroke will weaken as belief in winning the point lessens.

Scoring-Situation Strategy

Certain *scoring situations* in a match are vital to good strategy and success. In a game, a score of 30–15 is important because winning the next point will produce a score of 40–15. The leading player can use the 2-point difference as a lever to win the game within the next two points. If the 30–15 score becomes 30–30, either player may win the next two points.

A set score of 5–3 with the opponent serving is a crucial situation in the ninth game. If the opponent wins that game, the set is over at a 6–3 score. If the receiver of serve wins the ninth game, the score becomes 4–5 and the player who is behind serves with a tie set possible at 5–5 in the tenth game. Obviously, the 4–5 set score is also important, but the player behind is serving, and with a degree of serving skill, the server has the advantage. Other scores that are meaningful are the first point of any given game and the last point of a game, set, or match.

Game-Plan Strategy

The *overall game strategy and plan* are only as good as the skill of the player. The game plan for an early beginner is to do the best possible to return shots back across the net. By the time the player can hit with some consistency, percentage tennis becomes really important. It means the advanced beginner can work at hitting the ball back with depth and patience and begin to set up an opponent with subtle techniques to force an error. Continual maturation permits the player to understand that the mind is the most important part of the game. The ability to out-think the opponent becomes the key to victory. Changing pace, moving a player along the baseline, and moving the opponent to the net and back away from the net all begin to make sense.

The game plan and strategy for a player starts with the warm-up and ends with the last point of the match. In the warm-up, the player begins to assess the opponent's ability, being careful not to become overly confident of or intimidated by the opponent. During the warm-up, each player should determine the skills of the opponent and what strokes that opponent is capable of hitting effectively. The player who is assessing the other player should not change the game plan only to meet the opponent's skills. The assessing player must be able to react normally and not play as the opponent dictates. As an example of a game plan: If the opponent likes to serve and volley, the strategy might be to prepare to hit passing shots, lobs, and groundstrokes at the opponent's feet. Another example would be to stay at home base during a rally and force the opponent to rally from the baseline when the opponent lacks consistency in hitting groundstrokes. Game plans and strategy should be a combination of the player reacting to the opponent's weaknesses, and playing to the player's skill level.

Final game strategy thoughts include: (1) play every point and return every shot, (2) look for the short ball, and attack with an aggressive approach shot, completing the attack by continuing on to the net, (3) be consistent in play rather than hit the one spectacular shot, (4) use defensive lobs to "buy time," as most tennis players cannot hit solid overheads in reacting to a lob, (5) keep groundstrokes in play and deep, and (6) hit serves with pace and accuracy.

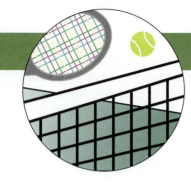

Learning Experience Reminders

Singles Strategy

1. Focus on playing *percentage tennis*.
2. Apply the *division line theory of play,* which simply stated is a division of a tennis court into two equal parts.
3. Effective placement of serve requires hitting down the center, wide, or directly at a receiver's body using both pace and spin.
4. Effective second serve placement requires accuracy with pace; no blooping the serve.
5. Return serves deep and back in line with the server's position.
6. Attack at the net after an effective serve, an approach shot, or off a firmly hit groundstroke that moves the opposing player.
7. Hitting winning volleys and overhead smash shots is a process. The winning shot is often the second or third shot rather than the first.
8. Beat the net player by either hitting at the feet, hitting a passing shot, or hitting a lob.
9. Overhead smashes should be hit deep or angled.
10. Basic groundstroke sequences, beyond hitting deep and straight back to the opponent, are a series of hitting down-the-line and cross-court shots, or an alternation of down-the-line and cross-court.
11. An important point to emphasize winning is at 30–15, and a set score of 4–5 with the opponent serving is a crucial game.
12. Strategy for singles should include playing your game and taking advantage of the weaknesses of your opponent.

Check Points

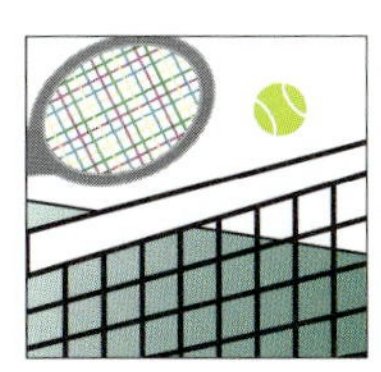

1. Percentage tennis is considered to be
   a. representative of who loses the most points.
   b. representative of who wins the most points.
   c. a strategy established to stay close in a match.
   d. none of the above.

2. The wasteland area is a non-official term used to describe
   a. a highly vulnerable area for a player to stand.
   b. another term for the service court area.
   c. the baseline area.
   d. none of the above.

3. The Division Theory of Play is related to
   a. dividing the court into four parts.
   b. dividing the court into two equal parts.
   c. dividing the strategy of play into two parts.
   d. all three of the above.

4. Service placement to be successful offensively must be
   a. 50% of all serves must be "in."
   b. 70% of all serves must be hit into the deep corners of the opponent's service court.
   c. at a level of no less than 60% accuracy.
   d. 80% accurate on a second serve.

5. Service returns are most effective when hit
   a. along the line of flight of the serve.
   b. down-the-line.
   c. along the line of flight of the serve at the feet of the server.
   d. cross court.

6. It is inadvisable to go to the net when
   a. a groundstroke has been returned with no authority.
   b. a ball has not been returned deeply to the opponent.
   c. the opponent has not been forced to move away from the net.
   d. any of the three exist.

7. The three ways to beat a player at the net are
   a. hit at the player's feet, pass the player, or lob.
   b. hit at the player, pass the player, or lob.
   c. lob, lob, and lob.
   d. rush the player at the net, pass the player, or lob.

8. Defensive lobs should be hit
   a. in order to attack the weakness of an opponent.
   b. to "buy time."
   c. whenever the opposing player is aggressive.
   d. rarely since they are basically limited in success.

9. Overhead smashes should be played when a lob has been returned
   a. high and anywhere on the court.
   b. in the middle of the court.
   c. between the service court line and the net.
   d. between the service court and the baseline.

10. A game score that is significant in order to gain an offensive advantage is
    a. 30-15.
    b. 30-30.
    c. 15-love.
    d. 40-30.

Answers to Check Points can be found on page 145.

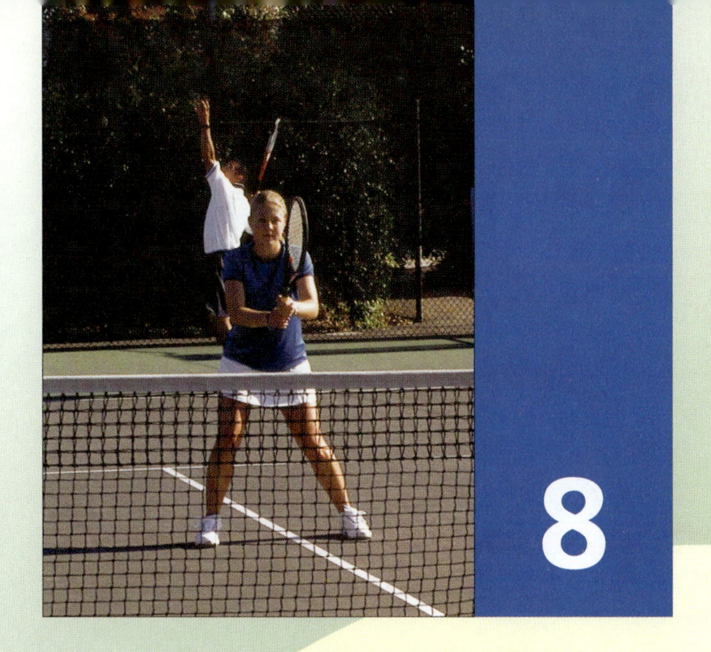

8

Doubles Strategy

With the exception of the strokes used, doubles strategy is entirely different from singles strategy. Doubles is an attacking game; singles tends to be a more passive defensive game. Doubles play is concentrated at the net or retreating from the net, whereas singles play is positioned at the baseline. The attacking concept of doubles provides an exciting type of match with quickly executed shots and good reactions. The beginner seldom experiences the challenge of doubles, yet this is the first situation a beginner may face if being taught in an instructional group.

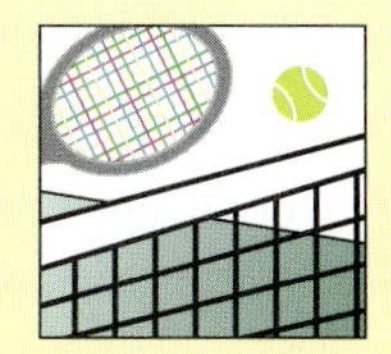

Basic Alignments and Formations

Numerous formations are found in doubles play, including club or recreational social doubles (usually college-class doubles), conventional doubles, and mixed doubles. Choosing a partner and deciding where each partner will be aligned on the court is the beginning to successful strategy.

Two-Back Formation

Beginning players should start from one of two formations, depending on how advanced the players are in executing strokes. These formations are associated with *social doubles*. If the players have yet to be introduced to net play, including volleying and overhead smashes, it is best to begin doubles at the baseline in a two-back formation. The *two-back formation* also is used by experienced players when the opposing team is at the net hitting overhead smashes while the two on the baseline team attempt to return lobs to defend against the overheads (Figure 8.1).

The weakness of the two-back formation is the defensive stature of the team and the lack of control at the net. A team that controls the net has an open court that will allow large areas in which to place the ball for winning shots. From the baseline, shots hit at players controlling the net have little potential for success because they involve only small target areas that the two players cannot cover at the net (Figure 8.2).

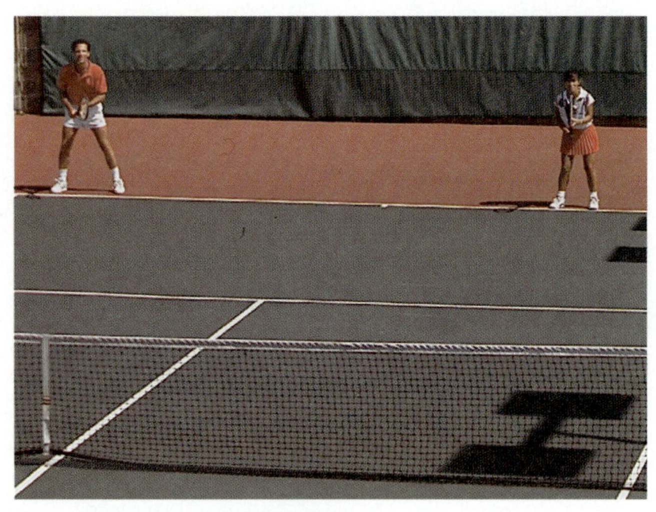

Figure 8.1 Two-back formation.

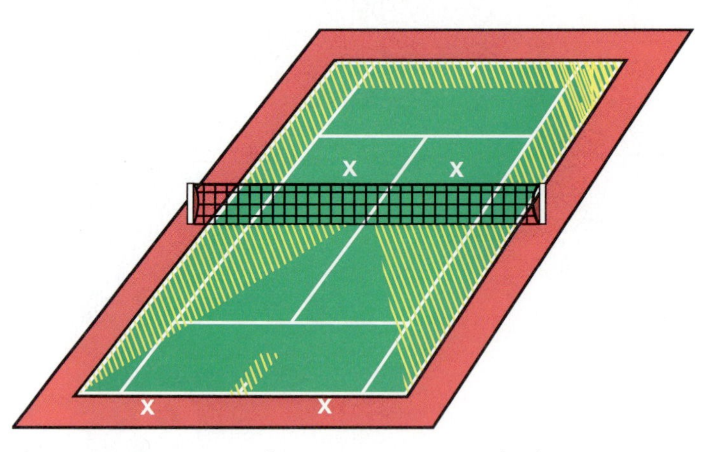

Figure 8.2 Target areas for two-up versus two-back.

One-Up, One-Back Formation

A second formation is *one up and one back*. This alignment is used when the players' net experience is at least adequate for protection at the net, and for execution of firmly hit volleys.

One player up and one player back stems from the original alignment of the players in the serving and receiving positions. The problem arises when the server doesn't have the confidence to serve and follow the serve to the net, or the return player does not follow the return to the net. Once the alignment holds at one-up, one-back, that alignment becomes vulnerable to open-area winning shots. (See Figures 8.3–8.5.)

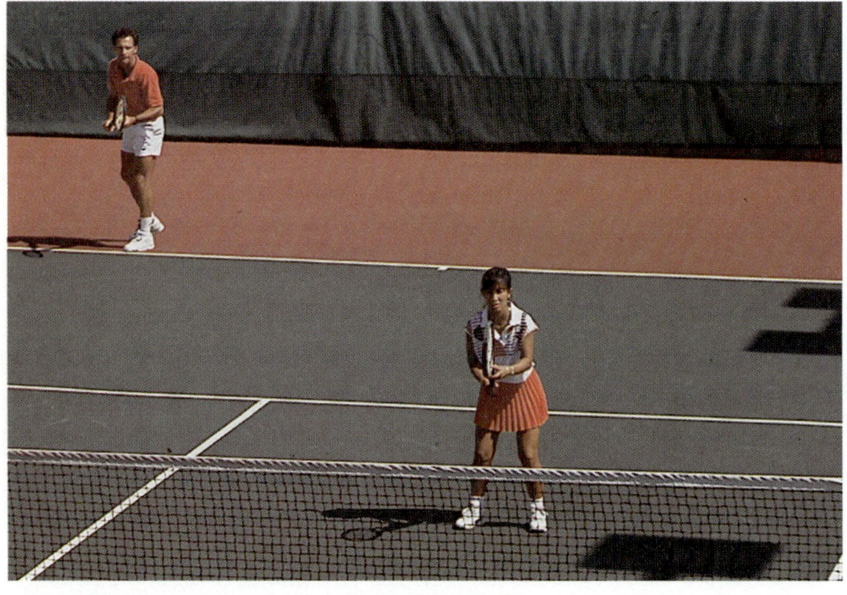

Figure 8.3 One-up, one-back formation (serving).

Conventional Doubles Formation: Two-Up in Tandem

Conventional doubles requires that a team attack the net, and, if need be, attack face to face with the opposing team. The key to good doubles play is to work together in tandem. If the ball is lobbed deep when the team is at the net, the two must retreat together, and when one player hits an overhead smash from the service court line, they both must advance to the net together. Playing conventional doubles means working as a team, knowing where the other player is located, and depending on the partner to hit the appropriate shot. When controlling the net, the doubles team attacks side by side, positioned in the middle of the two service courts. From that position, as if they were on a string, the pair moves up and back and side to side in a balanced position (Figure 8.6).

A conventional formation can produce a significant number of movement patterns on the court. First, a teammate may *poach* in doubles. The definition is

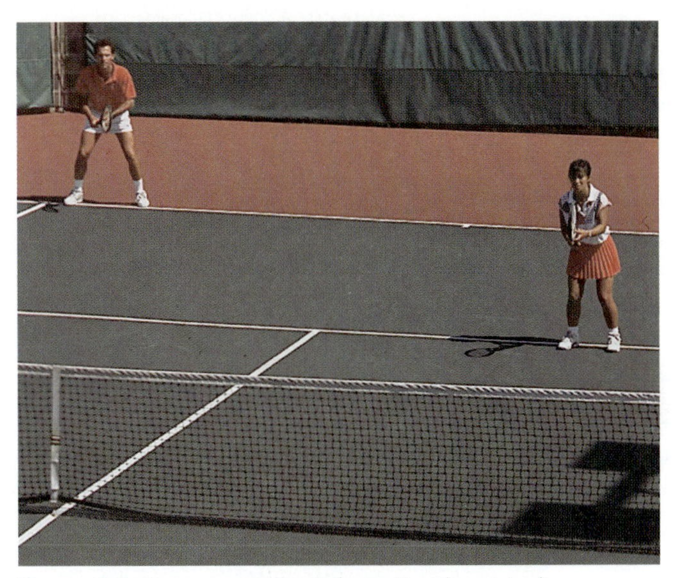

Figure 8.4 One-up, one-back formation (receiving).

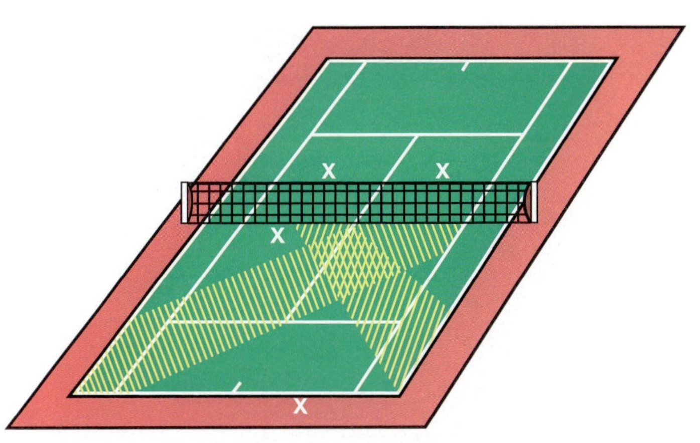

Figure 8.5 Target areas for two-up against one-up one-back.

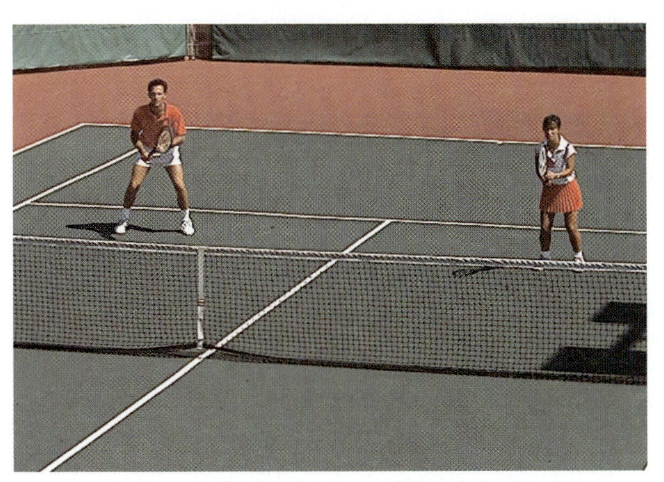

Figure 8.6 Two-up formation (conventional doubles).

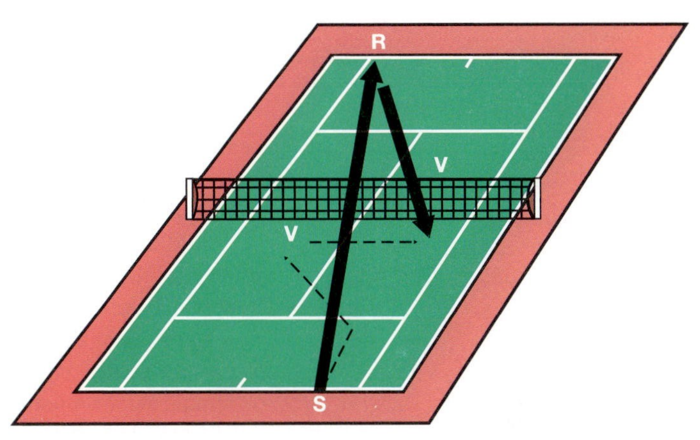

Figure 8.7 Poach movement patterns.

important. The poach is hitting a winning volley; it allows no margin for error. When poaching, the best target tends to be a volley directed at the feet of the net player. The net player steps across parallel to the net to hit a volley directed toward the partner at the baseline following a serve. The serving partner sees the poach attempt and veers to replace the position vacated by the poaching partner (Figure 8.7).

Another team movement pattern is to retreat to hit a lob, then recover for the next shot. The retreat incorporates a cross-action by team members to reach the ball. If the lob is to the left deep corner of the baseline, the partner on the right can see the ball and react to it better than the partner who would have to retreat in a straight line with the back to the opponents. At this point, the partners are at the baseline, where they will remain in a defensive posture until they can regain an advantage and return to the net (Figures 8.8 and 8.9).

Conventional Doubles Formation: Mixed Doubles

Mixed doubles combines one male and one female partner. The formation is the same as for conventional doubles. The only real change is related to the physical strength and skill of the female partner. If there is a strength and skill

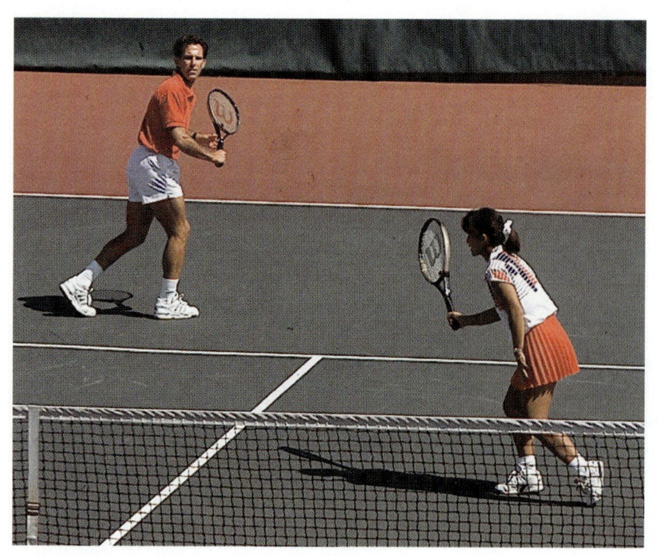

Figure 8.8 Retreat to return a lob (cross action).

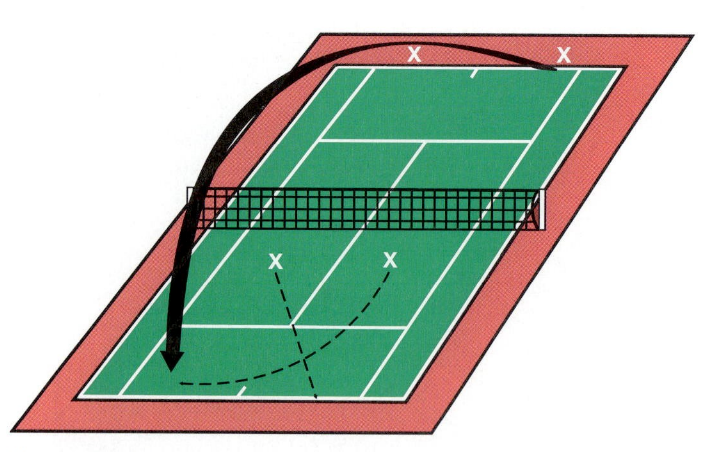

Figure 8.9 Movement pattern for retreating to return a lob.

difference (the differences also could be between two male or two female partners), the alignment may have to be adjusted. The reality of mixed doubles is that the opposing team typically attacks the female as often as possible. When a female player serves to a female opponent, the male at the net must poach whenever possible. With the female serving, the server's velocity or pace usually is not as great as when the male partner serves; consequently, the female server must stay in an up-back alignment. That alignment has been identified already as a weak formation, and it is the reason for the male partner poaching. A serve to the backhand of the return player will aid the serving team by making it easier for the male partner to poach, and easier for the female partner to respond to a groundstroke return.

When receiving against the female server, one response may be a direct return back to the male net player. If successful, the male partner eventually will retreat to the baseline to avoid being hit by a return of serve. A second strategy is to return serve cross-court. This subjects the server to returning a groundstroke from a defensive position, and it avoids the male partner at the net.

Mixed doubles is a delightful game, and it can be highly competitive. Each partner has a role to play and a responsibility to fulfill. Strategy for mixed doubles can be enlarged to cover any doubles in which the characteristics are similar. If one partner is a physically stronger partner but the players are of the same sex, the same approach to strategy should be used.

Special Formations

Variations of formations can help a team in special situations.

Australian Doubles

Australian doubles eliminates an opposing team's cross-court return. In this alignment the server and net player are situated in a perpendicular line to the net with both players on the same side of the server's court. If the server is serving to the opposing team's right service court, the server will be to the right of the center mark and the net partner will be set up on the inside center of the serving team's right service court (Figure 8.10). This alignment leaves the left service court of the serving team open during the serve. Following the serve, the baseline server moves to the left to cover the open court from the baseline. The partner at the net stays to create an up-back situation (Figure 8.11).

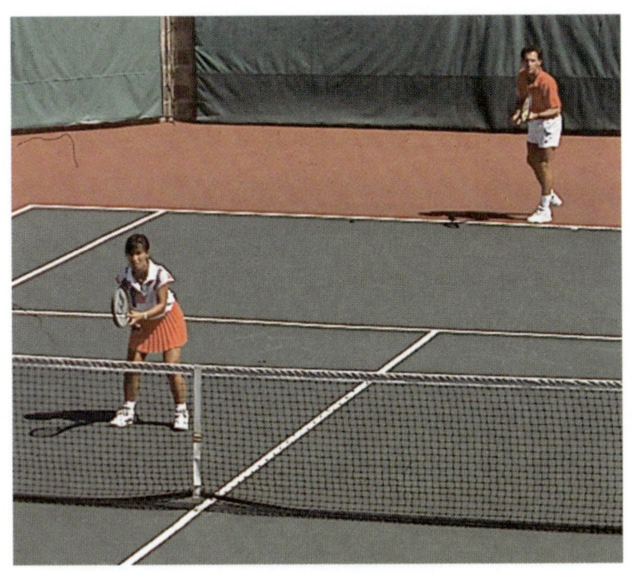

Figure 8.10 Australian doubles formation.

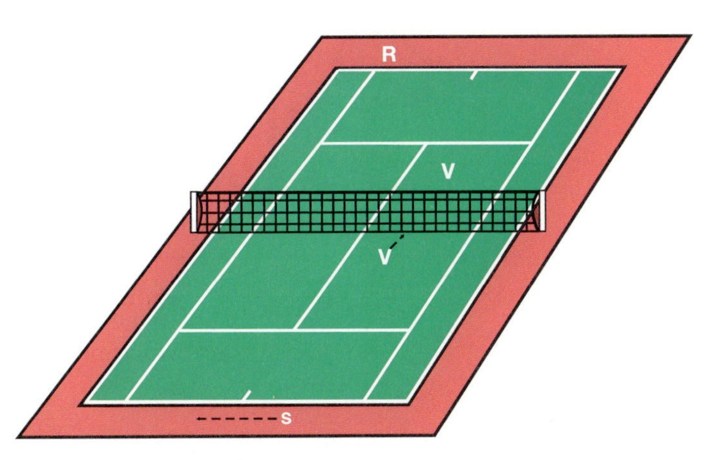

Figure 8.11 Movement pattern for Australian doubles formation.

The Australian formation has several options. The first is for the net player to cross to the left service court following the serve, while the serving partner moves farther to the right side of the baseline to protect that side of the court. A second option is for the team to crisscross following the serve, with the net player moving to the left and the server going straight to the net from the right side. A variation of the crisscross is for the server to follow the serve to the net on the left side, with the net player staying in the same position.

The more variations the Australian doubles formation can offer to the opposing team, the more confused those players can become. This formation is ideal for a team with one weak serving partner or a team with one partner who has a major skill weakness that the alignment can hide.

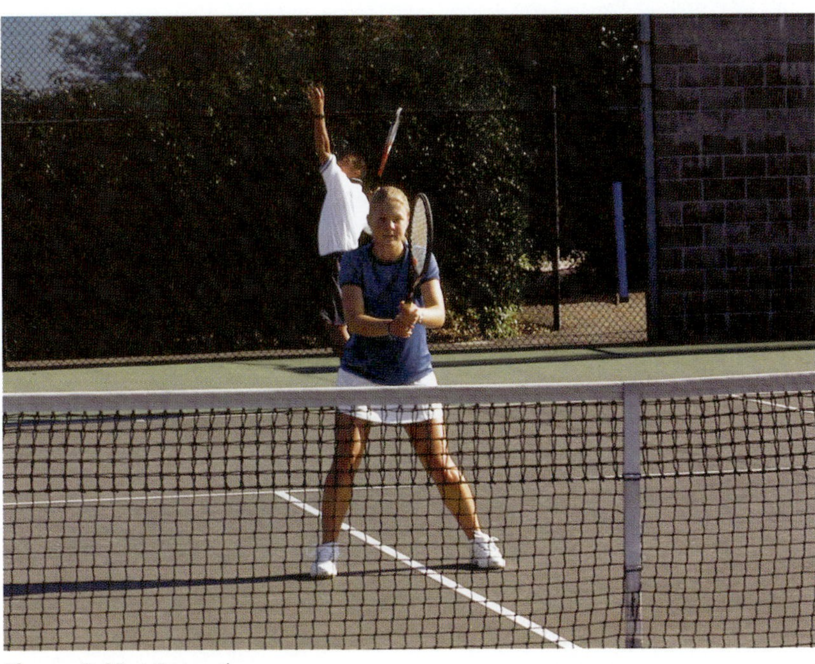

Figure 8.12 I Formation.

I Formation

Another special service formation is the I formation (Figure 8.12). It positions the net player at the net, straddling the middle service court line. Its strength is down the middle, and if the server serves wide, forcing a cross-court return, the net player is positioned to respond with a potential winning volley. Actually, any serve that forces a return down the middle is advantageous to the doubles serving team, but it also has a vulnerability that permits the receiving team to hit shots down the lines for winners.

The I formation gives the receiving team a different look from the serving team and forces the opposing team to make adjustments. Sometimes even a small adjustment creates mistakes by the team that is doing the adjusting and works to the advantage of the more creative I-formation team.

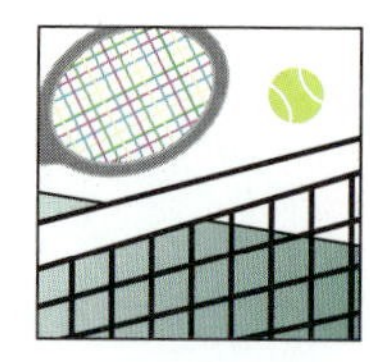

Service and Return-of-Service Strategy

Doubles play strategy is based on effective service and return of service. In addition, the full enjoyment of doubles play is realized when players are consistent in executing serves and returning service.

Service Strategy

The first service in doubles is extremely important. Three-fourths of all first serves should be hit successfully to give the serving team the leverage of moving to the net as a team in a two-up volley situation. Once the developing player has progressed beyond hitting flat services with pace to areas of the opponent's service courts, spin serves should be used in most situations.

A slice serve can be effective when serving to the opposing team's right service court, to force the receiver off the court and to allow the attacking serving team to overplay to the left to control the net. Once a topspin serve has been developed, a serve placement into the deuce service court inside corner is another effective serve. To reiterate, the service must be consistently accurate, and the placement, with spin, must be thoughtfully considered (Figure 8.13). In addition, the beginner must work hard at protecting the partner at the net during service. A soft, pushed serve will endanger that partner and compel the team to play two-back on the serve, thus defeating the advantage of the serving team in controlling the net.

Return-of-Service Strategy

Two considerations are attached to a *return of service* in doubles: first, to get the ball back over the net at the serving team's feet; second, to select the best target placement of the return, and then complete that task. The first consideration is an obvious strategy related to self-preservation. The second consideration requires more planning and assessment of at least four options for target areas (Figure 8.14):

1. Return the ball to the feet of the net player or the advancing server.
2. Pass the net player.
3. Lob the net player.
4. Hit cross-court angled toward the server.

The first three options were discussed with singles strategy as they relate to playing a net player. With a service

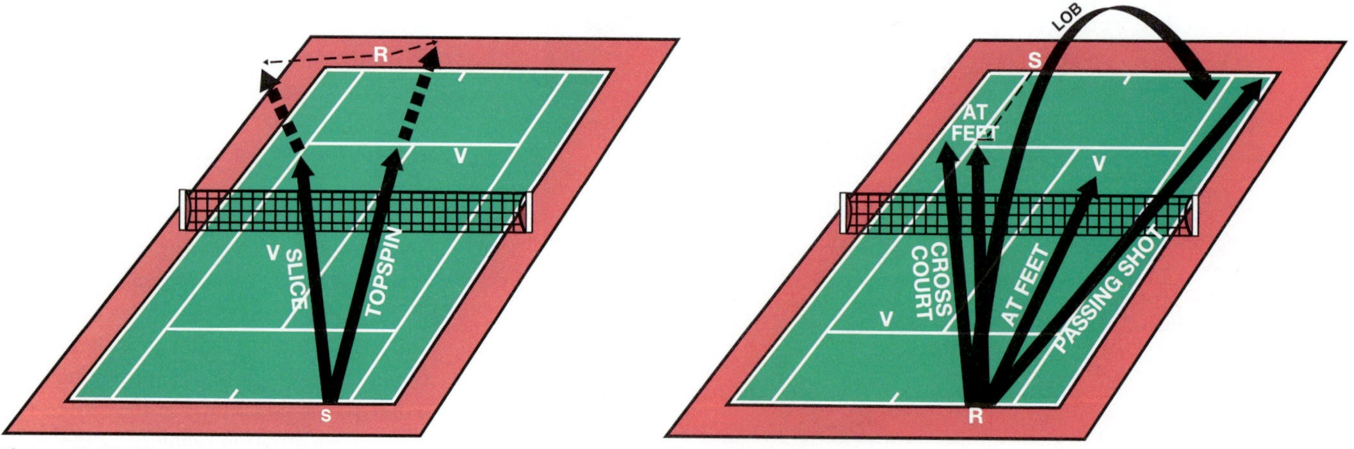

Figure 8.13 First-serve targets.

Figure 8.14 Options for return of service in doubles.

return, lobbing becomes difficult with a serve of any pace, but it is reasonably effective off a soft serve. If the net player does not advance on the net to within two steps from net position, the return at the net player can be effective also.

Passing the net player requires that the player at the net lean to the middle in anticipation of poaching, with the return shot directed down the alley. Being able to pass an opponent at the net down the alley is demoralizing, as that is the one area the net player must protect.

Angled cross-court returns and cross-court returns at the on-rushing server's feet are exceptional for hitting winning shots. The server cannot reach angled cross-court shots unless the server anticipates the shot or the angled return lacks crispness. Cross-court shots at the feet of the server moving to the net catch the server in a tentative position, and the final result is often a ball hit up for an easy return volley.

The choice of which return to hit is controlled to a large extent by placement of the serve in the service court, and by the velocity of the serve. A serve hit to the inside corner of the deuce service court usually eliminates the passing shot because of the central location of the ball. All other service returns from that location remain possible. The best choice is a return at the attacking server's feet. A serve placement to the inside of the ad service court has the same response as the serve to the inside corner of the deuce service court. Serves hit wide to the respective service courts permit all four service return options to be used.

The major lesson to be learned is that a good server will give the receiver only a limited number of options to select from during any given service situation. If a serve is well placed, the receiver will return serve to anticipated areas on the serving team's side of the court.

One last consideration of return of serve is for the receiving player to always get the racket on the ball. All strategy for a return of serve collapses if the receiver misses the return.

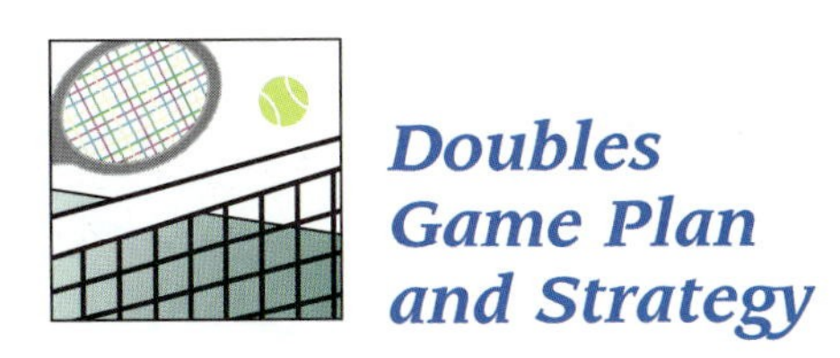

Doubles Game Plan and Strategy

The doubles plan of strategy is to execute strokes in an attacking manner, working to gain control of the net. All players at all levels of skill must do these two things. One of the easier skills in tennis is the volley shot. If a beginner can get to the net, play will be highly enjoyable from that position. Once the concept of taking control of the net is ingrained, the doubles team must remember to protect the alley and middle of the court. The two must learn to move as a team, in tandem, supporting each other and retreating or advancing together. The receiving team must return serves on a low trajectory with pace and attempt to hit a predetermined target area. The serving team should establish a relentless plan of attack with the server coming to the net following a well-paced serve.

Doubles play also requires specific responsibilities of each player during the serve. The server has the responsibility to get the first serve in play consistently to establish a flow, and to put pressure on the receiving team to return service effectively. The receiver of a serve in doubles must get the ball back across the net, in play. Once a beginner has developed the confidence to hit the ball back as receiver of a serve, it helps to think through a tactic or placement of the ball in advance, and to be ready for any type of serve. Net players on both the serving and receiving teams have similar responsibilities. Both have to be active and willing to poach. The players at the net also must have the courage to stand up and face a return of a shot and go on the attack rather than respond passively.

A final strategy is to communicate with the partner, out-think the opposing team, and out-reach the opponent.

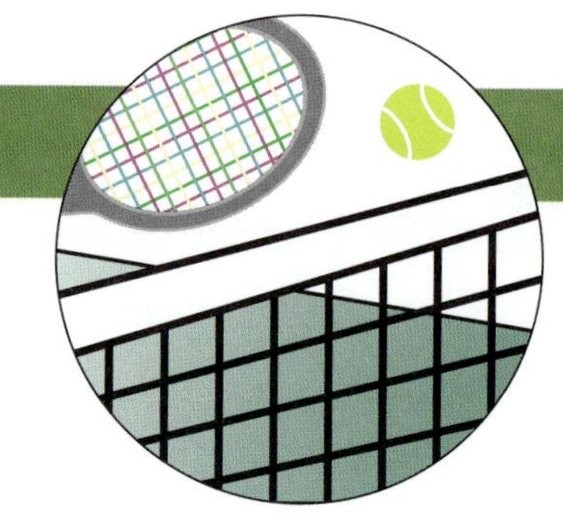

Learning Experience Reminders

Doubles Strategy

1. A two-back doubles formation is a defensive alignment that positions players behind the baseline when net skill is weak or the opponents are at the net hitting overheads.
2. Although a one-up, one-back formation is often used, it is highly vulnerable to open-area winning shots.
3. A two-up doubles tandem provides the most effective offensive alignment in doubles.
4. Australian formation and I doubles formation provide a different alignment for the opposing team to cope against.
5. Getting your first serve in is critical in doubles.
6. Return of service requires hitting at the feet of the net player or the in-rushing server, passing the net player, lobbing the net players, or hitting cross-court angled toward the server.
7. The key to successful doubles is gaining control of the net.

Check Points

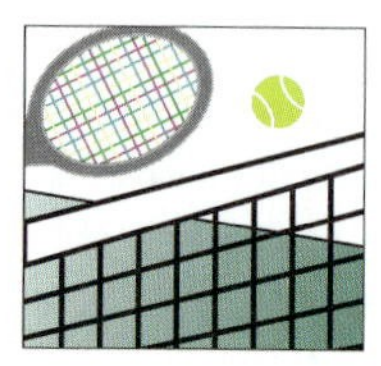

1. With the exception of one choice the two-back doubles formation is used
   a. as an offensive strategy by experienced players.
   b. as a defensive strategy by experienced players.
   c. as a beginning player alignment in doubles.
   d. by unskilled net players.

2. With the exception of one choice the one-up, one-back doubles formation is used by
   a. experienced players.
   b. social players.
   c. novice players.
   d. mixed-doubles players.

3. A poach shot is a movement pattern in doubles defined as
   a. attempting to hit a winning volley shot.
   b. hitting a winning overhead smash.
   c. hitting a winning volley shot.
   d. attempting to hit a winning overhead smash.

4. Tandem play in doubles requires that
   a players move to the net together in an attacking mode.
   b. players move to the baseline in a defensive effort to retrieve a lob.
   c. players cover for each other but remain balanced on the court.
   d. all three strategies are accurate.

5. The strength of using an Australian doubles formation is to
   a. protect the baseline.
   b. protect against the lob.
   c. eliminate a cross-court return by the opponents.
   d. eliminate a down-the-line return.

6. Return of serve requires the receiver in doubles to
   a. hit at the feet of the server.
   b. pass the net player.
   c. lob the net player.
   d. do none of the above.

Answers to Check Points can be found on page 145

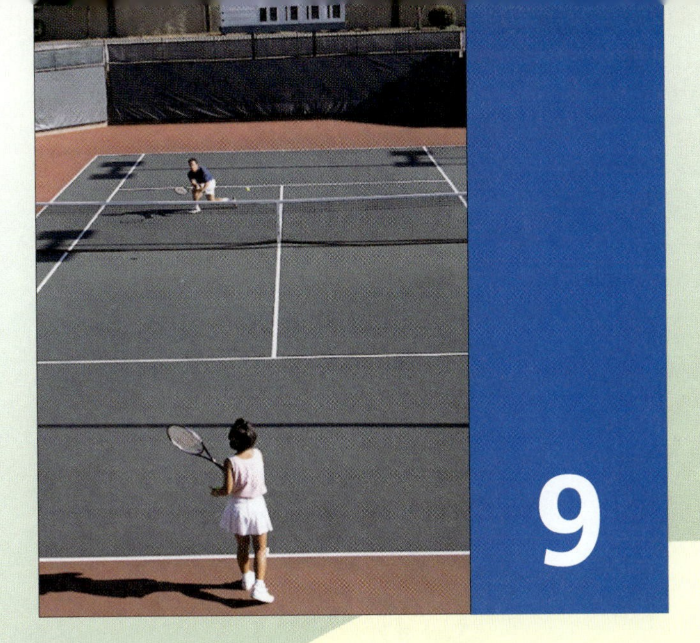

9

Tennis Practice

Practice in between playing matches is good for developing tennis skills and then applying them. Any group-instruction class uses numerous drills to develop skill. Reinforcement comes from playing in class and from suggestions during the performance of each drill-and-play situation. The beginning tennis player needs more work than can be provided in a group-instruction situation, however, and that work or practice can be achieved in additional practice time. In one type of practice you can do a series of drills by yourself; no partner is needed. A second series of drills is designed for use with a partner so you can engage in rally and skill development situations that provide you with the opportunity to test your skills and to learn from your mistakes.

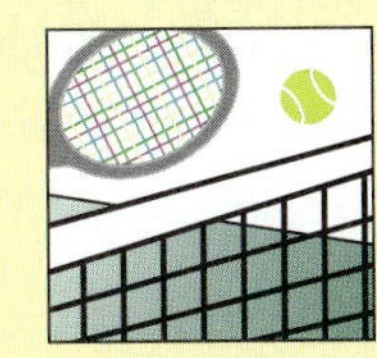

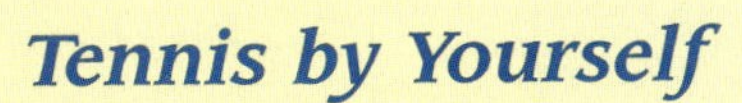

Tennis by Yourself

Tennis by yourself involves drills that require no partner, develops strokes with a checkpoint of mechanics reminders, and encourages variation in drill selection. On many occasions a player cannot find a suitable partner or one who wants to practice. The drills presented will take 45 minutes and will give you a good physical workout, plus provide you with a skill practice session that you can do on your own.

Serving Drill

The *serving* practice drill requires a player to use 30 tennis balls in serving to targets. The level of skill will establish the type of serves hit, and through a series of six sets, a player will hit 180 tennis serves.

Set #1

Serve 30 balls to the ad service court—inside corner.

Set #2

Serve 30 balls to the deuce service court—inside corner.

Set #3

Serve 30 balls to the ad service court—outside corner.

Set #4

Serve 30 balls to the deuce service court—outside corner.

Set #5

Serve 30 balls to the ad service court—10 to the outside, 10 to the middle, 10 to the inside.

Set #6

Serve 30 balls to the deuce service court—10 to the outside, 10 to the middle, 10 to the inside.

Movement Requirement

Player must run to the other side of the court and retrieve balls in a pickup run fashion.

Variations

Variations are quite acceptable, but only one type of serve per set should be initiated. A good variation is to serve and to go to the net for a volley, stopping as the ball strikes the service court.

Groundstroke Drill

The second drill—a simple *groundstroke*—uses a wall board, but goals must be set through the sequence. The drill has nine sets lasting 60 seconds each. After each stroke, the player must return to ready position and allow a distance to permit the ball to bounce twice before each stroke.

Set #1

Hit repetitive forehands.

Set #2

Hit repetitive backhands (remember to self-drop on the backhand side).

Set #3

Alternate forehand and backhand.

Sets #4, 5, and 6

Repeat sets 1–3 with slice.

Sets #7, 8, and 9

Repeat sets 1–3 with topspin.

SERVING DRILL CHECKPOINT OF MECHANICS

Counting successful serves might be insightful, but total concentration on mechanics will be more productive.

1. Am I looking at the tennis ball on the toss?
2. Is my toss accurate? high enough? in line?
3. Are my feet where they belong?
4. Do I have a full backswing? follow-through?
5. Is my grip appropriate to my serve?
6. Am I accurate? why? why not?

GROUNDSTROKE DRILL CHECKPOINT OF MECHANICS

1. Am I looking the ball into the racket?
2. Am I transferring weight into the ball?
3. Do I have a full backswing? follow-through?
4. Am I hitting with the appropriate grip?
5. Am I turning my shoulder early?
6. Is the ball at least 5' high on the wall board?
7. Am I accurate? why? why not?

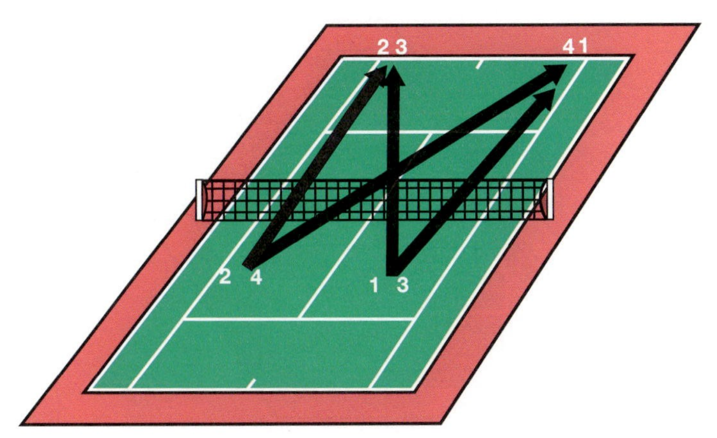

Figure 9.1 Approach shot movement drill.

APPROACH SHOT DRILL CHECKPOINT OF MECHANICS

1. Am I letting the ball drop, and am I timing my strokes?
2. Am I looking the ball into my racket?
3. Am I transferring my weight?
4. Is my backswing shortened?
5. Am I hitting into the court? why? why not?

Approach Shot Drill

The third drill is designed to develop confidence and eliminate overanxiety in players hitting *approach shots*. Approach shots seldom are executed in practice, so hitting four sets of 30 balls each will provide a good mental inset. Aim at the service court line for depth and 4 foot in from the sideline for accuracy. Drop the balls at least 2 feet away and at least waist high (Figure 9.1).

Set #1

From middle of the right service court, hit forehand down the line.

Set #2

From middle of the left service court, hit backhand down the line.

Set #3

From middle of the right service court, hit forehand cross-court.

Set #4

From middle of the left service court, hit backhand cross-court (Figure 9.1).

Movement Requirement

Player must run to the other side of the court and retrieve balls in a pickup run fashion.

Variations

The type of shot can be varied. The basic groundstroke pattern can be used, but as topspin and slice strokes are developed they should be incorporated in the drill. Hitting topspin down the line is another variation of the drill. Also, placing the ball on the drop in different areas of the service court and between the baseline and the service court line contributes to variation.

Moving Drill

A tennis player must *move*. Coupled with agility and quickness, movement can aid the player in getting to the ball in time. Three sets are designed to encourage agility and quickness and use of the racket in shadow boxing.

Set #1

Move to imaginary numbers and, in sequence, shadow box a groundstroke, an approach shot, or a volley. All balls stroked up to the service line require the players to return to ready position on the baseline, and all balls between the service line and the net require the player to assume a ready position at the net in the middle (Figure 9.2).

Set #2

The same drill as above except the shadow boxing should consist of lobs from the baseline and overhead smashes from the net. Player must assume ready position on each stroke (Figure 9.3).

Set #3

Eliminate shadow boxing, and move along the lines of the court, touching each junction between two lines (Figure 9.4).

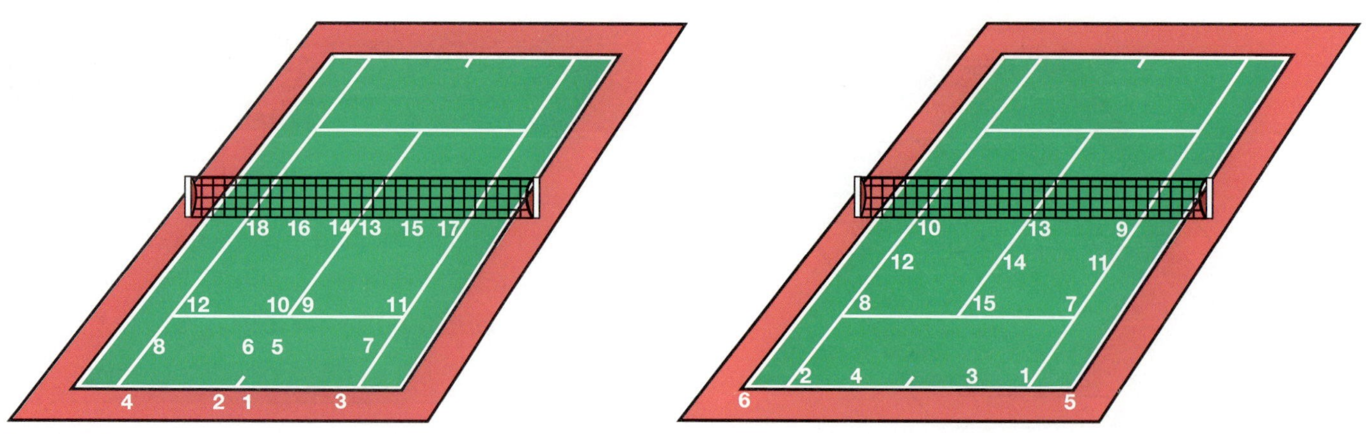

Figure 9.2 Shadow boxing movement, Set #1.

Figure 9.3 Shadow boxing movement, Set #2.

Overhead Smash Drill

The final drill is an *overhead smash.* The exercise requires a simple bounce of the ball off the court and above the head, providing time for the player to get set underneath the ball and hit an overhead smash.

Set #1

Hit 15 overheads from the right middle service court.

Set #2

Hit 15 overheads from the left middle service court.

Set #3

Hit 15 overheads from the right center position halfway between baseline and service line.

Set #4

Hit 15 overheads from the left center position halfway between baseline and service line.

Movement Requirement

After each pair of sets, the player must run to the other side of the court and retrieve balls in a pickup run fashion.

Variations

The player may locate other spots to hit the overhead and begin to identify the location of the target on the other side of the court.

The keys to executing the drills are to have a little self-discipline, become goal oriented, and build confidence that each skill can be performed. Beginning players who participate three times per week in "tennis by yourself" will see a marked change in their skill development.

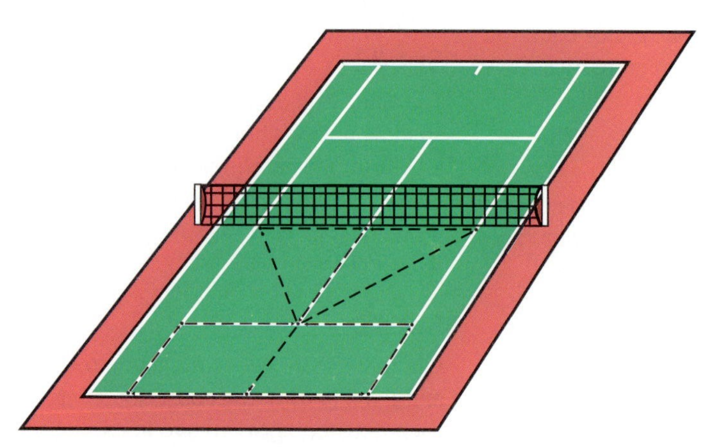

Figure 9.4 Fitness movement drill, Set #3.

OVERHEAD SMASH DRILL CHECKPOINT OF MECHANICS

1. Am I timing my stroke in a smooth, rhythmical motion?
2. Is my backswing in the middle of my shoulder blades and my elbow up at a right angle?
3. Is my non-racket hand pointing in reference to the ball?
4. Am I hitting into the court? why? why not?

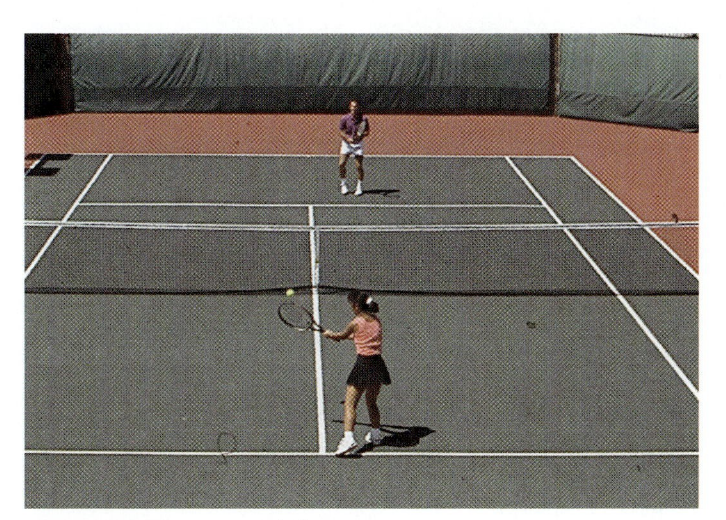

Figure 9.5 Short court drill.

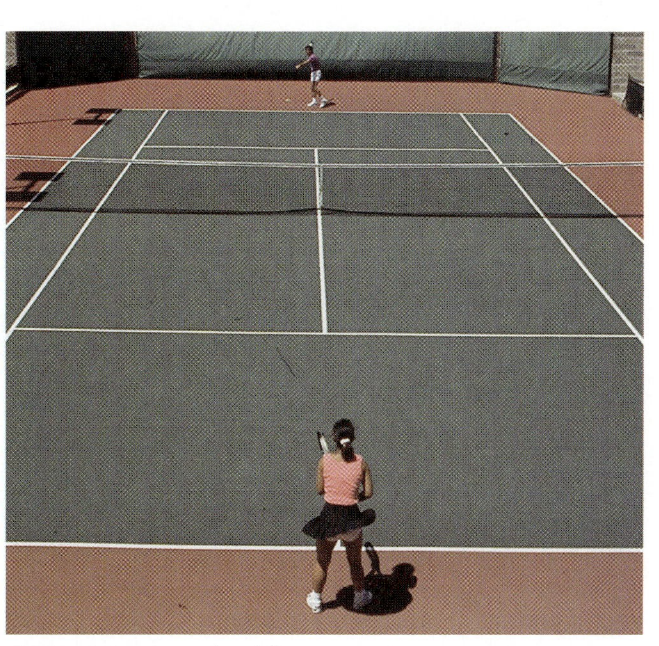

Figure 9.6 Bounce/hit drill.

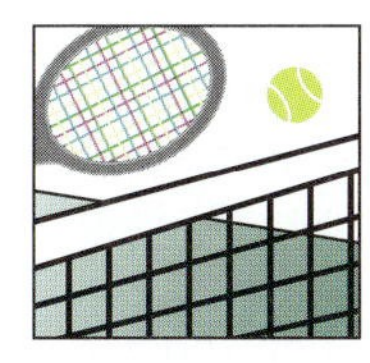

Partner Practice Drills

Partner practice drills supplement what you can practice on your own. Of the countless numbers of drills that involve two players, 14 are presented in this chapter to provide a beginning approach to practice. Five of the drills are groundstroke-oriented because groundstrokes are the base for the game. Additional drills will reinforce lobs, overheads, volley shots, and attacking the net.

Groundstroke Drills

Groundstroke drills progress from simple to fairly complicated.

Short-Court Drills

The short-court drill is a "touch" drill that requires the partners to stand in the service court of their respective side and hit groundstrokes with touch (Figure 9.5). The idea is to keep the ball within the confines of the service court and to assist the player in anticipation, shoulder turn, and sensing the "feel" of the stroke.

Bounce/Hit Drill

The bounce/hit drill (Figure 9.6) encourages focus and an inner feel for the groundstroke. The idea is for the partners to hit the ball from baseline to baseline without thinking about the mechanics of the stroke. By shouting "bounce" every time the ball bounces on the court and "hit" every time the ball is hit, the partners begin to focus on the ball and concentrate on the end result of hitting the ball to the other side of the court.

What is amazing is that form and mechanics of the groundstroke come about naturally when the partners really become involved in the drill. Two points to remember when executing this drill are: First, both partners must identify "bounce" and "hit," regardless of which side of the net the ball is on. Second, the verbal response must be loud enough for both partners to hear. Players tend to be self-conscious when doing this drill, and if there are players on adjacent courts, the etiquette of quiet on the courts might be disrupted. When

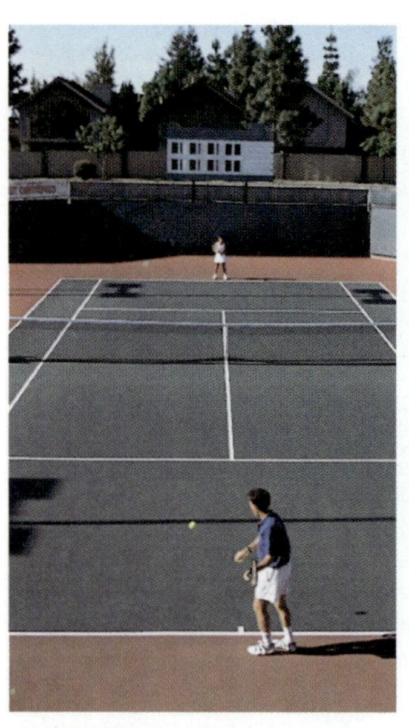
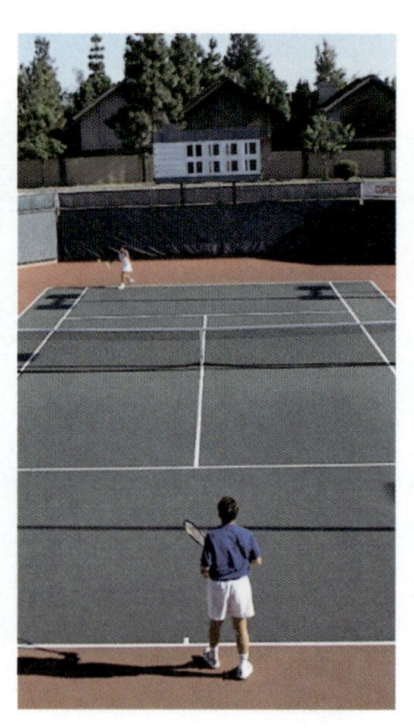
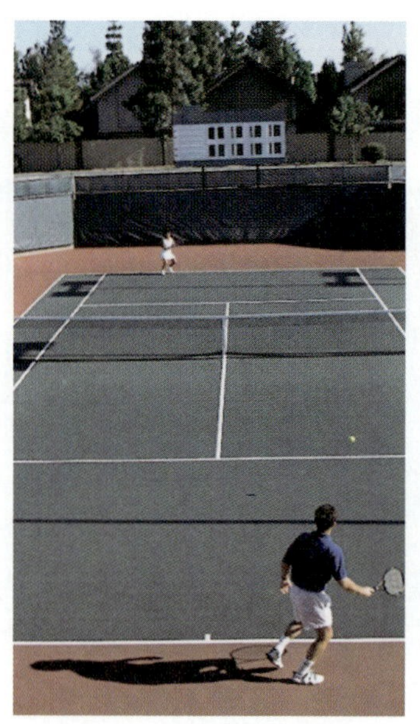
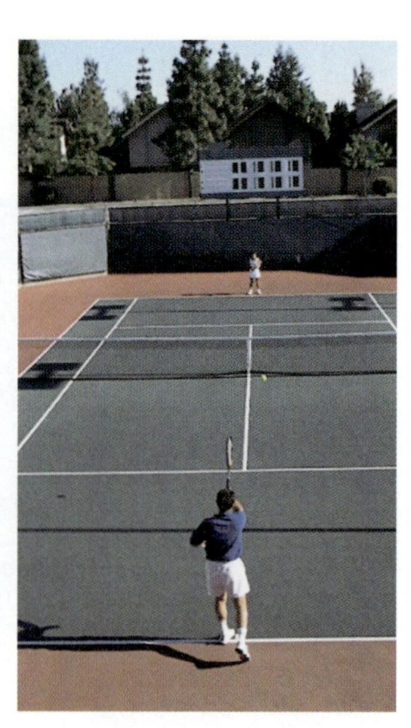

Figure 9.7 Homebase drill.

used properly, however, this drill will truly be of help in skill development.

Homebase Drill

The homebase drill is related to returning to the baseline center mark after hitting each groundstroke and to the concept that if the ball is hit deeply, it will keep the opposing player pinned to the baseline, restricting the player's ability to attack the net and forcing errors (Figure 9.7).

Both players are to use the area between the service court line and baseline as the target for each shot hit. After hitting the groundstroke, that player must return to the baseline center mark area and prepare for the next groundstroke.

The drill is played under gamelike situations in the sense that one player initiates play by self-dropping a groundstroke and hitting deep to the target area. A rally continues until one of the players hits a ball short of the target area. Play stops and the player who hits the short shot receives a negative point. Play then resumes with another self-drop, followed by a groundstroke rally to the target area. Play continues to a set negative score, with the player accumulating the greater negative score declared the loser (the concept with deep rallies is that it is not so much a player winning a point but, rather, the other player losing the point).

As skill develops, additional challenges can be added to the drill. One example is to play a homebase-approach-shot game. When a ball is hit short of the depth target, the receiving player moves up to hit an approach shot. Hitting an approach shot earns that player one point, but if the shot is missed, a 2-point negative penalty is assigned to the player.

Down-the-Line Groundstroke Drill

Hitting down-the-line groundstrokes encourages the player to establish a target when hitting the ball (Figure 9.8). The idea is to hit the ball down the sideline to the other partner. The ball should be positioned between the player and the sideline, forcing the player to hit a forehand or backhand, depending on which is the appropriate shot (with two right-handed players, one would be hitting with a forehand, the other with a backhand groundstroke). After hitting the ball, the player who has just hit returns to near the baseline center mark area. The idea is to have to move to hit the ball with the appropriate groundstroke rather than to stand in one spot, and eventually to play the ball so it is

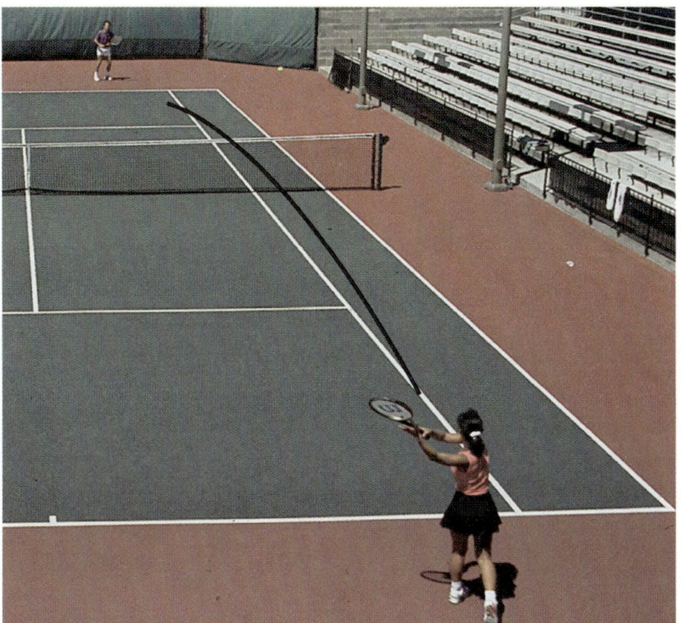
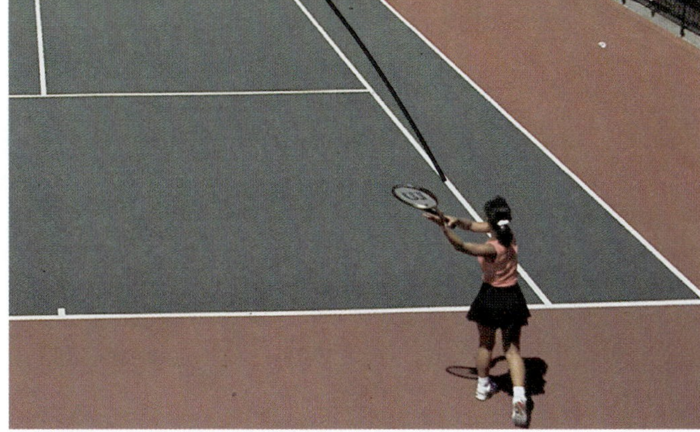

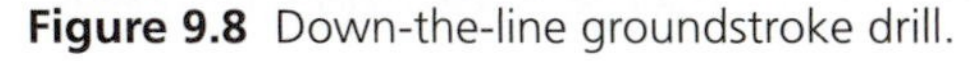
Figure 9.8 Down-the-line groundstroke drill.

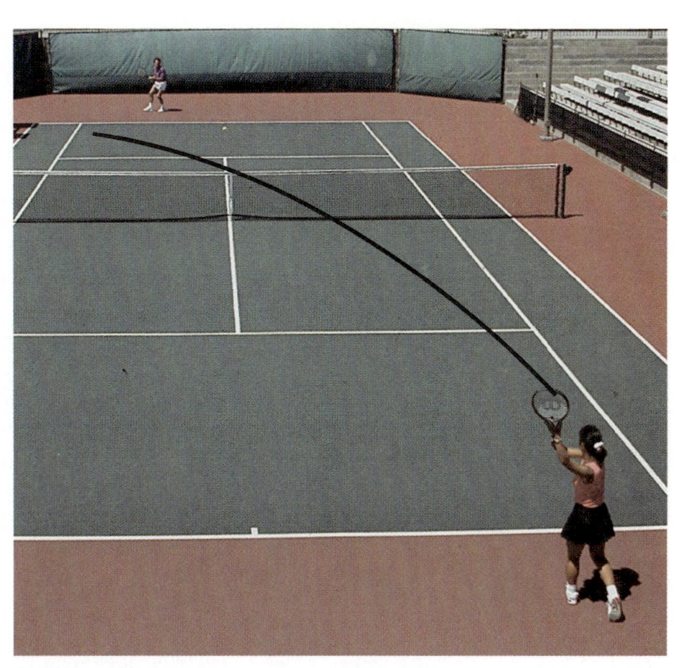

Figure 9.9 Cross-court groundstroke drill.

positioned for a choice of forehand or backhand.

Cross-Court Groundstroke Drill

The cross-court groundstroke drill has the same purpose of setting a target and the same organizational setup, but instead of going down the line, the ball is hit cross-court (Figure 9.9). Again, it is important to hit the ball and return to near the center mark.

For beginners, these last two drills are somewhat difficult. They tend to become frustrated because they are uncomfortable with hitting a backhand and reaching the intended target. Increasing the level of this skill is important, however, and you will not improve if you don't push yourself.

Down-the-Line/Cross-Court Groundstroke Drill

The final groundstroke drill adds to the progression of difficulty because it combines *down-the-line with cross-court.* The idea follows the sequence of: (1) Partner A hitting down the left sideline, (2) Partner B returning a cross-court shot to the right side court of Partner A, (3) Partner A then hitting down the right sideline to Partner B, who returns a shot cross-court to Partner A's left side court. (See Figures 9.10–9.13.) The sequence is repeated for development of consistency.

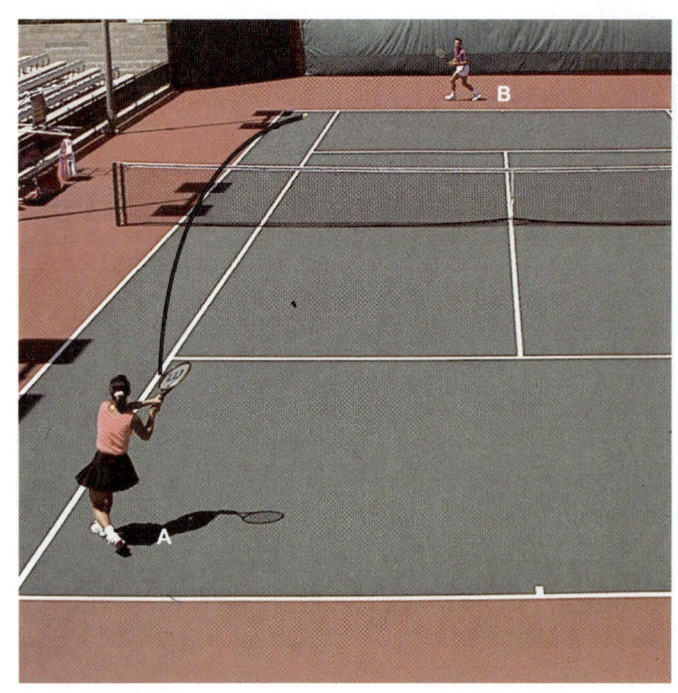

Figure 9.10 Down-the-Line/Cross Court Drill Sequence: Partner A hits down the left sideline.

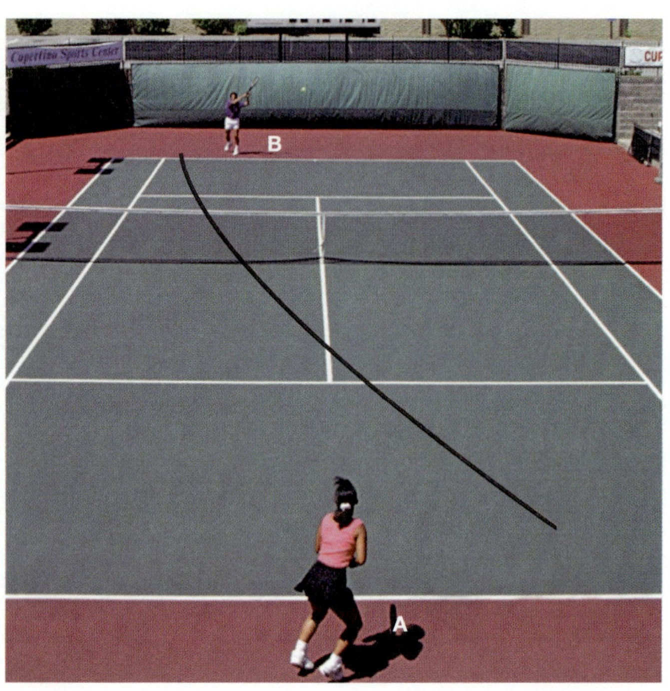

Figure 9.11 Down-the-Line/Cross Court Drill Sequence: Partner B returns a cross-court shot to the right side court of Partner A.

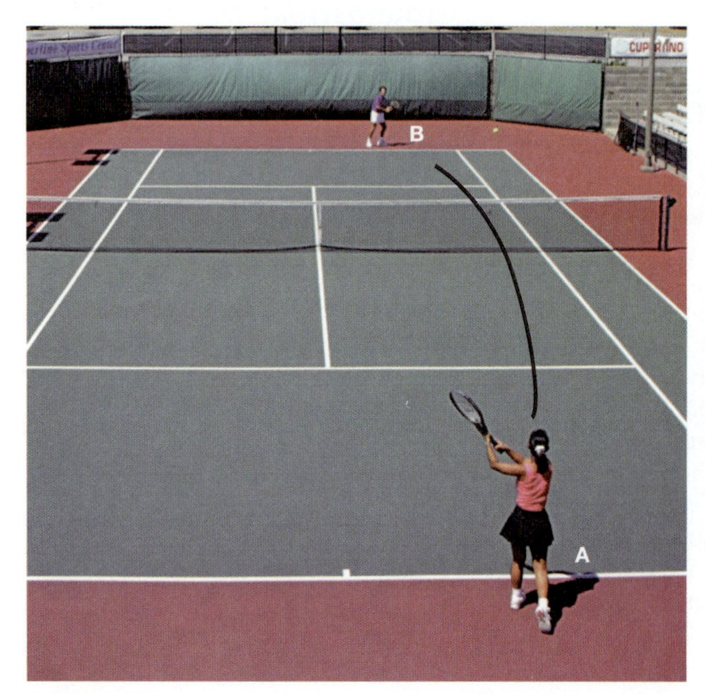

Figure 9.12 Down-the-Line/Cross Court Drill Sequence: Partner A hits down the right sideline to Partner B.

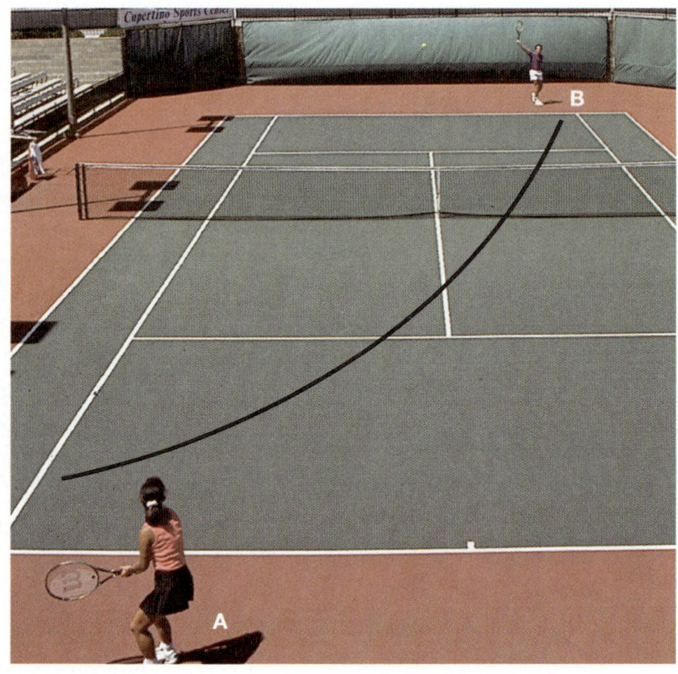

Figure 9.13 Down-the-Line/Cross Court Drill Sequence: Partner B returns a shot cross-court to Partner A's left side court.

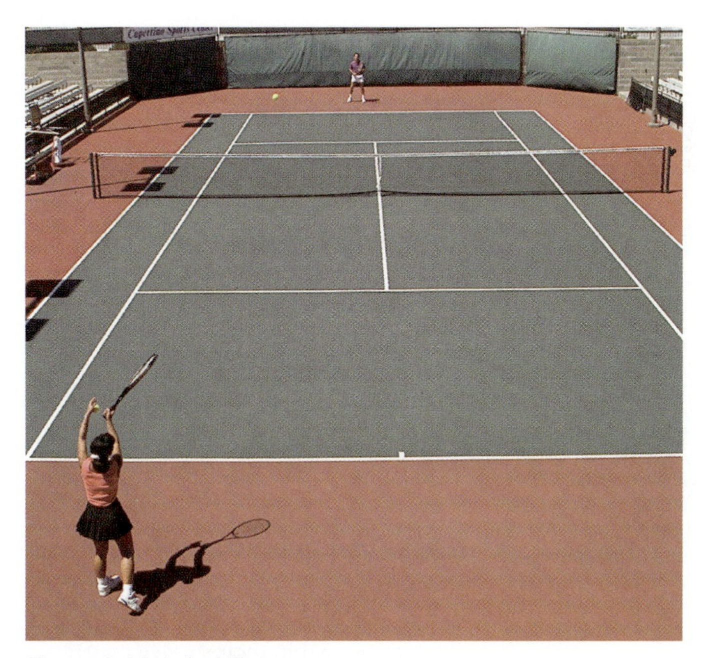

Figure 9.14 Lob drill.

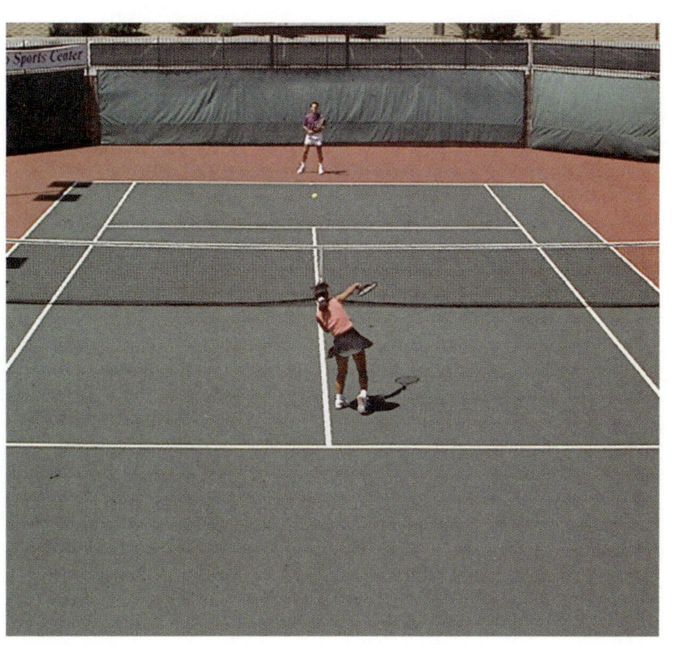

Figure 9.15 Overhead smash sequence drill.

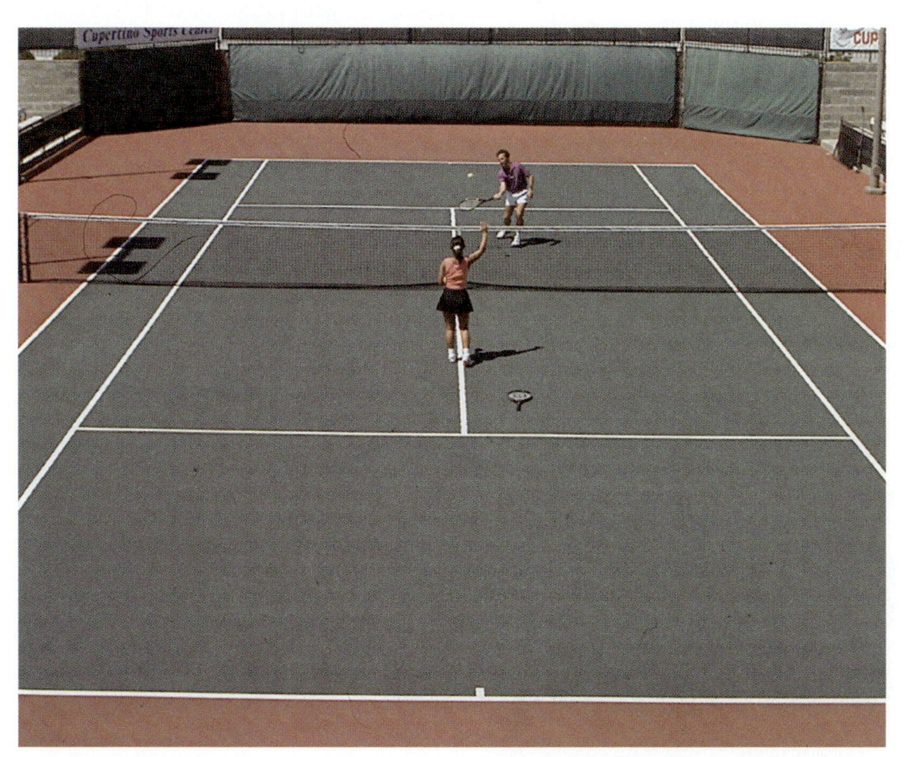

Figure 9.16 Toss/Volley drill.

Lob/Overhead Drills

Lobs and overhead smash practice fits nicely together. Two drills; one incorporating a lob sequence followed by a second drill consisting of a lob/overhead smash sequence assists in the development of these two skills.

Lob Sequence Drill

The *lob drill* simply requires the partners to exchange lobs (Figure 9.14). The emphasis should be on hitting deep with proper height for the selected lob. You should start with a defensive lob and experiment with ball height, and then continue by hitting topspin offensive lobs. Work on an equal number of forehand and backhand lobs, and as you progress, begin to place the lobs from corner to corner.

Lob/Overhead Smash Sequence Drill

The second drill is an extension of the lob drill. It consists of an *overhead smash at the end of the lob* with one partner self-dropping and lobbing short to the service court area and the other partner hitting overheads (Figure 9.15). As you improve, you should work on

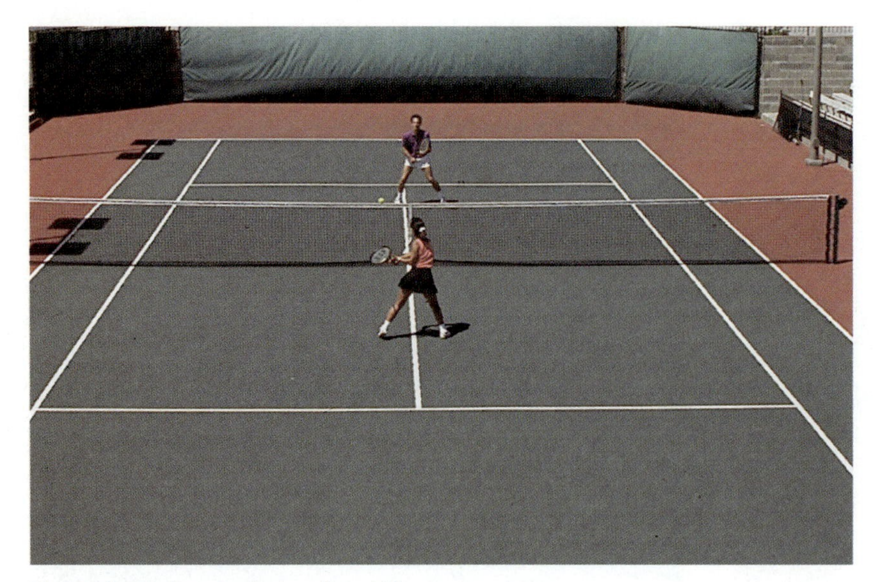

Figure 9.17 Face-to-face volley drill.

returning an overhead with a lob rather than self-dropping to initiate the overhead shot of the partner.

Volley Drills

Two volley drills can enhance the skill of all players, including beginners: the *toss/volley drill* and the *face-to-face volley*. As skill develops two additional drills that incorporate a *cross step volley* and a *cross court down-the-line volley* need to be added.

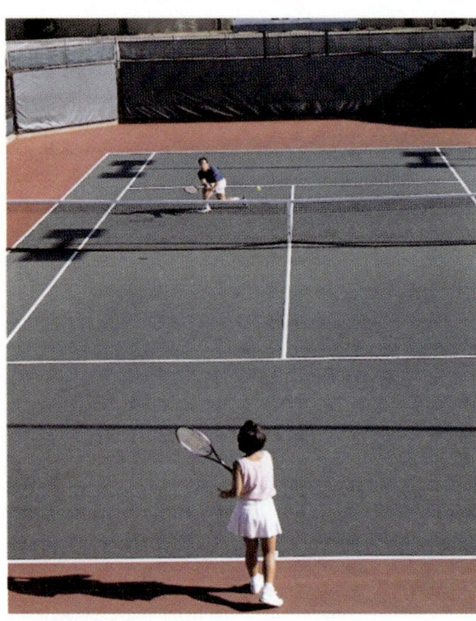

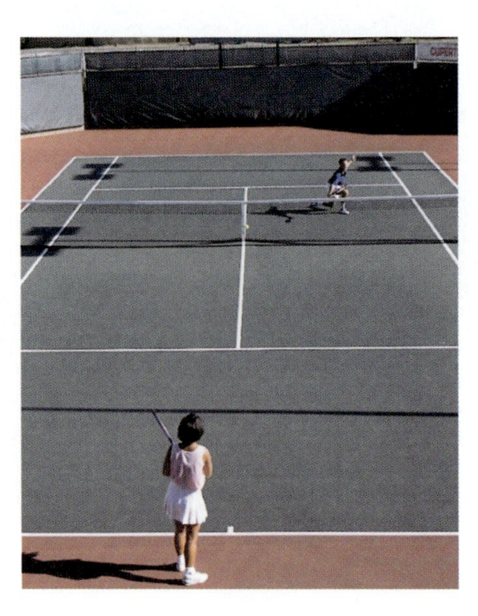

Figure 9.18 Cross-Step Volley.

Toss/Volley Drill

The toss/volley drill requires that one partner toss the ball to the other partner (Figure 9.16). The idea is to toss accurately to force the volleying partner to step into the ball with a short backswing and punch the ball back to the partner. This drill encourages good form, and it can progress with variations that force the volleying partner to hit low and high volleys plus adjust to a ball at the body. In addition, the partner's toss can force the volleying partner to cross-step and punch the ball deep to the baseline.

Face-To-Face Volley Drill

The face-to-face volley drill is a particularly fun drill because both partners face each other within their service courts and volley the ball back and forth (Figure 9.17). Progression again is important. Start with forehand-to-forehand volleys, then volley backhand to backhand. As your skill increases, you can alternate from forehand to backhand volleys, hit volleys at different elevations of the ball, and react to each placement of the ball that comes to you.

Cross-Step Volley Drill

The cross-step volley drill is designed to force the volleying player to cross-step rather than step with the inside foot (Figure 9.18). The baseline player hits a selected number of groundstrokes wide to the forehand of the net player, and the net player cross-steps to hit a deep volley return. Then the baseline player hits the same number of groundstrokes to the backhand side, forcing cross-step volley returns. All volley returns are to be hit deep between the service and baselines.

Down-the-Line/Cross-Court Volley Drill

The down-the-line/cross-court volley drill (Figure 9.19) has the same premise as the cross-step volley drill in Figure 9.18. The difference is that a select number of groundstrokes hit from the baseline are to be volleyed cross-court from the forehand side, then from the

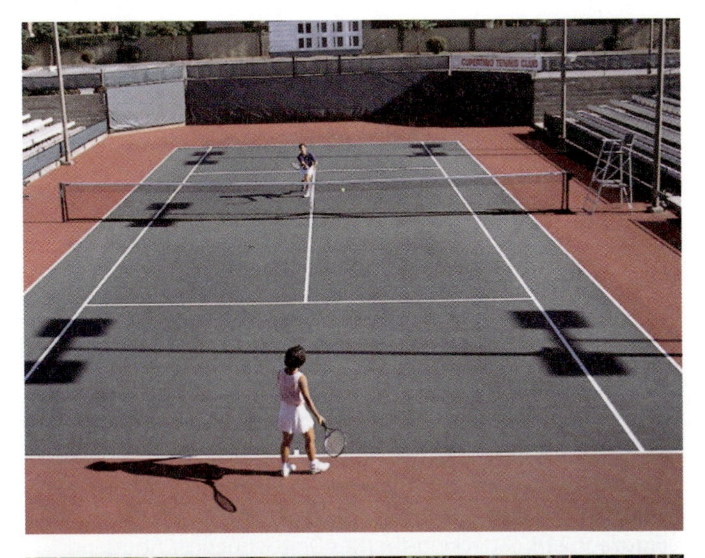

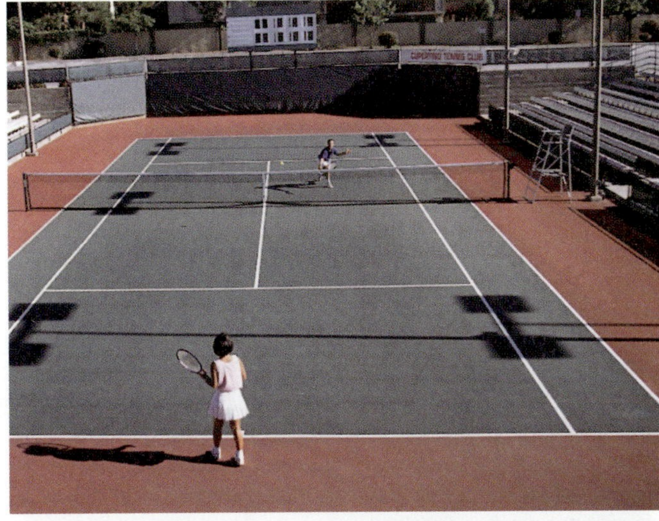

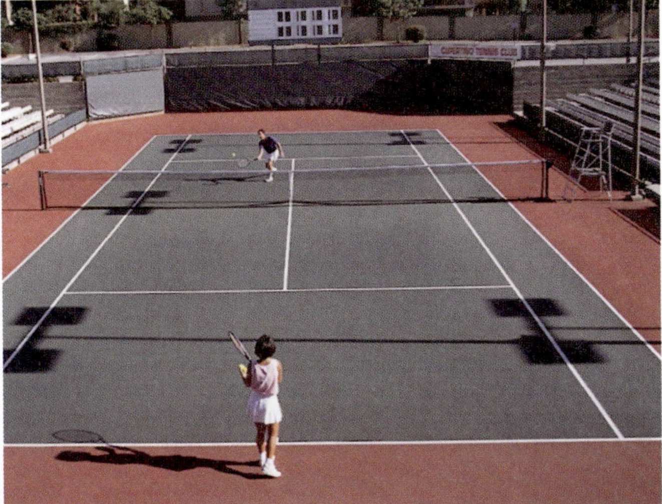

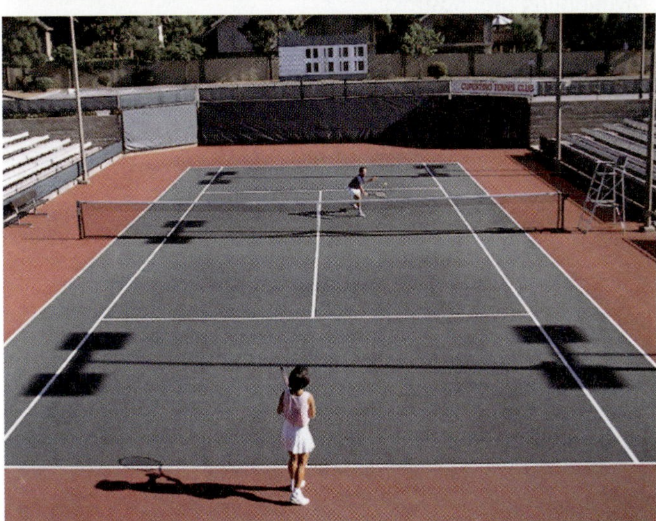

Figure 9.19 Cross-Court Down-the-Line Volley.

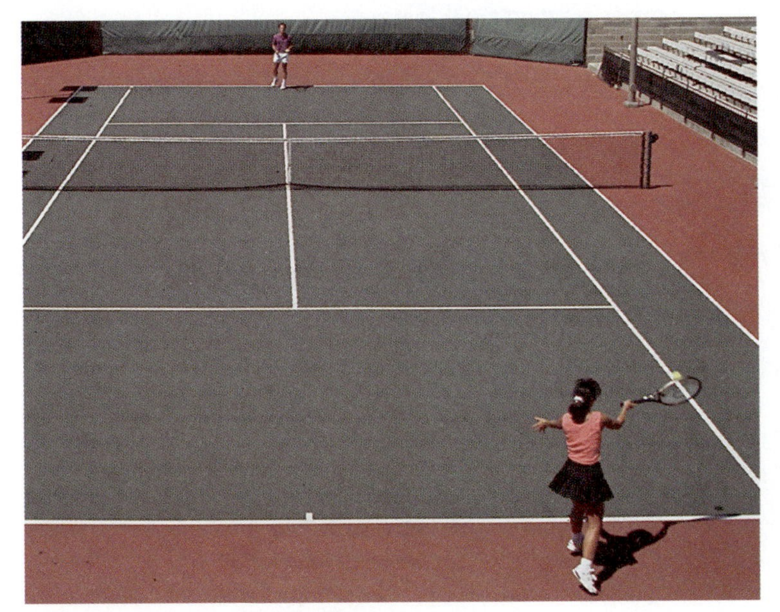

Figure 9.20 Service return drill.

backhand side, and repeated with forehand down-the-line and backhand down-the-line shots.

Service Return Drill

Service returns seldom are practiced and as a result, returns are neglected. The drill is simple: One partner serves and the other returns the serve (Figure 9.20). Focus on returns should be a first priority, with the main goal to hit each serve deep to the baseline. Then service returns can become more target-oriented by hitting both cross-court and down-the-line returns. To become really skilled in return of service, the return partner should have the opportunity to see different velocity serves with different spins. The drawback to practicing with another beginner is that neither of you is at the level to execute a variety of consistent serves. This is a drill that requires a skilled partner to deliver the serves.

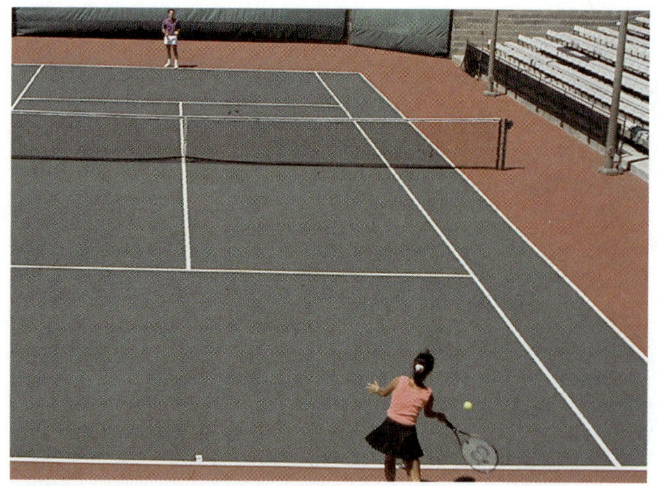

Figure 9.21A Attacking-the-Net Drill Sequence: Attacking player hitting groundstroke.

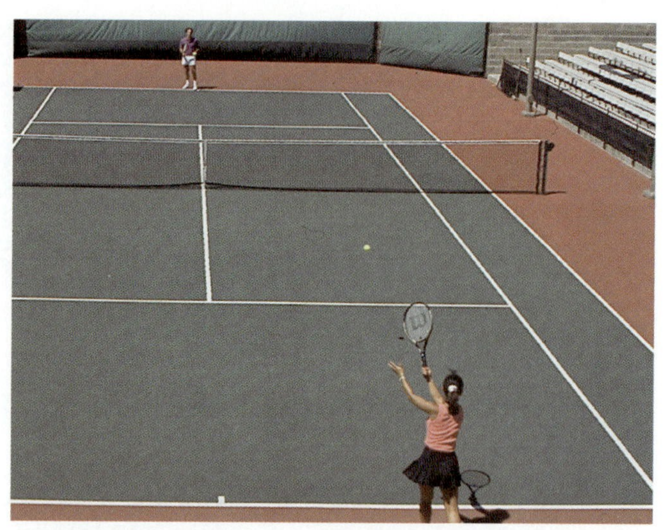

Figure 9.21B Attacking-the-Net Drill Sequence: Attacking player groundstroke follow through.

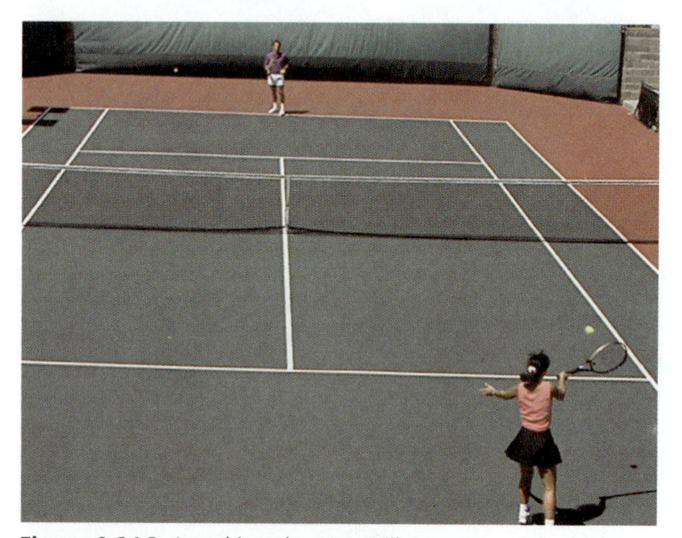

Figure 9.21C Attacking-the-Net Drill Sequence: Attacking player returning approach shot.

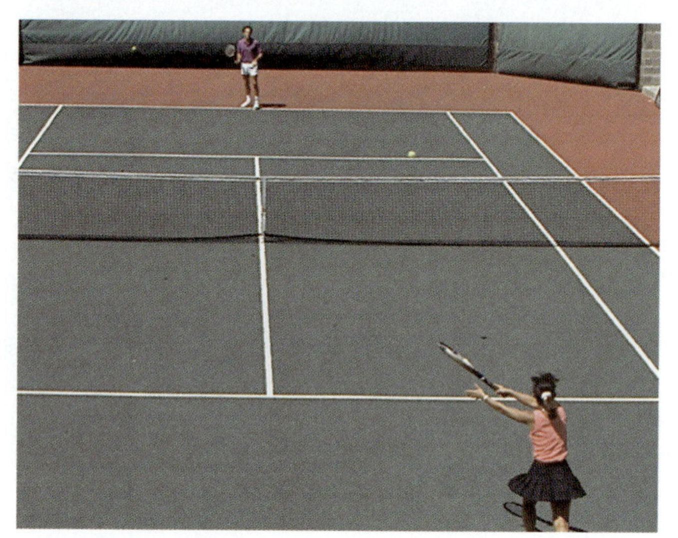

Figure 9.21D Attacking-the-Net Drill Sequence: Attacking player initiating move forward.

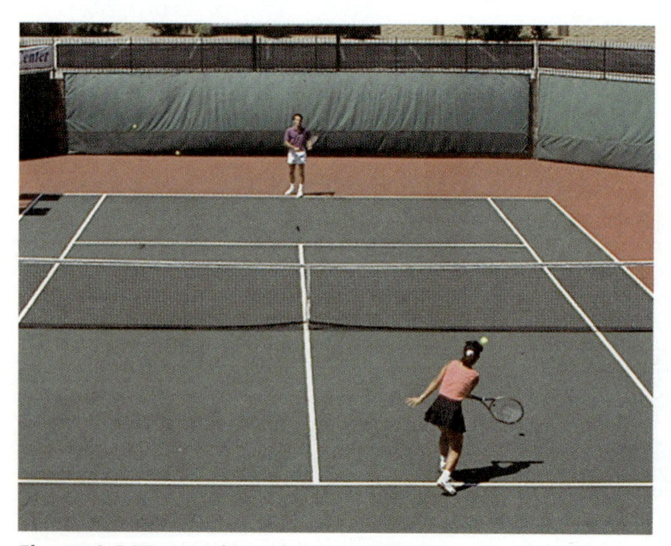

Figure 9.21E Attacking-the-Net Drill Sequence: Attacking player moving forward and returning volley shot.

Attacking-the-Net Drill

The final drill is an attacking-the-net drill that requires a partner to feed the ball to the attacking partner. The feeding partner holds three balls and places the first ball deep to the forehand of the attacking partner. The attacking partner hits a deep forehand groundstroke return and begins to advance to the net. The feeding partner then places the second ball to the attacking partner's forehand, forcing a forehand approach shot deep to the baseline. The attacking partner continues to advance to the net and receives a ball to the forehand side from the feeder that then is volleyed by the attacking partner. (See Figures 9.21 A–E.)

The sequence can be repeated to the backhand, mixed up with the attacking partner not knowing which direction the ball is being placed. Other shots, including a second volley and an overhead smash, can be incorporated into the drill as skill improves. The attacking player also can work on placement with depth and at angles to gain the best advantage at the net. This is not a particularly easy drill, but you will be surprised how well you do because you do not have time to think and because the ball is being placed to you.

Practice is important. The practice-by-yourself and partner-practice drills will enable you to progress and increase your skill level more rapidly than simply listening to instruction and practicing only during that instructional time. Tennis is an easy game once you gain the skills to play it. Practice enables you to gain the skills so you can have fun.

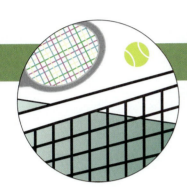

Learning Experience Reminders

Tennis Practice

1. It is critical to have meaningful practice following lessons and as a supplement to playing matches.
2. The Tennis by Yourself drills require effort and motivation to be meaningful. To make the drills work, make sure you read the Checkpoint of Mechanics boxes related to each skill area.
3. Partner Practice Drills require having a motivated partner and/or an advanced skill level partner who can return various shots with a degree of consistency.

Check Points

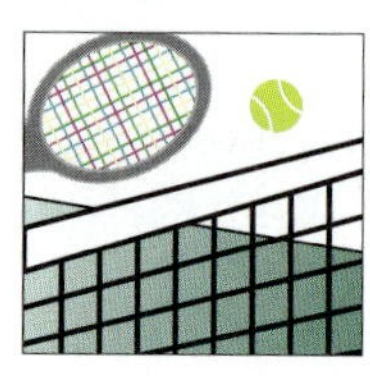

Select three specific skill related drills and describe how each drill will enhance your specific skill development.

Answers to Check Points can be found on page 145.

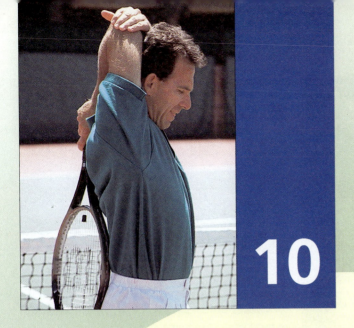

Physical Aspects of Playing Tennis

The physical aspects of playing tennis begin to play a major role in performance when you can maintain a rally—keeping the ball in play for a significant amount of time. In other words, you need to be physically fit to play tennis. You can do this by physically preparing to play, engaging in an overall fitness development program, learning how to prevent and care for tennis-related sport injuries, and understanding how to cope with problems on a tennis court related to heat, sun, and insects.

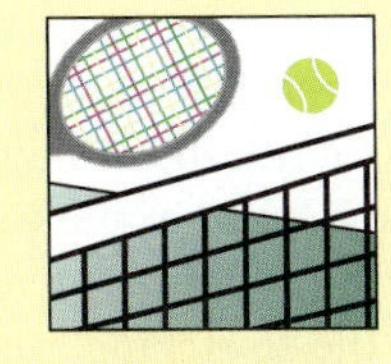

Physically Preparing To Play Tennis

The three phases involved in physically preparing to play are: (1) stretching as a warm-up to hitting the ball, (2) the basic tennis warm-up, and (3) the warm-down through stretching. The first two are designed to actually prepare the player to play, and the third enables the player to deactivate and decrease muscle stimulation.

When *stretching,* most young players give a cursory effort to preparation of the muscles. The young body, however, needs to establish a stretching routine that will be part of the total playing habit into middle age and beyond. It should be incorporated into the player's routine as that player continues to improve and place more stress on the body with extended rallies and overall court play development.

The recommended stretching includes some ballistic movement along with static stretching. If the player will devote just 5 minutes to these warm-up efforts, the risk of injury will be diminished, preparation for the hitting warm-up will be complete, and the body will feel relaxed and prepared to engage in a competitive situation.

Research indicates that, prior to stretching, the muscles should have engaged in some physical work. The work prescribed is an 8- to 10-minute warm-up including low-intensity jogging or cycling, which will increase blood flow,

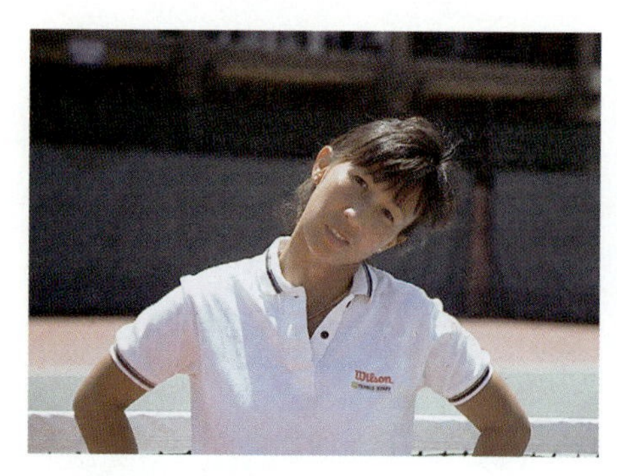

LATERAL HEAD TILT

Action: Tilt the head slowly and gently to one side and hold the stretch for a few seconds. Alternate to the other side and repeat.

Areas Stretched: Flexors and extensors and ligaments of the cervical spine.

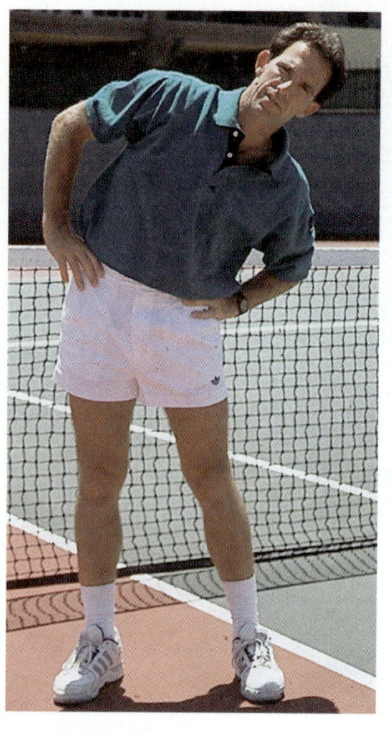

SIDE STRETCH

Action: Feet spread at shoulder width with hands on hips. Rotate the body to one side and repeat the process to the other side. Hold the stretch for a few seconds on each side.

Areas Stretched: Pelvis area muscles and ligaments.

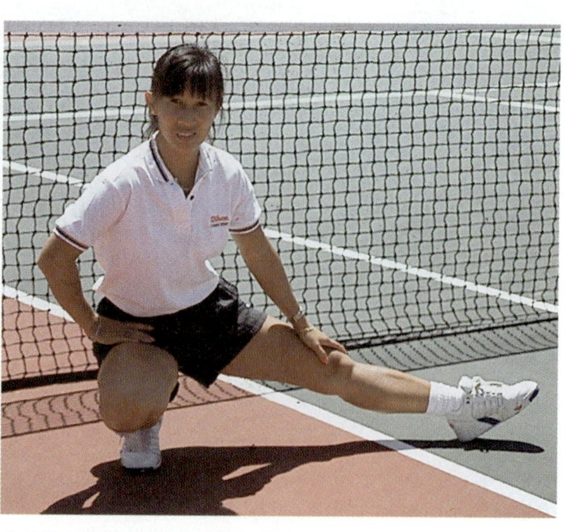

ADDUCTOR STRETCH

Action: Feet spread twice shoulder width with hands placed slightly above the knee. Flex one knee and go down to approximately 90 degrees. Hold the stretch and then repeat on the other side.

Area Stretched: Hip adductor muscles.

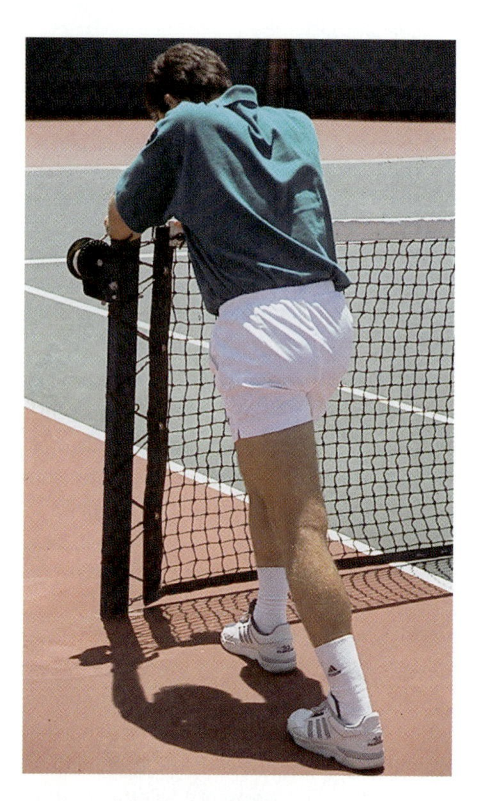

HEEL CORD STRETCH

Action: Stand against a solid object and stretch the heel downward. Hold the stretch for a few seconds and change legs.

Areas Stretched: Achilles' tendon, gastrocnemius and soleus muscles.

heart rate, and oxygen available to muscles. Following the brief running, stretching should begin with concentration on stretching neck flexors and extensors, ligaments of the cervical lumbar spine, ligaments of the shoulder joint, deltoid and pectoral muscles, abdominal muscles, muscles of the hip, muscles and ligaments of the pelvic area, quadriceps and hamstring of the upper leg, gastrocnemius and soleus muscles of the lower leg, and the Achilles tendon.

Eleven recommended stretching exercises for tennis are presented on the following pages. Each is described by the action required for execution and identified by the area to be stretched. The basis for most of these exercises is extrapolated from Werner W. K. Hoeger's *Lifetime Physical Fitness & Wellness: A Personalized Program* (Morton Publishing Company, 1999.)

A few final thoughts in regard to stretching prior to playing a tennis match: First is a second reminder that you must have already done some aerobic work to have warmed up before stretching. Second, the range of the stretch is to be done within your comfort zone. Third, the intensity of the stretch never should be painful. And fourth, the duration of a stretch should be for only a few seconds.

The *basic tennis warm-up* follows the stretching exercises. The warm-up is designed to increase circulation and respiration, and to provide a grooving of tennis strokes. A good warm-up should last 15 minutes, and at the conclusion, both players should be perspiring profusely. When warming up, the beginning player should always work on strokes to

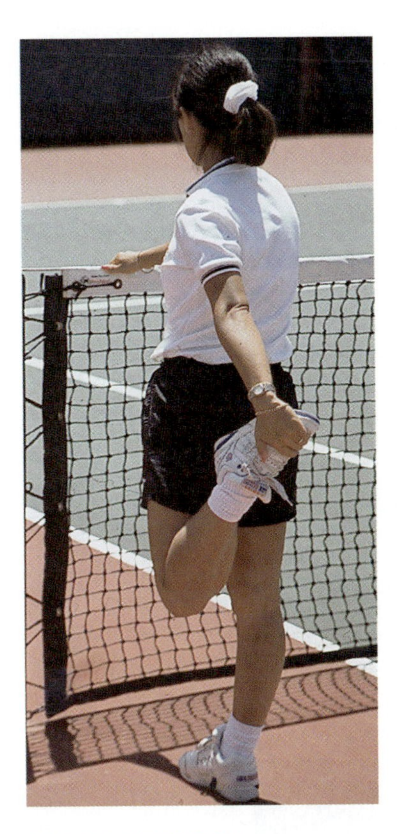

QUAD STRETCH

Action: Stand up straight, grasp the front of the ankle and flex the knee until the heel of the foot is touching the gluteal area. Hold the stretch for a few seconds and change legs.

Areas Stretched: Quadriceps muscle, and knee and ankle ligaments.

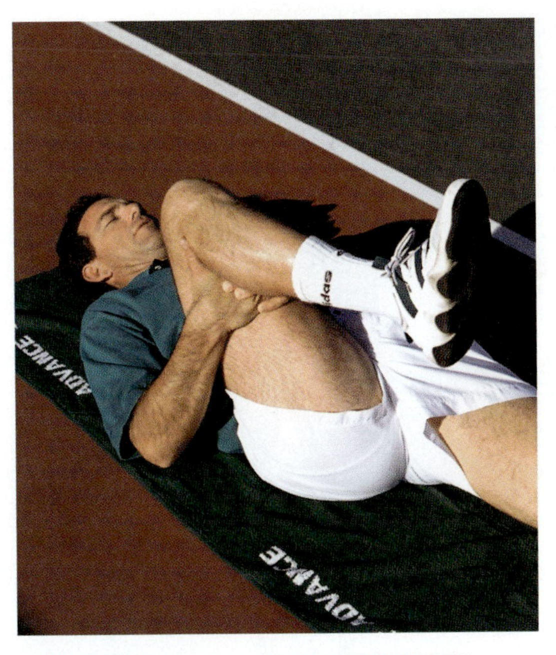

SINGLE-KNEE TO CHEST STRETCH

Action: Lie flat on a padded surface. Bend one leg at approximately 100 degrees and place both hands on the lower portion of the knee of the opposite leg, pulling that knee toward the chest. Hold the stretch at the chest level.

Area Stretched: Lower back and hamstring muscles, and the lumbar spine ligaments.

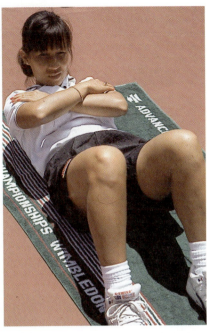

CURLS

Action: Lie flat on padded surface and bend knees at a 90 degree angle. Place arms across chest and curl the upper body to the knees. Repeat the process 15-20 times.

Area Exercised: Abdominal muscles.

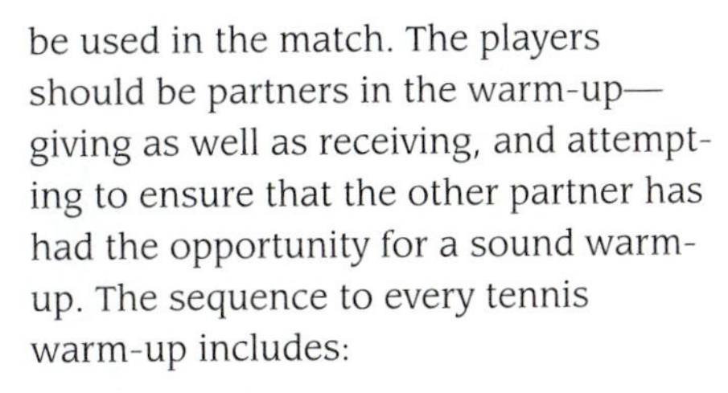

be used in the match. The players should be partners in the warm-up—giving as well as receiving, and attempting to ensure that the other partner has had the opportunity for a sound warm-up. The sequence to every tennis warm-up includes:

1. Groundstrokes
2. One player hits groundstrokes, the other volleys, then switch.
3. One player hits lobs while the other hits overheads, then switch.
4. One player hits serves while the other player retrieves the serves, then switch. (Note: there is no return of service; that takes time and detracts from the total warm-up effort.)

Although the sequence may differ depending on the location of the players geographically, the concept is reasonably standard.

Finally, at the conclusion of the match and while the players are talking to each other, they should complete a *warm-down stretching* activity. The stretching exercises identified include:

1. Side stretch.
2. Adductor stretch.
3. Heel cord stretch.
4. Quad stretch.

As part of the warm-down, assuming it is not extremely hot, you should put on a warm-up top and pants and cool down by stretching and walking for a period of time prior to sitting down for a rest. Besides stretching and walking, you should make sure you continue drinking liquids, and if you have an injury or feel muscle soreness it is advisable to apply an ice pack on that area for 15–20 minutes.

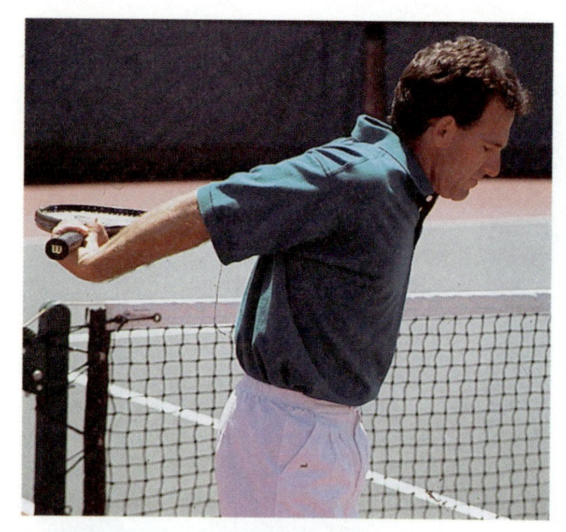

SHOULDER HYPEREXTENSION STRETCH

Action: Grasp the throat of the racket with hands close together. Slowly bring the arms up to as close to a perpendicular position to the shoulders as possible. Hold the stretch for a few seconds.

Areas Stretched: Deltoid and pectoral muscles and ligaments of the shoulder joint.

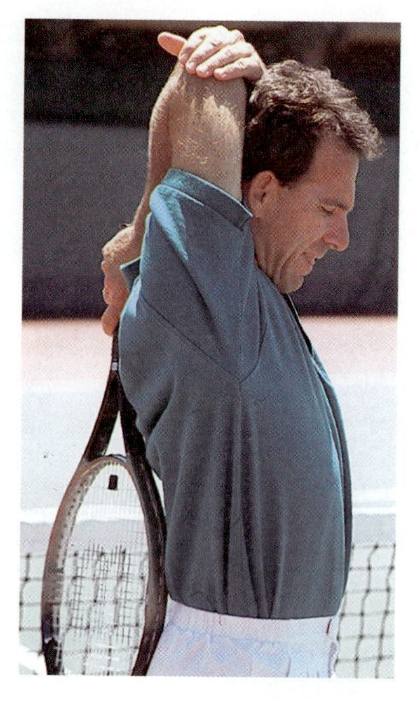

SERVING SHOULDER AND ARM STRETCH

Action: Place the tennis racket head in the small of the back with the elbow in an up position. Place the non-racket hand below the elbow and apply minimal pressure to place the shoulder area on stretch. Hold the stretch for a few seconds and repeat the process several times.

Areas Stretched: Ligaments of the shoulder joint and ligaments of the cervical and lumbar spine.

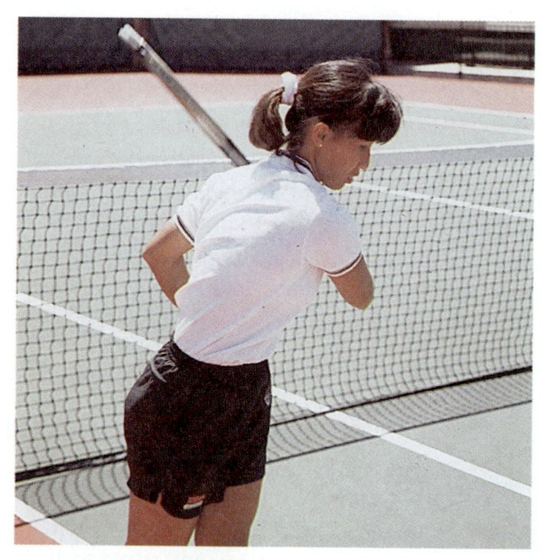

SERVING MOTION ROTATION AND STRETCH

Action: Start with the head of the tennis racket between the shoulder blades and rotate through the service motion. Hold the stretch on the follow through for a few seconds and repeat the process.

Areas Stretched: Upper and lower back area.

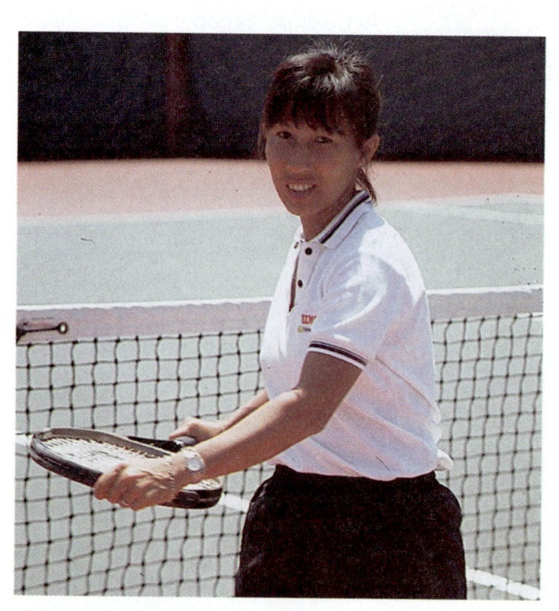

SEMI GROUNDSTROKE BODY ROTATION

Action: Place the feet approximately shoulder width apart, grasp the racket with your hands, and with the arms away from the body rotate the trunk as far as possible and hold the stretch. Repeat the rotation the other direction, and continue to follow the same process several times.

Areas Stretched: Hips, abdominal, chest, back, neck, shoulder muscles, and hip spinal ligaments.

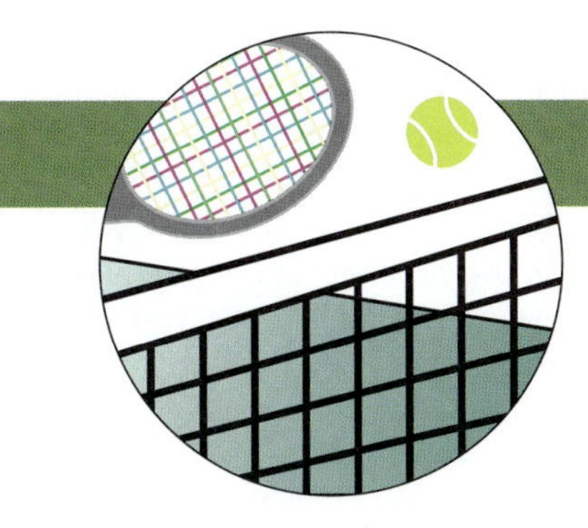

Learning Experience Reminders

Physically Preparing to Play

1. Do physical work for 8–10 minutes before stretching.
2. Stretching exercises should include both upper and lower body.
3. Tennis stroke warm-up includes a sequence of groundstrokes, volley, lobs/overhead smash, and service.
4. After a match make sure to warm down by walking, stretching, continual intake of liquids, and icing sore muscles.

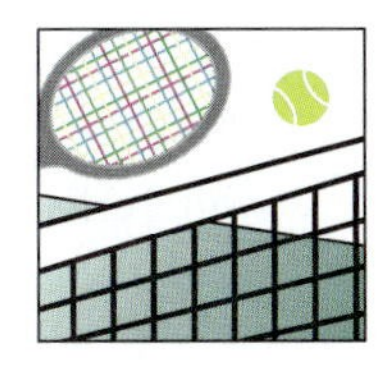

Overall Fitness Development

Fitness development for tennis can range from simplistic to sophisticated through the use of programs including aerobic exercise and strength training. Tennis players who are willing to run, incorporate a sensible exercise program, and work on tennis drills that incorporate agility and quickness will establish an advantage over individuals who neglect tennis fitness development.

Aerobic Fitness Development

Aerobic exercise contributes significantly to your success as a tennis player. You cannot use your skills and apply strategy to your best advantage if you are not in good physical shape. In addition, you are at risk for potential injury. During a tennis rally most of the energy the body uses is a product of anaerobic metabolism, the release of energy without the use of oxygen. Therefore, although energy needs during tennis play are not primarily aerobic ("with oxygen"), the more oxygen that can be used during a rally, the faster you can recover, and the less tired you will be during play. This means that you need to train your body to use large amounts of oxygen quickly. You can accomplish this through a number of physical activities, but a jogging program is recommended since tennis is a running form of activity.

For most people under age 35, an exercise intensity between 70 percent and 85 percent of *maximal heart rate* is adequate, and is called an *exercise heart rate range*. A maximal heart rate is the maximal speed a heart can beat when exercising as hard as you can. The typical way to predict your exercise heart rate range is to take the number 220 and subtract your age. After you have tabulated that number simply multiply 70 percent and 85 percent of that number (e.g., 220 − 20 years of age = 200. 200 × 70% = 140, 200 × 85% = 170). The calculation of these two numbers represent an exercise heart rate range (i.e., a 20-year-old's exercise heart rate range is 140 to 170). Providing you are in good health, this heart rate range will provide a guide for your level of exercise effort (before starting any exercise program it is advisable to have a physical exam).

Once you have a proper rate of exercise intensity, you need to determine the duration of your workout effort. Anywhere between 15 and 60 minutes will provide enough time to give your body sufficient practice at using oxygen. In general 20–30 minutes is recommended for the proper workout duration. This means 20–30 minutes of

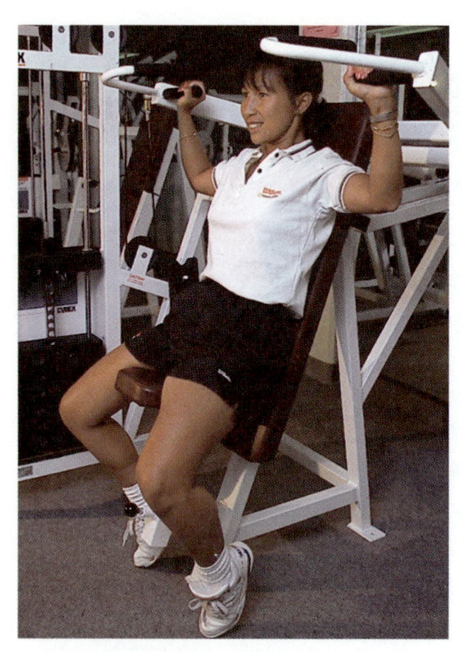

SHOULDER PRESS

Action: Sit upright and grasp handles. Press up until arms are fully extended and return to start.

Muscle Group: Triceps, deltoid, pectoralis major, trapezius, cervatus anterior

constant, nonstop exercise at your exercise heart rate. If you are just starting out, remember you need to progressively work into a full workout. It does you no good to start at a high level of effort and experience discomfort or injury the first day. Start slowly and progress to a more full workout. Try to do your aerobic work at least three to four times per week. Five times per week can be tolerated, but you need to also give your body a chance to rest. Typically you want to give your body a minimum of 24 hours between aerobic workouts. The less fit you are, the more time you need to set aside between your aerobic work and rest.

If you combine aerobic work with practice time on the tennis court using the drills as described in Chapter 9 — *Tennis Practice*, you will not only gain a positive level of fitness, but you will have also acquired improved quickness and agility for tennis play.

Strength and Fitness Development

There are several forms of *strength training* designed for further development of both muscular strength and endurance that can also enhance physical development for tennis. Basically, you can either use free weights or weight machines to accomplish this development. A variable resistance workout, using workout exercises on weight machines, is specifically recommended for tennis players. Each of these workouts includes an explanation of the workout and the muscle group developed. When you do these exercises you need to breathe, and lift in a smooth, slow action. These exercises are:

- Abdominal Crunch
- Tricep Extension
- Shoulder Press
- Arm Curl
- Chest Press
- Leg Press
- Back Extension
- Leg Extension
- Lat Pull Down
- Leg Curls

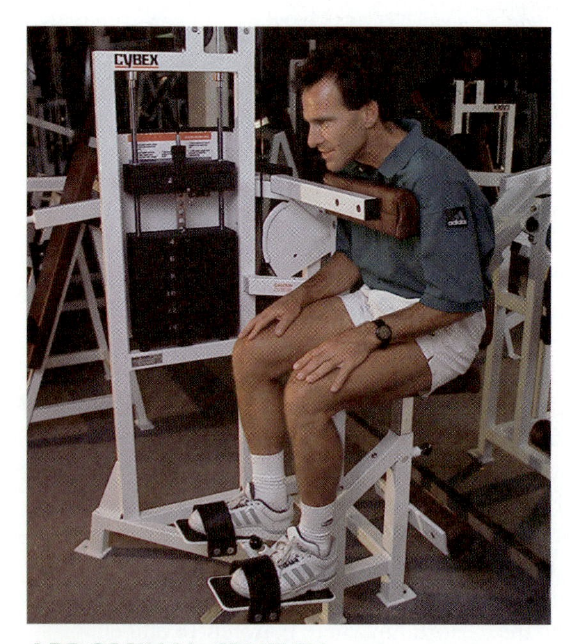

ABDOMINAL CRUNCH

Action: Sit in an upright position with chest against padded bar. Bring chest down toward knees.

Muscle Group: Abdominals

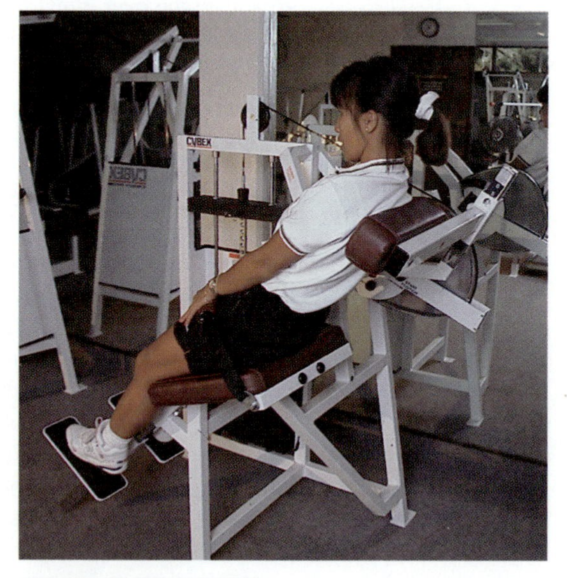

BACK EXTENSION

Action: Slowly press back until the back is fully extended.

Muscle Groups: Erector spinae, gluteus maximus

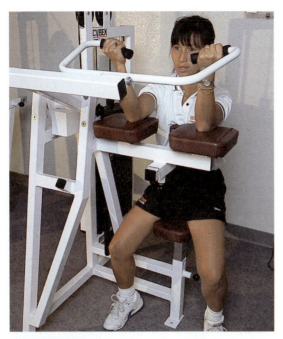

ARM CURL

Action: Sit upright and grasp grips with palms up and arms extended. Curl up as far as possible and return to start.

Muscle Groups: Biceps, brachiobrachialis, brachialis, and radialis

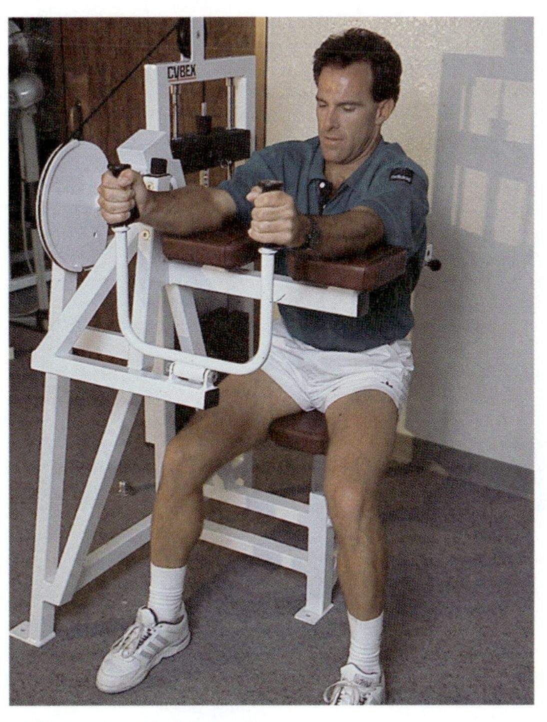

TRICEP EXTENSION

Action: Sit upright and grasp handles. Press down to full extension and return to start.

Muscle Group: Triceps

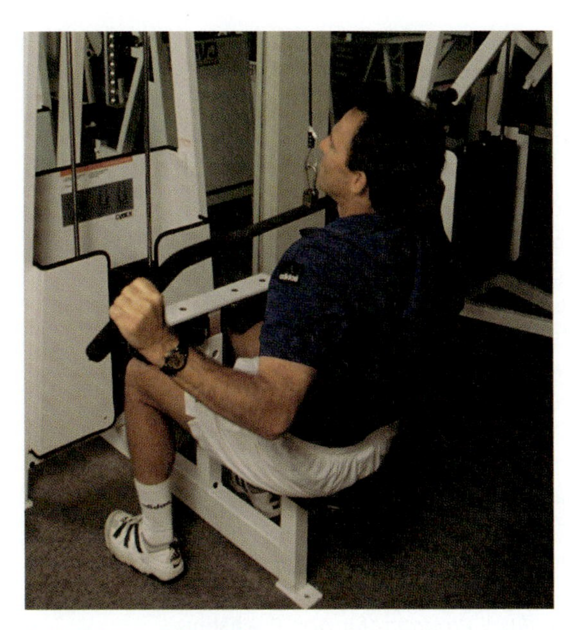

LAT PULL DOWN

Action: From a sitting position hold the bar with a wide grip and pull bar down until it touches the base of the neck.

Muscle Groups: Latissimus dorsi, pectoralis major

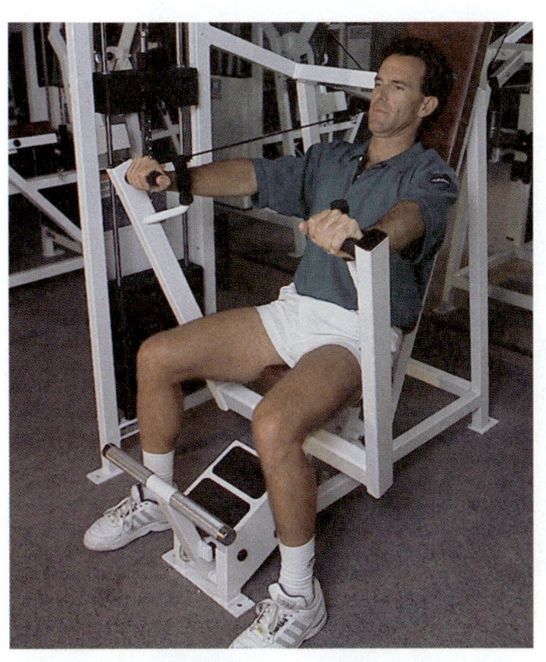

CHEST PRESS

Action: Sit upright and press arms forward until extended. Return to start.

Muscle Groups: Pectoralis major, triceps, deltoid

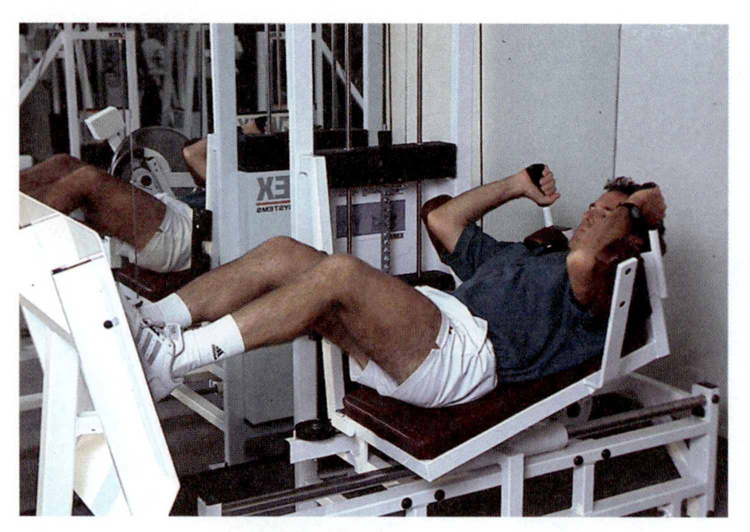

LEG PRESS

Action: Lie with flat back on surface, grasp handles and extend legs fully. Return to start.

Muscle Groups: Quadriceps, gluteals

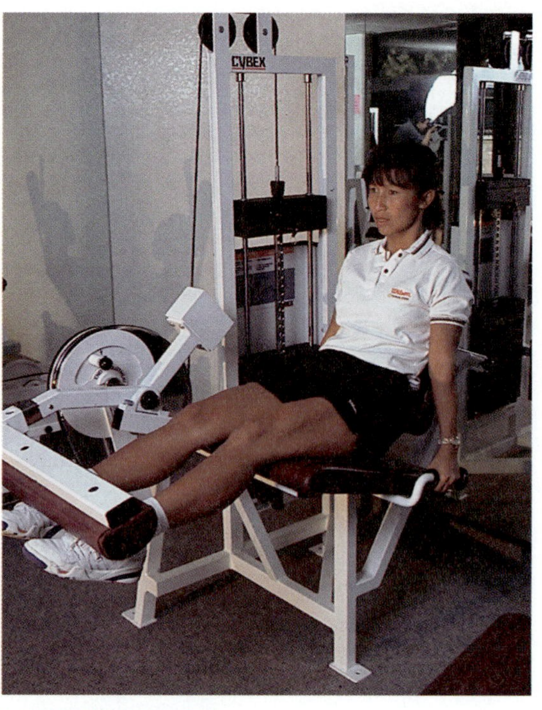

LEG EXTENSION

Action: Lie flat with feet under the bar and extend legs until straight.

Muscle Group: Quadriceps

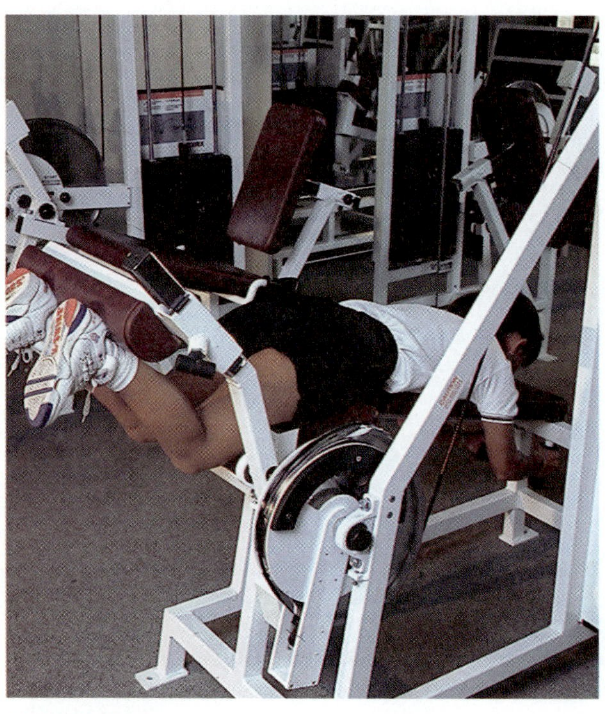

LEG CURLS

Action: Lie face down with legs under the bar. Curl up at least 90 degrees and return to start.

Muscle Group: Hamstring

Your workouts should consist of a minimum of three days per week with 2–3 sets of 10–15 repetitions. One of the exciting aspects of strength training programs is that most colleges and universities have facilities established for your choice of weight training workout, and many of these facilities have state-of-the-art equipment.

As with the various stretching exercises mentioned previously in this chapter, the basis for the weight training exercises has been modified for tennis and recommended from W. W. K. Hoeger's *Lifetime Physical Fitness & Wellness: A Personalized Program* (Morton Publishing Co., 1999) text. You are encouraged to review Hoeger's material for more in-depth information.

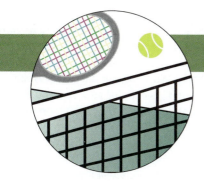

Learning Experience Reminders

Overall Fitness Development

1. Predict an exercise heart rate range by subtracting age from 220, and then multiply that number by 70% and 85% to determine a range.
2. Aerobic workouts should consist of 20–30 minutes for 3–4 times per week.
3. Strength training workouts using weight training machines should consist of 2–3 sets of 10–15 repetitions.

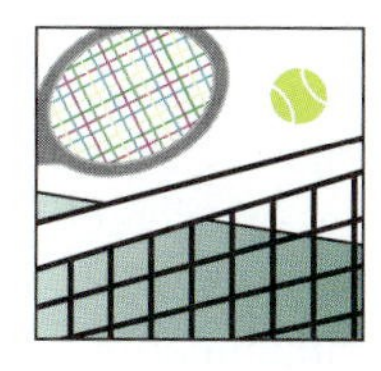

Preventing and Caring for Tennis Injuries

Of the numerous injuries associated with tennis, most can be prevented. Serious injuries related to contact sports, including concussions, cartilage and ligament damage of the knee, shoulder separations, and neck injuries, are seldom found in tennis. Knee, shoulder, and back injuries, however, are increasing in number, and most of the blame for these injuries can be placed on hard tennis court surfaces. As a general rule, injuries in tennis usually are mild and seldom restrict a player's participation. Those few serious injuries that do occur can be prevented in many cases.

Some *minor common tennis injuries are prevented* with a little attention. The blisters that often appear on hands and feet are caused by moisture, pressure, or friction. Feet that slide in a tennis shoe develop blisters. Prevention requires wearing a pair of cotton tennis socks with cushion insoles. Blisters on the racket hand often are caused by the racket turning in the player's hand. You can prevent this type of blister from developing by making sure you have the correct grip size. Usually a larger grip will enable a player to prevent the racket from turning in the hand. Blisters also occur on the racket hand from extensive play when the hand has not been accustomed to that amount of play. The wear and tear creates a "hot spot" that results in a blister. Prevention consists of being conscious of length of playing time and placing some limit on it.

Sometimes a player is bruised when hit by a ball or racket. The only way to avoid this injury is not to assume a position on the court that would provide an opportunity to be hit, or to avoid being hit in vulnerable spots of the body. For example, if you are on the direct opposite side of the net from the opposing player and the opposing player is about to hit an overhead smash in line with your position on the court, it is prudent for you to turn and duck. Also, bruising can occur when a player follows through with the racket and hits the shin when serving, or when doubles partners swing at the same ball and hit each other. These incidents can cause severe bruising, called a *hematoma*.

In unusually warm and humid weather, when body fluid and salt are lost rapidly, a player may get cramps. A muscle or muscle group contracts, causing spasms, usually in the abdominal area or gastrocnemius (calf muscle). To prevent a serious cramping problem, consume fluids in large quantities. Although water is the best choice of liquids, diluted fruit juices are an excellent alternative. Sports drinks (such as Gatorade®, Powerade®, and Exceed®), also are alternatives to dealing with cramps since they replace carbohydrates and electrolytes while also replenishing liquid. The key to liquid consumption on a hot and humid day is to drink, and then drink more (Drink a Sports Drink?, *Tennis,* July 1996 p. 99).

More *serious tennis injuries require professional care. Pulled muscles,* including the groin, hamstring, and gastrocnemius, generally occur as a result of poor stretching. They can often be avoided by going through a full warm-up. You will know when you have pulled a muscle simply from the pain and limited mobility allowed following the pull. Rest, ice, and other athletic training modalities are common for pulled muscle rehabilitation. If you pull a muscle it is important to see a sports-medicine-oriented physician for evaluation.

A *sprained ankle* is one of the most common injuries in tennis. They usually happen when the player tries to make a quick turn without the foot following in the turn. Sometimes a player will jump to hit a ball with a scissors kick on the overhead smash and land on the side of the foot, or a player will step on a ball during play. Pivoting incorrectly or landing on the side of the foot is a matter of not coordinating effort and physical skill. Stepping on the ball is controllable. Only three tennis balls should be available for play at any given point in a match. If one ball is in play during a rally, only two other balls can become a problem. Court awareness is important. You should keep your side of the court clean by picking up or pushing balls on the court to the net or fence. You also should be aware of a ball that comes from another court and stop play if the ball is in your court area. If a tennis player is lazy when it comes to picking up loose tennis balls, injury can be the result.

Ankle sprains are classified as Grade 1 (painful), Grade 2 (very painful), and Grade 3 (severe pain). Most ankle sprains occur to the outside of the ankle. With any significant discomfort see a physician for an x-ray, and once identified as a sprain it is recommended that you begin using ice in combination with rest, elevation, and compression (Twist and Shout, by A. Shaffer, *Tennis*, June 1999, pp. 93–96). You don't recover from an ankle sprain overnight. Give yourself time to rehabilitate.

Foot injuries are common for three out of four people, and if you play long enough you will sustain a tennis foot injury. Plantar Fasciitis is a high-risk foot injury. Symptoms are pain in the heel or arch experienced usually after you have rested after playing. Other foot injuries include inflammation of the sesamoid bone (the two metacarpal bones behind the big toe), capsulitis (an inflammation of connective tissue under the second toe), metatarsalgia (inflammation under the ball of the foot), tendonitis, stress fracture, and the common foot callus (Foot Faults, by A.L. Shaffer, *Tennis*, May 2000, pp. 80–82).

Tennis players are susceptible to *knee injuries* because of the weak anatomical structure of the knee, and due to the quick lateral movements and countless stops and starts required during play. Typically, most knee injuries are related to overuse and don't require surgery. Patellar tendonitis and patellofemoral pain syndrome are reflective of overuse, and are treated with ice, rest, compression, and elevation. Combined, they speed the healing process and reduce any tissue damage that might occur.

Wrist injuries are increasing in tennis. The most common injuries will most likely be tendonitis of the extensor tendons of the back of the hand, trauma to the soft tissue triangular fibrocartilage that encircles the wrist, or a carpal ligament sprain. These injuries happen because you are playing with a racket with limited shock absorption (tendonitis), applying too much pressure with spin strokes (slicing or topspin), or swinging late at the ball (trauma). You can manage wrist injuries by a few modifications. First, either lower tension on your racket strings or get a more flexible racket in order to have better shock absorption. Second, if you are experiencing discomfort hitting spin shots, back off and return to basic strokes. And third, work on stroke timing in order to make solid, timed contact with the ball. Wrist injuries "grow" on you. When you first feel pain, it is time to stop and check it out. If you let pain continue your wrist problems will expand. Rest and ice application are strategies to use with a wrist injury, and after 10 days without improving it is time for you to go to a doctor. If you must play with a wrist injury there are wrist braces available, but it is prudent to make sure you are not developing a chronic injury before you go to a wrist brace.

Shin splints are another injury that can be associated with tennis. The constant pounding, running, jumping, and landing on a hard court can create an inflammation of the soft tissues of the lower legs. A change of tennis court surfaces, high arches, tight calves, and intensity in your workouts and playing situations all can contribute to this injury. Prevention includes being aware of the causes, stretching, and using common sense regarding playing intensity and type of court you are playing on. Selecting the proper shoe with arch support and excellent shock absorption capabilities is also important. Recommended ways of dealing with a shin splint are rest and the application of ice when shin splints are in the acute stage (How to Prevent Shin Splints, by D. Higdon, *Tennis*, June 1992, p. 102).

Repetitive twisting and trunk rotation is a part of tennis. The trunk accelerating through on groundstrokes and executing the overhead arching motion in a serve or overhead increase the risk for *back injury*. In addition, hard court surfaces can be damaging. Preventive measures for back injury include aerobic conditioning, strength programs, and good stroke technique. Professional help following a back injury includes rehabilitation through an athletic trainer or a physical therapist who specializes in sports medicine (Oh, My Aching Back, by D. Squires, *Tennis USTA,* April 1993, p. 10).

Two injuries associated with tendonitis are somewhat common, but they occur for different reasons. The *Achilles tendon* sometimes is injured by simple physical actions such as jumping and landing on the ball of the foot without lowering the heel, or by pushing off the ball of the foot, thereby placing extreme pressure on the tendon. The tendon, when rupturing, sounds like a gunshot report, and the player becomes immobile immediately. Ridged, high-arched feet with heels that angle inward or flat feet that roll inward are most vulnerable to Achilles tendon problems.

The Achilles tendon often is chronically sore because players ignore persistent, tolerable pain and continue to play. The Achilles tendon and the sheath that surrounds it become inflamed, and soreness, swelling and pain are the outcome. Ignoring these signs can cause severe problems. The only way to address the injury is to stop playing and rest. Prevention, on the other hand, includes stretching the Achilles tendon in warm-up and warm-down. Orthotics for the shoe, or heel pads, also are used as a preventive measure, but elevating your heel also shortens the tendon when what is needed is to lengthen the tendon. As a result, stretching becomes even more important when using a heel pad.

Once an Achilles tendon injury has occurred, rehabilitation consists of rest and modality application. Modalities used in therapy include ice, massage, ultrasound, or electrical stimulation. They are used to reduce swelling and begin rehabilitation that brings the Achilles tendon back to a normal condition. A stiff or achy tendon is a sign of an impending rupture, and if you rupture an Achilles tendon, there is a very long process of rehabilitation following surgery or immobilization (Protecting Your Achilles, by A. McNab, *Tennis,* June 1993, p. 99).

The other common tennis injury is *tennis elbow*. There are several types of tennis elbow injuries, the main characteristic being an inflammation of the elbow area. The injury can be prevented if a player uses proper skill techniques and strokes. Hitting with the elbow leading on the backhand or hitting numerous slice or spin serves invites the injury. Prevention requires correcting poor mechanics and common sense regarding how many spin serves you are going to hit. Treatment of an elbow injury is restricted to rest or the application of a support. Elbow supports and splints are available to relieve minor pain from tennis elbow, but they will not eliminate the cause.

If an injury is perceived as serious, a physician should be consulted as soon as possible. If rehabilitation is recommended, it is advisable to seek out a sports medicine clinic. Most metropolitan areas have centers that work closely with physicians to rehabilitate injuries.

Home treatment should be limited to only minor injuries. Blisters usually dry up on their own; the main concern is to make sure that they do not get infected. For minor injuries, athletic trainers can develop devices to enable continuation of activity. For example, a trainer can devise a doughnut-shaped pad that will cover the blister, reduce pain at the pressure point, and prevent additional friction on the blister area. Bruises often can be treated with cold compresses or ice packs to reduce swelling. For injuries such as Achilles tendon, tennis elbow, and pulled muscles, rest may be the only solution.

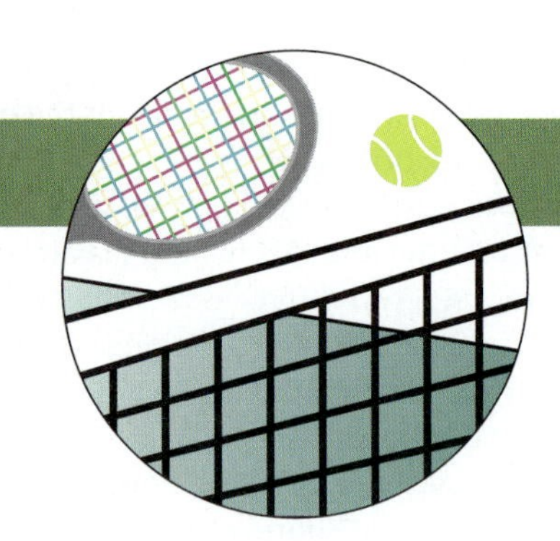

Learning Experience Reminders

Preventing and Caring for Tennis Injuries

1. Minor common tennis injuries include blisters, bruises, and cramps.
2. Serious tennis injuries include pulled muscles, sprained ankles, foot injuries, knee injuries, wrist injuries, shin splints, back injuries, Achilles tendon injuries, and tennis elbow.

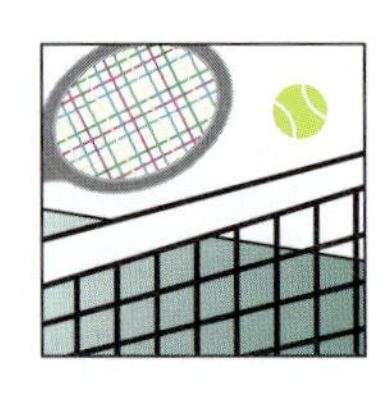

Coping with Heat, Insect Bites, and Sun when Playing Tennis

Additional problems that occur in tennis include hyperthermia, dehydration, sunburn, insect bites or stings. *Hyperthermia* (elevated body temperature) may lead to heat cramps, heat exhaustion, and heat stroke. Any of these conditions can occur when playing in hot weather for an extended period of time, since you lose large amounts of body fluids through sweating. Heat cramps can be painful, but they are not life threatening. Untreated heat stroke, however, may be fatal.

To prevent problems associated with *dehydration* make sure your clothing allows for good air circulation around your body. Avoid clothing that traps or absorbs heat. Dark shirts are an example of material that may absorb heat, while wearing light clothing reduces that absorption. Body fluids are important in regulating body temperature. If too many fluids are lost, your body is likely to overheat just like a radiator when its water level is low. Some sweating is necessary to keep the body cool, so you need to maintain an adequate level of body fluids by drinking appropriate liquids. To determine how much liquid to drink, a good guide is to drink a pint of water for each pound lost during play. Start replacing your body fluids by drinking small (3–6 ounces of water) amounts in 10–15 minute intervals prior to the beginning of your match and continuing throughout the match. Because water is being lost from the body, water is needed to replace body fluids. For most people, electrolyte replacement solutions (such as Gatorade®) are not needed during exercise, although they aid in recovery after play is complete. Avoid beverages with caffeine since they contribute to dehydration.

Sunburn can be avoided by applying sunscreen with a sun protection factor (SPF) of at least 15. PABA sunscreen offers even better protection. This type of sunscreen blocks both UVA and UVB rays. Wearing a hat is a prerequisite not only for avoiding sunburn but also for preventing heat stroke. Players often reject sunscreen because the lotion is applied by hand and then is transferred to the racket grip. By simply wiping your hands, you can avoid transferring the lotion to the grip of the racket. Some players also reject wearing a hat, suggesting that they can't see the ball on the serve toss and it gets in their way generally. These are just excuses.

One last potential physical problem deserves consideration. *Eyes exposed to ultraviolet rays* over an extended time are at risk for at least three eye diseases: cataracts (clouding of the lens), pterygium (a flesh-like growth on the white of the eye near the iris), and macular degeneration (breakdown of the retina with age). Pterygium is of particular concern, as the incidence of developing this eye disease is relatively high for those who are in the sun extensively (The Eyes Have It, by K. Chen, *Tennis*, May 1995, p. 74). A partial answer is to begin wearing sunglasses while playing tennis. New technology has produced a polycarbonate lens, in which the lens is wrapped around the head. It is recommended that the lens blocks 100 percent of UVA rays and 75–90 percent of visible light (Here Comes the Sun, by D. Sullivan, *Tennis*, July/August 1999, pp.113–115). A quality pair of sunglasses not only protects against the sun but also screens out peripheral light and wind while still providing clear visibility for the player.

Finally, depending on what part of the country you come from, *insect bites and stings* might bother you. Probably the most prevalent insect sting is from the bee or wasp. Avoiding being stung is an obvious preventive measure. When you are around bees and wasps, be especially alert. When you pick up a racket, make sure a bee is not lurking. Bees and wasps congregate at the opening of cans containing beverages with sugar. If you are stung, the recommended way of removing the stinger is to scrape the sac away and extract the stinger with a tweezer.

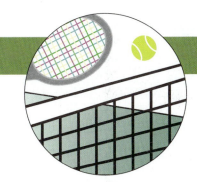

Learning Experience Reminders

Coping with Heat, Insects, and Sun when Playing Tennis

1. Drink water prior to playing and throughout a match.
2. Protect yourself from the sun by applying at least a 15 SPF sun block.
3. Protect your eyes from the sun by wearing sunglasses with a lens block of 100 percent UVA and a 75–90 percent block of visible light.
4. Be alert to insects that sting (i.e., bees, wasps, etc.).

Check Points

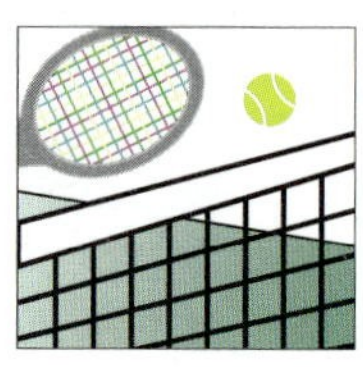

1. Warm-up requires
   a. an increase in blood flow.
   b. an increase in heart rate.
   c. a series of stretching activities.
   d. all of the above.

2. Select a stretch action for the upper extremity and describe the areas stretched:

   ____
   ____
   ____

3. Select a stretch action for the lower extremity and describe the areas stretched:

   ____
   ____
   ____

4. Select an upper extremity strength training action and describe the muscle groups that are developed for tennis.

   ____
   ____
   ____

5. Select a lower extremity strength training action and describe the muscle groups that are developed for tennis.

   ____
   ____
   ____

6. There are numerous possible injuries associated with tennis. Three significant injuries that are common are
   a. dehydration, tennis elbow, and back injuries.
   b. blisters, bruises, and dehydration.
   c. sprained ankles, shin splints, and Achilles tendon rupture.
   d. blisters, sprained ankles, and cartilage damage.

7. Determine your exercise heart rate by
   a. taking the number 220 and dividing by 70% and 85%.
   b. taking the number 220, divide by your age and multiply by 70% and 85%.
   c. taking the number 220, subtract your age, and multiply 70% and 85%.
   d. taking the number 220, subtract by 70 and 85.

8. Drinking liquids is important to do
   a. prior to and following a match.
   b. prior to, during, and following a match.
   c. prior to and during a match.
   d. during and following a match.

9. Tennis players are usually susceptible to knee injuries due to
   a. quick lateral movements and weak anatomical structure of the knee.
   b. sprinting and weak anatomical structure of the knee.
   c. jumping and weak anatomical structure of the knee.
   d. quick lateral movements and sprinting.

10. Sunglasses are recommended for tennis players. They should be designed to
    a. block out 15 percent of UVA.
    b. block out 75 percent of UVA.
    c. block out all UVA.
    d. decrease as much as possible UVA.

Answers to Check Points can be found on page 145.

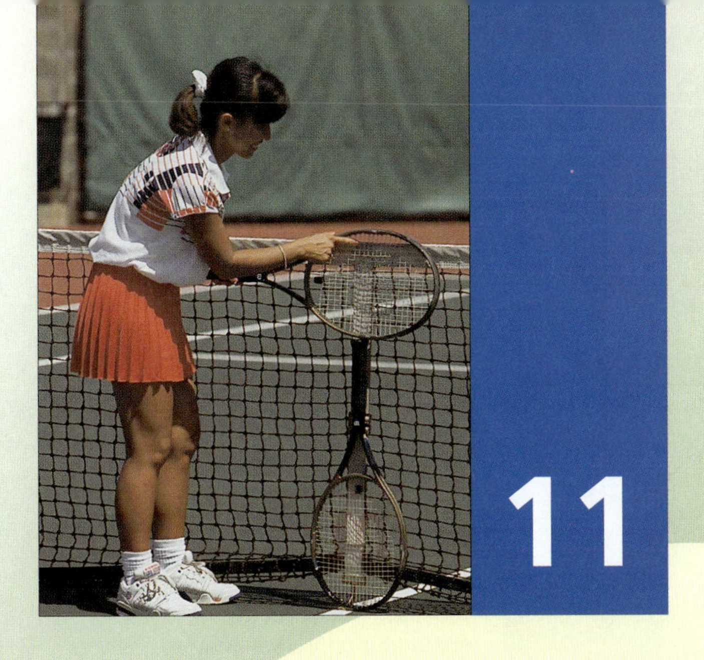

11

Tennis Behavior and Interpretation of Rules

Playing tennis requires understanding the written and unwritten rules of the game. Tennis has been played for centuries, and certain ways of behaving and interpreting rules have evolved over time.

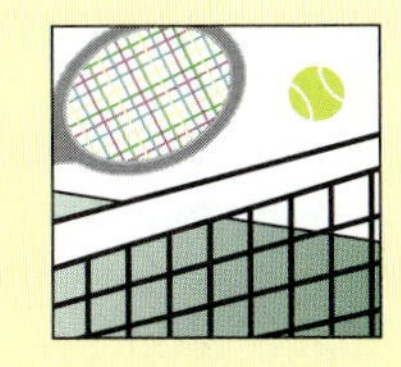

Behavior on a Tennis Court

The unwritten rules of tennis are associated with behavior on a tennis court. Most behavior rules have a logical purpose, and it is up to you to respect these rules.

Appropriate clothing for tennis does not require a major expenditure, but proper dress is part of the game. A tennis player must wear tennis shoes rather than track-type shoes or basketball shoes. Wearing proper shoes reduces the chance of injury, and it prevents marring of the tennis court surface (Chapter 12 has additional comments related to shoes as equipment). Municipal, private, and college courts have basic, general rules requiring proper footwear, and players are expected to wear shorts and a shirt to play on those courts. When playing at a private tennis club, clothing expectations are more conventional, consisting of tennis shorts or skirt and a tennis shirt or blouse.

Even the act of picking up a tennis ball is connected to expected behavior. Bending over and picking up the ball is, of course, one way to retrieve the ball. Other methods include a foot/racket pickup and a ball-bounce pickup. In the *foot/racket pickup* (Figure 11.1), the ball is positioned between the racket-side foot and the face of the tennis racket. Simultaneously lift the foot, ball, and racket to mid-calf level, and, as the ball becomes airborne, use the racket to bounce the ball to the court surface and catch it with your non-racket hand. The *ball-bounce pickup* (Figure 11.2) requires you to choke up on the racket handle and place the racket face on top of the ball. Then lift the racket slightly and contact the ball with a series of quick wrist movements that lift the ball off the court and into your non-racket hand.

Most tennis facilities consist of three or more courts enclosed by a

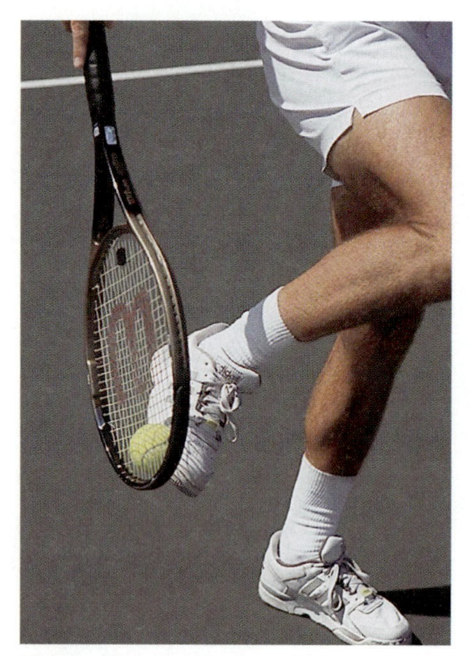

Figure 11.1 Foot/racket pickup.

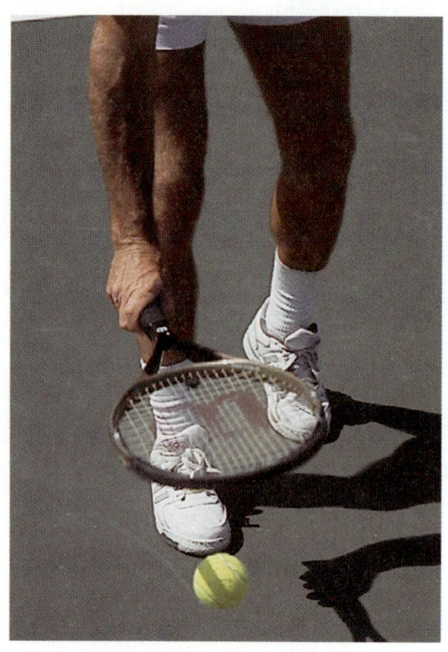

Figure 11.2 Ball bounce pickup.

fence, with one or two gates to admit players. When *walking on a tennis court,* you should wait until any play has stopped before proceeding to an assigned court, and you should walk along the fence as quickly as possible. *Talking on a tennis court* should be in normal voice tones, and conversation should be limited as much as possible to the match rather than to everyday visiting.

Warm-up is described in Chapter 10 as a part of physically preparing to play. Etiquette, or proper behavior, insists that each player be considerate during warm-up.

How to return tennis balls to another court, and *how to request a return of tennis balls* require court etiquette. When a tennis ball rolls across a court from an adjacent court while play is in progress, action should stop and the ball should be returned. The action should be stopped assuming that the rolling ball interferes with the play, and if it does, the point should be replayed. The ball should be returned to the adjacent court on a bounce to the requesting player. If a ball is hit onto another court, the requesting player should wait until play ceases on that court, and then with a raised hand request "ball please," followed by "thank you" upon receipt of the ball. Balls hit over the fence must be retrieved, and the retrieval must follow the same court behavior as when entering the court for the first time.

Once the *ball is in play* during a match, interruptions should cease. This includes practice serves. That practice is part of the warm-up and interferes with the flow of the game if it is done during the first or second games of the match. The server always must begin with two tennis balls. For convenience, one ball should be placed in the pocket of the tennis shorts and one in the hand for the toss. When receiving, the player should hit only a ball that is legally in play. It is poor form to return an "out" serve.

When a ball or other interference occurs during a match, a gesture of "play a let" is acceptable. A situation that might make the point is if a server hits the first serve as fault, followed by a ball rolling across the court. If the receiver responds by picking up the ball and returning it to the adjacent court, the receiver should immediately respond to the server, "take two."

Another form of court behavior is to communicate all calls to the opponents. Verbal forms of communication are "out" and "let." A ball that is "in" is assumed in by the continued play on the part of the player returning the shot. An index finger pointing up can be used as a sign language for a ball that is out, and a ball hit out of reach of a player that is good is signified by a flat, palm-down motion.

Emotion is to be left off the court! Throwing a racket, hitting an erratic shot after play has stopped, and verbal outbursts should not be tolerated. An easy way to cope with opponents who behave in such an unacceptable manner is to refuse to play them. Life is too short to accept that sort of behavior in an environment that is supposed to be fun. Other unacceptable responses include making excuses for losing while not acknowledging the good play of an opponent, and not keeping score accurately.

Perhaps the most misunderstood part of etiquette is related to a rules interpretation of *when a ball is called "in"*

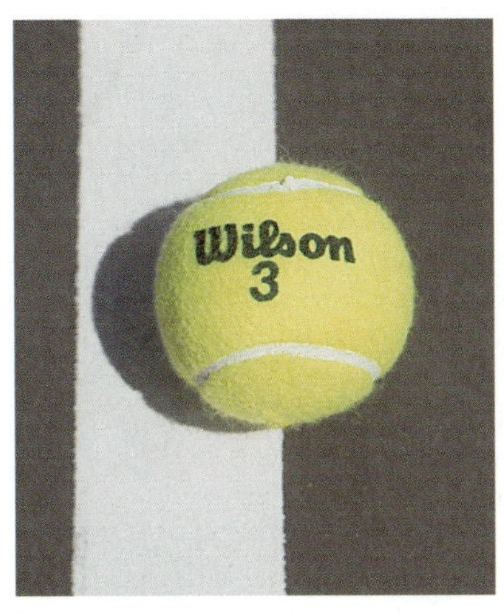

Figure 11.3 Ball on the line – "IN."

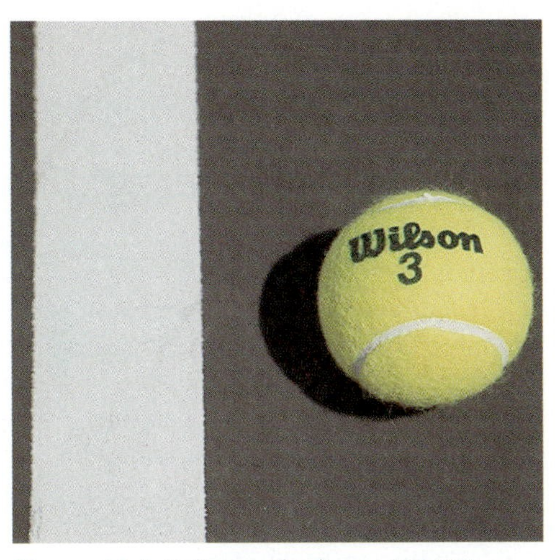

Figure 11.4 Ball near the line – "OUT."

or "out" on a line call. The rule and the etiquette application are simple. A ball that touches any part of a court boundary line is "in" (Figure 11.3) and any time a ball is wholly out by not touching any part of a boundary line, the call is "out" (Figure 11.4).

The problem arises when players don't see the ball and start guessing. There is no excuse for guessing; that call is specific! If a player does not see a ball as "out," the ball must be considered playable, and it is communicated as good by continued play. There never is a guess on a line call in tennis: The ball is always good unless it is seen to be out. When it is unknown if a ball is in or out on the last play of a rally or on a serve, there is an exception to the call with one option available. If a player does not see the ball, that player can request that the other player make the call. If the opposing player was *unsighted*, or doesn't wish to make the call, the call reverts to the original player, who then must accept the ball as being in bounds.

Besides playing a tennis match and acknowledging etiquette, *viewing a tennis match* requires certain behavior, as a spectator has the obligation to observe a match with respect for the players. No communication should take place between player and spectator, including the often asked question, "What's the score?" The spectator should be quiet, watch the play, and applaud a good point. Spectator disruptions are not approved at major tennis tournament matches (such as the U.S. Open, professional tour matches, and collegiate competition).

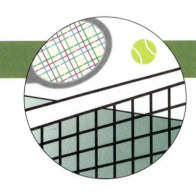

Learning Experience Reminders

Behavior on a Tennis Court

1. You must wear appropriate tennis shoes on a tennis court.
2. *Foot/racket pickup* and *ball-bounce pickup* are tennis skills related to picking a ball up off the court.
3. Wait until play has ceased on surrounding courts before walking onto your assigned tennis court.
4. *Ball please* and *thank you* are appropriate terms used to request a ball be returned from a court and for acknowledgment of the return.
5. A ball that is "in" play is acknowledged by continued play.
6. A ball that is "out" is acknowledged by stating OUT, or by pointing your index finger up.
7. A ball is always called in on any line call unless it is observed to be out.
8. If *unsighted,* it is appropriate to ask for an opponent to make a line call. If the opponent is *unsighted*, the ball must be ruled "in."

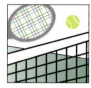

Interpreting Tennis Rules

The most applicable rules are interpreted on the following pages.

Tennis court dimensions are not important to know except in general terms, but the *terminology* of the court area is important. Key terms include baseline, center mark, back court, forecourt, right service court (deuce), left service court (ad), service line, and the alley. (See Figure 11.5.) Important differences in court dimension are the singles court size of 27' × 78' and the expanded doubles court size of 36' × 78'. The net is 3'6" high at the net supports and 3' high at the center. The net height at the center is of particular importance, because a lower or higher height would impact the rally between two players. The center net height is measured by placing one racket vertically at the center strap position and the other racket horizontally on top of the butt of the first racket's handle. Because most rackets today are oversized, the second string of the horizontal racket should be even with the top of the net for the net to be at the correct height (Figure 11.6).

36 ft
BASE LINE
CENTER MARK
BACK COURT
SERVICE LINE
RIGHT SERVICE COURT
LEFT SERVICE COURT
21 ft
4 ft 6 in
3 ft
ALLEY
SIDE LINE
POST
FORE COURT
NET
FORE COURT
POST
SERVICE
ALLEY
42 ft
LEFT SERVICE COURT
RIGHT SERVICE COURT
78 ft
13 ft 6 in
SERVICE LINE
27 ft
BACK COURT
18 ft
CENTER MARK
BASE LINE

Figure 11.5 Court dimensions.

The *choice of serve, side of court, and order of service* are significant choices to make at the beginning of a match. A decision on *choice of service and side of court* to begin play is made by spinning the racket or flipping a coin. A racket spin is done by placing the top of the racket head on the court. The opposing player calls either "up" or "down" to signify the position of the butt end of the racket when it falls to the court. The winner of the spin chooses, or requests the opponent to choose, the right to be the server or receiver. The player who doesn't have first choice then selects the end of the court to begin play. The choices may be reversed, with the winner of the spin choosing, or requesting the opponent to choose, the end to begin play, followed by the non-selecting player's choice of service or receiving serve.

A scenario might clarify the choices available: Player A wins the spin and states, "I will serve." Player B then states, "I will take the north side." A second scenario consists of Player A winning the spin and stating "your choice." Player B then states, "I will receive," followed by Player A's rejoinder of, "I will take the north side." The point is that the first player has the option of choosing service, receipt of serve, or end of the court, or of passing those choices on to the opponent.

The *order of serve* is a simple alternation of serves in either singles or doubles play. A player must serve through a full game, then exchange service with the opponent at the conclusion of that game. In doubles, the same situation exists except that teams alternate

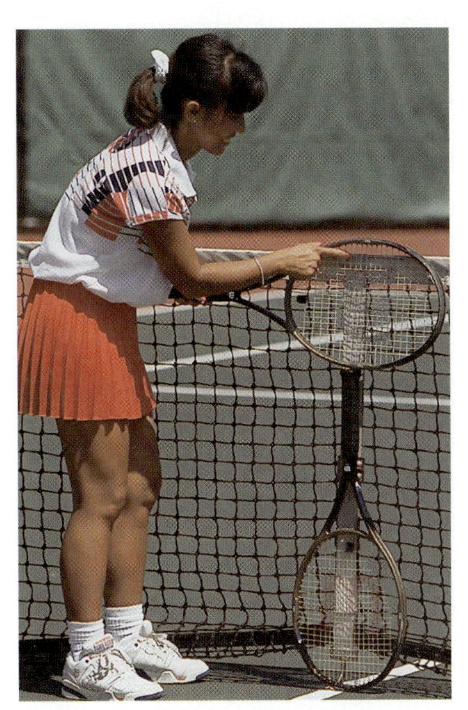

Figure 11.6 Measurement of the net.

serving following each game. If Team I serves the first game, Team II will serve game two, and the rotation continues. Player A of Team I serves the first game, Player A of Team II serves the second game, Player B of Team I serves the third game, and Player B of Team II serves the fourth game. The process repeats throughout the set, with Player A of Team I serving in game number five, etc.

Changing sides of the court has to be understood, as it has a significant effect on performance when playing outdoors. Without changing the side of court, one player always faces the sun or wind during play, giving the opponent an advantage. Rotation to different sides of the court occurs when the total number of games played is an odd number. If Player A (or Team I) serves from the north side of a court in game number one, sides will be exchanged for game number two. Player B (or Team II) then serves from the north side of the court, followed by Player A (or Team I) serving game three from the south end of the court. At the conclusion of game three, the players (or teams) again change sides of the court, with Player B (or Team II) serving from the south side of the court in game number four.

The sequence continues with players (or teams) exchanging sides of the court at the conclusion of the fifth, seventh, ninth, and eleventh, etc. total games played. At the end of a set, the players or teams change sides only if the total games are an odd number (such as 6-3 for a total of nine games). In singles, the rotation of server is continuous throughout play of a set. In doubles, the same principle applies with the rotation of each team in order of service.

Doubles play has rules to control the *location of players while serving and receiving*. As with singles once the serving rotation is determined for a team, as described, the rotation is permanent until a new set begins. The same is true for a team receiving the serve. One player always must receive from the right service court, and one player always must receive from the left service court. As with serving, a change in receiving order may occur only at the start of a new set.

Scoring a game, set, and match accurately is a major responsibility of both players. When viewed systematically, scoring is simple to understand. A tennis match is played in a sequence of points, games, sets, and match. It takes four points to win a game, (providing that the margin for victory is two points). A player must win six games to win a set, with a winning margin of two games. One exception to the rule is that if each player wins six games, a tiebreaker is played to determine the winner, and the final score always will be 7-6—a margin of only one game for the victory. In most situations, the winner of the match is the winner of two of three sets (professional players on the men's tour play three of five sets in some tournaments).

Each point won by a player is assigned a term, as given in Table 11.1. Scores to complete a set are one of the following: 6-0, 6-1, 6-2, 6-3, 6-4, 7-5, or 7-6. If a set score reaches 5-5 in terms of games won, two more games must be played. If one player wins both games, the final score is 7-5. If the players split games, the score will be 6-6, and a tiebreaker will be played. Examples of a match score are 6-2, 7-5, or 6-3, 1-6, 6-4. The winning player's scores are always identified first in a match; consequently, the 1-6 score of the second set

Table 11.1 Point Scoring

Point Number	Equivalent Term
First point	15
Second point	30
Third point	40
Fourth point	game (must win by two points)
No points	love
Tie score	deuce
After a tie at 4 points each—server leads	advantage in (AD IN)
After a tie at 4 points each—receiver leads	advantage out (AD OUT)

of the second match example indicates that the winner of the match lost the second set by a 6-to-1 game score.

A *tie-breaker* is played only when a set is tied 6-6. There are several forms of tie-breakers, including what are called 7, 9, and 12-point tie-breakers. The 12-point tie-breaker is the most popular. The winner of the tie-breaker is the first player to win 7 points with a winning margin of 2 points. If the score in a tie-breaker reaches 6-6 in number of points scored, the players must continue the game until one player has a winning margin of 2 points (8-6, 9-7, 10-8, etc.). A 5-5 point score can still produce a winner at 7 points if one player wins the next 2 points.

The server for the first point of a tie-breaker is designated by the continued rotation of serve per the normal rotation. The first server serves only one point—from the deuce service court. The second server then begins the serve from the ad service court. This server serves one point from the ad service court, then one point from the deuce service court. In singles, the service order now reverts to the first server, who begins service for one point from the ad service court, then moves to the deuce service court for the second point. The players exchange ends of court after a total of 6 points are played, with a continuation of the rotation.

In doubles play rotation, movement is the same as in singles except that four players are involved instead of two. Player A of Team I serves point number 1 to the deuce service court. Player A of Team II serves 2 points—one from the ad service court followed by one from the deuce service court. Player B of Team I then serves points 1 and 2 from the respective ad and deuce service courts, and the rotation continues to Player B of Team II, and so on. The tie-breaker singles and doubles rotation is presented in Table 11.2.

Placing the ball in play is sometimes misunderstood, so a clarification is in order. The start of every game is initiated with a service to the right service court. The service point, both in a regular game situation and in a tie-breaker, allows a maximum of two opportunities to hit a legal serve. The one exception is when a *let* is played. A let is a serve that is hit in all ways legally except that the ball touches the net on its path to the service court. A let permits the server to repeat that one serve, and any number of lets may be played in succession.

Once the *ball is in play*, a player must hit it over the net so it lands in the opponent's court. During a rally, players may hit the ball on the bounce or during flight (return of serve follows the bounce of the ball in the service court). A point is lost when a ball bounces twice before being returned, a ball lands out of the court boundaries on the fly, a ball hits the net and does not go over the net, and two serves (excluding a let) in a row do not fall into the appropriate service court.

A serve that does not strike the appropriate service court is called a *fault*. Servers also fault by swinging and missing a service toss and by stepping on the baseline during the serve. Touching the service line on a serve is called a *foot fault*. Many players have the habit of touching the baseline in this manner, and legally that is not accepted. If a player strikes the ball, then comes down on the baseline, the serve is legal. When the foot touches the line while the racket is in contact with the ball, or prior to hitting the ball, the serve is lost. In "friendly" play, foot faults usually are

Table 11.2 Tie-Breaker Server Rotation

Singles

Player Number	Service Court to Serve To	Number of Points
1	Deuce Service Court	1
2	Ad Service Court	1
2	Deuce Service Court	1
1	Ad Service Court	1
1	Deuce Service Court	1
2	Ad Service Court	1
change sides of court		
2	Deuce Service Court	1
1	Ad Service Court	1
1	Deuce Service Court	1
etc.		

Doubles

Team No.	Player No.	Service Court to Serve To	Number of Points
1	A	Deuce Service Court	1
2	A	Ad Service Court	1
2	A	Deuce Service Court	1
1	B	Ad Service Court	1
1	B	Deuce Service Court	1
2	B	Ad Service Court	1
change sides of court			
2	B	Deuce Service Court	1
1	A	Ad Service Court	1
1	A	Deuce Service Court	1
etc.			

ignored because they are difficult to see. But the server has a responsibility to avoid the illegal foot position.

Tennis has numerous rule infractions and interpretations. Some of them are listed below.*

1. Hitting a volley prior to the ball crossing the net is a loss of point except when a ball crosses the net and the wind blows or backspin carries the ball back across the net.
2. A ball that strikes the player or the player's clothing carries a loss of a point.
3. Throwing a racket at the ball carries the penalty of loss of the point.
4. If the ball strikes the net (excluding the serve) and continues on into the opponent's court, the ball is still in play.
5. If a doubles player hits the partner with the ball, the team loses the point.
6. A receiver of a serve must be ready for service or the serve must be repeated.
7. An opposing player may not hinder an opponent by distracting the opponent; however, partners on a doubles team are allowed to talk to each other when the ball is directed to their side of the court.
8. A player hit by a ball prior to the ball striking the court loses that point even if the ball is going to land out of bounds.
9. After the conclusion of a tie-breaker, the first server of the next set is the player who did not serve first in the previously played set.

The beginning tennis player should remember to treat the rules with respect and take them seriously so the game will be enjoyable.

* A review of tennis rules is found in the Appendix through permission of the United States Tennis Association, Publications Department, 70 West Red Oak Lane, White Plains, New York 10604.

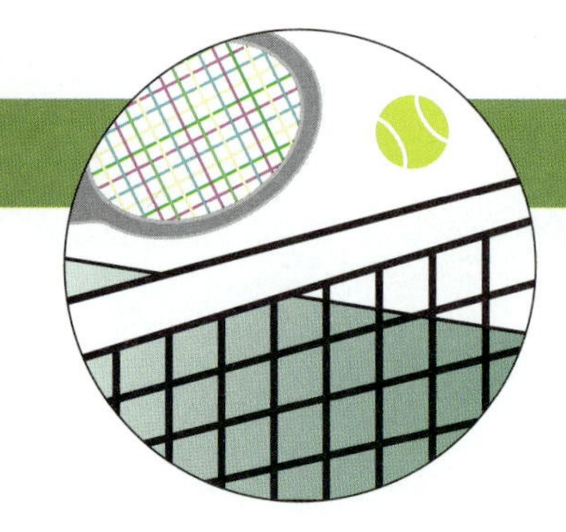

Learning Experience Reminders

Interpreting Tennis Rules

1. On the spin of the racket, the winner has the choice of electing to serve, receive, side of court, or to pass the choice to the opponent.
2. The order of service is a simple alternation of serves after each game is played.
3. Players change sides of the court on uneven total number of games.
4. A serve that doesn't strike the appropriate court is called a *fault*.
5. A set score is the first to six games with a winning margin of two games.
6. A score of 6–6 requires a 12-point tie-breaker.
7. A tie-breaker is played to seven points with a winning margin of two points.

Check Points

1. A ball that strikes the line of the court during play is considered
   a. a replay.
   b. out.
   c. in.
   d. none of the above.

2. Sides of the tennis court are changed by players after
   a. every third game.
   b. every odd total number of games accumulated by both players.
   c. every other game played.
   d. a player has an odd total number of games played.

3. Typically an official legal score of a match is
   a. 6-3, 3-6, 6-5.
   b. 7-6, 3-6, 6-3.
   c. 5-6, 7-6, 7-5.
   d. 7-5, 5-7, 7-1.

4. One of the scores used in a game as identified below is not a legal score:
   a. Deuce
   b. Advantage In (Ad In)
   c. 15-love
   d. 45-15

5. A let is a
   a. serve that is hit legally but touches the net before falling into the opponent's service court.
   b. replay of a point when a call is considered in doubt.
   c. term used to say "take two."
   d. fault.

6. Hitting a volley shot while the ball is on the opponent's side of the court is considered
   a. loss of point.
   b. fair play.
   c. a replay.
   d. a mistake.

7. A tie-breaker is
   a. played when the game score is tied 5-5.
   b. played when the game score is tied 6-6.
   c. played any time there is a tie score in a game.
   d. played until a player is ahead by two points.

8. It is poor etiquette to
   a. talk on the court.
   b. not wear appropriate tennis clothing.
   c. throw a tennis racket in anger.
   d. all of the above.

Answers to Check Points can be found on page 145.

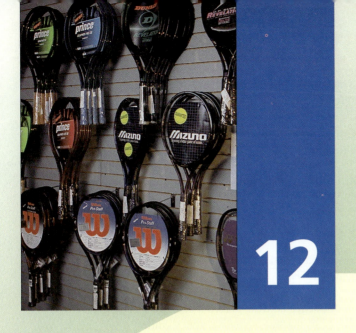

12

Tennis Courts, Equipment Design, Tournament Competition, and Resources

At the beginning of the new millennium tennis has experienced a modest renewal of participation. Sales of balls, a barometer of a sport's health, are up 4.8 percent within the tennis market (All in Favor, *Tennis*, December/January 2000, p. 18). This growth has included all ages, but the most dramatic is that 95 percent of newcomers to tennis are under 35 years of age and 54 percent of them are female (All in Favor, p. 18). As your tennis participation expands, your improvement of skills and knowledge base will be part of your overall continual development. Part of what is left in order to be totally informed regarding tennis is a coverage of intangibles related to how a tennis court is designed, which tennis racket to select, how to get involved in tennis competition, and what additional resources are available.

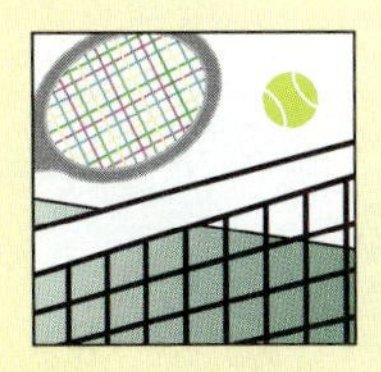

The Tennis Court

Tennis courts have five categories of *surfaces. Grass courts* are traditional but have outlived their usefulness. Wimbledon is the only major professional tournament still played on a grass court. For normal play, the upkeep and expense involved in maintaining the surface is nearly prohibitive. Few grass courts are found in the United States, and they are nearly extinct worldwide. Soft courts are popular throughout much of the world and east of the Mississippi River in the United States. The typical soft court is a *clay court*. Its surface provides a high bounce and a slow ball that encourage long baseline rallies. The term "clay court" is descriptive of what used to be the surface composition of a claylike material and coarse sand. A number of other claylike surfaces include shale and synthetic composites that play like clay.

Today a "clay court" is composed of a two-layer base of crushed limestone with ⅛" of brick dust, or a one-layer base of crushed and firmly packed stone material called "fast-dry." The clay surface poses a maintenance problem when reasonable play conditions are desired, because it requires watering and rolling, but the more recent surfaces are easier to maintain.

The *all-weather* or *hard court* surfaces are extremely popular in the United States. This is the surface with which most developing players are familiar. The surface may be composed of asphalt or cement topping, which contributes to ease of maintenance and cleaning. Courts with this surface are usually public, and they are easily recognized because they give a uniform, fast-bouncing action to the ball.

The *synthetic surface* is another type of hard surface that many players have used on their college campuses. The synthetic court surface usually is composed of a series of granulated rubber particles pulled together with an epoxy resin sprayed with a polyurethane coating and laid on a porous foundation. The court is designed to play like a naturally made court, but it is free of maintenance and cleaning problems. The synthetic court is called the Mercury Grassphalts Court, and it is one of several innovative courts.

Another court surface, called a *carpet,* is used for indoor tournaments on the professional tennis tour. The carpet is laid over whatever existing surface is available, and that combination produces a fast court that encourages a serve-volley game.

Hard and synthetic courts are smoothed or roughened depending on the amount of play and rally circumstances expected in a given geographical area. A high-altitude location will tend to have a roughened surface to provide more opportunity for baseline play. Courts in low altitudes will tend to have a smoother surface, as the density of the air allows for more rally situations.

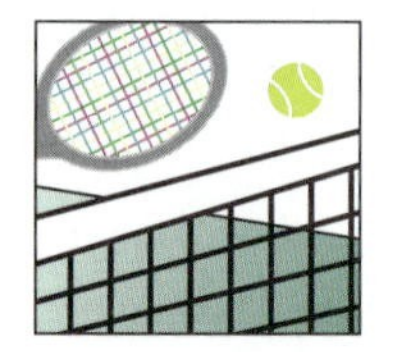

Tennis Equipment

At one time tennis rackets were made of various woods, including ash or beech and combinations of perhaps sycamore, obeche, or mahogany. The wood racket was handcrafted, and the number of wood laminations indicated the quality of the racket. Wood rackets now are obsolete, replaced by modern technology's new materials (Figure 12.1).

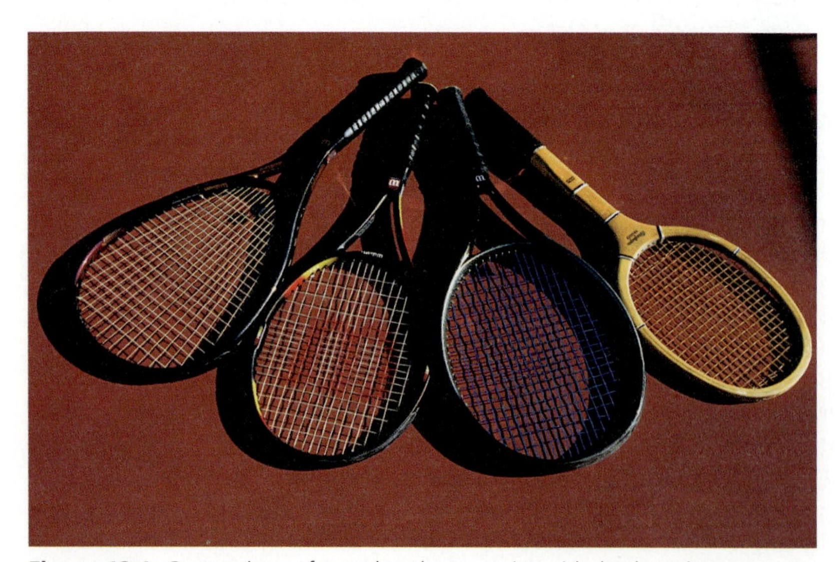

Figure 12.1 Comparison of wood and composite wide-body rackets.

Following wood, tennis rackets were designed with metal and aluminum materials, but these too are, if not obsolete, all but obsolete. The modern tennis racket of the 21st century is made of new materials like polyurethane, carbon, Kevlar, fiberglass, graphite, and titanium. These materials provide more power with control, reduced racket vibration and shock, and a lighter racket for quicker reaction for stroke readiness.

Wide-body rackets emerged as a popular racket just a few years ago.

They provided maximum power with increased control. They bent less at contact, providing more energy to the ball. The most recent technology has designed a racket that is more elongated than any previous racket. These long-body or *extra-long rackets* provide increased power, enhanced spin, and far more leverage when striking the ball. They enable a player to reach balls hit wide to them, and because they are so light they provide the player with the ability to move the racket more quickly in order to set up to hit a shot. The extra-long rackets (also called *stretch* rackets) are typically made of titanium and graphite, and they range from 27.5" to 29" in length (Figure 12.2).

Head size for today's rackets can range generally from 85 sq." to 125 sq." The larger the head size, the more power generated; the smaller, the more control. A mixture of power and control for head size should be between 100 sq." and 105 sq.". The heavier a racket the more power, but today's rackets are all basically light. Weight ranges from 8–9.8 oz. for super light-weight rackets, 9.9–10.8 oz. for light rackets, and 10.9 oz. and above for heavy rackets. A light racket provides greater maneuverability, while concealing shock and vibration. A typical example of a racket prototype might be 27.5 sq." in length, 105 sq." racket face, a weight of 9.25 oz., and the technology of a racket made of titanium mesh (this is titanium woven in with graphite). This prototype, as reflective of extra-long rackets, is now the most widely sold single type of racket.

Rackets also have changed in size over the last 15 years, ranging from a regular size to a mid-size to an oversize racket. The Prince racket was the first oversize racket, and now all companies are manufacturing oversize rackets. Shapes of racket heads range from pear-shaped to round to oblong.

Some terms used to describe the racket and what it is designed to accomplish are as follows. A *stiff* racket offers less control and more power than a flexible racket. A *flexible* racket will provide more control but less power. Twenty-seven-inch-length rackets often have more flexibility while wide-body and extra-long rackets tend to be more stiff, thus providing more power. A rule of thumb is that a racket length of 28.5" to 29" is a stiff, powerful racket; a length of 27.5" to 28" provides a combination of power and control; and a 27" length is designed more for control. Typically the beginner needs a flexible racket with some stiffness to provide a little power or zip to the ball. As skill is developed, a decision on more stiffness or more flexibility becomes a personal choice.

A flexible racket also tends to reduce vibration and shock, which decreases the potential for developing *tennis elbow* (tendonitis). *Vibration* is a term that defines a lingering back and forth motion of the racket frame and strings after the ball has been hit. Torque from vibration is then transferred to the elbow. *Shock* describes the contact of string to ball, and when a ball is hit off-center a twisting action occurs that also generates a torque action that is transferred to the elbow. In both cases the transfer of shock or vibration to the elbow is a contributing factor to tendonitis of the elbow.

Other terms applied to the function of a tennis racket are *power, control, feel, maneuverability, comfort, and stability*. These terms are also used in tennis publications and racket advertisements. Rackets are also characterized as head light, balanced, and head heavy. They are light, semi-light, and medium in weight.

The ideal area for contact with the ball is called a *sweet spot* (Figure 12.3). It can be located below center, above center, elongated, and wide across center. Most sweet spots are located at center and above center, but they do vary. Sweet spots basically allow for a shot that is hit not quite on center to still rebound effectively. The larger the oversize racket, the larger the sweet spot, so the more chance for success. A stiffer racket stretches the sweet spot, and lowering of the string tension increases a sweet spot's effectiveness (Sweet Talk About the Sweet Spot, by S. Chirls, *Tennis,* June 1992, p. 77). Racket grips are measured from $4\frac{1}{8}$" to $4\frac{7}{8}$", with the widely used grips ranging from $4\frac{1}{4}$" to $4\frac{5}{8}$". Grips are composed of

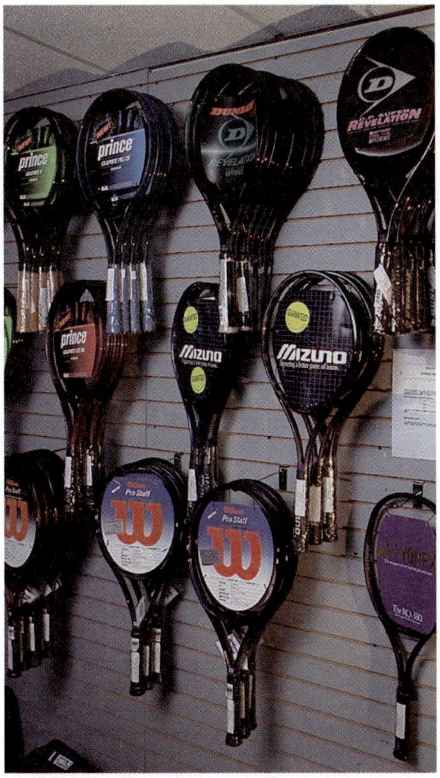

Figure 12.2 Assorted tennis rackets.

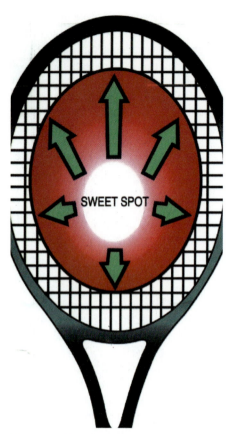

Figure 12.3 Sweet spot.

several types of material, but a good recommendation is to find a cushioned grip with a tacky feel that is perforated or embossed (Gear Guide 99 Rackets, by D. Dusek, *Tennis*, April 1999, p. 69). A grip should feel comfortable. Grip size is determined by a simple measure. Grasp the racket handle with an eastern forehand grip. When looking at your grip there should be a space between the fingertips of your hand and the palm. If you can place the index finger of your non-racket hand snugly between the fingertips and the palm of the racket hand, and the grip feels comfortable, you have a fit.

Rackets are purchased unstrung if they are of reasonable quality, and a decision has to be made regarding the type of string to use. When *selecting string*, you need to be aware that tennis rackets are strung with gut or synthetic nylon strings. Gut is a high quality string that has limited durability but great feel. Synthetic strings are designed to replace the feel of gut with a far more durable quality. There are a number of synthetic strings that provide a combination of durability and holding their tension. There are three types: monofilaments, multifilaments, and aramids. Monofilaments are composed of a single, solid-core string, encased in a thin outer cover. They are the most popular string for a tennis racket since they hold their tension and provide both durability and playability. Multifilaments consist of thousands of individual fibers woven together to form one piece of a string. They provide more power, but they are not as durable as monofilaments. Aramids are made of Kevlar or Technora and they are the most durable. However, they do not provide much in the way of feel or power (String Fever, by D. Dusek, *Tennis*, April 1999, pp. 64–65).

Racket strings also are defined by size, and when a racket is strung the string is measured in amount of tension applied to the racket. String size is measured in gauge. A thinner string (e.g., 16 gauge) increases power and spin, while a thicker 15 gauge is more durable, but generates less power and spin. String tension is measured in pounds of tension. The higher the tension the more control, but the less durability (string breaks). Lower tension enhances power (Figure 12.4).

Tennis rackets are expensive. So are strings. A high performance tennis racket usually retails for $135–300, and to string a racket is an added $18–35. Based on the above discussion regarding rackets, you have enough information to make a decision on what kind of racket to purchase. As a beginner you don't need a $300 racket. You don't even need a $135 racket. But you do need a racket that has as many qualities as possible that meet your needs, and one that is within your price range. Look for a racket with flexibility (control) and a good feel. Check to determine what features the racket may have that are similar to what has been described. And, check out the cost. Most sporting goods stores have "loaners," which allows you to try out their rackets. Take advantage of the loaner opportunity and play with different rackets. Pick one in your price range that meets your needs. When you buy a racket the chances are that you will also have to have it strung, so apply the information above to the choice of a string. You are best off with a monofilament string, but select one in your price range when first starting out as a player.

Tennis ball selection is another expense of tennis play. A can of tennis balls ranges from $2 to $4 and lasts only two to three hours of play (if play is continuous and skillful). Discount stores

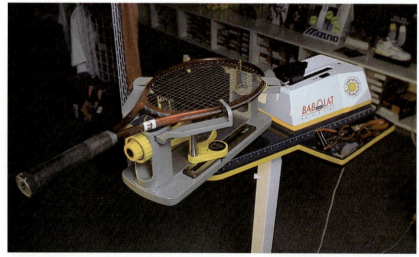

Figure 12.4 Tennis stringer.

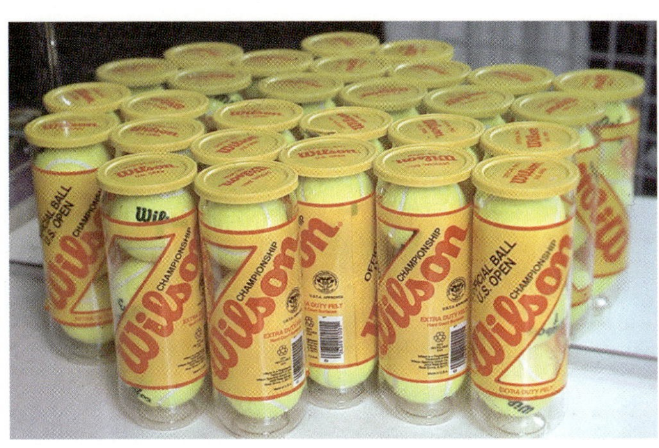

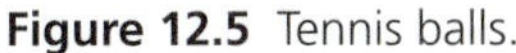
Figure 12.5 Tennis balls.

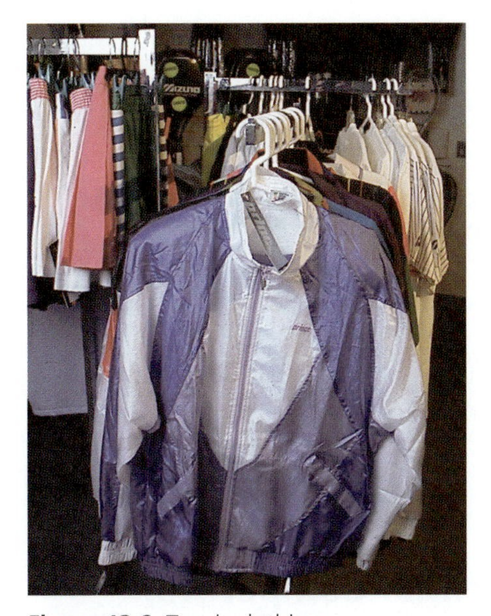

Figure 12.6 Tennis clothing.

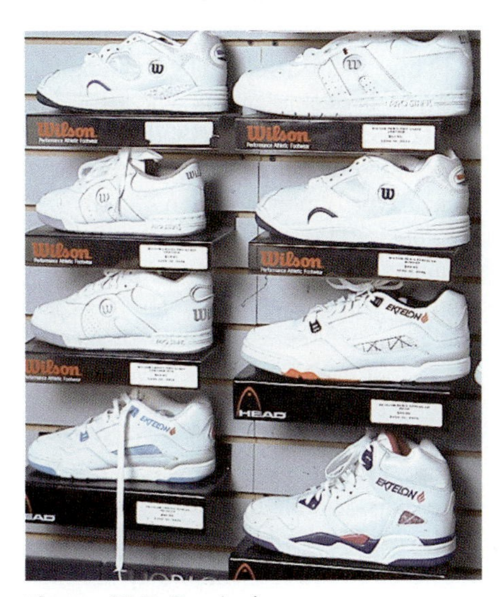

Figure 12.7 Tennis shoes.

and major sporting goods dealers often run specials for less than $2, but the player should be aware that there are many types of tennis balls for that price.

For true bounce and longevity, balls should be a name-brand (Figure 12.5), and flaws or unknowns should be ignored. Tennis balls are made of a molded rubber. Two cups are cemented together, covered with a wool material, and inflated with compressed air. They are then placed in a pressure-sealed container, ready to be used when you are ready to play with a new group of three tennis balls. Pressurized balls don't last as long as hard-core rubber tennis balls, but they are easier on elbows and they play with a true bounce. The hard-core ball has a greater life expectancy but begins to bounce too high after extensive play. If players live at high altitude, they should purchase only high-altitude balls. There is a difference in ball bounce when playing at sea-level and playing at 5,000 feet. Tennis balls designed for sea-level play bounce much higher at altitude, so a high-altitude ball allows for a bounce adjustment.

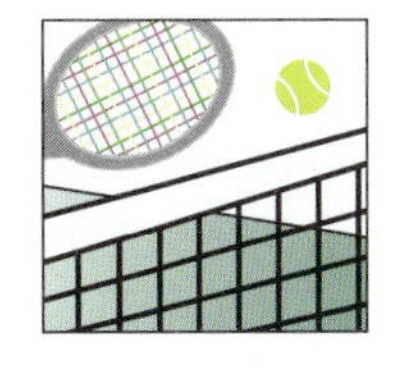

Tennis Clothing

The selection of *tennis shorts or skirt and a tennis top* is totally up to the player. An investment of $10 for a pair of shorts and a tee-shirt to an expenditure in excess of $200 for designer tennis shorts and top is the range for purchase of clothing (Figure 12.6).

Tennis shoes (Figure 12.7) are a different matter expense-wise. They are never inexpensive. The tennis shoe is designed for use on a tennis court and for the forward, backward, and lateral movement of the player.

Tennis shoes are sized like regular shoes, and some tennis shoes also are measured in widths of wide or narrow. A tennis shoe must have a firm insole and a good arch support. The back portion of the shoe that rests against the Achilles tendon has to be soft and pliable, with an absorbent heel cushion. A tennis shoe also should have durability, be comfortable, and have good traction.

The toe of a tennis shoe is vulnerable to dragging and wearing out. A check to determine how much abuse the toe of the shoe will take will help the player avoid a new purchase every 3 or 4 weeks. If the tennis shoe fits the player, if it provides good support, and if it won't wear out in a few weeks, it probably will cost $45 or more, but it is what a player ought to buy.

Socks are part of dressing for tennis. Tennis socks are not all that expensive, but they need to be selected carefully. You want a sock that leaves a little room for your toes, moves moisture away from your skin to an outer layer of the cotton of the sock, and has a cushion for the soles of your feet. Look for a tennis sock. One that is made of cotton has either a polyester fiber or a polyolefin fiber called Drylon to eliminate the excess sweat that contributes to blisters. Finally, in order to be fashionable, select either a low or below-the-calf length sock that is white.

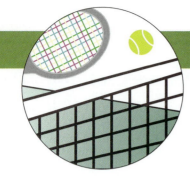

Learning Experience Reminders

Tennis Courts and Equipment

1. Tennis courts come in many surfaces, but the most popular is either an all weather (hard court) or a synthetic hard court surface.
2. Extra-long tennis rackets are the most popular and effective racket today. They are considered to be a stiff racket that allows the player more reach and greater power.
3. Stiff rackets offer less control and more power—flexible rackets provide more control and less power.
4. Rackets are rated based on such terms as control, maneuverability, vibration, shock, comfort, and feel.
5. The most durable, yet quality synthetic string designed for a tennis racket is a monofilament string, known for its durability and playability.
6. Tennis strings are measured by their gauge size and rackets are strung based on number of pounds of tension.
7. You can measure the fit of your tennis racket grip by placing your non-racket index finger in the space between the fingertips and the palm of your racket-hand grip.

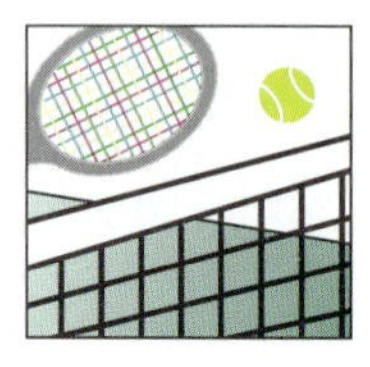

How to Get Started in Tennis Competition

A wide assortment of *tennis tournaments* take place in the United States. Those that are of most interest to the beginning player are associated with recreation programs, college campus recreation programs, city tournaments, and club programs. There are tournaments for all types of players, from the novice who is just learning to hit a volley shot without ducking to a highly skilled player. Tournaments usually are ladder tournaments, single-elimination or double-elimination tournaments, inter-club, or social round robin mixed doubles tournaments. Some are more competitive than others, and the player has to understand which are the more competitive and which are designed as social functions. With the proper perspective, all are fun to play.

Ladder tournaments are found in all situations, including most campus recreation programs. They allow players to play at their own level by challenging individuals of similar skill who are positioned higher on the ladder. Club competition is a highly competitive league-type of play in which records are kept and league standings are established. Rewards are given to the team finishing first and second in a league, with a team or teams advancing to another round of competitive play.

Many programs have single- and double-elimination tournaments with ratings, including novice, C, B, A, and open divisions. Most are sanctioned by the *United States Tennis Association* (USTA) and require membership in that organization to participate. Most USTA tournaments are identified by a rating scale, usually through the USTA National Tennis Rating Program. There are also age-division tournaments that have an open competition under 35 years of age, then age divisions, including 35 and over, 40 and over, 45 and over, 55 and over, 65 and over, etc.

Most single- or double-elimination tournaments are played through a period of a 3-day weekend, and a player may play five or six matches if the play continues all the way to the championship. The number of matches depends on the size of a draw for the tournament (a draw is the number of entrants).

The *USTA National Rating Program* has become a popular device for rating players, not only for tournament play but also for social play, to help people identify their level of skill so a match can be an equal competition. The rating scale is established from 1.0 through 7.0. The lower the rating classification, the closer to a beginner, and the higher the rating, the closer to a professional player. The classification of 3.0 to 5.0 seems to be the typical club player rating and is probably a major first goal for a developing player. The beginner usually starts at the 1.0 through the 2.5 level and progresses rapidly through the early classifications. The rating program provides a descriptive version of each classification, and many tennis teachers now are able to use the rating objectively and systematically. So you can rate yourself, Table 12.1 gives you a view of the National Tennis Rating Program categories.

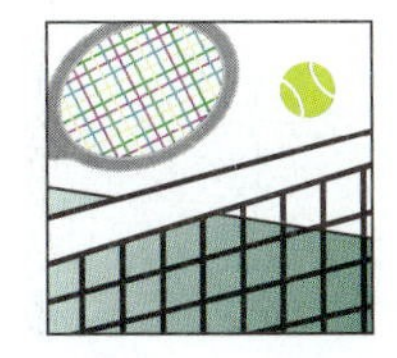

Tennis Resources

Numerous textbooks, periodicals, videos, and the internet are available to help you to learn to play tennis and to continue to develop skills and knowledge associated with the game. Also, tennis associations have been formed to promote the game in community and tennis club environments.

The USTA is the most well known agency or organization with the goal of promoting tennis at every level of play and competition. To play in sanctioned USTA tournaments, membership in the USTA is required. The same group sponsors the National Tennis Rating Program, mentioned earlier. The USTA also publishes *Tennis* and *Tennis USTA.* Other publications produced by the USTA include general textbooks, material for group instruction and for teaching tennis, strategy material, program planning, tennis information, and rules/ regulations.

A membership with the USTA is a small investment for the beginning player. Membership is inexpensive. The benefits for a serious player are excellent, and the organization really does function for the promotion of tennis. The USTA membership address is: USTA/Membership Department/ 70 West Red Oak Lane/ White Plains, NY 10604.

The USTA also has *sectional offices and state organizations.* The major role of these groups is to promote tennis. They also sponsor tennis tournaments. With a USTA membership, the member also receives newsletters from sectional and state organizations. The local, state, and sectional organizations also rate players and carry on the work of the USTA.

Tennis publications and the internet provide a plethora of instructional material for the avid tennis player. Of the many tennis books on the market, five that serve as a nice supplement to *Game, Set, Match* are:

1. *Tennis 2000-Strokes, Strategy, and Psychology* by Vic Braden and Bill Burns (1998, Boston: Little, Brown & Co., 284 pp.)

   The book covers a biomechanical analysis of tennis fundamentals through photos, and provides a complete analysis of tennis.

2. *International Book of Tennis Drills* produced by the U S Professional Tennis Registry (1998, Chicago: Triumph Books, 289 pp.)

   An extensive series of tennis drills to enhance tennis skill development and strategy insight.

3. *Sports Psychology Library: Tennis* by Judy L. Van Raalte and Carrie Silver-Bernstein (1999, Morgantown, WV: Fitness Information Technology, Inc., 135 pp.)

   Covers mental skills, building confidence, improving concentration, how to focus, how to play big matches, etc.

4. *The Inner Game of Tennis Revised* by W. Timothy Gallwey (1997, New York: Random House, 122 pp.)

   A revised version of Gallwey's classic tennis book on mind, body connection, and relaxed concentration.

5. *Tennis Injury Handbook: Professional Advice for Amateur Athletes* by Allan M. Levy, M.D. and Mark L. Feurst (1999, New York: John Wiley & Sons, 185 pp.)

   Includes techniques for stretching, conditioning, rehabilitation, how to avoid court-side aches and pains, and how to recognize and heal injuries.

Table 12.1 NTRP Rating Categories

Rating	Description
1.0	This player is just starting to play tennis.
1.5	This player has limited experience and is still working primarily on getting the ball into play.
2.0	This player needs on-court experience. This player has obvious stroke weaknesses but is familiar with basic positions for singles and doubles play.
2.5	This player is learning to judge where the ball is going although court coverage is weak. This player can sustain a rally of slow pace with other players of the same ability.
3.0	This player is consistent when hitting medium paced shots, but is not comfortable with all strokes and lacks control when trying for directional intent, depth, or power.
3.5	This player has achieved improved stroke dependability and direction on moderate shots, but still lacks depth and variety. This player is starting to exhibit more aggressive net play, has improved court coverage, and is developing teamwork in doubles.
4.0	This player has dependable strokes, including directional intent and depth on both forehand and backhand sides on moderate shots, plus the ability to use lobs, overheads, approach shots and volleys with some success. This player occasionally forces errors when serving and teamwork in doubles is evident.
4.5	This player has begun to master the use of power and spins and is beginning to handle pace, has sound footwork, can control depth of shots, and is beginning to vary tactics according to opponents. This player can hit first serves with power and accuracy and place the second serve and is able to rush net successfully.
5.0	This player has good shot anticipation and frequently has an outstanding shot or exceptional consistency around which a game may be structured. This player can regularly hit winners or force errors off of short balls and can put away volleys, can successfully execute lobs, drop shots, half volleys and overhead smashes and has good depth and spin on most second serves.
5.5	This player has developed power and/or consistency as a major weapon. This player can vary strategies and styles of play in a competitive situation and hits dependable shots in a stress situation.
6.0 to 7.0	These players will generally not need NTRP ratings. Rankings or past rankings will speak for themselves. The 6.0 player typically has had intensive training for national tournament competition at the junior level and collegiate levels and has obtained a sectional and/or national ranking. The 6.5 player has a reasonable chance of succeeding at the 7.0 level and has extensive satellite tournament experience. The 7.0 is a world class player who is committed to tournament competition on the international level and whose major source of income is tournament prize winnings.

Once you have determined your rating, write the appropriate rating number on your USTA membership card under "NTRP". In order to participate in USTA league or NTRP tournaments, you must get verified by a sectionally approved NTRP verifier. Your NTRP rating will help you find challenging opponents no matter where you play. (Printed with permission of the USTA)

The internet is a reference source that will continually change, but it is a fascinating option for finding information and instructional help regarding tennis. If you are interested in information associated with tennis results and stories you have an assortment of major choices that include:

ESPN. Sportszone
Excite Sports
CNN/SI
Foxsports.com
CBS.Sportsline
MSNBC - Sports
USA Today. Tennis
Nando-Tennis

If you are interested in websites with instructional analysis, general tennis information, and new ideas regarding tennis try:

1. *Welcome to Tennis One* (www.tennisone.com)

   An excellent tennis instructional site.

2. *The Tennis Serve* Center Court for Tennis on the Internet (www.tennisserver. com)

   A newsletter website that is a great source for just about any instructional or informational item that might be of interest.

3. *Tennis Links-The Ultimate Website* (www. tennislinks.com)

   An excellent source of tennis links for equipment, tournaments, and general tennis information.

4. *Tennis Direct* (tennisdirect.com)

   An on-line tennis catalog that includes an extensive list of videos, tennis instructional aids, equipment, and clothing. There is also a mailing address for a hard copy: Tennis Direct/1463 Premier/Troy, MI 48084.

5. *International Hall of Fame* (www.tennisfame.org)

   The official site for the Tennis Hall of Fame.

6. *United States Tennis Association* (www.usta.com)

   The official site for the USTA office that includes extensive information regarding membership, the organization, and countless other tennis related information.

Television also provides extensive coverage of major tennis events including the Australian Open, French Open, U.S. Open, and Wimbledon. In addition, smaller tournaments surface on television, along with an occasional collegiate tennis competition. These are also instructional in the sense that, by watching skilled players, you can pick up new techniques, skills, and a feeling for the game.

A final but important resource for a player who continues to develop after group instruction at the college/university level is a *teaching professional*. As an occasional review, or to have technique analyzed, a teaching professional is of value. The professional should be able to present the mechanics of stroke execution in an interesting and informative way, and should be able to analyze stroke mistakes.

Selecting of the proper resources is important and must be done with some insight. A player needs to keep up with changes in tennis, and to have enough knowledge to discuss tennis intelligently.

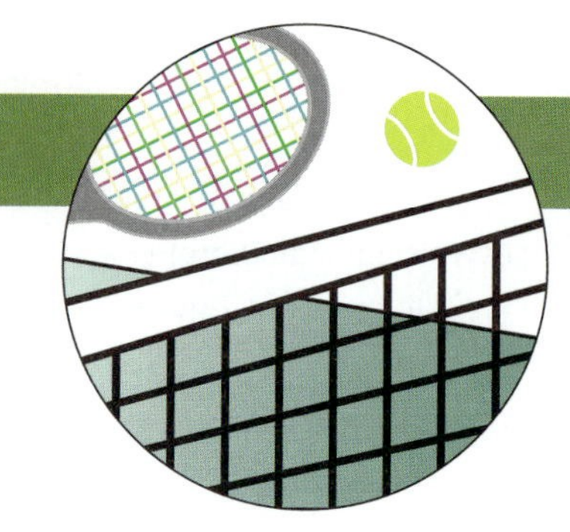

Learning Experience Reminders

Tennis Competition and Resources

1. Be sure to read and identify NTRP Rating Categories. Identify where you fit and use that rating as a measure for improvement.
2. Once you have acquired a skill level where you are comfortable with your play, seek out a tennis tournament that fits your skill level and play.
3. There are countless tennis resources. Refer back to the list of supplemental textbooks, and use the website addresses to explore the tennis internet.

Check Points

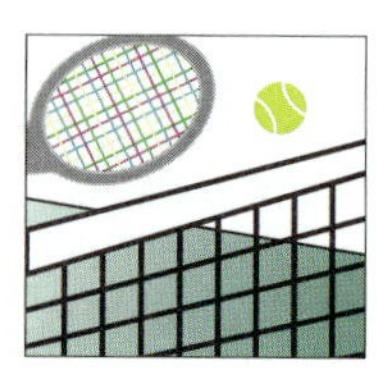

1. The most popular tennis court surface used by most players is
   a. clay.
   b. grass.
   c. all-weather (hard court).
   d. synthetic.
2. A stiff racket has
   a. more control and less power than a flexible racket.
   b. more power and less control than a flexible racket.
   c. both more control and power than a flexible racket.
   d. both less control and power than a flexible racket.
3. A typical racket grip size ranges from
   a. 4⅛ to 4⅝ inches.
   b. 4⅜ to 4⅞ inches.
   c. 4⅛ to 4⅞ inches.
   d. 4⅛ to 4⅜ inches.
4. The sweet spot of a tennis racket is found
   a. above center.
   b. in the center.
   c. wide across the center.
   d. all of the above.
5. Important characteristics to consider when buying tennis shoes include:
   a. Firm insole and good arch support.
   b. Aborsbent heel cushion and a soft, pliable heel cup.
   c. Neither a or b.
   d. Both a and b.
6. The most resilient, long lasting, and inexpensive string used for a tennis racket is
   a. synthetic gut.
   b. gut.
   c. nylon.
   d. none of the above.
7. A player who is consistent when hitting medium paced shots, but is not comfortable with all strokes and lacks control when trying for directional intent, depth, or power is rated as
   a. a 2.5 player.
   b. a 3.0 player.
   c. a 3.5 player.
   d. a 4.0 player.
8. The USTA's major publication is
   a. International Tennis Players.
   b. Tennis.
   c. Racquet.
   d. World Tennis.
9. Other tennis resources besides magazines include:
   a. Nando—Tennis
   b. www.tennislinks.com
   c. Gallwey's *The Inner Game of Tennis*
   d. All of the above
10. An instructional source for tennis players following taking a class is
    a. a teaching professional.
    b. playing matches.
    c. neither a or b.
    d. both a and b.

Answers to Check Points can be found on page 145

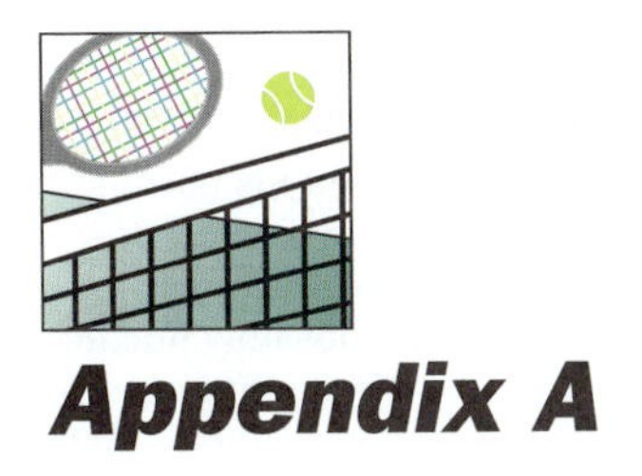

Appendix A

USTA's The Code: The Player's Guide for Unofficiated Matches

Preface

When your serve hits your partner stationed at the net, is it a let, fault, or loss of point? Likewise, what is the ruling when your serve, before touching the ground, hits an opponent who is standing back of the baseline. The answers to these questions are obvious to anyone who knows the fundamentals of tennis, but it is surprising the number of players who don't know these fundamentals. All players have a responsibility to be familiar with the basic rules and customs of tennis. Further, it can be distressing to your opponent when he makes a decision in accordance with a rule and you protest with the remark: "Well, I never heard of that rule before!" Ignorance of the rules constitutes a delinquency on the part of a player and often spoils an otherwise good match.

What is written here constitutes the essentials of The Code, a summary of procedures and unwritten rules which custom and tradition dictate all players should follow. No system of rules will cover every specific problem or situation that may arise. If players of good will follow the principles of The Code, they should always be able to reach an agreement, while at the same time making tennis more fun and a better game for all. The principles set forth in The Code shall apply in cases not specifically covered by The Rules of Tennis and USTA Regulations.

Before reading this you might well ask yourself: Since we have a book that contains all the rules of tennis, why do we need a code? Isn't it sufficient to know and understand all the rules? There are a number of things not specifically set forth in the rules that are covered by custom and tradition only. For example, if you have a doubt on a line call, your opponent gets the benefit of the doubt. Can you find that in the rules? Further, custom dictates the standard procedures that players will use in reaching decisions. These are the reasons why we need a code.

—Col. Nick Powel

Note: This edition of The Code is an adaptation of the original, which was written by Colonel Nicholas E. Powel.

General Principles

1. Courtesy. Tennis is a game that requires cooperation and courtesy from all participants. Make tennis a fun game by praising your opponents' good shots and by not:
   - conducting loud postmortems after points;
   - complaining about shots like lobs and drop shots;
   - embarrassing a weak opponent by being overly gracious or condescending;
   - losing your temper, using vile language, throwing your racket, or slamming a ball in anger; or
   - sulking when you are losing.
2. Counting points played in good faith. All points played in good faith stand. For example, if after losing a point, a player discovers that the net was four inches too high, the point stands. If a point is played from the wrong court, there is no replay. If during a point, a player realizes that a mistake was made at the beginning (for example, service from the wrong court), he shall continue playing the point. Corrective action may be taken only after a point has been completed.

The Warm-up

3. Warm-up is not practice. A player should provide his opponent a five-minute warm-up (ten minutes if there are no ball persons). If a player refuses to warm-up his opponent, he forfeits his right to a warm-up. Some players confuse warm up and practice. A player should make a special effort to hit his shots directly to his opponent. (If partners want to warm each other up while their opponents are warming up, they may do so.)
4. Warm-up serves. Take all your warm-up serves before the first serve of the match. Courtesy dictates that you not practice your service return when your opponent practices his serve. If a player has completed his warm-up serves, he shall return warm-up serves directly to his opponent.

Making Calls

5. Player makes calls on his side of the net. A player calls all shots landing on, or aimed at, his side of the net.
6. Opponent gets benefit of doubt. When a match is played without officials, the players are responsible for making decisions, particularly for line calls. There is a subtle difference between player decisions and those of an on-court official. An official impartially resolves a problem involving a call, whereas a player is guided by the unwritten law that any doubt must be resolved in favor of his opponent. A player in attempting to be scrupulously honest on line calls frequently will find himself keeping a ball in play that might have been out or that he discovers too late was out. Even so, the game is much better played this way.
7. Ball touching any part of line is good. If any part of the ball touches the line, the ball is good. A ball 99% out is still 100% good.
8. Ball that cannot be called out is good. Any ball that cannot be called out is considered to have been good. A player may not claim a let on the basis that he did not see a ball. One of tennis' most infuriating moments occurs after a long hard rally when a player makes a clean placement and his opponent says: "I'm not sure if it was good or out. Let's play a let." Remember, it is each player's responsibility to call all balls landing on, or aimed at, his side of the net. If a ball can't be called out with certainty, it is good. When you say your opponent's shot was really out but you offer to replay the point to give him a break, you are deluding yourself because you must have had some doubt.
9. Calls when looking across a line or when far away. The call of a player looking down a line is much more likely to be accurate than that of a player looking across a line. When you are looking across a line, don't call a ball out unless you can clearly see part of the court between where the ball hit and the line. It is difficult for a player who stands on one baseline to question a call on a ball that landed near the other baseline.
10. Treat all points the same regardless of their importance. All points in a match should be treated the same. There is no justification for considering a match point differently than the first point.
11. Requesting opponent's help. When an opponent's opinion is requested and he gives a positive opinion, it must be accepted. If neither player has an opinion, the ball is considered good. Aid from an opponent is available only on a call that ends a point.
12. Out calls corrected. If a player mistakenly calls a ball "out" and then realizes it was good, the point shall be replayed if he returned the ball within the proper court. Nonetheless, if the player's return of the ball results in a "weak sitter," the player should give his opponent the point. If the player failed to make the return, his opponent wins the point. If the mistake was made on the second serve, the server is entitled to two serves.
13. Player calls his own shots out. With the exception of the first serve, a player should call against himself any ball he clearly sees out regardless of whether he is requested to do so by his opponent. The prime objective in making calls is accuracy. All players should cooperate to attain this objective.
14. Partners' disagreement on calls. If a player and his partner disagree about whether their opponents' ball was out, they shall call it good. It is more important to give your opponents the benefit of the doubt than to avoid possibly hurting your partner's feelings by not overruling. The tactful way to achieve the desired result is to tell your partner quietly that he has made a mistake and then let him overrule himself. If a call is changed from out to good, the point is replayed only if the out ball was put back in play.
15. Audible or visible calls. No matter how obvious it is to a player that his opponent's ball is out, the opponent is entitled to a prompt audible or visible out call.
16. Opponent's calls questioned. When a player genuinely doubts his opponent's call, the player may ask: "Are you sure of your call?" If the opponent reaffirms that the ball was out, his call shall be accepted. If the opponent acknowledges that he is uncertain, he loses the point. There shall be no further delay or discussion.
17. Spectators never to make calls. A player shall not enlist the aid of a spectator in making a call. No spectator has a part in the match.
18. Prompt calls eliminate two chance option. A player shall make all calls promptly after the ball has hit the court. A call shall be made either before the player's return shot has gone out of play or before the opponent has had the opportunity to play the return shot.

    Prompt calls will quickly eliminate the "two chances to win the point" option that some players practice. To illustrate, a player is advancing to the net for an easy put away when he sees a ball from an adjoining court rolling toward him. He continues his advance and hits the shot, only to have his supposed easy put away fly over the baseline. The player then claims a let. The claim is not valid because he forfeited his right to call a let by choosing instead to play the ball. He took his chance to win or lose, and he is not entitled to a second chance.
19. Lets called when balls roll on the court. When a ball from an adjacent court enters the playing area, any player shall call a let as soon as he becomes aware of the ball. The player loses the right to call a let if he unreasonably delays in making the call.
20. Touches, hitting ball before it crosses net, invasion of opponent's court, double hits, and double bounces. A player shall promptly acknowledge if:
    - a ball touches him;
    - he touches the net;
    - he touches his opponent's court;
    - he hits a ball before it crosses the net;
    - he deliberately carries or double hits the ball; or
    - the ball bounces more than once in his court.

21. Balls hit through the net or into the ground. A player shall make the ruling on a ball that his opponent hits through the net and on a ball that his opponent hits into the ground before it goes over the net.
22. Calling balls on clay courts. If any part of the ball mark touches the line on a clay court, the ball shall be called good. If you can see only part of the mark on the court, this means that the missing part is on the line or tape. A player should take a careful second look at any point-ending placement that is close to a line on a clay court. Occasionally a ball will strike the tape, jump, and then leave a full mark behind the line. The player should listen for the sound of the ball striking the tape and look for a clean spot on the tape near the mark. If these conditions exist, the player should give the point to his opponent.

Serving

23. Server's request for third ball. When a server requests three balls, the receiver shall comply when the third ball is readily available. Distant balls shall be retrieved at the end of a game.
24. Foot Faults. A player may warn his opponent that the opponent has committed a flagrant foot fault. If the foot faulting continues, the player may attempt to locate an official. If no official is available, the player may call flagrant foot faults. Compliance with the foot fault rule is very much a function of a player's personal honor system. The plea that he should not be penalized because he only just touched the line and did not rush the net is not acceptable. Habitual foot faulting, whether intentional or careless, is just as surely cheating as is making a deliberate bad line call.
25. Service calls in doubles. In doubles the receiver's partner should call the service line, and the receiver should call the sideline and the center service line. Nonetheless, either partner may call a ball that he clearly sees.
26. Service calls by serving team. Neither the server nor his partner shall make a fault call on the first service even if they think it is out because the receiver may be giving the server the benefit of the doubt. But the server and his partner shall call out any second serve that either of them clearly sees out.
27. Service let calls. Any player may call a service let. The call shall be made before the return of serve goes out of play or is hit by the server or his partner. If the serve is an apparent or near ace, any let shall be called promptly.
28. Obvious faults. A player shall not put into play or hit over the net an obvious fault. To do so constitutes rudeness and may even be a form of gamesmanship. On the other hand, if a player believes that he cannot call a serve a fault and gives his opponent the benefit of a close call, the server is not entitled to replay the point.
29. Receiver readiness. The receiver shall play to the reasonable pace of the server. The receiver should make no effort to return a serve when he is not ready. If a player attempts to return a serve (even if it is a "quick" serve), then he (or his team) is presumed to be ready.
30. Delays during service. When the server's second service motion is interrupted by a ball coming onto the court, he is entitled to two serves. When there is a delay between the first and second serves:
    - the server gets one serve if he was the cause of the delay;
    - the server gets two serves if the delay was caused by the receiver or if there was outside interference.

    The time it takes to clear a ball that comes onto the court between the first and second serves is not considered sufficient time to warrant the server receiving two serves unless this time is so prolonged as to constitute an interruption. The receiver is the judge of whether the delay is sufficiently prolonged to justify giving the server two serves.

Scoring

31. Server announces score. The server shall announce the game score before the first point of the game and the point score before each subsequent point of the game.
32. Disputes. Disputes over the score shall be resolved by using one of the following methods, which are listed in the order of preference:
    - count all points and games agreed upon by the players and replay only the disputed points or games;
    - play from a score mutually agreeable to all players;
    - spin a racket or toss a coin.

Hindrance Issues

33. Talking during a point. A player shall not talk while the ball is moving toward his opponent's side of the court. If the player's talking interferes with his opponent's ability to play the ball, the player loses the point. Consider the situation where a player hits a weak lob and loudly yells at his partner to get back. If the shout is loud enough to distract his opponent, then the opponent may claim the point based on a deliberate hindrance. If the opponent chooses to hit the lob and misses it, the opponent loses the point because he did not make a timely claim of hindrance.
34. Feinting with the body. A player may feint with his body while the ball is in play. He may change position at any time, including while the server is tossing the ball. Any movement or sound that is made solely to distract an opponent, including but not limited to waving the arms or racket or stamping the feet, is not allowed.
35. Lets due to hindrance. A let is not automatically granted because of hindrance. A let is authorized only if the player could have made the shot had he not been hindered. A let is also not authorized for a hindrance caused by something within a player's control. For example, a request for a let because the player tripped over his own hat should be denied.
36. Grunting. A player should avoid grunting and making other loud noises. Grunting and other loud noises may bother not only opponents but also players on adjacent courts. In an extreme case, an opponent or a player on an adjacent court may seek the assistance of the referee or a roving official. The referee or official may treat grunting and the making of loud noises as a hindrance. Depending upon the circumstance, this could result in a let or loss of point.
37. Injury caused by a player. When a player accidentally injures his opponent, the opponent suffers the consequences. Consider the situation where the server's racket accidentally strikes the receiver and incapacitates him. The receiver is unable to resume play within the time limit. Even though the server caused the injury, the server wins the match by retirement.

    On the other hand, when a player deliberately injures his opponent and affects the opponent's ability to play, then the opponent wins the match by default. Hitting a ball or throwing a racket in anger is considered a deliberate act.

When to Contact an Official

38. Withdrawing from a match or tournament. A player shall not enter a tournament and then withdraw when he discovers that tough opponents have also entered. A player may withdraw from a match or tournament only because of injury, illness, personal emergency, or another bona fide reason. If a player cannot play a match, he shall notify the referee at once so that his opponent may be saved a trip. A player who withdraws from a tournament is not entitled to the return of his entry fee unless he withdrew before the draw was made.
39. Stalling. The following actions constitute stalling :
    - warming up for more than the allotted time;
    - playing at about one-third a player's normal pace;
    - taking more than the allotted 90 seconds on the odd-game changeover;
    - taking a rest at the end of a set that contains an even number of games;
    - taking more than the authorized ten minutes during an authorized rest period between sets;
    - starting a discussion or argument in order for a player to catch his breath;
    - clearing a missed first service that doesn't need to be cleared; and
    - bouncing the ball ten times before each serve.

    Contact an official if you encounter a problem with stalling. It is subject to penalty under the Point Penalty System.
40. Requesting an official. While normally a player may not leave the playing area, he may visit the referee or seek a roving official to request assistance. Some reasons for visiting the referee include:
    - stalling;
    - chronic flagrant foot faults;
    - a medical time-out
    - a scoring dispute; and
    - a pattern of bad calls.

    A player may refuse to play until an official responds.

Ball Issues

41. Retrieving stray balls. Each player is responsible for removing stray balls and other objects from his end of the court. A player shall not go behind an adjacent court to retrieve a ball, nor shall he ask for return of a ball from players on an adjacent court until their point is over. When a player returns a ball that comes from an adjacent court, he shall wait until their point is over and then return it directly to one of the players, preferably the server.
42. Catching a ball. Unless you have made a local ground rule, if you catch a ball before it bounces, you lose the point regardless of where you are standing.
43. New balls for a third set. When a tournament specifies new balls for a third set, new balls shall be used unless all the players agree otherwise.

Miscellaneous

44. Clothing and equipment malfunction. If clothing or equipment other than a racket becomes unusable through circumstances outside the control of the player, play may be suspended for a reasonable period. The player may leave the court after the point is over to correct the problem. If a racket or string is broken, the player may leave the court to get a replacement, but he is subject to code violations under the Point Penalty System.
45. Placement of towels. Place towels on the ground outside the net post or at the back fence. Clothing and towels should never be placed on the net.

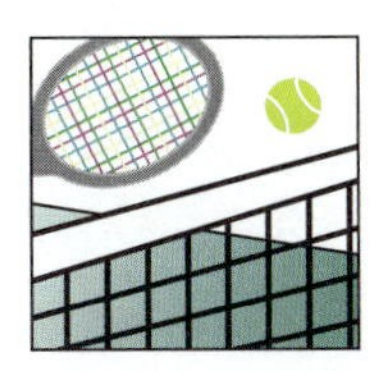

Answer Key to Check Points

Chapter 1

1-a, 2-c, 3-d, 4-a, 5-a, 6-b, 7-d, 8-c

Chapter 2

1-b, 2-a, 3-c, 4-b, 5-d, 6-d, 7-a, 8-b, 9-c, 10-d

Chapter 3

1-d, 2-a, 3-a, 4-c, 5-d, 6-a, 7-a, 8-d

Chapter 4

1-d, 2-a, 3-a, 4-d, 5-c, 6-b, 7-c, 8-a, 9-d, 10-c

Chapter 5

1-c, 2-c, 3-a, 4-d, 5-a, 6-a, 7-c, 8-b

Chapter 6

1-b, 2-d, 3-c, 4-b, 5-a, 6-c

Chapter 7

1-a, 2-a, 3-b, 4-b, 5-c, 6-d, 7-a, 8-b, 9-c, 10-a

Chapter 8

1-a, 2-a, 3-c, 4-d, 5-c, 6-d

Chapter 9

Refer to the various skill drills in the chapter and your skill level

Chapter 10

1-d, 2-Refer to the stretching section pp. 110–112, 3-Refer to the stretching section pp. 110–112, 4-Refer to the strength training section pp. 114–116, 5-Refer to the strength training section pp. 114–116, 6-a, 7-c, 8-b, 9-a, 10–c

Chapter 11

1-c, 2-b, 3-b, 4-d, 5-a, 6-a, 7-b, 8-d

Chapter 12

1-c, 2-b, 3-a, 4-d, 5-d, 6-c, 7-b, 8-b, 9-d, 10-c

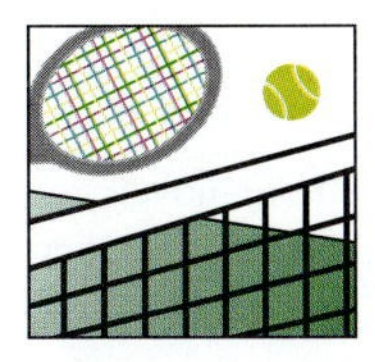

Glossary of Terms

Ad: Advantage of one point to the server or receiver in a tie game.

Ad court: The left service court.

Ad in: Advantage to the server.

Ad out: Advantage to the receiver.

Aerial game: Overhead smashes and defensive and offensive lobs as part of the total tennis game.

American twist service: Serve that has a reverse side spin applied to the ball.

Anxiety: Mental pressure that reduces physical performance.

Approach shot: A groundstroke hit inside the baseline toward the net.

Australian doubles formation: A two-player alignment in doubles that places the net player in a position perpendicular from server to the net.

Backhand: Balls hit on the non-racket side of the body.

Ballistic warm-up: Physically moving the body to prepare for a match.

Baseline: The end of the court, located 39 feet from the net.

Center mark: The division line on the baseline that separates the right side from the left side.

Center strap: The strap that anchors the middle of the net to the court at a 3-foot height.

Chop: An exaggerated slice stroke.

Closed face: Position of the racket face as it is turned down toward the court.

Complex overhead smash: Includes a scissors kick in addition to the orthodox overhead smash as the player jumps to hit the ball.

Control: The measure of how effectively the racket permits the player to place the ball on various shots.

Conventional doubles: Two players in a doubles match who are positioned as one up (at net), one back (at baseline).

Close in: Move in on the net following an approach shot, an overhead smash, or a volley.

Cross court: Hitting the ball at an angle across the width of the court with the net as the central boundary.

Defensive lob: A ball hit to give the defending player a chance to recover from an opponent's offensive shot.

Deuce: A tie score in games at 40-40 or beyond.

Dink shot: A sidespin drop shot hit at an angle from the net to the other side of the court.

Division of play: The division of the court between the opponent's position and the other player's position that provides an equal distance to reach a forehand or a backhand shot.

Double fault: Serving two illegal serves during one service point.

Down the line: A shot hit down a sideline in a direct line from the player.

Drive: A ball hit with force.

Drop shot: A ball hit from a groundstroke position that barely clears the net and dies on the opponent's side of the court.

Drop volley: Same shot as drop shot but from a position of hitting the ball before it bounces on the court.

Dump shot: A push action that guides the ball to an open area beyond the opponent's side of the court.

Etiquette: Rules of behavior on a tennis court.

Feel: The general kinesthetic sense of how a racket feels in the hand of the player.

Fault: An illegally hit serve.

Flat serve: A serve hit with little spin and with a basically flat trajectory.

Flexible racket: A tennis racket that has more control and less power.

Forecourt: Area of the tennis court between the net and the service court line.

Forehand: Balls hit on the racket side of the body.

Groundstroke: The act of hitting a ball following the bounce of the ball on the court.

Half volley: A ball hit immediately following the bounce on the court.

Homebase: The position assumed by a player who prefers to play from the baseline and rally.

Let: A point played over because of interference or a serve replayed because of an otherwise legal serve touching the net.

Lob: A ball hit up over the net player, driving that player back away from the net.

Longbody: An extra long racket.

Love: A zero score.

Match: The best two of three sets in most play situations.

Moonball: A lofted topspin shot intended to change the pace of a rally; halfway between a lob and a groundstroke.

Net play: Generally, offensive play near the net with volley shots and approach shots characteristic of the shots hit.

Non-racket shoulder: The shoulder of the arm on which the racket is not grasped (right-hand player's non-racket shoulder is the left shoulder).

Non-racket side of the body: The same description as for non-racket shoulder, but refers to the whole side of the body (right-handed player's left side of the body).

Offensive lob: A lofted shot hit deep to opponent's baseline with topspin ball action used to chase opponent away from the net.

Open face: Position of racket face as it is turned up to the sky.

Orthodox overhead smash: An overhead smash that requires no foot position exchange.

Overhead smash: An offensive throwing action stroke similar to a serve in motion but delivered at the net back to the baseline.

Pace: A ball hit with the same consistency, usually with some degree of velocity.

Percentage tennis: A philosophical strategy based on forcing the opponent to make the error rather than one's hitting all winning shots.

Playability: A subjective measure of how the racket responds in general during play.

Power: Also described as a "sweet spot," the measure of the "power zone" of the racket.

Punching action: Hitting the ball with little backswing or follow through.

Racket face: The strings of the racket as they face the oncoming ball during a stroke sequence.

Racket head: The total racket area including the string and the material around the face.

Racket shoulder: The shoulder of the arm with which the player grasps the racket.

Racket side of the body: Same description as for the racket shoulder but including the whole side of the body.

Rally: Sustained play of a point, usually associated with hitting only groundstrokes from the baseline area; never refers to hitting a ball on the fly, as in a volley.

Return of serve: The act of hitting a ball back off a serve.

Service court line: The line that is the base of the service courts and that is parallel to the net and baseline.

Set: Represents the winning of six games with a margin of 2 games, or winning by a score of 7-5 or 7-6.

Sidespin: Spin action imparted on a tennis ball so the ball will land on the court and kick away from the person hitting the ball; ball is hit on the backside portion to give the sidespin effect.

Slice serve: A serve hit with sidespin.

Social doubles: Tennis played in a friendly atmosphere with a player alignment usually of one up, one back.

Stability: Ability of a racket to resist the twisting motion when the ball is hit off center.

Stiff racket: A tennis racket that has less control and more power.

Strategy: The planning of an attack when competing against another player or a doubles team.

Stretch racket: An extra long racket or long-body racket.

Stretch warm-up: Static stretching of muscle groups to prepare for a match.

Sweet spot: Surface area of the racket face that provides a functional rebound area as the ball strikes the racket at contact.

Swinging action: A groundstroke movement that represents the motor pattern of swinging as in a baseball bat swing.

Throwing action: A serving or overhead smash motion that represents a throwing pattern as in throwing a baseball.

Timing: The coordinated effort of hitting a ball at the right synchronized point.

Topspin: A ball hit with an overspin rotation action.

Topspin serve: A serve that has a forward or overspin rotation applied to the ball; end result is a high-bouncing, quick rebound from the tennis court.

Underspin: A ball hit with backspin rotation; the ball will have a tendency to float and slow down when striking the tennis court.

Vibration: The measure of how well a racket absorbs vibration at contact with the ball.

Warming up: The act of physically preparing for a tennis match.

Warming down: The act of cooling off the body in a sequential, logical order upon finishing a tennis match.

Wasteland: The area between the baseline and the service court line where a player never should set up to begin a rally.

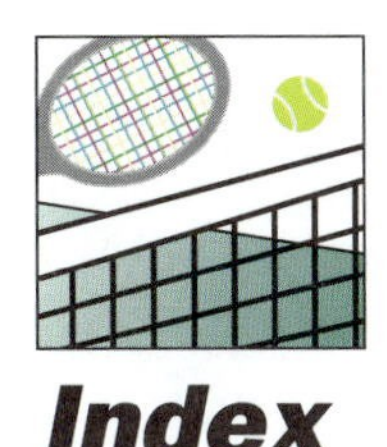

Index

Visual Basic® 6 Programming

Business Applications with a Design Perspective

Visual Basic® 6 Programming

Business Applications with a Design Perspective

Jeffrey J. Tsay

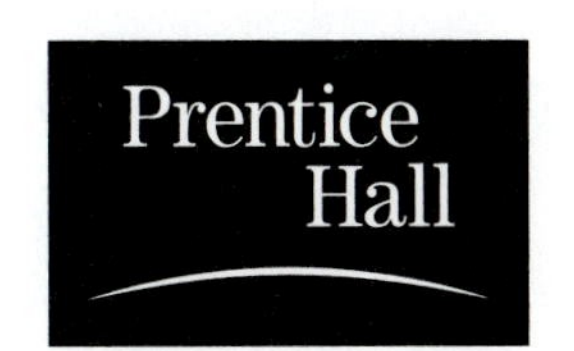

Upper Saddle River, New Jersey

Visual Basic® 6 Programming: Business Applications with a Design Perspective

International Standard Book Number: 0-13-026199-8

03 02 01 00 4 3 2 1

Interpretation of the printing code: the rightmost double-digit number is the year of book's printing; the rightmost single-digit number, the number of the book's printing. For example, a printing code of 00-1 shows that the first printing of the book occured in 2000.

Library of Congress Cataloging-in-Publication Data

Tsay, Jeffrey.
Visual Basic 6 programming : business applications with a design perspective / Jeffrey Tsay.
p. cm.
Includes index.
ISBN 0-13-026199-8
1. Microsoft Visual Basic for Windows. 2. BASIC (Computer program language) 3. Business--Computer programs. I. Title.

HF5548.5.B3 T79 2000
005.26'8--dc21

00-027874

Editor-in-Chief: Mickey Cox
Managing Editor: Melissa Whitaker
Assistant Editor: Kerri Limpert
Senior Marketing Manager: Kris King
AVP/Director of Production & Manufacturing: Michael Weinstein
Production Manager: Gail Steier de Acevedo
Project Manager: Tim Tate
Senior Manufacturing and Prepress Manager: Vincent Scelta
Manufacturing Buyer: Natacha St. Hill Moore
Cover Designer: Marjory Dressler
Book Designer: Graphic World Inc.
Full Service Composition: Graphic World Inc.

Brief Contents

Contents

Preface

Dedication

To My Parents

Introduction

I have been looking for a Visual Basic textbook that:

- **Helps students clearly see the practical applications of Visual Basic (VB) features.** Because of the voluminous number of features available, students new to VB programming tend to get lost as to how to best use a particular VB feature. For example, VB provides a number of controls that allow the developer to quickly design a visual interface. Introducing the student to each of these controls is one matter. Whether the student will be able to properly choose a control in a given application scenario, however, is another.
- **Provides proper coverage in both programming topics and design issues.** As a programming textbook, it should not only introduce VB language elements but also properly discuss programming logic and algorithms. In addition, a proper attempt to teach the application context of programming will inevitably involve a discussion of design choices. Thus, design issues must also be properly considered in all applicable areas.
- **Enables the instructor to focus on important topics.** The textbook should provide sufficient technical information to which students can refer. This allows the instructor to emphasize key points without spending a tremendous amount of class time explaining details.
- **Reinforces important topics effectively.** The textbook should provide plenty of examples to illustrate how important VB features can be applied and how programming logic and algorithms can be implemented. In addition, it should provide a sufficient number of exercises for the student to practice in order to hone his or her programming skills.
- **Provides a guide for the student to use the VB integrated development environment (IDE) not only as a programming tool but also as a learning device and as a source of technical information.** Many of the VB features can be learned by simply "playing" with the VB IDE. In addition, the Help file contains a wealth of technical information and is available at the student's fingertips. The textbook should provide pedagogical devices that guide the student toward using these resources. A student equipped with this learning skill will be able to continue to develop as a programmer after the course without relying on additional books.

While existing textbooks satisfy some of these needs, none appear to meet all these criteria. As an attempt to satisfy the needs of my class, I wrote some handouts, which were met with enthusiastic responses from my students. My efforts evolved into a complete textbook.

Features

This book has been written with the aforementioned goals in mind. It contains the following features.

Application Context

While retaining the typical organizational structure of presenting VB topics, this book provides clear application contexts. For example, Chapter 3, "Some Visual Basic Controls and Events," introduces many VB controls. Instead of beginning with introducing the features of each control one by one, the chapter first discusses an application scenario then presents the control that is most suitable given the application requirement(s). All chapters are written with a similar flavor. For example, Chapter 9, "Arrays and Their Uses," includes a discussion of practical array uses, which call for different programming logic and techniques. Most chapters include application examples, which help the student see how the materials learned in that particular chapter can be put together in an application. Most of them also involve discussions of programming logic and/or algorithms. They serve to reinforce and integrate what the student has just learned.

Design Orientation

Chapter 3 also serves as an example of the design orientation that this textbook emphasizes. In the process of introducing each VB control for the application context, the chapter provides a guide to the design choice for the visual interface. Of course, design issues are not limited to the visual interface. Given a set of application requirements, many different code elements (e.g., statements or object's methods) and code structures (including the placement of code in different modules) can be assembled to obtain the same result. Wherever more than a single plausible alternative can accomplish the same goal, this textbook attempts to point out the difference and suggest a choice, if applicable. For example, as early as Chapter 2, "Introduction to Visual Basic Programming," the text suggests that the Unload statement is preferred to the End statement to terminate a program.

While most textbooks appear to shy away from discussing design issues probably as an attempt for simplicity, proper discussion of the issues helps the student gain a clearer understanding and prepares him or her to be a better software developer.

Code Examples: Step-by-Step

This textbook provides many code examples to illustrate the uses of various VB features. Good code examples help students learn more effectively for several reasons. They show the programming context for the code, illustrate good programming practice, and also serve as an "analogy" by which the student can extend the code application.

Most of the code examples are not just code fragments but complete procedures. Although an experienced programmer may be able to place a code fragment in a problem context easily, a beginner can be faced with countless uncertainties as to how to use the code fragment properly. For example, a beginner can be very uncertain about whether a method of a control can be used only in an event of the same control. A code example with a control's event procedure that includes the use of yet another control's method can easily clarify the doubt in the beginner's mind without any additional words.

Although it is desirable to give code examples in complete procedures, it is also important that the key point is not buried in tedious details and countless lines of code. The code examples have been carefully structured to illustrate the point without being unnecessarily complex.

In presenting most of the code examples, wherever the meaning of the code is less than apparent to the beginner, the text provides the thinking process behind the code. Only after the logic of developing the solution is fully explained is the "complete" code presented. Thus, the student learns not only how the code works, but also the code development process step-by-step. This approach emulates the effective teacher's presentation in the classroom. The student should be able to gain a taste of this process as early as in Chapter 2 when working with "Revising the First Program."

Attention to Interactions Among Control Interfaces

VB is an event-driven language. Event procedures are executed when events occur. Most events are triggered by user actions, but the same events can also be triggered by code. Therefore, some event procedures can be executed for no "obvious" reasons, causing unexpected results. For example, while clicking a list box will trigger its Click event, assigning a value to its ListIndex property will also fire the same event. Thus, whatever code is placed in the Click event will be executed in both situations. However, the beginner may never realize that the event procedure has been executed because of an assignment statement.

To the beginner, these unexpected results are mysterious and can be frustrating in an attempt to trace the source of error. This textbook calls particular attention to these potential problems and suggests ways to avoid the problems. The instructor should benefit from not having to help the student hunt for the mysterious bug.

Special Boxes

Three types of special boxes are used throughout the textbook: ***Tip*** boxes, ***Try This*** boxes, and ***Look It Up*** boxes. Tip boxes alert the student to special coding tips and/or potential programming pitfalls. They draw the student's attention to some particular programming techniques. Try This boxes encourage the student to experiment with code and observe the outcomes. These hands-on experiments help the student retain knowledge. Look It Up boxes guide the student to additional technical information in the MSDN Help file on a particular VB feature. Students who follow the instruction will gradually develop the habit and capability of searching for answers from this valuable resource.

End-of-Chapter Assignments

Starting from Chapter 2, each chapter contains three types of assignments: Visual Basic Explorer, Exercises, and Projects. Visual Basic Explorer includes hands-on exercises that allow the student to explore, experiment, and inspect results. They are designed to be a "learn by doing" tool. Students who perform these exercises will learn more than what the chapter covers and retain the knowledge more easily. Innovative students should also be able to follow the pattern and devise their own "tools" to make their own discoveries when no answer is readily available.

The Exercises are designed for the student to practice and expand what they learn in the chapter. Each chapter contains many exercises with a wide range of varieties. Instructors should be able to choose and assign the exercises they deem most suitable for the course objectives. The student is encouraged to work on as many as his or her time allows to become truly proficient. The Projects require the assembly of concepts and techniques from the current chapter as well as previous chapters. These projects will require major efforts by the student and can be considered as devices for integration of the learned programming knowledge.

Background of Students

The contents of this book have been successfully field-tested with two groups of students: business graduate students without programming background and undergraduate students who have taken one or more programming courses. Both groups of students should have some exposure to the Windows operating system as a user. They should have a good understanding of the Windows' basic terms and concepts. For example, they should know how to start a program, how to use the mouse to navigate, and how to create a file or folder.

Regardless of previous experience, if you are a student inspired to be a proficient software developer, you should find this book worth studying and keeping as a reference. It discusses many intriguing programming problems and design issues not found in a typical textbook.

Organization

There is a consensus among VB instructors that students have a harder time understanding and developing programming logic than designing the user interface. The proposed treatment, however, varies. Two alternatives have emerged: (1) introducing programming elements (e.g., flow of execution control) first and (2) introducing almost all essential VB controls at the beginning. The latter approach appears to produce better results.

Although students may have difficulty with developing programming logic, their hardest challenge is the clear understanding of the context of their code in the VB environment. VB is an event-driven language. Its code behaves in quite a different manner from that in the procedure-oriented language. Students can see the effect of their code only after they clearly understand the relationship between the actions of the user/system and the code they place in the event procedure. That is, they can see the complete picture only after they have a good understanding of "events" and event procedures.

Introducing more controls at the beginning does not hinder students' progress in developing the ability to handle programming logic. On the contrary, with the broad exposure to VB controls, they become acquainted with events more readily. In addition, they are better able to design a user interface that is more efficient for data entry and for code. (Students with limited exposure to VB controls tend to use exclusively the text box for data entry, even when other controls can be much more efficient.)

Because of this consideration, Chapter 3 introduces many controls in the context of data entry. It emphasizes the design choices for different controls. Other controls are introduced in the chapters where the controls are needed. Students' responses to this approach have been very positive.

Chapter 1, "Introduction," provides an overview of the book. Topics in Chapter 2, "Introduction to Visual Basic Programming," through Chapter 7, "Repetition," are considered "essential" and should be studied in sequence. Chapters 8, "Database and the Active X Data Objects," through 11, "Menus and Multiple-Form Applications," however, are fairly "modular." Any chapter can be studied without the background of the other, although some assignments at the end of the chapters do assume the knowledge of previous chapters. (Also, an example in Chapter 10, "Special Topics in Data Entry," relies on the knowledge of Chapter 9.) A flowchart in the Instructor's Manual provides further details of chapter background requirements of previous chapters.

The current structure is based on the consideration of the topics' relative importance and level of difficulty. Databases are discussed in Chapter 8 before arrays (Chapter 9) because of their importance. The introduction to ADO (ActiveX Data Objects) instead of DAO (Data Access Objects) in that chapter is based on the consideration that the former appears to be the thing of the future.

Instructors who want to teach files can use Appendix A, "Data Management Using Files," any time after Chapter 7. The appendix contains summary tables that compare different file structures. The student should find them helpful in understanding different VB file modes. Instructors who want to teach graphics should be able to use Appendix B, "Graphics, Animation, Drag and Drop," after Chapter 8 (or Chapter 7 if the drag-and-drop example using the MS HFlexGrid is omitted).

As a special note, topics covered in Chapter 10 are seldom found in a typical textbook. However, many instructors consider these topics important. The chapter can be deemed as an application of VB programming techniques. The student may be intrigued by the "tricks" used to minimize code and to generalize its applicability in performing data validation. Hopefully, the student will be inspired to develop code in a similar fashion.

Instructor Resources

- *Online Instructor's Manual*—This manual contains teaching objectives and lecture notes to aid the instructor in classroom presentations, solutions to all exercises, and tips to projects found at end of each chapter.
- *Web Site (www.prenhall.com/tsay)*—For instructors, this site contains the Online Instructor's Manual, code examples from each chapter, and data files required for exercises and projects. For students, this site includes solutions to selected exercises and data files required for exercises and projects. This site also contains updated information on the textbook contents and links to other Visual Basic sites.

- *Instructor's CD-ROM*—The CD (0-13-031074-3) contains the Online Instructor's Manual, test questions and answers, and student data files.
- *Smart**Force** Systems Visual Basic Training CD-ROM*—Instructors who desire to have additional hands-on training for their students can elect to include Prentice Hall & Smart**Force** Systems' Visual Basic Training CD-ROM with this textbook. This CD-ROM contains tutorials that are certified to the Expert level of the Microsoft User Specialist Program. It provides students with concept reinforcement via a hands-on simulation of the application with performance exams at the end of each module. When combined with this textbook, students have a complete learning and reinforcement package.

Acknowledgments

This book would not have been possible without the enthusiasm and support of Alex von Rosenberg, Executive Editor at Prentice Hall. Also, Managing Editor Susan Rifkin, one of the most capable people I have ever met, provided all the necessary coordination, which ensured smooth progress for the completion of the manuscript. Her attention to details and schedules is sincerely appreciated. Melissa Whitaker provided additional coordination after the completion of the manuscript. Kerri Limpert, Assistant Editor, contributed a lot of thought and positive energy to ensuring that this book is supported by a rich supplement package.

Tim Tate, Project Manager at Prentice Hall, coordinated the design and production activities and helped ensure the quality of the final product. In addition, his cheerful manner made the interactions with him truly enjoyable. Suzanne Copple of Graphic World helped edit the manuscript as well as handle the actual production. Also, her accommodation of several last-minute changes is sincerely appreciated.

I want to thank my assistant, Ampapat Suchiva for her continuous and tireless efforts in proofreading several versions of the manuscript and for her suggestions for improvement of the contents. I feel extremely lucky to have an assistant as dedicated as she has been.

A special thank you goes to a generous friend, whom I got to know via the Internet and have not had the pleasure of meeting in person: Ben Wu of Indiana University. He reviewed the draft of the entire manuscript and provided many constructive comments and suggestions.

I am grateful to the following reviewers whose constructive suggestions help shape the contents and writing style of this textbook:

Larry Andrew	Western Illinois University
Kelly J. Black	California State University at Fresno
David Cooper	New River Community College
Marvin Harris	Lansing Community College
Paul C. Jorgensen	Grand Valley State University
Susan K. Lippert	George Washington University
Pati Milligan	Baylor University
Paula Velluto	Bunker Hill Community College
John F. Walker	Dona Ana Branch Community College - New Mexico State University

I am also indebted to the following colleagues, students, and friends for their contributions in various ways to this book: Dan Burns, Mark Eakin, Doug Allison, Bruce Campbell, Phawinee Chaiwattana, Li-Ju Christine Chen, Meei-Ling Chen, Iris Shihyin Chien, James Garth Dimock, Christine Ding-tsyr Gau, Yi-Hsien Huang, Aygun Sarioglu, Jeffrey Nevin Scroggins, and Ada Wang (Yu Yin).

I have been on an Internet VB discussion group since it began at Texas A&M University. The group moved to a server hosted by L-Soft, International and has since become two. The addresses are as follows:

VISBAS-L@PEACH.EASE.LSOFT.COM and
VISBAS-BEGINNERS@PEACH.EASE.LSOFT.COM

I benefited much more from the discussions than I have contributed. To those active participants, I sincerely express my thanks.

Dr. David Leuthold, professor emeritus of political science at the University of Missouri-Columbia has been my inspiration, mentor, and role model. His advice and encouragement are deeply appreciated. My good friend and an experienced book author Professor Lanny Solomon of the University of Missouri-Kansas City also provided advice in the development and writing process.

To say that writing this book is a family endeavor is not an exaggeration. My daughters Carolyn and Angela helped with editing the prospectus and the first few chapters of the manuscript. My son, Jonathan, helped with capturing the screens for production. My wife, Nora, read and tested the hands-on instructions of the first few chapters. During this intensive book-writing period, she single-handedly shouldered various responsibilities and obligations so that I could remain focused on the book. Without you, Nora, I know I would have not progressed this far. Writing this book reminds me of the good old days when I was writing my dissertation. Nora, Thank you!

Jeff Tsay

1 Introduction

This book introduces you to Visual Basic (VB) programming. It is oriented toward business applications, with a design perspective. Many business applications involve data-entry operations. On appearance, data entry appears to be a fairly simple programming problem. However, once you start to develop this type of application program, you will encounter many intriguing issues. For example, as soon as you start to design the data-entry screen, you will wonder how to best design the visual interface. (Thus, you will be faced with interface design issues.) In addition, you will have to develop code to validate the data entered by the user because data accuracy is of the utmost importance to any business. Here, you may find a lot of duplicate code. (Thus, you will need to design the code structure to minimize duplication.) Business applications also involve data storage and processing. Therefore, you will need to deal with data management issues and develop algorithms to process data efficiently. This book is oriented toward handling these issues.

This chapter gives an overview of VB programming. Naturally, when you are learning VB programming, your first question is, "What is Visual Basic?" The first section, 1.1, provides some explanations. In Section 1.2, we consider what constitutes a sound application program. We also discuss the steps involved in developing a program. Section 1.3 provides some suggestions on how to use this book.

After completing this chapter, you should be able to:

- Explain what Visual Basic is.
- Contrast the operating environment of Visual Basic with that of programs developed using procedure-oriented languages.
- Set forth the criteria for a sound application program.
- Enumerate the steps to develop a program.
- Understand the importance of hands-on experience in learning a programming language.

1.1 What Is Visual Basic?

Evolution of Visual Basic

Visual Basic evolves from ***BASIC*** (an acronym for ***B***eginner's ***A***ll-Purpose ***S***ymbolic ***I***nstruction ***C***ode), which was created in the 1960s. Its syntax is similar to FORTRAN (another programming language that was developed to handle ***For***mula ***Tran***slation). However, BASIC primarily was used for interactive computing, whereas FORTRAN was used in the batch-processing environment where each program was run as a job without human interaction or intervention. When microcomputers were introduced, BASIC was the language available in nearly all makes (e.g., Tandy, Apple). Its power was fairly limited because of hardware limitations. When the personal computer (PC) became available, Microsoft introduced GW-Basic with its disk operating system (DOS).

As you may be aware, programs written in BASIC (any version) need to be processed by a ***language processor*** (a ***program*** that "processes" the BASIC program) before their instructions can be understood and executed by the computer. The BASIC language processors up to that point were "***interpreters***," which read one line of BASIC code at a time, "interpreted" the code, and carried out the activities called for by the instructions. Because of the overhead associated with interpreting the code, the execution is very slow.

To improve execution speed, BASIC "***compilers***" were introduced. A version of the BASIC compilers by Microsoft is ***Quick Basic***. A compiler is another kind of language processor that translates a ***source program*** (e.g., a program written in Quick Basic) into the machine language (or some pseudocode that is fairly close to the machine language). The resulting program is recognized as the ***object program***. Because of the elimination of the overhead of "interpretation," the object program runs much faster than a source program under an interpreter.

As you can see from the diagram in Figure 1.1, the key difference between an interpreter and a compiler is the output. The interpreter takes the source program along with the data as input and produces the results that the source program calls for. In contrast, the compiler takes only the source program as input and produces an object program in a lower-level language. The object program must be executed along with required data in order to produce the results. As an analogy, imagine you are in a hotel in a foreign country requesting room service. The only language you know is English. Your requests begin with "Bring me an apple," among other things. An interpreter (who understands English) will read your first line, bring you an apple, and proceed to the next line. A compiler, on the other hand, will just translate your requests into the native language, leaving the remainder to someone else to execute.

FIGURE 1.1
Difference Between Interpreter and Compiler

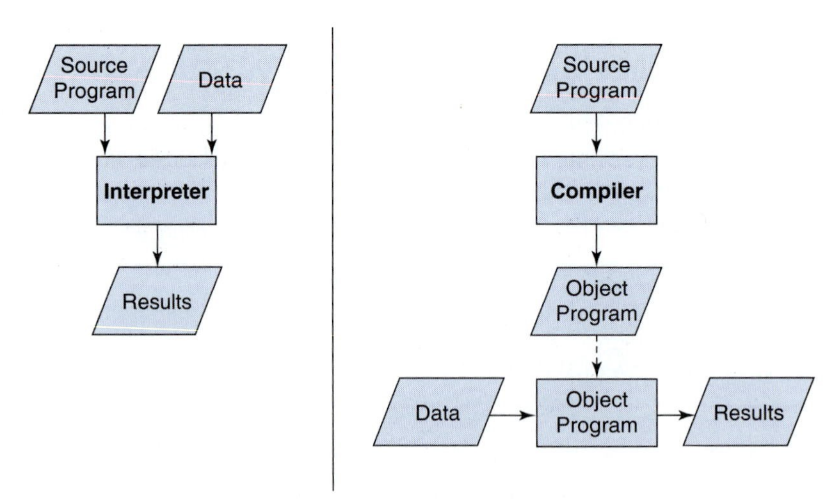

Difference between interpreter and compiler: the former produces results of computations; the latter produces an object program, which needs to be loaded into the memory to run in order to obtain the results.

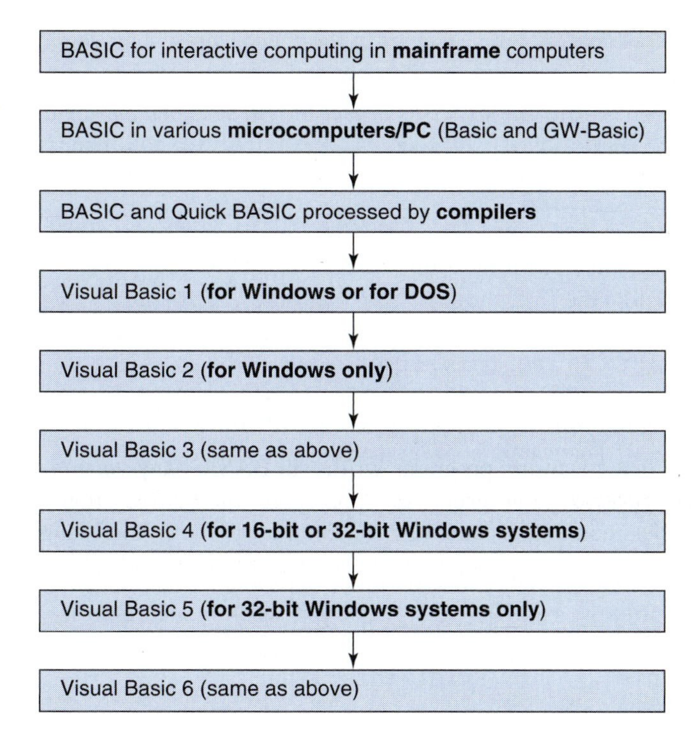

FIGURE 1.2
Milestones of the Evolution of Visual Basic

Despite its speed, Quick Basic has its drawbacks, especially by today's standards:

- It is a procedure-oriented language. When it runs, the program, instead of the user, dictates the sequence of activities to be carried out. The user is not allowed any flexibility.
- Its interface is text based instead of graphics based. The appearance is not very attractive. The keyboard is used nearly exclusively to obtain user input or commands. In many cases, text-based input is more susceptible to errors and may not be as efficient as other "gadgets" that are available in the graphics-based environment.
- Programs take a long time to develop and are difficult to change, especially when the change involves the visual interface. The programmer needs to track all the details relating to the location, size, and color of all boxes and texts drawn on the screen. A minor change can call for painstaking efforts by the programmer to ensure that everything is done correctly.

After the graphic user interface (***GUI***)-based Windows operating system was introduced for PCs, ***Visual Basic*** arrived in 1991. The first version of VB had two editions: one for DOS and another for the Windows system. As the Windows system gained in popularity, the later versions of VB were designed only for the Windows operating systems. Earlier versions of VB were written for 16-bit operating systems because 32-bit operating systems were not yet available. There were two editions of VB in version 4: one for 16-bit operating systems (e.g., Windows 3.0) and another for 32-bit operating systems (e.g., Windows NT, Windows 95). Since version 5, all editions have been made exclusively for 32-bit operating systems. The newest version at this time is version 6. Figure 1.2 provides a diagram that briefly depicts the *milestones* of the evolution of VB.

Characteristics of Visual Basic

The vocabulary and syntax of VB are derived from BASIC. However, VB differs significantly from BASIC in several respects:

- VB provides a set of ***visual objects*** (recognized as "***controls***") that can be drawn easily onto a window (called a *form*). These controls eliminate the need to develop the code to construct the visual interface. The layout of the windows that contain the controls can be changed easily by dragging and dropping the controls to a new location, without necessitating a change in the code. Thus, the process for program development and revision becomes much easier and requires much less time and effort.

- The code structure of VB is ***object based***, whereas that of BASIC is not. In BASIC, there is no "object." Its code usually follows the following syntax:

  ```
  Verb Operand List
  ```

  For example, to print a line of text in BASIC (e.g., "Print this line"), the code will look like the following:

  ```
  Lprint "Print this line."
  ```

  Although some VB code still retains this form, most of its code is structured around objects. The syntax appears as follows:

  ```
  Object.Method parameter list
  ```

  Where the so-called method is the action or activity to be carried out.
  To print the same line using VB, you would code the following:

  ```
  Printer.Print "Print this line."
  ```

  As you can see, "Printer" is recognized as an object. Its "Print" method will print the line on the object, the printer.
  Object-based coding is easier because the object and the action are identified separately, resulting in a more concise set of vocabulary. In BASIC, you must remember to use "Lprint" to print on the printer and "Print" to print on the screen. In VB, you use the same "Print" method to print on different objects. It is also more consistent with the user's activity in the GUI environment. For example, when you are editing a document with a word processor, you highlight a block of text (identify the object) and then instruct the computer what to do with it (indicate an action such as cut or paste).

- VB is an *event-driven* rather than procedure-oriented language. As discussed previously, when a procedure-oriented program runs, it dictates the sequence of operations. This means the programmer must predefine the sequence when developing the program. In addition, changing the sequence of operations requires revising the program. On the other hand, an event-driven program does not dictate the sequence of operations. The user can instruct the computer to perform whatever operations the program is capable of, in any sequence he or she desires. This offers the user flexibility. Any changes in the sequence of operations will not call for revising the program. In this sense, an event-driven program is easier to develop and requires fewer revisions.

  However, event-driven programs present the programmer with a different kind of challenge. In many instances, an activity can be carried out only after some "prerequisite" actions have been taken or data are ready. (For example, when the user clicks the Send button in an email application, the target email address, the subject line, and the body of message must all be filled in.) When the user initiates the activity, there is no guarantee that the prerequisites have been met. As a programmer, you must find ways to ensure that the prerequisites are there.

Visual Basic as a Language and as a Processor

From the previous discussion, you understand that VB is a programming language used to write programs to make the computer perform desired tasks. A programming language is a medium of communication with the computer. It is used to communicate to the computer what needs to be done. It has its own vocabulary and grammatical rules (syntax). These elements can be combined to form a program, which is the complete set of instructions designed to perform the defined tasks.

You have also learned that the program you write in VB (the language) will need to be processed by a VB language processor, which is also a computer program. In most instances, we also refer to the VB language processor as Visual Basic. When we say that we write a program in VB6, we are actually expressing that we are writing a VB program that VB6 (the processor) can understand and process. Thus, the term *Visual Basic* can actually mean two different things (the language and the processor) in different contexts or the two things at the same time.

When you develop a VB program, you will work with a software program that does more than just "process" your program. It provides an environment in which you can draw the visual interface, write the code, compile and test the program, and make additional changes. This VB "processor" is recognized as the ***VB Integrated Development Environment (IDE)***. Its significance is explored further in Chapter 2, "Introduction to Visual Basic Programming."

Statement and Code. A VB program can consist of many instructions. An instruction that is "complete" in meaning and can stand alone like a "sentence" is recognized as a ***statement***. Usually, you will use a line to write a statement. Some statements are very long. In such cases, the statement can be spanned over several lines. The mechanic of spanning a statement over multiple lines is explained in Chapter 2. Statements in a program are collectively recognized as ***code***. The following sample code fragment comes from Chapter 7, "Repetition":

```
Do Until EOF(NameFile)
    'Read a name from NameFile
    Line Input #NameFile, TheName
    'Add the name to the list box
    lstNames.AddItem TheName
Loop
```

Each line in this code is complete in meaning and, therefore, is a statement.

Editions of Visual Basic 6

In this book, you will learn the VB language pertaining to the features available in version 6 of the VB language processor (compiler). There are actually three different editions of VB6:

1. *The Standard Edition.* This edition consists of the "basic" (standard) features of the language. It is designed for beginners who want to learn the language for the first time.
2. *The Professional Edition.* In addition to all the features in the standard edition, this edition includes various ActiveX objects that experienced programmers can use to develop sophisticated applications (including Internet applications).
3. *The Enterprise Edition.* As the name implies, this edition is designed for corporations that develop applications internally or as commercial software vendors. It includes all the features of the professional edition. In addition, it provides utility programs (tools) that can be used to facilitate the development of large projects, which can involve several members in a team.

This book focuses on the professional edition.

1.2 Overview of Visual Basic Program Development

Before you get involved in the details of actually developing a VB program, it is desirable that you become aware of the criteria for a sound program. These criteria provide benchmarks against which the quality of your programs can be compared and thus serve as the guide for your application development. In addition, you should also be acquainted with the program development cycle. A good understanding of the cycle will equip you with a step-by-step roadmap to developing your program so that you can be more efficient and effective in carrying out your programming endeavor. This section discusses these two aspects.

Criteria for a Sound Application Program

How do you judge the soundness of an application program? As a programmer, you examine the program in two completely different perspectives: ***external*** and ***internal***. First, you inspect the program from an external perspective and judge it in terms of the application requirements. The criteria include the following:

- *Functionality.* The program must meet the requirements of the application; that is, it must deliver the functionality called for by the application. For example, if an order-processing application needs to update both the customer records and the on-hand quantities of all products ordered, the program must be able to carry out both. The program cannot be considered complete until it can perform both functions. In short, the question is, "Can the program do what it is supposed to do?"
- *Efficiency.* The program should also perform the required functions efficiently. By efficiency, we mean the program should minimize the consumption of computer resources, including computer time and storage space. I have seen a general ledger package that takes several minutes of computer time to post 10 transactions from a general journal to a general ledger, almost as fast (slow) as a person can handle the task manually. Such a program obviously fails the efficiency test.
- *User-Friendliness.* The concept of user-friendliness is not new. The "ancient" concept stipulated that the message to the user be clear, meaningful, and in a friendly tone. However, with the GUI environment, this concept encompasses a much wider variety of user expectations. Briefly, a user-friendly program should do the following:
  - Provide the user with maximum mobility around the user interface.
  - Be consistent in appearance and behavior among different windows.
  - Provide the user with supports in using the program to perform his or her task. Examples of support include providing dialog boxes for lookup and online help.
  - Be flexible in accommodating user's tastes and preferences.
  - Guard the user against errors and mistakes. If not handled carefully in the program, some errors caused by the user can crash the application, resulting in loss of data. All errors and mistakes by the user should be handled in the program properly to prevent accidental loss of data or causing any inconvenience to the user.

From the perspective of the programmer, the program not only should satisfy the external requirements as outlined previously but also should be developed with a set of ***internal standards***. The code developed for a program should have the following characteristics:

- *Consistency in Coding Style.* There is a set of coding conventions that the programmer should follow when developing code. These conventions include coding mechanics such as properly indenting blocks of code (for visual clues to the code structure) and naming objects with predefined prefixes (for easy identification of the types of objects involved). Code developed with a consistent style is much easier to read and understand. As an illustration, look again at the code fragment on page 5. It is properly indented, providing a clue that it is a code "block." The name *lstNames* also follows the naming convention; it contains a three-letter prefix, lst, indicating the type of object it represents.
- *Code Clarity and Readability.* In addition to the consistent coding style, there are other factors that make code clearer and easier to understand. For example, if the names used to represent data in your program are meaningful, your program will become much easier to read and follow. The person who reviews the code can easily associate the names with the data they represent, making the tracing of programming logic much easier. As an example, you also might have inferred that lstNames in the preceding code sample contains "names." In many cases, the purpose (meaning) of some code

may not be clear. Adding comments can make the program easier to understand. In the preceding code example, the lines that start with a single quote are comment lines.

- *Modularity in Code Design. Modularity* refers to the design of code structure so that each block of code is isolated from the rest of the program; that is, each block can perform its designated task without depending on the state of other blocks and without being interfered with by the actions of other parts. In this way, each block of code is independent of the others. Thus, program logic and flow of execution are "localized" and much easier to trace. Such a code structure is easier to debug (correct errors), review, and revise.
- *Elegant Algorithms.* An algorithm is a systematic approach to solving a programming problem. It usually involves the iterative application of a group of defined steps to arrive at the solution. An algorithm is said to be elegant when its logic is easy to trace and implement and is efficient in terms of its speed and storage requirements. Given a fairly complex problem, an infinite number of algorithms can be constructed to solve it. Some are efficient; some are not. For example, the sorting problem (arranging data elements in order) has a simple goal. Yet literally hundreds of algorithms for sorting exist. For a fairly large volume of data, the difference in speed between the best and the worst algorithm is a factor of several hundred times. Thus, careful identification and selection of algorithms for your program can make it perform much more efficiently.
- *Code Maintainability.* Often, the requirements of a program change over time. A change in the requirements necessitates revision of the program; thus, efforts are involved in maintaining the program. All the internal factors mentioned previously have an impact on code maintainability. However, code maintainability is not limited to the aforementioned factors. This is particularly true in VB. Some code by nature is more "generally applicable" than other code. *General applicability* refers to the attribute of certain code blocks that will not necessitate any revision, even when the program requirements are changed. For example, in many cases, you may need to clear the content of the controls (visual objects) in the visual interface. One way to perform this is to refer to the controls by name and assign a certain value to these controls. In VB, you can assign the same value to these controls without referring to their specific names. The latter approach is more generally applicable because no matter how the names of the controls are changed, you can still use the same code to perform the task. The use of the more generally applicable code will undoubtedly result in a program that is much more maintainable. (An example is provided in Chapter 7.)

The diagram in Figure 1.3 summarizes this discussion.

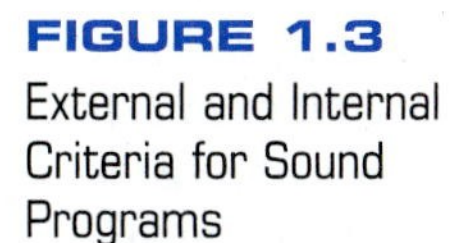
FIGURE 1.3
External and Internal Criteria for Sound Programs

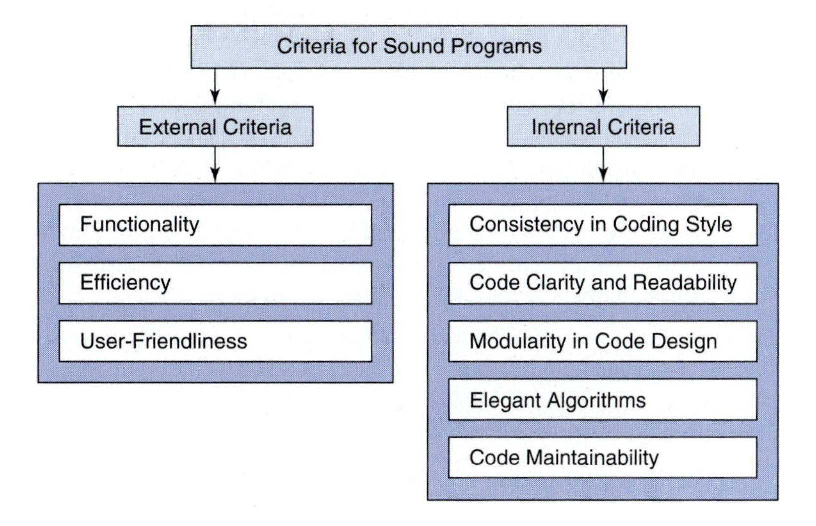

How are these criteria for sound programs treated in this book? The functionality issue depends on the programmer's understanding of the application requirements. All the other issues are considered throughout the book where applicable. In most cases, we call your attention to why a certain problem is solved with a particular block of code instead of other alternatives. The performance implications of different code structures and algorithms are considered where applicable. In addition, a significant portion of Chapter 9, "Arrays and Their Uses," is also used to present different sorting algorithms. We believe this will stimulate your mind and you will become more critical in selecting and devising a suitable algorithm to solve the problem at hand. The user-friendliness criterion is very important, especially in the context of data-entry screens and user interfaces. Chapter 10, "Special Topics in Data Entry," is devoted in particular to treating this topic thoroughly.

Steps in Program Development

When you are ready to develop an application program, there is a fairly standard set of steps you should follow. Your progress will be much smoother when you observe these steps, which can be outlined as follows:

1. *Analyze and Define the Problem.* As already discussed, the first requirement of a sound program is that it must meet the needs of the application. Thus, a clear understanding of the problem and goals is the first step in developing the program. Only when the needs and requirements of the program are clearly understood can you determine how the program is to look and act.

When developing a program, you can save a lot of time, headaches, and effort in revision if you know its exact requirements/specifications at the very beginning. Analyze the problem carefully and define the requirements clearly before proceeding.

2. *Design the Visual Interface.* Based on your analysis and understanding of the problem, you will be able to design the visual interface for the program. You will start to work with the VB IDE. You will need to decide what data fields should appear on a form. This process can become quite involved. VB provides various visual objects (controls) that you can use to represent these data fields. It takes a careful analysis to determine which VB control will be the best given the nature of a data field. Chapter 3, "Some Visual Basic Controls and Events," provides an analytical framework for this purpose.
3. *Define User-Program Interaction.* The user interface consists of the ***visual aspect*** as described previously and the ***behavior*** in which your program responds to the user's actions and to what happens in the computer internally. You will need to determine what your program should do in detail. The user's actions and system activities are recognized as "***events***." User actions that can trigger events include such things as pressing a key, clicking a control, or making a selection from a menu. System activities can also trigger events. Examples of these activities include loading and unloading a form. You must first be aware what "events" will be triggered when each of these actions occurs. Based on how you decide your program should react, you will place the code in the pertinent event to respond accordingly. Some of those commonly seen events are discussed in Chapter 3. Additional events are discussed in other chapters, where the events need to be handled.
4. *Design the Code Structure.* On appearance, the code you will develop to respond to an action should be placed in the event that the action triggers. Thus, your code structure will simply be dictated by the responses you want your program to carry out. In reality, however, it can be much more complex. You will be introduced to various complex situations. Suffice it to say, it pays to analyze the complex situation thoroughly before writing any code. As your program grows into multiple modules (a module is a code window that contains your code), you will also discover that many

code blocks can be shared. Thus, the appropriate module(s) in which to place these blocks can become an issue. Your design of the code structure can have far-reaching implications on the maintainability of your code. The importance of this design phase cannot be overemphasized. Some authors maintain that most (more than 60%) of your time and effort should be expended on this endeavor to produce a sound program. Some of these design issues are discussed in Chapter 10; Chapter 11, "Menus and Multiple Form Applications"; and Chapter 12, "Object-Oriented Programming." The context of the discussions in these chapters pertains to minimizing code duplication and dealing with the issues associated with large projects.

5. *Write Code.* Based on your design, you will then develop the code to perform the activities that your program requires. In addition to ensuring that the code performs what is called for, you should pay particular attention to your coding style. As mentioned, this includes the mechanical aspects of indenting and following the naming conventions. You will start to learn about this aspect beginning in Chapter 2.
6. *Test and Edit the Program.* Unless a program is very short, it is rare that the program anybody develops will run correctly the first time. The program can have various kinds of errors:

   - It can have syntax errors, resulting from the failure to follow the rules to put various code elements together.
   - It can also have semantic errors, resulting from the difference between what the programmer codes and what he or she actually means (the failure to say what the programmer means). For example, the programmer may code a "Print" statement thinking it will output on a printer. However, the statement actually means to display output on a form.
   - Finally, it can have logic errors, resulting from the differences between what the programmer believes a block of code will do and what the program actually does. This type of error is the trickiest and can take days or even weeks to resolve in some complex situations. Thus, in most cases, you will test run your program and discover some unexpected problems or results. You will then modify your code to solve the problems you have identified and test it again. You will repeat the process until no problem or unexpected result is encountered.

   Testing and editing code constitute most of your effort in the coding activity. To minimize the possibility of encountering "mysterious" logic errors, it is advisable to break the code into small steps and test it often. This makes it easier to identify the range of code that causes the error. A smaller number of statements make the error source easier to track down and correct.
7. *Place the Program into "Production."* After a program is thoroughly tested, it is ready to be placed in actual use. A program that works with live data and produces "real" results is called a ***production program***. When you are developing and testing the program, you work in the VB IDE. A program to be placed in production should be compiled to produce a separate object program. This object program (an executable file) can then run without the IDE. Additional explanations of the IDE and the step to compile and generate the executable file are discussed in Chapter 2.

Figure 1.4 summarizes the steps of program development.

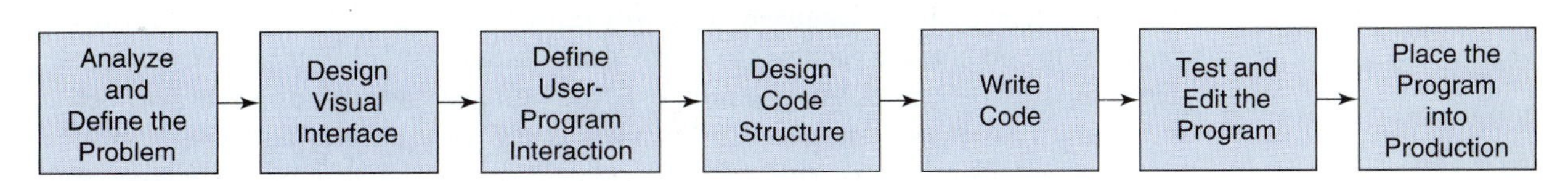

FIGURE 1.4
Steps of Program Development

When a beginner is working on a programming exercise, some of these steps may be combined (or not applicable). For example, the exercise may be so simple that it requires little analysis of the problem or design of code structure. Thus, once the goal is understood, you can start to work on designing the visual interface, write the code, and test the program. However, as you proceed and the problems become more complex, it pays to revisit this complete "roadmap." You will appreciate the importance of those steps that you initially could do without.

1.3 How to Use This Book

This section offers a few suggestions on how to use this book. We would like to stress that hands-on practice (actually writing and testing the program rather than just reading and thinking about it) is the key to successfully learning a programming language. That is, you learn to program by programming, just like you learn to swim by swimming, not by observing. Perhaps, another analogy can help illustrate the point.

Learning the Language: An Analogy

In many ways, learning a computer language is no different from learning a human language. We use a language to convey ideas. Before you can speak a language fluently, you must build a wide vocabulary. You will also need to know the rules to put the vocabulary together to convey an idea. The sentences must be structured correctly. Without the correct structure, these sentences will be hard to understand. (In the case of computer languages, the computer will simply refuse to understand.)

It is also important to note that a correctly structured (grammatically correct) sentence may not necessarily convey exactly the idea that you have in mind. For example, the two sentences, "You like a dog" and "You are like a dog" are both grammatically correct. But you know how different the reactions can be from your listener. In VB, the statement A = B = C may have quite a different meaning from what you may think. (Wait until Chapter 5, "Decision," for the answer.) You must also choose the right vocabulary to express the right ideas. Furthermore, even if the sentences convey the correct meaning, you may find that there are better ways to convey the same thing; that is, different sentences may have different effectiveness in conveying the same idea.

The previous discussion suggests that there are four aspects of "speaking a language" (writing a VB program):

1. Vocabulary
2. Grammar (syntax rules)
3. Semantics (meaning)
4. Effectiveness

To express yourself well in a language as a speaker or writer (not just as a reader or listener), you need to build a large vocabulary, follow the syntax rules, understand clearly the meanings of the vocabulary, and find the proper expression to convey the ideas effectively. It takes a lot of practice to learn to speak a new language fluently and convey ideas effectively. At the beginning, even a very simple sentence bears repetition to gain the desired level of familiarity.

The Case for Hands-On

When you are developing a VB program, you will be the "speaker or writer" of the language, not just a reader or listener. To be good at VB programming, you will do exactly as you would to learn a new (human) language. You will learn the "vocabulary" of VB. You will also learn the rules to combine the elements to form expressions and statements that express what you want the computer to perform. As you progress, you will also discover different ways of getting the same result. In many instances, the "different ways" may have different performance implications. You will be faced with "design choices" and select the more effective and efficient approach.

From learning the vocabulary to making an intelligent design choice, the development of your proficiency takes a lot of hands-on practice, which enables you to do the following:

- Gain familiarity not only with the VB IDE but also with the vocabulary and syntax rules of VB without exerting stress on your memory. Many details are involved in each code line. They do not stand out in your memory until you actually write the code. Familiarity will make you much more efficient in handling the same (or a similar) problem. You will find your second attempt takes much less time than the first one. Familiarity improves your efficiency and enhances your confidence.
- Gain a more indepth understanding of the interrelationship between different parts of the code. You will be able to see the effect of the code you place in different "events" more readily. This level of understanding allows you to develop and trace programming logic more easily.
- Identify opportunities for code improvement. Some programming problems can appear different in their context but call for the same or similar solution. The first time you encounter the problem, you might just be glad that you have a solution. The second time, you may see some faults of your original solution and attempt to improve on it. In the process, you will explore, experiment, and discover new solutions. As a result, you will gain even more knowledge. You will be able to write programs that perform effectively, much like a speaker delivering an effective speech.

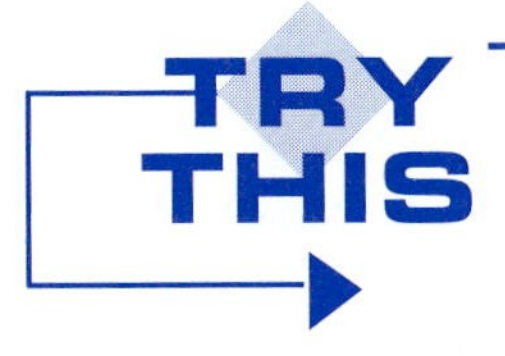

You have seen how to make the printer print a line of text. Write a line of code in VB to print the following text.

```
Practice makes perfect.
```

How do you feel? As easy as the code may be, you should find that there are details to pay attention to. Only hands-on experience can provide this additional insight. The solution is given at the end of the Summary section.

To repeat, merely reading the text is not enough. You may gain some knowledge of VB by reading, but you still need the hands-on practice to obtain the familiarity, the deep understanding, and the skills for effective delivery. This book provides many devices that facilitate your hands-on practice with VB. We suggest that you do the following:

1. Try the examples in each chapter, and ensure that all the results are as expected. In most cases, you can try the examples as you read. As you work with the examples, you become familiar with the code structure and its use.
2. Test the code in the "Try This" boxes. These boxes allow you to see the effect of the code and provide you with a deeper understanding. The benefit of these exercises can be immense.
3. Complete the VB explorer exercises. These exercises deal with topics that are not discussed in detail in the text and broaden your working knowledge of VB. They are designed so that you find answers to VB questions in a fun way. They serve to illustrate how you can explore VB on your own. Hopefully, by working with this group of exercises, you will become more adventuresome and daring, trying anything without being afraid of encountering an error. Once you develop this "mental capacity" toward VB (and the computer), whenever you have an intriguing question, you will be able to (1) devise your own code strategy to test your question, (2) discover the answer, and (3) figure out how and why your code works out the way it does. You will be able to learn a lot on your own.

4. Work on the exercises and projects suggested by your instructor (and even more if you can find time). These assignments give you an opportunity to put together what you learn from the text in a meaningful way. The acid test of your VB programming skill rests in whether you can successfully develop the code to perform the requirements of these assignments. These assignments vary in difficulty and fields of applications. They challenge you in different ways and can be very interesting and intriguing. The ample exercises offer plenty of choices in taking on the challenge.
5. Have a thorough understanding of a chapter before proceeding to the next. This is particularly important for the first seven chapters. Each chapter is built on the preceding ones. Together, the seven chapters form the foundation for the remainder of the book. This also means that *the first few chapters deserve a lot of your study time.* I have had some students who thought that the first few chapters were fairly easy and thus devoted relatively little time to studying this material. These students had to work twice as hard later just to catch up, while those who worked hard initially had a much easier time and more fun with the later chapters.

Keep this in mind: Programming is more of an art than a science. The more you do, the better and the faster you can program. Hands on. Hands on. And more hands on.

Beyond the Content Coverage

There is so much to learn about VB. It includes many controls and objects, which can be used in a wide range of applications. These controls and objects have many features. It takes several books just to document all the features. As a result, it is impossible for a textbook to cover all aspects of this language.

However, this book provides a special feature that can help equip you to explore, learn, and expand your knowledge in VB on your own. Starting from Chapter3, each chapter contains several special boxes titled "Look It Up." These boxes show you what types of information on VB you can obtain from the online help file. These boxes serve as a reminder that a lot of valuable information is available at your fingertips. These boxes are intended to help you build a habit of looking up your questions in the online help file. Follow the instructions and perform all the suggested "lookups." You will learn a lot more by just doing this. Better yet, getting familiarized with the help file can be the best resource in your study of VB.

Once you become acquainted with the help file, you will be able to appreciate the wealth of information that is readily available. While you are writing your program, the help file is right there for your use. It provides many details that textbooks may not have. Above all, it covers *all* the features of VB. Thus, if you decide to pursue a topic not covered in this book, you will be able to proceed comfortably by browsing the file for the needed information. Chapter 2 has a section that shows you how to browse the online help file.

Summary

This chapter provides an overview of VB programming. We explained what VB is from various aspects: its evolution, its operating environment, and the various editions of VB6. In the process, we also differentiated between the two types of language processors: interpreters and compilers.

We also discussed the criteria for sound application programs. Programs can be evaluated from an external perspective by such criteria as functionality, efficiency, and user-friendliness. As a programmer, you will also evaluate a program internally by looking at its code. The criteria include coding style, code readability and clarity, modularity in design, algorithmic elegance, and code maintainability. It is important to keep all these criteria in mind when developing programs. By observing these criteria faithfully, you can build good habits that facilitate your development of sound programs.

We also discussed the set of steps that you should follow in developing applications:

1. Analyzing and defining the problem
2. Designing the visual interface

3. Defining the user-program interaction
4. Designing code structure
5. Writing code
6. Testing and editing code
7. Placing the program into "production"

This procedural outline gives you a development roadmap. By following these steps, you can avoid duplicate time and effort in your programming endeavor.

Finally, this chapter urges you to have a lot of hands-on practice. This book offers you various ways to facilitate your practice. We suggest that you:

1. Try all the examples in each chapter.
2. Do all the experiments in the "Try This" boxes.
3. Work on the VB explorer exercises in each chapter.
4. Complete all assignments suggested by your instructor.
5. Understand the materials thoroughly in one chapter before proceeding to the next. This is particularly important for the first seven chapters.

We also suggest that you build a habit of browsing the online help file for any needed information. The "Look It Up" boxes in this book serve as reminders and facilitators for this purpose. You should take full advantage of them.

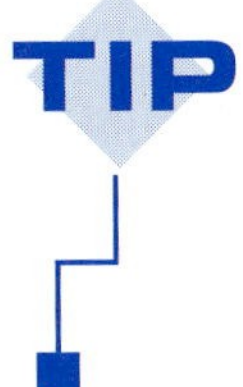

The solution to the "Try This" box on page 11 is as follows:

```
Printer.Print "Practice makes perfect."
```

Common mistakes include (1) failing to include a dot (.) between Printer and Print and (2) failing to enclose the text in a pair of double quotes (not single quotes).

Review Questions

1-1. What is Visual Basic? Is it a language or is it a program?

1-2. What is an interpreter? a compiler? Based on the discussion in the text, if both are available (separately) to process a source program, which one will you use? (*Hint:* your choice should depend on the stage of your program development because one is more convenient but the other is more efficient in execution. Note also that fortunately, you do not have to make such a choice for VB. Chapter 2 explains why.)

1-3. How is Visual Basic different from its predecessor, BASIC?

1-4. What is an "event"? How is programming in an event-driven language such a Visual Basic different from that in a procedure-oriented language?

1-5. Explain the following terms:

Program
Statement
Code

1-6. Computers are becoming faster and faster in speed and bigger and bigger in memory and storage size. Why should the programmer still be concerned about program efficiency in speed and in storage usage? (*Hint:* Your computer may be performing more than one task at a time.)

1-7. What does *user-friendliness* mean? What constitutes a user-friendly program?

1-8. Why is it important to observe consistency in coding style?

1-9. What factors can enhance code clarity and readability?

1-10. What does *modularity* mean? Why is it an important consideration in code design?

1-11. How do you judge whether an algorithm is elegant?

1-12. What factors affect the maintainability of a program?

1-13. Enumerate the steps that a programmer should follow in developing a program. What can happen if these steps are not followed?

1-14. Why is hands-on practice important to learning Visual Basic? What benefits can you gain by doing a lot of hands-on practice?

1-15. What benefits can you gain by developing a habit of browsing the online help file?

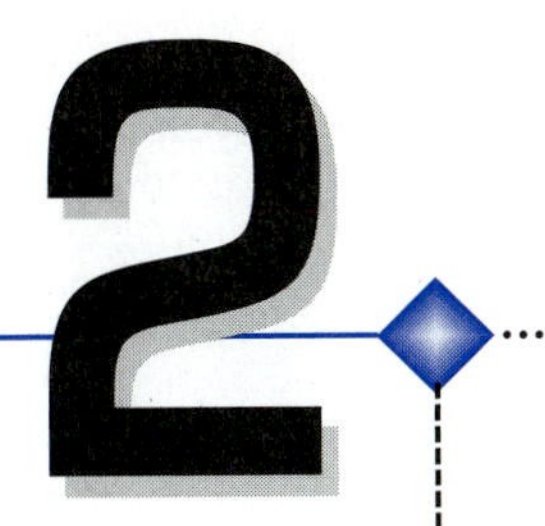

2 Introduction to Visual Basic Programming

This chapter provides a hands-on overview of the Visual Basic (VB) program development cycle. Chapter 1, "Introduction," enumerated the steps involved in the cycle. There we also mentioned that in developing a simple VB program, several of those steps could be combined. Once you understand the programming goal, you design the user interface, develop the necessary code, and then run and test your code. You will revise the code and repeat the run-test process until the program works exactly as wanted. All these activities are carried out in the VB Integrated Development Environment (IDE). A thoroughly tested program to be used in "production" (to perform the "real" work) should be compiled into an executable. You subsequently can use that program without the VB IDE. We will begin by introducing the VB IDE and conclude by showing the steps to compile a program and run an executable.

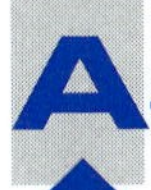

After completing this chapter, you should be able to:

- Navigate the VB IDE.
- Appreciate the use of a form.
- Create controls on a form and adjust their sizes.
- Understand the events, properties, and methods of controls.
- Understand how the code and events work in a VB program.
- Open and save a VB project.
- Understand the coding mechanics and the naming convention.
- Get help from the MSDN help system.
- Enumerate the types of statements in a program.
- Compile a program into an executable and run it without the VB IDE.

2.1 Navigating the Integrated Development Environment

This section introduces the VB IDE. You will learn how to start the IDE and will have a brief visit of the important parts in it.

Starting the VB IDE

To start the VB IDE, perform the following steps:

1. Click the Start icon at the lower-left corner of the desktop (screen). A menu should appear (Figure 2.1).
2. Highlight the Programs option by resting the mouse pointer on the item. Another menu should appear (Figure 2.1).
3. Highlight the Microsoft Visual Basic 6.0 option. A third menu should appear (Figure 2.1).
4. Click the Microsoft Visual Basic 6.0 option. The ***New Project dialog box*** (Figure 2.2) should appear.

FIGURE 2.1
Sequence of Menus to Invoke VB IDE

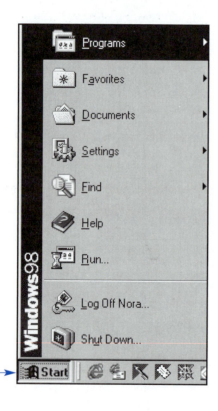

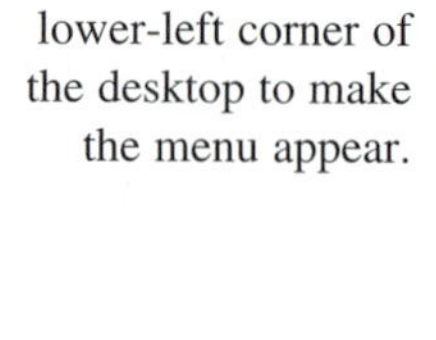

Click this icon at the lower-left corner of the desktop to make the menu appear.

Rest your mouse pointer on this item. It will be highlighted. Its submenu will appear.

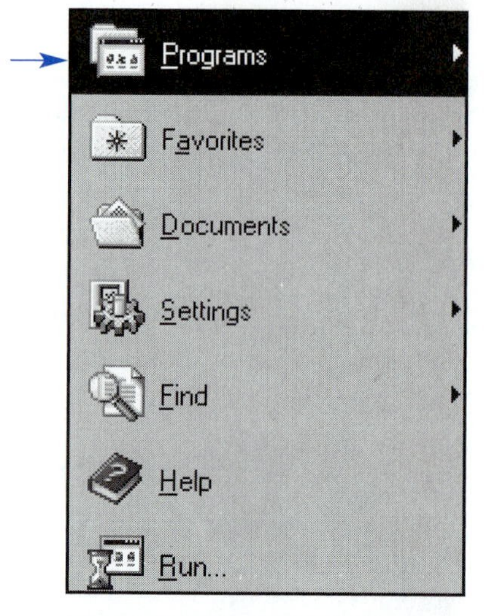

Look for this item in the Program submenu and highlight it; you should see another submenu as shown on the right.

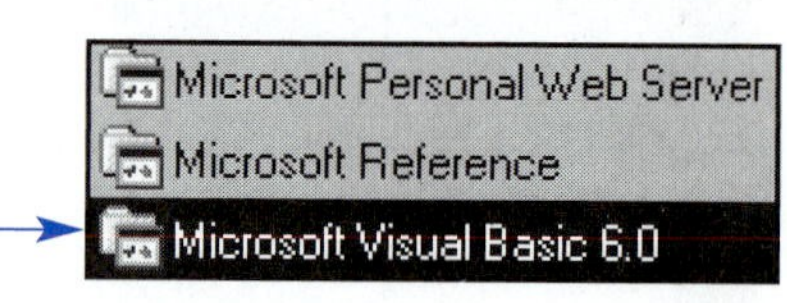

Click this item. You will see the New Project dialog box.

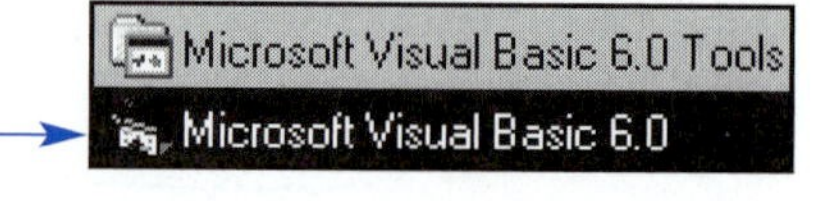

TIP

If your system has the entire Microsoft Visual Studio installed, the menu sequence will be slightly different. Look for the "Microsoft Visual Studio 6.0" in the Programs submenu. Then look for Microsoft Visual Basic 6.0.

FIGURE 2.2
The VB New Project Dialog Box

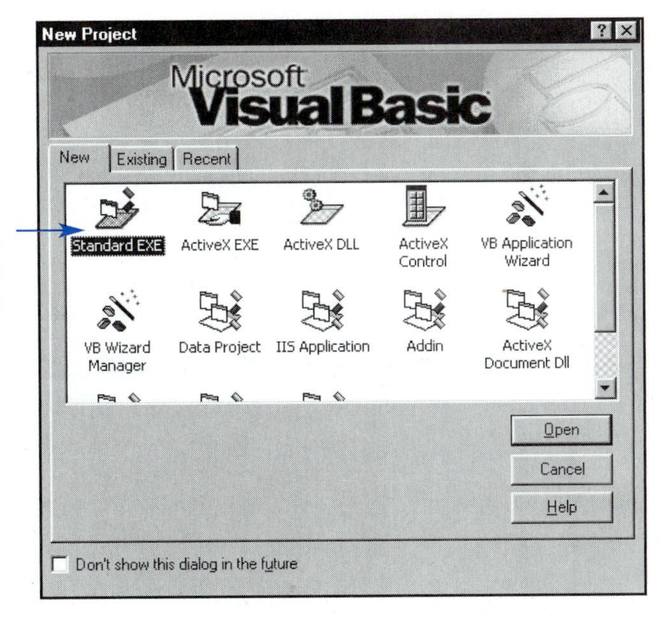

This is the VB New Project dialog box. Make sure that the Standard EXE icon is highlighted before clicking the Open button.

Note that the Standard EXE icon is highlighted. If it is not, click the item to select it. Then click the "Open" button. The VB IDE will come into action. You will see a window with the title bar showing "Project 1 – Microsoft Visual Basic [Design]". (See top of Figure 2.3.)

The Menu Bar and the Toolbar

The menu bar and the toolbar are found under the title bar of the VB IDE, as shown in Figure 2.3.

FIGURE 2.3
The Menu Bar and Toolbar

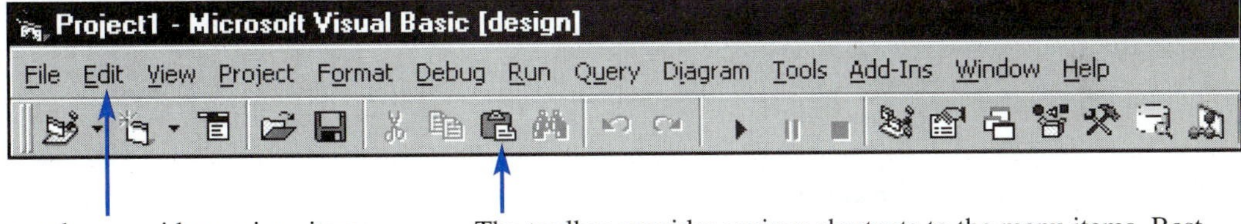

The menu bar provides various items that you need to use while working on your VB project.

The toolbar provides various shortcuts to the menu items. Rest the mouse pointer on one of these icons and a ToolTip text will appear.

The ***menu bar*** provides many menu items. These items are fairly similar to most of the Windows applications. For example, the edit menu contains options such as the familiar Cut, Copy, Paste, and Select All options found in word processing applications. Click on some of these menu items and explore the available options. We will refer to these menu items when they are needed.

The ***toolbar*** provides shortcuts to the menu bar. All the options available here are also available in the menus. However, the items on the toolbar allow you to gain quick access to the options. If you need to know what option an icon on the toolbar represents, simply rest the mouse pointer on the icon. A ToolTip text will appear to indicate what the icon is for (see Figure 2.3).

The Toolbox

On the left side of the IDE is the ***toolbox***, which contains various icons (see Figure 2.4). These icons represent various VB controls, which are visible objects that can be drawn on the form. Again, if you want to know what control a particular icon represents, rest the mouse pointer on the icon and a ToolTip will appear. We will see some of these controls in action in the next section. (*Note:* If you do not see the toolbox, click the View menu and select the Toolbox option. Or, click the toolbox icon on the toolbar.)

The Form and Code Window

In the center of the IDE, you should see a form with a title bar, Form1 (Figure 2.4). The form is what you use to develop the visual interface in VB. Behind the form is the code window in which you write your code. If you double-click the form, the code window will appear. If you click the "x" (close) button on the upper-right corner of this window, it will disappear and the form will reappear on top. Another way to toggle the appearance/disappearance of the form and the code window is to use the ***Project Explorer.***

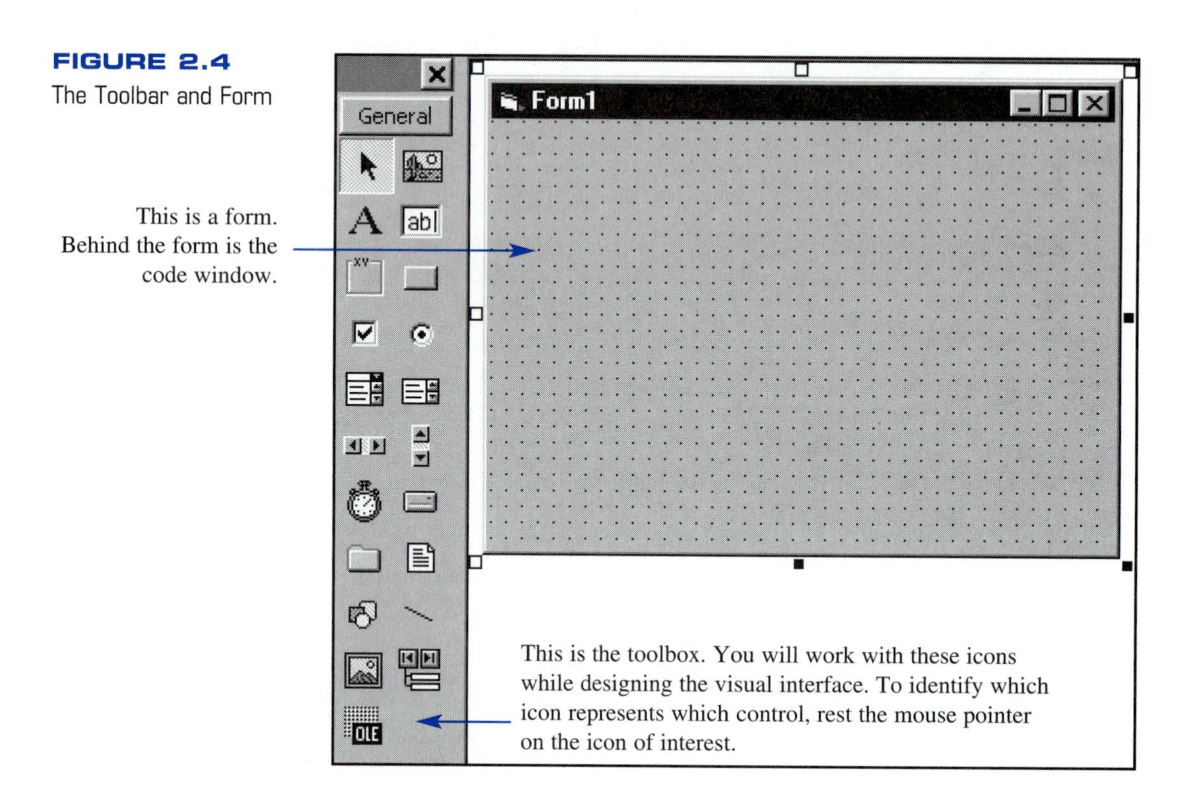

General
Form1
This is a form. Behind the form is the code window.
This is the toolbox. You will work with these icons while designing the visual interface. To identify which icon represents which control, rest the mouse pointer on the icon of interest.

FIGURE 2.4
The Toolbar and Form

The Project Explorer

On the upper-right corner of the IDE is the project explorer. This window shows all the forms and modules that your current VB project contains (Figure 2.5). (*Note:* If you do not see this window, click the View menu and select the Project Explorer option. Or, press Ctrl+R.)

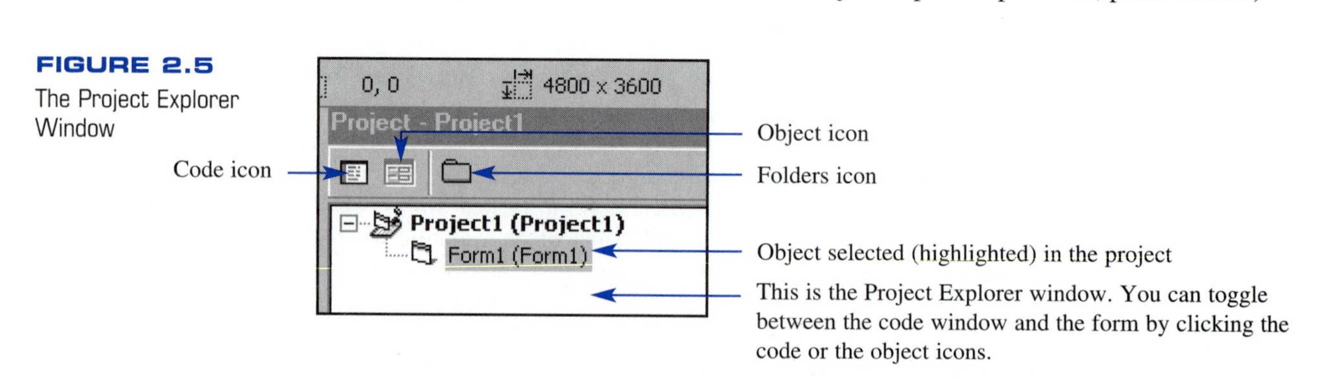

FIGURE 2.5
The Project Explorer Window

There are three icons at the top of this window: the Code, Object, and Folders icons (see Figure 2.5). Clicking the Code icon will make the code window appear in the middle of the IDE screen over the form. Clicking the Object icon will make the IDE display the form over the code window. When developing a project, you will use these two icons often because you will need to toggle between the Code and Object views from time to time. If you have more than one form in your project, the form displayed is the one that is highlighted and the code is the one associated with this form. The Folders icon toggles the Folders view and can be useful when you have many forms and modules in a project.

The Properties Window

The ***Properties window*** (Figure 2.6) lies below the Project Explorer window on the right side of the screen. Immediately below the title of the Properties window is an Object box, which shows the object being displayed. (Forms and VB controls are collectively referred to as objects.) There is a drop-down button on the right side. If you click that button, a drop-down list will display all objects on the form. You can select an object from the list by clicking the item of interest. *(Note:* If you do not see this window, click the View menu and select the Properties window option. Or, press F4.)

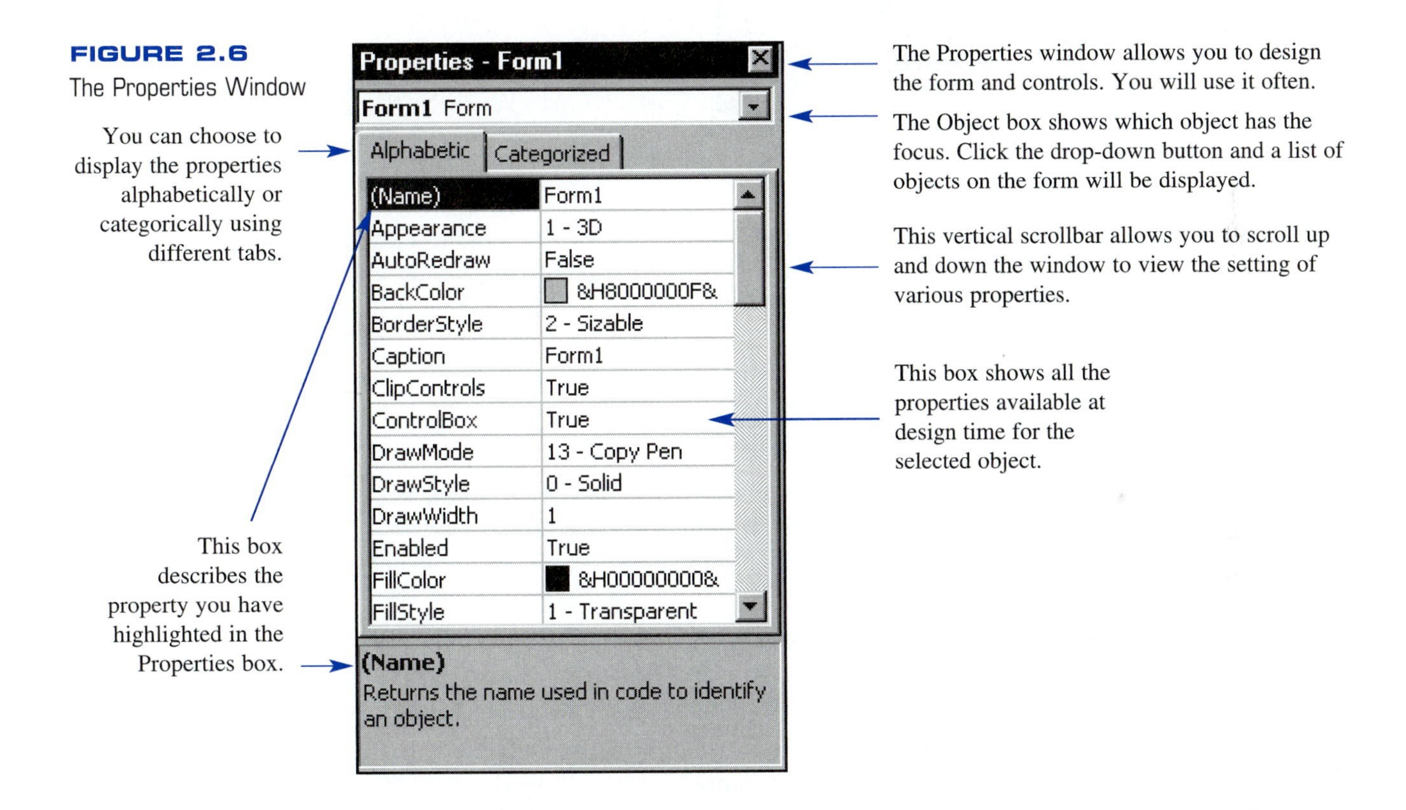
You can choose to display the properties alphabetically or categorically using different tabs.
This box describes the property you have highlighted in the Properties box.
Properties - Form1
Form1 Form
Alphabetic
Categorized
(Name) Form1
Appearance 1 - 3D
AutoRedraw False
BackColor &H8000000F&
BorderStyle 2 - Sizable
Caption Form1
ClipControls True
ControlBox True
DrawMode 13 - Copy Pen
DrawStyle 0 - Solid
DrawWidth 1
Enabled True
FillColor &H00000000&
FillStyle 1 - Transparent
(Name)
Returns the name used in code to identify an object.
The Properties window allows you to design the form and controls. You will use it often.
The Object box shows which object has the focus. Click the drop-down button and a list of objects on the form will be displayed.
This vertical scrollbar allows you to scroll up and down the window to view the setting of various properties.
This box shows all the properties available at design time for the selected object.

FIGURE 2.6
The Properties Window

In the middle of this window is the ***Properties box***, which displays the properties of the selected object. You can use this window to set the value for various properties of the object. *A property is a special type of data associated with the object.* The object acts, behaves, and/or appears differently depending on the values of its various properties. On the right side of the Properties window, there is a vertical scrollbar, which you can use to scroll up and down the window to view the Property settings. Below the list of properties is a small window that explains the property selected in the window. If you select (click) a different property, different explanatory text will appear in this area. Note that different types of objects have different properties. You can explore and learn a lot about the properties of an object by clicking different properties in this window and viewing the text in this area.

Between the Object box and the Properties box, there are two tabs: Alphabetic and Categorized. These tabs determine the order in which the properties are displayed. When the Alphabetic tab is selected, properties are displayed in alphabetic order. If you would rather that they be displayed by categories, you can select the Categorized tab. In this case, properties will be displayed in groups by their effect on appearance, behavior, etc., of the object.

The Form Layout Window

Below the Properties window is the ***Form Layout*** window (Figure 2.7). You can use this window to set the position of your form. If you want to view more items of the Properties window, you can click the "x" (close) button on the Form Layout window's upper-right corner. This window will disappear and the Properties window expands vertically. To bring the Form Layout window back, click the Form Layout icon in the toolbar or the Form Layout window option of the View menu.

FIGURE 2.7
The Form Layout Window

The Form Layout window allows you to set the runtime position of the form.

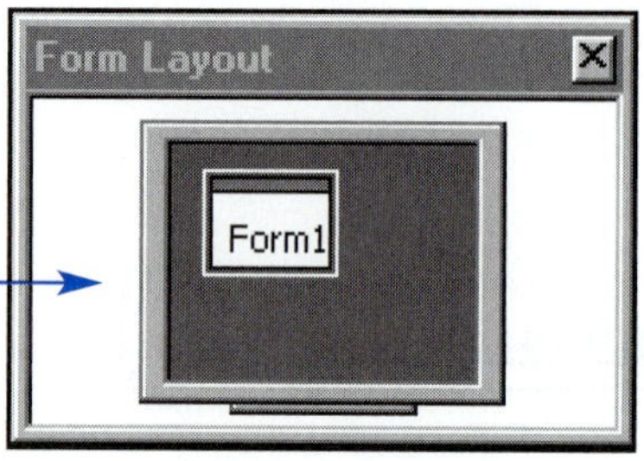

Exiting the VB IDE

You have completed a brief tour of the VB IDE. To exit the software, click the Close (x) button on the upper-right corner of the IDE window or click the File menu then click the Exit option.

2.2 Your First Visual Basic Program

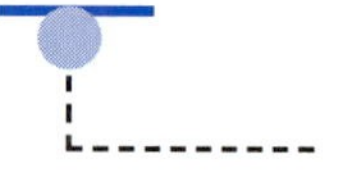

You have just completed a brief tour of the VB IDE. As explained at the beginning of this chapter, the VB IDE is where you work to develop a VB program (project). You are probably eager now to learn to write your first VB program. We will first walk through a program development cycle so that you can get a hands-on feel. We will then explain the concepts behind all the work.

A Simple Program Walkthrough

This program displays "Welcome To Visual Basic!!!" in a label on a form when you click on a button with the caption "Say Welcome." This project involves three VB objects: a form, a label, and a command button. As you recall, a form is readily available in the VB IDE when you start a new project. However, you will need to bring the label and the command button from the VB's toolbox, which is located on the left side in the VB IDE. Now, let's walk through the following steps to develop the "Welcome" project.

1. Start your VB6 IDE with a new standard EXE project. Follow the steps outlined in the preceding section.
2. Resize the form so that its width is about one-quarter of the screen width and its height is also about one-quarter of the screen height. You can resize the form by dragging one of the sizing handles on the sides and corners of the form. (You "drag" by holding down the mouse button and moving away from the original point.) Figure 2.8 shows the sizing handles of the form.
3. Draw a label on the form. Double-click the label icon in the toolbox (Figure 2.9). You should see the label with a caption "Label1" at the center of the form (Figure 2.10). Drag a sizing handle on the right to the right so that the label will look wide enough to hold about 30 characters.
4. Draw a command button on the form.

FIGURE 2.8
Sizing Handles

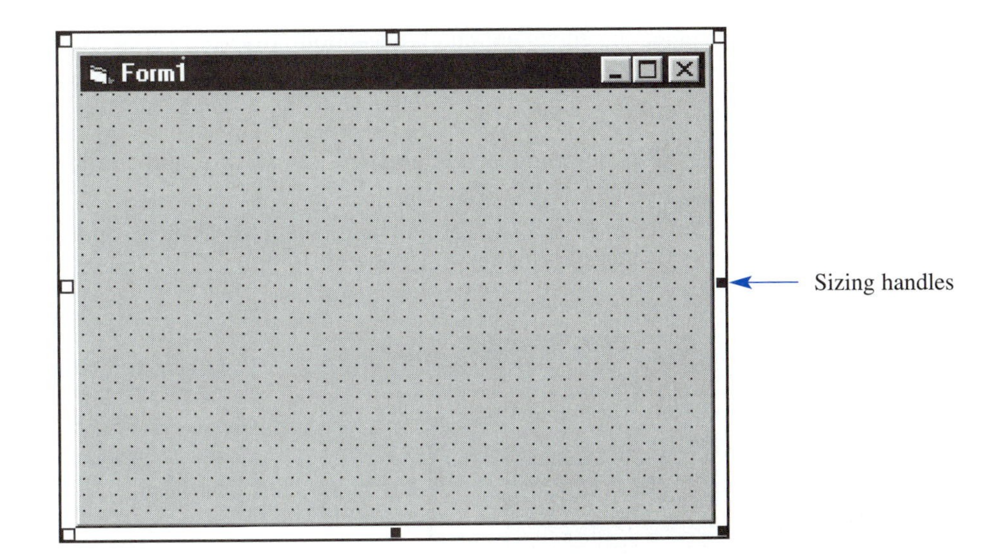

FIGURE 2.9
The Label Icon and Command Button Icon

Label icon in the toolbox

General

abl

Command Button icon in the toolbox

4.1 Click the command icon on the toolbox.

4.2 Point the mouse on the form below the label control and drag down and to right corner for about $\frac{1}{3} \times 1$.

4.3 Release the mouse. You will see the shape and size of the button (Figure 2.10).

FIGURE 2.10
Drawing a Command Button

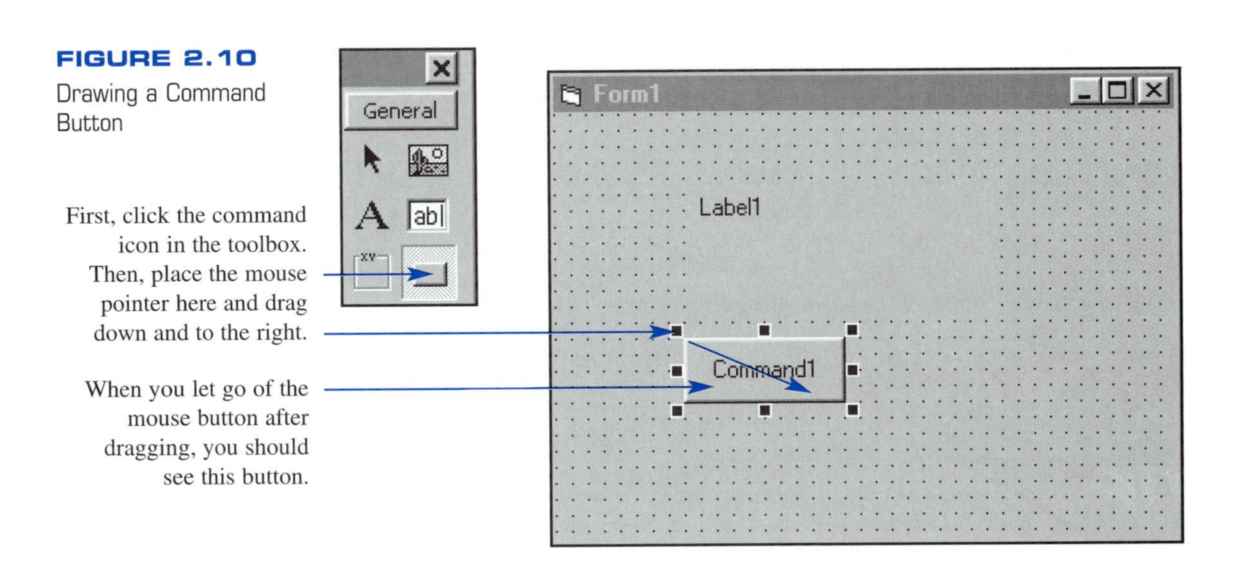

First, click the command icon in the toolbox. Then, place the mouse pointer here and drag down and to the right.
When you let go of the mouse button after dragging, you should see this button.
General
abl
Form1
Label1
Command1

You can resize the command button by dragging one of the button's sizing handles, the same way you resized the form and the label.

5. Change the command button's caption property to "Say Welcome." You change the property setting through the Properties window. (If you do not see the window on your screen, click the Properties window option in the VB View menu or press F4.)

   5.1 Click the command button on the form so that the Properties window shows the properties of this button.

   5.2 Use the scrollbar of the window to find the Caption property. Type "Say Welcome" to replace "Command1" in the box (Figure 2.11).

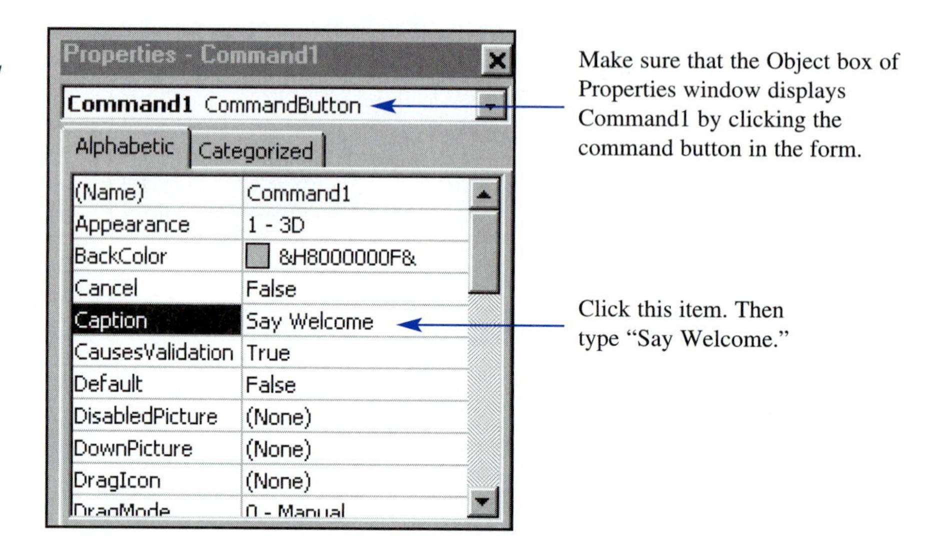

FIGURE 2.11
The Properties Window for Command Button

6. Add code to the code window.

   6.1 Double-click the command button on the form (not the icon in the toolbox, nor the form itself). The code window will appear in place of the form. You should see some code lines in the code window as shown in Figure 2.12.

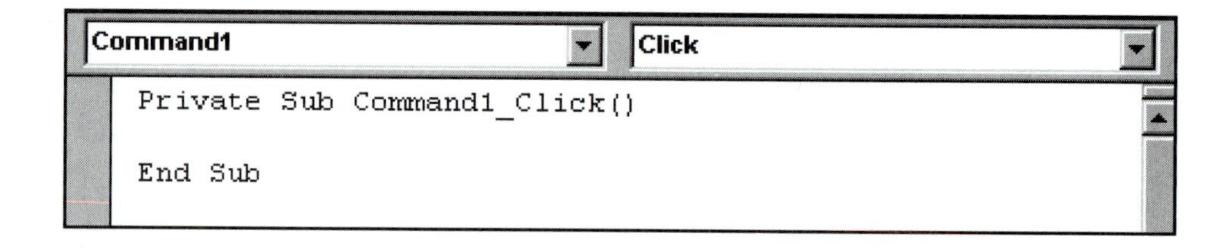

FIGURE 2.12
The Code Window

   6.2 Add two lines of code as shown below:

```
Private Sub Command1_Click()
  ' Make the label display the Welcome message
  Label1.Caption = "Welcome to Visual Basic!!!"
End Sub
```

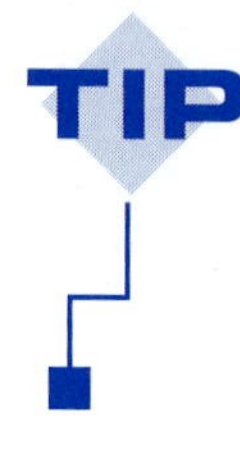

TIP

Beware of the difference between the lowercase L and the number 1. To human eyes, l (lowercase L) and 1 (numeral 1) look very similar. To the computer, they are completely different. Some beginners tend not to be careful in distinguishing the two. The consequence can range from an obvious syntax error with an immediate fix to days of searching for a "mysterious" bug in the program. A similar situation exists between the letter O (or its lowercase o) and the number 0.

7. Run the program. Click the Start button in the Toolbar or click the Start option in the Run menu.
8. Click the "Say Welcome" button. You should see the screen now displays, "Welcome to Visual Basic!!!" instead of its original "Label1" (Figure 2.13).

Congratulations! You have successfully completed a VB project. Click the close (x) button on the form's title bar to end the project.

FIGURE 2.13
Your First Project Action

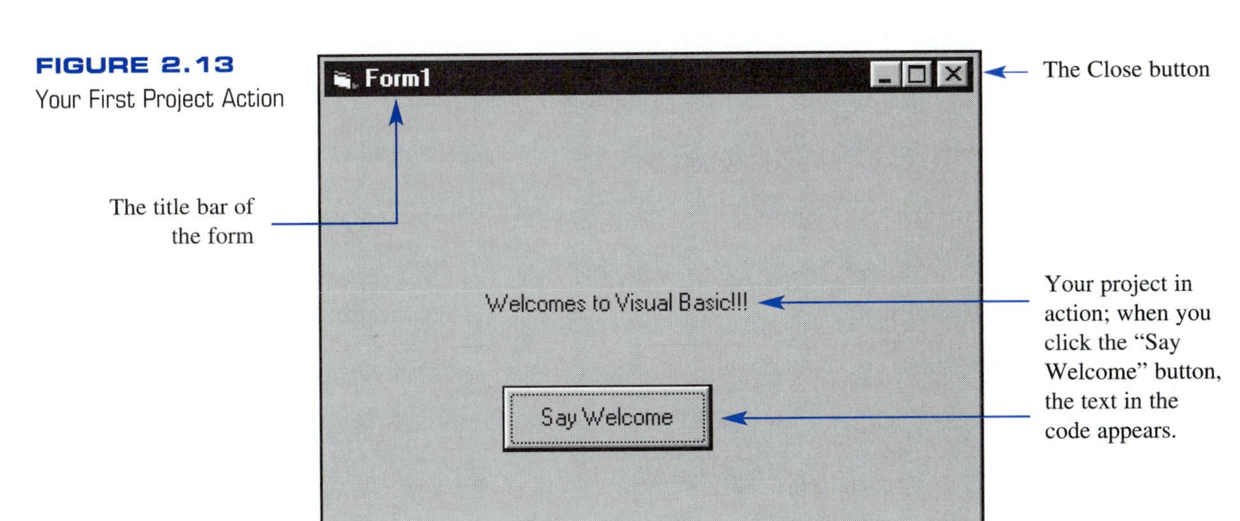

To move a control on a form, click the control and drag it from inside to the desired location.

Handling VB Program Files

When you complete a program, you should save it on the disk. (Realistically, you should save more often than that.) The saved work can be retrieved later for execution and additional testing and editing. Let us take a look at this file-handling aspect here.

Saving the Files. To save your project, click File in the menu bar, then click the Save Project option. Alternatively, click the Save icon on the toolbar (see Figure 2.14).

FIGURE 2.14
The File Menu and Save Icon

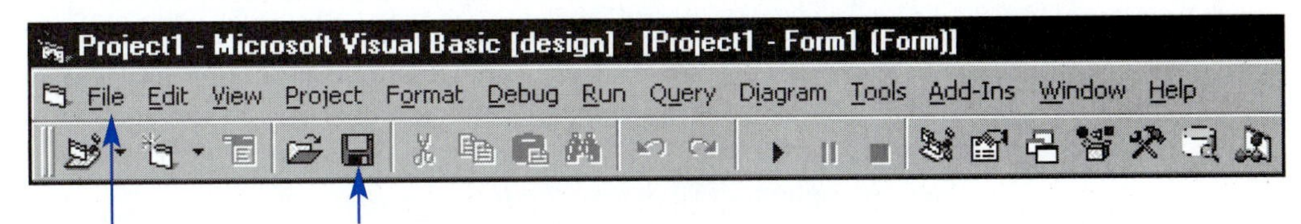

Because this is the first time you are saving the project, a Save File As dialog box will appear to prompt you for the file name to use for the form (see Figure 2.15). Before you actually save the file, consider where you want to save it. At this point, the dialog box shows the default folder (which is where the VB IDE is located) to save your work. If you save the current project as well as all the future projects in this folder, you will eventually have difficulty identifying which file(s) belong to which projects. Worse yet, you may accidentally write over some files. *It is advisable that each project be saved in a separate folder.*

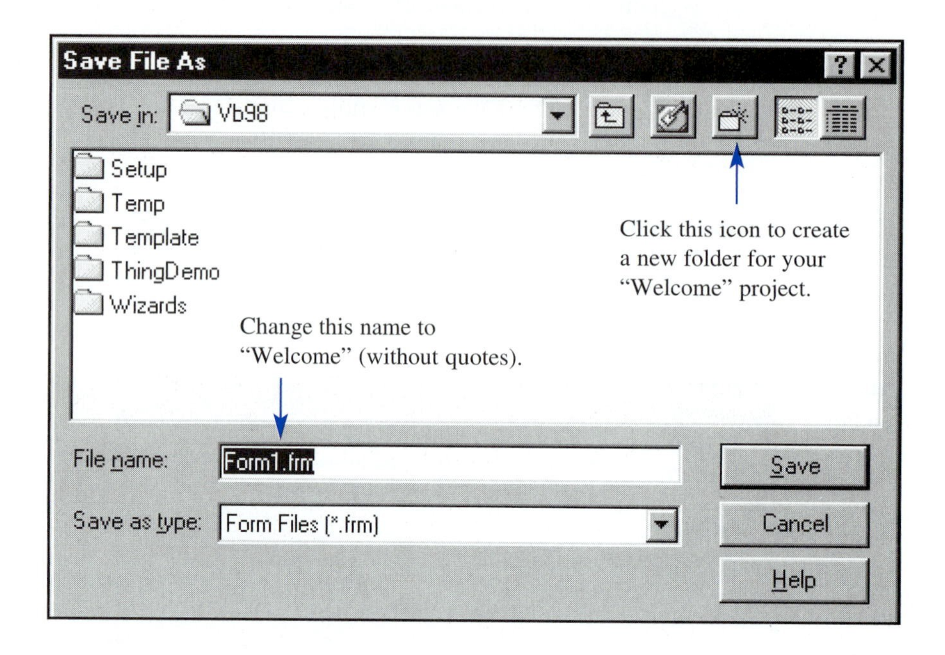

FIGURE 2.15
The Save File As Dialog Box

You can create and open a new folder with the dialog box by performing the following steps:

1. Click the "Create New Folder" icon on the upper-right side of the dialog box. A folder with the name "New Folder" will appear.
2. Change "New Folder" to a more meaningful name, for example, "Welcome."
3. Double-click the folder to open it.

With the "Welcome" folder open, you can save the form file in it:

1. Change "Form1" in the file name box to "Welcome" to make it descriptive. Note that the form file has the extension "frm." You should not change it.
2. Click the Save button in the dialog box.

Another dialog box will prompt you for the name to save for the project (with the extension "vbp"). Change the default name, Project1.vbp, to Welcome and click the Save button to save the project file. (Notice that you can use the same name for both the form and the project files because they have different extensions.) The Save File As dialog box will not appear if you are saving files that already exist and you use the Save option in the file menu (or the Save icon in the toolbar).

The previous file-saving exercise indicates that *there are two files for your project*: the form file and the project file. The form (frm) file contains information on the controls and the code on the form. The project (vbp) file contains information on forms (e.g., their names and locations) and other resources the project requires. If you save your form in a different location, the content of the project file will change. In the future, when you are saving these files using the Save As option, *always save the form file first*.

A "Save" Reminder by the IDE. One good way to ensure that your work is saved is to use the "reminder" or automatic saving feature of VB when you test your program. To use this feature, do the following:

1. Click the Tools menu.
2. Click the "Options" option. The Options dialog box will appear.

Save your VB files often while working on your project to avoid accidental loss. In addition, you should copy your files to another location for backup. Experienced programmers know how easy it is to lose their work by neglecting to save. The backup provides a convenient means to fall back on when the current copy is accidentally destroyed.

3. Select the Environment tab (see Figure 2.16).
4. Select "Save changes" or "Prompt to save changes" in the frame labeled "When a program starts." If you select the latter, you will be asked whether to save the changes each time you start your program. I like this choice because I can decide whether to save when it reminds me, although I usually choose to save the work anyway.

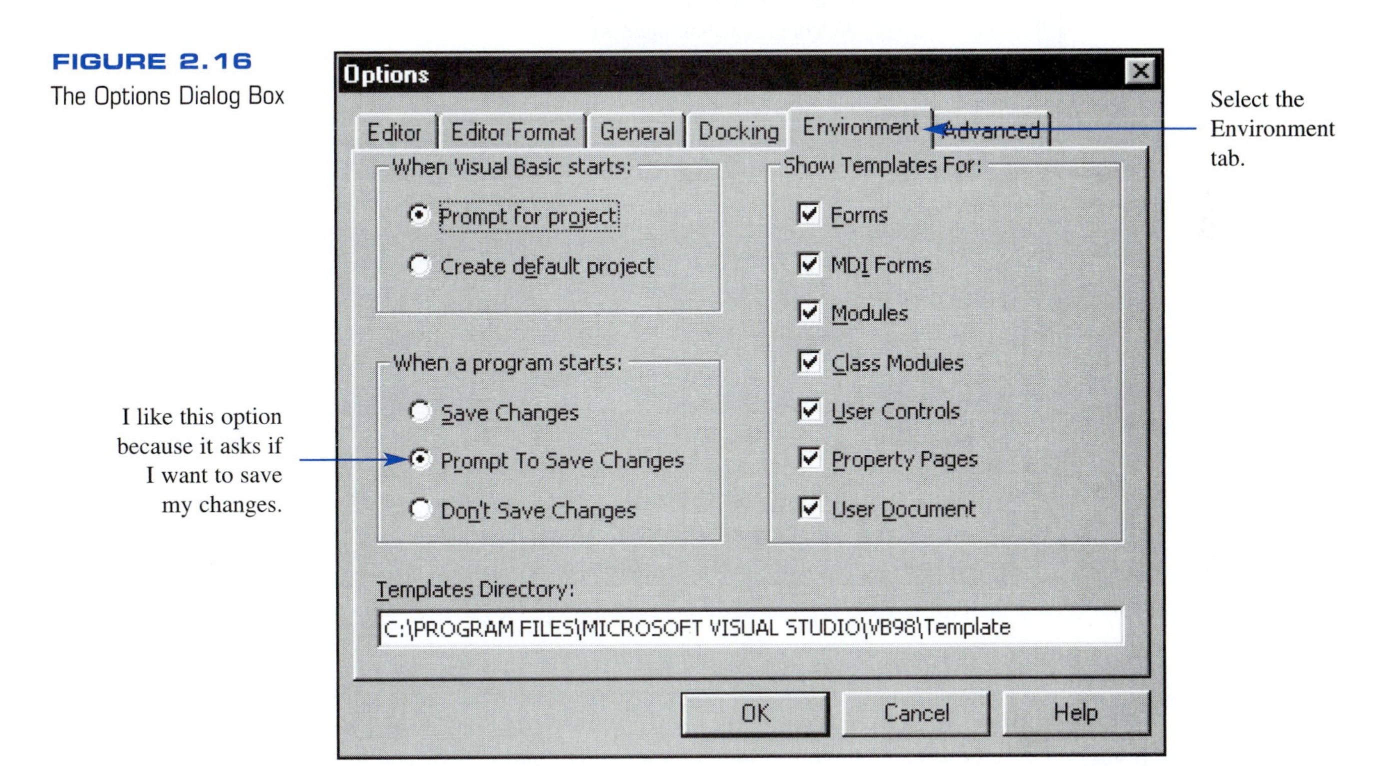

FIGURE 2.16
The Options Dialog Box

Reopening a Project. Often, you will need to reopen a project that you have worked on previously. To open an existing project while in the VB IDE, do the following:

1. Click the File menu. A drop-down File menu will appear (Figure 2.17).
2. Click the Open Project option. An Open Project dialog box similar to the Save File As dialog box shown previously will appear.
3. Browse through your computer system to find your project.

Alternatively, *you may find your project at the bottom of the File drop-down menu* (see Figure 2.17). If you do, you can simply click the project name to open the project.

Opening a Project While Starting the IDE. If you are starting the VB IDE when you need to open an existing project, you can also find the project by selecting either the Existing or Recent tab (see Figure 2.18). Browsing through the Existing tab is similar to browsing the Open Project dialog box, whereas selecting the project from the Recent tab is similar to finding the name at the bottom of the drop-down File menu.

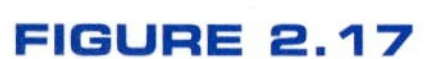

FIGURE 2.17
Reopening a Project

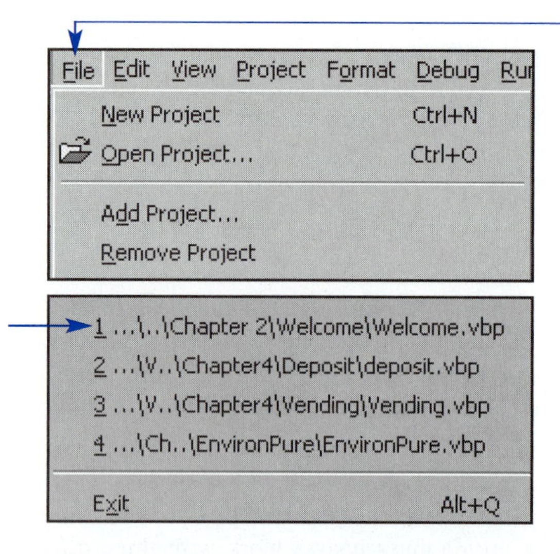

Click the File menu. Then click the Open Project option. The Open Project dialog box will appear.

At the bottom of the drop-down file menu, you may just find this project. Click it to open.

FIGURE 2.18
Using Different Tabs in the New Project Dialog Box to Locate a Project

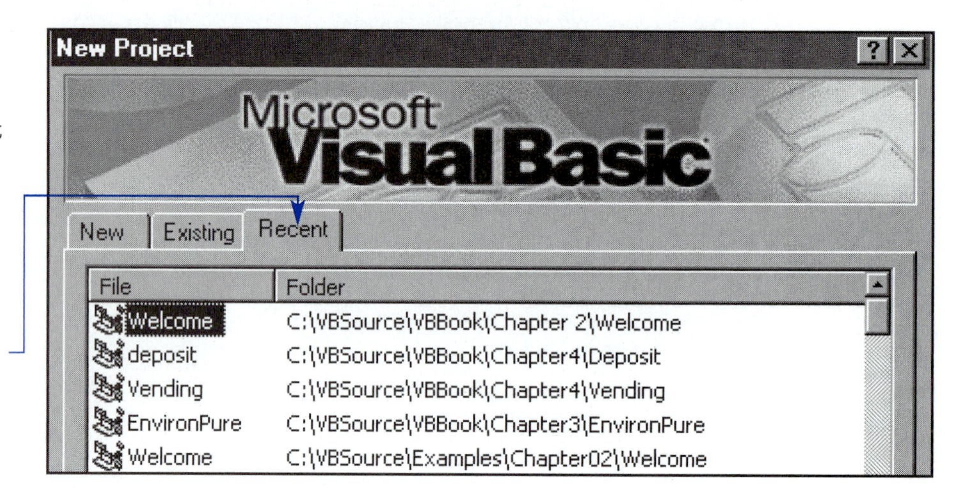
New Project
Microsoft
Visual Basic
New
Existing
Recent
File
Folder
Welcome C:\VBSource\VBBook\Chapter 2\Welcome
deposit C:\VBSource\VBBook\Chapter4\Deposit
Vending C:\VBSource\VBBook\Chapter4\Vending
EnvironPure C:\VBSource\VBBook\Chapter3\EnvironPure
Welcome C:\VBSource\Examples\Chapter02\Welcome

In the New Project dialog box at the start of the VB IDE, you can click the Recent tab to find a project recently worked or the Existing tab to browse the system for an existing project.

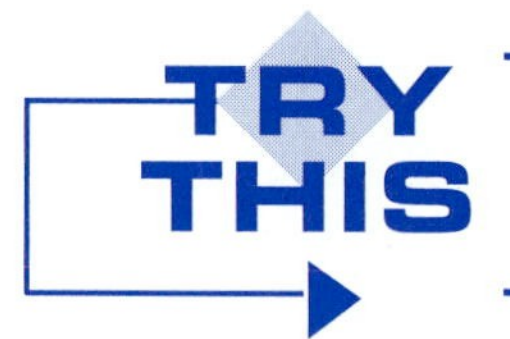

After you have saved your first project, exit the IDE. Then restart the IDE. Reopen your project using different methods outlined in this subsection. You will reopen a project often in the future. Gain hands-on experience now.

2.3 Some Basic Concepts

Understanding the Integrated Development Environment

Let us take another look at the steps we just took to develop the "Welcome" project. When you were resizing the form and bringing both the label and the command button to the form, you were in the "design phase" of your project. This phase is called ***design time.*** At design time, you work with the visual aspect of your project. The elements that you bring from the toolbox onto the form are called *controls.* When you run the project by clicking the Start button on the toolbar, your project enters ***runtime.*** In this phase, the code in your project actually comes to life, responding to events triggered by either the user's or the system's actions. When you clicked the "Say Welcome" button, the command button's "Click" event occurred.

The code you wrote in Sub Command1_Click was then triggered in response. The line you typed,

```
Label1.Caption = "Welcome to Visual Basic!!!"
```

tells the computer to move the text string "Welcome to Visual Basic!!!" to the caption of Label1. The ***Caption property*** of Label1 is then changed and displayed on the label. When your program quits, you still remain in the development environment, ready for another round of modification to the project.

Back in the Good Old Days. In the old DOS environment, when programs were developed in procedure-oriented languages (e.g., COBOL), all the visual aspect of a program was written in code. Additional code was (as is now) also needed to handle computations. The code was written with some text editor and saved as a file. The file was then input into a language processor, recognized as a compiler, which translated the source program into machine executable code (in machine language), which was saved as a separate file. This executable file was then run to produce the results that the developer desired. (*Note:* Quick Basic worked a bit differently.) In effect, a programmer had to work with three different programs at different phases of the program development activities to obtain results: an editor at design time, a compiler at compile time, and the compiled program at runtime (see Figure 2.19). You can imagine how long it could take (and how tedious it was) to develop a bug-free program that could be used formally for business data processing.

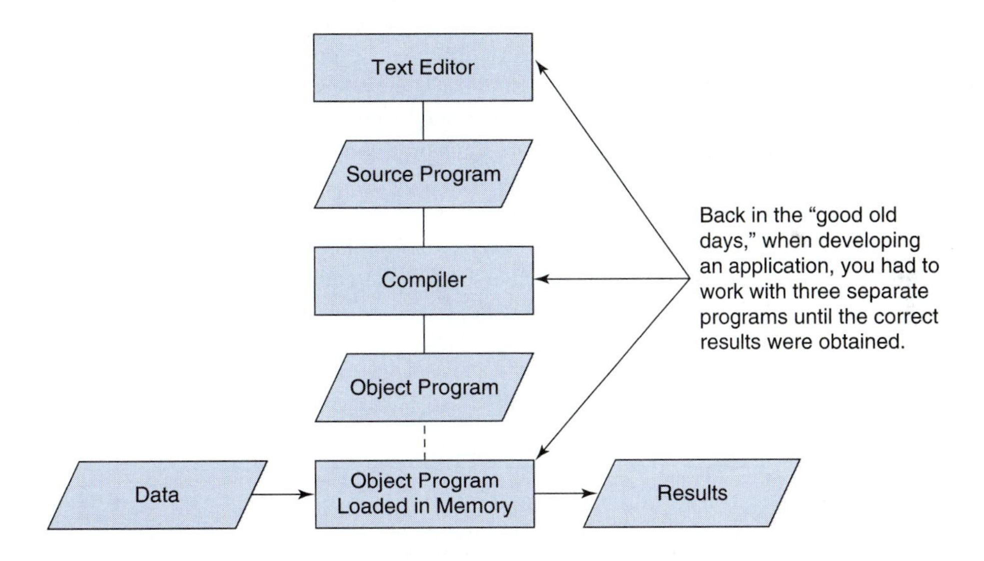
Text Editor
Source Program
Compiler
Object Program
Data
Object Program
Loaded in Memory
Results
Back in the "good old days," when developing an application, you had to work with three separate programs until the correct results were obtained.

FIGURE 2.19
The Three Interfaces of an Object

Now in the VB IDE. In contrast, when you are developing a program in VB, all the activities in visual design, code editing, and testing can be carried out in a single environment, as you have already experienced. While you are entering code, VB checks for apparent syntax errors. In addition, it compiles your code. When you run your program, VB makes your program execute without having to leave the development environment and is thus recognized as the Integrated Development Environment (IDE).

Coding Mechanics

You may have noticed that there are two lines of code inside the preceding Command1_Click event procedure:

```
' Make the label display the Welcome message
Label1.Caption = "Welcome to Visual Basic!!!"
```

However, only the second line causes an action. The first line is a comment statement.

Comments on Code. A comment statement starts with a tick (') mark or a Rem keyword. When VB sees a line beginning with a tick mark (apostrophe) or Rem, it ignores the line. The following line will have the same effect as the line with a tick mark above:

```
Rem Make the label display the Welcome message
```

You can also write comments at the end of a code line as shown below:

```
Label1.Caption = "Welcome to Visual Basic!!!" 'Show Welcome
```

Or

```
Label1.Caption = "Welcome to Visual Basic!!!" Rem Show Welcome
```

Why should we use comment lines? Comments usually are used by the programmer to provide clues to the purposes of the code. They enhance the readability and understandability of the program. They are an indispensable part of the program documentation. A well-documented program is much easier to maintain. You should use comments for your program whenever applicable. Someday, when you come back to your programs, you will appreciate your own thoughtfulness if your code is accompanied by plenty of comments.

Furthermore, if you write a program for a company, another programmer may have to update your code in the future. If it is properly commented, he or she will have a much easier time figuring out what your program does and how it should be changed.

Indenting Code Lines. VB has relatively few restrictions on how the code is written. As long as the syntax is correct, each code line can start practically in any position. For readability, it is advisable to indent the code within a procedure. We have observed (and will observe) this convention on all the code presented.

You can also insert blank lines between any code lines. If your procedure consists of several blocks of code, each dealing with a specific task, inserting blank lines between these blocks can make each block stand out, thus providing a visual cue to the logical structure of your procedure.

Line Continuation. Sometimes, you may have to code a long, complex statement. You may find it desirable to break such a statement into several lines. You can do this by using a space followed by an underscore (_) at end of the line and continue the remainder of the code in the next line as illustrated next:

```
Label.Caption = _
"Welcome to Visual Basic"
```

There are actually some restrictions on code. For example, a single line of code cannot exceed 1023 bytes. In addition, you are not allowed to have more than 256 blank spaces in a line before you start code. Also, you cannot have more than 25 continuation lines for one statement. Practically, however, such restrictions are not very restrictive and you probably will never encounter them.

Multiple Statements on a Line. You can have more than one statement on a line by inserting a colon (:) between statements. For example, you can code the following:

```
HourlyPay = 10 : Area = Height * Width
```

Although there is nothing wrong with the syntax, you may not want to code your program this way. Statements are harder to read. Sometimes, you can miss the flow of your program logic when reviewing the code.

Interfaces of VB Objects

You have worked with a form and two controls. Forms and controls are collectively recognized as objects. Each type of object provides different functionality. For example, forms serve as containers for other objects and as windows for the visual interface. Labels are used to display texts, which are usually simple messages or instructions for the user. Command buttons are used to initiate specific actions when the user clicks on them. All objects provide interfaces for your code. These interfaces include properties, events, and methods (Figure 2.20). Let us have a closer look.

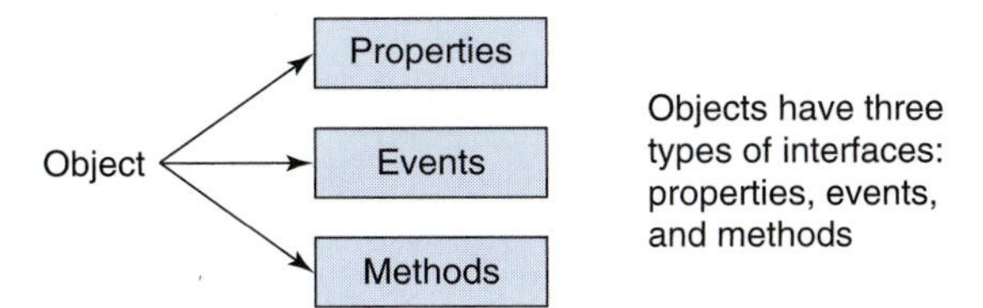
Object
Properties
Events
Methods
Objects have three types of interfaces: properties, events, and methods

FIGURE 2.20
The Three Interfaces of an Object

Properties. Objects have ***properties***, most of which relate to the appearance of the objects. Properties are just special types of data that are associated with an object. Other properties decide how an object behaves. Many properties can be set at either design time or runtime. Other properties can be set only at design time. Still others can be set or available only at runtime. In code, you refer to a property of an object by the following syntax:

```
Object.Property
```

The object name and the property name are separated by a dot (.). There should be no spaces in between. For example, you can refer to the background color property of the label named Label1 by coding:

```
Label1.BackColor
```

Thus, to set its background color to red, you will code:

```
Label1.BackColor = vbRed
```

Where vbRed is a constant name recognized by VB and represents the red color. Many controls have common properties. We will explore some of them in the next section.

Events. In addition to properties, objects also have events, which are user or system actions recognized by the object. As you can see from the "Welcome" project, the command button has a Click event. When the user clicks on the button, the ***Click event*** is raised (triggered). Different objects recognize different events. As discussed in Chapter 1, VB is an event-driven language. When a VB project starts to run, it waits for events to occur and responds by executing the code written to handle these events accordingly. You write code for each of the events that you want the program to handle. The procedure written to handle an event is called an ***event procedure***. Event procedures have the following syntax structure:

```
Private Sub ObjectName_Event(parameter list)
    <Code to handle the event>
End Sub
```

The first line of the procedure starts with "Private Sub," which is used to indicate the beginning of a ***Sub*** procedure. The object name identifies the object of interest. The object and event are separated by an underscore (_). The event name is followed by a pair of parentheses that

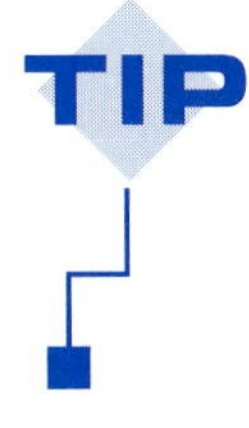

You might have discovered some confusing terminology in the previous discussion. The term *control* has been used in two different contexts. Initially, we introduced those objects dragged into the form from the toolbox as *controls*. The flow of execution in a program, however, is also referred to as *control* in the previous paragraph. For clear differentiation, we use (and will continue to use) the term *execution control* to refer to execution flow. Unless the context is very clear, we will use the term *VB control* to refer to VB objects.

enclose a list of parameters if they exist for the procedure. Not all event procedures have parameters. For example, the Command1_Click event procedure has none.

The ***End Sub*** line physically defines the end of the procedure; that is, any lines beyond this point have nothing to do with this procedure. When execution control drops down to this line, it will return to the point where this procedure was triggered. In most cases, this means the computer will be waiting for another event to trigger another event procedure.

Exploring Available Events of an Object. You can find what events an object can recognize and what parameters each event procedure has by exploring the code window (see Figure 2.21).

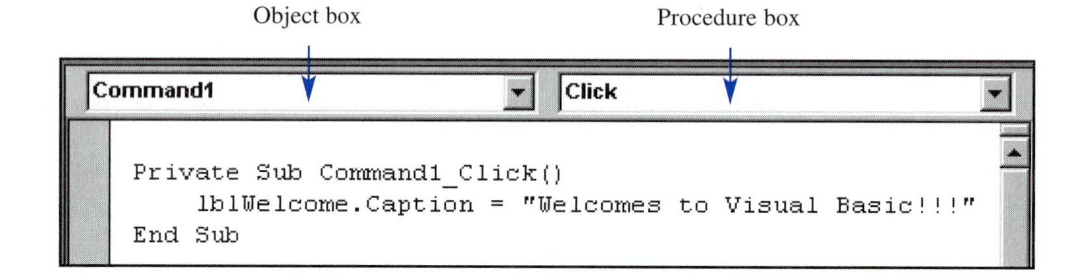

FIGURE 2.21
The Code Window

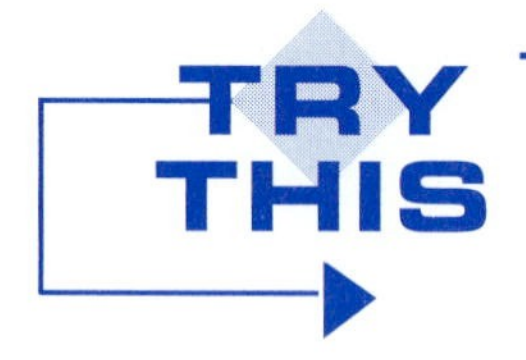

In the code window of your current project, select Form from the Object box on the left. You should see a Form Load event procedure template in the code window:

```
Private Sub Form_Load()
End Sub
```

Then select the KeyPress from the Procedure box on the right. You should see the following event procedure template in the code window:

```
Private Sub Form_KeyPress (KeyAscii as Integer)
End Sub
```

You may want to try a few more, just for fun and to gain familiarity. Remove these lines to continue.

The Object box at the upper-left corner has a list of all the objects on the form. You can see the names of these objects by clicking on the drop-down button. The Procedure box on the right side shows the list of events the object on the left recognizes. If you click on an event in this list, an event procedure template will appear in the code window. This is the easiest (and the standard) way to start writing code to handle a particular event.

Always use the procedure template provided by VB to code an event procedure. When in the code window, first select the object name from the Object box. Then select the event from the Procedure box. The event procedure template will appear in the code window.

A project can have many event procedures. *The relative position of these procedures is not important.* Procedures get invoked by the events and are not executed by the order they are placed in the code window. In contrast, *the order of the code lines within the procedure is very important*. In general, these lines are executed top down, line by line (or more accurately, statement by statement). The result of executing a line may depend on the results from the previous lines. Thus, any lines that are placed "out of order" can cause an erroneous result.

Methods. Finally, objects have ***methods***, which are actions that objects are capable of performing. For example, Move is a method that many objects have. The following code will move the label you have created to a random location on the form. (For the time being, do not worry about how the code works.)

```
Label1.Move (Rnd * ScaleWidth), (Rnd * ScaleHeight)
```

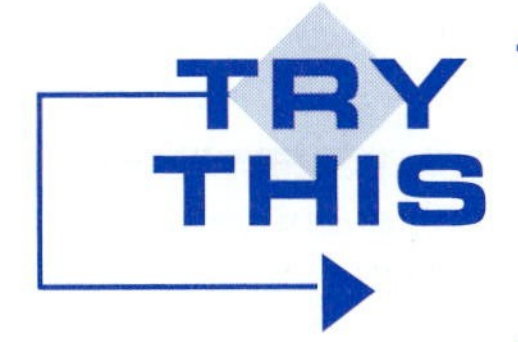

Insert the preceding code into the Command1_Click event procedure you created in the preceding section. Run the program and click the "Say Welcome" button as many times as you enjoy. You should see the welcome label move all over the form. Remove this line to continue.

The syntax to use a method is as follows:

```
Object.Method [first parameter], [second parameter] . . .
```

Notice that there is a dot (.) between the object and the method (as is the case in the code for the property). Some methods have required parameters. Some have optional arguments. Still other methods require no parameters.

These parameters provide information for the method to perform proper actions. For example, the Move method just shown requires at least one parameter. However, it can take up to four parameters. Its syntax appears as follows:

```
Object.Move Left, [Top] [Width] [Height]
```

Where Object = a control or form.
Left, Top = a number indicating the coordinate at which the left side (top) of the object should be aligned.
Width, Height = a number giving the width (height) of the object.

Note that only the Left parameter is required. If omitted, there will be no change to the original settings for these properties.

The preceding Move statement tells the label to move to a position in which its upper-left corner is at the point as defined by the two given parameters.

Defaults

Sometimes, you may encounter code that is not explicit in its expression. Yet, it can still be acceptable to VB. This occurs because when VB encounters missing (unspecified) elements in an expression, it "fills in the blank" by assuming a certain default element. Here are some defaults worth noting.

Default Object. You sometimes see methods or properties used without explicitly referring to the object; that is, the code shows only the method without being preceded by an object and a dot. In this case, we say the method has a default object. For example, the following code will move the form, aligning itself to the upper-left corner of the screen. The form is the default object of the Move method.

```
Move 0,0
```

The "complete" statement should be as follows:

```
Me.Move 0, 0
```

Where *Me* is a special name that represents the form. When the code needs to reference to the form itself, the keyword *Me* can be used in its place.

Default Property. In addition, an object can have and usually does have a default property. For example, the following two lines will have the same effect.

```
Label1 = "Welcome to Visual Basic!!!"
Label1.Caption = "Welcome to Visual Basic!!!"
```

The Caption property is the default property of labels. Although there are reasons to write code using default objects and properties, the code is not as clear as when the defaults are explicitly stated. In some cases, the programmer may erroneously assume a default property, causing unexpected problems in the program. *It is advisable to avoid coding with defaults.* Explicit code is more readable and understandable.

Default Property Setting. Most objects have many properties. When an object is initiated, each of these properties is assigned with an assumed setting (value). This setting is referred to as the default setting of the property. For example, you may have already discovered that the default settings (values) of the Caption property for the first label, command button, and form are Label1, Command1, and Form1, respectively. In most cases, default property settings are the proper settings for your project. In addition, not all the properties of an object have significant bearings on the performance of the project. These default property settings are usually left untouched.

2.4 Exploring More Properties

Let us now explore some more properties of the three objects (form, label, and command button). We have mentioned that all three objects have the Caption property. Indeed, you have changed the Caption property of the command button from "Command1" to "Say Welcome" at design time by using the Properties window. You also have used code to change the Caption property of the label from "Label1" to "Welcome to Visual Basic!!!" Why not try to change the form's caption property to "My First VB Project"? You can do this either at design time using the Properties window (follow the same steps for the command button) or by code (double-click the form to obtain the form load code template and place the code in that event). Which way do you prefer? In general, if you do not anticipate the property setting to change when your program runs, it is easier and more efficient to set it at design time.

Common Properties

Forms and Labels have many common properties. If you carefully examine the Properties window of each object, you should be able to identify quite a few. The following is a short sample list of these common properties and their uses:

Property	Uses	Default Setting
Appearance	How the object will look: flat or three-dimensional	3-D
BackColor	Background color	Gray; standard color for buttons
Font	Font displayed in the object	MS San Serif 8
ForeColor	Foreground (text) color	Black; standard text color
Top	Vertical position of the object	
Left	Horizontal position of the object	
Width	Width of the object	
Height	Height of the object	

Of course, any of these property settings can be changed. You may have noticed that as you move the objects around, their Left and Top properties change. Furthermore, as you resize the objects, their Width and Height properties also change. You can also set a numeric value for any of these properties in the Properties window. When you do, their size or position on the screen will change accordingly.

Changing the Font for the Label: An Exercise

As an exercise, let us change the font size of the label in your project to 12. Follow these steps:

1. Click the label's Font property in the Properties window. An ellipsis (. . .) button should appear in the property box.
2. Click the Ellipsis button. A Font dialog box will appear (Figure 2.22).
3. Click "12" in the Size window on the right.
4. Click the "OK" button.

FIGURE 2.22
The Font Dialog Box

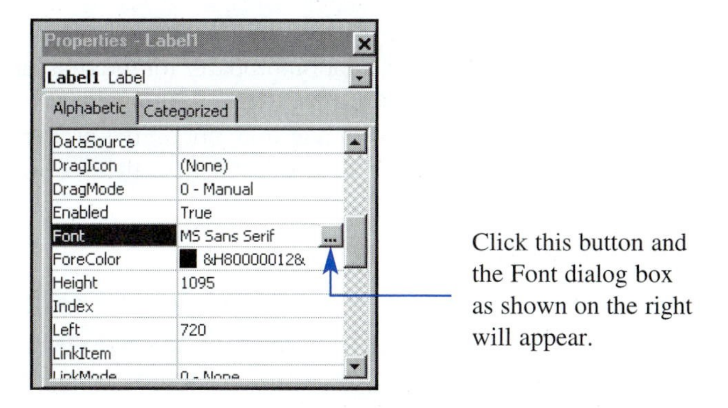

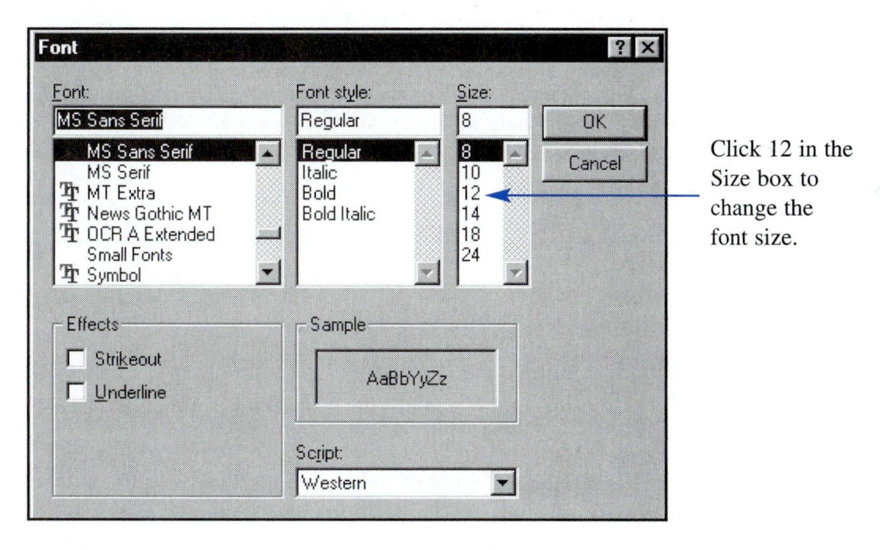

The AutoSize Property

Now, you might discover that the size of the label that you previous drew is not big enough to hold the text. Of course, you can resize the label by using its sizing handle as you did with the form before. However, there is another way that is much more convenient. You can set the label's ***AutoSize property*** to "True." The label automatically adjusts its size based on its caption content.

2.5 Getting Help from the Help Menu

At this moment, you might find the large number of properties of these objects overwhelming. However, understand that they are made available to make your job as a programmer easier.

Once you become familiar with them, you will "look for their help" actively. Most of the time, you may wonder what features a newly encountered property provides. The answer is most likely at your fingertips. VB6 comes with a comprehensive online help system. To find out more about the AutoSize property of the label control, you can do the following:

1. Click the Help menu on the menu bar. You will see a drop-down list with many options, among them at the top are Contents, Index, and Search.
2. Click the "Index" tab. You will see an MSDN (Microsoft Developers Network) Library Visual Studio 6.0 Help dialog box (Figure 2.23).

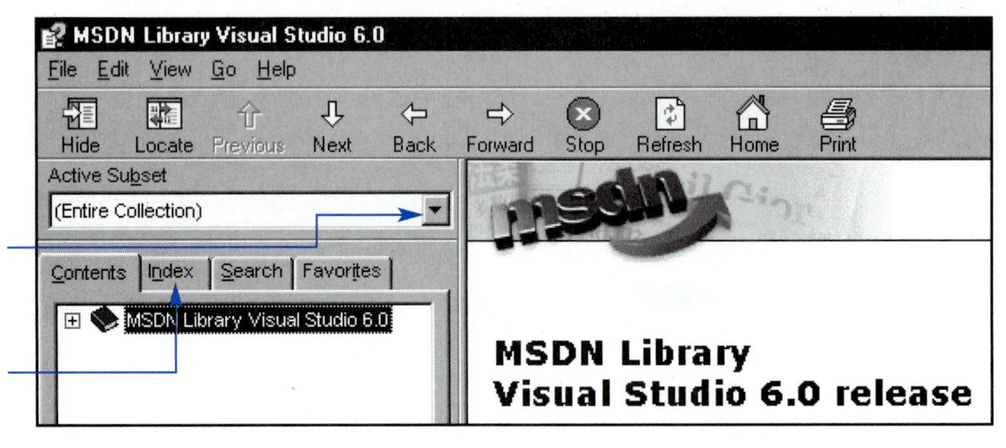

FIGURE 2.23
The MSDN Help Dialog Box

You can limit your search to only Visual Basic by selecting "*Visual Basic Documentation" from this box.

Different tabs will show different contents in the window below.

TIP

You can get many of your VB questions answered by browsing the Help file. Get acquainted with the online help screen as soon as you can. When you have a question about a control, property, event, or method, look it up from the online Help file first.

The Index Tab

You can explore this facility in various ways. For now, we will focus on how we can use the Index tab to find the answer to our question: What is the AutoSize property of the label control? To search, do the following:

1. Type "label control" in the text box labeled "Type in the keyword to find." As you enter a keyword or phrase in the text box, the content of the list box below changes, showing the topics most closely matching your keyword. You will see "Label Control" highlighted in the list box after you type in the keyword.
2. Double-click the highlighted "Label Control" in the list box. You will see a "Topics Found" list box in which many titles related to label controls appear (Figure 2.24). The right column indicates where the title (topic) is located.
3. Select the item with "Visual Basic Reference" on its right.
4. Click the Display button.

The text box on the right of the Help screen will display the explanation for label control (Figure 2.25).

Help Text and Hyperlinks

Between the heading "Label control" and the explanation, there is a line with several keywords underlined and in light blue color. These keywords are hyperlinks to additional information, much like the hypertext you see when browsing Internet Web pages.

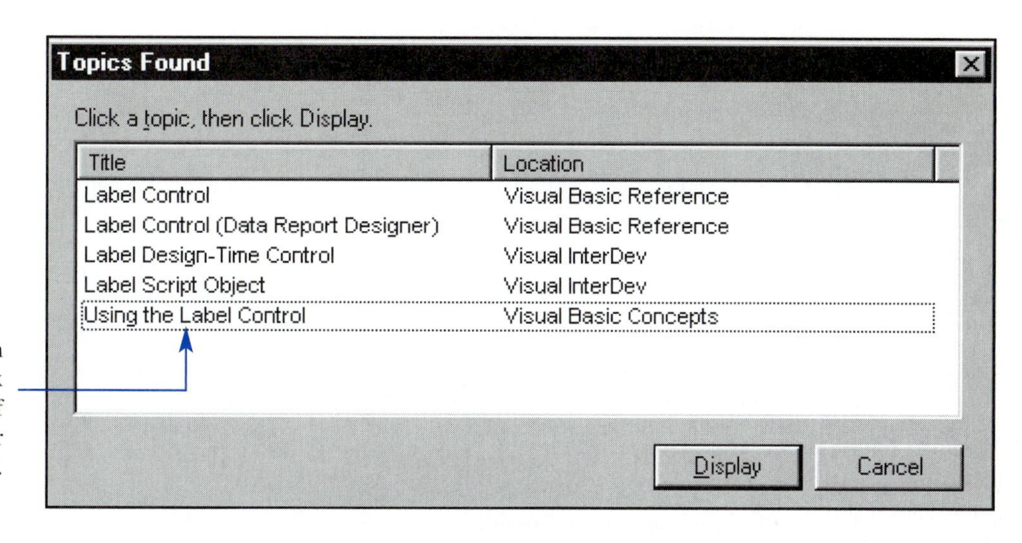

FIGURE 2.24
The Topic Found Dialog Box

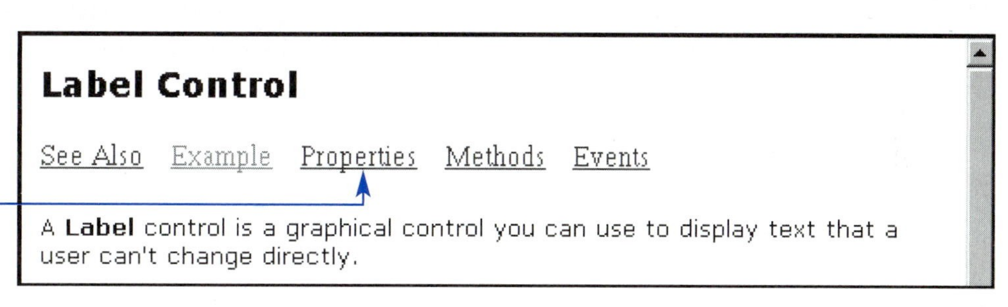

FIGURE 2.25
Help Screen for Label Control

Click the word "Properties." You will see a Topics Found dialog box that shows a list box of topics. You can browse down the list to find the topic of your interest. For example, if you double-click "AutoSize property" (or click that item and click the Display button), a window explaining the use and available settings of the property will appear.

A quick way to find an explanation for the AutoSize property of the label control is to highlight the AutoSize property in the Properties window and then press F1. The context-sensitive help screen will display the help page for the property.

Another Way to Explore

There are other ways to explore the MSDN Help file. For example, if you click the Content tab, next to the Index tab on the left side of the Help dialog box, you will see a book icon labeled "MSDN Library Visual Studio 6.0." Click the book icon and an array of book icons with various topics will appear. One of these is the Visual Basic Documentation icon. Click this icon, and from there, you should be able to explore various VB topics. This is a convenient way to get general information about a specific VB topic. If you have a specific question such as a method, a property, or an event, using the Index tab can make your search easier.

In this book, you will be reminded of the help file from time to time by a special "Look It Up" box. You can learn more on your own by reading the help text. You will also know what specific type of knowledge you can gain by following the pointer in the box. Because these pointers are related to specific topics, most of the time we will refer to the Index tab just presented.

However, you should be aware that the MSDN help file is not prepared exclusively for VB, as the file name implies. Thus, you may run into topics that you are totally unaware of. If you want to limit your search to only topics related to VB, you can select "*Visual Basic

Documentation" in place of "Total Collection" from the combo box above the four search tabs (see Figure 2.23).

2.6 Naming Objects

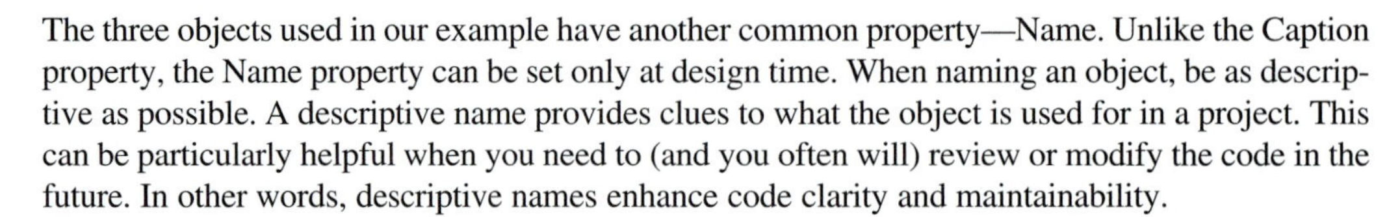

The three objects used in our example have another common property—Name. Unlike the Caption property, the Name property can be set only at design time. When naming an object, be as descriptive as possible. A descriptive name provides clues to what the object is used for in a project. This can be particularly helpful when you need to (and you often will) review or modify the code in the future. In other words, descriptive names enhance code clarity and maintainability.

Object Naming Convention

Companies also adopt naming standards for their projects. These standards typically include rules on how objects should be named. A commonly used standard in this regard is to use the first three letters in lowercase to indicate the type of object, followed by a descriptive name. For example, the three objects we have used in this chapter have the following name prefixes:

Object Type	Prefix	Example
Form	frm	frmWelcome
Label	lbl	lblWelcome
Command	cmd	cmdQuit

A more complete list of these prefixes is given in the next chapter. We will continue to mention the name prefix whenever we encounter a new object. In this book, this standard will be followed to help you develop a sound naming habit.

TIP

When naming objects, make the names as distinct as possible. Include the standard three-letter prefix as part of their names. Code clarity and maintainability are greatly enhanced with this practice.

Changing the Object Names in the Project

Let us now implement the aforementioned naming standard in our example project. Here are the steps to take:

1. Change the form's name to frmWelcome. You can do this by using the Properties window. The steps are as follows:

   1.1 Click the form.

   1.2 Select the Name property in the Properties window.

   1.3 Type "frmWelcome" (without quotes) in the box.

   It is a good habit to test the program whenever a change is made. After you have changed the form name, start the project by clicking the Start button. Then click the "Say Welcome" button. The project should execute without any problem.

2. Change the label's name to lblWelcome. Then start the project. This time, you get an error message "Object Required" (Figure 2.26) displayed in a message box. Click the Debug button in the message box. You should see the following line highlighted:

```
Label1.Caption = "Welcome to Visual Basic!!!"
```

This occurs because after you change the label's name, there is no label or anything on the form with the name Label1. To correct this error, change this line as follows:

```
lblWelcome.Caption = "Welcome to Visual Basic!!!"
```

(*Note:* Your error message will be different if the computer automatically inserts the "Option Explicit" line into the code. Ignore the difference for the time being. We will discuss this statement in Chapter 4, "Data, Operations, and Built-In Functions.") After making this correction, run the project again. This time the project should run without any problems.

FIGURE 2.26

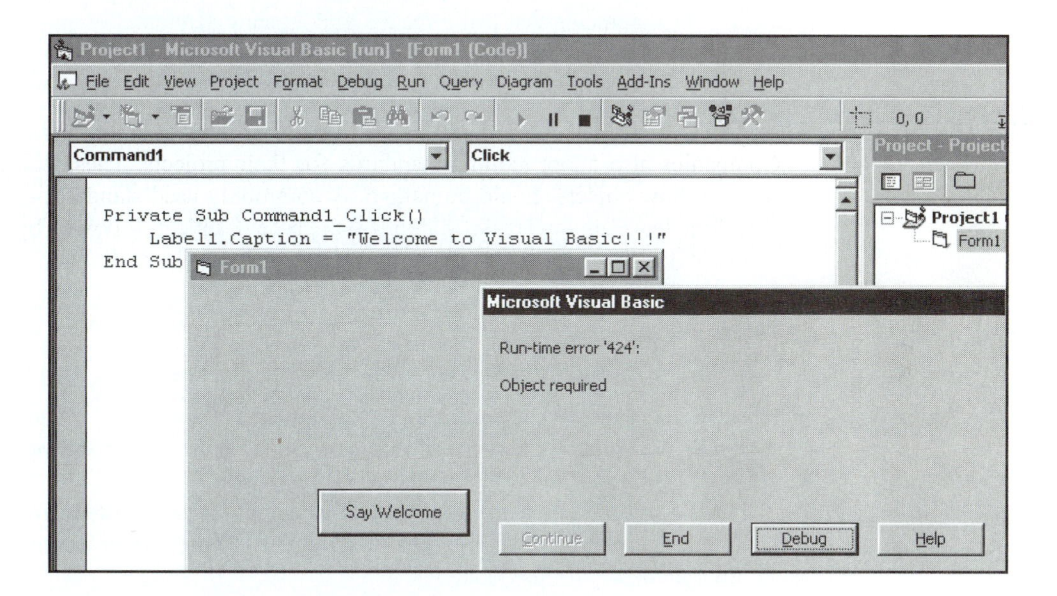

3. Change the command button's name to ""cmdWelcome." Start the project and click the command button. This time nothing happens; that is, "Welcome to Visual Basic!!!" is not displayed on the screen. The code in the Command1_Click event procedure was not executed because the command you clicked is no longer named command1 but cmdWelcome. When you clicked the command button, the system was looking for the event procedure, cmdWelcome_Click. With no procedure of that name, the system ignored the click. The procedure's name in the code should be changed. To correct, replace "Command1" in the procedure header to "cmdWelcome." The corrected event procedure should appear as follows:

```
Private Sub cmdWelcome_Click()
    ' Make the label display the Welcome message
    lblWelcome.Caption = "Welcome to Visual Basic!!!"
End Sub
```

From this exercise, you have learned:

- To become aware of observing sound naming standards.
- To test the code as often as possible.
- To name all the objects before placing any code in the code window.

When developing a project, always make sure that all objects have been named properly before starting to place any code in the code window. This helps eliminate the possibility of encountering various "mysterious" errors in code associated with the names.

2.7 Overview of the Code Structure

You have learned that the code in event procedures handles the events and that when developing code for them, you should use the event procedure templates provided by the IDE. You have also learned that the order of the procedures in the code window is not important because they are invoked by the event, not by the order in which they appear. Also, in general, code in a procedure is executed top down. But is there some kind of code in a procedure that will not get executed in sequence?

In terms of the order in which statements are executed, there are basically two types of statements: (1) statements that bring results and execute sequentially and (2) statements that direct flow of execution control. We will study each of these types in detail in later chapters. Let's take a brief look at each here.

Statements That Bring Results and Execute Sequentially

Most statements bring results such as relocating an object on the screen or moving data from one location to another in the memory. For example, we have seen the following statement, which moves the form to the upper-left corner of the screen.

```
Me.Move 0, 0
```

We have also seen the statement:

```
lblWelcome.Caption = "Welcome to Visual Basic!!!"
```

This statement moves the text string, "Welcome to Visual Basic!!!" to the caption of the label, named lblWelcome. Statements of this type are recognized as ***assignment statements***. They are the most commonly seen statements in VB programs.

These types of statements are executed sequentially in the order they appear in a procedure. There are many more of these types of statements. You will encounter many of them throughout the remainder of this book.

Statements That Direct Flow of Execution Control

From time to time, you will encounter situations in which you need to change the sequence of execution in your code. For example, you may need to execute a block of code only if a certain condition is true, you may need to repeat the execution of a block of code for a certain number of times, or you may want to leave (jump away from) a block of code when your program reaches a certain point of execution.

Conditional Execution. If you need to execute a block of code that depends on a certain condition, you may need to use the If block. Its syntax appears as follows:

```
If Condition Then
    Statements to be executed when Condition is True
Else
    Statements to be executed when Condition is False
End If
```

Where *Condition* is an expression that can be evaluated to either True or False.

For example, suppose you want to set the BackColor property of the label lblWelcome to either blue or green depending on the value of the random number given by the Rnd function. You can code the following:

```
If Rnd <.5 Then
    lblWelcome.BackColor = vbBlue
Else
    lblWelcome.BackColor = vbGreen
End If
```

Rnd is a random number generator that returns a fractional number in the range of 0 and 1. vbBlue and vbGreen are named constants that VB recognizes to be values for the blue and green colors. The preceding code block will set the background color of the label to blue if the random number has a value less than .5; otherwise, it will set it to green. There are other code structures to handle execution of different statements based on certain conditions. Chapter 5, "Decision," discusses these in more detail.

Repetition. In many other situations, you may need to execute a block of code repetitively. One way to handle this is to use the ***For . . . Next loop***. The code syntax for this structure is as follows:

```
For Counter = Starting Value To Ending Value
    Statements to be repeated
Next Counter
```

Suppose you need to print 10 numbers, 1 to 10, on the form. You can use this structure in the following manner:

```
For Counter = 1 To 10
    Me.Print Counter
Next Counter
```

When this block of code is executed, Counter will start with a value 1. Then the statement inside the For block (i.e., Me.Print Counter) is executed, resulting in the number 1 being printed on the form. (Recall that *Me* refers to the form.) The next statement (Next Counter) will send the execution control back to the For statement. Counter is then increased by 1 to 2, which is in turn printed when the Print statement is executed. The "loop" will continue until Counter is greater than 10. Then the execution control is transferred to the statement immediately below the block. Other variations and ways of coding repetitions are discussed in detail in Chapter 7, "Repetition."

Code That "Jumps." Still yet, there are statements that can jump (skip) the remainder of code in a block or a procedure. These statements include GoTo (which results in execution flow that is hard to trace and *should be avoided by all means*), Exit Do, Exit For, Exit Sub, and Exit Function. We will wait until there is a need to use each of these statements to explain their uses.

An event procedure that contains various code structures discussed previously is given in Figure 2.27.

FIGURE 2.27
A Sample Procedure with Various Code Structures

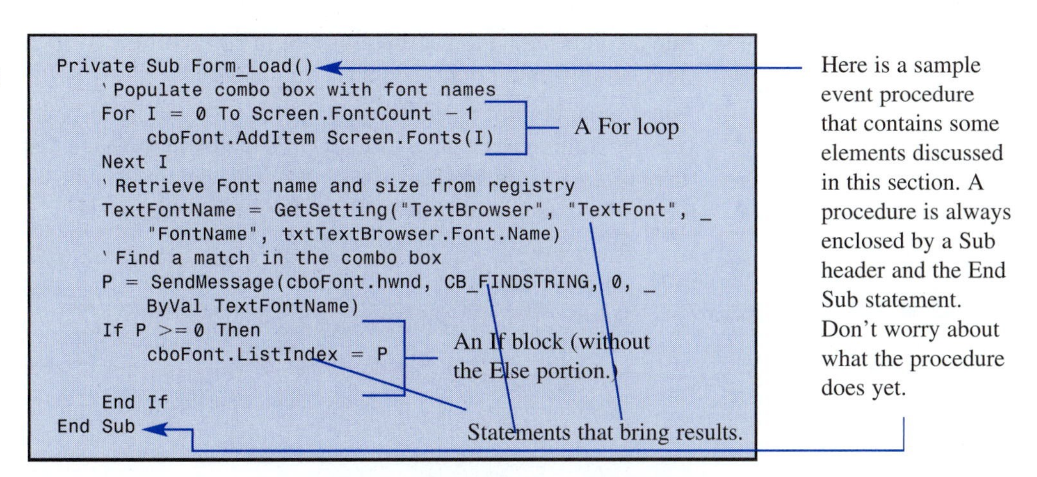

2.8 Revising the First Program

Let's make our first program a bit more dynamic and lively. This revision should allow you to explore more code and better understand the relationship of all parts in VB. The revised project will involve the use of the If block and will also involve a new control, the ***timer.*** We will revise the program to appear and behave as follows:

1. The "Welcome to Visual Basic!!!" sign will automatically appear when the program starts and will have a bigger font and more lively colors: blue foreground and red background.
2. When the program starts, the Welcome sign (the label) will appear from the right margin of the form and move "smoothly" across the form. After it completely disappears from the form, it will reappear from the right margin again. This will continue on and on.
3. The program will end when you click a command button with the caption "Quit."

The Visual Interface

The first thing to do is to revise the visual interface as shown in Figure 2.28. Follow these steps:

1. Change several properties of the label control.
   1.1 Set its Caption property to "Welcome to Visual Basic!!!" by using the Properties window. (Notice the extra space at the end of the string. It is intended for the red area to look balanced.) The steps involved should be similar to those used to change the Caption property of the command button to "Say Welcome."
   1.2 Set its AutoSize property to True.
   1.3 Set its Font property to Coronet, 24, Bold, and Italic. If your computer does not have this font, set it to your favorite font. The steps to set the font have been presented in a previous section.
   1.4 Set its BackColor property to red. Use the Properties window. When you click this property in the Properties window, you will see a drop-down button. The drop-down window shows the available colors. Click the Palette tab to find red.
   1.5 Set its ForeColor to Blue in the same manner as in Step 1.4.
   1.6 Make sure the label is placed in the middle of the form vertically.
   1.7 Make sure its name is lblWelcome.
2. Make sure the form is named frmWelcome. Set its caption to "Welcome."
3. Delete the "Welcome" command button from the form. Click the button. Then press the Delete key.
4. Add a command button at the lower-right corner of the form. Set its Name property to cmdQuit and its caption to "Quit."
5. Add a timer control to the form. Its position is not important. It will not appear when your program runs. Change its name to tmrWelcome. (Note that the name prefix for the timer is *tmr*.) Set its interval to 250. We will explain what this number means later. The form should appear like the one shown in Figure 2.28.

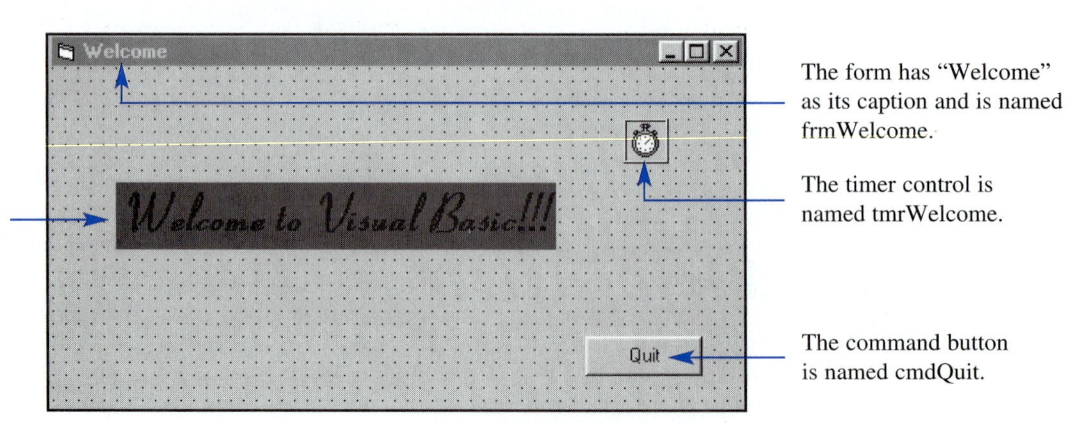
Welcome
Welcome to Visual Basic!!!
Quit
The form has "Welcome" as its caption and is named frmWelcome.
The timer control is named tmrWelcome.
The command button is named cmdQuit.
The label has its ForeColor set to blue and BackColor set to red. Its caption is also set at design time. It is named lblWelcome.

FIGURE 2.28
The Visual Interface for the Revised Project

Coding the Revised Project

Before considering how to code the revised project, you need to remove all existing code from the code window:

1. Highlight all the text in the code window.
2. Press the Delete key.

Now, let's turn our attention to what code we need for this revised project. Because all the required properties of all controls have been set, our main focus here is to make the label move across the form. Here is the list of questions we need to answer:

1. How do we place the label on the right margin of the form?
2. How do we move the label across the form "smoothly"?
3. How do we know the label has disappeared from the form?

Placing the Label on the Right Margin of the Form. Recall that the label has a Left property, which locates the label's left side on the form (as discussed in the preceding section on exploring additional properties). The right margin of the form should have the value of the entire width of the form (Figure 2.29). Thus, we can set the Left property of the label to the form's width. This should place the label on the right margin of the form. The code should be as follows:

```
lblWelcome.Left = Me.Width
```

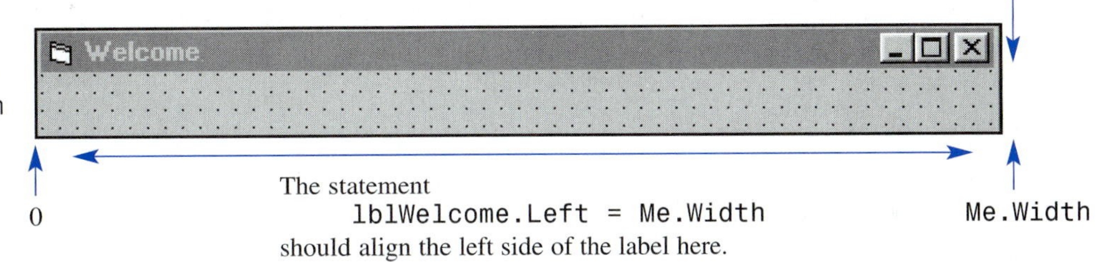
Welcome
0
The statement
lblWelcome.Left = Me.Width
should align the left side of the label here.
Me.Width

FIGURE 2.29
Aligning the Label on the Right Margin of the Form

In which event procedure should we place the preceding statement? We want this line to be executed as soon as the project starts. The event that is raised when the project starts is the ***Form Load event***, which occurs when the form is being loaded into memory. This event is where we can place code that sets initial values for various properties and data before the occurrence of any other events. Therefore, we will place the previous statement in this event. To get the event code template from the code window, do the following:

1. Select Form from the Object box.
2. The Form Load event procedure template should automatically appear. Make sure this is the event procedure that appears in the code window. If not, select Load from the procedure box.

The code should appear as follows:

```
Private Sub Form_Load()
    'Place the label on the right margin of the form.
     lblWelcome.Left = Me.Width
End Sub
```

TIP

Another way to obtain the Form Load procedure template is to double-click the form when it (rather than the code window) appears in the center of the IDE. When there is no existing event procedure for the form in the code window, Form Load is the default event.

Moving the Label Across the Form. How can we move the label? We can use the Move method discussed previously. Or, we can set the label's Left property. Each time this property changes, the label repositions itself accordingly. For example, we can use the following code:

```
lblWelcome.Left = lblWelcome.Left - lblWelcome.Width / 10
```

This statement will subtract one-tenth of the label's width from its current Left property value and assign the result to that property, causing the label to move to the left by one-tenth of the label's width. Notice that the equal sign (=) in the statement does not mean "equal" but to move data from the right hand side to the left hand side of the equal sign.

Now, imagine that you have a command button and place the previous statement in its Click event. Each time you click the command button, the label will move to the new position. If you can click the button at an even tempo, the label will move smoothly across the form. It is, of course, hard for anybody to click the button evenly. (And even if you can, you will get tired quickly!) That's why we use the timer.

The ***timer control*** keeps track of time. At design time, you can see its appearance on the form and set its properties. At runtime, it disappears from the form. When enabled, all it does is to keep track of time. The timer has one event, the Timer event, which is similar to a Click event in that when the Timer event is raised (triggered), the code in its event procedure is executed. However, the Timer event is not raised by a click but by the time interval you set for its Interval property. An interval value of 1 is equivalent to one-thousandth of a second. Thus, if you set its interval property to 250, the Timer event will be raised every quarter of a second. Therefore, if you place the line to set the label's Left property in this Timer event, the label will move left every quarter of a second by one-tenth of the label's width. The code should appear as follows:

```
Private Sub tmrWelcome_Timer()
    lblWelcome.Left = lblWelcome.Left - lblWelcome.Width / 10
End Sub
```

To enter the code just shown, do the following:

1. Make sure that the timer's name has been set to tmrWelcome. Click the timer control on the form and check its name in the Properties window. (Also check the Interval property to ensure that it is set to 250.)
2. Double-click the timer control. The Timer event procedure should appear in the code window.
3. Type in the previous code line.

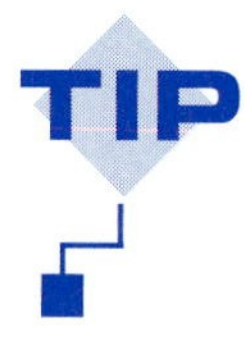

If you are already in the code window, you can obtain the Timer event procedure template by simply selecting tmrWelcome from the Object box.

Determining Whether the Label Has Completely Disappeared. If you test the program now, the label will appear from the right margin of the form and move to the left gradually until it disappears. However, it will not reappear. It is time for us to answer the question: How can we tell if the label has completely disappeared from the form? The Left and Top properties of all the controls on the form are set relative to the upper-left corner of the form, which has a coordinate value (0,0). Thus, when the label's Left property has a value zero, the label's left margin is aligned with the left margin of the form (Figure 2.30). At that time, the entire width of the label still appears on the form. This means when the label's Left property plus its width is less than 0, the entire label has moved out of (disappeared from) the form. Therefore, it will be time to move the label to the right margin of the form again. So, an If block can be coded as follows:

```
If lblWelcome.Left + lblWelcome.Width <= 0 Then
    lblWelcome.Left = Me.Width
Else
End If
```

FIGURE 2.30
Welcome Banner on the Left Margin of the Form

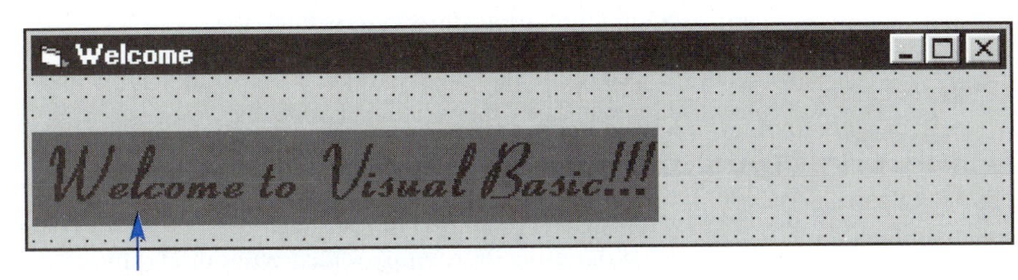

The label's Left property is 0 at this point. When it moves farther left for its entire width, its Left property plus its width will be 0.

The If statement tests whether the Left property plus the Width property is less than zero. If so, the line below it (the assignment statement) will be executed. The assignment statement moves the label to the right margin of the form, as explained previously.

What code should we place between Else and End If? This will be the situation that the label can still be seen on the form. That's when the label should move in the normal way. Thus, the complete Timer event procedure should appear as follows:

```
Private Sub tmrWelcome_Timer()
    If lblWelcome.Left + lblWelcome.Width <= 0 Then
        ' Label has disappeared from the form.
        ' Place it on the right margin.
        lblWelcome.Left = Me.Width
    Else
        ' Label can be seen. Keep moving to the left.
        lblWelcome.Left = lblWelcome.Left - lblWelcome.Width / 10
    End If
End Sub
```

Modify your timer procedure to match the preceding code.

Ending the Program. We have answered all the questions we raised at the beginning of coding this revised project. All that is left now is to consider how the program should end. Like all Windows-based programs, your project unloads when the user clicks the Close (x) button in its control box. Although many users will click the Close button to quit, it is a good practice to provide the user with a "formal" way. The Quit button is used for this purpose. You can use the Unload statement to terminate the program. The code should appears as follows:

```
Private Sub cmdQuit_Click()
    Unload Me
End Sub
```

Recall that "Me" is a special name for the current form. Because the form name is frmWelcome, the code "Unload frmWelcome" and "Unload Me" will have the same effect.

TIP

Another way to quit a program is to use the End statement:

```
Private Sub cmdQuit_Click()
    End
End Sub
```

There are some differences in the effects of Unload and End statements. We discuss this in more detail in Chapter 11 when we work with multiple forms. Suffice it to say that *the Unload statement is considered less abrupt and a better method.*

Revised Project in Summary. The complete code should include three event procedures:

1. The Form Load procedure to place the banner (label) on the right margin of the form
2. The tmrWelcome Timer procedure to move the banner across the form and replace the banner on the right margin again
3. The cmdQuit Click procedure to terminate the program

Test your project. You can also try to click the form's Maximize button so that the form will cover the entire screen. Enjoy the welcome banner as it moves across the form to say "Welcome!!!"

Completing the Development Cycle

All the aforementioned steps in revising the example program enable us to develop a working program. Once a program is thoroughly tested without any problem, it can be placed into "production." As you may recall from Chapter 1, this should be the last step of the application (program) development cycle. In this step, the program is compiled into an executable file. From then on, you use the compiled version (the executable) to process live data. You will no longer need to use the IDE to run that program.

To illustrate, let's compile the revised example into an executable file. Here are the steps:

1. Save your project. Make sure the project is saved as Welcome.vbp.
2. Click the File menu in the IDE. You should see a "Make Welcome.exe" option in the menu (see Figure 2.31).
3. Click the "Make Welcome.exe" option. A Make Project dialog box should appear to prompt for the filename for the executable (see Figure 2.31). The text box should show "Welcome.exe" (without the quotes).
4. Click the OK button. The VB IDE will proceed to compile and show you the progress. When it is done, your Welcome program is compiled and ready to run on its own without the IDE.

FIGURE 2.31
Steps to Compile a Program

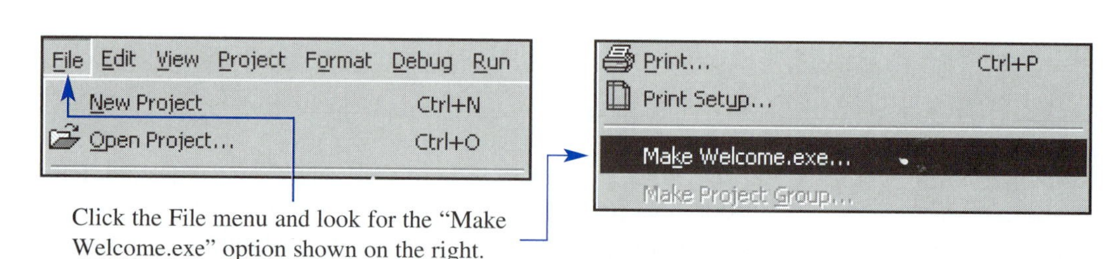

Click the File menu and look for the "Make Welcome.exe" option shown on the right.

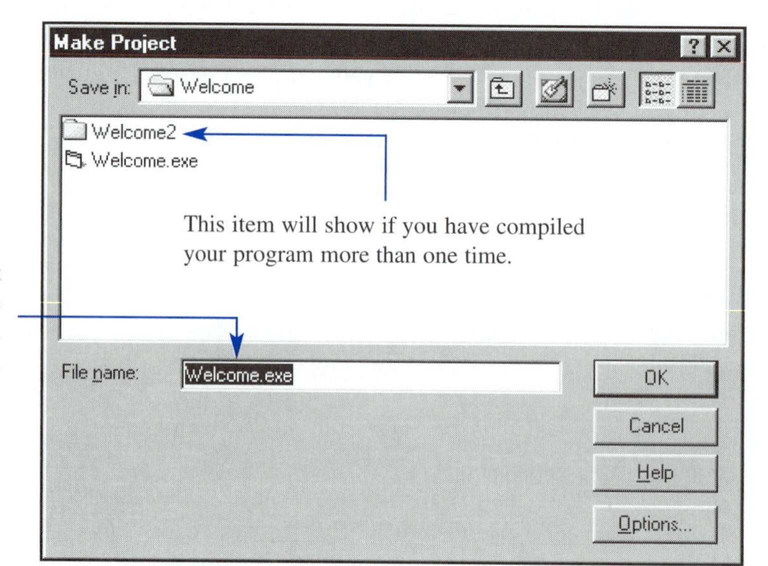

This item will show if you have compiled your program more than one time.

Here is the Make Project dialog box. Make sure the File Name box shows Welcome.exe.

How do you run the compiled program? Once the program is compiled, its executable will run in exactly the same way as all other executables. You can use the Run option of the Start menu to start the program. This will be similar to the way you run the Setup program to install your VB6 into your system. Alternatively, if you would rather have the program appear in the Program submenu of the Start menu so that it can be run like some of your major applications such as Word, Excel, or VB6, you will need to create a "shortcut" in your system. The steps for both alternatives are described briefly next.

To run the Welcome executable using the Run option of the Start menu:

1. Click the Start button on the desktop.
2. Click the Run option. A Run dialog box will appear.
3. Type the path of your Welcome executable into the Open combo box. Or, use the Browse button to find the Welcome executable.
4. Click the OK button to run.

To add the Welcome executable to the Programs submenu:

1. Click the Start button on the desktop.
2. Highlight the Settings option. A submenu will appear.
3. Click the "Taskbar & Start Menu" option. A Taskbar Properties dialog box will appear.
4. Click the "Start Menu Programs" tab.
5. Click the Add button. A Create Shortcut dialog box will appear.
6. Enter the path for your Welcome executable in the Command Line text box (e.g., C:\VbSource\VBBook\Welcome\Welcome.exe). Or, use the Browse button to locate your Welcome executable.
7. Click the Next button. The Select Program Folder dialog box will appear.
8. Select a folder in which you would like the Welcome executable to be included (e.g., Programs or Accessories) and Click the Next button. (You can also create a new folder for your executable by clicking the New Folder button.) The Select a Title for the Program dialog box will appear.
9. Enter a title for the executable in the text box, for example, "Say Welcome."
10. Click the Finish button.

Summary

This chapter began with a brief tour of the VB IDE. You have become acquainted with the menu bar, the toolbar, the toolbox, the form, the Code window, the Project Explorer window, the Properties window, and the Form Layout window. Getting familiar with their locations in the IDE and their proper uses can make your programming endeavor much easier.

You then walked through the development cycle of a simple VB program. Through that process, you have gained hands-on experience with VB6's IDE. You worked with three VB objects (form, label, and command button) and the three interfaces of VB objects: properties, methods, and events. You now understand that you can do the following:

- Set various properties of an object to certain values so that the object will appear or behave the way you want it to.
- Use the object's methods to make it perform certain desired actions.
- Place code in the object's event procedure to handle the event, that is, to make the computer do what you want it to when the event is "triggered."

After the program development walkthrough, you have also learned what the term *IDE* means. You have also had a first look at the online help file, which is very informative and can be a useful learning and exploring tool. You have also learned several programming tips. Among these, two are most worth repeating: (1) name all objects before coding and (2) save your project often.

We have mentioned several times the concept of code readability and maintainability. Three important suggestions follow:

1. Insert many comments as a part of your code documentation.
2. Indent the code lines inside a procedure.
3. Give all objects names that are as meaningful as possible.

The revised project introduces you to one more control, the timer. The project also shows you the use of the If block. Finally, we show you how to compile a project when it is ready to be placed into production. You should be able to appreciate the power of VB as demonstrated in this project. With only a few lines of code, you can see a banner moving across the form. Hopefully, this project not only provides you the additional hands-on experience but also stimulates your interest in VB programming.

Visual Basic Explorer

2-1. Border Property of the Label. Draw a label onto a new standard form. Look for the BorderStyle property in its Properties window. (If you do not see this window, press F4.) What is the setting currently? Change this setting to 1 (fixed single). How does the label appear now? It should look like a three-dimensional box.

2-2. BackColor Property of the Label. Use the label created in 2-1. Click the BackColor property in the Properties window. You should see a down-arrow button. Click that button. You should see a window with two tabs: Palette and System. Click one tab, then another. What do you see under each tab? Select white color from an item of either tab. Now, the label should look like a text box in a typical window.

2-3. Alignment Property of the Label. Use the same label in 2-2. Make sure the AutoSize property is set to False. Resize the label wider so that there is extra space beyond the text "Label1." Now, set the alignment property to right justified (1). Check the position of "Label1" in the label. Where does it appear? Change the alignment property to Center (2). Check the position of the text again. Where does it appear?

2-4. Font Property of the Command Button. Draw a command button on a new form. Can you change the font to Courier 12? (Yes, the command button has the Font property. Follow the steps discussed in this chapter.)

2-5. BackColor Property of the Command Button. Use the command button in 2-4. Change its BackColor property to red. (Refer to 2-2 for additional clues. Look for the color in the Palette tab.) Do you see any change in color in the command button? Why? (You will get the answer if you work on 2-6.)

2-6. Style Property of the Command Button. Use the same command button in 2-5. Change its Style property from "standard" (0) to "Graphical" (1). Do you see any change in color now? If you set the BackColor to red as instructed in 2-5, you should see the command button turn red.

2-7. Picture and Icon Properties of the Form. (This exercise assumes that the VB's graphics folder has been installed.) Click the form's Picture property in the Properties window. You should see an ellipsis (. . .) button indicating choices. Click that button. You should see the Load Picture dialog box. Find and select the Balloon.bmp file in your system. In a typical installation, the file should be located in the following folder:

Microsoft Visual Studio\Common\Graphics\Bitmaps\Assorted\

You should see a balloon in the upper-left corner of the form.

Now set this property to . . .\graphics\Metafile\Business\Check.wmf. What do you see?

Set the icon property to . . .\Graphics\Icons\Mail\Mail16a.ico

(*Note:* The icon property can only accept files with an ico name extension.) What change do you see on the form?

2-8. WindowState Property of the Form. The form's WindowState property can be set to one of the three values: 0 (normal), 1 (minimized), and 2 (maximized). Run the project each time after you change the setting to one of these values.

Run the project with its WindowState property set to normal. You should see the Minimize ("–"), Maximize ("+"), and Close ("x") buttons on the right side of the form's title bar. Click each of these buttons. What happens?

The form also has the MaxButton and MinButton properties. Set one of these properties to False. Run the project. Inspect the right side of the form's title bar. See any change?

2-9. ControlBox Property of the Form. Set the form's ControlBox property to False and inspect its title bar. Run the project. You can no longer end the project by clicking the Close button on the title bar—it is no longer there. Terminate the project by clicking the End button on the toolbar or the End option in the Run menu.

2-10. Cancel and Default Properties of the Command Button. Draw a text box and two command buttons on the form. Set the Name property of the text box to txtShow. Set the Caption property of one command button to Default and its name property to cmdDefault. Set the caption of the other command button to Cancel and its Name property to cmdCancel. Enter the following code in the code window. (*Hint:* Obtain the event procedure templates by the steps discussed in the text.)

```
Private Sub cmdCancel_Click()
    txtShow.Text = "Cancel button has been clicked."
End Sub

Private Sub cmdDefault_Click()
    txtShow.Text = "Default button has been clicked."
End Sub
```

Run the program. Click the text box. Then press the return key followed by the Esc key. You should hear the beep (or ding) but nothing else. Click the Close ("x") button.

Now, set the Cancel property of the Cancel button to True and the Default property of the Default button to True. Run the program and click the text box again. Press the Enter key. You don't hear anything. Look at the text box. "Default button has been clicked" should appear. Press the Esc key. What do you see now? What can you conclude about the Cancel and Default properties of the command button?

2-11. Change Event of the Label—Using the Help File. Bring a label into a new form. Switch to the Code window. (You can do this by clicking the Code View icon in the Project Explorer window, using the Code option in the View menu, or just double-clicking the form.) Select Label1 in the Object box at top left. Browse the procedure box at top right. You should see an event name, "Change." Question: When does a change event occur for a label? (*Hint:* Use the Help file. Roadmap: Click the Help menu, the Index option, enter "label control" as the keyword, double-click "label control." double-click "Visual Basic Reference" in the Topics Found list box, click the "events" hyperlink in the Label Control explanation box on the right, and double-click "change event." Then look for "label" in the explanation window.)

To see how it works, place the following code in the code window (*Hint:* Again, obtain the event procedure templates by using the steps explained in this chapter):

```
Private Sub Label1_Change()
    MsgBox "Caption of Welcome label has changed."
End Sub
Private Sub Form_Click()
    Label1.Caption = "Hello!"
End Sub
```

Run the project. Click the form. When is the above message displayed?

Exercises

In the following exercises, make sure that all objects in your projects are named properly before you start your coding.

2-12. Beeper. Set a new form's caption to "Beeper" and name the form frmBeeper. Give the code such that with no VB control on your form, when the user click on your form, the computer will make a sound. (*Hint:* The event is Form_Click. The command to make a sound is Beep.)

2-13. Say Yes, Say No. Use a label control and two command buttons. One command button has a caption, "Say yes," the other, "Say no."

Provide the code so that when your program runs, the label will display "Yes!" when the "Say yes" command button is clicked; and "No!" when the "Say no" button is clicked. (*Hint:* Name the commands cmdYes and cmdNo and the label lblYesNo. Set the Caption property of the label in the Click event of each command button.)

2-14. Move Left, Move Right. Use one label and two command buttons. Set the Label's Caption property to "I can move!," Font property to MonoType Corsiva 24, Border style property to fixed single (1), and background color to Blue. (*Note:* If your computer does not have MonoType Corsiva, use your favorite font as a substitute.) Set one command button's caption to "Move Left" and name to cmdMoveLeft. Set the other command button's caption to "Move Right" and name to cmdMoveRight.

Provide the code so that as the program runs, the label will move to the left by one-half of the label's width if the "Move Left" button is clicked and will move to the right by the same distance to the right if the "Move Right" button is clicked. (*Hint:* The line below will move the label named lblMover to the left by one-half of its width.)

```
lblMover.Left = lblMover.Left - lblMover.Width / 2
```

2-15. Showing Intention of Move. Modify project 2-14 to handle the keyboard. At runtime, when the user uses the Tab key to move the focus to the "Move Left (Right)" button, the label (lblMover) will display, "I will move left (right)." When the user presses the return key, the label will move as promised. (*Hint:* When the user tabs to a control, the control's GotFocus event is raised. When the user presses the Return key on a command button, the Click event is raised.)

2-16. Move Up, Move Down. Use one label and two command buttons. Set the Label's caption to "I can move!." font to Bookman Old Style Bold Italic 20, Border style to fixed single (1), and background color to Green. (*Note:* If your computer does not have Bookman Old Style, use your favorite font as a substitute.) Set one command button's caption to "Move Up" and name to cmdMoveUp. Set the other command button's caption to "Move Down" and name to cmdMoveDown. Provide the code so that as the program runs, the label will move up by twice the height of the label when the "Move Up" button is clicked, and will move down by the same distance when the "Move Down" button is clicked. (*Hint:* The property to set an object's vertical position is "Top." You can get more hints from 2-14.)

2-17. Random Movement. Use one label and one command button. Set the label's Caption property to "I don't necessarily move." Also set its color, font, and border style to make it look attractive. Set the command button's caption to "Move." Provide the code so that as the project runs, the label will move to a random location only about half of the time when you click the "Move" button. (*Hint:* Use an If statement:

```
If Rnd >= .5 Then
     'the statement to move the label
End If
```

An example to move a label to a random location is given in the text.)

2-18. Make It Red, Make It Blue. Use one label control and two command buttons. Set the form's caption to "Color Exercise." Set the label's caption to "Show My Color," border style to fixed single (1), and font to Times New Roman 20. Set one command's caption to "Make it Red"; set the other to "Make it Blue." When the program runs, the label will change its background color to red and foreground color to green or background color to blue and foreground color to white, depending on which command button is clicked. (*Hint:* The names for colors red, blue, green, and white are vbRed, vbBlue, vbGreen, and vbWhite, respectively.)

2-19. Change Color or Not. When the user clicks on the form, its background will be red if the random number (VB's Rnd function) is less than .5; otherwise, it will be blue. (*Hint:* Use an If statement with the following structure:

```
If Rnd < .5 Then
     ' set the form's background color to Red
Else
     ' set the form's background color to Blue
End If
```

The event is Form_Click.)

2-20. Floating Banner. Modify the revised "Welcome" project in the text so that the "Welcome" sign (label) will appear from the bottom center of the form and move up every half of a second by one-quarter of the label's height until it disappears from the form. Then make it reappear from the bottom center again and repeat the movement. The program should quit when the user clicks a command button with the caption "Quit."

2-21. Changing Mood. Draw two image controls and a timer on a new form. Name them imgHappy, imgSad, and tmrMood, respectively. Place imgHappy in the center of the form. Set the Visible property of imgSad to False. Then set the picture property of imgHappy and imgSad to Happy.bmp and Sad.bmp, respectively. The two files are located in the following folder:

Microsoft Visual Studio\Common\Graphics\BitMaps\Assorted\

Provide code so that at runtime, the picture at the center of the form will show the happy face for one second and change to sad face for another second, alternately.

(*Hint:* In the Form Load event, use the Move method to move imgSad to overlap imgHappy. Set the timer interval to 1000. In its Timer event, reverse the Visible property of each image, that is, from True to False and vice versa. If you enjoy this exercise, modify the problem to animate traffic lights. The pictures are available in the Graphics\Icons\Traffic\ folder.)

Projects

2-22. The Rotating Banner. Modify the Welcome project in this chapter so that as soon as the left margin of the banner disappears from the form's left side, it reappears from the right as shown in Figure 2.32.

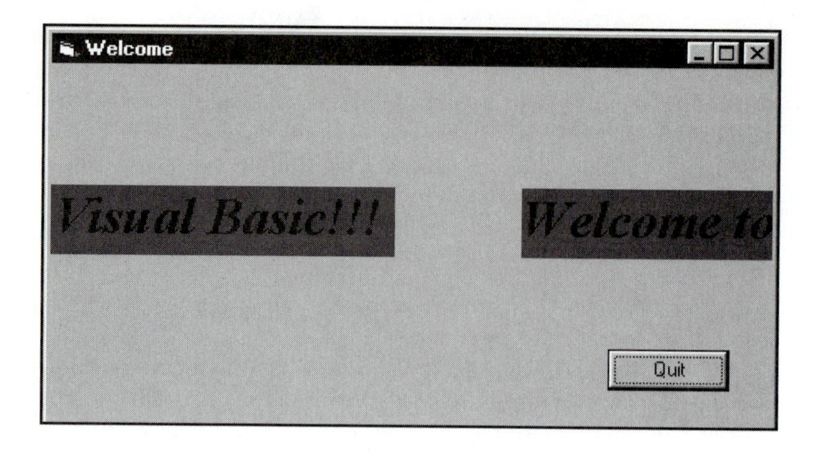

Figure 2.32
The Rotating Banner

(*Hint:* This involves a trick. You need to set up two identical labels. Call them lblWelcome1 and lblWelcome2. Start the first label the same way as the example project in the text. Then, in the Timer event procedure, allow it to move in the same manner without the If block. Make the second label follow the first label with the distance between the left margins of the two labels equal to the form's width. Then when the second label starts to disappear from the form, assign its Left property to the first label's [use an If block to handle this].)

2-23. Random Position, Random Size, Random Color. Use one label control and one command button. Set the form's Caption property to "Randomizer." Set the label's border style to fixed single (1) and caption to "I change as I wish." Place the command button at the upper-left corner of the form.

Provide the code so that when the program runs and the user clicks on the command button, the form will move to a random location and its size will change simultaneously. Its background color will be red or blue depending on whether the value of the random number (VB's Rnd function) is greater than .5. The label will move to a random location within the form. Its background color will be white if the form's background is blue; otherwise, it will be green.

(*Hint:* The following statements will move the form to a random location in the screen and will have the form's size changed as well.

```
X = Rnd * Screen.Width
Y = Rnd * Screen.Height
W = Rnd * Screen.Width
H = Rnd * Screen.Height
Me.Move X, Y, W, H
```

But beware that W must be wide enough to accommodate the widths of the label and the command button. H must be high enough to accommodate the height of the label and the command button. For the form and the controls to stay visible, X must be less than Screen.Width ñ W and Y must be less than Screen.Height – H. Use the If statement to adjust these values.

The code to move the label randomly is available in the text. Use the If block to set the color for the form and the label.)

2-24. Random Changes at Regular Time Intervals. Modify the project in 2-23 so that the form will change its position, size, and color every half of a second. When the user clicks the command button with the caption "Stop," the program quits.

3 Some Visual Basic Controls and Events

In the preceding chapter, four Visual Basic (VB) objects (the form and three controls) and some of their capabilities were explored. There are, of course, many more VB objects and controls. Many of the controls have features that can make your design of a data-entry screen more powerful and user-friendly. This chapter presents various data-entry/user-interface situations. For each situation, you will learn the appropriate VB control(s) to use. In addition, when you place many VB controls on a form, you may discover that the sequence of controls is not exactly the way you want. This chapter also shows how this sequence can be modified.

As explained in Chapter 2, "Introduction to Visual Basic Programming," each VB control has its events. These events are "raised" when something happens in the system or when the user takes an action. You can place code in the procedures that are associated with these events so that the computer behaves exactly as you would like. Thus, these events are where you give your program "life" and "personality." We will explore a few of the events most commonly used in data-entry operations. All the code you place in your project will directly or indirectly relate to one or more of these events. It is thus very important that you have a clear understanding of them.

After completing this chapter, you should be able to:

- Have a clear understanding of the important features and the role each of the following VB controls plays in the user interface for data-entry operations:
  - Text box
  - Masked edit box
  - Frame
  - Tab
  - Option button
  - Check box
  - List box
  - Combo box
  - Picture box
  - Image control
- Set the tab order for the controls placed on the form.
- Understand the nature and uses of the following events:
  - Form load
  - KeyPress
  - Click and DblClick (double-click)
  - GotFocus and LostFocus

3.1 Obtaining Open-Ended Input from the User: Text Box and Masked Edit Control

Let's begin with a simple example. Suppose you would like to have a VB program to keep track of your friends' names and phone numbers. Your first step, as explained in Chapter 2, is to design the visual interface. In this process, you will need to place VB controls onto the form for the user to enter the name and phone number. What VB control(s) can we use for this purpose? A VB control that enables us to enter any type of data is the text box. As its name suggests, the text box "specializes" in handling text data.

Text Property of the Text Box

The text box control has a property called ***Text***. At design time, you can set this property to any text, which will then be displayed at runtime, much like the label control you saw in Chapter 2. Unlike the label control, however, the text box also allows the user to enter and edit its content at runtime. The text so obtained can then be further processed or simply saved for future use.

As an exercise, place a text box control in a new form by double-clicking the text box icon in the toolbox. You will see "Text1" displayed in the box (Figure 3.1). Because we are interested in using it for inputting the friend's name, you should name the control txtName and clear the text to make it a blank. You can change the control's name by typing "txtName" (without quotes) in the Name property in the Properties window. To clear the text box, delete "Text1" from the control's Text property.

FIGURE 3.1
Bringing a Text Box to a Form

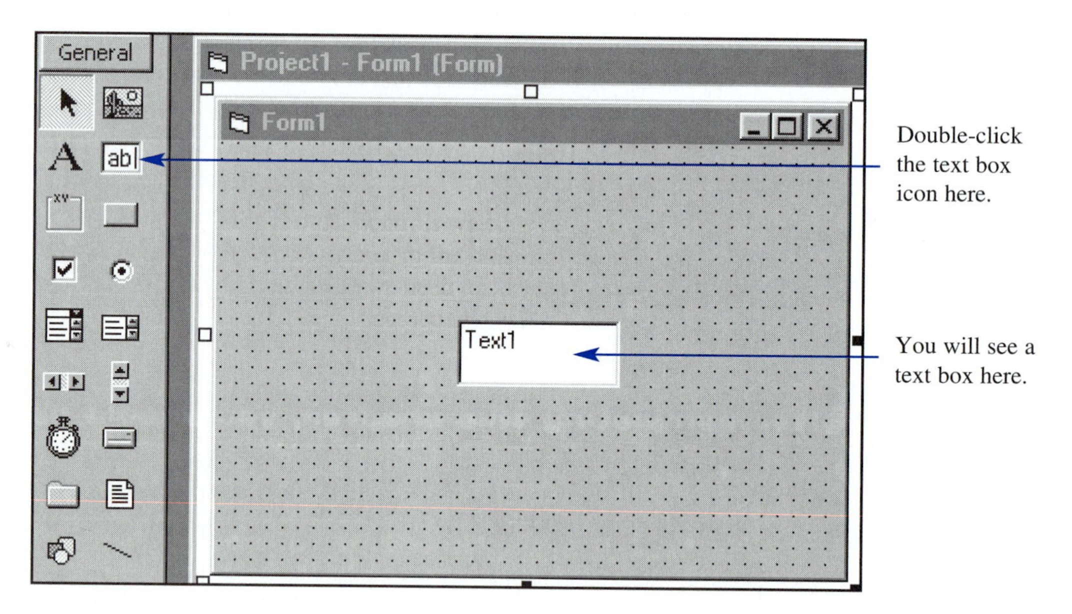

If you glance over the form again, you certainly realize that a blank box in a form means little to the user. It provides no clue as to what we are supposed to do with it. Here, we are immediately reminded of the label control. We can place a label with a proper caption such as "Name (Last, First Init.)" by the text box. Such a clue is indispensable. We come to realize that text boxes are almost always accompanied with labels when used for input purposes. Your result should look like that shown in Figure 3.2.

FIGURE 3.2
Making Label and the Text Box Work Together

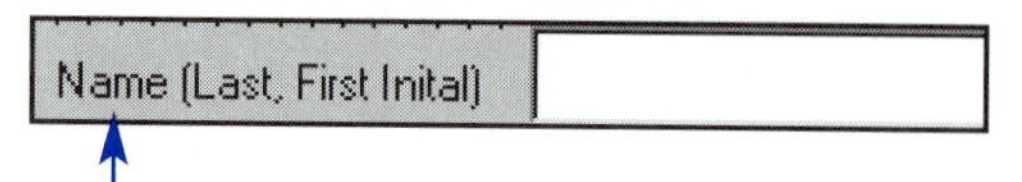

A text box should always be accompanied by a label to provide clues as to what is to be entered.

After you have the label and the text box in the form, run the program. Enter your name into the text box. You should encounter no problem. You may be wondering what the computer knows at this point. Therefore, we will make the computer display the content of the text box when you click on the form. The form has a Click event. This is where we will place the code to display the message. End the program. Enter the following code:

```
Private Sub Form_Click()
    MsgBox "Your name is" & txtName.Text
End Sub
```

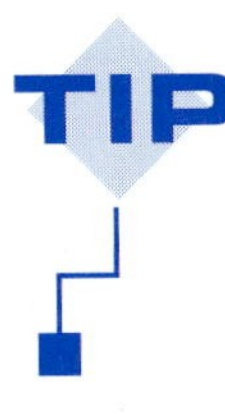

Both the label and text box controls can be used to display text. So, how do you decide which one to use? If you don't want the user to change its content, use the label control. If you need the user's input, use the text box. You can make a label control look like a text box by setting its Back Color property to "Active Title Bar Text" (white) and Border Style property to 1 (fixed single).

Now, run the program again. Enter your name and click the form. You should see a message box displaying the message, "Your name is" along with your name. (End the program before proceeding.) In the preceding code, the "&" operator concatenates the text string "Your name is" with the content of the text box named txtName. If you enter "Smith, John" as your name in the text box, the resulting text string will be "Your name is Smith, John." Figure 3.3 shows the result. We discuss string operations in more detail in Chapter 4, "Data, Operations, and Built-In Functions." The MsgBox displays the text in a dialog box and waits until the user acknowledges the message by clicking the OK button. We discuss more about the MsgBox in Chapter 6, "Input, Output, and Procedures."

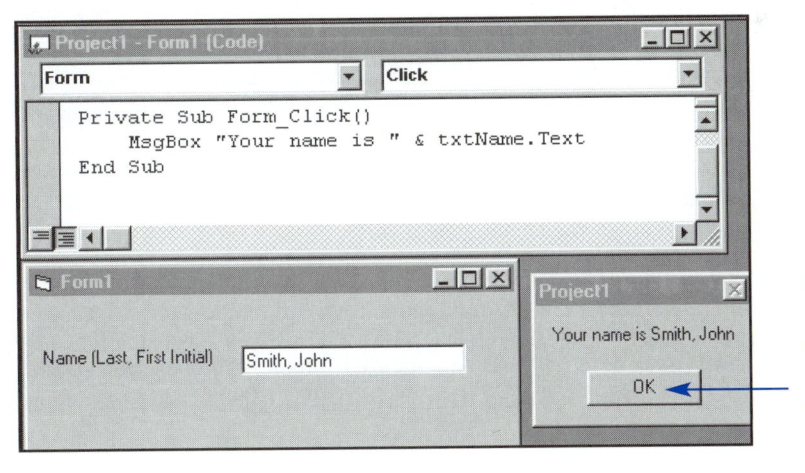

FIGURE 3.3
Showing What's Entered in the Text Box

We can create the phone number field on the form in the same manner:

1. Add a label and change its caption to "Phone."
2. Add another text box. Change its name property to Phone and clear its box by clearing its Text property.

The user interface is now ready for another test. Start the program and try to enter a friend's name and phone number. A sample result is given in Figure 3.4.

The Focus. Notice that because you have more than one control to accept input, *you can enter data into a control only when it has the focus.* A user can set the focus of a control by clicking on it or by pressing the Tab key repetitively until the focus reaches that control. When the text box gets the focus, a blinking cursor will appear in its box.

You can also use the SetFocus method to set focus on a particular text box control. For example, the following statement will set the focus on txtName:

```
txtName.SetFocus
```

This method can be useful when you find a need to set the focus on some control after certain operations. For example, suppose the user has just clicked the Save command button, thus triggering the Click event procedure to save data on the screen. However, after the data are saved, the focus will remain on the command button. By including the statement, you can make it convenient for your user to continue the data-entry operation. The code structure should appear as follows:

```
Private Sub cmdSave_Click()
     ' Statements to save data
     ' Reset focus on the first control
     txtName.SetFocus
End Sub
```

Something to Be Desired. Back to our original project. Keying in the name should be simple and smooth. However, you should notice that the phone number field has a defined pattern; that is, the area code (enclosed in a pair of parentheses) is followed by a hyphen, a three-digit prefix, another hyphen, and the four-digit number. Is there a way to show the parentheses and hyphens automatically since they are in fixed positions? This will not only automatically force the user to follow the pattern but also save the user four keystrokes, a nearly 30% improvement in keying efficiency.

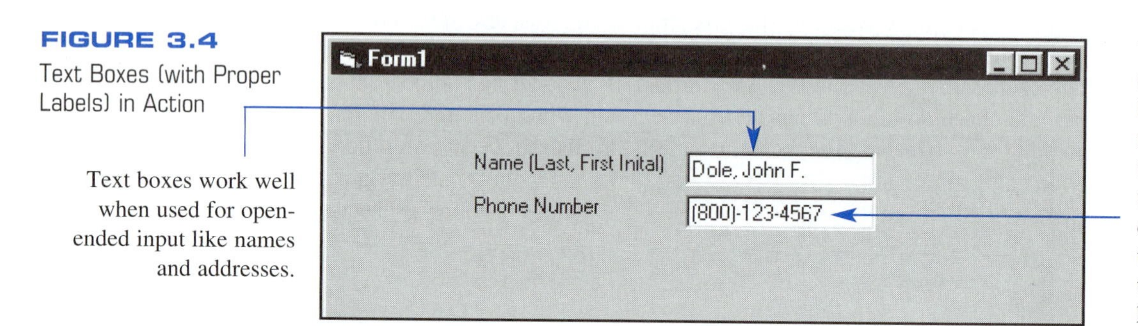
Form1
Name (Last, First Inital)
Dole, John F.
Phone Number
(800)-123-4567
Text boxes work well when used for open-ended input like names and addresses.
When a text box is used as an input box for the phone number, it is hard to ensure that the user will always enter the same pattern. In addition, it takes several extra keystrokes.

FIGURE 3.4
Text Boxes (with Proper Labels) in Action

The Masked Edit Box Control

There is a VB control that can handle this defined pattern, the masked edit control. This control has a ***Mask property,*** which, when left blank, will cause the control to act like a standard text box. However, the property can be set to expect and conveniently enforce a desired input pattern.

Adding the Masked Edit Box Control. This control is not a standard (intrinsic) VB control but can be added to the project. To add, do the following:

1. Click the Project menu then select the Components option (Figure 3.5). The Components dialog box will appear.

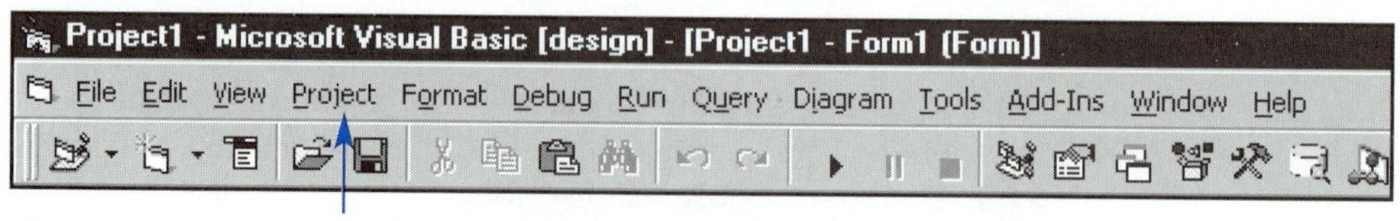
Project1 - Microsoft Visual Basic [design] - [Project1 - Form1 (Form)]
File Edit View Project Format Debug Run Query Diagram Tools Add-Ins Window Help
Click here, then look for "Components" in the drop-down menu.

FIGURE 3.5
Project Menu in the Menu Bar

2. Make sure the Controls tab in the Components dialog box is selected. Otherwise, click this tab.
3. Locate "Microsoft Masked Edit Control 6.0" and click on its check box to check the box (Figure 3.6).
4. Click the OK button.

FIGURE 3.6
The Controls Tab in the Components Dialog Box

Be sure this tab is selected.

Check this one.

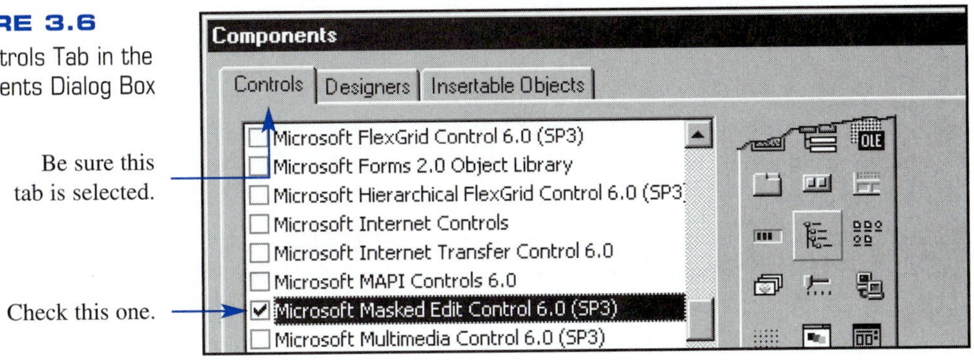

The masked edit control icon "##|" will appear in VB's toolbox. To include this control in our project:

1. Delete the text box for phone number. Click on the text box on the form and press the Delete key.
2. Place a masked edit control in place of the text box.
   - 2.1 Click the masked edit icon in the toolbox.
   - 2.2 Draw this control in the same place where the text box was. Adjust its size and position properly.
   - 2.3 Change its Name property to mskPhone.

The Mask Property. As mentioned, the masked edit box has a Mask property. Set this property to "(###)-###-####"; you should see the mask appear in the control's box in the form (Figure 3.7).

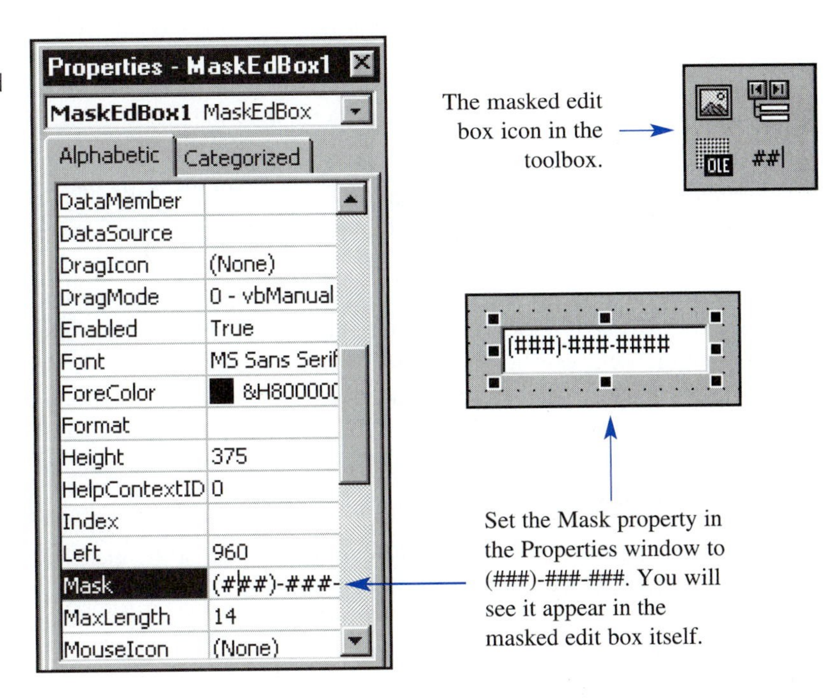

FIGURE 3.7
The Masked Edit Box and Its Mask Property

Start the program and try it. A sample is shown in Figure 3.8.

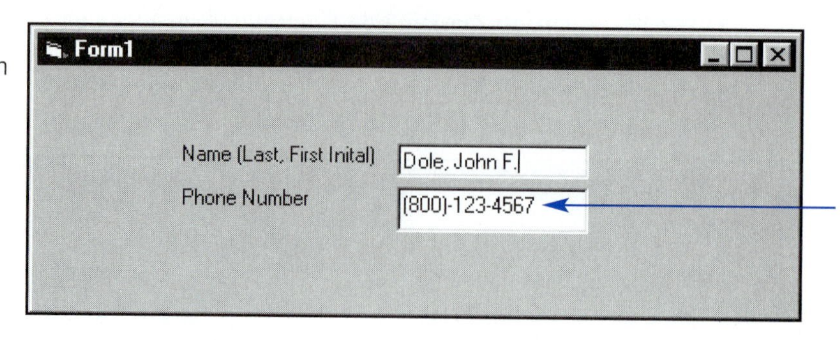

FIGURE 3.8
Masked Edit Box in Action

Here's a masked edit box in action. The parentheses and dashes are automatically displayed. With its Mask property set as above, the box will not accept any nonnumeric keys.

The "#" symbol in the mask is a placeholder for a required digit, and the parentheses and hyphens are literals. At runtime, the literals present themselves in their respective positions, but the # signs disappear. Many more mask characters are available for different uses. For example, an "A" mask character is a required alphanumeric character placeholder. Explore the Help file for many additional mask features of this control as suggested in the "Look It Up" box that follows.

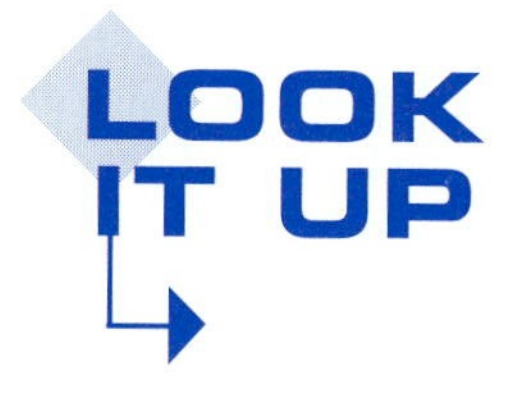

Search the online Help screen using "Mask property" as the keyword in the Index tab. The page provides a complete list of mask characters used in the Mask property of the masked edit box. Take a good look at the page now. You will need to visit the page from time to time in the future when you have a special requirement for the masked edit box.

Comparing the Text Properties of the Two Controls

Both the text box and masked edit box have the Text property, which holds the exact content of the box. However, there are some differences in the property between the two controls. The Text property of the text box is available at both design time and runtime; that is, you can set this property at both design time and runtime by code. In addition, the user can key anything into the text box at runtime.

In contrast, the Text property of the ***masked edit box*** is not available at design time. You can set its value only by code or by the user's key input at runtime. If you assign its value by code, the value must conform to the pattern dictated by the box's mask. For example, if you have set the Mask property for a masked edit box named mskPhone as "(###)-###-####", then your code to assign a phone number to this control must be in the same pattern as shown in the following assignment statement:

```
mskPhone.Text = "(123)-456-7890"
```

Otherwise, a runtime error will result. When the user enters a key that does not conform to the expected pattern by its mask, the masked edit box will not accept the key, and the cursor stays at the same position as if nothing had happened. For example, if you try to enter a letter into mskPhone, it will ignore your attempt because its mask expects only numbers. In real applications, most of the data errors are introduced by the user. The Mask property ensures that only the proper type of key is entered. Thus, the masked edit box can help enhance data accuracy.

Clearing the Text Property

You often may find it desirable to clear the text box or the masked edit box. You can clear the text box easily by assigning a zero-length string (a string that contains nothing) to the Text property as follows:

```
txtName.Text = ""
```

You cannot do exactly the same for the masked edit box because this control expects an exact match of the pattern as specified in the mask. However, you can clear the mask first. *Without the mask, the masked edit behaves exactly like a text box.* Thus, it will allow you to assign a zero-length string to its Text property. Once this is done, you should restore the mask so that the user can enter data only with the expected pattern. The following code shows how this is done:

```
mskPhone.Mask = ""                     'To clear the mask
mskPhone.Text = ""                     'To clear the edit box
mskPhone.Mask = ""(###)-###-####"      'To restore the mask
```

SelStart and SelLength Properties

Sometimes, when a control gets the focus, we would like to highlight its content. Both the text box and masked edit box have an event, GotFocus, which occurs when a control gets the focus. Highlighted text can be replaced by any key entered and can be erased easily by pressing a Backspace key or Delete key. Both the text box and masked edit box have SelStart and SelLength properties. The ***SelStart property*** sets or returns the current cursor position in the control, with the first position being zero (0). Thus, if you want to place the cursor at the beginning of the control, you will assign a zero (0) to its SelStart property. The ***SelLength property*** sets or returns the length (the number of characters) of the text being selected. The selected text is highlighted (Figure 3.9). The following code will highlight the content of a text box named txtName when it gets the focus:

```
Private Sub txtName_GotFocus()
    txtName.SelStart = 0 'Set the cursor at the beginning
    'Highlight the text from the beginning
    txtName.SelLength = Len(txtName.Text)
End Sub
```

FIGURE 3.9
Highlighted Text Box

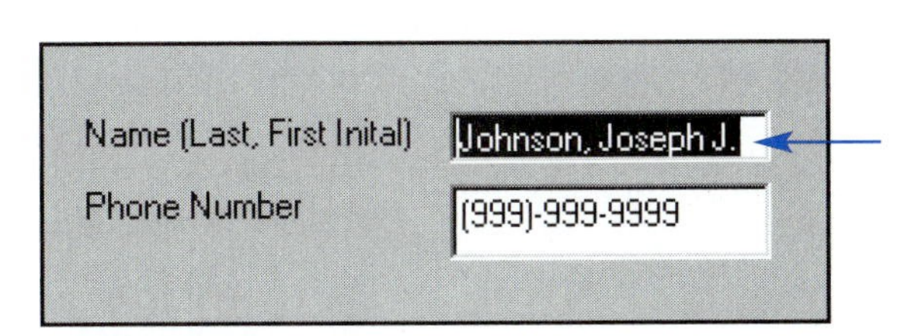

When you tab into this text box, named txtName, the statements in the GotFocus event will cause the control's content to be highlighted. The user can easily replace or delete (or perform cut or copy) the highlighted text.

The code is placed in the txtName's ***GotFocus event*** procedure, which is triggered when txtName gets the focus. Its SelStart property is set to 0 to place the cursor at the beginning of the text. The following expression:

```
Len(txtName.Text)
```

involves the use of the ***Len function***, which returns the length of the parameter enclosed in the pair of parentheses (txtName.Text). The SelLength property of txtName is then set to this returned value. (We discuss more on functions in Chapter 4.) Because the SelLength property highlights the text starting from the current cursor position (which is currently at the beginning as set by the SelStart property), the entire text in txtName will be highlighted. As you may have learned from other Windows applications, highlighted texts will be replaced by whatever you type over them.

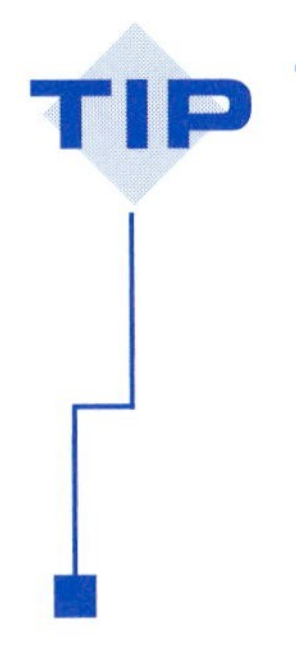

In general, the key you enter into a text box is inserted into the existing text. Because the highlighted text is replaced by the key you enter, you can make your text box act in the "type over mode" (instead of the default "insert mode") by highlighting the character where the cursor is. The text box has a change event that occurs when its text changes. You can use this event to effect the "type over mode":

```
Private Sub txtName_Change()
'highlight the character where the cursor is
    TxtName.SelLength = 1
End Sub
```

The ClipText Property

In addition to the Text property, the masked edit box also has the ***ClipText property***. The difference between the two properties is that the Text property has the exact content (including the literal characters in the mask) in the box, whereas the ClipText property has only the text without the literal. Usually, this is what the user actually enters. In the preceding code example, which assigned "(123)-456-7890" to mskPhone.Text, the control's ClipText property will be "1234567890" and its Text property will be "(123)-456-7890."

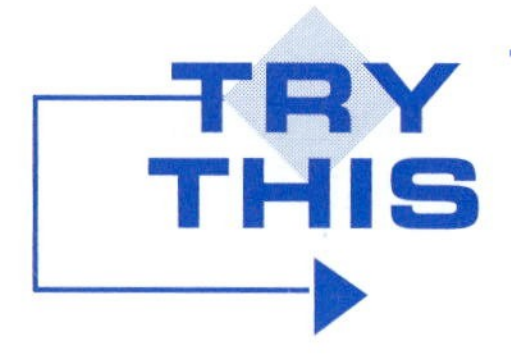

Bring one text box, one masked edit box, and a command button to a new form. Name them txtName, mskBirthDate, and cmdShow, respectively. Set the Mask property of mskBirthDate to *##-##-####*. Set the Caption property of cmdShow to "Show." Then double-click the command button in the form to show the code window. Give the following lines of code:

```
Private Sub smdShow_Click()
     MsgBox "Name is " & txtName.Text
     MsgBox "Birthdate text is " & mskBirthDate.Text
     MsgBox "Birthdate clip text is " & mskBirthDate.ClipText
End Sub
```

Run the program. Key in some data and click the Show button. In addition to gaining the experience and proficiency of working with the VB IDE, you should be able to get a good feel about what these Text and ClipText properties mean as well as how the code works.

The following table provides a summary of the new properties discussed in this section.

Property	Applicable Object	Use/Remark
Text	Text box	For the user to enter data; value can be set at design time or assigned by code at runtime; for example, txtName.Text = "John Smith."
	Masked edit box	For the user to enter data; not available at design time; entered data or value assigned must be in accordance with the mask pattern.
Mask	Masked edit box	To define the pattern for the expected data type; for example, a "#" will expect a number for the corresponding position in the Text property.
SelStart	Text box, masked edit box	To set the cursor position in the field (control); for example, the code mskDate.SelStart = 1 will place the cursor at the second position of the field.
SelLength	Text box, masked edit box	To select a portion of the text; for example, the statement txtName.SelLength = 3 will select (highlight) three characters in the field beginning from the current cursor position.
ClipText	Masked edit box	Gives the data that is not a "literal" part of the mask; for example, a masked edit box with the mask "##-##-####" and that contains a text string of "12-31-1999" will return a value 12311999.

3.2 Arranging Many VB Controls on a Form: Frame and SSTab Controls

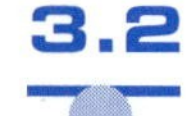

Let's expand our consideration. Suppose we are designing an entry screen for an account file used by a hospital. The screen will be used to collect not only personal data about the account holder and his or her employer but also information on the holder's health insurance. One obvious difference from the previous situation is the number of data fields on the form. How does this affect our design? As the number of fields increases, we need to ensure that the form layout looks neat, logical, and uncluttered. That is, VB controls placed on the form should be aligned neatly with each other and be grouped properly. Furthermore, the grouping of these fields should appear to be logical and "natural" to the user.

The Frame Control

A VB control often used to help group related data fields is the ***frame control.*** As its name suggests, the frame control provides a frame within which various controls can be placed (Figure 3.10). It has a Caption property, which can be used to indicate its content. When used properly, the frame control not only provides a means of grouping controls logically but also facilitates a neat arrangement of the form layout.

FIGURE 3.10
Frame Control: Icon and Appearance

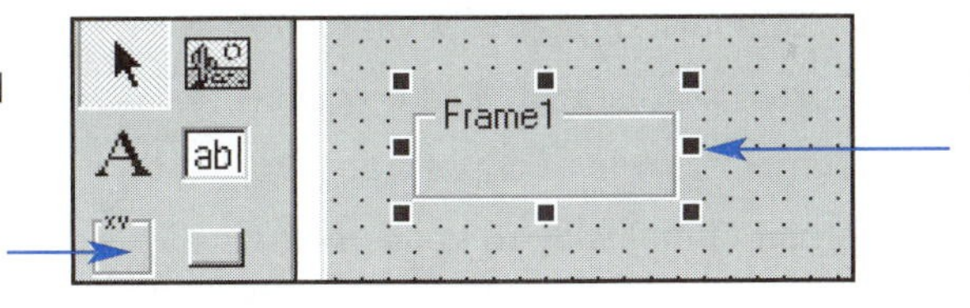

Frame icon in the toolbox

Frame control in a form. You can adjust its size in exactly the same way as other controls.

Design Time Behavior. Controls within the frame are treated as one logical unit. When the frame is moved, all controls in it move with it. If you delete the frame control, all controls within it are also deleted. Because the frame control has the capability to hold other controls, it is recognized as a type of ***container***.

Placing Controls in a Frame. At design time, to place a control in the frame, the control must be drawn in the frame; that is, you must click the control icon in the toolbox first and then point and drag inside the frame. If you first draw a control onto the form and then drag it into the frame, the control is not a "logical" part of the frame and will not be handled accordingly. When you move the frame, the control will stay at its original location rather than move with the frame.

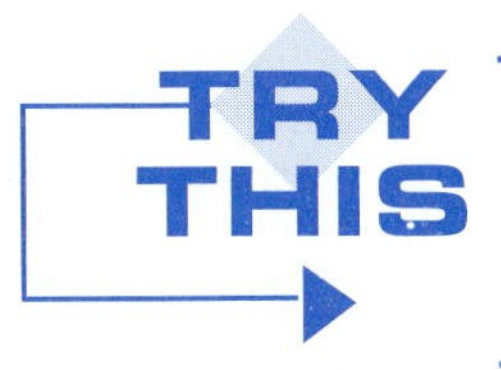

Place a frame in the center of a new form. Then double-click the text box icon in the toolbox. The text box should appear in the frame. Move the frame. You should notice that the text box does not move with the frame. The text box is not a logical part of the frame because it was not actually drawn into the frame.

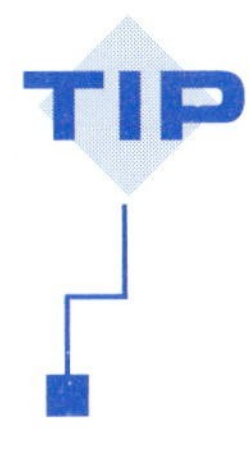

You can make an existing control become a logical part of the frame by first cutting it from the form and then pasting it onto the frame. A simple way to do this is to right-click on the control to get the pop-up context menu and click the Cut option. Then right-click on the frame to get the pop-up context menu again and select the Paste option. The pasted control appears on the upper-left corner of the frame. You can drag it to its desired position.

A simplified form layout with two frames is presented in Figure 3.11 as an illustration.

FIGURE 3.11
Frames Containing Other Controls

Form1

Name and Address
Name
Address
City
State
Zip Code

Insurance
Insured ID
Insurance Co.
Program/FECA ID
Program Name
Employer Name

Here are two frames in action with other controls drawn inside each. Controls in a frame are treated as a logical unit. You can set each frame's caption property to show the contents.

The steps to draw a control onto a form were discussed in Chapter 2. The added layer of the frame makes drawing the controls in the frames a bit more complex. To create the interface in Figure 3.11, follow these steps:

1. Draw two frames on a new form. Adjust the size and position of the frames so that they will look like those in the figure.
2. Draw five labels inside the left frame. Notice that *you must first click the label icon in the toolbox and then place the mouse pointer inside the frame and drag.* That is, you can no longer just double-click a label and make it show in a frame. Once a label is drawn into the frame, you can adjust its position so that it will be located properly.
3. Draw five text boxes onto the left frame using the same steps as for the labels. Adjust their sizes and positions so that they will look like the five text boxes in the figure.
4. Set the Caption property for the left frame to "Name and Address."
5. Set the Caption properties for the labels so that they will appear as Name, Address, City, State, and Zip Code, respectively. You may want to set the AutoSize properties to True for all labels before setting their Caption properties.
6. Clear the text in the text boxes.
7. Repeat steps 1 through 6 to draw the right frame and the controls inside it.

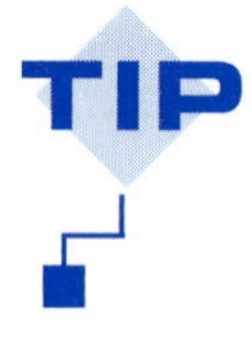

When setting various properties of several controls of the same type, work with one property at a time, instead of with one control at a time. As you switch from one control to another, the same property you have just worked on will be highlighted in the Properties window, making it easy to locate the property and change its setting.

As a reminder, before you start to write any code for the project, set the Name properties of all the controls to be referenced in the code.

Runtime Behavior, Visible Property, and Enabled Property. At runtime, all controls contained in the frame control are also treated as a single unit. For example, assuming the left frame control in Figure 3.11 is named fraAcctHolderAddr, executing the following code will make the entire frame invisible. None of the controls in the frame can be seen.

```
FraAcctHolderAddr.Visible = False
```

Similarly, the following code will make all controls in that frame disabled. That is, none of the text boxes in the frame can receive focus or accept any input from the user.

```
FraAcctHolderAddr.Enabled = False
```

Most of the VB controls have the Visible and Enabled properties. The default values of these properties are True. They can be set at design time or by code. At runtime, a control with its ***Visible property*** set to False will be invisible as if it did not exist. Once the property is changed to True, the control will appear again. You can manipulate this property with your code to hide the control when it is not needed in your program context and to show it only when it is needed.

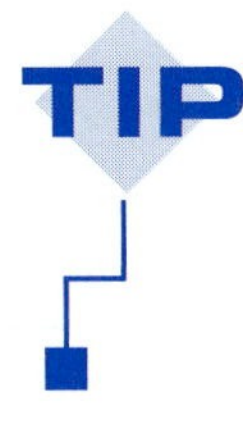

Occasionally, you might find that when you run your program, you see nothing but the code window. This means you have accidentally set the form's Visible property to False. This error can easily occur when you concentrate so much on setting the Visible property without realizing that the object in the Properties window is the form, not the control you have in mind.

When a VB control (e.g., text box) has the focus, the user can key in data. A control can receive focus only when it is enabled. A disabled control (with its Enabled property set to False) cannot receive focus or input. Its appearance will also change to a light gray to indicate its disabled status. Figure 3.12 shows this contrast.

FIGURE 3.12
Label: Enabled and Disabled

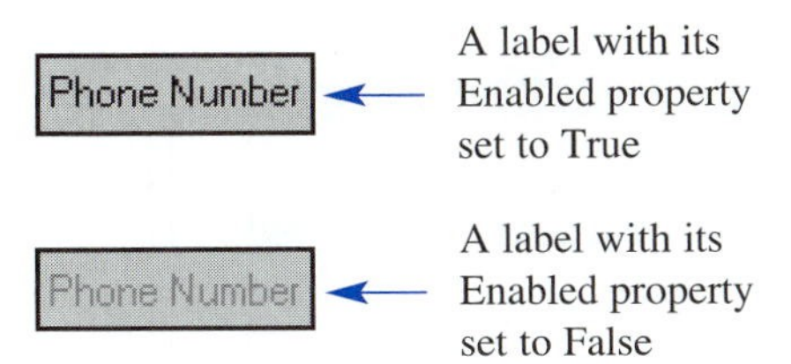

The SSTab Control

Let's further consider the hospital account screen. The data to be collected are far more detailed than what we have just presented. For example, concerning personal data, the hospital needs not only the account holder's name and address but also additional identification (e.g., gender and date of birth), phone numbers, spouse, and so on, not to mention additional information on the holder's insurance. It is impractical, if not impossible, to include all these data elements in one screen. However, it is highly desirable to treat all these data as one single logical unit. That is, you want to save, retrieve, and update all these data in a single operation. What VB control can help handle this situation? Believe or not, you have already seen that control in action in the VB IDE. Recall the Components dialog box that we worked with to bring the masked edit box into the toolbox. It consists of several tabs, each containing logically related data elements. The VB control that presents tabs and allows the user to view among these tabs is called the ***SStab control.***

However, this control is not one of the standard (intrinsic) controls. To add it to the toolbox:

1. Click the Project menu and select the Components option.
2. Check the box for "Microsoft Tabbed Dialog Control 6.0."
3. Click the OK button.

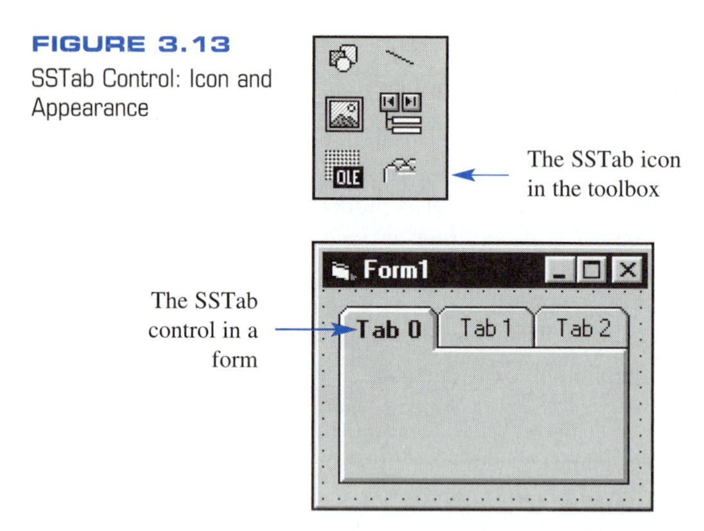

FIGURE 3.13
SSTab Control: Icon and Appearance

Figure 3.13 shows the SSTab icon and its appearance on a form. The number of tabs and each tab's individual caption can be changed in the Property Pages dialog box. You can access this dialog box by double-clicking the (Custom) property of the Properties window. With this dialog box, you can also specify the number of tabs per row as well as where you want the tabs to show on the control (Figure 3.14). The tabs can be "oriented" at the top (0—ssTabOrientationTop) as shown here, the bottom (1—ssTabOrientationBottom), the left (2—ssTabOrientationLeft), or the right (3—ssTabOrientationRight). You can also set the font for all tabs. To change the font, click the Font tab of the same dialog box. You can then select the desired font and size.

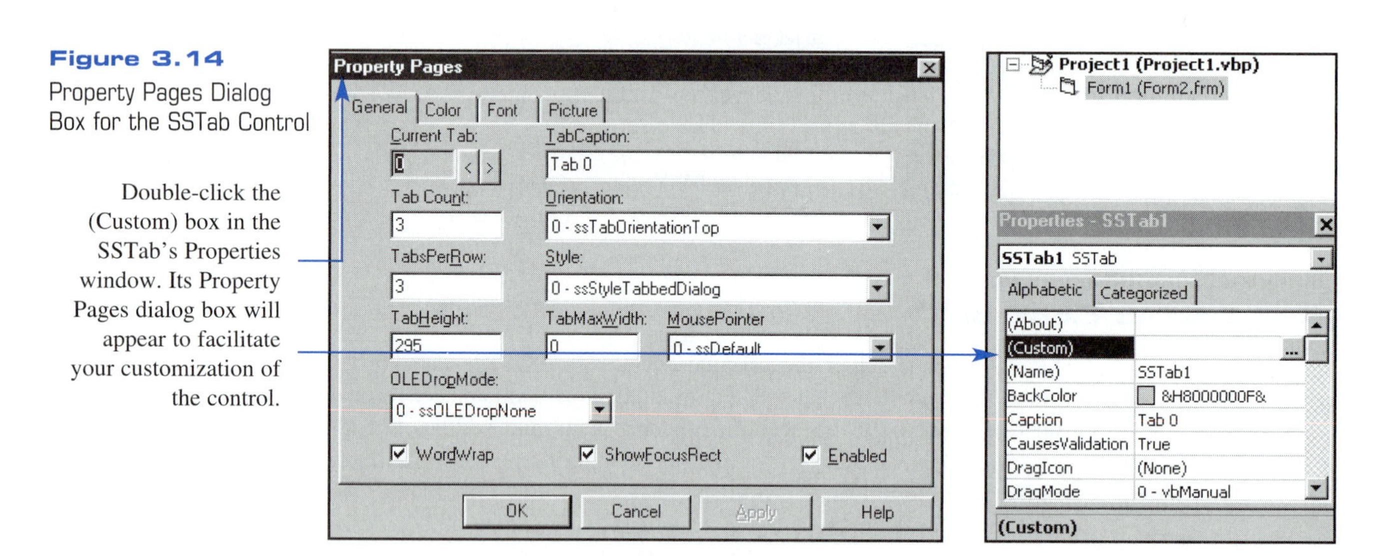

Figure 3.14
Property Pages Dialog Box for the SSTab Control

Like the frame control, each of these tabs serves as a container. Various VB controls, including the frame, can be drawn in it. At runtime, the user can move between these tabs by clicking the tab captions or by pressing Ctrl+Tab. The control's Tab property value tells you which tab your user is working on. (The first tab has a Tab property value of 0.) You can also use code to change the tab by assigning a value to the control's Tab property. For example, the following statement will make a tab control named sstAcctInfo show its third tab. (Note again the Tab property for the first tab is 0.)

```
sstAcctInfo.Tab = 2
```

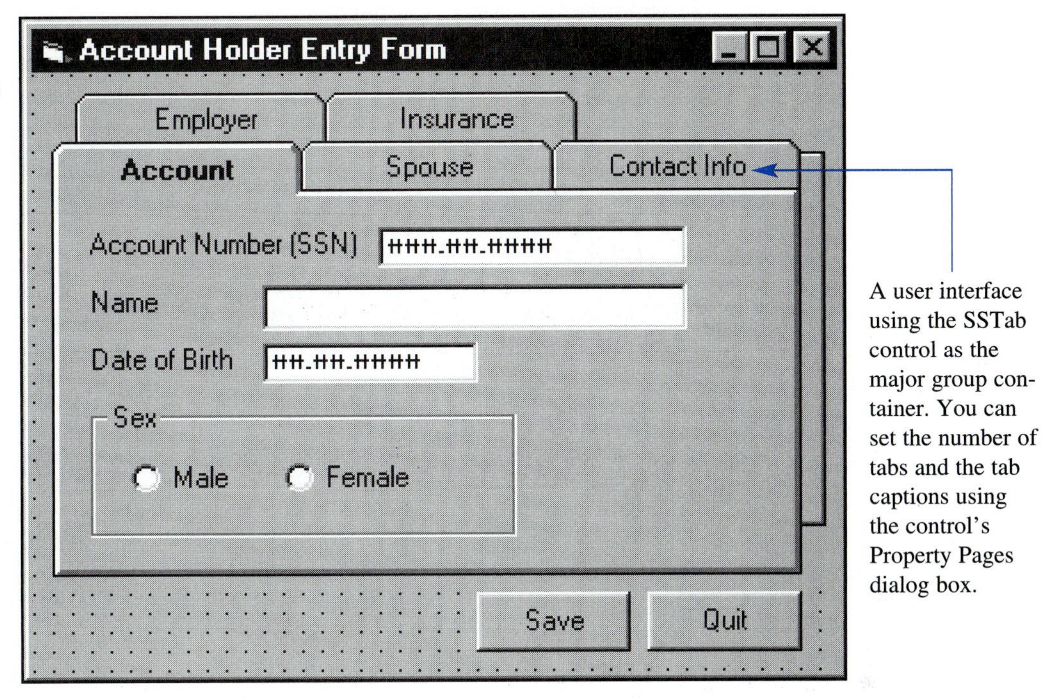

FIGURE 3.15
A Sample of Using the SSTab for Visual Interface

Figure 3.15 shows the redesigned (but still simplified) hospital account holder entry form, using the SSTab control as the main grouping device.

To create the interface from a new form, follow these steps:

1. Add SSTab and masked edit box controls to your project by using the Component option of the Project menu. The steps to add a nonstandard control are explained in Section 3.1.
2. Draw a SSTab control onto the form. Adjust the size of the tab control.
3. Customize the SSTab using its Property Pages dialog box, as illustrated in Figure 3.14. Using the dialog box, you can do the following:

    3.1 Change the number of tabs to five by setting the tab count to five in the General tab.

    3.2 Set the tab captions. You can do the following:

    3.2.1 Ensure the Current Tab box shows 0.

    3.2.2 Replace "Tab0" with "Account" in the TabCaption box.

    3.2.3 Enter 1 in the Current Tab box. (Or you can click the > button to effect the change.) Then replace "Tab1" with "Spouse."

    3.2.4 Set all other tab captions in the same manner.

4. Draw controls into the first tab. Notice that there is a frame used to group the option buttons for gender. You may want to draw this frame first.
5. Draw controls onto the other tabs. The details (including fields to include) are left to you as an exercise.
6. Draw the command buttons onto the form. (Notice that they are not drawn inside the tab control.) Then change the captions of these buttons as well as the form.

More discussion on the SSTab control is presented in Chapter 10, "Special Topics in Data Entry." The following table lists the new properties discussed in this section.

Property	Applicable Object	Use/Remark
Visible	The form and all controls that can appear during runtime	The object will be visible if this property is set to True; invisible, if False. For example, the code `lblAddress.Visible = False` will make the label lblAddress disappear.
Enabled	Same as above	To enable or disable a control; a disabled control cannot receive focus and thus cannot accept any user input; an object is enabled if this property is set to True; disabled, if False. The code `fraID.Enabled = False` will disable all controls in the frame named fraID.
Tab	SSTab	To set or return the Tab position; for example, the code `sstAccount.Tab = 1` will show the second tab of the tab control named sstAccount.

3.3 Data with Limited Number of Choices: Option Buttons and Check Boxes

Let's consider the hospital account holder information screen again. One "blank" to be filled in for identification purpose must be "gender." We can add another text box and ask the user to fill in either M (for male) or F (for female). However, this choice is not really "optimal." A careless user might enter O (for other). An interface designed this way will require additional code to ensure the validity of entered data.

The Option Button

One VB control that can be conveniently used for this purpose is the ***option button*** (Figure 3.16). This control has Caption and Value properties. The text in the ***Caption property*** is displayed next to the button and is typically used to show the choice. Its ***Value property*** is set to either True or False to indicate whether this option is chosen. An option button with a value True will show a dot bullet in its button. Otherwise, the button will be empty.

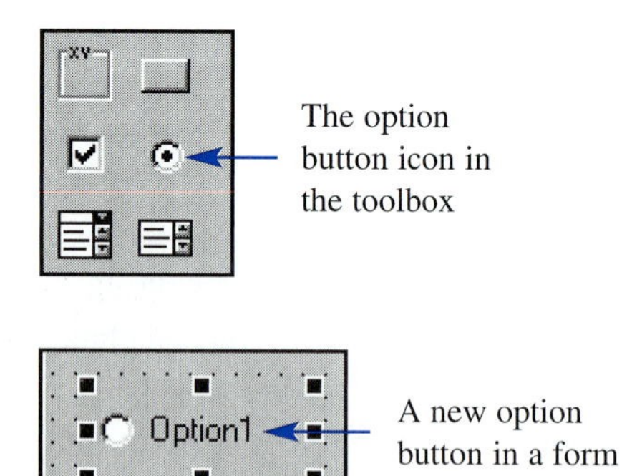

FIGURE 3.16
Option Button: Icon and Appearance

Option Buttons Work in Group. When the Value property of one option button is set to True, the same properties of all other option buttons in the same group will automatically be set to False. If one button is clicked "On," all others in the group will be turned "Off." For the gender question, two option buttons can be brought into the frame. One can be captioned Male; the other, Female. At design time, you can also set a default choice by setting the Value property of either button to True. Figure 3.17 shows the gender option buttons as a part of the account holder identification frame.

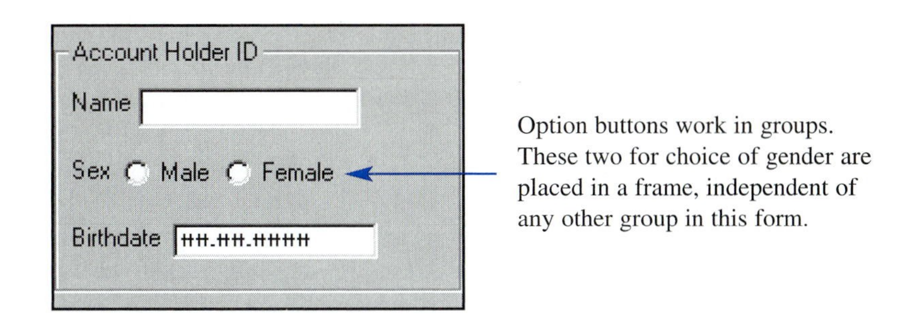
Account Holder ID
Name
Sex Male Female
Birthdate ##-##-####
Option buttons work in groups. These two for choice of gender are placed in a frame, independent of any other group in this form.

FIGURE 3.17
Option Buttons in a Frame

Notice that *all* option buttons on a form constitute a single group. Only one option button can be selected from a group. To have more than one group of option buttons in a form, you must place each group in a different container, such as a frame or a picture box (to be introduced in Section 3.5).

At runtime, when an "Off" button is clicked, it will be turned "on" and its value will be set to True. Clicking an "On" button will not result in any change. You can presume the "On" status in the Click event. As an illustration, assume that the two buttons used for gender are named optFemale and optMale. The following code will cause a message box to display "Female button is clicked" or "Male button is clicked" when you click on the button that is initially off.

```
Private Sub optFemale_Click()
    MsgBox "Female button is clicked"
End Sub

Private Sub optMale_Click()
    MsgBox "Male button is clicked"
End Sub
```

Notice again that clicking on an option button that is already on will not turn it off. Nor will it raise the Click event. Thus, there is no need to check the value of the button in the Click event.

In data-entry operations, usually no immediate response by the computer is needed when the user makes a choice among the option buttons. You may wonder then: When the user is ready to save the result (say by clicking a Save command button), how does the computer know which button is on? Your code must test the Value property of the option button. For example, the following code shows which button is on at the time the command button named cmdSave is clicked (Figure 3.18).

```
Private Sub cmdSave_Click()
    If optMale.Value Then
        MsgBox "Male button is on."
    Else
        MsgBox "Female button is on."
    End If
    ' Place the code to save data here
End Sub
```

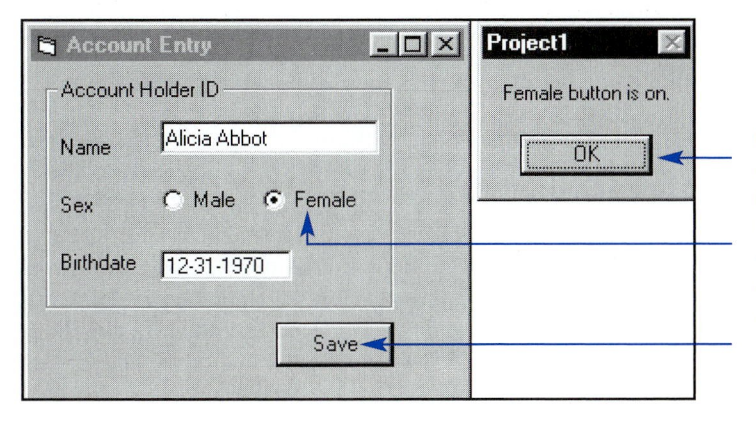
Account Entry
Account Holder ID
Name Alicia Abbot
Sex Male Female
Birthdate 12-31-1970
Save
Project1
Female button is on.
OK
Clicking the Save command button (cmdSave) while the Female option button (optFemal) is on will cause the computer to display the message "Female button is on" with the above code.

FIGURE 3.18
Option Buttons in Action

As explained in Chapter 2, the If statement can have the following structure:

```
If condition Then
    Statements to execute if the condition is true
Else
    Statements to execute if the condition is not true
End If
```

Recall that the Value property of an option button is either True or False. The If statement will test to see whether this value is True for optMale. If it is, the computer displays "Male button is on." Otherwise, it will display "Female button is on." An If block structured this way must be closed with the "End If" statement. Chapter 5, "Decision," discusses the If statement in more detail.

Check Boxes for Independent Choices

For data with a limited number of items that are mutually exclusive, option buttons are ideal. However, what if these choices are not mutually exclusive, but rather are independent? For example, a health survey questionnaire may ask the respondent whether he or she regularly has breakfast, lunch, and dinner. The respondent may regularly have all or skip any of the three meals. In such situation, the check box control will be suitable.

FIGURE 3.19
Check Boxes: Icon, Appearance, and in Action

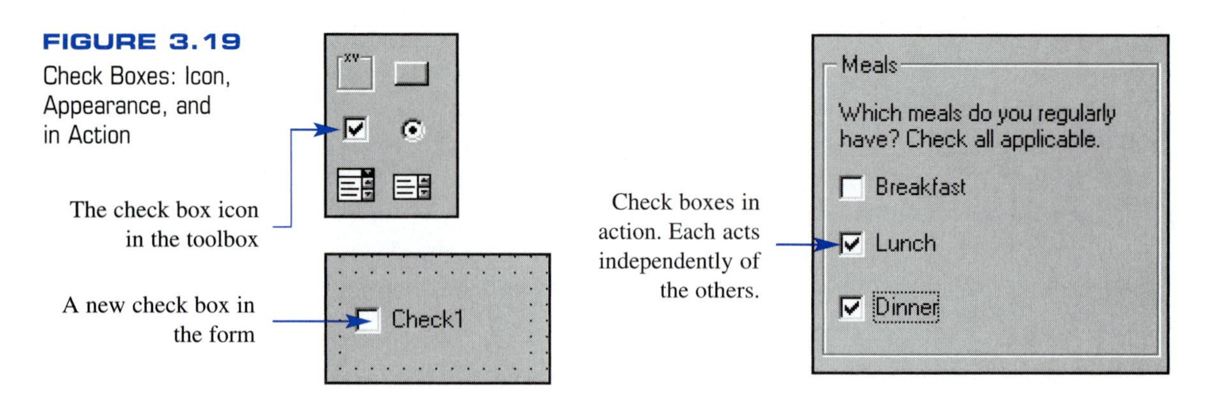

Check boxes appear very similar to the option buttons (Figure 3.19). The Caption property can display text in a manner similar to the option button. However, as noted, the check boxes work independently of each other. Any number of them can be set "on" at the same time regardless of the value (status) of the other check boxes. When clicked "on" (value set to 1, vbChecked), its squared box shows a check mark (√). If you click it again, the check mark disappears, suggesting it is turned "off" (value set to 0, vbUnChecked). This behavior differs from that of the option button, which once clicked on will stay on until another button in the same group gets clicked on. Thus, in the check box's Click event, you cannot assume that the box is on. Your code must test its value. The following code tests if a check box named chkBreakfast is on.

```
Private Sub chkBreakfast_Click()
    If chkBreakfast.Value = vbChecked Then
        MsgBox "The respondent regularly has breakfast!"
    Else
        MsgBox "The respondent does not eat breakfast regularly."
    End If
End Sub
```

Note how the If statement is expressed. The Value property of chkBreakfast is compared with vbChecked (1). The equal sign between the two operands is not an assignment but an instruction to compare to see whether the two are equal. If they are, the result is True. Just like "True," the symbol vbChecked is a ***named constant*** (i.e., a constant with a given name) recognized by VB and has a numeric value 1, which is the value of the check box's Value property when the box is turned on. For code clarity, always choose a named constant over a literal constant.

Theoretically, a check box with a caption "Male?" (or "Female?") will suffice to ascertain a person's gender. However, such a design choice will not be politically correct, albeit efficient. As a software developer or systems designer, you should be concerned about not only efficiency but also other factors such as users' needs, corporate policy, and various systems environmental considerations.

Difference in the Click Event Between the Check Box and the Option Button. Note also, when you click a check box that is off, it will be turned on and vice versa. In either case, the Click event is raised. Therefore, you need to test the Value property of the check box in the Click event. This differs from the way the option button responds. As explained previously, if you click on an option button that is already on, the Click event will not be raised.

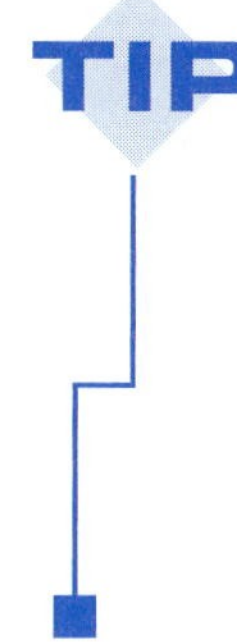

Never code an option button's Click event as follows:

```
Private Sub optMale_Click()
    If optMale Then
        MsgBox "Male button is clicked."
    Else
        MsgBox "Female button is clicked."
    End If
End Sub
```

Why? An option button can only be turned on when it is clicked. Thus, the Else portion of the code will never be executed. Refer to the preceding subsection for the correct code.

The Value Property in Brief. We discussed only one new property, the Value property, in this section. Notice, however, the settings for the Value properties of the option button and the check box are different.

- For the option button, valid settings include True and False. An option button that is set "on" (selected) has the value True; otherwise, False.
- For the check box, valid settings include 0 (vbUnchecked), 1 (vbChecked), and 2 (vbGrayed; seldom used). A check box with its box checked (on) will have its Value property set to vbChecked. When its box is not checked (off), it will have its Value property set to vbUnchecked.

3.4 Longer List of Known Items: List Boxes and Combo Boxes

A principle that we implicitly stated in the preceding section is that whenever the expected data are known with a limited number of items, your program should provide these items for the user to select, rather than prompting the user to enter (into a text box, for example). Such design reduces the number of keystrokes, thus improving the data-entry accuracy and efficiency. In addition, there won't be a need to check for entry errors, thus making the program simpler and faster.

What if the number of known items is not just "a few" but "quite a few"? For example, a college can have a large number of departments. But the departments are known and seldom change. Using option buttons to identify a department may not sound practicable, but we should still resist the use of text boxes for this purpose. The data that the user enters can contain errors. Furthermore, it can take the user many keystrokes to complete the entry. One possible solution is to use data codes (call it department ID) in place of the complete department names. However, your program will still need to verify the accuracy of entered data, even though such a design should reduce the number of keystrokes. Solution? Use the list box or combo box.

The List Box Control

The list box is a box that contains a list, such as department names in the college of business, names of students in a VB class, or fixed assets a company owns (Figure 3.20). When the list of elements in the box is longer than the physical height of the list box control, the list box shows a vertical scrollbar, which the user can use to scroll up and down to browse its content. The item that the user clicks is identified as the list's Text property. The list box's ***ListIndex property***, also set in the Click event, indicates the position of the item clicked. For example, suppose the list box in Figure 3.20 is named lstMonths. If the user clicks March in the list, then lstMonths.Text will show "March," whereas lstMonths.ListIndex will give a value of 2. Note that the first position in the list has a ListIndex value of 0, not 1. You can also use code to select an item. For example, the following code will "select" the first item in the list and thus set the Text property to "January."

```
LstMonths.ListIndex = 0
```

FIGURE 3.20
List Box: Icon and Appearance

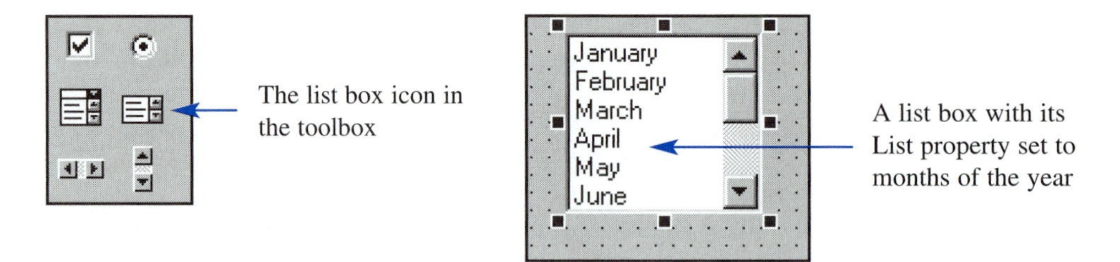
The list box icon in the toolbox
January
February
March
April
May
June
A list box with its List property set to months of the year

Populating the List Box. How do you build a list for the list box? If you have a short list with known data, you can create the list at design time. Follow these steps:

1. Click the list box in the form.
2. Click the List property in the Properties window; a drop-down arrow button appears.
3. Click that button. An empty list will appear (Figure 3.21).
4. Key in your list into this small window. At the end of each list item, press Ctrl+Enter to enter the next item.
5. Press the Enter key when the list is complete.

FIGURE 3.21
The List Property of the List Box in the Properties Window

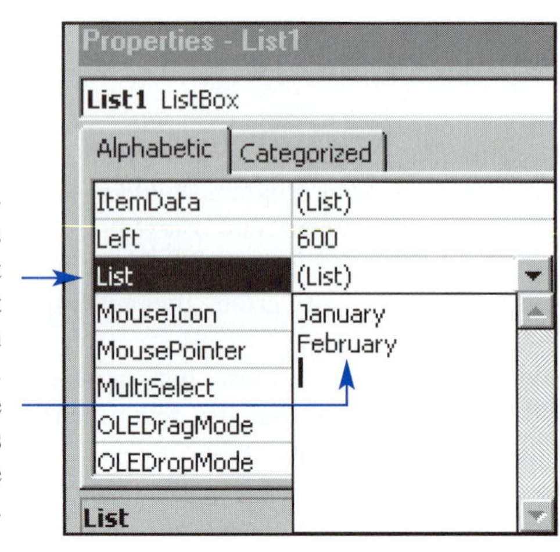
You can use this property in the Properties window to create a list for the list box at design time. Key in your items in the box. Press Ctrl+Enter at the end of each item. Press the Enter key when the list is complete.
Properties - List1
List1 ListBox
Alphabetic
Categorized
ItemData
(List)
Left
600
List
(List)
MouseIcon
January
MousePointer
February
MultiSelect
OLEDragMode
OLEDropMode
List

If you create the list for the list box at design time, there will be an .frx file associated with the form file. When you forward your source project (say, turn it in as an assignment), be sure to include this file. Otherwise, the project cannot be opened successfully on the target computer.

If you have a fairly long list or the data items are not known at design time, you will need to build the list by code using the ***AddItem method***. This method has the following syntax:

```
Listboxname.AddItem ItemToAdd, position
```

For example, the following code will add "John Wayne" to the list box named lstMyFriends in the second position. (The position count starts at zero.)

```
lstMyFriends.AddItem "John Wayne", 1
```

If you omit the position parameter, the name will be added at the end of the list.

The RemoveItem Method. You can also use the code to remove any item from the list box using the ***RemoveItem method***. For example, the following code will remove the third item from the list.

```
lstMyFriends.RemoveItem 2
```

The ListCount Property. The list box has a ***ListCount property*** that gives the number of items in the list box. At any time, its value represents the actual count. Because the list's ListIndex starts at zero, the highest ListIndex value is ListCount – 1. Thus, the ListCount property of lstMonths shown previously will give a value 12, and its highest ListIndex value should be 11.

The MultiSelect Property. The list box has an interesting property, the MultiSelect property. The default value of this property is None (0), meaning only one item can be selected from the list box. If the property is set to Simple (1) or Extended (2), the list box will allow multiple selections from its content (Figure 3.22). The difference between these two settings lies in the way the list box responds to the mouse click and combinations of keys.

FIGURE 3.22
List Box with Different Settings for the MultiSelect Property

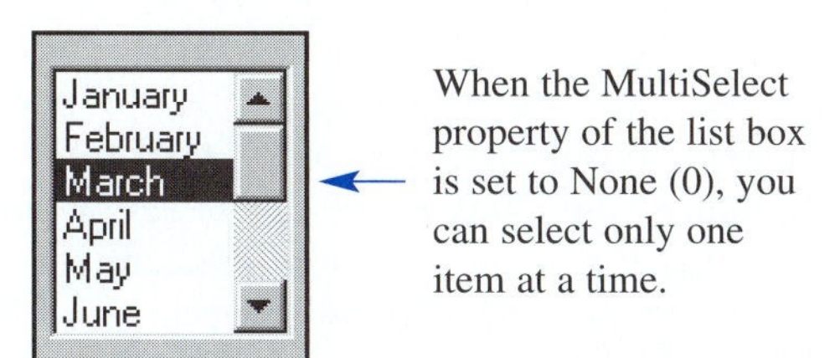
January
February
March
April
May
June
When the MultiSelect property of the list box is set to None (0), you can select only one item at a time.

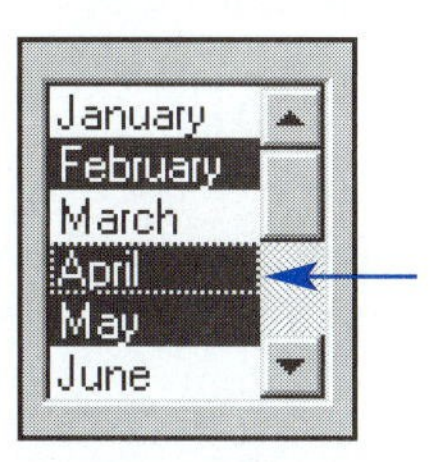
January
February
March
April
May
June

When the MultiSelect property is set to either Simple (1) or Extended (2), you can select more than one item.

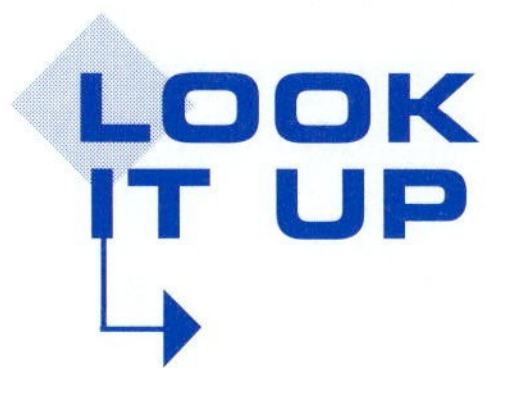

The keyword "MultiSelect property" (Visual Basic Reference) in the Index tab of the VB online Help menu will lead you to a detailed explanation on how you can use different key-mouse combinations to select or deselect an item in the list box with different settings of the MultiSelect property.

The Style Property. Another interesting property is the Style property, which can be set to Standard (0, default) or Checkbox (1). With the default setting, each item appears in the list box as plain text. With the Checkbox setting, a check box is placed in front of each item, making it look like a check box (Figure 3.23). *When the Style property is set to Checkbox, the list allows multiple selections from the list, regardless of the MultiSelect property setting.*

FIGURE 3.23
List Box with the Style Property Set to Checkbox (1)

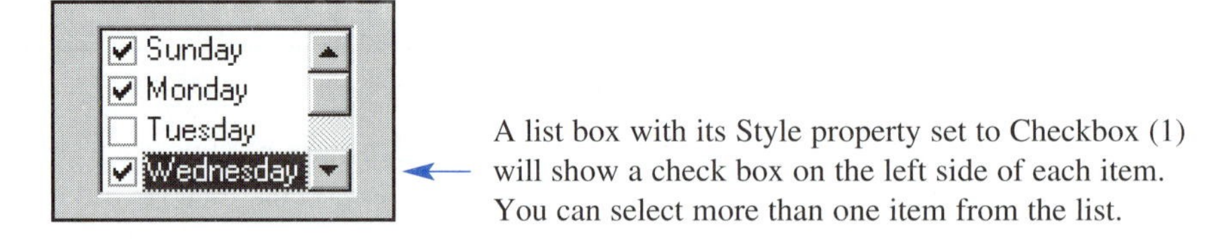
Sunday
Monday
Tuesday
Wednesday
A list box with its Style property set to Checkbox (1) will show a check box on the left side of each item. You can select more than one item from the list.

The Sorted Property. At design time, the Sorted property of the list box can be set to False (0; default) or True. When the property is set to False, items in the box will appear in the order as originally set. If the property is set to True, then at runtime, items will appear in ascending order regardless of when the item is added to the list. This can be very convenient for the user when searching for an item.

Versatility of the List Box. By now you must have been impressed with the versatility of the list box. But how does this relate to data entry? Recall that we introduce the list box as an alternative to option buttons and check boxes when there are too many known items to show on the screen. The list box has the capability to hold many items but requires only limited space because its vertical scrollbar can be used to browse various parts of its content. When its MultiSelect property is set to 0 (None), it is a good alternative to option buttons. When its MultiSelect property is set to Simple or Extended or when its Style property is set to Checkbox, it becomes a good alternative to check boxes. In addition, the list box has the flexibility to add items to the list either at design time or at runtime without the need to adjust its visual appearance.

The Text and ListIndex Property. How does your program know which item in the list box is selected? As explained previously, the list box's Click event sets its Text and ListIndex properties. When the MultiSelect property is set to None (0) and the Style property is set to Standard (0), the item clicked is also the item selected and is highlighted. Thus, your program can use either the Text property or the ListIndex property to identify what is selected.

The Selected Property. When the MultiSelect property is set to either Simple (1) or Extended (2) or when its Style property is set to Checkbox, the list box behaves pretty much like the check box; that is, the Click event can select or deselect an item. Thus, the Text and the ListIndex properties give the last item clicked, but this item may be a deselected item. These properties can no longer be relied on to identify whether the item itself is selected.

In this situation, you will have to rely on the ***Selected property*** of individual items to decide whether a particular item is selected. This property is available only at runtime and is indexed for all items in the list. It is set to True when the particular item is selected; False, otherwise. For example, the following code shows how you can decide whether the first item of a list box named lstMajors is selected.

```
If lstMajors.Selected(0) Then
    MsgBox "The first item is selected."
Else
    MsgBox "The first item is not selected."
End If
```

Notice that the Selected property is followed by a pair of parentheses that enclose a number, zero. This is the way to index an item. The index begins with 0. Thus, Selected(0) refers to the first element in the list. Note that the value in the pair of parentheses does not have to be a constant. It can also be a variable (a name that represents some value). Recall that in Chapter 2, we showed a code structure for the For loop:

```
For Counter = 1 to 10
    Statements to be executed
Next Counter
```

Statements inside the structure will be executed 10 times. The first time, Counter will have a value 1; second time, 2; and so on until Counter is greater than 10. Also, as mentioned previously, the first item in the list box has an index of 0 and the last item will have an index of ListCount – 1. Thus, if you are interested in inspecting whether each item in the list is selected, you can code the following:

```
For I = 0 to lstMajors.ListCount - 1
    If lstMajors.Selected(I) Then
        MsgBox "Item no. " & I & " is selected."
    Else
        MsgBox "Item no. " & I & " is not selected."
    End If
Next I
```

Again, as mentioned in Chapter 2, the "&" operator concatenates two strings into one. Thus, if the first item is selected, the message box will display the following:

```
Item No. 0 is selected.
```

Chapter 7, "Repetition," discusses loops in more detail.

The List Property. The list box has the List property that sets or returns the items in the list box. This property is indexed in the same manner as the Selected property. In the previous example, if the first item in the majors list is accounting and if it is checked, you can make the computer display "Accounting is selected." by coding the following:

```
If lstMajors.Selected(0) Then
    MsgBox lstMajors.List(0) & " is selected."
End If
```

To display all selected items, you can code the following:

```
For I = 0 to lstMajors.ListCount - 1
    If lstMajors.Selected(I) Then
        MsgBox lstMajors.List(I) & " is selected."
    End If
Next I
```

The Need for the Combo Box

Like the option button and the check box, the list box provides a fixed set of choices for the user and does not allow the user to add additional items directly into the box. There are cases in which it is necessary for the user to add more items at runtime. For example, you may provide a list of zip codes in a list box for your user to choose from, but a new customer may have a zip code different from any existing ones. This is a case in which the combo box comes in handy. The ***combo box***, as the name suggests, provides a combination of a text box and a list box (Figure 3.24). Under certain Style property settings (discussed later), its text box area can be used to enter data, just like a typical text box control, whereas its list box can be used to select an item like a list box.

FIGURE 3.24
Combo Box: Icon and Appearance

The combo box icon in the toolbox

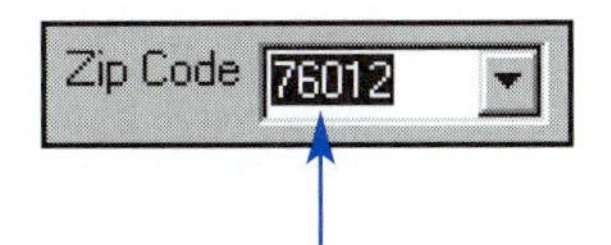

Here is a combo box in action when its Style property is set to either Dropdown Combo or Dropdown List. If the setting is Dropdown Combo, the user can also enter data in this box just as in a text box.

Similar Properties. The combo box control has many properties that behave exactly the same way as those of the list box:

- It has the Text and ListIndex properties, which identify the item that the user clicks. When the ListIndex property is set by code, the Text property is automatically set to the associated item.
- It has the Sorted property and behaves the same way as the list box.
- It has the List property, whose items are indexed in exactly the same manner as the list box.
- It has the ListCount property that gives the number of items in its list, just like the list box.

Similar Methods. The Combo box also has the AddItem and RemoveItem methods to add and remove items from its list. Note that an item that is entered into its text box area will not be automatically added to its list; that is, when another item appears in the text box, whatever was previously entered will be lost. Thus, if you need to keep the entered text in its list box, you will need to write code to handle it. Suppose you have a combo box named cboZipCode in your project. To add (to its list) the item that has just been entered into its text box area, you can code the following:

```
cboZipCode.AddItem cboZipCode.Text
```

As you can see in the code, the text area is recognized as its Text property. The AddItem method will add whatever appears in the combo box's text box into its list.

The Style Property. Its Style property, however, is quite different from that of the list box. The available settings include the following:

- Dropdown Combo (0; default): under this setting, the combo box will show a fixed-height text box with a drop-down button, which when clicked, will drop down to display the list. The user can either make a selection from the list provided or type in the data.
- Simple Combo (1): under this setting, you can adjust its height like the list box. Both the text box and the list will show. The user can either make a selection from the list or type in the data.
- Dropdown List (2): In this setting, the combo box looks exactly the same as the Dropdown Combo setting. However, the user can only make a selection from the list and is not allowed to enter any data.

Figure 3.25 shows combo boxes with different Style settings.

Notice that when its Style is set to Dropdown Combo or Dropdown List, it requires only as much space as a single-line text box. Its text box clearly shows what has been selected or entered. In contrast, the list box requires more space to meaningfully display the list and has no capability to accept items the user may desire to key in.

FIGURE 3.25
Different Style Settings of Combo Boxes

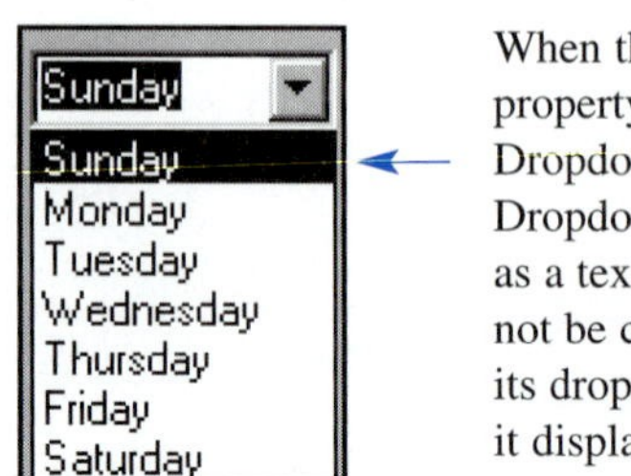
Sunday
Sunday
Monday
Tuesday
Wednesday
Thursday
Friday
Saturday
When the combo box's Style property is set to either Dropdown Combo or Dropdown List, it will appear as a text box. The height cannot be changed. You can click its drop-down button to make it display the list content.

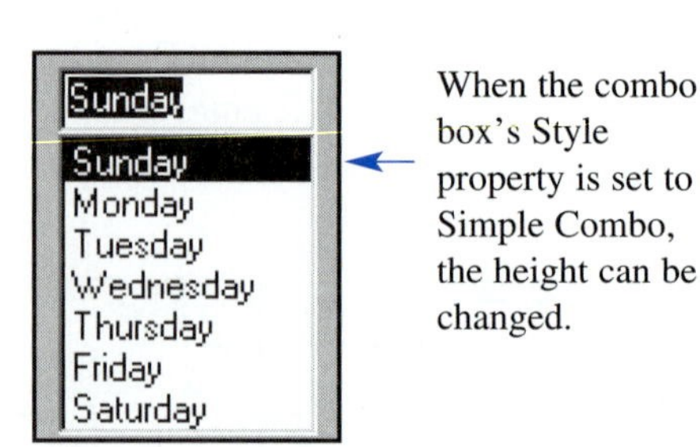
Sunday
Sunday
Monday
Tuesday
Wednesday
Thursday
Friday
Saturday
When the combo box's Style property is set to Simple Combo, the height can be changed.

Finally, the list box also has some properties that are not available in the combo box. For example, the combo box does not have the MultiSelect property. Only one item can be selected from its list. Thus, *the combo box can be used as an alternative only to option buttons, not to check boxes.*

Between the List Box and Combo Box. Because there are many similarities and some differences between the list box and the combo box, how do you decide which control to use given a certain circumstance? Here is a list of decision rules you can consider:

1. Does the situation involve multiple selection? If so, the list box is the clear choice. Otherwise, consider factors listed next.
2. Is the available space in the form an important issue? If so, the combo box is the clear choice.
3. Is the list complete? If the user has to be given the opportunity to enter an item not already in the list, the combo box is the clear choice.
4. How important is it to show the "result" (choice) clearly and explicitly? If it is very important, then the combo box is the choice.

If you cannot decide from these guidelines, then consider how each control will affect the layout of your form. The control that will give a more pleasing look in your form layout should be your choice.

The following table summarizes the new properties discussed in this section.

Property	Applicable Object	Use/Remark
ListCount	List box, combo box	Gives the number of items in the list.
ListIndex	List box, combo box	Returns or sets a number pointing to the position of the item clicked or "selected" by code; for example, the code: `cboWeekDays.ListIndex = 3` will select the fourth item in the combo box named cboWeekDays. The item (Wednesday) will appear in the "box."
MultiSelect	List box	When this property is set to None (0), only one item can be selected from the list box (assuming the Style property is set to Standard); otherwise, multiple items can be selected.
Sorted	List box, combo box	When the property is set to True, items in the list will appear in ascending order at runtime.
List	List box, combo box	Gives the text of a particular item in the list; for example, `lstMonths.List(3)` will give the fourth item (April) in the list.
Selected	List box	A True or False value that indicates whether a particular item in the list box is selected; for example, lstMonths.Selected (0) will give a value True if the first item (January) is selected.
Style	List box	Can be Standard (0) or Checkbox (1); if this property is set to 1, each item in the list box will show a check box.
	Combo box	Can be Dropdown Combo (0), Simple Combo (1), or Dropdown List (2). Refer to the text for details of behavior under each setting.
Text	List box, combo box	Gives the item selected (clicked) from the list; in the case of the combo box, data can also be entered if the Style property is set to 0 (Dropdown Combo) or 1 (Simple Combo).

3.5 Picture Boxes as Containers and Image Controls for Pictures

The Picture Box

In a preceding section, we mentioned that the picture box can be used as a container; that is, it can be used to contain other VB controls. Its icon and appearance are shown in Figure 3.26. When used as a container, it functions very similarly to the frame. You can draw VB controls into a picture box. These controls are then handled as a single group; that is,

- When you move the picture box, all controls in it are moved.
- When you delete the picture box, all VB controls inside the control are deleted.
- When you disable or make invisible the picture box, all controls in it are also disabled or invisible.
- Option buttons included in a picture box are treated as a logical group; that is, when one is clicked on, all the others are automatically turned off.

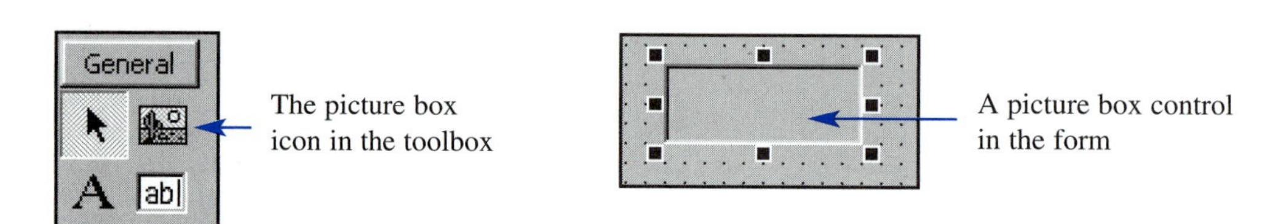

FIGURE 3.26
Picture Box: Icon and Appearance

Setting the Picture Property. The picture box can be used to show a picture. How do you bring a picture into the picture box? At design time, you can set its ***Picture property***. Double-click that property in its Properties window, and a dialog box appears for you to specify a file containing a picture. This control supports files with various formats such as bitmap (bmp), icon (ico), metafile (wmf), JPEG (jpg), and GIF (gif). If you decide to remove the picture, you can click the Picture property in its Properties window then press the Delete key. At runtime, you can use the LoadPicture function to load a picture. For example, you can code the following:

```
picFamily.Picture = LoadPicture("C:\Windows\Clouds.bmp")
```

You can remove the picture using the same function by specifying a zero-length string for the picture file path:

```
picFamily.Picture = LoadPicture("")
```

The size of the picture box drawn into the form sets the boundary for the picture brought into the picture box. If the picture is smaller than the box, it shows in the upper-left corner of the box. On the other hand, if the picture is larger than the picture box, only its upper-left portion will be shown in the box. The metafile, however, always adjusts itself to the size of the box drawn on the form.

Picture boxes use more system resources than frames. So why use them? The answer is that you may need them because of their additional features. For example, you might find it desirable to have some special background for the container to provide a cue. By the use of its Picture property, the picture box can have a picture as the container's background, whereas the frame cannot. Also, in some applications, the picture box is the only control allowed as the container (see Chapter 11, "Menus and Multiple Form Applications").

The Image Control

If you want to use pictures in your user-interface design but are hesitant because of the picture box's system resource requirements, the image control provides an alternative. This control also has a picture property, which can be set in exactly the same manner as the picture box. The image control has a ***Stretch property***, which, when set to False, causes the control to adjust its own size to that of the picture; when set to True, it stretches the picture's size to fit in the control's size.

Like most of the VB controls, the image control has Click and DblClick events. If you are a fan of icons, you can use an image control in place of a command button. Fill it with an icon, then use the Click event to handle whatever you want the icon to perform. Used in this manner, the image control is a graphic alternative to the command button. To make this substitution more complete, you can set the image's ***ToolTipText property*** with some descriptive text for the icon. At runtime, when the user rests the mouse pointer on the icon for a short moment, the ToolTip text will be displayed. Note that the command button can also handle graphics. The differences between the two controls in this respect are left to you as an explorer exercise.

Compared with the picture box, the image control requires fewer computer resources. However, you should be aware that it does not have all the capabilities of the picture box. For example, the picture box can be used as a container, whereas the image box cannot.

3.6 VB Controls in the Design of a Data-Entry Interface: Recapitulation

We have seen quite a few VB controls in this chapter. We have considered them in the context of data-entry interface design. In the process, we have presented a few design principles, including the following:

1. Minimize the number of user keystrokes to improve data-entry efficiency as well as to minimize potential errors.
2. Present the layout of the form neatly (uncluttered).
3. Group logically related data fields together.

The text box is considered the most versatile control in accepting any kind of text or numeric data from the user. However, the user must key in every character the data field is expected to contain. The longer the data field, the higher the possibility that the user enters a wrong key, in addition to the lengthier time for the entry. Whenever the text box is used as a field for data input, you should be prepared to write code to check for data validity. Thus, alternatives to the text box should be considered when applicable. One such situation is when the input fits a specific pattern such as dates and Social Security numbers. In such cases, masked edit boxes should be used. They help reduce the number of keystrokes and filter out keys that do not fit the expected pattern.

Another situation in which alternatives to the text boxes can be considered is when the data elements are known before the program starts. In this case, if the number of available choices is very small, such as gender or names of meals, option buttons and check boxes should be used. The key criterion in choosing between these two types of controls is whether the known choices are mutually exclusive or independent of each other. If the choices are mutually exclusive, you should use option buttons. On the other hand, if the choices are independent of each other, you should use check boxes.

As the number of available known items grows or if the items can change, the list box or combo box should be considered. The choice between the two depends on several factors, such as the nature of the choice (mutual exclusiveness), space availability in the form, possibility that data have to be added by the user, and their visual effect on the form layout. If the available known choices are not mutually exclusive, you can use only the list box, which has the MultiSelect property and the Checkbox Style property. Otherwise, you can decide between the two VB controls based on additional characteristics of the data. If at runtime the list of known data is not exhaustive (i.e., the user may still have to enter data not already included in the list), you should use the combo box. In addition, if space on the form is limited, the combo box will be preferred; otherwise, whichever gives a better fit for the layout should be chosen.

Containers such as frames and picture boxes are presented as a necessity to group logically related option buttons in order for the latter to function properly. Containers are also desirable and needed to group logically related data fields together. They not only make the layout of the form neater but also make it easier for the user to anticipate the type of data fields in the group. This can enhance data-entry efficiency. As the number of data fields for a data-entry "screen" becomes too big, the SSTab control can be used. In such case, each tab should contain data of the first level major grouping. Other containers can then be used for the subgroupings.

We noted that the picture box as a container uses more system resources than the frame. However, there are cases in which the picture box may be called for, as explained previously. The picture box can also be used to display pictures on the form. We presented the image control as an alternative for simple picture display. The image control is also presented as a possible alternative to the command button when you prefer to use an icon to start an action such as open or save. (Note that the command button can also display icons when its Style property is set to graphic, as shown in an exercise in this chapter.)

3.7 Naming the Controls and Setting the Tab Order

Naming Convention: Suggested Name Prefixes

We have introduced many VB controls in this chapter. In Chapter 2, we strongly recommended that all VB controls be named with three letter prefixes to enhance code clarity. We have observed this standard wherever we used a VB control. We believe this is important in developing a good coding habit. To refresh your memory and for your convenience, we tabulate all the controls we have met so far with their prefixes.

VB Object	Prefix
Check box	chk
Combo box	cbo
Command button	cmd
Form	frm
Frame control	fra
Image control	img
Label	lbl
List box	lst
Masked edit	msk
Option button	opt
Picture box	pic
SSTab control	sst
Text box	txt
Timer	tmr

Setting the Tab Order

The order in which a VB control in a form receives its focus when the user presses the Tab key is recognized as the tab order. This order is determined by the control's TabIndex property, which is set by VB in the order the control is brought into the form. The first control brought to the form will have its TabIndex value set to 0. When you test your program, you may find the tab order not in accordance with your original design. In addition, when you are designing an interface with many data elements, you may have to insert controls into or delete controls from the form, making it necessary to adjust the tab order again.

You can reset the TabIndex property of these controls to the proper value. The typical procedure is to start with the first control, setting its TabIndex to 0; the second to 1; and so on. When the form contains many controls, the task can become tedious and memory-intensive (yours, not the computer's). The Tip box that follows provides a trick used by the experienced programmer to make the job easier.

When resetting the TabIndex properties for the controls, start with the last control first. Go backwards and set each TabIndex to zero (0). This is much easier. It works because as the TabIndex of a control is set to zero, all the TabIndexes previously set will be increased by 1.

3.8 Some Commonly Used Events

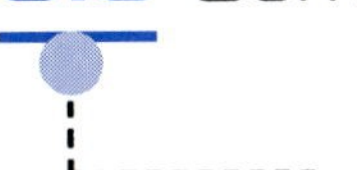

Our preceding discussion has focused on which VB controls to use and how to arrange them on a form. We will still need to place the code in the project before it will work the way we want. You have had a general idea that the code should be placed in certain events. The next question, naturally, is in which event to place specific code. This, of course, depends on what you want to accomplish. The following discussion considers various programming requirements and the proper events in which to place code.

Setting the Initial State at Runtime: The Form Load Event

In many cases, when your program starts, before the computer shows your form, you want various controls and variables to be in a certain state. For example, you may want to populate a list box with data that are not available until runtime. Or, you may want a combo box to show an initial choice. In what event should we place the code for this purpose? It is the Form Load event.

The ***Form Load event*** occurs when the form is loaded into the memory and before the form is displayed. At this stage, all the controls' properties are set to their initial states (i.e., their default settings or the settings that you made for them during design time). You may want to change some of these settings so that the controls will appear the way you want when the form first appears.

For example, assume that your form has a combo box named cboWeekdays with its list set at design time to Sunday, Monday, and so on. You would like for this box to show Sunday (the first element in its list) as soon as the program starts. How can you do this? Because you want to show the setting as soon as the program starts, the code should be placed in the Form Load event.

How should it be coded? This depends on the setting of the control's Style property. If it is set to Dropdown Combo (0), you can assign a value to its Text property directly as follows:

```
cboWeekDays.Text = "Sunday"
```

However, this setting of the Style property is not really the best for the current situation. It allows the user to enter the text into the box. Weekdays are known and will never change. To eliminate the possibility of any data-entry error, you should allow the user only to select an item from the combo box's list (and not to enter his or her own). Thus, the Style property should be set to Dropdown List. Recall that under this setting, the user is not allowed to enter the text. Nor can you use the code to set its Text property. However, you may also recall that when its ListIndex property is set to a certain value, its Text property is automatically set to the item corresponding to the ListIndex property. Thus, we can set the ListIndex property to 0 to indirectly set its Text property to Sunday (because Sunday is the first item in the combo box's list). The code should appear as follows:

```
Private Sub Form_Load()
'Set default Text for the combo box to first element (Sunday)
    cboWeekDays.ListIndex = 0
End Sub
```

Various Uses of the Click and DblClick (Double-Click) Events

In many instances, you can place the code in a Click event to perform some specified task when the user clicks or double-clicks on an object. These events are most often used in conjunction with the command button, option button, check box, list box, and combo box.

Command Buttons. The Click event procedures most often seen are related to the command button, whose caption typically indicates to the user what to expect. For example, you may have a program for the user to enter certain data required for certain computation, for example, the net present value of an annuity. When the user is ready for your program to compute, he or she will click a command button on the form with a caption "Compute." In this case, it is certainly clear to you that you will place your code to perform the computation in the command button's Click event. As another example, in most forms, a command button is used for the user to end the program. Typically, the button is named cmdQuit and its caption property is set to "Quit." Remember how the code was presented previously? Here it is again:

```
Private Sub cmdQuit_Click()
    Unload Me
End Sub
```

Option Buttons and Check Boxes. When the user clicks on an option button or a check box, the Click event is raised. You can place code in the control's Click event if a certain response is expected. For example, in a mailing label printing application, the user has a choice of printing all members or only those in the zip code areas selected from a list box named lstZipCode. The user indicates his or her option by clicking one of the two option buttons, optAll or optSelected. It is obvious that when the user opts to print all members, any selections made from the list box will be meaningless. Thus, the list box should be disabled. On the other hand, when the user opts to select zip codes from the list box, the latter should be enabled. In short, depending on which option button is clicked, the list box is enabled or disabled. Figure 3.27 shows a sample visual interface with such a design. The code should be placed in the Click event of each option button and should appear as follows:

```
Private Sub optAll_Click()
' All members should be printed; disable the list box
    lstZipCode.Enabled = False
End Sub
Private Sub optSelected_Click()
' Only members in selected zip code areas should be printed.
' Enable the list box
    lstZipCode.Enabled = True
End Sub
```

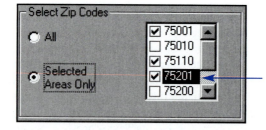

FIGURE 3.27 Conditionally Enabling the List Box by Selection of Option Buttons

List and Combo Boxes. As you may recall, the list box and combo box also have the Click event. The use of the Click event in conjunction with these two controls varies. As you have already seen, when the user clicks on these two controls, their ListIndex and Text properties are set to the item clicked. Thus, you can use this event to retrieve the selection made by the user. For example, you may want to show the current choice in the text box txtName as soon as the user clicks an item in the list box lstName. The event to place the code will be lstName_click, and you will assign the list's text property to that of the text box. Thus, the code will appear as follows:

```
Private Sub lstName_Click()
'Show the item selected in the textbox
    txtName.Text = lstName.Text
End Sub
```

Beware, however, that *the Click event can be triggered not just by the user's action.* It is also raised when your code sets the ListIndex property. This can create problems if you want the Click event procedure to respond only to the user's action. For this reason, experienced programmers typically use the Double-Click (DblClick) event to avoid unexpected problems.

As an illustration, if you want the user to indicate which item to delete from a list box, named lstCandidate, you may instruct the user to double-click the item to remove. In this case, the event in which to place the code will be lstCandidate_DblClick. The item to be removed from the box is indicated by the ListIndex property. (Recall again when the user clicks an item, the ListIndex and Text properties are set to this item. Note also the Click event is always raised before the Double-Click event.) Thus, the code will appear as follows:

```
Private Sub lstCandidate_DblClick()
    lstCandidate.RemoveItem lstCandidate.ListIndex
End Sub
```

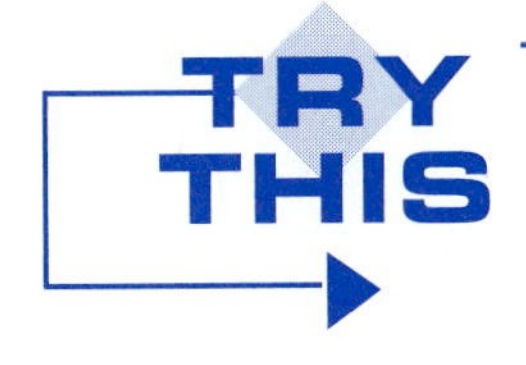

Bring a combo box into a new form. Name the combo box cboTest. At design time, set its list property to contain Sunday, Monday, ... , Saturday. Place the following in the code window:

```
Private Sub cboTest_Click()
    cboTest.RemoveItem cboTest.ListIndex
End Sub

Private Sub Form_Load()
    cboTest.ListIndex = 0
End Sub
```

Run the program. Check the list in the combo box. Do you see Sunday in it? No. It has been removed because when your program starts, the Form Load event sets the list index of the combo box, which triggers the box's Click event. In the Click event procedure, the item pointed to by the current ListIndex is removed. All these happen without any clicking by the user. Pretty tricky. That's why you may want to avoid using the (single) Click event for the combo or list box to handle user actions. However, notice that you can use the combo box's Double-Click event only when its Style property is set to 1 (Simple combo).

Viewing the Key Entered: The KeyPress Event

In many cases, you may want to inspect the key that the user enters into a control for various purposes. For example, you may want your program to perform a series of actions when the user presses the Enter key. Or, you may want to ensure that only certain types of keys (e.g., numeric keys) are entered into a text box. When the user presses a key, the control's ***KeyPress event*** is raised. This event occurs after a key is pressed but before the key is shown in the control. When the event is triggered, the system also passes the code value (recognized as the ASCII value) of the key pressed to the event procedure. You can inspect its content and do whatever you deem appropriate with it. For example, suppose you want to ensure that none of the keys the user enters into a text box named txtAddress are question marks. Your code will most likely appear as follows:

```
Private Sub txtAddress_KeyPress(KeyAscii as Integer)
    If KeyAscii = 63 Then
    ' This is a question mark
        MsgBox "No question mark, please." 'Display a message
        KeyAscii = 0 'Suppress the key
    End If
End Sub
```

In this event procedure, the ASCII value that the user presses (KeyAscii) is passed to the procedure and is compared with 63, the ASCII value for the question mark. If they are equal, the message "No question mark, please." is displayed. In addition, KeyAscii is set to zero. This, in effect, suppresses the key pressed because a key with a zero ASCII value is just a null key. You will learn more about key codes in later chapters.

The KeyPress event procedure includes a KeyAscii parameter. It is worth repeating that when you code an event procedure, *you should always use the procedure template provided by VB rather than create your own event procedure header.* All the parameters in an event procedure are predefined and are automatically provided in the procedure template. (You should never change any part of the parameter list.) This way you will never have to figure out what parameters the event header should have and the proper way to include them. The steps to obtain a procedure template have been explained in Chapter 2. You can find the use (or meaning) of each parameter from the Help file by searching for the event name in question.

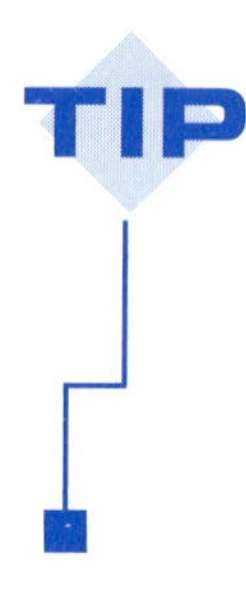

When you double-click a control on a form, a default procedure template for the control is automatically given in the code window. This provides a convenient shortcut to the code window and the event procedure. However, you must be aware that the event procedure template obtained this way may not be exactly the one you want. For example, when you double-click a text box, its Change event procedure template will appear. But you may actually want to use the KeyPress event. Check the event name before entering any code. *Placing the code in a wrong event procedure unintentionally is a common error for beginners.* Pay extra attention to avoid this type of mistake.

Before the User Does Anything in a Control: The GotFocus Event

Sometimes when the user tabs into a field or clicks the field to set the focus, you want your program to perform some preparatory activities, such as keeping the current content of the control in a variable (as a backup) or highlighting the content to facilitate editing. What event is triggered when the user tabs into a control? The control's GotFocus event. The code placed in this event will be executed as soon as the control gets the focus. For example, you want to keep the current content of a text box named txtName before the user starts doing anything on the field (so that when the user presses the Esc key, you can restore the content). You can code the following:

```
Private Sub txtName_GotFocus()
    PreviousName = txtName.Text
End Sub
```

Note that the preceding code keeps only the content of the text box in a variable named PreviousName. To restore the content when the user presses the Esc key, more code will be needed. You should be able to complete this exercise by the time you finish Chapter 4.

As the User Leaves the Field: The LostFocus Event

When the user finishes working with a field (VB control), he or she leaves that field. Usually, this is the moment you want to perform additional operations on a field, such as converting all letters in the field to uppercase letters. When the user leaves a field, the LostFocus event is triggered. As with all previous events, you can place code in this event to perform any operations you deem desirable. For example, if you want all characters entered into a field named txtUser to be converted to the uppercase, you can place the code in the control's LostFocus event as shown here:

```
Private Sub txtUser_LostFocus()
    txtUser.Text = UCase$(txtUser.Text)
End Sub
```

In the preceding code, UCase$ is a built-in function that converts a string into uppercase letters. The statement instructs the computer to convert the content of txtUser to the uppercase and then assign the result to the text property of txtUser.

Before VB6, LostFocus was also the event in which the field level data validation code was placed. There are, however, potential problems with placing the data validation code in this event. For the convenience of data validation, VB6 introduces a new event, Validate, which occurs before the LostFocus event. We discuss data validation in Chapter 10.

The following table summarizes the events discussed in this section:

Event	Applicable Objects	Trigger	Uses
Form Load	Form	When the form is loaded into memory	To initialize values of variables and properties
Click	Form, command button, option button, check box, list box, combo box	1. When the user clicks the object 2. When the code assigns a value to the Value property of option button or check box 3. When the code assigns a value to the ListIndex property of the list box or combo box	To carry out some activities initiated (usually) by the user
Double-Click	List box, combo box	When the user double-clicks the object (the Click event is always triggered with this event)	To carry out the activities initiated by the user (exclusively)
KeyPress	Text box, mask edit box, form	When the user presses a key	To carry out certain activities or verify the validity of the key
GotFocus	Text box, masked edit box	When the object receives focus as a result of tabbing to or clicking the object	To perform some "preparatory" activities such as highlighting the text
LostFocus	Text box, masked edit box	When the object loses focus as a result of tabbing from the object or clicking another object	To perform "finishing touch" activities such as converting to uppercase letters or checking field level validity

Notice that the "Applicable Objects" column lists the objects that are most commonly seen with the event, rather than all the objects that recognize the event. Some events (e.g., GotFocus and LostFocus) are recognized by almost all objects. However, these events are usually used in conjunction with only a few objects.

3.9 An Application Example

You have been introduced to many VB controls and several of their related events. You may be wondering how all these "pieces of puzzles" can be put together to perform a task. Here, let's consider an example for this purpose. The example pertains to an order-entry screen for a manufacturer of water filters. Before we proceed further into any details, please note that the main purpose of the example is to show which controls should be used in a given situation and where (in which event) a particular segment of code should be placed. So that our attention can be focused on our key interest, it is necessary to simplify the problem. Please ignore some potential ramifications as we proceed. In addition, please work along as you read. You will have a much better understanding of the subject if you actually work on the problem while reading.

The Project

The Environ-Pure Company manufactures two models of water filters (Puri-Clear and Environ-Safe). Models are added and deleted as new technology evolves and the company's market strategy shifts. The products are sold through three distributors who redistribute the products to the retailers. The company is negotiating with several potential distributors as additional channels of distribution. Typically, the distributors place a purchase order for one model at a time, with a quantity ranging from 500 to 2,500 units. Regular orders are delivered by the company's own trucks. Occasionally, some orders need to be rushed. In such cases, the company ships them either through U.P.S. or through a special carrier arranged by the distributor.

You are assigned to design a user interface to take orders from the distributors. The screen should capture the following data elements:

1. Date of the order
2. Distributor number
3. Model number
4. Quantity ordered
5. Whether this is a rush order
6. If so, how the order should be delivered (U.P.S. or a special carrier)

You should also provide code that makes the program behave properly.

The Visual Interface

As we have repeated several times, the first step in developing a VB project is to design the visual interface. Let's consider what VB control should be used for each of the required data elements.

Once you understand the requirements for your project, carefully analyze the nature of the data field so that you can use the best control for its purpose. Using the most suitable control for the data field can make both the data-entry operation and your code efficient and effective.

Date of Order. A date field has a specific format. The masked edit box appears to be the best choice. We will name this control mskDate. In addition, we should set its mask property to "##-##-####" at design time.

Distributor Number. As the project description states, there are only two distributors. The data field under consideration has a limited number of choices. Controls that may be appropriate would seem to be either the check box or option button. Notice that an order can be placed by only one distributor. Thus, the control that comes to mind immediately is the option button. However, in this case, the option button is probably not the best choice. Why? The number of distributors can change over time, as the project description implies. If we use the option buttons, each time the company adds or deletes a distributor, the visual interface will need to be revised. Obviously, this is not an ideal solution.

As discussed previously, the other possible VB controls for known choices are the list box or combo box. In the real-world application, the names of the distributors can be added to these controls from a file (or database) maintained by the user. The use of either the list box or combo box can eliminate the need to revise the program as a result of any change in distributors.

Should we use the list box or the combo box? If you go through the list of criteria for determining the appropriate control between the two, you should find the two controls tie almost all the way. This suggests that the appearance of the control is the determining factor. We would like for the control to appear as a "box" for a single line input. Thus, we choose the combo box for this purpose. We will name it cboDistributor.

Model Number. The factors to consider for the control for the model number are similar to those for the distributor number. The dynamic nature of known items (adding and dropping models) and the appearance consideration suggest that we should also use the combo box. We will name this control cboModel.

Note that the model number should be selected from the list of existing models, not keyed in by the user. This means that the Style property of cboModel should be set to Dropdown List, not the default setting, Dropdown Combo. The model numbers should be added to the combo box using the AddItem method when the program starts (and not set at design time by editing the List property). In real applications, these models should be read from a file or database maintained by the user. (We discuss database and files in later chapters.)

All these same considerations also apply to the distributor number. Thus, the Style property of cboDistributor should also be set to Dropdown List.

Quantity Ordered. The main consideration here is that keys entered into this data field should be numeric. There is a range of values (500 to 2,500) that is considered typical. It appears that the number entered should not exceed 4 digits. Either a text box or a masked edit box should be suitable. We will use the text box for this purpose and name it txtQuantity. In addition, we should also set the ***MaxLength property*** of this control to 4. Setting the maximum length will ensure that the user will not accidentally enter a number that far exceeds the reality.

Use the MaxLength property to limit the number of characters the user can enter into a text box when the number can be determined at design time. Doing so can help eliminate unexpected extra keys being entered into the box, which could cause problems for your program.

Special Instructions. Finally, we need to determine whether the order is a rush order. Because this is a yes-or-no question, it appears that the check box will serve as a good visual interface. We will name it chkRush. In addition, when it is a rush order, we should also record the type of delivery: U.P.S. or special carrier. Because the user will be choosing between the two types of carriers (mutually exclusive choices), option buttons appear to be the most appropriate. We will name them optUPS and optSpecialCarrier.

As a side note, you may argue that the combo box can be a better choice than the option buttons in this case based on the same considerations given to distributor numbers and model numbers. Yes, you are right. Our choice here is based more on the interest to demonstrate how option buttons can be used.

Command Buttons and the Form. In addition to the data fields already considered, we should also provide a means for the user to save data and end the program. This can be done by adding two command buttons to the form. One will be named cmdSave and captioned "Save"; another, named cmdQuit and captioned "Quit."

We should also set the proper Caption and Name properties for the form. We will name the form frmSalesOrder and set its caption to "Environ-Pure Sales Order Entry Form."

Grouping and Layout. Once we have decided what VB controls to use for all required data fields, we can consider how these controls should be arranged. The VB controls for special delivery instructions are logically related. Thus, they should be grouped together, perhaps within a frame. The other fields all pertain to the order itself; thus they can be grouped in another frame. All these fields should have proper labels to indicate the nature of the field. The command buttons are usually placed at the bottom or the right side of the form. In this form, the layout should look very neat when the two command buttons are placed at the bottom.

When you have to place quite a few controls on a form, be sure to take advantage of the frame control. Frames can help your form layout appear neat and logical.

With all these considerations, we can now draw two frames and all labels onto a form. We will also set captions for all controls properly as shown in Figure 3.28.

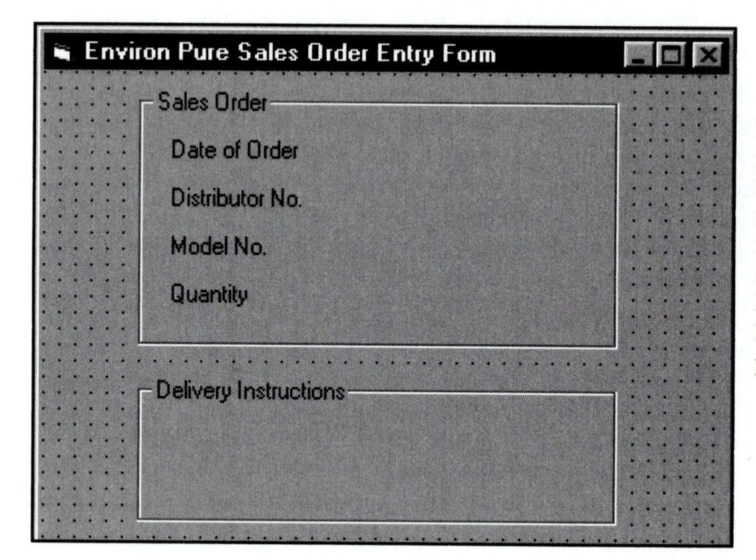

FIGURE 3.28
Initial Visual Framework for the Project

The initial layout for the project should have (1) the form's caption property properly set, (2) two frames with captions set to Sales Order and Delivery Instructions, and (3) four labels with their caption properties properly set.

Then, we will add the other controls we considered. Notice that the masked edit control needs to be added to the toolbox. (Refer to the discussion of the masked edit box at the beginning of this chapter for specifics.) Here we need to set several properties of each control properly. These properties have already been discussed and are summarized in the following table.

Field/Button	Type of Control	Property	Setting
Date of Order	Masked edit box	Name	MskDate
		Mask	##-##-####
Distributor No.	Combo box	Name	CboDistributor
		Style	2-Dropdown List
Model No.	Combo box	Name	cboModel
		Style	2-Dropdown List
Quantity Ordered	Text box	Name	txtQuantity
		Text	(blank)
		MaxLength	4
Rush Order?	Check box	Name	chkRush
		Caption	Rush Order?
U.P.S.	Option button	Name	optUPS
		Caption	U.P.S.
Special Carrier	Option button	Name	optSpecialCarrier
		Caption	Special Carrier
Save Command	Command button	Name	cmdSave

Field/Button	Type of Control	Property	Setting
		Caption	Save
Quit command	Command button	Name	cmdQuit
		Caption	Quit
Form	Form	Name	frmSalesOrder
		Caption	Environ-Pure Sales Order Entry form

The resulting layout of the form appears as Figure 3.29.

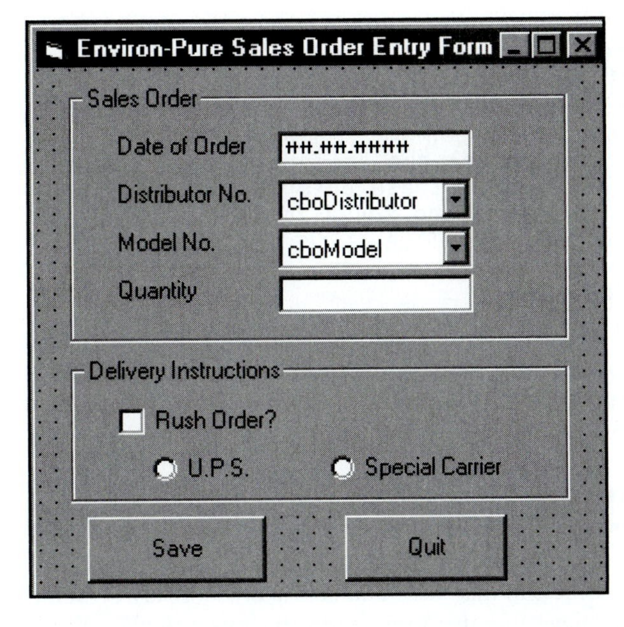

FIGURE 3.29
The Visual Interface for Environ-Pure

The completed visual interface should contain one masked edit box, two combo boxes, one textbox, one check box, two option buttons, and two command buttons. Make sure these controls are properly named. Also notice that the mask for the masked edit box should appear. In addition, the names of the combo boxes should appear if their Style properties are set to Dropdown List (2).

Pay particular attention to the appearance of the masked edit box and the two combo boxes. The string "##-##-####" should appear in the date field if the Mask property of the masked edit box is set properly. Also, the names of the combo boxes should appear in the controls if their Style properties are set to 2-drop-down list.

Setting the Tab Order

After all controls are placed in proper position, you should test their tab order. You can do so by running the program, verifying that the focus is on the masked edit (date of order) when the program starts, then pressing the Tab key repetitively to see if the focus is set on the controls in the order you want. That is, the focus should go in the order of: Date, Distributor Number, Model Number, Quantity, Rush Order, U.P.S. (or Special Carrier), Save, and finally, Quit. (Note that at runtime, you can tab to only one of the option buttons. Thus, you should also test their tab order at design time.)

If the tab order is not exactly the way you desire, you can set the TabIndex property of all controls to zero in reverse order, that is, from Quit, Save,..., and finally Date of Order. This technique is explained in a Tip box in the section dealing with setting the tab order.

Coding the Event Procedures

With the visual interface in place, we can now focus on the "action" aspect of the project. We need to consider in which events to place what code. This, of course, depends on what we would like for the program to do. Let's consider one VB control (data field) at a time.

Date of Order. Our main concern here is the accuracy of the date entered by the user. One possibility is for the computer to fill the date into the control automatically. For simplicity, we will not do it this way now. Notice that the masked edit box with the proper mask in place will automatically check to ensure that all keys are numeric. However, numeric data do not guarantee that the entire field is a valid date. Thus, at some point, we will need to check that the masked edit box has a valid date.

Which event should we use? We can decide whether the masked edit box has a valid date only when the field is complete, that is, when the user leaves the field. As explained previously, VB6 provides an event purely for the field level data validation, the Validate event. We will place the code in this event. How do we check for a valid date? There is a built-in function, ***IsDate***, that checks exactly whether a string is a valid date. If the string is a valid date, the function returns a True value; otherwise, False. (We discuss built-in functions in more detail in Chapter 4.) Thus, we can use this function to perform the test. The code appears as follows:

```
Private Sub mskDate_Validate(Cancel As Boolean)
    If IsDate(mskDate.Text) Then
    ' the control has a valid date; do nothing
    Else
    ' the control has an invalid date; display a message
        MsgBox "Please enter a valid date."
        ' Reset the focus to this control
        Cancel = True
    End If
End Sub
```

In the code, when an invalid date is found in the masked edit box, a message is displayed. The event also includes a parameter, Cancel. When this parameter is set to True, the focus will be reset to the current control. Otherwise, the focus will move to the next control. Additional issues concerning error checking are discussed in Chapter 10.

Distributor Number. As explained previously, we need to add the list of distributors to the combo box by code. For simplicity, we will assume that these distributor numbers are 100 and 101. We also know that the AddItem method can be used. The question is where the code should be placed. Recall that these numbers should already be in the combo box as soon as the program starts, suggesting that form load is the event to place the code. Thus, the code should appear as follows:

```
Private Sub Form_Load()
' Add distributor numbers to cboDistributor
' In real applications, numbers are read from a file or database
    cboDistributor.AddItem 100
    cboDistributor.AddItem 101
End Sub
```

Model Number. Like the distributor numbers, model numbers should be added to the combo box as soon as the program starts. Thus, the Form Load procedure presented previously should be modified as follows:

```
Private Sub Form_Load()
' Add distributor numbers to cboDistributor
' In real applications, numbers are read from a file or database
    cboDistributor.AddItem 100
    cboDistributor.AddItem 101
' Add model numbers to cboModel
' In real applications, models are read from a file or database
    cboModel.AddItem "Puri-Clear"
    cboModel.AddItem "Environ-Safe"
End Sub
```

In addition to getting model numbers into the combo box ready for selection, let's also assume that the Puri-Clear model is the most commonly ordered model. To save the user from having to make the selection, we would like to set the model as the user's choice whenever the user moves to this field. Note that this model is the first item in the list. Thus, we can set the combo box's ListIndex to 0 to effect the choice. But where should we place the code? Again, recall that we would like for this to happen as soon as the user moves to this field, that is, when the control gets the focus. Thus, the event to use is this control's GotFocus event. The code appears as follows:

```
Private Sub cboModel_GotFocus()
    ' set the first item as the choice
    cboModel.ListIndex = 0
End Sub
```

Quantity Ordered. This is a text box. We would like to ensure that the user enters only numeric keys. In what event should the code be placed? As explained, as soon as the user presses a key, the KeyPress event is triggered. Thus, the proper event to place the code is the KeyPress event of this control, txtQuantity. For simplicity, we leave out the code but simply indicate the key-error-checking routine should be placed in the template presented next (you will learn more about error checking in Chapter 10):

```
Private Sub txtQuantity_KeyPress(KeyAscii As Integer)
    ' Place key error checking routine here
End Sub
```

Special Delivery Instructions. When the user clicks the check box for "Rush Order?" the check box is checked or unchecked. The ensuing selection of types of delivery (U.P.S. or special carrier) makes sense only when the check box is checked. Thus, we should not allowed the user to make any selection between the two option boxes when the check box is unchecked; that is, we should enable (disable) the two option buttons when the check box is checked (unchecked). As implied in the opening statement, the code should be placed in the check box's Click event:

```
Private Sub chkRush_Click()
    If chkRush.Value = vbChecked Then
    ' the check box is checked, enable both option buttons
        optUPS.Enabled = True
        optSpecialCarrier.Enabled = True
    Else
    ' the check box is unchecked, disable both option buttons
        optUPS.Enabled = False
        optSpecialCarrier.Enabled = False
    End If
End Sub
```

If you test the program at this point, you should notice that when the program starts, the check box is unchecked (a good thing because most orders are not rush orders). However, the two option buttons are also enabled (not a good condition because we want to disable them when the rush order check box is unchecked). We should go back and set (at design time) the Enabled properties of both option buttons to False.

Always disable the controls for input purposes that do not require any user input or action in the context. This saves the user's time and eliminates confusion by the user. Be sure to enable these controls again when the context requires the user's input.

Command Buttons. As you recall, it is customary to place code in the Click event to handle all expected activities when the user clicks a command button. Although we show the Save command button, for simplicity, we will simply note that code to save the screen should be placed in the command's Click event without providing the actual code. We would, however, place a line of code to display the message, "Data saved."

```
Private Sub cmdSave_Click()
     ' Place the routine to save data here
     ' then display the following message
     MsgBox "Data saved."
End Sub
```

The code to terminate the program has been presented in this chapter as well as the preceding chapter; it is left for you to complete as an exercise.

Testing the Project

Now, you have completed the project. It's time to test it to see whether it works as expected. If everything goes correctly, you should be able to see that the visual layout looks like Figure 3.29. In addition, when you run the program, you should able to verify the following:

1. The date of order field does not accept any nonnumeric keys (although no message is displayed). Furthermore, it will display an error message when you leave the field with an invalid date.
2. When you click the distributor number field and the model number field, you should be able to see their proper contents.
3. When you tab to the model number field, it should automatically display the "Puri-Clear" model.
4. The quantity field will not allow you to go over four digits. (Check its MaxLength property if it lets you enter more than that.)
5. When the rush order check box is unchecked, the two option buttons are disabled; but when the former is checked, the two are enabled.
6. When you click the Save button, the computer displays the "Data saved" message.
7. When you click the Quit button, the program ends. (You are to provide the code to handle this.)

In the process of testing the program, you may find some typing errors. You may even find that you have placed code in a wrong event. If you believe that you have done everything correctly but the program still does not work properly, you may want to check the names of the controls you use in the code against those in the form. Unmatched names for the "presumably" same control can give you a source of "unsolved mystery."

Summary

In this chapter, we have presented three related VB topics: (1) controls commonly found in data-entry applications; (2) how they are chosen, arranged, and presented; and (3) what events are commonly used.

Six controls are commonly used for the user to either enter or specify input. These include the text box, the masked edit, the option button, the check box, the list box, and the combo box. When the input in question is open ended, your choice of controls should be limited to the text box or the masked edit, depending on whether the input field has a predefined pattern. On the other hand, if your input items are known at either design time or runtime, you should consider the other four controls as an alternative to the first two. The criteria for the choice of controls include the following:

- The number of known items
- Whether the items are known at design time
- Whether the items will change over time
- Whether the selections are mutually exclusive
- Whether there is a possibility that the user will have to add items while entering data

The frame control, the picture box, and the tab control are introduced as containers for other controls (including themselves). They facilitate the arrangement and grouping of other controls into a neat, uncluttered and logical layout of the form (the visual interface). We have also introduced the image control as an alternative to the picture box when you need to use pictures in a form. Once every control in the form is in place, you should verify that the tab order of all controls is as expected. Techniques to adjust the tab order have been presented.

Finally, we have explained various events, including Form Load, KeyPress, Click, DoubleClick (DblClick), GotFocus, and LostFocus. These events are often used to handle various data-entry requirements/specifications. Therefore, it is important to understand their proper use.

The example near the end of the chapter should help you understand how pieces in VB are put together to form a "project." You should work on the example diligently. Once you have a clear understanding of the example, you will be able to handle the many more details and the complexity of programming logic to be introduced in later chapters.

Visual Basic Explorer

3-1. How Does the Text Box Handle It? Draw a tall text box in your form (e.g., 1355 × 720). Run your project. Type a paragraph from the textbook into this text box. How many lines of the text do you see? What happens to the "extra" characters that you cannot see in the box? Press the Home key. What do you see? Press the End key. What do you see? Press each of the arrow keys until it reaches the beginning or end of the text. You should have a pretty good idea how each key works with the text box. Notice that the left-arrow key and up-arrow key behave the same way. So do the right-arrow and down-arrow keys.

3-2. The PasswordChar Property of the Text Box. Set the PasswordChar property of the text box to "*" (You can try to enter "**" and see what happens.) Run the project. Enter some words in the text box. What is displayed?

3-3. The MultiLine Property of the Text Box. Continued from 3-1. Set the Multiline property of the text box to True. Run the project again. Type the same paragraph into the text box. How many lines of the text do you see? What happens to the "extra" characters that you could not see in the box? Press the Home key. What do you see? Press the End key. What do you see? Press each of the arrow keys until it reaches the beginning or end of the text. You should have a pretty good idea how each key works with the text box. Do the left-arrow and up-arrow keys behave the same way now? How about the right-arrow and down-arrow keys?

3-4. The Scrollbars Property of the Text Box. Continued from 3-3.

A. Set the Multiline property to False. Set the Scrollbars property to 1 (Horizontal). Run the program and enter the same paragraph. How many lines of text do you see?

B. Set the Multiline property to True. Set the Scrollbars property to 1 (Horizontal). Run the program and enter the same paragraph. How many lines of text do you see? In addition to arrow keys, you should also be able to navigate the text box with the scrollbar.

C. Set the Multiline property to False. Set the Scrollbars property to 2 (Vertical). Run the program and enter the same paragraph. How many lines of text do you see? Does the scrollbar help you navigate the text box?

D. Set the Multiline property to True. Set the Scrollbars property to 2 (Vertical). Run the program and enter the same paragraph. How many lines of text do you see? Does the scrollbar help you navigate the text box?

E. Set the Multiline property to True. Set the Scrollbars property to 3 (Both). Run the program and enter the same paragraph. Press the Return key to move to the next line.

3-5. The Alignment Property of the Label Control. Bring a label control to the form. Make it wider than enough to show a caption, "Testing for Justification." Change the alignment property to right justify (1). Inspect the effect. Then change the alignment property to center (2) and inspect the effect again.

3-6. The Alignment Property of the Text Box Control. The text box control also has the alignment property. However, it works a bit differently from the label. Bring a text box to the form. Leave "Text1" as its default text property.

Experiment the following setting: Change the alignment property to left justify (0), right justify (1), and center (2). Notice any change in behavior in the text box? For each alignment property setting, start the program. Erase "Text1" from the box. Enter "123." Notice any change in behavior?

(*Note:* If the alignment property does not seem to work properly, set the Multiline property to True.)

3-7. Clicking the Option Button and the Check Box. Bring a check box and an option button into a new form. Run the project. Click the check box repetitively. Then click the option button repetitively. Do you observe the same response?

3-8. The PromptChar Property of the Masked Edit Box. Bring a masked edit box into a new form. (*Note:* you may need to bring this VB control into the toolbox as explained in this chapter.) Set its Mask property to "##-##-####" and start the program. When the control gets the focus, what is displayed in the box? (You should be able to see underscores and dashes ["-"].) Change the PromptChar property to a space. Run the project again. You can see only the dashes. (This fine point can be important when you need to check the number of characters the user has entered.)

3-9. The Align Property of the Picture Box. Bring a picture box into a form. Set its Align property to 1 (Align Top). Where and how does it appear now? Set the property to other values (Align Left, Align Right, and Align Bottom). See how the Align property works?

3-10. The Picture Box as the Container. Continue from 3-9. Draw a few image controls into the picture box you have aligned in 3-9. Place pictures into these image controls. Recall that the image control has a Click event. Now, align the picture box at the top of the form. What have you created? (A toolbar.) Align the picture box on the left. What have you created? (A toolbox.)

3-11. Checking the Check Boxes in a List Box. Use a command button and a list box. Name the command button cmdCheck and set its Caption property to "Check." Name the list box lstWeekDays. Set its Style property to Checkbox (1) and its List property to Sunday, Monday,… and Saturday. Give the following code in the cmdCheck Click event procedure. Run the project. Click the command button. What do you see in the list box? Which days are checked? Can you still check and uncheck every item?

```
Private Sub cmdCheck_Click()
    lstWeekDays.Selected(0) = True
    lstWeekDays.Selected(2) = True
    lstWeekDays.Selected(4) = True
End Sub
```

3-12. Image Control versus Command Button. Draw an image control and a command button in a form. Make both appear to be about the same size. Set the image control's Stretch property to True. Set the Picture property of both controls to Phone03.ico, which is located in the subfolder \Microsoft Visual Studio\Common\Graphics\Icons\Comm. What do you see? Any picture in the command button? Set its Style property to Graphical. Now, do you see the picture? Set its Caption property to "Call." Set the ToolTip Text property of both controls to "Make a phone call." Then place the following line in the Click event of both controls:

```
Beep
Beep
Beep
```

Run the program. Click on both controls. Which one looks better to you? Try other pictures in other folders on both controls. Which one looks better?

Exercises

3-13. Most Suitable Control for Each Data Element. For each of the following data elements, determine what is the most suitable VB control to use for input. If more than one control can be suitable, state the conditions under which each will be better.

A. Address
B. Description of a product
C. Inventory ID (No.)
D. Eye color of a person
E. Hair color
F. Nationality
G. Course and section number
H. A series of questions in a hospital admission questionnaire such as:

- Have you been hospitalized before?
- Have you had any major surgery before?
- Are you allergic to any medicine?
- Has anybody in your family had a heart condition?

3-14. Which Event to Use? For each of the following situations, determine in which event procedure you should place your code:

A. When the user clicks a command button captioned "Save," your program need to save the data on the screen.
B. As soon as the user makes a selection among four option buttons, your program needs to display an appropriate message.
C. As soon as the user checks on or off a check box, your program needs to make another VB control visible or invisible.
D. As soon as the user enters a key into a masked edit box, your program needs to check to see whether it is a Return key.
E. As soon as the user enters a key into a text box, your program needs to determine whether it is an Esc key.
F. As soon as the user enters a key into a combo box, your program needs to determine whether it is an uppercase letter.
G. When the user tabs into or clicks a combo box, your program needs to highlight the content of the entire box.
H. Your program needs to determine whether the Social Security number in a masked edit box represents a valid employee when the user leaves the box.
I. As soon as the user makes a selection in a list box, your program needs to know if it is the fifth item in the list.
J. As soon as the user clicks on an item in a combo box, your program will need to move that item to a text box.

3-15. Make It Double. Here's a project that will double a number entered by the user.

1. Draw a label onto a new form. Change the Caption property of the label to "Enter a number."
2. Draw a text box by the right side of the label. Change its Name property to txtNumber. Clear its Text property.
3. Add another label below Label1. Change the second label control's Name property to lblResult and clear its Caption property.

4. Add a command button below the text box. Change its Caption property to "Double" and name property to cmdDouble.
5. Add the following code to the code window. (*Hint:* Use the code template provided by VB before adding the statement inside the procedure.)

```
Private Sub cmdDouble_Click()
    lblResult.Caption = "Twice of " & txtNumber.Text & _
    " is " & Val(txtNumber.Text) + Val(txtNumber.Text)
End Sub
```

Run the program and make sure the results are as expected.

3-16. Make It Do More. Modify the preceding project as follows:

1. Add two more command buttons. Change the Caption property of the first button to "Half" and the Name property to cmdHalf. Change the Caption property of the second button to "Square" and the Name property to cmdSquare.
2. Add code so that:

- When the user clicks the Half button, your program will display in lblResult the following message (assuming the user enter a number 10):

```
Half of 10 is 5
```

- When the user clicks the Square button, your program will display in lblResult the following message (assuming the user enter a number 10):

```
Square of 10 is 100
```

Hint: To obtain one half of a number, code:

```
Val(txtNumber.Text) / 2
```

To obtain the square of a number, code:

```
Val(txtNumber.Text) * Val(txtNumber.Text)
```

3-17. Hello! Text Box for Input. Use a label, a text box, and two command buttons. Set their properties as follows:

Control	Property	Setting
Label	Caption	Enter a Name
Text box	Text	(cleared)
	Name	txtName
Command button	Caption	Hello
	Name	cmdHello
Command button	Caption	Quit
	Name	cmdQuit

Provide the code to perform the following:

When your project runs, you will enter a name into the text box. When you click the Hello button, the computer will display a message showing "Hello!" followed by the name you've just entered in the text box. After you click the OK button in the message box, the computer clears the text box and waits for further actions. When you click the Quit button, your program quits.

3-18. Checking for Date Validity, Use of Masked Edit Box. Use a label, a masked edit box, and two command buttons. Set their properties as follows:

Control	Property	Setting
Label	Caption	Enter a Date
Masked edit box	Mask	##-##-####
	Name	MskDate
Command button	Caption	Check
	Name	cmdCheck
Command button	Caption	Quit
	Name	cmdQuit

When your project runs, the user will enter a date into the masked edit box. When you click the Check button, the computer will check to see whether the date entered is valid. If it is a valid date, the computer displays a message, "It's a valid date." Otherwise, the computer displays a message, "Please enter a valid date." After you click the OK button in the message box, the computer clears the masked edit box and waits for further actions. When you click the Quit button, your program quits. (*Hint:* Refer to the application example for code to check date validity. The way to clear a masked edit box has also been presented in the text.)

3-19. Events and Messages. Use a label, a text box, and a masked edit box. Align them vertically down. Set the label's AutoSize property to True and clear its caption. Set the Mask property of the masked edit box to "##-##-####." At runtime, when the user tabs to (or clicks) the text box, the label will display "Enter your name." When the user tabs to (or clicks) the masked edit box, the label will display "Enter your birth date." (*Hint:* Place code in the GotFocus event procedure of each of the two controls.)

3-20. Practicing Form Layout and Use of Container. Draw your favorite credit card on a new form. (*Hint:* Use a picture box as the container. Set the Picture property to your favorite picture as the background. Also, use the line control to draw horizontal or vertical lines.)

3-21. Practicing Form Layout and Use of Container. Draw your driver's license on a form. (*Hint:* Use an image control to hold your own picture.)

3-22. Practicing Form Layout and Use of Container. Draw a check of your bank account in a form. (*Hint:* Use a picture box as the container. You may want to include a picture as the background. Use the line control to draw lines. Use the text box for the user to enter payee and amount and to sign. You may have to change the background color and the border style of the text boxes to make them transparent.)

3-23. Setting Colors in Different Events. Use two text boxes and one command button. Name the text boxes txtName and txtAddress. Name the command button cmdQuit. Set the BackColor property of the command button to red. At runtime, when each of the text boxes receives focus, the text color is black. When it loses focus, its text color turns to blue. (*Hint:* The relevant events for the text boxes are GotFocus and LostFocus. The names of the colors are vbBlue and vbBlack. If you do not see the red color expected of the command button after setting its back color, make sure its Style property is set to Graphic.)

3-24. Adding Items to Combo Box. Use a combo box and a command button. Set the caption of the command button to "Add." Provide the code such that at runtime, when you click the Add button, whatever you have typed in the combo box is added to the combo list. Give proper names to these controls.

3-25. I Give You. You Give Me. List Boxes. Use two list boxes. Call them lstEast and lstWest. Use the List property to add the following 12 oriental zodiac symbols to lstEast. Provide the code such that at runtime, whichever symbol you click in one list box moves to the other list box; that is, it appears in the other box while disappearing from the list box the user clicks. (*Hint:* Code in the Click event and use the AddItem and RemoveItem methods.)

Rat	Rabbit	Horse	Rooster
Bull	Dragon	Sheep	Dog
Tiger	Snake	Monkey	Boar

3-26. Invitation to the Party. Checkbox Style List Box. Use one list box and a command button. Use the List property of the list box to add five of your friends' names. Set the list box's Style property to Checkbox. Set the Caption property of the command button to "Invite." Then provide the code to do the following:

At runtime, click the names of your friends who you plan to invite to your birthday party. When you click the "Invite" button, the program will display a message box for each friend who will be invited; for example, "Jerry will be invited to my birthday party."

3-27. Passing Data Between Controls. Use a combo box, a list box, and a command button. Set the Caption property of the command button to "Add." At runtime, when you click the command button, whatever you have typed in the combo box is added to the list box (not the combo box). But when you double-click the list box, the item gets transferred to the combo box; that is, it appears in the list of combo box and disappears from the list box. Give each control a proper name. (The event name for double-click is DblClick.)

3-28. Enabling and Disabling Controls Depending on the Check Box. First, bring a picture box into a new form. Set its Picture property to plane.ico (The icon file is located in the Microsoft Visual Studio\Common\Graphics\Icons\Industry folder.) Draw inside the picture box a check box, a label, and a text box. Name the check box chkFreqFlier. Set its Caption property to "Are you a frequent flier of our company?" Name the label lblFreqFlier. Set its Caption property to "Frequent Flier Number." Place the text box on its right side. Clear its Text property. Name it txtFlierNumber. Set the Enabled property of both the label and the text box to False. When your project runs, if the check box is checked on, both the label and the text box will be enabled. If the check box is clicked off, both the label and the text box will be disabled. (*Hint:* The event to code is chkFreqFlier_Click. Compare its Value property with vbChecked.)

3-29. Enabling and Disabling Controls Depending on Option Buttons. First, bring a frame into a new form. Set its Caption property to "Payment Method." Next bring three option buttons into the frame. Name them optCash, optCheck, and optCreditCard. Set their Caption property to Cash, Check, and Credit Card, respectively. Place a label and a combo box below the three option buttons but still within the frame. Name the label lblCreditCard. Set the label's Caption property to "Credit Card Type." Name the combo box cboCreditCard. Set its List property to hold Visa, Master Card, American Express, Diner's Club, and Discover. Set the Value property of optCash to True. Set the Enabled property of lblCreditCard and cboCreditCard to False. Then provide code to perform the following:
When your project runs, if the credit card option button is clicked, your program will enable both the label and the combo box. In addition, the combo box's ListIndex property is set to zero (0). Otherwise, both the label and the combo box are disabled. (*Hint:* Beware. You have more than one event to take care of the requirement. That is, the event[s] that the credit card option button is turned off is not this option button's Click event.)

Projects

3-30. The Jury Selection Questionnaire. A jury selection system has the following questionnaire.

Have you had any major injury?

Are you the citizen of the United States?

Your place of birth _________
Date of birth __________
How many years have you lived in this county?
Driver license number_________
List counties and states you have lived since 1985
Are you or your relatives in law enforcement?
    If so, Who?
Your occupation __________
Work phone ____________
Employer________________
    How long_______ years
Spouse's name__________________
Spouse's employer______________
Spouse's occupation_____________
    How long______ years
Number of children _____
Home phone_____________

Required: Design a form for this questionnaire, using the most suitable VB control for each question. (*Hint:* Add containers wherever appropriate. Give each control for input purposes a meaningful name.)

3-31. The Alumni Association Database. Your school would like to maintain a database for its alumni association. The database will include information on the alumnus' personal identification such as name, gender, date of birth; academic records such as major, highest degree, and year and term of last degree; contact information such as address, home phone, and email address; spouse's name and work phone; work-related data such as position, company name, address, and work phone number; and association history such as the year the alumnus joining the association, date, and amount of the last association dues paid.

Required: Design a form for such purpose. Add additional data elements wherever you see fit. Use the most suitable VB control for each data element. (*Hint:* Add containers wherever appropriate. Give each control for input purposes a meaningful name.)

3-32. The Account Holder File. A clinic needs a data-entry screen to enter account holder data. The following data elements must be entered.

Insured's (account holder's) name
Insured's address (number, street)
City, state, and zip code
Insured's telephone number
Insured's policy group or Feca Number
Insured's date of birth
Sex
Employer's name
Insurance plan name or program name
Type of insurance
    Medicare, Medicaid, Champus, Champva, Group health plan, Feca, or Others
Is there another health benefit plan?

If so, give the following:

Other insured's name

Other insured's policy or group number

Other insured's date of birth

Sex

Employer's name

Insurance plan name or program name

Required: Design an interface for such purpose. When the question, "Is there another health benefit plan?" is answered affirmatively, all controls used to take input for the other insured should be all enabled. Otherwise, they should be disabled. (*Hint:* Use the SSTab control. Separate data between the primary insured and the other insured. Also use frames wherever applicable.)

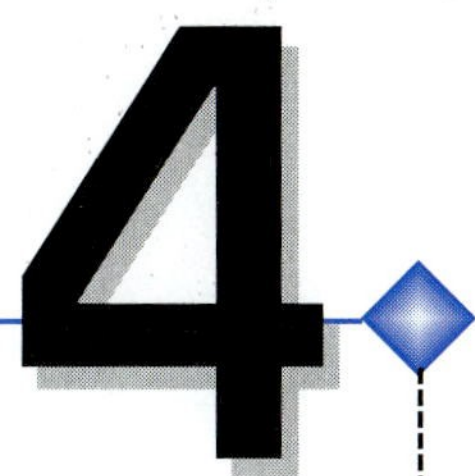

4 Data, Operations, and Built-In Functions

Thus far, you have learned more than a dozen Visual Basic (VB) controls and have explored their important features. They present themselves as great tools for building an elegant graphic user interface. However, data obtained from the interface usually need to be further handled before they become truly useful. In many cases, complex computations must also be performed. The results are then displayed. In this chapter, we study various aspects of data and the operations/computations that the computer can perform on them.

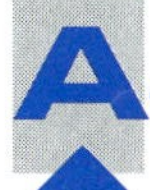

After you complete this chapter, you should be able to:

- Differentiate among different types of data.
- Declare data types properly for constants and variables.
- Appreciate the importance of having the VB IDE check for variable declarations and make VB insert "Option Explicit" automatically for your projects.
- Differentiate and appreciate the implications of the scope and duration of variables under different declarations.
- Gain an understanding of different number systems.
- Understand the nature of the assignment statement.
- Recognize and use various arithmetic expressions and functions.
- Recognize and use various string functions.
- Understand better how data and VB controls are used together in a project.

4.1 Classification and Declaration of Data

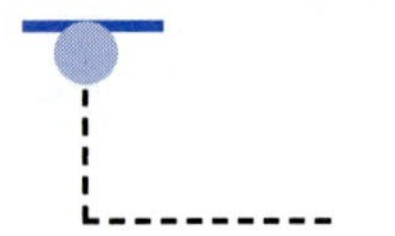

Consider the following code:

```
MsgBox "Your age is " & 24
```

What types of data have you used? Two different types of data are involved in the preceding statement. The text enclosed in a pair of quotation marks is a ***string***, whereas the number, 24, is ***numeric*** data. A string consists of zero or more characters, whereas numeric data are numbers, which can be used for various computations and can be further classified into many different types. The first level of data classification by type can be depicted as in Figure 4.1.

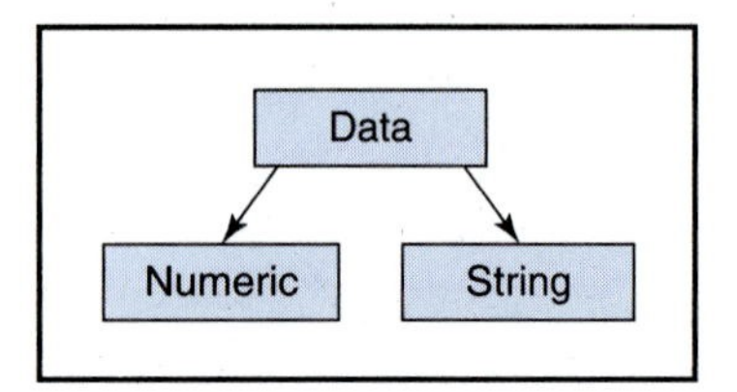

FIGURE 4.1
Classification of Data by Type

All data must be stored somewhere in the computer memory before they can be retrieved for additional manipulation or display. If a memory location with some data is expected to change as a result of operations, it is recognized as a ***variable***. A variable must be given a name so that you can refer to it. Data that present themselves "as is" and are never expected to change are recognized as ***constants***. A constant can go without a name but can also be given a name. A constant without a name has to be presented and used as literal. A constant that is given a name and is referenced accordingly is recognized as a ***named constant***. This classification can be depicted as in Figure 4.2.

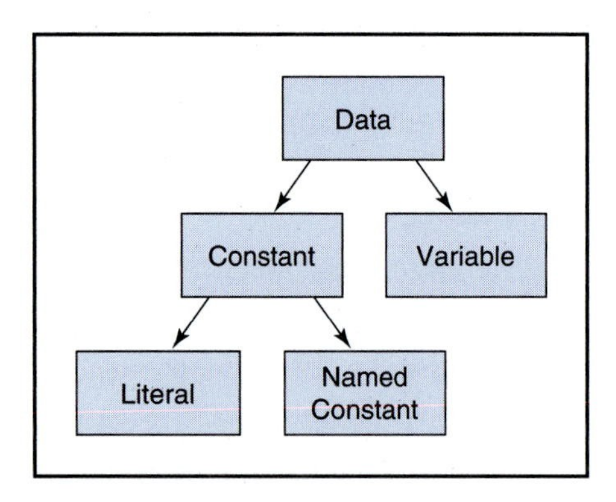

FIGURE 4.2
Classification of Data by Variability

To summarize, data can be classified by type into numeric and string and by variability into constant and variable. The following table shows the classifications:

	Numeric	String	Name Required?
Constant	Numeric constant	String constant	Optional
Variable	Numeric variable	String variable	Required

Declaring Constants

Before a named constant can be used in your program, you must make sure that VB can recognize it. Some named constants are predefined and automatically recognized. They are called ***system constants***. You have seen some of these constants in the preceding chapters. For example, you have seen named constants for colors such as vbGreen, VbBlue, and vbRed. You have also seen true or false named constants, True and False. Other named constants must be declared before VB can recognize them. These are called ***symbolic constants***. You use the ***Const statement*** to declare a symbolic constant. The general syntax is as follows:

```
Const name [as data type] = literal
```

For example, the following statement declares the named constant Zero to have a constant value of 0. As the syntax in the preceding example suggests, you can also omit "as Integer" from the declaration without affecting the result.

```
Const Zero as Integer = 0
```

Why Name Constants? Properly named constants can enhance the understandability of the code. When reviewing code, you may not recognize the specific meaning of a particular value such as 0 or 1. This is particularly true when the constants are used as the property setting of a VB control. Instead, if you code these constants as vbUnChcked (for 0) and vbChecked (for 1) in setting the property value of a check box, anyone, including yourself, should be able to follow the code much more easily. In addition, in some cases, you may find it necessary to later change the value of a constant. Using a named constant, you need to make the correction in only one place: where the constant is declared. In contrast, you will have to search the entire program for the constant to change if the constant literal was used.

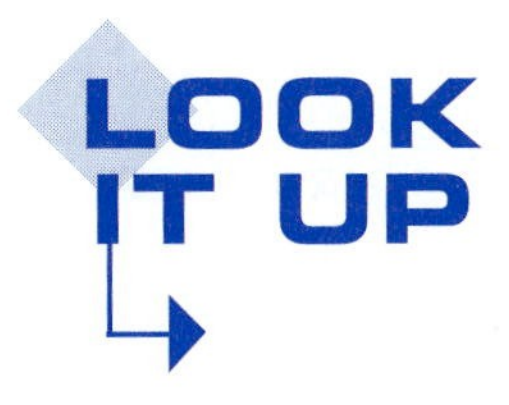

The keyword "Visual Basic Constants" in the Index tab of the Help screen provides a long list of constants (classified into groups) recognized by VB. For example, you can find all system constants for colors as well as for properties of various controls. Look over the Help page now, and refer to it often in the future when you find a need for a named constant.

Declaring Variables

A variable can be used without being declared. However, it is a good habit to declare all variables used in a project. The reasons for this are given later in the section "Why Force Yourself into Declaring All Variables?" You use the ***Dim statement*** to declare a variable. The syntax is as follows:

```
Dim Variable1 [As data type][, Variable2 [As data type]]...
```

For example, you can code the following:

```
Dim TheName as String, SSN as Long
```

This statement declares a variable, TheName, as the String type variable and another variable named SSN as a Long integer. (Numeric data types are explained in Section 4.3 and the String type is discussed in Section 4.5.)

However, note that for code clarity, it is advisable to declare *only one variable per line*. (Many companies adopt this coding standard.) Thus, a better way to code the preceding line is as follows:

```
Dim TheName as String
Dim SSN as Long
```

Using Type Suffixes. A variable or symbolic constant can also be declared with a trailing special character that signifies a data type. These special characters (e.g., $, %, and &) are called *type-declaration characters* (or *type suffixes*) and are listed in Section 4.3. The following statement with type-declaration characters will have the same effect as the previous example.

```
Dim TheName$
Dim SSN&
```

Recall in Chapter 2, "Introduction to Visual Basic Programming," we emphasized the importance of using meaningful names for VB objects. This observation can certainly be extended and applied to all types of names, including constants and variables. As you can see, declarations using type suffixes are not as easy to understand as those using data type names. For code clarity, *always use data type names instead of type suffixes.*

For program readability, always give your variables and constants meaningful names. Declare only one name per line. Also, use the data type names instead of type suffixes to declare the data types for the variables and constants.

Checking for Variable Declarations

You can have VB check to see whether all the variables used in your program have been declared properly. To accomplish this, you code the following in the general declaration area of the code window:

```
Option Explicit
```

You can even have VB automatically add this line for you. To implement this, do the following:

1. Click the "Options" option in the Tools menu. The Options dialog box will appear (Figure 4.3).
2. Select the Editor tab.
3. Check "Require variable declaration."
4. Click the OK button.

Once you do this, VB will automatically add the "Option Explicit" statement to any new project. When you run a project with this statement, VB will display an error message for any variable not declared.

FIGURE 4.3
The Editor Tab of the Options Dialog Box

VB will automatically add the "Option Explicit" statement in your project when this one is checked.

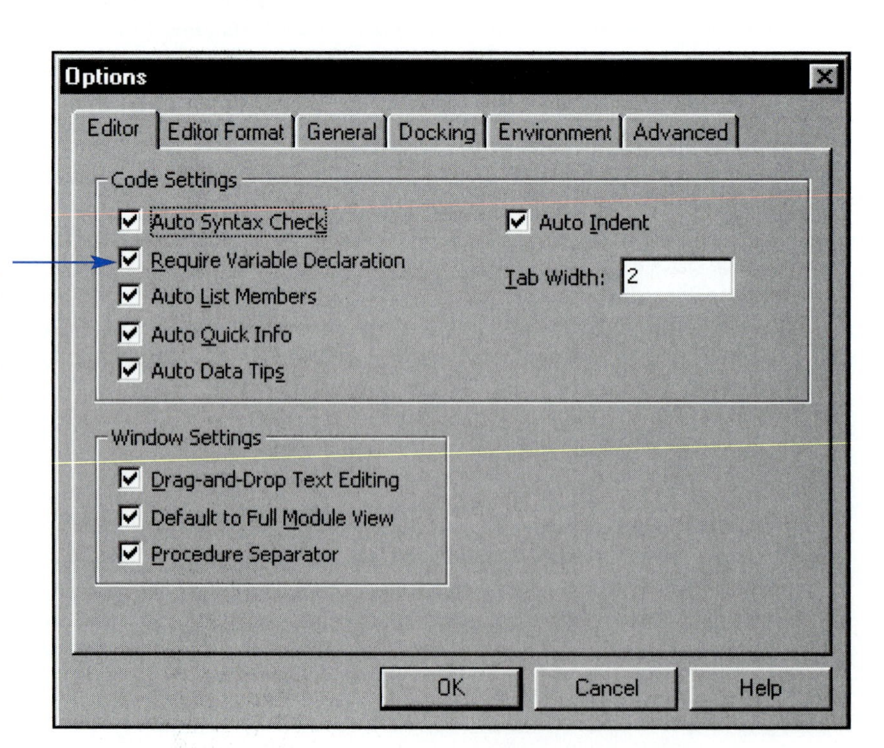

Why Force Yourself into Declaring All Variables? The following are some advantages to declaring all variables:

- A variable not declared may give you unexpected results. This kind of error is hard to uncover.
- This practice helps identify misspelled variables, which can cause unexpected results.
- If you declare a variable with proper capitalization, the same capitalization will be maintained automatically by VB throughout the program. For example, if you declare a variable, HourPay with a Dim statement, then in your program, regardless of how you type the variable (e.g., hourpay or HOURPAY), VB will change it to HourPay, the way you initially declared the variable. This enables you to check immediately whether you have typed in a name properly. Proper capitalization also enhances the readability of your program.

Experienced programmers know the importance of having all the variable names correctly spelled. A minor error in spelling a variable name sometimes can result in "mysterious" errors in the program, causing numerous hours of hunting for the bug. *Always include the "Option Explicit" statement in your project.*

Rules for Variable Declaration

When you are declaring variables or named constants, some rules must be observed:

- A variable or constant name can contain any combination of letters and numbers. However, it must begin with a letter and it cannot be longer than 255 characters.
- It must not be a reserved keyword used by VB.
- It must not contain any embedded period (e.g., Your.Name) or embedded special characters used for data type declaration (e.g., The%Completed).

4.2 Scope and Lifetime of Variables

Variables and constants have their scope and lifetime (duration). *Scope* refers to how "widely" a variable is recognized, whereas *lifetime* refers to how long a variable remains in computer memory. The placement of a variable declaration can affect both the scope and the duration of that variable. Let's now consider this aspect.

Form-Level Declaration

The code window associated with the form is recognized as the ***form module***. Variables and constants declared with a Dim statement in the general declaration area (right after the Option Explicit statement) are the ***Module (Form)Level*** variables and constants. They are recognized by all procedures in the form module. In addition, they exist as long as the form module does; that is, their values are preserved until the form is "destroyed." In a single form application, the form is destroyed when the project ends. We discuss the life of a form in more detail in Chapter 11, Menus and Multiple Form Applications."

Procedure-Level Declaration

Variables and constants declared in a procedure are recognizable only in that procedure. They are said to be the ***Procedure Level*** (or ***Local***) variables and constants. The same names used in other procedures refer to different memory locations and have nothing to do with those in the current procedure. Because these variables are independent of each other, you can declare different data types in different procedures even for the same name. For example, it is legitimate to have the following declarations for I:

```
Private Sub cmdTest1_Click()
Dim I as Integer
    ' additional code lines
End Sub
Private Sub cmdTest2_Click()
Dim I as Long
    ' additional code lines
End Sub
```

However, such a practice can create confusion even for yourself when you review the code later. *Avoid this practice by all means.*

Lifetime of Variables Declared in a Procedure with Dim. Variables declared with a Dim statement in a procedure exist for as long as the procedure is in action. When the procedure ends, these variables are said to be "out of scope" and disappear. When the procedure is called again, these variables are reinitialized; that is, they no longer have their previous values. They will be reset to zero if they are numeric variables or to a zero-length string if they are string variables.

Static Declaration

If you want a local variable to preserve its value for the duration of the form module, not just of the procedure, you can use the "Static" statement for the declaration. When you declare a variable with the ***Static statement,*** the value of that variable will be preserved and will not be reinitialized between each call of the procedure. The following example illustrates the difference between a variable declared with a Dim statement and one with a Static statement:

```
Private Sub Form_Click()
Dim I as Integer
Static J as Integer
    I = I + 1
    J = J + 1
    MsgBox "I = " & I & ". J = " & J
End Sub
```

When you run this program and click on the form repetitively, you will notice that the message box continues to display 1 for I but increases the value for J each time (see Figure 4.4).

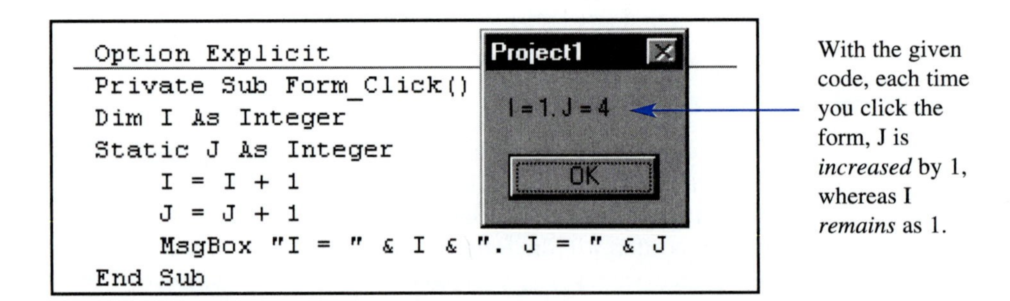

FIGURE 4.4
Effect of Static Declaration

Scope of Static Variables. If a static variable lives as long as the form, how then is it different from a module level variable? They differ in scope. A static variable (which can be declared only inside a procedure) is a local variable, recognized only in the procedure. On the other hand, a module level variable is recognized by all procedures in the same form. For example, suppose you have a form with a command button named cmdTest. Consider the following code:

```
Option Explicit
Dim K as Integer

Private Sub Form_Click()
Static J as Integer
    K = K + 1
    J = J + 1
    MsgBox "K = " & K & ". J = " & J
End Sub

Private Sub cmdTest_Click()
    MsgBox "K = " & K
    MsgBox "J = " & J
End Sub
```

When you run the program and click the form repetitively, you will see both K and J increase by 1 each time. However, when you click the "Test" button, the computer displays a "compile error" message stating "variable not defined" with the variable J in the cmdTest Click procedure highlighted (Figure 4.5). This indicates that J is not recognized in this procedure.

FIGURE 4.5
Effect of Variable Scope

Declaring J as Static in another procedure results in an error when you click the command button named cmdTest because J is not a form level variable and is not declared in this procedure.

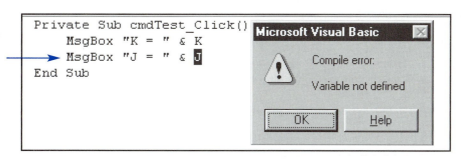

Overlapping Declarations in Form and Procedure. What happens when a module (form) level variable is also declared in a procedure? The one declared in the procedure is a different variable, a local variable with the same name. VB recognizes the variable of the narrowest scope. Thus, this procedure recognizes only the local variable, not the module level variable, whereas other procedures where no variable of the same name is declared recognize the module level variable. To see the effect, draw a command button in a new form. Name it cmdTest and set its Caption property to "Test." Then enter the following code:

```
Option Explicit
Dim K as Integer

Private Sub Form_Click()
    K = K + 1
    MsgBox "K = " & K
    'You will see a different K each time you click the form.
End Sub

Private Sub cmdTest_Click()
Dim K as Integer
    K = K + 1
    MsgBox "K = " & K
    'You will always see 1 when you click the command button.
End Sub
```

Run the project. You should see that each time you click the form, K is increased by 1. The module level variable K is recognized. However, when you click the command button repetitively, you will continue to see K equal to 1. In this procedure, the local (procedure level) variable is used.

You are not allowed to declare two variables with the same name in the same procedure. Nor are you allowed to do the same in the general declaration area. You will have a "duplicate declaration in current scope" error. The computer will not be able to tell which variable you are referring to if it allows you to declare variables this way. Always use unique names to avoid confusion.

Scope and Lifetime: A Recap

To recapitulate, variables have different scopes and lifetimes, depending on where and how they are declared. A variable declared at the form level is recognized by all procedures, whereas a variable declared in a procedure is recognized only in that procedure. If the same variable name is declared in different contexts (in the form and/or in different procedures), *the variable declared in the procedure is the one recognized inside the procedure.*

Besides its scope, a variable also has its lifetime. A form level variable has its value preserved until the form is destroyed. The value of a procedure level variable is reinitialized each time the procedure is called if the variable is declared with a Dim statement. However, if it is declared with a Static statement, the procedure level variable's value is preserved until the form is destroyed.

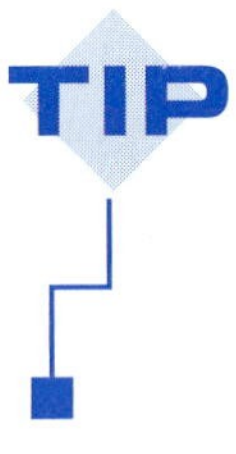

If you would like all your variables in a procedure to be static, you can use the following syntax:

```
Private StaticSubprocedurename(parameter list)
```

As you recall, static variables behave differently. They are not reinitialized each time the procedure is called. Beware of the potential side effect that may result.

The following table provides a summary of the scope and duration of variables.

Declaration	Scope	Duration
Dim A As Integer (in the general declaration area)	Form (module) level variable recognized by all procedures	The value is preserved for as long as the form exists.
Dim B As Integer (inside a procedure)	Procedure level (local) variable recognized only in that procedure	As soon as the procedure ends, the value is gone.
Static C As Integer (allowed only inside a procedure)		The value is preserved for as long as the form exists.

Declaring Constants. The value of named constants cannot be changed. Although they have similar scope and lifetime as variables, it would seem more appropriate to use the same names for the same types and values throughout the project. This practice enhances the consistency and maintainability for the project. Thus, *you should declare named constants at the form (project) level.*

Scope and Program Modularity

As you can see from the previous discussion, a variable declared in the general declaration area is recognized by all procedures in the form module. This also means that only one memory location is used to handle the variable. Thus, you may be tempted to declare all variables at the form level for convenience and to conserve memory. However, this is poor programming practice.

Why? When a variable is recognized by all procedures, it is shared by all procedures. When the value of this variable is changed in one procedure, the result affects *all* procedures. In some cases (and too often), such a change may not be expected when you write your code. This coding practice makes the resulting program difficult to maintain. In addition, because of the duration of the form level variables, the memory use is not necessarily minimized. Thus, *the general rule is to declare each variable with a scope as narrow as possible*; that is, to the extent possible, declare the variables you need to use in the procedures where you need them and declare variables at the form level only if they absolutely have to be shared by more than one procedure. By declaring variables with the narrowest scope possible, you keep procedures independent of each other, which is the basic foundation of modular design.

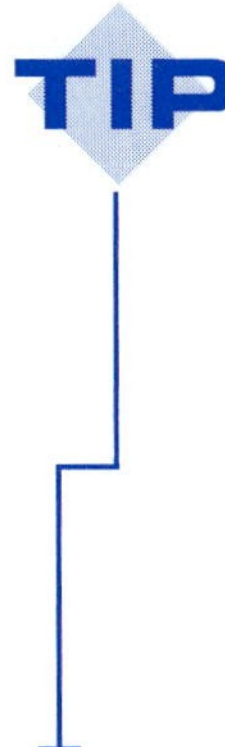

TIP

When you absolutely need procedures to share certain variables, declare them at the form (module) level. However, try to design your code such that each of these variables is assigned/changed in as few procedures as possible. This makes it easier to trace the source of the change when a problem occurs. If the value of a variable needs to be changed to perform some operations within a procedure and such a change is not intended for all other procedures, you should take care to restore the original value of the variable. This can be done by the use of a temporary variable (e.g., a properly declared variable named TempVar) as shown in the following code fragment:

```
TempVar = YourVariable 'Save the original value
YourVariable = New Value 'Change the variable to a new value
' Your code that uses the New value
YourVariable = TempVar 'Restore the value at the end
```

Constant and Variable Naming Convention

Some companies also adopt naming conventions for constants and variables, in addition to those that they use for controls. The rules for variables typically stipulate that there should be a one-character prefix for the scope, followed by another three-character prefix for the data type. For example, a module (form) level integer variable can have a prefix "mint," where "m" indicates the scope (modular level) and "int" represents its data type. This naming notation is recognized as the Hungarian notation. The purpose of such rules is to enhance the readability of the code.

Some well-known authors, however, maintain that such a practice appears to be an overkill and can make the code extra long, adding an overhead to the coding effort. This textbook will not follow this convention in using variables and constants. However, you should be aware that such a convention does exist. You can find additional details of this convention in the Help file by searching the Search tab (not the Index tab) for the keyword "constant and variable naming convention" (ranked 21 in the list of topics found).

4.3 Numeric Data and Types

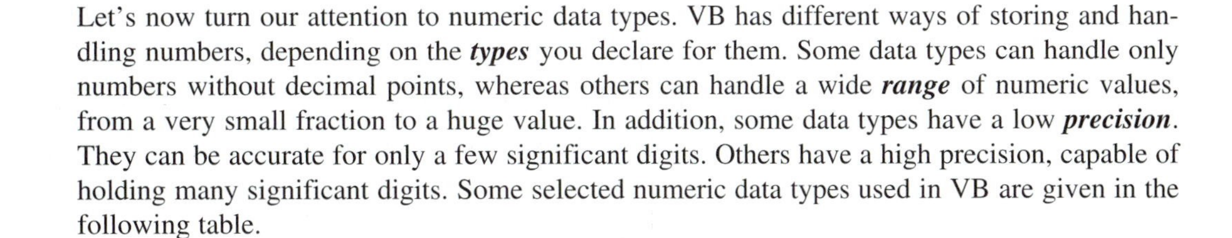

Let's now turn our attention to numeric data types. VB has different ways of storing and handling numbers, depending on the ***types*** you declare for them. Some data types can handle only numbers without decimal points, whereas others can handle a wide ***range*** of numeric values, from a very small fraction to a huge value. In addition, some data types have a low ***precision***. They can be accurate for only a few significant digits. Others have a high precision, capable of holding many significant digits. Some selected numeric data types used in VB are given in the following table.

Data Type	Storage Size in Bytes	Type Suffix	Value Range
Byte	1	(none)	0 to 255
Boolean	2	(none)	True or False
Integer	2	%	-32,768 to 32,767
Long	4	&	-2,147,483,648 to 2,147,483,647
Single	4	!	1.401298E-45 to 3.402823E38 (in magnitude)
Double	8	#	4.94065645841247E-324 to 1.79769313486232E308 (in magnitude)

As noted previously, declaring data with type suffixes makes the code less readable. Do not use them in your own code. They are listed here for your reference in case you encounter them when reviewing someone else's code.

Byte and Boolean Types

As you can see from the preceding table, ***Byte*** type data can handle only a small range of values with a very narrow range and low precision (fewer than three "complete" digits). It cannot handle negative values. Thus, its use is rather limited for computational purposes. ***Boolean*** type data are used to store the logical state, True (-1) or False (0). In contrast to Byte data, Boolean data are often used, although there are only two values. Many properties of VB controls can accept only Boolean data. These properties (e.g., Visible or Enabled) must be set to the desired state for the VB controls to work properly. Also, If statements always involve the use of Boolean data.

Integer and Long Types

The ***Integer*** type, sometimes also called ***Short integer,*** uses two bytes to store data. This data type is often used as counters, which seldom exceed several thousands. It is also used as the index for elements in a list. The ***Long*** type uses exactly the same internal coding scheme as the Short integer type, but it uses four bytes instead of two for storage and is therefore often called the ***Long integer*** type. As shown in the table, it has a wider range and higher precision than the Short integer.

When the result of a numeric operation exceeds the capacity that a data type can handle, an ***overflow error*** will occur at runtime. In those cases in which you are not sure how big an integer may be, you should use Long integer to be on the safe side.

Single and Double Types

In contrast to the short and Long integer types, the ***Single*** and ***Double*** types can handle data with fractional numbers and decimal points. These two data types use the ***floating point*** coding scheme to store data. This coding scheme breaks the stored data into two portions: One portion is used to keep track of the exponent, while the other portion stores the base value (mantissa) of the data. As an illustration, the number 123.45 can be expressed as 1.2345×10^2. The mantissa value, 1.2345, is stored in one part of the storage area, while the exponent, 2, is stored in another part. This form of representation can also be used in code, where the mantissa is presented first followed by a symbol E (for "exponent") and the exponent value. Here are some examples:

Actual Value	Floating Point Representation
34500	3.45E4
-34500	-3.45E4
.0002345	2.345E-4
-.0002345	-2.345E-4

Both the Single and Double data types can handle a wide range of values, as shown in the previous table. However, the Single type has a precision of approximately 7 significant digits. This means if you have an amount like 1234567.89 that must be stored accurately, then you should not use the Single type because the last few digits of the amount will be lost. If you need to use a floating point type to handle your data, you should keep this in mind.

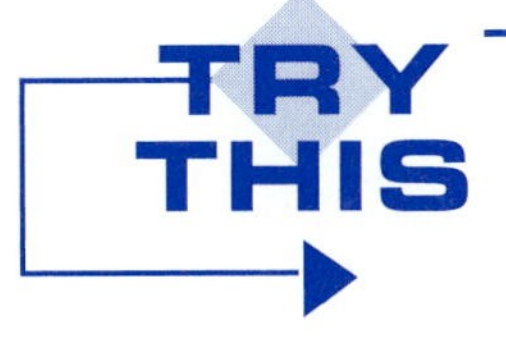

Type the following code in the code window of a new project without any VB control. Run the project and click the form. What does the message box display? Change "Single" to "Double" in the Dim statement. Run the program again. What do you see this time?

```
Private Sub Form_Click()
Dim Amount as Single
    Amount = 1234567.89
    MsgBox "The amount is " & Amount
End Sub
```

We can summarize the characteristics of the six numeric data types discussed in this subsection as follows:

Data Type	Value Range	Precision	Speed	Remark
Byte	Small	Low	NA	Seldom used for computation purposes
Boolean	Small	Low	NA	Often used to represent "state," such as True or False (On or Off)
Integer	Small	Low	2	Often used as counters
Long	Medium	High	1	Used for integer computations; cannot handle decimal point
Single	Large	Medium	3	Can be accurate for about seven significant digits
Double	Very large	Very high	4	Requires twice the storage of the Long or Single type

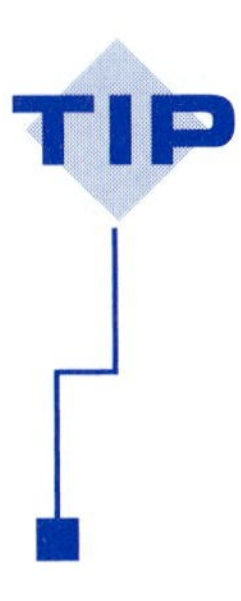

When you are uncertain about how many significant digits the actual data may have, use the data type with the higher precision for the variable. Your program may become slower and will consume more storage space. (Between Integer and Long, the latter is faster, however.) Nevertheless, you are assured that your program will not encounter a serious problem unexpectedly. Story has it that the stock market once crashed because a computer program used by a large bank in New York City failed to process all transactions when the assumed maximum number of transactions was exceeded on that day. *Program robustness should outweigh the efficiency consideration.*

Other Numeric Data Types

In addition to the numeric data types just described, there are also data types of Currency, Decimal, and Date. They use 8, 14, and 8 bytes of storage, respectively. The Currency type always reserves four decimal places for data. The Decimal type can handle 28 significant digits, and you can place the decimal point anywhere in this range (e.g., 123456789.0123456789). The Date type is used to handle date/time data, as the name implies. Basically, it uses the double floating point representation to handle the data. Its fractional part is used to keep track of the time, whereas the integer part is for the date value.

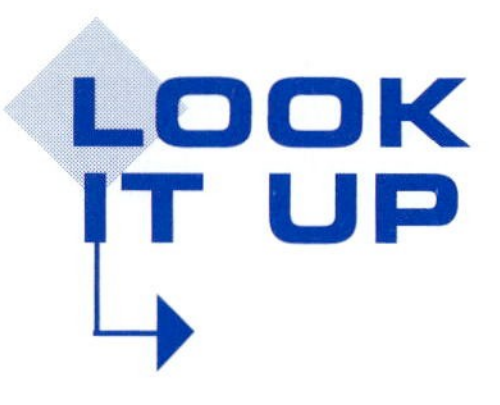

Search for the keyword "Data types" in the Index tab of the Help screen. Then select "Data Types Keyword Summary—Visual Basic Reference" in the Topics Found dialog box. The list under "Set intrinsic data types" gives you additional data types and descriptions. For example, it lists Currency, Decimal, and Date types among others. It also discusses String and Object types.

Declaring Numeric Data Types

As explained in Section 4.1, you can declare a numeric variable using the following syntax:

```
Dim name as data type
```

Or

```
Dim name+type suffix
```

You probably have noticed in the first table that not all data types can be declared with a type suffix. Besides the four types listed in the table, the only other numeric data type that can be declared with a type suffix is Currency, with an "@" symbol. Again, for code clarity, avoid declaring variables with type suffixes.

Here are some examples of variable declarations:

```
Dim NewRec as Boolean              'Declare NewRec as Boolean type
Dim NumberOfEmployees as Integer 'Declare # of employees as integer
Dim RecordCount as Long            'Declare RecordCount as long
Dim HourPay as Single              'Declare hour pay as single
Dim BillsIncome as Double          'Declare Bill's income as double
Dim Amount As Currency             'Declare Amount as currency
```

The Variant Data Type

What if you declare a variable without explicitly giving its type? The variable is then given a Variant data type. This is also the data type that VB assumes for you if you use a variable without declaration and you do not have an "Option Explicit" statement. The Variant data type can take on any type of data, numeric or string. Thus, in a way, it is a versatile type with a lot of flexibility and capability. However, this versatility can also cause unexpected results and a lot of confusion. Consider the following code:

```
Dim V as Variant
    V = "1.23"
    V = V + "45"
```

What result do you expect? V will contain a string "1.2345" because both V and "45" are strings and the "+" symbol is considered a string concatenation operator (see the string section that follows for more explanation). But what do you expect from the following?

```
V = "1.23"
V = V + 45
```

The answer is 46.23. Because 45 is a number, VB considers "+" as an addition operator. It thus converts the string "1.23" to the number 1.23 and then performs the addition. What's more: After the last statement, V is no longer a string but a floating point double type! See the confusion that the Variant type can cause?

In addition to the potentially unexpected result and confusion, the Variant type also uses more computer memory to store and is slower because of the additional complexity involved in handling this data type. *Stay away from this data type as much as possible.*

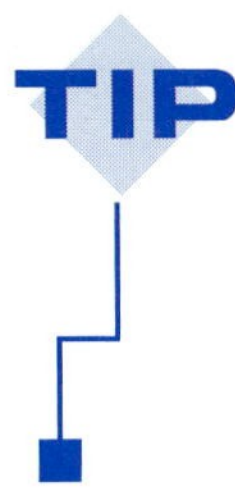

Beware of a coding mistake as shown below:

```
Dim Counter1, Counter2 As Integer
```

Some might think that Counter1 has been declared as an integer. It is *not*! It is a Variant type. VB expects an explicit declaration of data type for each individual variable. Because no data type is declared for Counter1 (e.g., no "As Integer" immediately following it), it treats the variable as a Variant.

A Bit of Number Systems

Before we discuss the operations of numeric data, let's take a brief look at the number systems. This discussion should help build a foundation for a deeper understanding of numeric operations.

Human beings use the decimal system for numbers. We count from 0 to 9 before adding another digit in presenting the number. Computers, on the other hand, operate on bits (binary digits) and bytes. A number is represented internally in the computer by setting various bits on or off. For example, the number zero is represented by setting off all bits used for that number; and one, the lowest bit, on. Because a bit has only two states (on and off), to go to the next number (2), the lowest bit is turned off, while the next lowest bit is turned on. Such a system is recognized as the binary number system. This coding system can be depicted as follows:

Binary system	Decimal system
0000	0
0001	1
0010	2
0011	3
0100	4
0101	5
0110	6
0111	7

Converting Between the Two Systems. If you examine the binary system closely, you may discover that each bit position represents a value of two raised to a certain power. For example, the lowest bit and the second lowest bit represent 2^0 and 2^1, respectively.

This can be depicted as follows:

```
Binary number   1  1  1  1  1  1  1  1
Decimal value   2⁷ 2⁶ 2⁵ 2⁴ 2³ 2² 2¹ 2⁰
```

From Binary to Decimal. To find the corresponding decimal value for any binary representation, multiply the bits by their corresponding positional value and sum the total. For example, a binary number, 10101, can have its decimal value computed as follows:

```
Binary value    1    0    1    0    1
multiply by     2⁴   2³   2²   2¹   2⁰
Results        16 +  0 +  4 +  0 +  1 = 21
```

From Decimal to Binary. Conversely, to find the binary value for a decimal number, divide the number by two and find the remainder, which is the bit value for the lowest position. Then divide the integer quotient by two again to obtain the bit value for the next higher position. Repeat this process to find the bit value for each successive position until the resulting quotient is zero. The following table shows how the binary representation for 13 can be obtained.

Step	4	3	2	1
Value To Be Divided by 2	1	3	6	13
Integer Quotient	0	1	3	6
Remainder (Binary Equivalent)	1	1	0	1

As the table shows, in the first step (last column), 13 is divided by 2, resulting in a quotient 6 and a remainder 1. Then, in step 2, 6 (the previous quotient) is divided by 2, resulting in a quotient 3 and a remainder 0. This process continues until step 4, when the resulting quotient is 0. The remainder row shows the bit representation for 13, that is, 1101.

The Hex Decimal Representation. Although the binary number system corresponds to the internal coding exactly, it is inconvenient to show a long number with this system. To simplify the representation, the hex decimal system has been introduced. Under this system, each digit has 16 possible values (0 to 15), as opposed to 2 in the binary system and 10 in the decimal system. The numbers are represented as shown in the following table:

Decimal	Binary	Hex
0	0000	0
1	0001	1
2	0010	2
3	0011	3
4	0100	4
5	0101	5
6	0110	6
7	0111	7
8	1000	8
9	1001	9
10	1010	A
11	1011	B
12	1100	C
13	1101	D
14	1110	E
15	1111	F

As you can see from the table, the letters A, B, C, D, E, and F are used to represent 10, 11, 12, 13, 14, and 15, respectively, so that each of the 16 numbers in the hex decimal system is one digit. The next number after F will be 10 because we have exhausted all symbols to represent a number in one hex digit.

Notice that the letters used in this context have no direct association with the letters we use in any text. They are simply "symbols" used to represent the numbers in the hex system. Notice also a hex decimal digit can be conveniently used to represent four bits in the binary system. For example, a hex number F0 will indicate that the lower four bits are zeros (off), while the upper four bits are 1s (on).

Converting Between Hex and Decimal Numbers. Converting numbers between the two systems is similar to converting between decimal and binary numbers. Each position, p, in the hex system presents a value of 16 raised to the power of p – 1, beginning from the lowest. To convert a hex decimal number to a decimal value, multiply each hex digit by its positional value and sum the total. For example, the hex number F3D can be converted to a decimal value as follows:

Hex number	F	3	D
Decimal equivalent	15	3	13
Multiply by	16^2	16^1	16^0
Result	3840 +	48 +	13 = 3901

To convert a decimal number to a hex representation, divide the number by 16 to find the integer quotient and the remainder, which gives the value at the lowest position. Divide the quotient by 16 again to obtain the remainder for the value at the next lowest position. Continue this process until the integer quotient is zero. For example, the following table illustrates how a decimal number, 3901, can be converted to a hex number:

Step	3	2	1
Number To Be Divided by 16	15	243	3901
Integer Quotient	0	15	243
Remainder	15	3	13
Result: Remainder in Hex	F	3	D

As you can see from the table, in step 1 (last column), the number 3901 is divided by 16, giving an integer quotient of 243 and a remainder of 13, which can be represented in the hex system as D. In a similar fashion, the previous quotient, 243, is divided by 16 to obtain the quotient and remainder for the second round. The process continues until the resulting quotient is zero in step 3. The remainder in hex representation F3D gives the solution.

Representing Hex Numbers in VB. VB allows a direct representation of hex numbers. You can code a hex number by preceding it with an "&H." For example, to represent a hex number F, you code &HF. If the number is fairly big, attach an "&" at the end to indicate it is a Long integer. For example, code &HABCD0& instead of &HABCD0.

Why Discuss Number Systems? Usually, VB shows results with decimal values. After all, the decimal system is what we are most familiar with. So, why discuss the number systems? Here are some reasons:

- In some cases, it is much easier to think in terms of bits. In VB, many "states" (e.g., which mouse button is pressed) are represented by "flags," which are collectively represented by an integer with its specific bits set on or off. An understanding of the binary number system will make it easier for us to see the relationship between "setting a bit on" and an integer value. Incidentally, a Boolean value is stored as a two-byte integer. The value False has all its bits off (&H0000), whereas True has all its bits on (&HFFFF). You can easily see that False has a numeric equivalent of 0. Also, when an integer's highest bit is on, it is a negative number. Its complement (a value that adds that number to make it zero) is the number's negative value. Because adding 1 to &HFFFF will clear all its bits, making it zero, you can see why True has a numeric value of –1. (See Explorer Exercise 4-1.)
- Some "operators" operate bitwise. For example, the logical operators (e.g., And, Or) operate by bit. When you understand the binary number system, you will be able to understand the results of the operations much more easily. The logical operators are discussed in Chapter 5, "Decision."
- Some numbers are more conveniently represented by hex numbers. Each hex digit can represent a certain state more readily. You may have noticed that the number used in representing colors (as shown in the BackColor and ForeColor properties) are in hex representation. For example, the white color is coded as &H00FFFFFF&, and the black color is coded as &H00000000&.

- Some constants are traditionally represented by hex numbers. For example, the parameter constants used in API (an acronym for Application Program Interface) calls are all in hex representation. Getting acquainted with the hex number system will alleviate your "fear" of the mystery associated with this representation. (We discuss API calls in Chapter 14, "Beyond the Core.")

The Assignment Statement

We are now ready to discuss numeric operations. Before doing so, however, let's take another look at the assignment statement. Consider the following statement:

```
HourPay = 12.50
```

The equal sign (=) in the statement instructs the computer to move data resulting from the operation(s) on the right side to the variable on its left side. Statements with this structure are recognized as "assignment statements" and are the most common statements in nearly all programs. In addition to assigning a constant to a variable, you can also assign the value of a variable to another variable:

```
HourPay = StandardHourPay
```

It is important to note that because the result on the right side will be moved to the left, *any variables appearing on the right side must have been assigned with proper values* before execution reaches the statement. In the previous statement, we assume StandardHourPay is another variable and has been declared and assigned some value before execution reaches this line.

You can also assign data entered in the VB control to a variable. For example, the following code will assign to the variable HourPay whatever number the user enters into the text box named txtHourPay (Figure 4.6).

```
HourPay = txtHourPay.Text
```

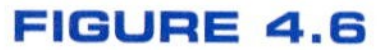
FIGURE 4.6

Moving Data Between Text Box and Variable

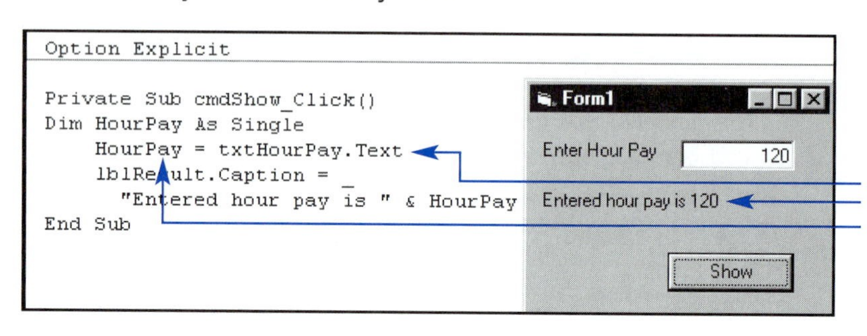

This illustration shows that you can assign data entered into a text box to a variable, whose content can then be displayed.

Notice that the left side of an assignment statement must be a variable or a control property whose value can be set at runtime. Notice also that the equal sign in the statement does not mean "equal" but represents an instruction to move the result on the right side to the variable on the left. Thus, you can write a statement such as the following:

```
I = I + 1
```

This statement says to add 1 to the value of I and then move the result to I. The effect is that I is increased by 1.

TIP

Keep in mind that the language has strict syntax rules that govern how each type of statement should be constructed. In the case of the assignment statement, only one variable can be on the left side. Thus, the following statements will result in ***compile errors***:

```
I, J = 1
I and J = 1
```

Also, the result of the following statement may not be what you expected:

```
I = J = 1
```

In some languages, this may mean I and J both are assigned a value 1. However, in VB, this line means to compare whether J is equal to 1. If so, assign a value True to I; otherwise, assign False.

Swapping Two Values. Once assigned a new value, the variable loses its previous content. Thus, it is important to remember that if you still need the original value of the variable, you will have to keep it in another variable before assigning a new value to it. For example, suppose you need to swap the values for two variables, named AdamsPay and JonesPay. The following code will *not* get the desired results:

```
AdamsPay = JonesPay
JonesPay = AdamsPay
```

This code fails because the first line assigns JonesPay (e.g., 5000) to AdamsPay. AdamsPay now has the value of 5000, no matter what it had previously. This in effect results in both variables containing the same value, JonesPay. The second line assigns 5000 to JonesPay, which was the original value of JonesPay anyway.

How do we solve this problem? As suggested, because we will need the original value of AdamsPay, we should find a way to keep its value before the variable is assigned with another value. You can do this by introducing a temporary variable to hold the original value of AdamsPay. Once this is done, JonesPay can be assigned to AdamsPay and the value in the temporary variable (Adams' original value) can then be assigned to JonesPay. The diagram in Figure 4.7 shows how this algorithm works.

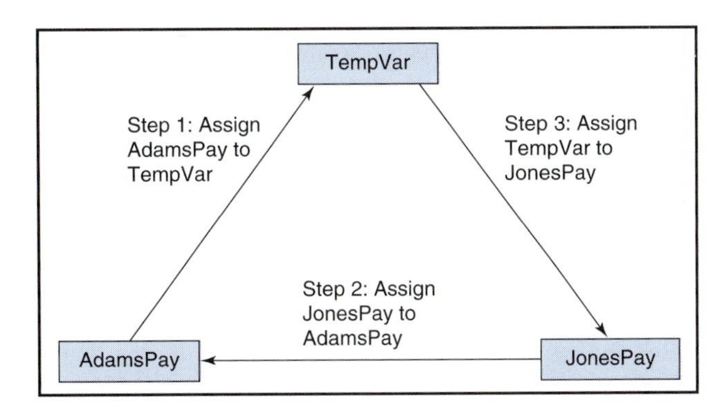

FIGURE 4.7
Swapping Data Between Two Variables

The following code accomplishes swapping the values of the two variables:

```
TempVar  = AdamsPay
AdamsPay = JonesPay
JonesPay = TempVar
```

In the future, you may see many situations where at the first glance, the problem appears pretty hard to tackle. In such cases, your solution may lie in an introduction of an additional variable. Please remember this point.

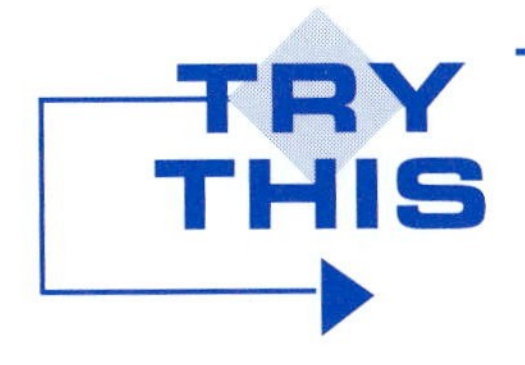

Draw a command button onto your new form. Set its Name property to cmdSwap and its Caption property to "Swap." Enter the following code. Run the program, click the button, and observe the result. You should be able to verify the swap.

```
Private Sub cmdSwap_Click()
Dim TempVar As Single
Dim AdamsPay As Single
Dim JonesPay As Single
    AdamsPay = 5000
    JonesPay = 7500
    TempVar = AdamsPay
    AdamsPay = JonesPay
    JonesPay = TempVar
    MsgBox "After the swap, AdamsPay is " & AdamsPay & _
        " JonesPay is " & JonesPay
End Sub
```

Numeric Operations

Back to our discussion of the assignment statement. The code that appears on the right side of the equal sign (=) is recognized as ***expression***, which can be a constant, a variable, or any operations on any combinations of constants and variables that result in a value. The symbols used to express ***arithmetic operations*** in VB are similar to our daily arithmetic symbols and are listed in the following table.

Symbol	Arithmetic Operations	Example	Meaning
-	Negation (unary)	-A	Negative value of A
+	Addition	A + B	A plus B
-	Subtraction	A – B	A minus B
*	Multiplication	A * B	A times B
/	Division	A / B	A divided by B
^	Power	A ^ B	A^B
Mod	Modulus	A Mod B	The remainder of A divided by B

The following are examples of valid expressions:

```
Salary + Commission
Mph * Hours
(Fahrenheit - 32) * 5 / 9
3.1416 * R ^ 2
20 Mod 3
```

The Mod operation divides the first operand by the second operand and returns the remainder. Thus, the last expression, 20 Mod 3, will give 2 as a result because the remainder of 20/3 is 2.

Operational Precedence. When you combine several arithmetic operations in one expression, the order of execution resembles the ordinary arithmetic rules of precedence as follows (from highest to lowest):

1. The unary negation (-); that is, a negative sign followed by an expression, such as -3 or –X
2. The exponential operation (^)
3. Multiplication, division, and Mod (*, /, and Mod)
4. Addition and subtraction (+ and -)

When the expression involves two or more operations of the same level of precedence, the execution goes from left to right.

Use of Parentheses. In many cases, you may find this order not exactly what you want. You can use parentheses to change the order of execution. An operation enclosed in a pair of parentheses will always be performed first. You can place as many pairs of parentheses as you want in an expression. You can also nest the parentheses. In this case, operations in the innermost pair will be performed first. Here are some examples of expressions using parentheses:

```
(7 + 8) * 3
(1 + Rate) ^ N ' compound interest for n periods
H * (A * X ^ (1 + B)) 'total costs for the learning curve effect
```

Data Type Conversions

If an arithmetic operation in an expression has two operands that are of different data types, VB will have to perform conversion to make them the same type before it can proceed with the computation. In addition, if the result of the expression has a different data type from that of the variable on the left side of the assignment statement, VB will also make a conversion before moving the result to the variable. For example, consider the following code:

```
Dim I As Integer
I = .5 * 20
```

There will be two conversion operations in executing the preceding code. In the code, .5 is a floating point constant, whereas 20 is an integer constant. To make the two operands compatible, the number with smaller range or precision will be converted to the one with higher range and precision. Thus, before the multiplication operation, 20 must be converted to a single floating point number. The multiplication is then carried out in a single floating point operation. The result is a single floating point value (10), which is then converted back to an integer number before it can be stored in an Integer variable.

Sometimes, unexpected results may occur. Consider the following code:

```
Private Sub Form_Click()
Dim A As Long
    A = 1000 * 1000
    MsgBox "1000 x 1000 = " & A
End Sub
```

What result do you expect when you run the program and click the form? It gives a runtime error—overflow! You know the Long variable A can certainly handle the resulting value (1,000,000) in the assignment statement. What caused the problem? Both of the constants (1000) are treated as integers. Thus, the multiplication is done as an integer operation. As you recall, the highest value an integer can take on is 32767, which is certainly much smaller than the result of the multiplication! To avoid problems of this nature, always use the same data type for all operands and the variable on the left side of the assignment.

Sometimes, you may have to use operands that are of different type from the variable on the left side. In such a case, you can explicitly use VB's built-in data conversion functions to perform the conversion. These built-in functions are discussed later in this section. For our problem, you can use one of the following lines as the assignment statement to avoid the overflow error:

```
' make one of the operands Long, forcing the other to convert
A = 1000 * 1000& '& is the type suffix for Long integer
A = 1000& * 1000& ' Make both Long, same type as the variable
A = CLng(1000) * CLng(1000) 'use the "convert to Long" function
```

Computing Net Sale: An Application Example

You have learned a lot about numeric data in this chapter. These are in addition to those VB controls you learned in Chapter 3, "Some Visual Basic Controls and Events." Have you been wondering how all these can be put together into an application? The purpose of this example is to show you how VB controls and numeric data can be used together for a simple but practical application. Please work along as you read.

The Project. A retailer's gross receipts consist of cash and credit cards. Both cash and credit card receipts are deposited in the bank daily. Before making the deposit, the owner needs to figure out her net receipts (which will be her actual amount of deposit). Cash is deposited on a one for one basis; that is, there is no discount or fee. However, she has to pay the bank a processing fee of 2.5% for all credit card receipts. You are to develop a project to compute the net receipts that she can use to prepare her deposit slips.

Input, Process, and Output. One way to analyze the project is to examine the input, process, and output of the project. It is usually easier to consider the output first. What the retailer needs to know is the net receipts that include both cash and net credit card receipts. It would also be nice to show the amount of credit card processing fees. The input should include the amount of cash and gross credit card receipts.

The process (computation) should be fairly simple. There will be no change in cash receipts between the gross and net amount. The credit card processing fee can be computed from the gross credit card receipts. The formula should be as follows:

```
ProcessingFees = GrossCreditCardReceipts x .025
```

This analysis can be shown as in the following table.

Input	Processing	Output
Cash receipts	None	Cash receipts
Gross credit card receipts (GCCR)	GCCR × .025	Credit card processing fees (CCPF)
	GCCR – CCPF	Net credit card receipts

In addition, it will be nice to show total gross and net receipts. The retailer can use the total gross amount to verify the entered data. The total net receipt amount can be used for the preparation of deposit slips.

The Visual Interface. What VB controls should we use to obtain input from the user? Both cash receipts and credit card receipts are numeric. The exact amounts vary from day to day. It would appear that text boxes are the most suitable VB controls to use. Output can also be displayed in text boxes. However, we do not want the user to accidentally change the results. Thus, label controls would be a better choice. In addition, we can make the labels look like text boxes by properly setting their BackColor and BorderStyle properties. We can also set both text boxes and all labels to display amounts right-justified so that they will feel and appear "right." For code clarity, we can use a named constant for the processing fee rate. We will also use variables to store computational data before the values are displayed in the output labels.

When should the computation be carried out and displayed? For simplicity, the computation will be done when the user clicks on a command button with a caption "Compute." It would also be nice to provide the user a command button to quit. A sketch of the interface design is presented in Figure 4.8.

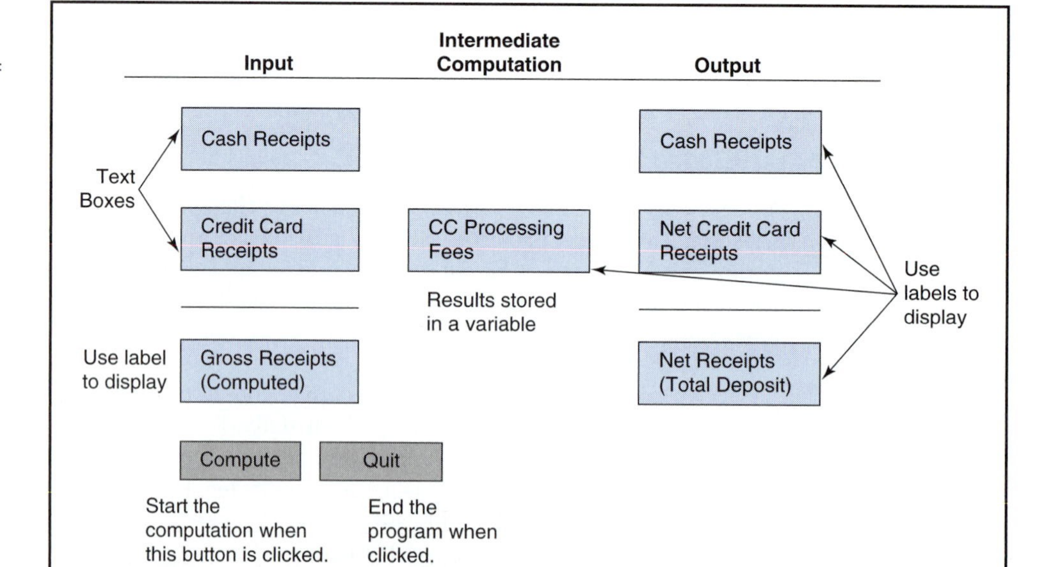

FIGURE 4.8
A Sketch of Input, Process, and Output of the Receipts Project

As you may recall, we learned in Chapter 2 that text boxes by themselves give no clues to the user about what they are or what the user should do. Thus, when we translate this sketch into a VB form layout, we must also add proper labels. The resulting visual interface appears as in Figure 4.9.

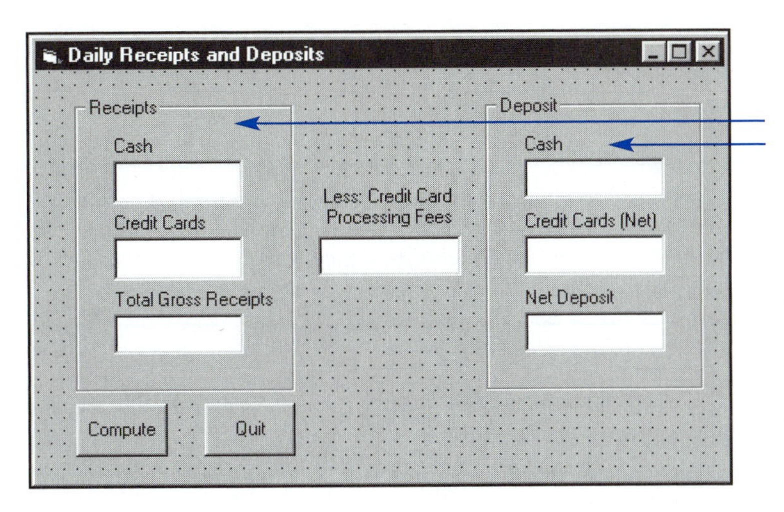

FIGURE 4.9 Visual Interface for the Receipts Project

In this application, the user will enter cash and credit card receipts on the left column. When the user clicks the Compute button, all other amounts will be computed and displayed. The "boxes" for all the computed amounts are label controls to prevent accidental alterations by the user.

The settings of selected properties of the VB objects used are summarized in the table that follows.

Named Object	Description	Property	Setting
txtCash	For cash input	Alignment MultiLine	Right Justify True (to make right alignment work; you may not need this)
txtCreditCards	For credit card input	Alignment MultiLine	Right Justify True (to make right alignment work; you may not need this)
lblGrossReceipts	To display gross receipts	BackColor BorderStyle Alignment	White Fixed single Right Justify
lblProcessingFees	To display processing fees	BackColor BorderStyle Alignment	White Fixed single Right Justify
lblNetCash	To display cash receipts	BackColor BorderStyle Alignment	White Fixed single Right Justify
lblNetCreditCards	To display net credit cards	BackColor BorderStyle Alignment	White Fixed single Right Justify
lblNetReceipts	To display net receipts	BackColor BorderStyle Alignment	White Fixed single Right Justify
cmdCompute	To perform computations	Caption	Compute
cmdQuit	To end the program	Caption	Quit

Declaring the Variables and Constant. Before writing any code, let's try to identify the variables to use and their data types. In addition, we should also consider whether to name any constant to be used in the project. From our analysis:

- We know cash and credit cards entered will be used in computations. We can use variables to hold the data entered into the text boxes. For computations, variables are faster and easier to reference than the properties of controls.

- We also need variables to hold credit card processing fees and the net credit card receipts.

If you need to refer to a property setting several times in a procedure, assign it to a variable first. From then on, use the variable. The code executes faster with a variable than with a property of an object. Of course, if the property setting changes, the variable will need to be reassigned with the new setting.

The next question is: What data type should each variable be? Recall in our previous discussion, we suggested that the same data type be used for all the variables in a statement to avoid the problem with conversion. Because all these variables will be used to handle amounts, they will involve decimal points. This excludes the Integer and Long types from consideration. The floating point (Single and Double) and Currency types are the potential candidates. You may recall that the Single type can handle only about six or seven significant digits. If the retailer has a gross sale in excess of $100,000.00, the Single type will not have enough precision (or, call it field width) to handle the amount. Thus, the choice should be between Double and Currency. The Currency type has the advantage of being accurate but is slower in speed than the Double type. Assume that the processing speed is the most important criterion for this project. Our choice will then be the Double type for all variables. With all these considerations, we will now place the following code in the ***cmdCompute Click event*** procedure:

```
Dim Cash As Double
Dim CreditCards As Double
Dim ProcessingFees As Double
Dim NetCreditCards As Double
```

Because a variable should be declared before it is used, it makes sense *to place all the preceding lines at the beginning of the procedure*. Doing so also has another advantage. When you need to check the declaration for a particular variable, it is much easier to locate at a "predetermined" location.

How do we handle the credit card processing rate? Using a named constant for the rate appears to have some advantages. First, the name itself can give a clear purpose for the computation. More important, if the rate literal is used in several places in the project, when there is a change in the rate, you may have to search over the entire project to make the corrections. On the other hand, if you use a named constant, you define it at only one place and therefore revise the rate only once at the same place. With this consideration, we will place the following line in the general declaration area in the code window:

```
Option Explicit
Const CreditCardRate As Double = 0.025
```

Again, the constant is declared as the Double type to be consistent with all the variables used to avoid data type conversion. Placing the declaration in the general declaration area will make the constant recognizable in all procedures.

Computations. Once we have the variables declared, we can assign the content of the text boxes to them:

```
'Store user entered data in variables
Cash = txtCash.Text
    CreditCards = txtCreditCards.Text
```

These variables can then be used in the computations. The credit card processing fees are computed by multiplying the (gross) credit card receipts by the processing fee rate:

```
' Perform fees computations
ProcessingFees = CreditCards * CreditCardRate
```

The net credit card receipts is the difference between the gross credit card receipts and the processing fees.

```
' Find net credit card deposit
NetCreditCards = CreditCards - ProcessingFees
```

Displaying the Results. We are now ready to display the results. "Net" cash will be the same as its original amount. Both the computational results will be displayed in their corresponding labels.

```
' Display results
lblNetCash.Caption = Cash
lblProcessingFees.Caption = ProcessingFees
lblNetCreditCards.Caption = NetCreditCards
```

The totals can be displayed by adding cash and gross/net credit card receipts.

```
' Display totals
lblNetReceipts.Caption = Cash + NetCreditCards
lblGrossReceipts.Caption = Cash + CreditCards
```

Finally, we also need to provide code to end the program execution. This is done in the cmdQuit Click event procedure. As explained in Chapter 2, a good way to handle this is to unload the form:

```
Unload Me
```

The Complete Code. Putting everything together, the complete code appears as follows:

```
Option Explicit
Const CreditCardRate As Double = 0.025

Private Sub cmdCompute_Click()
Dim Cash As Double
Dim CreditCards As Double
Dim ProcessingFees As Double
Dim NetCreditCards As Double

'Store user entered data in variables
    Cash = txtCash.Text
    CreditCards = txtCreditCards.Text

    ' perform fees computations
    ProcessingFees = CreditCards * CreditCardRate
    ' find net credit card deposit
    NetCreditCards = CreditCards - ProcessingFees

' Display results
    lblNetCash.Caption = Cash
    lblProcessingFees.Caption = ProcessingFees
    lblNetCreditCards.Caption = NetCreditCards
'Display totals
    lblNetReceipts.Caption = Cash + NetCreditCards
    lblGrossReceipts.Caption = Cash + CreditCards
End Sub

Private Sub cmdQuit_Click()
    Unload Me
End Sub
```

An Issue of Presentation. Have you been actually working on our example? If you have (and you should), it is time to test run the program to see if it gives the correct and desired results. The program should work. However, you might discover one minor problem. When the credit card receipts have a fractional number, the resulting amounts on the form do not appear to be neatly presented; some may have no decimal points, and others may have a decimal point with several digits to the right. Is there a way to force the computer to display two decimal places for all amounts so that they appear neatly aligned by the decimal point? The answer lies in the Format function.

The Format Function

The Format function provides a wide variety of formatting capabilities. The syntax is as follows:

```
Format$(Expression, Formatting String)
```

where *Expression* represents any valid expression that evaluates to either a string or a number to be formatted and *Formatting string* represents a string that specifies the format.

The formatting string can be a user-defined string or a name recognized by VB. For example, VB recognizes the name "Standard," which will show the number with commas (as thousand separators) and a period with two decimal places; for example, Format$(3000, "Standard") will give the result: 3,000.00. The following table lists selected additional named numeric formats.

Format Name	Meaning	Example Code	Result
Currency	Display the dollar sign before the number with thousand separator and two digits to the right of the decimal point.	`Format$(3000, "Currency")`	$3,000.00
Fixed	Display at least one digit to the left and two digits to the right of the decimal point.	`Format$(3000.1, "Fixed")`	3000.10
Percent	Display number multiplied by 100 with a percentage sign (%) appended to the right with two digits to the right of the decimal point.	`Format$(0.25, "Percent")`	25.00%
Scientific	Use standard scientific notation.	`Format$(1234, "Scientific")`	1.234E+03

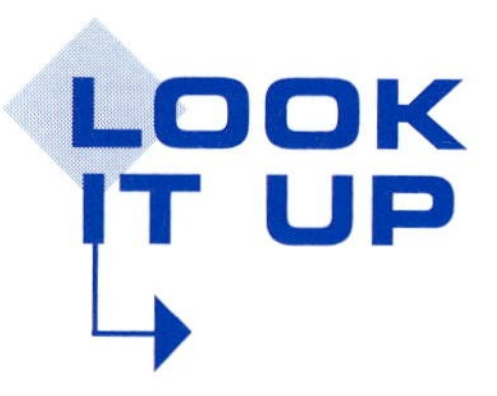

Search the Index tab of the online Help file with the keyword "Number formats." You should see many additional named formats for numbers and date/time data. It also shows special symbols that can be used to define your own format. Remember this keyword. You may have to visit that Help page often in the future.

We can use the Format function with the Standard format to display all the amounts in the form. To do so, the statement to display (net) cash should be changed to the following:

```
lblNetCash.Caption = Format$(Cash, "Standard")
```

All other statements to display the amounts should be changed similarly. You will notice that "Standard" appears in several lines of code. You can, instead, use a symbolic constant (e.g., FmtStandard) in place of all the literal "Standard." You can declare the constant right next to the declaration of credit card processing rate:

```
Const FmtStandard as String = "Standard"
```

Then the statement to display (net) cash can be changed to the following:

```
lblNetCash.Caption = Format$ (Cash, FmtStandard)
```

All other amounts, including the two text boxes, can be formatted in a similar fashion. In case you decide to change the format (e.g., to Currency) later, all you will have to do is to change the constant value.

A Side Note on Design. In the previous example, the credit card rate was treated as a constant. In a real application, this may not be a good design. The rate can change. Each time the change occurs, you will need to change and recompile the program. A careful design should call for the rate to be saved in some file/database and read in when your program starts. I have seen a commercial program with the Social Security tax rate hard-coded in the program. When the client company called for an update, the software company charged the client "service fees." Don't you think this practice is taking advantage of their own poor design?

4.4 Built-In Numeric Functions

VB also provides many built-in functions that can be used to handle conversion, mathematical, and financial operations.

Mathematical Functions

The following table outlines mathematical functions.

Function	Use	Code Example	Result
Abs(*x*)	Returns the absolute value of x	`Abs(-3.2)`	3.2
Cos(*x*)	Returns the cosine value of x, where x is an angle in radians	`Cos(3.14159265359)`	-1
Exp(*x*)	Returns the value of e^x	`Exp(1)`	2.71828182845905
Fix(*x*)	Returns the integer portion of x by truncation	`Fix(3.6)`	3
Int(*x*)	Returns the integer portion of x by truncation	`Int(3.6)`	3
Log(*x*)	Returns the natural logarithm of x	`Log(2.71828182845905)`	1
Rnd	Returns a random number in the range of 0 to 1 (but less than 1)	`Rnd`	Fractional random number
Sgn(*x*)	Returns the sign (1, 0, or –1) of x	`Sgn(-9)`	-1
Sin(*x*)	Returns the sine value of x, where x is an angle in radians	`Sin(0)`	0
Sqr(*x*)	Returns the square root of x	`Sqr(100)`	10

Fix and ***Int*** differ in their way of handling negative values. Fix truncates the fraction, whereas Int gives the next negative integer smaller than the parameter; for example, Fix(-3.3) will return –3, whereas Int(-3.3) will return –4.

Rnd is a random number generator, which returns a random fractional number between 0 and 1 each time it is called. Rnd uses a seed to start the random number sequence. To avoid repeating the same sequence each time you run a program, you can use the ***Randomize statement*** to set a different seed as follows:

```
Randomize
```

The Randomize statement uses the system timer as the seed for the random number sequence. Because it is virtually impossible to have the same timer value repeated, there is no chance that the same sequence of random numbers will be generated.

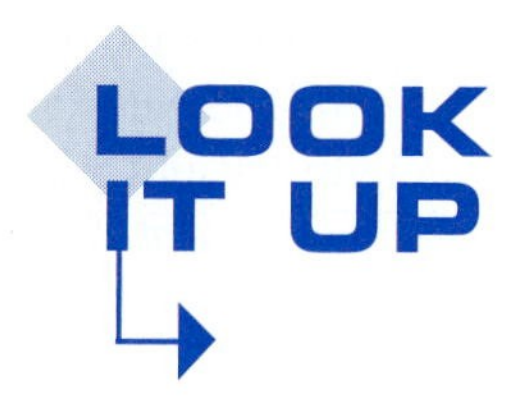

The Rnd function can also take an optional parameter. Depending on the value of the parameter, Rnd can behave differently, ranging from giving the same number every time to providing the most recently generated random number. Check the Rnd function in the Index tab of the online Help file for details.

Conversion Functions

The following table lists some conversion functions.

Function	Use	Code Example	Result
CBool(*x*)	Returns a Boolean type value; all nonzero values converted to True	`CBool(1)`	True
CByte(*x*)	Returns a Byte type value	`CByte("12")`	12
CCur(*x*)	Returns a Currency type value	`CCur("12.34")`	12.34
CDate(*x*)	Returns a Date/Time type value	`CDate("31-Dec-98")`	12/31/98
CDbl(*x*)	Returns a Double type value	`CDbl("12.34")`	12.34
CDec(*x*)	Returns a Decimal type value	`CDec("12.34")`	12.34
CInt(*x*)	Returns an Integer type value	`CInt("12.34")`	12
CLng(*x*)	Returns a Long type value	`CLng("12.34")`	12
CSng(*x*)	Returns a Single type value	`CSng("12.6")`	12.6

In all the conversion functions listed in the table, *x* is an expression that can be evaluated to a numeric value. These functions typically are used to convert from one numeric data type to another. However, they can also be used to convert strings that appear to human beings as numbers. For example, the expressions CLng("3,456") and CLng("$3,456") will both yield a result of 3456. However, the expression CLng(" ") will result in a "type mismatch" error because a blank space is not considered to be a number.

You may have noticed that the preceding example program to compute net receipts behaves exactly as described here, although the content of the text box is assigned to the numeric variable directly without calling any conversion function. The Text property of the text box is of the Variant type. However, those variables are declared to be the Double type. As noted previously, when the data type of the expression (source) is different from the variable on the left side (target) of an assignment statement, a data conversion will occur. Thus, one of these conversion functions is automatically called.

Note also, the Int and Fix functions differ from CInt and CLng in that the former pair truncate the fractional portion from the result, and the latter round the number. Thus, using the number 5.5 in Int or Fix will have a result of 5 but will have a result of 6 with CInt or CLng.

Date/Time Functions

Date/Time functions are listed in the following table.

Function	Use	Code Example	Result
Date	Returns (sets) current date as set in the computer	`Date`	Today

Function	Use	Code Example	Result
Now	Returns current date and time as set in the computer	`Now`	Current date and time
Time	Returns current time as set in the computer	`Time`	Current time
DateSerial(*year,month,day*)	Returns a date given the year, month, and day in the parameter	`DateSerial(00, 5, 31)`	5/31/00
DateValue(*Date*)	Returns a date given a string such as "02-28-1998" as the parameter	`DateValue("May-31-00")`	05/31/00
DateAdd(*interval, number, date*)	Returns a Date/Time value after adding the specified date by the specified number of intervals	`DateAdd("m", 2 , "03-31-00")`	05/31/00

The DateAdd function is a versatile function in handling Date/Time data. The interval parameter can take on different strings representing different intervals such as year ("yyyy"), month ("m"), week ("ww"), hour ("h"), minute ("n"), and second ("s"). The number parameter requires a Long integer, while date can be any Date/Time value. For example, the following expression:

```
DateAdd("s", 5, Now)
```

will return a Date/Time value that represents 5 seconds from now. You can use the result to trigger an action, such as starting a screen capture program.

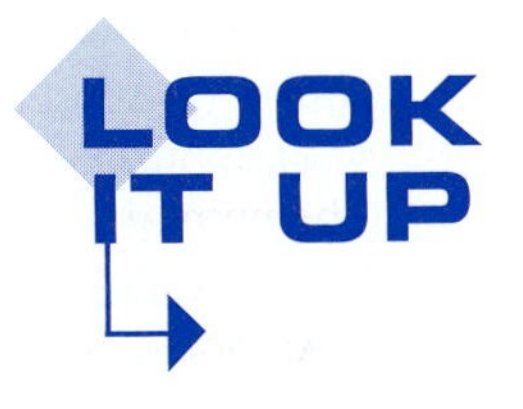

If you need to perform Date/Time calculations, use the keywords "DateAdd function" and "DateDiff function" to search the Index tab of the online Help file. These two pages provide details and fine points for various computations. For example, it shows that the expression, DateAdd("m", 1, "31-Jan-1995") will return "28-Feb-1995" and DateAdd("m", 1, "31-Jan-1996") will return "29-Feb-1996."

VB also provides financial functions that can be used to compute annuity, mortgage payments, and depreciation amounts. You can find these functions by searching the online Help file with the keyword "Financial functions."

Using Functions

You can use functions in any expressions in the same the way you use a constant or variable. Here are some examples, assuming all variables involved have been properly declared and assigned with proper values:

```
TheWidth = Abs (X1 - X2) 'width of a rectangle
GrossPay = CDbl (HourRate) * CDbl(HoursWorked) 'compute gross pay
' Compute total time under the learning curve model
```

```
TotalTime = InitTime * Units ^ _
    (1# + Log(LearningRate) / Log (2#))
Sample = Sqr(100 * Rnd) 'square root of 100 times a random number
MsgBox "Today is " & Date ' Display today
```

4.5 String Data

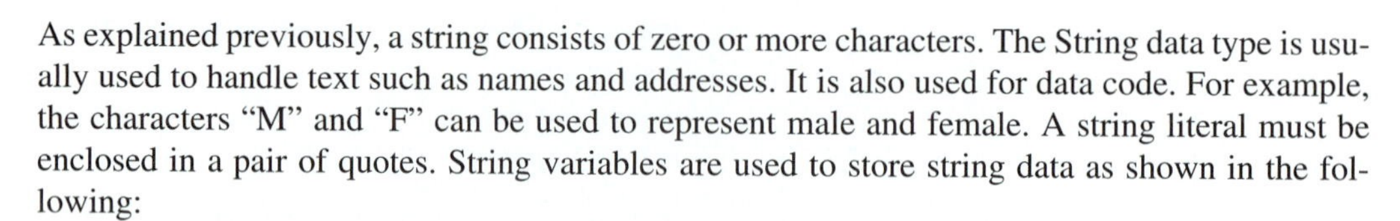

As explained previously, a string consists of zero or more characters. The String data type is usually used to handle text such as names and addresses. It is also used for data code. For example, the characters "M" and "F" can be used to represent male and female. A string literal must be enclosed in a pair of quotes. String variables are used to store string data as shown in the following:

```
LastName = "Smith"
```

The code moves the string literal "Smith" to the variable named LastName. You can also assign data in a control or a variable to another variable. For example, the following code will assign to the variable LastName with the text the user has entered in the text box control named txtLastName.

```
LastName = txtLastName.Text
```

Declaring String Variables

You can declare a string variable with one of the following syntax forms:

```
Dim Name As String
```

Or

```
Dim Name As String * n
```

For example, you can code:

```
Dim Address As String
```

Or

```
Dim Address As String * 32
```

You can use the syntax in the first line to declare a ***variable-length string*** and the second line to declare a ***fixed-length string*** with a length of 32 characters. A variable-length string variable can contain any number of characters. Its length depends on what is assigned to it. A fixed-length string variable contains exactly the number of characters as declared. If you assign a string longer than its length, the excess on the right is truncated. If you assign a string shorter than its length, its remaining portion is padded with blank spaces.

String Operations and Built-In Functions

You cannot perform computations on string data. However, you can perform concatenation on strings. The concatenation operation joins two separate strings. You can use either "+" or "&" as the symbol for the concatenation operation. Here are two examples of concatenations:

```
EmployeeName = "John " + "Smith"
EmployeeName = txtFirstName.Text & " " & txtLastName.Text
```

The first line will result in the string "John Smith" being assigned to the variable EmployeeName. In the second line, the content of the text box named txtFirstName is first concatenated with a blank space (" "). The result is then concatenated with the content of the text box named txtLastName. Finally, this result is assigned to the variable EmployeeName. If txtFirstName contains the string "John" and txtLastName contains the string "Smith," EmployeeName will have the string "John Smith" as the result.

The Ambiguous "+" Operator. Both "+" and "&" symbols can be used for the concatenation operation. However, the "+" operator can be ambiguous. This is particularly true when one of the operands involved is a string, and the other is a number. Consider these lines:

```
Dim Text as String
Text = "123" + "123"
Text = "123" + 123
Text = "ABC" + 123
```

The first line will result in Text containing the string "123123" as expected. However, the second line will result in Text containing a string value of "246." Because 123 is a number, VB considers "+" an addition operation, instead of concatenation. Thus, "123" is first converted to a number 123. The two numbers are then added together. The resulting value is then converted to a string before it is assigned to the variable Text.

The third line will cause a runtime "type mismatch" error. Again, VB treats the expression as a numeric addition first. When it is unable to successfully convert the string "ABC" to a number, it issues a type mismatch error message.

If you mean to have string concatenations for the previous examples, the following lines will produce the correct results:

```
Dim Text as String
Text = "123" & "123"
Text = "123" & 123
Text = "ABC" & 123
```

Because VB knows the "&" operator is only used for string concatenation, it will first convert 123 into a string "123" in the last two lines. The first two lines will result in a string of "123123," and the third line results in "ABC123."

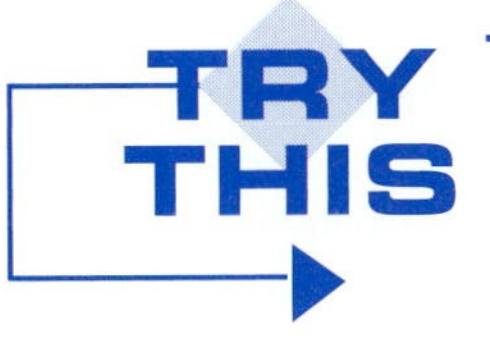

Type the following code in the code window of a new project. Run the project and click the form. Observe the results. Then replace the "+" symbol with the "&" symbol. Repeat the test. You should be able to get a good feel about how VB treats the two symbols.

```
Option Explicit
Private Sub Form_Click()
Dim Text123 As String
Dim TextABC As String
   Text123 = "123" + 123
   MsgBox "Text123 is " & Text123
   TextABC = "ABC" & 123
   MsgBox "TextABC is " & TextABC
End Sub
```

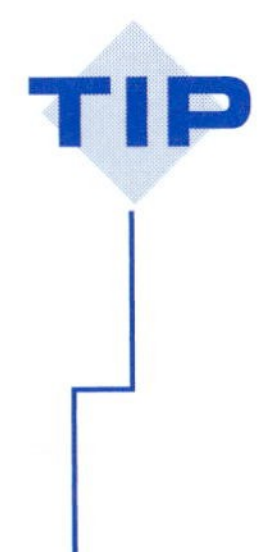

Because the "&" symbol is also used as a type suffix, you must be sure that there is a space between this symbol and the variable before it to avoid a syntax error. For example, the following expression:

```
FirstName& " " & LastName
```

will cause an error. But the following expression (notice the space before "&"):

```
FirstName & " " & LastName
```

will produce no error.

Built-In String Functions. In addition to the concatenation operation, many built-in string functions can be used to manipulate string data. The following table lists selected functions.

Function Name	Syntax	Use
Asc	Asc(*char*)	Returns the ASCII key code value of a character; for example, Asc("A") returns "65."
Chr$	Chr$(*n*)	Returns a character with an ASCII value n; for example, Chr$(65) returns "A."
Val	Val(*S*)	Converts the string S to a numeric value; for example, Val("-23.5") returns "–23.5."
Str$	Str$(*n*)	Converts a number n into a string; for example, Str$(-23.5) returns "–23.5."
StrReverse$	StrReverse$(*S*)	Returns a string of the mirror image of the string S; for example, StrReverse$("AB") returns "BA."
LCase$	LCase$(*S*)	Returns the lowercase of the string S; for example, LCase$("AbC") returns "abc."
UCase$	UCase$(*S*)	Returns the uppercase of the string S; for example, UCase$("AbC") returns "ABC."
Space$	Space$(*n*)	Generates a string with n blank spaces; for example, Space$(1) returns " ".
String$	String$(*n, char*)	Generates a string with n repetitive characters; for example, String$(3, "A") returns "AAA."
Left$	Left$(*S, n*)	Returns a string with the first n characters of the string S; for example, Left$("My Name", 2) returns "My."
Right$	Right$(*S, n*)	Returns a string with the last n characters of the string S; for example, Right$("My Name", 4) returns "Name."
Mid$	Mid$(*S, b,* [*n*])	Returns a string of n characters that starts at the bth position in S; for example, Mid$("My Name", 2, 3) returns "y N."
InStr	InStr([*p*],*S, c*)	Returns the position in S at which the content matches the string c. The comparison will start at position p. If p is omitted, it will start at position 1; for example, InStr("My Name", "y") returns "2."
InStrRev	InStrRev(*S,c,*[*p*])	Returns the position in S at which the content matches the string c. The comparison goes backward from position p. If p is omitted, it will start from the end; for example, InStrRev("02-02-43", "-") returns "6."
Len	Len(*S*)	Returns the length of the string; for example, Len("My Name") returns "7."
LTrim$	LTrim$(*S*)	Returns a string with all leading blank spaces trimmed off; for example, LTrim$(" My ") returns "My."
RTrim$	RTrim$(*S*)	Returns a string with all trailing blank spaces trimmed off; for example, RTrim$(" My ") returns "My."
Trim$	Trim$(*S*)	Returns a string with all the leading and trailing spaces trimmed off; for example, Trim$(" My ") returns "My."

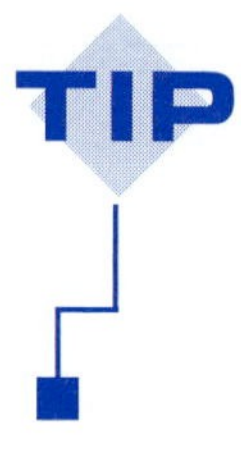

All the functions with a $ suffix have their counterparts without the suffix; for example, Trim$ and Trim both are valid function names performing basically the same function. The difference is that a function with a $ suffix returns a string, whereas the function without the suffix returns a Variant type. According to some empirical tests, the functions without the $ suffix take approximately 50% more time than their respective counterparts. *Always use the function with the $ suffix when the expected result is a string.*

Asc and Chr$ Functions. The Asc function returns the ASCII key code value of a character. For example, the ASCII key code value for "A" is 65. Thus, Asc("A") will return a value of 65. The Chr$ function converts a key code value to a character and can be considered the complement of the Asc function. Chr$(65) returns a character "A."

What do we need this pair of functions for? These functions provide a convenient way to perform computation on characters, which can become pretty tedious otherwise. For example, suppose you are developing a Scrabble game; you probably would need to provide a capability to generate a string of random letters. The Chr$ function makes this fairly easy.

First, you know there are 26 letters. Thus, you need to generate a random number within the range of 26 so that each number will correspond to a letter. The following code should accomplish this:

```
Int(Rnd * 26)
```

Because the Rnd function returns a fractional number in the range of 0 to 1 (but less than 1), multiplying the returned number by 26 should produce a number between 0 and 25.9999. The Int function will truncate the fractional portion, giving a result between 0 and 25. Because "A" has an ASCII value of 65, Int(Rnd * 26) + 65 should produce the ACSII value of the random letter. You can then use the Chr$ function to convert this ASCII value to display the letter.

```
MsgBox "The next random letter is " & Chr$(Int(Rnd * 26) + 65)
```

As another illustration, suppose you want to display the next letter following the one that the user has entered in a text box named txtLetter when the user clicks a command button named cmdNext. What code will you provide in the command button's Click event procedure? You will first obtain the ASCII value of the current letter (using the ASC function). Add 1 to that value to get the ASCII value of the next letter and then convert the result to the letter (using the Chr$ function). The code can appear as follows:

```
Private cmdNext_Click()
Dim KeyAscii As Integer
     'Get the ASCII value of the letter
     KeyAscii = ASC(txtLetter.Text)
     MsgBox "The next letter is " & Chr$(KeyAscii + 1)
End Sub
```

In this illustration, we assume the user will not enter the letter "Z" or more than one letter in the text box.

Val and Str$ Functions. The Val function converts a string into a numeric value. For example, Val("123") will return a value 123. The Str$ function does the opposite. It converts a number into a string. For example, Str$(123) will return a string " 123." Note that there is a leading blank space before the string "123." This can be very important if you intend to check the length of the resulting string. If you do not want the leading blank space for any reason, you should use the Format function instead. For example, Format$(123,"General Number") will return a string "123."

Note that the Val function ends its attempt to convert a string as soon as it encounters a nonnumeric character. Thus, Val(" ") will return a 0 with no error. In addition, Val("3,456") will return a value 3. Recall that CLng(" ") results in an error, whereas CLng("$3,456") will return a value of 3456. In a text box (e.g., txtUnitsSold), you may expect that the user will enter numbers with commas. Thus, one of the conversion functions should be used. However, you may also anticipate that the user will leave the box blank if the value to enter is zero. In such a case, the Val function will be "safer." Thus, you are faced with a dilemma of choosing the appropriate function to use. One possible solution is to use yet another function to decide which function to use. The function ***IsNumeric(S)*** can be used to test whether the string parameter S is a valid numeric string. If it is, the function returns a value True; otherwise, False. Thus, your solution can look like the following:

```
If IsNumeric(txtUnitsSold.Text) Then
    UnitsSold = CLng(txtUnitsSold.Text)
Else
    UnitsSold = Val(txtUnitsSold.Text)
End If
```

Or, you can even insist that the user enter a valid number before accepting the data. In this case, your code in the Else block will be a message requesting the user to enter a valid number.

LCase$ and UCase$ Functions. The LCase$ function returns a lowercase string. For example, LCase$("ABC") will return a string "abc." The UCase$ function returns the uppercase string. Thus, UCase$("abc") will give "ABC."

Space$ and String$ Functions. The function Space$(n) will generate a string with n blank spaces. The String$(n, char) function returns a string with n repeated characters, char. For example, String$(16, " ") will produce a string with 16 blank spaces. Note that the second argument in String$ can also be an ASCII code instead of a character. Thus, String$(16, " ") and String$(16, 32) will produce the same result because the ASCII code for the blank space is 32.

Left$, Right$, and Mid$ Functions. The Left$, Right$, and Mid$ functions deal with the substring of a string. Left$(S, n) returns the first n characters of the string S. Thus, Left$("Upper",2) returns "Up." Right$(S, n) returns the last n characters in string S. Thus, Right$("Upper",3) will return "per." The Mid$(S, b, n) returns a string of n characters in S beginning from the bth position. Mid$("Upper", 2, 3) will return "ppe." If the third parameter is omitted, all the remaining string starting from the Bth position will be returned. For example, Mid$("Upper", 2) will return "pper."

Mid$ can also be used as the target of a string assignment. For example, assume the string variable MyStr contains a string "Uppercase." The following code will change the string to "Upper hand":

```
Mid$(MyStr, 7, 4) = "hand"
```

In this statement, the four characters in MyStr starting from the seventh position are replaced with a string "hand." The last argument in Mid$ is an optional argument. If it is omitted, either the remaining length of MyStr or the length of the expression on the right side of the assignment (whichever is shorter) is used. The following table summarizes the examples discussed concerning these functions.

Code	Result (Value of A)
`A = Left$(''Upper'', 2)`	"Up"
`A = Right$(''Upper'', 3)`	"per"
`A = Mid$(''Upper'', 2, 3)`	"ppe"
`A = Mid$(''Upper'', 2)`	"pper"
`A = ''Uppercase'' Mid$(A, 7, 4) = ''Hand''`	"Upper Hand"

The InStr and InStrRev Function. The InStr(S, ss) function returns the position in S where its substring matches the string ss. For example, InStr("ABCDE", "CD") will return a value 3. Actually, the complete syntax for the function is as follows:

```
InStr([p],S,ss,[Compare])
```

where *p* = the position in S at which to begin the search
S = the string to be searched on
Ss = the substring to search for
Compare = a value to specify the type of comparison; for example, the named constant vbTextCompare will cause the search to not be case sensitive

You can find additional constants for different comparisons by searching the Index tab of the online Help file with the keyword "InStr function."

Using this syntax, the expression InStr("12-31-1999", "-") will return a value 3 and the expression InStr(4, "12-31-1999","-") will return a value 6. The InStrRev function has the following syntax:

```
InStrRev(S,ss,[p],[Compare])
```

Where all the parameters have exactly the same meaning as those parameters in the InStr function. However, the positions in which the parameters are placed in the two functions are different. Also note that to specify the fourth parameter for the InStr function, you must also provide the value for the first parameter, as shown in the second through fifth code examples in the following table.

Code	Result (Value of Pos)
`Pos = InStr("Containing", "in")`	6
`Pos = InStr(1, "Containing", "in")`	6
`Pos = InStr(7, "Containing", "in")`	8
`Pos = InStr(7, "Containing", "In")`	0
`Pos = InStr(7, "Containing", "In", vbTextCompare)`	8
`Pos = InStrRev("Containing", "in")`	8
`Pos = InStrRev("Containing", "In", ,vbTextCompare)`	8

These functions and the substring functions (Left$, Right$, Mid$) together form a very useful group of functions in parsing strings. An illustration is provided in the next subsection.

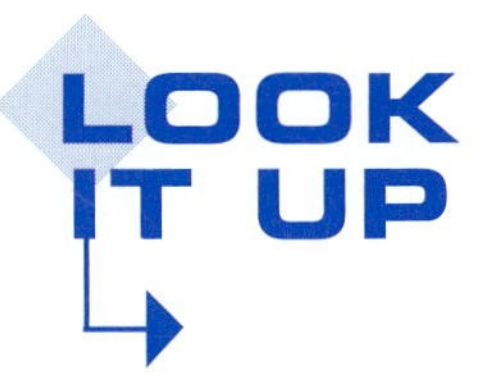

Search the Index tab of the online Help file for the keyword "InStr function" to find additional explanations of the function. The page provides a list of the available settings for the compare parameter. The "See Also" link will lead you to the Help page for the InStrRev function.

The Len Function. The Len function returns the length of the string. For a variable-length string, Len returns the string's actual length, including blank spaces. The string " " containing nothing between the quotes has a length zero. Thus, Len(" ") will return a value of 0. In contrast, if a zero-length string is assigned to a fixed-length string, the Len function will still return the length of the string, not zero. For example:

```
Dim MyString as String * 6
MyString = ""
MsgBox "Length of MyString is " & Len(MyString)
```

The message box will still display the length as 6. As explained previously, the length of a fixed-length string will not change. The string is padded with spaces when it is assigned with a zero-length string.

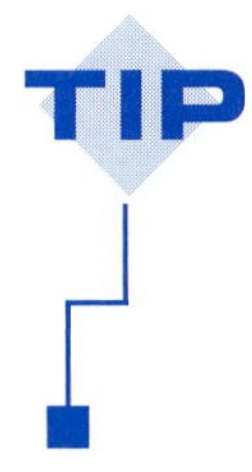

If you need to check whether a string (e.g., MyStr$) is of zero length, your code is more efficient with the following:

```
If Len (MyStr$) = 0 Then
```

than with:

```
If MyStr$ = "" Then
```

Trim$, Ltrim$, and Rtrim$ Functions. If you are interested in the length of the visible characters in the fixed-length string, you can use the Trim$ function to trim off the spaces and obtain the length accordingly. Len(Trim$(MyString)) should give the length of the string with no leading or trailing spaces. If you are interested in trimming off only the leading spaces of any string, you can use the LTrim$ function to do the job. Furthermore, if you are interested in trimming off only the trailing spaces, you should use the Rtrim$ function.

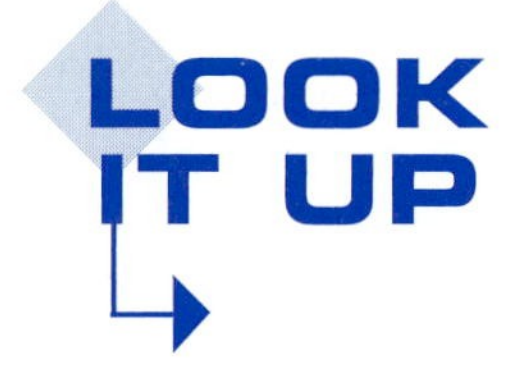

Search the keyword "String functions" in the Index tab of the online Help file. The box will display two "String functions." There are several items under the second one. Among the list is "new in Visual Basic 6.0." Double-click that item and scroll down the page and you will see a list of more than a dozen new string functions. These functions can really make your job of manipulating strings much easier. Look in particular for Replace, Split, and additional Format functions.

The Calculating Vending Machine: An Example

To illustrate how some of the aforementioned string handling functions can be used to solve a programming problem, let's consider an example. In this project, a list box is used as the display of a vending machine. The customer buys an item by clicking on it. The visual interface of the project in action is given in Figure 4.10. At runtime, this program behaves in the following manner:

- When the user clicks an item in the list box (named lstVending), he or she buys it. (No confirmation. No refund. It's a vending machine after all.) The price is added to the total. *Note:* Do not change the settings for the MultiSelect or Style property.
- When the user finishes the purchase, he or she clicks a button (named cmdShow) captioned, "That's all." The computer will then display all the items purchased as well as the total, as shown in Figure 4.10.
- When the user clicks another button (named cmdQuit) captioned "Quit," the program ends.

Setting Up the Vending Machine. The list box will display the items available as the program starts. How do we add the items to the "Vending Machine"? We can use the list box's AddItem method to add the food items along with their prices. (In a real application, items and their prices can be read from a file or database.) We would also like to align the prices in a column. This can be accomplished by inserting a ***tab character*** between the food item and its price. The key code constant for the tab character (Chr$(9)) is defined in VB as vbTab. We will have six items in the vending machine. The code should be placed in the Form Load event procedure:

```
Option Explicit
Private Sub Form_Load()
    lstVending.AddItem "New York Top Sirloin" & vbTab & "16.95"
    lstVending.AddItem "Boston Red Lobster" & vbTab & "26.95"
    lstVending.AddItem "Alaska King Salmon" & vbTab & "15.95"
    lstVending.AddItem "Home Made Sandwich" & vbTab & "12.95"
    lstVending.AddItem "Washington Red Apples" & vbTab & "4.95"
    lstVending.AddItem "Florida orange Juice" & vbTab & "5.95"
End Sub
```

Figure 4.10
The Vending Machine in Action

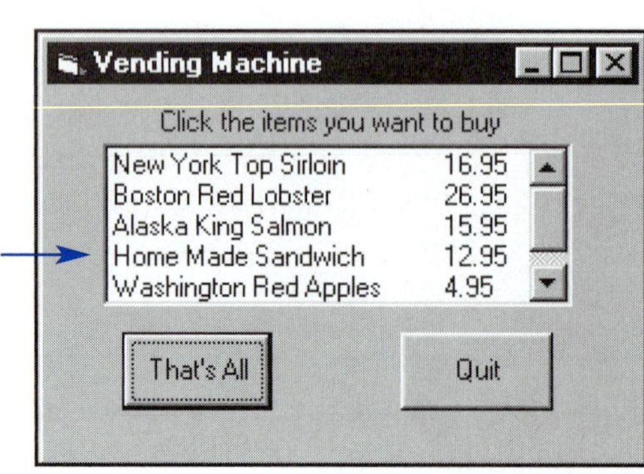

The vending machine offers expensive food. A list box is used to display menu items. What you click is what you get.

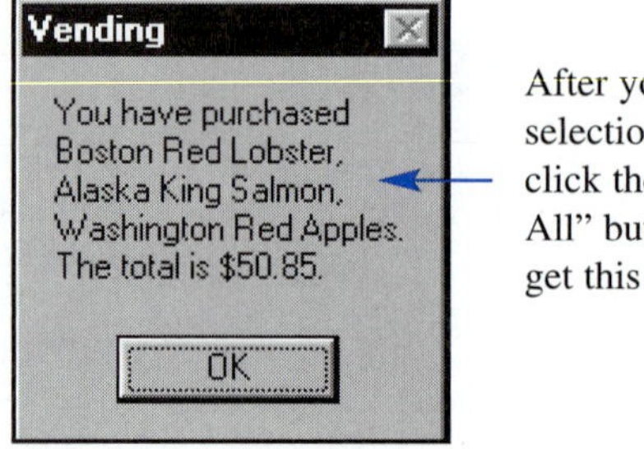

After you make the selections and click the "That's All" button, you get this message.

Notice that the length of each item varies slightly. The price of each item has a slightly different length, too. However, the use of the tab character (vbTab) helps align the prices fairly evenly.

A Side Note on Coding Mechanics. Notice the repetitive references to lstVending in the previous procedure. A coding structure exists that allows you to use a "shorthand" reference to the same object. This involves the use of the With...End With structure, which has the following syntax:

```
With Object
     Statements
End With
```

Inside the With block, any statement that begins with a dot (.) will be automatically qualified with the object. For example, the preceding Form Load event procedure can be rewritten as follows:

```
Private Sub Form_Load()
     With lstVending
          .AddItem "New York Top Sirloin" & vbTab & "16.95"
          .AddItem "Boston Red Lobster" & vbTab & "26.95"
          .AddItem "Alaska King Salmon" & vbTab & "15.95"
          .AddItem "Home Made Sandwich" & vbTab & "12.95"
          .AddItem "Washington Red Apples" & vbTab & "4.95"
          .AddItem "Florida orange Juice" & vbTab & "5.95"
     End With
End Sub
```

All the .AddItem statements will be interpreted as "lstVending.AddItem" because the With statement refers to lstVending. This structure is not only convenient for coding but also efficient for execution. The reference to the object is set for all statements in the block, thus avoiding the need to locate the object for each statement individually.

When you have a block of code that refers to an object several time, use the With...End With structure to reference the object. Your coding will be more efficient, the code will execute faster, and the code will also be easier to read.

Determining the Item the Customer Has Chosen. Next, when the user makes a selection by clicking an item in the "vending machine," what does the computer know? You may recall that the item is identified by the list box's Text property (as well as the ListIndex property). This item will be referenced several times in the program. Thus, we will assign the text to a variable, which we will name TheItem. We can code the following:

```
TheItem = lstVending.Text 'store the clicked item in a variable
```

Obtaining the Item Name. How do we get the name of the item from this text? (Recall that the text has both the name and the price.) We know that the item and its price are separated by the tab character. If we know the position of the tab character, we should be one step closer to solving our problem. We can use the InStr function to find this position. If we use the variable TabPos to keep track of the position, we can code the following:

```
' Find the position of vbTab in the selected item
TabPos = InStr(TheItem, vbTab)
```

The item name starts at the beginning of the string and ends one position before the tab character position. Thus, it can be computed as follows:

```
Left$(TheItem, TabPos - 1)
```

Putting Items Bought Together. The question then is what should we do with this result? Consider this list:

One, two, three, …

When you have only one item like "One," you will show only the item "One." If you have more than one item, you want to insert a comma (,) between the two items; that is, in addition to adding the item, you also add a comma and a space. Thus, if you use a variable named ItemsBot to track the items purchased, you will assign the item name to ItemsBot when this item is the first one; that is:

```
ItemsBot = Left$(TheItem, TabPos - 1) 'For the first item
```

If the item is not the first one, you will add a comma (with a space) and the item name to the existing string. Thus, the code should be as follows:

```
ItemsBot = ItemsBot & ", " & Left$(TheItem, TabPos - 1)
```

Showing Items on Separate Lines. Here is an additional thought. What if we want to show each item on a separate line? This ensures that the text to be displayed is wrapped properly. The character combination Chr$(13) & Chr$(10) (recognized as carriage return and line feed) will make the computer display what follows it in the next line. This constant has a predefined name vbCrLf. Thus, to make each item appear on a separate line, we can insert this named constant to the preceding code:

```
ItemsBot = ItemsBot & ", " & vbCrLf & Left$(TheItem, TabPos - 1)
```

Telling the First Item from Others. Finally, you can tell whether the current item is the first item purchased or not by checking the length of ItemsBot. If the current item is the first one, nothing has been bought before. The length of ItemsBot will be zero. Thus, the code to add the item name to the list ItemsBot should be as follows:

```
If Len(ItemsBot) = 0 Then
    'First item, just keep the item name
    ItemsBot = Left$(TheItem, TabPos - 1)
Else
    'Not the first item; add a comma, and concatenate the new item
    ItemsBot = ItemsBot & ", " & _
        vbCrLf & Left$(TheItem, TabPos - 1)
End If
```

Obtaining the Price. So far, we have taken care of the list of items bought. How do we get the price from TheItem? Recall that the price starts from one position beyond the tab character and extends to the end of TheItem. The Mid$ function can be used neatly to find the price string:

```
Mid$(TheItem, TabPos + 1)
```

Recall that the Mid$ function takes three parameters. When the last parameter is omitted, it returns the remainder of the string beginning with the position specified in the second parameter.

Accumulating the Total. We will use the variable called Total to keep track of the total purchases by the customer. The price string obtained previously should be converted to numeric data before it is added to Total. We can use the Val function to convert the price string. Thus:

```
' Add the purchase price to total
Total = Total + Val(Mid$(TheItem, TabPos + 1))
```

The Complete Code for a Selected Item. As described in the project requirements, the customer buys an item when he or she clicks on it. Thus, all the preceding code should be placed in the lstVending Click event procedure. The complete lstVending Click event procedure appears as follows:

```
Private Sub lstVending_Click()
Dim TabPos As Integer
Dim TheItem As String
```

```
        TheItem = lstVending.Text 'store selected item in a variable
        ' Find the position of vbTab in the clicked item
        TabPos = InStr(TheItem, vbTab)
        If Len(ItemsBot) = 0 Then
            ' first item, just keep the item name
            ItemsBot = Left$(TheItem, TabPos - 1)
        Else
            'Not the first item; add a comma, a CrLf
            'and concatenate the new item
            ItemsBot = ItemsBot & ", " & vbCrLf & _
            Left$(TheItem, TabPos - 1)
        End If
        ' add the purchase price to total
        Total = Total + Val(Mid$(TheItem, TabPos + 1))
    End Sub
```

Declaring the Variables Used. Notice that four variables have been used: ItemsBot, Total, TheItem, and TabPos. We need to consider their data types and scope. In terms of their data types:

- Both ItemsBot and TheItem are used to handle string data. They should be declared as the String type.
- Total is used to accumulate the purchase amount. Because the total does not require a number of many digits but can be a fractional number, it can be declared as a single floating point variable.
- TabPos is used to keep the position of vbTab in the string, TheItem, which does not have many characters. Thus, TabPos can be declared as an integer variable.

In terms of their scope:

- Both TheItem and TabPos are used only in the lstVending Click event procedure. We should declare (and have declared) them in that procedure.
- However, both ItemsBot and Total are used in both lstVending Click procedure and cmdShow Click procedure (discussed next). They should be placed in the general declaration area right after the Option Explicit line:

```
Option Explicit
Dim ItemsBot As String
Dim Total As Single
```

Handling "That's All." Finally, let's consider handling the event when the user clicks the button captioned "That's all." This is the event where your program should tell the user what he or she has purchased and the total amount. The list of purchased items has been collected in the lstVending Click procedure. We'd like for the computer to show a message like the following:

```
You have purchased
Boston Red Lobster,
Florida Orange Juice.
The total is $32.90.
```

More Text on Separate Lines. If you examine the tentative output carefully, you should notice that both the first line and the last line of output are on separate lines from the purchase list. In addition, at the end of the purchase list as well as the end of the total there is a period. This means the key code vbCrLf and the period should be added at the proper places. Notice also the amount displayed has a "$" sign and there should two decimal places, suggesting that the total should be formatted with the Currency format. The code should appear as follows:

```
MsgBox "You have purchased" & vbCrLf & ItemsBot & "." & _
vbCrLf & "The total is " & Format$(Total, "Currency") & "."
```

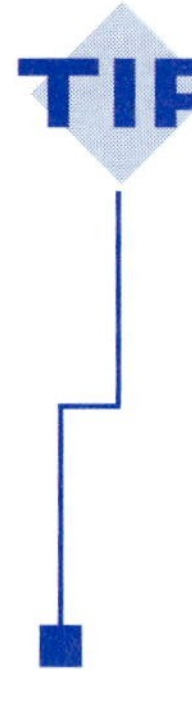

Be aware that you are not allowed to break a string constant into multiple lines as shown below:

```
lblDemo.Caption = "This is a demonstration of _
    an extremely long string message"
```

In the first line, the compiler considers the space and the underscore as a part of the string literal (because the string has not yet been closed with a double quote), thus fails to recognize it as an underscore for line continuation. The *correct code* should be as follows:

```
lblDemo.Caption = "This is a demonstration of " _
    & "an extremely long string message"
```

Um..., Not Yet. There is another fine point we should consider. What if the user clicks the "That's all" button before clicking any item? Using the previous line will result in the following message:

```
You have purchased
    .
The total is 0.00.
```

Although that's not too bad, it does not appear very neat. We'd rather inform the user that he or she has not yet selected any item. Recall that we can test whether any item has been purchased by checking the length of ItemsBot. Thus, the more complete code is as follows:

```
If Len(ItemsBot) = 0 Then
    MsgBox "You have not selected any item yet."
Else
    MsgBox "You have purchased" & vbCrLf & ItemsBot & "." & _
    vbCrLf & "The total is " & Format$(Total, "Currency") & "."
End If
```

Reinitializing Data for the Next Customer. Once the message is displayed, we should also clear ItemsBot and Total so that the vending machine will be ready for another customer. To do this, we can assign a zero-length string to ItemsBot and a value 0 to Total:

```
ItemsBot =""
Total = 0
```

Complete Code, "That's All." Recall that the name of the command button is cmdShow. The complete procedure to handle the event when the customer clicks the "That's all" button should appear as follows:

```
Private Sub cmdShow_Click()
    If Len(ItemsBot) = 0 Then
        MsgBox "You have not selected any item yet."
    Else
        MsgBox "You have purchased" & vbCrLf & ItemsBot & "." & _
          vbCrLf & "The total is " & _
          Format$(Total, "Currency") & "."
        ItemsBot = ""
        Total = 0
    End If
End Sub
```

Finally, we should also take care of the event when the user clicks the "Quit" button:

```
Private Sub cmdQuit_Click()
    Unload Me
End Sub
```

Additional Remarks. This example involves four event procedures:

1. The Form Load event procedure to prepare the list box to show food items
2. The lstVending Click procedure to accumulate the customer's purchases
3. The cmdShow Click procedure to display the result
4. The simple cmdQuit Click procedure to unload the form

Run and test the program. If everything works correctly, you should be able to verify that the computer:

- Displays in the list box all the items with their prices as soon as the program starts.
- Displays a "reminder" message if you click the "That's All" button before making any selection.
- Accumulates and displays correctly the items and the total prices you have "purchased" when you click the "That's All" button after you have made selections.

Ends the project when you click the Quit button.

Summary

The computer operates on data. In terms of their modifiability, data can be classified into constants and variables. Constants remain unchanged throughout the duration of the program, whereas variables vary as a result of operations or assignments. In terms of their uses, data can be classified as numeric or string. Numeric data are used for mathematical computations or logical operations (which are discussed in Chapter 5). Depending on the format in which they are stored, numeric data can be further classified by type into Byte, Boolean, Integer, Long, Single, Double, Currency, Decimal, and Date/Time. Each data type varies in speed and storage requirements. It therefore pays to understand the nature of each type.

There are various operations and built-in functions to handle numeric data. Most of the symbols used in mathematical operations (and even their precedence of execution) correspond well with the daily use. Many built-in functions are introduced in this chapter; some relate to mathematical operations, and others deal with data conversion. There are also Date/Time functions that can be useful. Many financial functions (including depreciation methods) have also been built into the VB system. Although we have not discussed any of them, if you have a special need for some financial computations, you should explore the online Help file. Chances are you will find some that can help you in solving your problems.

String data are used to handle texts and data code. There are also many built-in functions to handle string data. With these functions, you can easily extract or change a portion of a string. You can convert data between numeric and string easily. Such power and flexibility make it easy to develop useful applications such as string search, highlighting, replacing, and encrypting operations.

The Variant data type can take on any data type. With such flexibility, it can be used to handle tricky situations. However, it has greater storage requirements. Operations using Variants are much slower than those using any other data type. In addition, it is easy to run into unexpected results using this data type. Beginners are advised to stay away from it.

We also discussed the scope and lifetime of variables. Variables declared at the form (module) level are recognized by all procedures. Variables declared in a procedure are recognized only in that procedure. In general, you should declare a variable with as narrow a scope as possible. Such practice keeps your project free from unexpected data and code entanglement in which a change in one procedure affects the result or operation of another procedure.

Variables declared at the module (form) level remain "alive" for the entire duration of the form. Their values are preserved until the form is destroyed. Variables declared within a procedure with the Dim statement are reinitialized (as 0 for numeric data and as zero-length string for string data) each time the procedure is called. To keep the value of a procedure level (local) variable for the entire duration of the form, declare the variable with the Static statement.

Several examples have been provided in the text to help you understand and integrate the material better. Work on all of them. You can benefit immensely from such exercises.

Visual Basic Explorer

4-1. Some Hex Values of Interest. Type in the following code in a new form's Click event procedure. Run the project, click any part of the form, and examine the results.

```
Private Sub Form_Click()
     Print &HFF
     Print &HFF&
     Print &HFFFF
     Print &HFFFF&
End Sub
```

What values do you get? The first two values should give you no surprises. But what about the last two values? Why are they different? The value &HFFFF is of the Integer type. The two bytes holding the value have all the bits on. The highest bit of a number represents its sign. When it is on, it is a negative number. Its complement (whatever is required to add the value to zero) is the number's negative value. Adding 1 to &HFFFF will clear all bits, making it zero. Therefore, &HFFFF is –1.

The value &HFFFF& is a Long integer (because an "&" type suffix is attached). Its lower two bytes are all on, but its higher two bytes are all zero; that is, its internal coding is actually &H0000FFFF&. Therefore, it is a positive number and is 65535. (Perform the conversion as discussed in the text to verify.)

4-2. Numeric Value of True and False. Type in the following code in a new form's Click event procedure. Run the project, click any part of the form, and examine the results. What numeric values do True and False have?

```
Private Sub Form_Click()
     MsgBox "10 times True is " & 10 * True
     MsgBox "10 plus True is " & 10 + True
     MsgBox "10 times False is " & 10 * False
     MsgBox "10 plus false is " & 10 + False
End Sub
```

True is internally coded as a two-byte integer with all its bits on: &HFFFF, which is –1 as shown in 4-1. False is internally coded as a two-byte integer with all its bits off: &H0000. Thus, it is numerically zero.

4-3. Data Type in Numeric Operations. Type in the following code in a new form's Click event procedure. Run the project and click any part of the form. Overflow? Why? Now, change the line to A = 1000 * 1000& and try again. No problem? Why?

```
Private Sub Form_Click()
Dim A As Long
     A = 1000 * 1000
     MsgBox "A =" & A
End Sub
```

4-4. Data Type: Comparing Single, Double, and Currency Types. Type in the following code in a new form. Run the project and click any part of the form.

```
Option Explicit

Private Sub Form_Click()
Dim D As Double
Dim C As Currency
Dim S As Single
```

```
        D = 1234567890
        S = D
        C = D
        Print "D = "; D
        Print "S = "; S
        Print "C = "; C
    End Sub
```

What results do you see? Especially, what value does S have?

Now change the line for D to:

```
    D = 0.0000123456789
```

Repeat the testing process. What results do you see? Particularly, what value does C have?

4-5. The Rnd Function. Draw three command buttons on a new form. Name them cmdForward, cmdRecent, and cmdSeed. Set their Caption properties to Forward, Recent, and Seed, respectively. Then type in the following code:

```
Option Explicit

Private Sub cmdRecent_Click()
    Print Rnd(0)
End Sub

Private Sub cmdForward_Click()
    Print Rnd(1)
End Sub

Private Sub cmdSeed_Click()
    Print Rnd(-1.23)
End Sub
```

Run the program. Click each button repetitively a few times. Then click each button once. Have you got a good feel about the effect of each of the parameter values for Rnd? If not, look up in the Index tab of the online Help file using "Rnd" as the keyword.

4-6. Some Date/Time Functions. Draw a command button on a new form. Name it cmdToday and give it the caption "Today." Then type in the following code:

```
Option Explicit

Private Sub cmdToday_Click()
Dim D As Date
    D = Now
    Print "Year = "; Year(D)
    Print "Month ="; Month(D)
    Print "Day ="; Day(D)
End Sub
```

Run the project and click the command button. What do you think the following functions do? Now, Year, Month, and Day.

4-7. The DateAdd Function. Draw a command on a new form. Name it cmdNextMonth and give it the caption "Next Month." Then type in the following code.

```
Option Explicit
Dim D As String
Private Sub Form_Load()
    D = "07-01-1998"
End Sub
Private Sub cmdNextMonth_Click()
    D = DateAdd("m", 1, D)
    Print D
End Sub
```

Run the project. Click the Next Month button repetitively. What results do you see? Isn't this a convenient way to find the same day of the next month? (e.g., 07/01/98, 08/01/98, 09/01/98, and so on).

But now, change the D line to:

```
D = "07-31-1998"
```

Repeat the experiment. What results do you get? Does everything turn out to be what you expected? (Were you expecting to see month end dates?)

There are many other uses of the DateAdd function, depending on the first parameter you specify. Check out the online Help file, using the keyword "DateAdd function."

4-8. The String$ Function. As explained in the text, the String$(n, c) function generates n repeated characters of c. Try each of the following lines (individually) in the Form Click event, click the form after you start the program each time, and observe the result.

```
Print String$(10,"A")
Print String$(10,65)
Print String$(10,"AB")
Print String$(10,6566)
```

What do you conclude from your experiments?

4-9. The SelText Property of the Text Box. Draw a text box and a command button on a new form. Place these controls on the right side of the form. Name the text box txtTest and set its HideSelection property to False. Name the command button cmdHighLight and set its Caption property to "Highlight." Enter the following code:

```
Private Sub Form_Click()
    Print txtTest.SelText
End Sub
Private Sub cmdHighLight_Click()
    txtTest.SelStart = 2
    txtTest.SelLength = 3
End Sub
```

Run the program. Enter some long text into the text box. Then do the following:

A. Click the form. See anything? (No.)
B. Highlight a portion of the text box. Click the form. What do you see? Whatever you highlight should be printed on the form. Highlight a few different portions and click the form to get a good feel.
C. Click the Highlight button. What do you see in the text box? (The setting of the HideSelection property makes the highlight show.)
D. Click the form. What do you see?

You should have a good feel about the "read" capability of the SelText property.

4-10. The SelText Property of the Text Box (continued). Add a command button to the preceding project. Name it cmdInsert and set its Caption property to "Insert." Enter the following code:

```
Private Sub cmdInsert_Click()
    txtTest.SelText = "***Inserted***"
End Sub
```

Run the program. Enter some text into the text box. Then do the following:

A. Place the cursor anywhere in the text box and then click the Insert button. What do you see?
B. Highlight a portion of the text and then click the Insert button. What do you see this time? Is the highlighted text still in the text box?
C. Click the Highlight button and then click the Insert button. What do you see?

The "write" capability of the SelText property can be conveniently used to replace or insert text into a text box.

4-11. **Scope of Variables.** Type in the following code:

```
Option Explicit
Dim A As Integer
Dim B As Integer

Private Sub Form_Load()
    A = 1
    B = 2
End Sub

Private Sub Form_Click()
Dim B As Integer
    MsgBox "A =" & A
    MsgBox "B =" & B
End Sub
```

Run the program. Then click the form. Why is A equal to 1 but B equal to 0?

4-12. **Scope and Lifetime of Variables**. Enter the following code. Run the program. Click the form a few times. What do you observe? Why is B always 1, while A and C have different values after each form click?

```
Option Explicit
Dim A As Integer

Private Sub Form_Click()
Dim B As Integer
Static C As Integer
    A = A + 1
    B = B + 1
    C = C + 1
    MsgBox "A =" & A
    MsgBox "B =" & B
    MsgBox "C =" & C
End Sub
```

4-13. **Scope of Variables.** Enter the following code. Run the program and click the form. What does the computer say? Change the keyword "Static" to "Dim" and try again. What happens? A variable declared in a procedure is not recognized in another procedure.

```
Option Explicit

Private Sub Form_Load()
Static A As Integer
    A = 10
End Sub

Private Sub Form_Click()
    MsgBox " A=" & A
End Sub
```

Exercises

4-14. **Converting Numbers Between Systems.**

A. Convert the following numbers to binary values:

- 41
- 255
- 4095

B. Convert the following numbers to hex values:

- 1000

- 255
- 32768 (*Hint:* Check results in C below for verification.)

C. What are the decimal values of the following hex numbers? (*Hint:* To verify your computation, write simple code to obtain the results; e.g., Print &HFF will print 255.)

- &H1000
- &HFFFE
- &H10000
- &H10000&

4-15. Converting Temperature. The relationship between the two measurement systems of temperature can be expressed as follows: Fahrenheit = 32 + Celsius * (9/5). Design a project with two text boxes (with proper labels) and two command buttons. When the user clicks the "Convert to Fahrenheit" command button, your program will convert the data in the text box containing the Celsius data into Fahrenheit degrees and show the result in the text box for the Fahrenheit data. When the user clicks the "Convert to Celsius" command button, the opposite conversion takes place.

4-16. Converting Measurements. A mile is equal to 1.60935 kilometers. One kilogram is equal to 2.20462 pounds. One acre is equal to 4046.85 square meters. Draw six text boxes (with proper labels such as Miles, Kilometers, and so on) and two command buttons on a new form. Set one command button's Caption property to "Convert to Metric." Set the other command button's Caption property to "Convert to British."

Provide the code so that when the user clicks the "Convert to British" button, your program will convert the data in the text boxes containing the metric data into British/American measurements and show the results in the proper text boxes. When the user clicks the other button, the opposite conversion occurs.

4-17. The Area and the Length of the Hypotenuse of a Right Triangle. The area of a right triangle is computed by multiplying the two sides of the right angle, divided by 2. The length of the hypotenuse is equal to the square root of the total of the sides squared.

Design a project to compute the area and the hypotenuse. The user is expected to click a "Compute" command button after entering the values of the sides. There should also be a "Quit" command button.

4-18. Testing Divisibility. Develop code to test whether or a number, N, can be evenly divided by another number, D. Use two text boxes for the user to enter N and D, respectively, with a proper label for each. After the user has entered the numbers, he or she clicks a command button with the caption "Test." Your program will display a message indicating whether N can be evenly divided by D. (*Hint:* Use the Mod operator.)

4-19. Last Day of the Previous Month. Write an expression that will give the last day of the previous month. Show the result in a text box. (*Hint:* You will need to use the following date/time functions: DateSerial, Date, Month, and Year. The last day of the previous month is one day before the first day of the current month.)

4-20. Julian Date. The Julian date represents a date by a five-digit number. The first two digits represent the year, and the last three digits represent the date sequence number in that year. For example, 99001 represents January 1, 1999. Write two short routines: one to convert a Julian date to a date/time value and another to convert a date/time value to a Julian date. (*Hint:* You should find DateAdd and DateSerial useful.)

To test your routines, draw two text boxes and two command buttons onto a new form. Set the Caption property of one command button to "Julian" and another to "Date." Use one text box (with a "Julian Date" label) to enter a Julian date; the other (with a "Regular Date" label) to enter the date in the mm/dd/yyyy format. When the user clicks the Date button, your program will convert the Julian date in the "Julian Date" text box and display in the "Regular Date" text box a date in the mm/dd/yyyy format. Conversely, when the user clicks the Julian button, the regular date is converted to a Julian date.

4-21. Rotation Encryption. A plain text string can be encrypted by rotating each letter in the text by 13 positions in the alphabet. For example, "A" (first position in the alphabet) will be "rotated" into "N" (fourteenth position in the alphabet); and "N" to "A" (13 + 14 = 27, which goes back to 1).

An interesting feature of this encryption algorithm is that you can use it to both encrypt and decrypt. For example, the string "POKE" will be encrypted into "CBXR," but applying the same algorithm on "CBXR" will result in "POKE."

Draw a text box and a command button onto a new form. Provide the code so that when the user enters a text string in the text box and clicks the command button, the text will be encrypted by the rotation algorithm just described. The result should be displayed in the same text box. The text should be "restored" when the user clicks the button again (if your routine works properly). Assume the user is allowed to enter only uppercase letters. (*Hint:* Use a For loop. You should find the functions Mid$, Asc, Chr$, and the Mod operator useful.)

4-22. Activity Monitor. Suppose you have a data-entry screen. For security reasons, you don't want it to stay inactive for a long period. (Your user is probably away from the desk. Somebody else can peek or even poke the data.) So, you decide that if the computer is inactive for 5 minutes, the program should automatically quit. Write the code to handle this requirement. (*Hint:* When some user activity occurs, either the mouse will move or the keyboard will be pressed; that is, use the form's KeyDown and MouseMove events to compute the time to quit. Use a timer to check whether the current time (Now) is beyond the time to quit. Check the time every second. The variable TimeToQuit should be recognized by all three event procedures. For test run purposes, set the time to quit at 5 seconds instead of 5 minutes. Also, set the form's KeyPreview property to True.)

Efficiency: Checking for the time to quit every second seems too often. You can make the program more efficient. (*Hint:* The timer's interval property can be changed at runtime. Its maximum interval is 65535.)

4-23. The Name Enforcer. Nearly all words in a name (e.g., personal name, street name) starts with an uppercase letter. Let's also assume that you will not accept any uppercase letter after the first in a word. Provide the code to enforce this rule while the user is entering the name for a text box named txtName (i.e., perform the uppercase to lowercase conversion automatically no matter what case [upper or lower] the user enters the letter). Note that there can be more than one word in the text box. (*Hint:* Place the code in the KeyPress event. The first letter of a word is either the first character in the text box or one whose left side is a space. You need to use the built-in functions Asc, Chr$, Ucase$, and Lcase$.)

Incidentally, there is a function, StrConv, that can perform this process on an entire string. But here, the problem requires the immediate conversion as each character is being entered.

4-24. Computing the Economic Order Quantity. The economic order quantity can be computed by the following formula:

Q* = Square Root of (2*P*D/S)

Where P = cost to place an order

D = annual demand

S = annual cost to carry an item

Design a project that will take P, D, and S as input (use text boxes), compute the EOQ, and display the result (in a label, because you do not want the user to enter any number here.) (*Note:* Include two command buttons: one to handle computation and another to quit.)

4-25. Future Value of a Deposit. The future value of a deposit (loan) compounded annually can be computed as follows:

$F = D (1 + Rate)^n$

Where D = amount of deposit (loan)

Rate = annual percentage rate

N = number of years

Design a project to compute the future value of a deposit.

Question: Can the user use your program to determine how long it will take to double his or her money? How?

4-26. Finding Last Name and First Name. A label has a caption "Name (Last, First)." A text box is on its right for the user to enter the name. When the user clicks the "Show" button, your program will "compute" the last name and first name and display the results using the MsgBox statement (e.g., "Your name is John Smith."). (Note that the user is expected enter a name in the format like, "Smith, John.") When the user clicks the "Quit" button, your program unloads.

4-27. Searching and Highlighting. Set up a form with two text boxes with proper labels. The first one will be used to enter the search word, and the second one will contain a long string of text to be searched on (name it txtLongText). This text box has several lines. (Set its MultiLines property to True.) When your program starts, the user enters a long text into the second box. Then each time he or she enters a search word and clicks on the "Find Next" button, your program will look for that word in the second text box. If the search word is found, it is highlighted in the second text box. Otherwise, the message "Word not found" will be displayed (use the MsgBox statement). (*Hint:* Set the HideSelection property of the second text box to False. Use vbTextCompare as the fourth parameter for the InStr function to make the search not case sensitive.)

4-28. Repetitive Searching and Highlighting. (Continued from 4-27.) We would like to allow the user to click the "Find Next" button repetitively. Each time he or she clicks the "Search" button, your program will find and highlight the next matching word in the second text box. When there are no more matches, the message "Word not found" will be displayed. (*Hint:* Use the first optional parameter to specify the position to start searching. If the current search is a new search, it should start from position 1; otherwise, it should start from the previous position plus the length of the word being searched. You will need static variables to keep track of the previous position and word being searched.)

4-29. Repetitive Search and Replace. Modify the preceding project. Add a text box (with proper label) and a command button. Set the command button's Caption property to "Replace."

Provide the code so that when this button is clicked, the text found in txtLongText will be replaced with the text in the new text box. Make sure that when no matching text is found or when the new text box contains no replacement text, a proper error message is displayed. (*Hint:* See 4-10 for string replacement.)

Projects

4-30. Computing Daily Receipts. At the end of each day, a restaurant owner needs to determine the amount of sales, credit card processing fees, sales taxes, and net receipts. The cash register gives a tally of the amounts received by category. A sample of the tally appears as follows:

Cash	$1,569.82
American Express	4,031.99
Other Credit Cards	5,903.22
Total	11,505.03

Food	$8,135.03
Liquor	2,320.00
Beer	1,050.00
Total	11,505.03

American Express (AE) credit card receipts are mailed to AE, which will deduct a 4.25% of processing fee and make a direct deposit in the restaurant's bank account in 2 weeks. (Statements are mailed to the restaurant.) Cash and other credit card receipts are deposited in the bank the same night. These credit cards are subject to a 2.45% processing fee, which will be subtracted from the restaurant's account balance and shown in the monthly bank statement.

The food sales include a 7.25% sales tax. The liquor sales are subject to 10% liquor tax, and beer sales are subject to a 7% beer tax. Both liquor and beer taxes are expenses of the restaurant, whereas sales taxes are withholdings. Thus, the amount of food sales to be reported for this sample should be $8,135.03/(1 + .0725). The restaurant owner will report and remit all these withholdings and taxes to the state tax authorities every month.

Required: Design a project to compute the net receipts (monetary), bank deposit, credit card processing fees, net sales, net revenues (net of fees and taxes), and taxes (withholdings and expenses) owed to the state tax authorities. Your visual interface should be neat, clear, and uncluttered.

4-31. The Virtual Vending Machine. Imagine that on the third floor of the Business Building there is this "Do-It-Yourself Vending Machine." On the top row of its display (screen), it clearly identifies itself as the "Almighty Virtual Vending Machine." This sign is shown as blinking light. (Make it look like a neon sign.) On the left side of this sign, there's a picture (image of your choice). On the right side of the sign, there's a clock that shows the current date and time, which ticks every second. (*Hint:* Use one timer for the blinking light and another timer for the date/time clock. Set the fonts of the labels to make them look really "neat.")

In the middle of the screen is a list of the menu choices. It shows six of your favorite dishes with prices. However, this list box is tall enough to show only four items. From this list, a customer can select any number of items to purchase. (*Note:* Use the Checkbox Style property for the list box. Set its foreground and background colors such that it will look like a vending machine. Use the AddItem method to create the menu list. Concatenate a tab character between each item and its price. The tab character has a predefined constant name, vbTab. Using this character, if all the item names are about the same length, the prices will line up in the same column.)

On the left side of this list box, there's a check box for the customer to indicate whether he or she is a student at your college. If so, the box (with proper label) below the check box is enabled so that the customer can enter his or her student ID. Otherwise, this box and its related label are disabled. (*Hint:* Use a frame to contain the check box and the ID field, which should be the user's Social Security number.)

On the right side of the list box, two option buttons allow the customer to identify the payment method: cash or credit card. If the choice is "credit card," the combo box below it (with proper label) is enabled to allow the customer to indicate the type of the credit card: Visa, Diners Club, Master Card, Discover, or American Express. Otherwise, the combo box and its label are disabled. (*Hint:* Use another frame to contain the option buttons and the combo box. Set the default credit card to Visa. The combo box should not accept any other kind of credit cards.)

At the bottom of the screen, there are two command buttons. The left one has a caption "Buy"; and the right one, "Bye." When the "Buy" button is pushed (clicked), the computer should display the items the customer has chosen, total purchase, and indicate the payment method. If the customer is a student at your college, he or she is entitled to have a 20% discount. Below is a sample display (use the message box for this purpose):

```
You have purchased chicken noodle soup, cheesecake, and beer.
The total purchase is $12 with a 20% discount. Net amount is $9.60.
You paid with a Visa credit card.
```

If the customer is not a student of your college, the middle line will read as follows:

```
The total purchase is $12 with no discount.
```

The machine will "reset" to its original state after the message is displayed. When the "Bye" button is clicked, the program ends. (*Note:* This project is different from the example in the chapter. You can no longer use the list box's Click event to keep track of what the customer has bought. Instead, you figure out what has been selected in the Buy button's Click event. You will need to use a For loop to test what have been checked in the list box.

5 Decision

Beginning with Chapter 2, "Introduction to Visual Basic Programming," you have often seen the need for an If statement (or block) to make a program work properly. It is not an exaggeration to claim that you just cannot write a program without the use of the If block. This is true because however simple a programming problem may be, it is bound to involve some "decisions"; that is, depending on the condition of one thing, something else will have to be handled differently. For example, suppose your program has a check box, which is used to ascertain whether a patient of a clinic is insured. If so, you want to enable a frame control for the user to enter insurance information; otherwise, the frame will be disabled. You will need to use the If block in the check box's Click event to determine whether the check box is checked or unchecked and to execute the proper code accordingly.

When we used the If block previously, we basically looked at the syntax. It is now time to take a closer look at its structure and additional details. Sometimes, various alternative actions need to be taken depending on the result obtained from a single expression, a situation commonly referred to as *branching*. In such a case, coding with the If block structure can become cumbersome. VB provides an alternative structure, the Select Case block, to handle this situation more concisely. We also study this structure in this chapter.

Both the If block and the Select Case block structures involve the use of logical expressions, which are expressions that can be evaluated to a Boolean value, True or False. In order for you to thoroughly understand both structures, it is desirable that we study logical expressions first.

After you finish this chapter, you should be able to:

- Understand relational and logical operators and use them in logical expressions.
- Use logical operators in bit-wise operations.
- Code the If block structure to solve various programming problems that involve decisions.
- Appreciate and design various alternatives to the If block.
- Understand and use the Select Case block structure.

5.1 Logical Expressions

As you may recall, a simple If statement has the following syntax:

```
If Condition Then Statement
```

Where *Condition* represents an expression that can be evaluated to True or False and *Statement* represents a VB statement such as the assignment statement explained in previous chapters.

This type of conditional expression is recognized as the logical expression. Two types of operators are used to construct a logical expression: relational operators and logical operators. Let's take a look at relational operators first.

Relational Operators

Relational operators are used to compare the operands and decide whether the relation is true. For example, you can use the equal (=) operator to test whether two variables, A and B, are equal by coding:

```
If A = B Then MsgBox "A and B are equal"
```

When A is actually equal to B, the expression is True and the message, "A and B are equal" will be displayed. Otherwise, the expression will be False, and the message will not be displayed. The following table provides a list of the relational operators.

Relational Operator	Example	Remark/Explanation
=	A = B	The result is True when A is actually *equal* to B; otherwise, False.
<>	A <> B	The result is True when A is *not equal* to B; otherwise, False.
>	A > B	The result is True when A is *greater than* B; otherwise, False.
>=	A >= B	The result is True when A is *greater than or equal to* B; otherwise, False.
<	A < B	The result is True when A is *less than* B; otherwise, False.
<=	A <= B	The result is True when A is *less than or equal to* B; otherwise, False.

Numeric Comparisons. Typically, relational operators are used to compare numeric data. For example, the following code checks whether the hours worked in a week entered by the user is greater than or equal to 168. If so, a message box is displayed.

```
If Val(txtHoursWorked.Text) >= 168 Then
    MsgBox "Have you ever slept?", vbQuestion
    TxtHoursWorked.SetFocus
End If
```

In the code, if the number of hours worked is found to be greater than or equal to 168, the message box displays a question mark with a message teasing the user. (Additional details concerning the use of the MsgBox statement are presented in Chapter 6, "Input, Output, and Procedures.") The text box's SetFocus method is then used to reset the focus on the text box so that the user can correct the number.

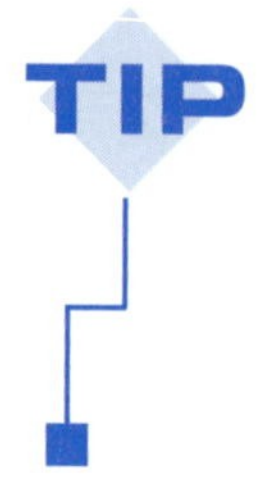

Recall that the minimum requirement for a user-friendly program is that the message should provide concise information in a friendly tone. The message displayed in the preceding code is not really a good example. A better message would be as follows:

```
MsgBox "The maximum number of hours allowed per week is 60.",_
  VbInformation
```

In addition, if the upper limit is 60, the hours worked should be compared with 60, not 168.

Potential Problem with Conversion. When the operands involved are of different data types, a conversion will have to take place before the comparison is done. Occasionally, a conversion can result in some unexpected result. Consider this example:

```
Option Explicit
Const RateS As Single = 0.095
Const RateD As Double = 0.095

Private Sub cmdCompare_Click()
Dim A As Single, D As Double
    A = RateS * 99895
    D = RateD * 99895
    If A = D Then
        MsgBox "A and D are equal."
    Else
        MsgBox "A and D are not equal."
    End If
End Sub
```

You can test the code by placing a command button in a new form, naming it cmdCompare and setting its Caption property to "Compare." Then type in the preceding code and click the command button after you start the project. The message "A and D are not equal" is displayed when you click the "Compare" button. Why? If you inspect the computational results, D has a value of 9490.025 but A has 9490.024. A is less accurate because its data type is Single and is unable to represent the data with the exact precision.

Although the advice is to always use the same data type to avoid data conversion in any operations (including comparisons), you occasionally may be faced with a situation when it is necessary to perform mixed-data type comparisons. In such a case, instead of comparing for equality, you can avoid the problem by allowing a very small difference between the two values. For example, you can work around the problem with the previous example by modifying the code for the comparison as follows:

```
If Abs((A - D) / D) < 0.0000001 Then
```

In this statement, we assume that we are willing to accept a relative difference of 10^{-7} as "virtually" equal. However, this approach will do well only if D is not close to zero. If D is anywhere near zero, you should check the absolute difference, that is, Abs(A – D), instead of the relative difference.

String Comparisons. The familiar relational operators can also be used to compare string data. For example, you can compare to see whether a name entered in a text box (e.g., txtName) is the same as the variable, CustName, by coding the following:

```
If txtName.Text = CustName Then . . .
```

Notice that all the six relational operators can be used in string expressions. The question is how are the string data compared? For example, is "A" greater than "a"? No. The comparison is based on the ASCII value of the characters. Because "A" has an ASCII value of 65 and "a" has a value of 97, "a" is greater than "A."

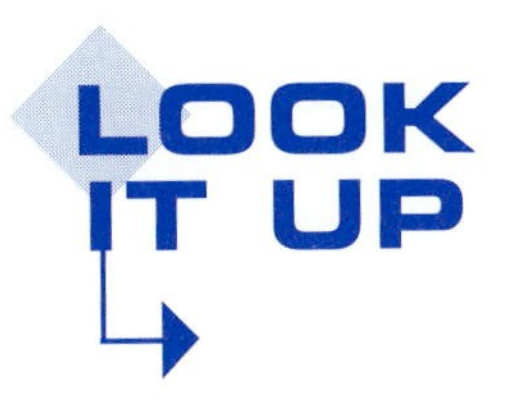

Search the VB online Help file using the Index tab for the keyword "Key code constants." It shows not only the ASCII value of each key but also the predefined name (named constant) of the key. However, not all keys are shown in this table. On the other hand, the keyword "ASCII character codes" gives a complete list of the character values with the corresponding characters without showing any corresponding predefined names. You will need to refer to both tables to handle programming problems that involve key code values.

Comparing Strings with Unequal Lengths. What happens when two strings are not of the same length? Basically, the comparison is carried out from left to right in pairs one character after another until an inequality is found or one of the strings runs out of characters.

Thus, the string "b" is greater than "abcd" because the first character in the first string, "b" is greater than the first character in the second string. As another example, the string "ab" is greater than "a." The latter string runs out of characters before an inequality can be determined.

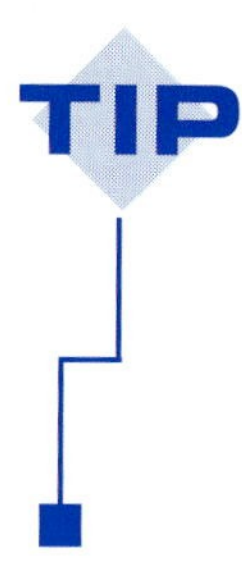

In some cases, you may want the character comparison to not be case sensitive; that is, you want to consider the uppercases and lowercases of the same letter equal. You can make the comparison not case sensitive by using the UCase$ or LCase$ functions before the comparison is performed. For example, the code:

```
If UCase$(txtName.Text) = UCase$(CustName)  Then . . .
```

will result in True for a name McCord and MCCORD or any variations of uppercase or lowercase spellings on either side of the equality comparison.

Assignment Statements

Notice that in addition to being used in If statements, the logical expression can also be a part of an assignment statement. That is, you can assign the result of a comparison (or logical operation, explained in the following section) to a numeric variable such as follows:

```
D = A = B
```

In this statement, the first "=" represents the assignment operation (move the result of the operation on the right side to the variable on the left), and the second "=" is the equality comparison operator that compares whether A and B are equal. In this example, assuming D is a Boolean variable, it will have a value True if A is indeed equal to B; otherwise, it will have a value False. If D is of any kind of numeric data type other than Boolean, it will have a value –1 if A is equal to B; otherwise, it will have a value of 0.

Of course, just like any typical assignment statement, the result of a comparison can also be assigned to a property setting of any VB control that expects True or False. For example, suppose you would like to enable or disable a check box, named chkDorm, depending on whether the variable, Score, is greater than or equal to 80. You can code the following:

```
chkDorm.Enabled = Score >= 80
```

This statement will enable the check box, chkDorm, when Score is greater than or equal to 80; otherwise, the check box will be disabled.

Logical Operators

Logical operators are primarily used in logical expressions to perform operations on Boolean data. For example, the following code tests whether the conditions that the purchase amount (named Purchase) is greater than $10,000 and that the account has no previous balance (named Balance) are both true:

```
Status = Purchase > 10000 And Balance = 0
```

Note that there is the "And" logical operator between the two comparisons. The And operator requires both of the comparisons to be True to produce a result of True; that is, the variable, Status, will have a value True if the purchase amount is greater than $10,000 and the previous balance is equal to zero.

The following table provides a list of the logical operators often used in programs.

Logical Operator	Example	Remark/Explanation
Not	Not (A = B)	The Not operator negates the operand on its right. Thus, in the example if A is equal to B, the entire expression will be False.
And	Purchase > 10000 And Balance = 0	When the expressions on both sides of the And operator are True, the result is True; otherwise, False.

Logical Operator	Example	Remark/Explanation
Or	Purchase > 10000 Or Balance = 0	When either expression on both sides of the Or operator is True, the result is True; otherwise, False.
Xor	Purchase >10000 Xor Balance = 0	When exactly one of the two expressions on both sides of the Xor (exclusive Or) operator is True, the result is True; otherwise False. That is, when both sides are True or when both are False, the result is False.

Uses of Logical Operators. Here are two examples of using the logical operators:

Example 1. A clinic patient who is insured and who assigns the right to claim the insurance will be charged a co-payment, while his or her insurance company will pay for the remaining charges. Assume that the variables, Insured and Assigned, have a value "Y" if the patient is insured and has assigned the insurance claim to the clinic. To compute the charge to each party, you can code the following:

```
If Insured = "Y" And Assigned = "Y" Then
    ChargeToPatient = CoPay
    ChargeToInsurance = TotalCharge - ChargeToPatient
End If
```

Example 2. A store will give a 20% discount to a customer who is either a student or has purchased at least $1,000 worth of goods. Assume that the check box, chkStudent, is used to identify whether a customer is a student, and the variable, Purchase, represents the amount of purchase. The computation of discount can be coded as follows:

```
If chkStudent.Value = vbChecked Or Purchase >= 1000 Then
    Discount = Purchase * .2
End If
```

The Xor Operator. Although the first three logical operators correspond well to our daily life connotation, the Xor operator may call for some additional explanation. As explained in the table, this operator sets the result to *True only if exactly one of its two operands is True*. An easy way to understand how it works is to think of it as an inequality operator; that is, when its two Boolean operands are not equal, the result is true. (Additional fine points are considered later.) As its name implies, *this operator is most useful in handling a situation where the conditions are mutually exclusive*. For example, when making a journal entry in accounting records, the user can enter only a debit or credit amount for an account involved in that transaction. Assume the two text boxes, txtDebit and txtCredit, are used for the user to enter the amount and only positive amounts can be entered. The following code can be used to check that one and only one amount is entered:

```
If Val(txtDebit.Text) > 0 Xor Val(txtCredit.Text) > 0 Then
' Only one amount has been entered; OK
Else
'Either both are zero or both amounts are entered.
'Display a message
    MsgBox "Please enter one amount for the account."
End If
```

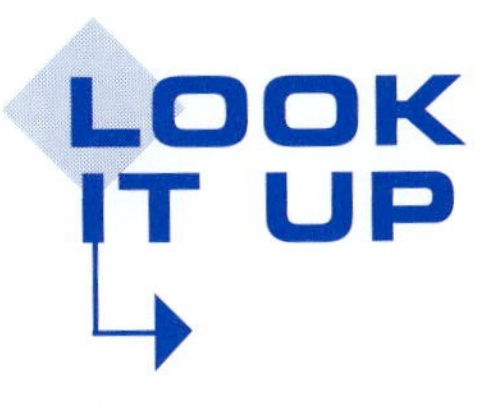

The "logical operators" keyword in the Index tab of the VB online Help file lists two more logical operators Eqv (Equivalence) and Imp (Implication). It also provides additional explanations on how each of the logical operators works. Be sure to read over the material. It should enhance your understanding of the discussion presented in this section.

Bit-Wise Operation of Logical Operators. Logical operators actually operate on data on a bit-by-bit basis and can be used to perform operations not only on Boolean data but also on Integer (Long and Short) data (Figure 5.1). In this context, a bit is considered True when it is on (with a value 1) and False when it is off (with a value 0). (Notice that the context is a bit not a data field.)

Figure 5.1
Bit-Wise Operation of Logical Operators

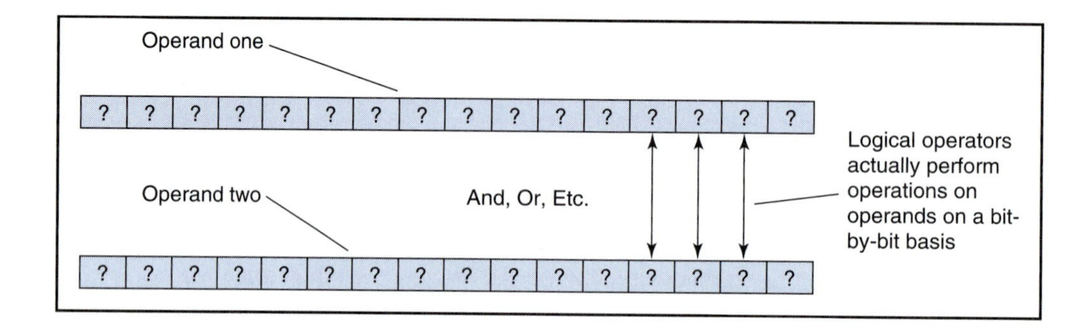

Specifically, the ***Not operator*** will reverse the on or off state of each bit; that is, an on bit will become off, and an off bit will become on, as shown in Figure 5.2.

Figure 5.2
The Not Operation

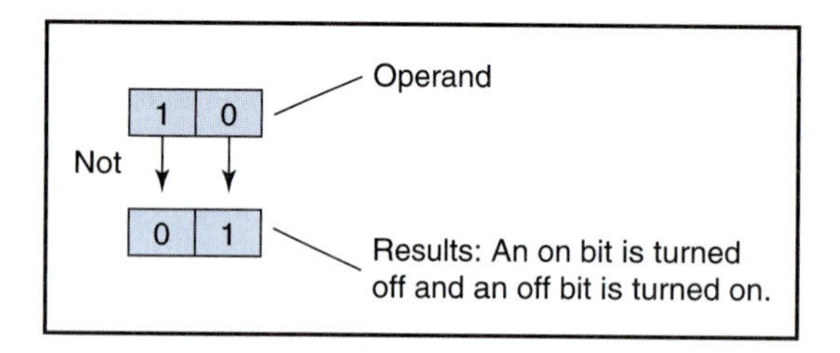

Incidentally, recall that a Boolean variable takes two bytes of storage. False is coded with all the bits turned off. Thus, in the hex decimal representation, it is &H0000, which, if assigned to an Integer variable, should have a value of 0. Applying a Not operation on the value will result in all bits being turned on to become &HFFFF, representing True, equivalent to a value -1.

The ***And operator*** will produce a result of 1 (on) for a bit if both its operands' corresponding bits are 1 (on); otherwise, the result will be 0 (off), as shown in Figure 5.3.

Figure 5.3
The And Operation

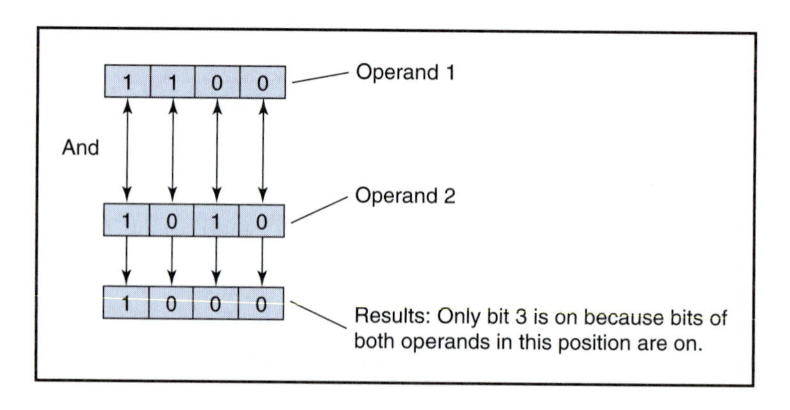

The ***Or operator*** will produce a result of 1 for a bit if either of the corresponding bit operands is 1 (on); otherwise, the result will be 0 (off), as illustrated in Figure 5.4.

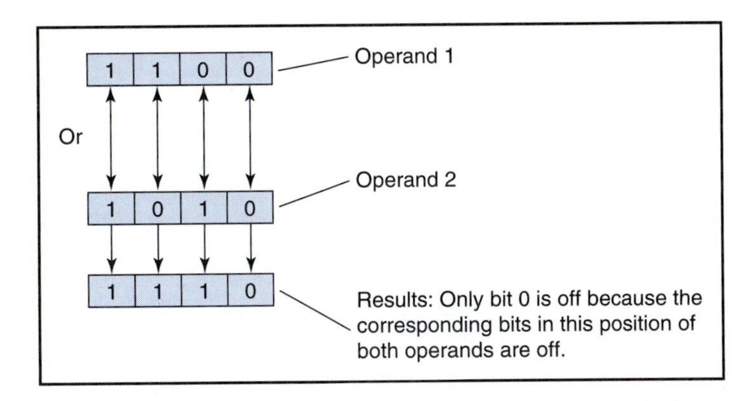

Figure 5.4
The Or Operation

The ***Xor operator*** will produce a result of 1 (on) for a bit if only one of the two bit operands is on; otherwise, the bit will be 0 (off), as shown in Figure 5.5.

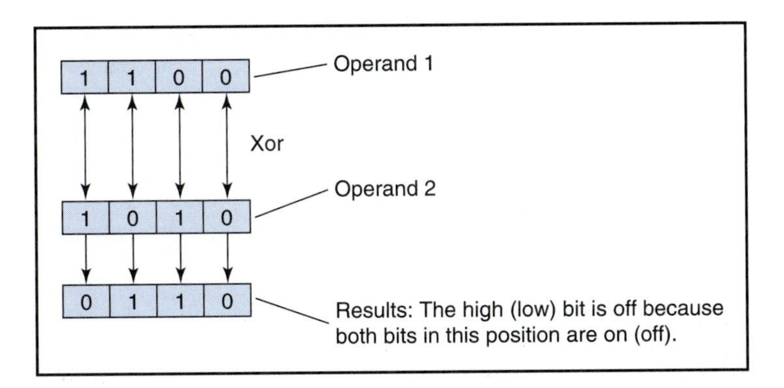

Figure 5.5
The Xor Operation

Setting a Flag. These operators can be used to set, test, or toggle flags. A ***flag*** is a bit of data representing the on/off state of something. A flag is on when that particular bit is set to 1, and off when it is set to 0. Because an Integer variable has 16 bits, it is often used to hold a group of flags. As an illustration, assume you have an Integer variable, Flags, that you want to use to represent several classifications of an account. You want to use the lowest bit to represent whether the account affects cash flow and the second lowest bit to represent whether the account is a control account. As you may recall from Chapter 4, "Data, Operations, and Built-In Functions," the lowest bit has a numeric value of 1 when it is on; and the second lowest bit has a numeric value of 2 when it is on. Thus, if you want to set the lowest bit on, you can code the following:

```
Flags = Flags Or 1
```

Recall that the Or operator will set the resulting bit to 1 when either of the operands (bits) is 1. In our case, the second operand has only its lowest bit set on (to 1). Thus, when the two operands are "Ored," the result will be exactly the same as that for Flags, except that its lowest bit will be on regardless of its previous status. This result can then be assigned to Flags to reflect the Flags' new state. This operation is illustrated in Figure 5.6.

By the same token, to set the second lowest bit on, you code the following:

```
Flags = Flags Or 2
```

Testing a Flag. To test whether the lowest bit of Flags has been set on, you can use the And operator. For example, you can code the following:

```
Test = Flags And 1
```

Again, recall that the result of an And operation will be 1 (on) for a bit only if both corresponding operands are 1 (on). Thus, the result will be 1 only if Flags' lowest bit is also on, as illustrated in Figure 5.7.

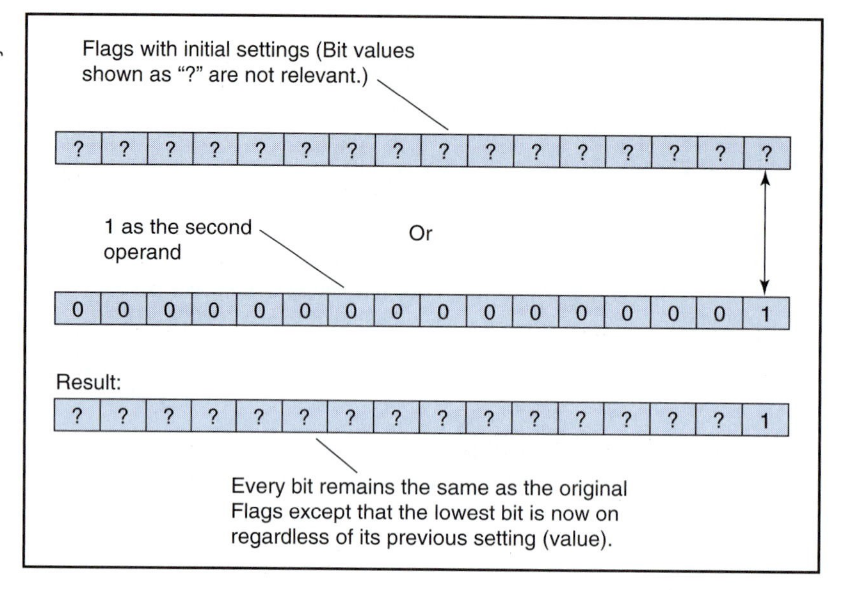

Figure 5.6
Setting a Flag with the Or Operator

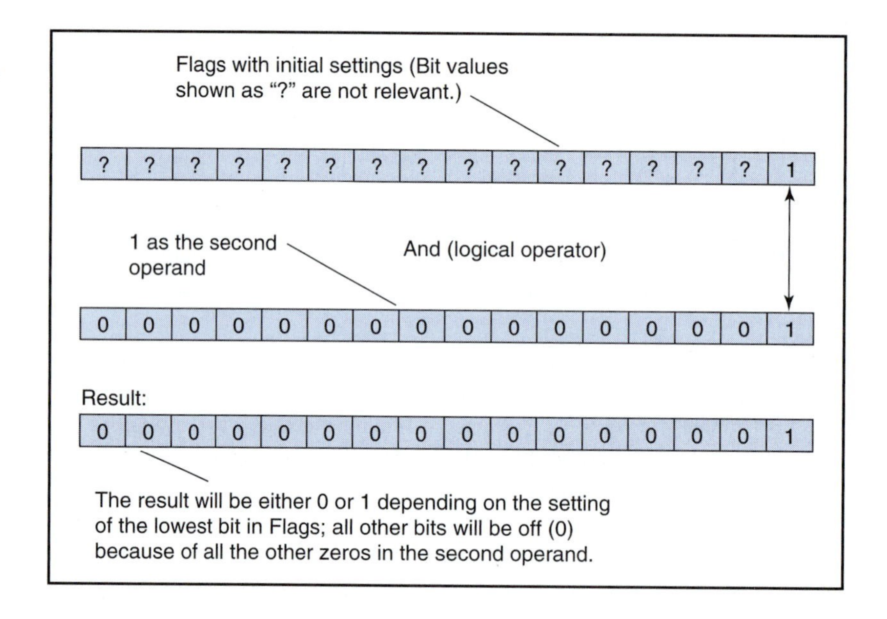

Figure 5.7
Testing a Flag with the And Operator

By the same token, you can test whether the second lowest bit is on by coding the following:

```
Test = Flags And 2
```

Testing for an Odd or Even Number. The previous illustration of testing whether the lowest bit of Flags is on has an additional interesting application. You may be aware that *all odd integers have the lowest bit on, whereas even integers have it off*. Thus, the same code can be used to test whether a number is odd or even. To experiment and verify, place a text box and a command button on a new form. Name the text box txtNumber and the command button cmdTest. Also set the Caption property of the command button to "Test." Then, type in the following code:

```
Option Explicit
Private Sub cmdTest_Click()
Dim Test As Integer
    Test = Val(txtNumber.Text) And 1
```

```
        If Test = 0 Then
        'The lowest bit is off. This is an even number.
            MsgBox txtNumber.Text & " is an even number."
        Else
        'The lowest bit is on. This is an odd number.
            MsgBox txtNumber.Text & " is an odd number."
        End If
    End Sub
```

Once you run the project, enter a number and click the Test button. The program should be able to tell you whether you have entered an odd or even number.

Toggling a Flag. The Xor operator also has a very interesting application. Often, it is used to toggle a flag, that is, to turn a flag from one state to the other. As explained earlier, this operator sets the result of a bit to 1 only when one of the two operands is 1 (on). Thus, if you repetitively perform the Xor operation with a constant "on" bit to another operand, this latter operand will be off when it was originally on and on when it was originally off. That is, you can use the following code to change the setting of its lowest bit:

```
Flags = Flags Xor 1 'Toggle the lowest bit
```

In addition, if you execute the same line of code again, the setting of its lowest bit is restored to its original value. The Xor operation is illustrated in Figure 5.8.

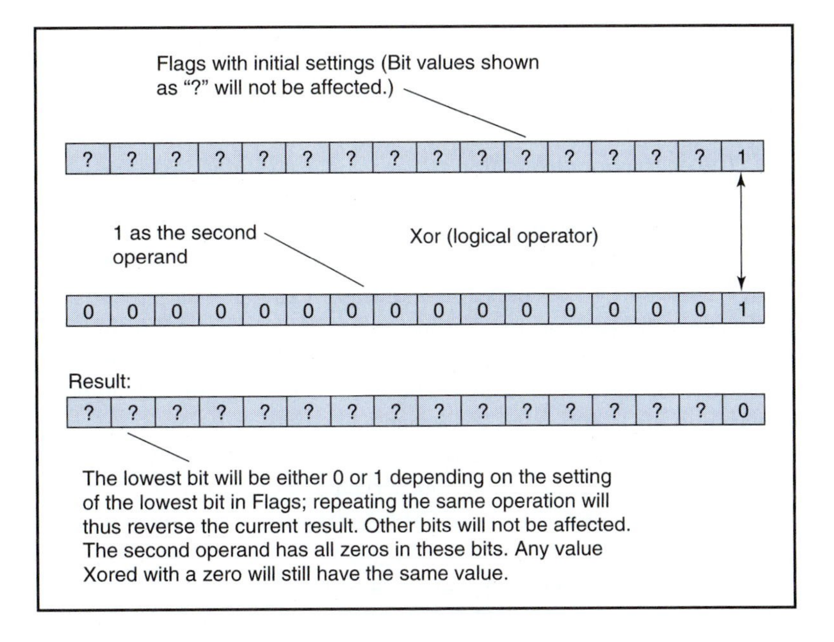

Figure 5.8
Toggling a Flag with the Xor Operator

Again, by the same token, you can toggle the second lowest bit by coding the following:

```
Flags = Flags Xor 2 'Toggle the second lowest bit
```

Use of the Xor Operator for Encryption. The toggling capability of Xor makes it a popular operator to perform encryption operations. If some data is Xored with a "password" (or key), the data changes its original value. However, when the encrypted data is Xored again with the same password, the data is restored to its original value.

Here is a highly simplified example. Set up a new project as follows:

1. Place a text box and two labels on a new form.
2. Name the text box txtOriginal, the first label lblEncrypted, and the second lblDecrypted.
3. Clear the Text property of the text box and set the properties of the two labels so that they look like blank text boxes (by setting BackColor to white and BorderStyle to fixed single).

The visual interface should appear as in Figure 5.9.

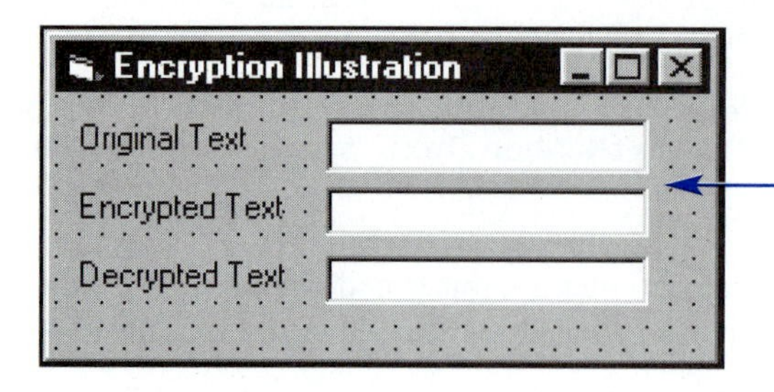

Figure 5.9
Visual Interface for Encryption Illustration

With the code below, whatever the user types into the text box (txtOriginal) will be encrypted and shown in the second blank (lblEncrypted), which is then decrypted and displayed in the third blank (lblDecrypted).

Assume you want to use the letter "X" as the "password" for encryption. Type the following code into your new project:

```
Option Explicit
Private Sub txtOriginal_KeyPress(KeyAscii As Integer)
Dim Encrypted As Integer
Dim Restored As Integer
    ' Encrypt the key being entered with "X"
    Encrypted = KeyAscii Xor vbKeyX
    ' Add the encrypted key to the encrypted label
    lblEncrypted.Caption = lblEncrypted.Caption & _
        Chr$(Encrypted)
    ' Restore the encryption by applying the same "password"
    Restored = Encrypted Xor vbKeyX
    ' Add the restored key to the restored label
    lblDecrypted.Caption = lblDecrypted.Caption & Chr$(Restored)
End Sub
```

The encryption/decryption routine is placed in the text box's KeyPress event, which is triggered when the user enters a key into the text box. This event procedure has a parameter, KeyAscii, that gives the ASCII value of the key pressed. The code first encrypts this value by Xoring it with the ASCII value of "X." (Note that the named constant for the ASCII value of "X" is vbKeyX.) The encrypted character (along with all previously encrypted characters) is displayed in the label named lblEncrypted. The encrypted ASCII value is then performed with another Xor operation with the same password (vbKeyX). This operation should restore the key to what was originally entered. The restored key (along with all previously restored keys) is displayed in the label named lblDecrypted.

Run the project and enter some text into the text box. As you enter a key, you should be able to see the encrypted result in lblEncrypted. You should also be able to verify that the restored text in lblDecrypted is the same as the text you originally entered.

Note that this routine ignores the possibility that the user may press a control key such as the Enter key or the Backspace key. You should be able to fine-tune the program before finishing this chapter. The refinement is left to you as an exercise.

An interesting application of encryption/decryption is the swapping of two values of the same data type. Assume both A and B are integers. Consider the following code:

```
A = A Xor B
B = A Xor B
A = A Xor B
```

What have you done? You have just swapped the values of A and B. How does the code work? The first line has both A and B encrypted and the result is stored in A. Now, think of B as the key. Applying the key to the encrypted data (A), you obtain the decrypted result, A from line 2. But the result is stored in B. Using B (with the original value of A now) as the key and applying it to the encrypted data (still stored in A), you obtain the original value of B, which is assigned to A in line 3. Tricky. But the code is very efficient. It involves the use of the (fast) logical operator without any extra storage space. Note, however, that the logical operators work properly only on Integer data. Fractional numbers are truncated.

The following table summarizes the use of logical operators in bit-wise operations.

Operator	Operation	Example	Result	Remark
Not	Reverse the content	Not &HFFFF	&H0000	Not –1 = 0; that is, Not True is False.
And	1 only if both corresponding bits are 1	&H0F And &F03	3	Can be used to test whether certain bits are on and to mask off certain bits.
Or	1 if either (or both) of the corresponding bits is 1	&H0F Or &F03	&H0F	Can be used to turn on certain bits.
Xor	1 only if either (but not both) of the corresponding bits is 1	&H0F Xor &H03	&H0C	Can be used to toggle certain bits and to encrypt data.

Operational Precedence

In Chapter 4, we listed the operational precedence of various numeric operators used in an expression. All these rules still hold for all conditional expressions used in an If statement, but now there are two more types of operators: relational and logical operators. How are these new operators "ranked"? These new operators rank lower in their operational precedence than any of the numeric operators. In addition, the relational operators have precedence over the logical operators, among which Not has the highest precedence followed by And. Here is the list of operators again, ranking from the highest to the lowest in operational precedence:

1. Unary negation
2. Power (^)
3. Multiplication, division, and Mod (*, /, Mod)
4. Addition and subtraction (+, -)
5. Relational operations (=, <>, >, >=, <, <=)
6. Not
7. And
8. Or and Xor

Too many rules to remember? If you think so, use parentheses to explicitly express the order of operations. Parentheses help add clarity to what needs to be done first.

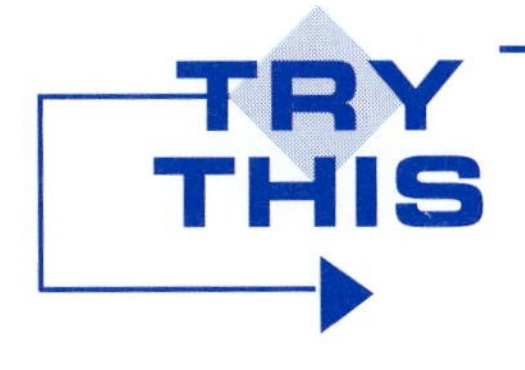

Want to verify that the And operator actually takes precedence over the Or operator? Test this code:

```
Private Sub Form_Click()
    Print True Or True And False
End Sub
```

If Or and And rank equal in precedence, the result should be False. If And has the precedence, the result should be True. Enter the code and click the form. What do you see?

Now, you have seen how relational and logical operators work. These operators are used to construct logical expressions, which most likely are used in If statements. It is time to take a closer look at the If statement (block).

5.2 The If Block

Recall that a simple If statement has the following syntax:

```
If Condition Then Statement
```

When the expression in the condition portion is True, the statement portion is executed; otherwise, it is ignored. For example, you can code the following:

```
If Score > = 90 Then Grade = "A"
```

This statement says if Score is greater than or equal to 90, an "A" is assigned to Grade. If Score is less than 90, nothing is assigned to Grade because the statement portion is ignored.

Note that the condition can be any logical expression or even numeric expression because the latter can be converted to either True or False. *Any nonzero value will be converted to True.* In addition, recall that an expression can be as simple as a variable, control property, or constant, as explained in Chapter 4. Thus, it is correct to code the following:

```
If optMale.Value Then Sex = "M"
```

This statement says if optMale.Value is True, then assign "M" to the variable, Sex. Since the Value property of the option button optMale is either True or False (which is what the computer is checking for), there is no need to code:

```
If optMale.Value = True Then Sex = "M"
```

Indeed, any numeric data can be placed in the condition portion:

```
If A Then cboZipCode.ListIndex = 0
```

We assume that A is a numeric variable in this line. The ListIndex property of the combo box, cboZipCode, will be set to 0 when A is any value but zero. Recall again that a numeric expression is considered True when it is nonzero and False when zero.

Simple If Block

Often, when a condition is true, you may need to execute more than one statement. In such cases, the previous simple structure would appear to be deficient. The following simple If block will serve the purpose better:

```
If Condition Then
    Statements to be executed
End If
```

Notice that the first line of the block starts with an If and ends with the keyword Then. No other expression (except for comments) can be coded after Then; otherwise, the line will be interpreted as a simple If statement explained previously. Also notice that the block ends with an "End If" statement. All statements within these two lines will be executed when the condition in the If line is True. Consider the following code in an event procedure:

```
Private Sub chkSort_Click()
    If chkSort.Value = vbChecked Then
        cboSortField1.Enabled = True
        cboSortField2.Enabled = True
    End If
End Sub
```

The If statement checks to see whether the check box, chkSort, is checked. If so, both the combo boxes containing sort field 1 and sort field 2 are enabled. (*Note:* To test the preceding code, set the Enabled property of the two combo boxes to False at design time.)

What happens to the two combo boxes in the previous example if the check box is clicked off? Nothing inside the If block will be executed. Both can be either enabled or disabled before the event procedure is triggered. However, once enabled, no code inside the procedure will disable the two combo boxes.

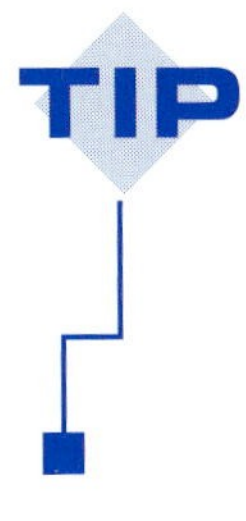

When coding If blocks, it is a good idea to code the If structure first before putting in any statements to be executed in the block; that is, write the If line and the End If line first then insert all the statements in the block afterward. It is easy to be too preoccupied with all the details involved in coding the statements within the If block to remember to close the block with the End If line. It will be even harder later to figure out where the proper place should be to insert the End If line when you are informed by the compiler of a missing End If statement (or even statements).

What if you really mean to disable the two combo boxes when the check box is clicked off? Given what we have learned in this chapter so far, one way to solve this is to code the procedure as follows:

```
Private Sub chkSort_Click()
     cboSortField1.Enabled = False
     cboSortField2.Enabled = False
     If chkSort.Value =vbChecked Then
          cboSortField1.Enabled = True
          cboSortField2.Enabled = True
     End If
End Sub
```

In the preceding code, the two combo boxes will always be disabled first (regardless of the check state of the check box) and then enabled if the check box is found checked.

The If...Then...Else...End If Block

Although the previous code gives the correct result, you probably feel awkward about it. Apparently, it is not completely efficient because it always disables the combo boxes even when they will be enabled immediately inside the If block. Is there an If block structure that allows the execution of a group of statements when a condition is True, and another group when the condition is False? Yes, there is and you have seen it in Chapter 2. The syntax structure appears as follows:

```
If Condition Then
     Statements to be executed when condition is True
Else
     Statements to be executed when condition is False
End If
```

With this structure, we can code the preceding example as follows:

```
Private Sub chkSort_Click()
     If chkSort.Value =vbChecked Then
          cboSortField1.Enabled = True
          cboSortField2.Enabled = True
     Else
          cboSortField1.Enabled = False
          cboSortField2.Enabled = False
      End If
End Sub
```

This code will not only produce correct results but literally do what we expect it to: enable the combo boxes when the check box is clicked on and disable them when the check box is clicked off.

Beware of the code structure. Some VB beginners may fail to see the ***syntax error*** in the following structure:

```
If A > B Then Print A
Else Print B
End If
```

continues

When an If statement ends with an executable statement (as in the first line), VB considers the If block complete. Thus, the Else and End If statements below will have no context. The *correct structure* should be as follows:

```
If A > B Then
     Print A
Else Print B
End If
```

Note that the "Print B" statement can be placed in the same line with Else as shown in this box or be placed below Else (the preferred way) as shown in the text.

Leaving One Side Out. Note that with this syntax structure, it is okay to omit statements from either the True or False side of the block. For example, the following code should cause no syntax problem:

```
Private Sub chkCitizen_Click()
     If chkCitizen.Value = vbChecked Then
     'Respondent is a citizen. No problem.
     Else
     'Respondent is not a citizen. Reject the service.
          MsgBox "You are not qualified to serve as a Juror."
     End If
End Sub
```

This event procedure is triggered when the user clicks the check box that asks whether the respondent is a citizen. As you can imagine, the check box is used in a data-entry screen for the jury selection questionnaire. If the box is checked off, the "qualification" message is displayed. In this example, a statement is provided only on the False side of the block. You may wonder why not directly test whether the check box is unchecked as follows:

```
If chkCitizen.Value = vbUnChecked Then
'Respondent is not a citizen. Reject the service.
     MsgBox "You are not qualified to serve as a Juror."
End If
```

Both blocks of preceding code should work properly. Indeed, the second block appears to be more concise. However, some companies have coding standards that require all conditions in the If statement be expressed in affirmation. They maintain that such a coding standard makes the code easier to review because of code logic uniformity.

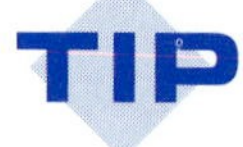

Avoid using If statements with negative conditions. Combining Not with Or can be confusing. As an illustration of negative conditions with the Or operator, consider the following code:

```
If lstTest.Style <> vbListBoxStandard Or _
     lstTest.MultiSelect <> vbMultiSelectNone Then
'Statements to handle multiple selections
End If
```

The code tests whether the list box allows multiple selection (figure it out for yourself). The following code alternative should be easier to understand:

```
If lstTest.Style = vbListBoxStandard And _
     lstTest.MultiSelect = vbMultiSelectNone Then
'The list box does not allow multi-selection
Else
'Statements to handle multiple selections
End If
```

It is also perfectly acceptable to provide code for only the True side of the If block as illustrated in the following code:

```
Private Sub txtName_LostFocus()
    If Len(Trim$(txtName.Text)) = 0 Then
        MsgBox "Please enter name before proceeding further."
        txtName.SetFocus 'Reset focus on txtName
    Else
    End If
End Sub
```

This event procedure is invoked when the user moves away from a text box named txtName. The If statement checks whether the VB control is blank. If so, an error message is displayed and the focus is reset on txtName, using the SetFocus method. As discussed in Chapter 3, "Some Visual Basic Controls and Events," this is the "traditional" way of performing field-level data validation. Data validation is discussed more thoroughly in Chapter 10, "Special Topics in Data Entry."

Note that the previous If block can actually do without the Else line. You can think of the Else statement as being there as a reminder that no statement has been coded on the False side.

The If...Then...ElseIf...Then...Else...End If Block

Many times, a decision can be much more complicated than that in the previous example; that is, several conditions, rather than just the "either or" situation, will determine the "conclusion." For example, a teacher may assign an A to any score greater than or equal to 90, a B if the score is greater than or equal to 80, and a C to all other scores. Is there an If block that can handle this situation conveniently? Yes! The syntax appears as follows:

```
If Condition1 Then
    Statements to be executed when condition1 is True
ElseIf Condndtion2 Then
    Statements to be executed when condition2 is True
ElseIf Condition3 Then
    Statements to be executed when condition3 is True
Else
    Statements to be executed
    when none of the above conditions are True
End If
```

In this structure, you can have as many ElseIf statements as desired following the If statement. You can then code a "catch all" Else statement after all of the ElseIf statements. It is an error to place an ElseIf after an Else statement. Again, the entire block is closed with an End If statement.

When the block is executed, the conditions in the If block are tested one after another top down (condition1 then condition2, and so on) until one condition is true. At that point, those statements under that condition are executed and the remainder of the If block is skipped. If none of the conditions are true, the statements in the Else portion (if any) are executed.

Using this structure, the teacher's grade assignment problem can be coded as follows:

```
If Score >= 90 Then
    Grade = "A"
ElseIf Score >= 80 Then
    Grade = "B"
Else
    Grade = "C"
End If
```

The code will first check whether Score is greater than or equal to 90. If so, A is assigned to Grade and the remainder of the If block is ignored. If the first condition is not true, the ElseIf statement checks to see whether Score is greater than or equal to 80. If so, B is assigned to Grade and the remaining part of the If block is ignored. On the other hand, if the condition in the ElseIf statement is not true, the statement in the Else block will be executed; that is, C is assigned to Grade.

Varying the Criteria. Of course, this structure can be used to handle more complex situations. Consider this investment decision example. An independent oil exploration company will invest in an oil exploration project if a pretest indicates that the probability of finding oil is at least 50%. Otherwise, the net present value of the project will have to be greater than $1 million. If not, the company will invest only if the project will cost less than $100,000. The decision rule can be depicted as in Figure 5.10.

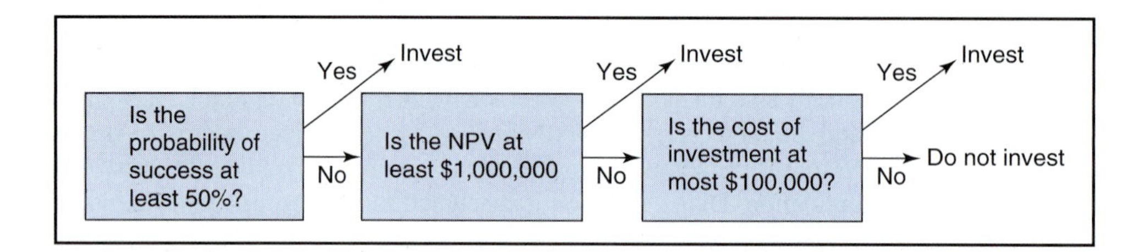

Figure 5.10
Decision Rules for the Investment Decision

Note that unlike the previous example, at each stage of the decision, a different factor is involved in this problem. This, however, poses no problem to this If structure. Assume Invest is a Boolean variable indicating whether to invest. Also, the variables, Probability, NPV, and Cost, have been assigned proper values. One way to solve the problem is to code the following:

```
If Probability >= .5 Then
    Invest = True 'Invest when the probability of success is high
ElseIf NPV >= 1000000 Then
    Invest = True 'Invest when the expected return is high
ElseIf Cost <= 100000 Then
    Invest = True 'Invest when the cost risk is low
Else
    Invest = False ' don't invest if none of the above is true
End If
```

An Error-Checking Procedure: Another Example. Like the previous "If Then Else" block, any part of the "If Then ElseIf Then" structure may leave out statements without causing a syntax problem. To illustrate, consider a data-entry error-checking routine. You would like to be sure that keys entered into a text box named txtNumber are numbers. If not, you want to display an error message and suppress the key. How do you code this?

As you recall, when the user presses a key, the KeyPress event is triggered and the KeyAscii value of the key is also passed as a parameter to this event procedure. In coding this event, you should do the following:

- Inspect the key to see if it is numeric.
- Be aware that not all the keys that are nonnumeric are "bad keys" for this error-checking purpose. The control keys, such as the Enter key and the Backspace key, are also captured in the KeyPress event. All these control keys have an ASCII value lower than 32 (the ASCII value of the space key, a constant named vbKeySpace).
- Display an error message and suppress the key if it does not belong to either of the previous two groups of keys.

How do you check for a numeric key? The system constant names for the ASCII values of the keys 0 and 9 are vbKey0 (48) and vbKey9 (57), respectively. You can compare the KeyAscii value of the key pressed to see if it is in this range. One way to implement the error-checking procedure will be as follows:

```
Private Sub txtNumber_KeyPress(KeyAscii As Integer)
    If KeyAscii < vbKeySpace Then
    ' These are control keys, ignore.
    ElseIf KeyAscii >= vbKey0 And KeyAscii <= vbKey9 Then
    ' These are numeric keys, ignore.
```

```
        Else
        ' These are neither control keys nor numeric keys.
        ' Display an error message
            MsgBox "Please enter numeric keys only."
            KeyAscii = 0 ' Suppress the key
        End If
    End Sub
```

In this code example, no statement appears in either the If or the ElseIf portion of the If block. However, the code works exactly the way you want it to. The KeyAscii value is first compared with vbKeySpace (32). If the value is less than 32, the key is a control key. Otherwise (the ElseIf block), the value is checked to see whether it is within the range of numeric keys. If not (the Else block), an error message is displayed. In addition, the KeyAscii parameter is assigned a value of zero. This will suppress the key. As a result, no key will appear in the text box.

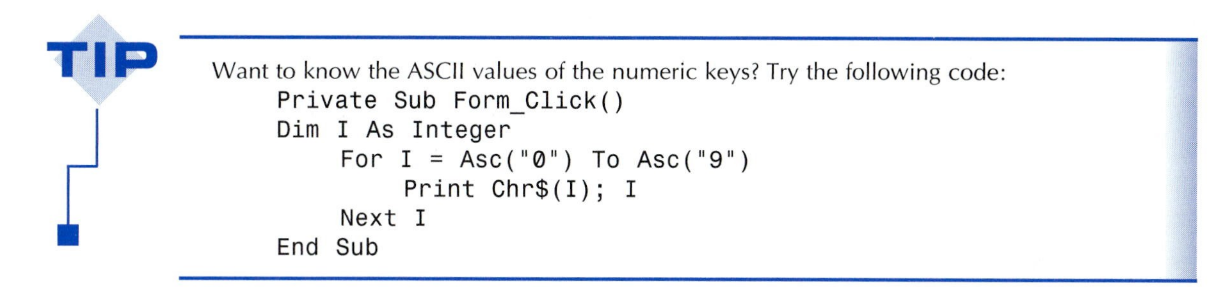

TIP

Want to know the ASCII values of the numeric keys? Try the following code:

```
Private Sub Form_Click()
Dim I As Integer
    For I = Asc("0") To Asc("9")
        Print Chr$(I); I
    Next I
End Sub
```

Nesting If Blocks

Any of the If blocks can be further nested to handle complex conditions. As an illustration, assume a teacher's grading system requires that a student must have not only a score of 90 or better but also a perfect attendance to earn an A; otherwise, a B is given. A student with a score in the range of 80 to 89 must have at least a 90% attendance record to earn a B. All other students will get a C. These decision rules are depicted in the flowchart in Figure 5.11.

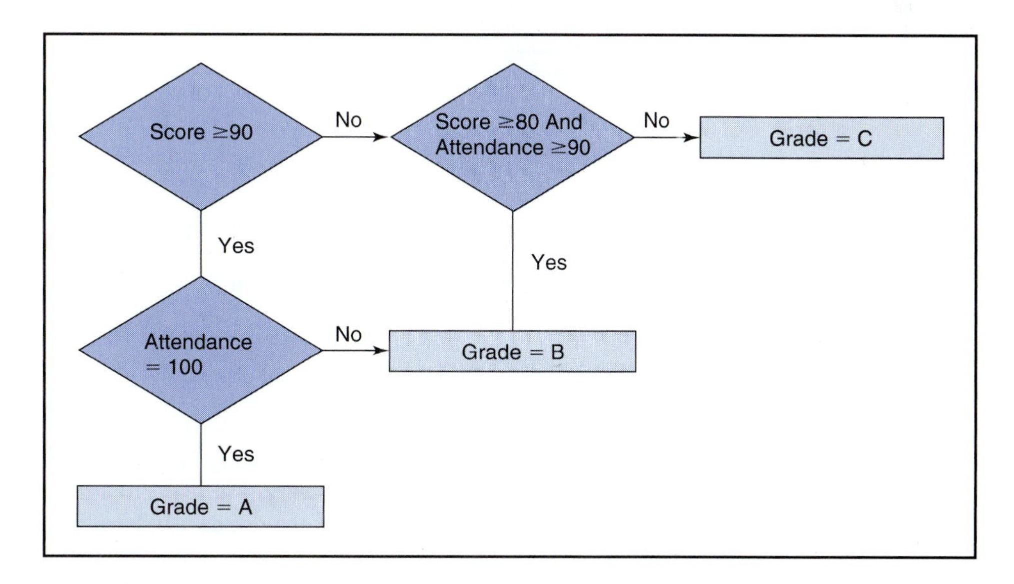

Figure 5.11
Flowchart of Grade Assignment

The two text boxes in the user interface shown in Figure 5.12 are used to enter both the score (txtScore) and the attendance percentage (txtAttendance). When the user clicks on the "Show Grade" button (cmdGrade), the grade is displayed in the label named lblGrade. The following code provides a solution:

```
Private Sub cmdGrade_Click()
Dim Score As Integer
```

```
Dim Attendance As Integer
Dim Grade As String
    Score = Val(txtScore.Text)
    Attendance = Val(txtAttendance.Text)
    If Score >= 90 Then
        If Attendance = 100 Then
            Grade = "A"
        Else
            Grade = "B"
        End If
    ElseIf Score >= 80 And Attendance >= 90 Then
        Grade = "B"
    Else
        Grade = "C"
    End If
    lblGrade.Caption = Grade
End Sub
```

In the preceding code, the score and attendance percentage are obtained from the two text boxes, txtScore and txtAttendance, respectively. The score is first compared with 90. If it is greater or equal to 90, the second-level If statement checks whether the attendance value is equal to 100. If so, an A grade is assigned; otherwise, a B grade is assigned. The ElseIf statement checks whether the score is greater than or equal to 80 and the attendance is at least 90. If so, a B grade is assigned; otherwise, a C grade is assigned. The resulting grade is displayed in a label, named lblGrade.

Figure 5.12
The User Interface for Grade Assignment

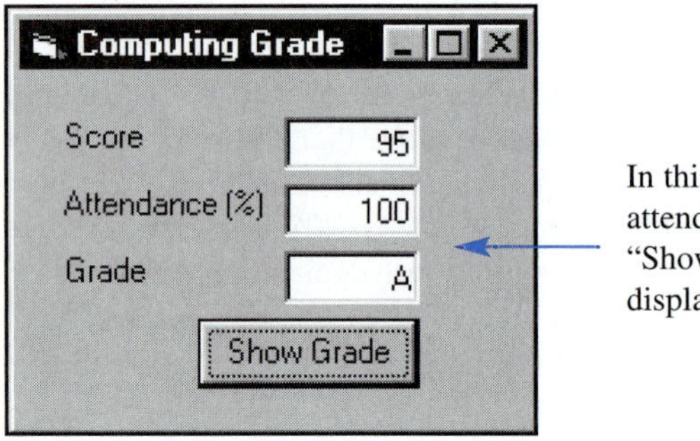

In this project, the user enters the score and attendance percentage and then clicks the "Show Grade" button. The resulting grade is displayed in a label named lblGrade.

Will This Work? You may wonder why not just code as follows to solve the previous problem:

```
If Score>=90 And Attendance = 100 Then
    Grade = "A"
ElseIf Score >= 80 And Attendance >= 90 Then
    Grade = "B"
Else
    Grade = "C"
End If
lblGrade.Caption = Grade
```

This would appear much simpler. But *the modified code would not work correctly*. The initial problem states that if a student has a score of at least 90 and perfect attendance, he or she will earn an A. Without perfect attendance, he or she will earn a B. The original solution produces the correct result. The modified code will assign a C to a student who has a score of 100 but with an 80% attendance! The 80% attendance will fail not only the If test but also the ElseIf test, thus falling into the "catch all" Else block for an assignment of a grade C.

Rule for Nesting. When If blocks are nested, one rule to keep in mind is that one block should enclose the other, constituting a relationship of the inner and outer blocks. It is not logical (and therefore not allowed) to intertwine any If blocks. Figure 5.13 shows both the acceptable and unacceptable nesting blocks.

Figure 5.13

Legitimate and Illegitimate Nesting of If Blocks

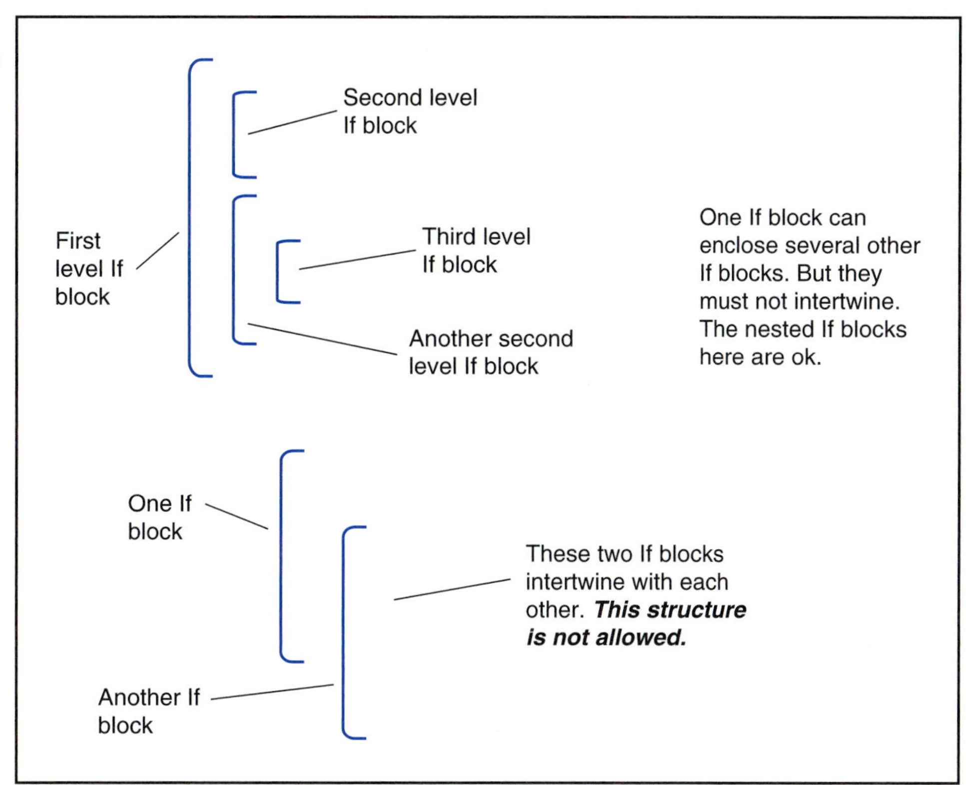
Second level If block
First level If block
Third level If block
Another second level If block
One If block can enclose several other If blocks. But they must not intertwine. The nested If blocks here are ok.
One If block
Another If block
These two If blocks intertwine with each other. ***This structure is not allowed.***

If Blocks: A Summary of Syntax. In terms of syntax, the If block can be structured several ways. The following table provides a summary.

Syntax Structure	Example	Remark
If *condition* Then *statement*	If optMale.Value Then Sex = "M"	This is not a preferred coding structure.

If *Condition* Then
  Statement(s)
End If
	If Len(txtName.Text) = 0 Then
	  MsgBox "Must have a name"
	  txtName.SetFocus
	End If
		Use this structure to handle situations in which one or more statements must be executed when a certain condition is True, but no action is required when the condition is False.

If *Condition* Then
  Statements
Else
  Statements
End If
	If chkPrintAll.Value = vbChecked Then
	
	  lstZipCode.Enabled = False
	Else
	  lstZipCode.Enabled = True
	End If
		Use this structure to handle situations in which a group of statements need to be executed when the condition is True, otherwise another group of statements are to be executed.

If *Condition1* Then
  Statement group 1
ElseIf *Condition2* Then
  Statement group 2
ElseIf *Condition3* Then
  Statement group 3
Else
  Statement group 4
End If
	If optBreakfast.Value Then
	  Charge = 4.50
	ElseIf optLunch.Value Then
	  Charge = 7.50
	ElseIf optDinner.Value Then
	  Charge = 10. 50
	Else
	  Charge = 0
	End If
		Use this structure when a series of mutually exclusive conditions will require different actions or cause different results.

Additional Notes on Coding the If Block

If blocks are used extensively in programs because most programming problems involve many decisions. We need to consider several issues before leaving the topic.

Indenting. When If blocks are used, the programming logic becomes less than straightforward because some statements may or may not be executed based on the result of the If expression. Keeping track of all possible results can become challenging. Thus, it is important to provide as much "visual aid" as possible in the code to facilitate future review and current logic development/tracing.

One important aspect of this is to indent the code properly. In addition to observing the normal rule of indenting inside a program, all statements in each portion of the If block should be indented. In a nested block, the inside If block skeleton (If, ElseIf, Else, and End If) should be indented just like the inside statements. However, the statements inside the inner If block should be further indented. Such a layout clearly indicates the level of logical nesting. You probably have noticed that all code in the previous examples has followed this standard. To refresh your memory, here is a layout:

```
If Condition1 Then '(level 1 If block)
    Statements may appear here (level 1)
    If Condition2 Then      '(level 2 if block)
        Statements may appear here (level 2)
        If Condition3 Then '(Level 3 if block)
            Statements (level 3)
        ElseIf Condition4 Then '(Level 3)
        Statements (level 3)
        Else
        Statements (level 3)
        End If
        Statements may appear here (level 2)
    ElseIf Condition5 Then '(level 2)
        Statements may appear here
        (Several levels of nested If similar to above can appear)
    Else
        Statements may appear here
        (several levels of nested if blocks can appear here)
    End If
    Statements may appear here
ElseIf Condition6 Then '(Level 1)
    Statements including nested If statements can appear
Else '(level 1)
    Statements including nested If statements can appear
End If
```

Note, however, that indenting the code does not affect its execution. It only enhances code readability. You still need to exercise care in ensuring that:

- All open If statements are properly matched with the End If statements.
- Right statements to execute are placed in the right block.

Use of Comments. The importance of using comments (remarks) in programs cannot be overemphasized. Comments can be especially helpful to people who review code that contains many If statements. In many cases, the meaning of the expressions (conditions) in the If statement is not very self-explanatory. Comments help you and the reviewer follow the logic of the code much more easily. Consider the following statement:

```
If KeyAscii < vbKeySpace Then
```

Without any comments with it, it may take a while for a beginner to figure out what the If statement is attempting to accomplish. Adding a remark similar to the following line can make it much easier for anybody who reads the code:

```
' These are control keys and can be ignored
```

Efficiency and Clarity. Another issue concerning the use of the If block relates to the efficiency (speed of execution) versus the clarity of code. Consider this line of code (used in some countries to determine whether a person is a candidate for military draft):

```
If Sex = "M" And Age >=16 Then
```

Although the line of code is very clear, it is not as efficient as the following code:

```
If Sex = "M" Then
    If Age >= 16 Then
```

In the first approach, three operations are always involved in the expression: First, Sex is compared with "M." Second, Age is compared with 16. Finally, an And operation is performed on the results from the two comparisons. On the other hand, the second approach may take only one operation to reach a decision, thus is much more efficient. Because the probability of a person being a male is approximately 50%, the chance that the second If statement is tested is only one half. In addition, there is no need to perform an "And" operation. Thus, there is clearly a conflict between code clarity and code efficiency.

Which way do you prefer? Apparently, there should be a proper balance. In general, as long as the code clarity is not inhibited too badly, the second approach should be used. In addition to being faster, there are cases in which only the second approach will work. For example, assume that an individual investor will consider whether to invest in a stock only if the company's earnings per share (EPS) is positive and its price:earnings ratio is less than 20. The following statement may result in execution error:

```
If EPS > 0 And Price / EPS < 20 Then
```

Why? Because EPS may be equal to zero, resulting in a "divide by zero" error when the computer attempts to evaluate Price/EPS. A code structure as shown next will not have the problem because the second condition will be evaluated only if EPS is greater than zero.

```
If EPS > 0 Then
    If Price / EPS < 20 Then
```

We have just considered the case of the And operator. How about the Or operator? There are situations in which you can easily break a statement involving Or operations into several lines. For example, assume that you have a routine that you do not want to execute if A > B Or C > D Or A*C > 100. You certainly can code it as follows:

```
If A > B Or C > D Or A * C > 100 Then Exit Sub
```

where *Exit Sub* is a statement to leave the Sub procedure without further executing any statements below that line. Its effect is the same as if the execution has reached the End Sub statement.

However, the following code will be faster (for the same reason as explained earlier) and probably clearer:

```
If A > B Then Exit Sub
If C > D Then Exit Sub
If A * C > 100 Then Exit Sub
```

There are, however, situations in which breaking a statement with the Or operator can result in many more lines of code. Consider the following If block:

```
If A > B Or C > D Then
    Many statements here to be executed (block 1)
Else
    Many statements here to be executed (block 2)
End If
```

This structure can be rewritten as follows:

```
If A > B Then
    Many statements here to be executed (block 1)
Else
    Many statements here to be executed (block 2)
End If
```

```
If C > D Then
    Many statements here to be executed (block 1)
Else
    Many statements here to be executed (block 2)
End If
```

Apparently, breaking the If statement into two separate blocks will result in repeating both blocks of statements in each of the newly constructed If blocks. The code will not appear to be concise.

Code Clarity and Alternatives. As we have pointed out several times, when the code involves too many If blocks (especially nested ones), it can become challenging to trace the logic. The effects of the code can become much harder to figure out. Are there any alternatives? Yes, the possibilities include the following:

1. ***Use of the IIf (immediate If) function***: The IIf function has the syntax:

   ```
   IIf(Condition, expression 1, expression 2)
   ```

   This function returns the value of expression 1 when the condition is evaluated to be True; otherwise, it returns the value of expression 2. For example, in the following statement:

   ```
   A = IIf(X > 0, Y, Z)
   ```

   A will have a value Y when X > 0; otherwise, it will have a value of Z.

   The IIf function is known to be slow. All three arguments passed to the functions are evaluated before a value is returned. In addition, some potential problems exist. For example, suppose you would like to assign the result of Y/X to A when X is positive; otherwise, a zero. The following code will result in an error when X is zero because Y/X will be always evaluated whether X is 0 or not.

   ```
   A = IIf(X > 0, Y/X, 0)
   ```

   In summary, IIf can be used in certain situations to shorten the code. However, because of the concern of its efficiency and some potential problems, it may not truly be a good alternative to the If block.

2. ***Computations:*** With careful analysis, many of the apparent needs for the If block can be converted into computational formulas. Consider the following code that we used in one of the previous illustrations.

   ```
   Private Sub chkSort_Click()
       If chkSort.Value =vbChecked Then
           cboSortField1.Enabled = True
           cboSortField2.Enabled = True
       Else
           cboSortField1.Enabled = False
           cboSortField2.Enabled = False
       End If
   End Sub
   ```

   The procedure enables or disables the combo boxes, cboSortField1 and cboSortField2, depending on whether the check box chkSort is checked. An alternative way to code the procedure is given as follows:

   ```
   Private Sub chkSort_Click()
   Dim OnOff as Boolean
       OnOff = chkSort.Value = vbChecked
       cboSortField1.Enabled = OnOff
       cboSortField2.Enabled = OnOff
   End Sub
   ```

   In the preceding code, the Boolean variable is assigned a value True when the Value property of chkSort is equal to vbChecked (when the check box is checked) and False when the check box is checked off. This result is then assigned to the Enabled property of the two combo boxes, causing the two combo boxes to be enabled or disabled, depending on the value of OnOff. (Again, to test the code, set the Enabled property of the two combo boxes to False at design time.)

As another example, assume that a bookstore sells only three book titles. A customer can buy only one copy of each book but can buy any combination of the three books. The check boxes chkBook1, chkBook2, and chkBook3 are used to represent whether the customer wants each of the books. Their prices are represented by the variables Price1, Price2, and Price3, respectively. When the customer is ready to check out, the cashier clicks on the check boxes and the command button cmdCompute to compute the total purchase. The result is displayed in the label lblTotal. The visual interface appears as in Figure 5.14.

Figure 5.14
Visual Interface for "Only-Three" Bookstore

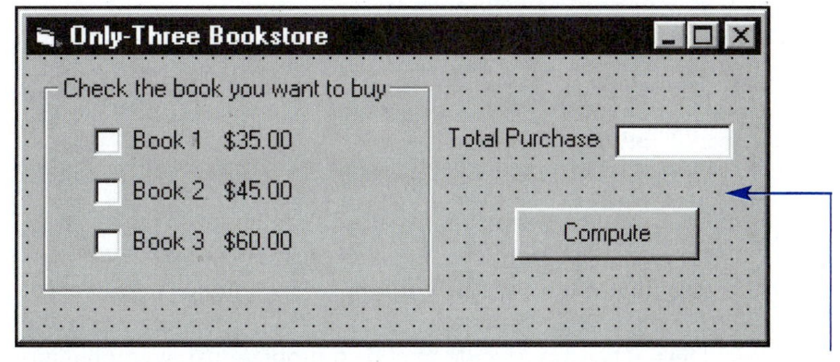

This bookstore sells only three books. After the customer makes the selections, the cashier clicks the Compute button to get the total purchase. The "text box" is actually a label, named lblTotal. You can make it appear this way by setting its BackColor to white and BorderStyle to 1 (Fixed Single).

One possible solution to this problem is as follows:

```
Private Sub cmdCompute_click()
Dim Total as Currency
   Total = 0
   If chkBook1.Value = vbChecked Then
      Total = Price1
   End If
   If chkBook2.Value = vbChecked Then
      Total = Total + Price2
   End If
   If chkBook3.Value = vbChecked Then
      Total = Total + Price3
   End If
   lblTotal.Caption = Total
End Sub
```

Because the value of a check box is 1 (vbChecked) when it is checked and zero otherwise, the preceding code can be converted into a computational formula. The modified code can appear as follows:

```
Private Sub cmdCompute_click()
Dim Total as Currency
    Total = chkBook1.Value * Price1 + chkBook2.Value * Price2 _
       + chkBook3.Value * Price3
    lblTotal.Caption = Total
End Sub
```

How does the code work? Consider the first book. If its check box is checked, chkBook1.Value will be 1. Thus, the following expression:

```
chkBook1.Value * Price1
```

will result in a value of Price1. If the check box is off, the result will be zero. The same is true for the expressions for the other two books. Thus, adding the results of the three multiplication expressions should yield the correct total. As in the previous example, the computational alternative has much shorter code and the If condition is embedded in the formula.

In the previous code, we focused on computing the total and did not show how Price1, Price2, and Price3 obtained their values. They should be declared as form level variables and can be initialized in the Form Load event. So that we can focus on our current discussion, a simple solution is given here. A better solution is given in the exercise.

```
Option Explicit
Dim Price1 As Currency
Dim Price2 As Currency
Dim Price3 As Currency
Private Sub Form_Load()
    Price1 = 35
    Price2 = 45
    Price3 = 60
End Sub
```

Let's return to our discussion of computing the total. Although the alternative appears to be more concise, you must not get carried away with this approach. The meaning of the code may not be as apparent or intuitive as the If block. Sometimes, this alternative approach may not produce the correct result or execute efficiently. Thus, when you decide to code a problem using computational formulas in place of the If block, be sure that you test the code thoroughly. In addition, provide comments in the code to explain how the formula works so that the formula will not become a mystery when you review it in the future.

3. ***Use of the Select Case Block:*** If the conditions in the "If, ElseIf" block depend on the different results of the same expression, one good alternative to the If block is the Select Case Block. This is explained in the next section.

5.3 The Select Case Block

As explained in the Section 5.2, an alternative to the If block is the Select Case block, which is particularly useful when the decision depends on the result of one single expression. Consider the previous example of assigning a grade based strictly on the student's score. The grade will be A, B, or C if the score is at least 90, 80, or below 80, respectively. This problem can be conveniently solved by the use of the Select Case block.

Syntax Structure

The Select Case block has the following syntax structure:

```
Select Case Expression
Case Criterion 1
    Statements (group1) to be executed when criterion 1 matches _
    the result of expression
Case Criterion 2
    Statements (group 2) to be executed when criterion 2 matches _
    the result of expression
.
.
Case Criterion n
    Statements (group n) to be executed when criterion n matches _
    the result of expression
Case Else
    Statements (group n+1) to be executed when none of the _
    above criteria match the result of expression
End Select
```

Where the expression can be any kind: numeric, string, or logical; and the criteria should have the same type as the expression. Each criterion can consist of a list of single values and ranges.

As an illustration, using the Select Case block, the grading problem discussed in the preceding section can be coded as follows:

```
Select Case Score
Case Is >= 90
     Grade = "A"
Case 80 To 90
     Grade = "B"
Case Else
     Grade = "C"
End Select
```

As you can see from the illustration, Score is the expression whose value will be evaluated against the criteria stated in the "Cases." The first Case (Is >= 90) has an open range; that is, any Score value greater or equal to 90 will belong to this Case and will result in the statement Grade = "A" being executed. The second Case has a closed range (where both ends are specified) and is expressed with the keyword "To." A score in the range of 80 to 90 will result in the statement Grade = "B" being executed. Finally, if none of the cases are true, the statement(s) in the catch all Case Else will be executed.

When specifying the range in the Case statement, always specify the lower value first. Otherwise, the criterion will never be True. In checking the range, the computer assumes the first number is the lower end of the range and the second value is the higher end. That is, the following Case *will never be True*:

```
Case 90 To 80
```

Mutual Exclusiveness of Cases. Notice that the cases are considered mutually exclusive; that is, only one of the case blocks will be executed. The testing of cases starts from the top and proceeds down. As soon as a criterion (Case) is found true, no more comparisons will be performed. Thus, in the previous example, when a score is 90, "A" will be assigned to Grade. The second case will never be tested (even though 90 is also a value in the second case), resulting in a correct assignment decision.

Why not just code the second case "Case 80 to 89"? This will work correctly as long as Score is an Integer (Long or Short) variable. However, if Score is a variable that can take on a fractional value, a score of 89.99 will not belong to this case and thus become a "Case Else."

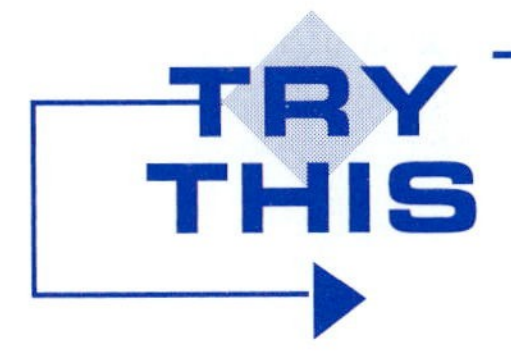

Draw a text box on a new form. Enter the following code:

```
Private Sub Form_Click()
     Select Case Val(Text1.Text)
     Case 0 To 60 'First message
          MsgBox "The number is in the range of 0 to 60."
     Case 50 To 100 'Second message
          MsgBox "The number is in the range of 50 to 100."
     End Select
End Sub
```

Enter a number in the range of 50 to 60; you will always see the first message displayed. The second message is displayed only when you enter a value greater than 60. See how the block works when the criteria in the Case statements are not mutually exclusive?

Detailed Syntax Rules. When coding the criteria, observe the following syntax rules:

- To specify a value to test for equality, give the value. For example, "Case 80" would mean to compare whether the expression in the Select Case statement (the expression; e.g., Score) is equal to 80.
- To specify several values to test for equality, separate the values in the list with commas. For example, "Case 80, 81, 85" would mean to compare whether the expression is equal to 80, 81, or 85.
- To specify a closed range, insert the keyword "To" between the lower- and upper-end values. For example, "Case 80 To 90" would mean to test whether the expression is within the range of 80 to 90 (inclusive).
- To specify an open range, use the keyword "Is." For example, "Case Is < 0" would mean to test whether the expression is negative.
- You can combine all these situations in one Case statement by separating the criteria with commas. For example, you can code the following:

```
Case 50, 80 To 90, Is < 0
```

Variations in the Case Structure. Just like the If block, you can omit statements from any of the cases. For example, in the preceding section, we used the If block to check for numeric keys for a text box, txtNumber. That routine can be replaced by the use of the Select Case block as follows:

```
Private Sub txtNumber_KeyPress(KeyAscii as Integer)
     Select Case KeyAscii
     Case Is < vbKeySpace
     ' These are control keys; ignore
     Case vbKey0 To vbKey9
     'These are numeric keys; ignore
     Case Else
     ' These are neither control keys nor numeric keys;
     ' display an error message and suppress the key
        MsgBox "Numeric key only, please."
        KeyAscii = 0
     End Select
End Sub
```

This code allows only numeric keys. What if you also expect a decimal point to be entered? The ASCII value for period (decimal point) is 46. (There is no predefined named constant for this key.) To accommodate this, you can insert the following line:

```
Case 46
```

Without any statement following this Case, no message will be displayed; just like the previous two Cases.

Because all three cases are handled in the same way (do nothing), we could indeed combine the three cases together:

```
Select Case KeyAscii
Case Is < vbKeySpace, vbKey0 To vbKey9, 46
' Legitimate keys; do nothing
Case Else
' Unexpected keys; display a message and suppress the key
     MsgBox "Numeric key only, please."
     KeyAscii = 0
End Select
```

Note that in the first Case statement, commas are used to separate the three criteria. It is interesting to point out that this Case provides a good example of a list of all types of criteria allowed by the syntax: open-ended range, closed range, and single value. Of course, you can add more to the list. For example, if you also expect negative numbers, you can also include 45 (ASCII code for "-") in the Case line:

```
Case Is < vbKeySpace, vbKey0 To vbKey9, 45, 46
```

Note that when coding individual values in the list, their order does not really matter. However, for convenience and clarity, you should list them in the order that gives you the clearest meaning.

Dealing with Constants. The use of the numeric values 45 and 46 in the previous code should cause you to be concerned about code clarity. When you come back to review the code after a while, you may not be able to understand what these two values represent. One possible solution is to use the Asc function. Recall that this function gives the ASCII value of a key. Thus, in place of 45 and 46, you can code the following:

```
Case Is < vbKeySpace, vbKey0 To vbKey9, Asc("-"), Asc(".")
```

The code will be clearer. However, it will execute a bit slower because the Asc function will need to be called to give the ASCII values of the two keys. Another alternative is to declare two constants for the two keys and use them wherever they are needed. For example, you can declare the following:

```
Const KeyMinus As Integer = 45
Const KeyPeriod As Integer = 46
```

Then code the Case statement as follows:

```
Case Is < vbKeySpace, vbKey0 To vbKey9, KeyMinus, KeyPeriod
```

This approach takes a bit more code, but the code is both efficient and clear.

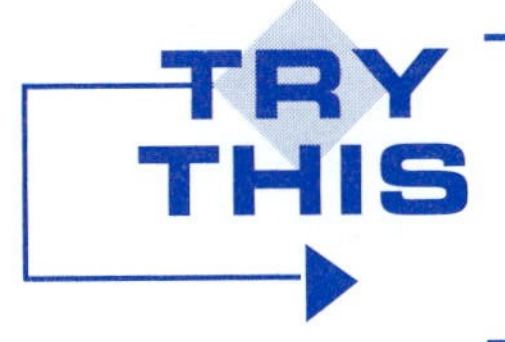

Enter "Case < vbKeySpace" in the code window for the previous example. Then move the cursor to another line. You will see the line you have just entered is changed to "Case Is < vbKeySpace." The IDE does more than we expect, doesn't it? This also indicates that the IDE checks the syntax of each line you enter as soon as you move away from it.

Nesting Select Case Blocks

You can nest Select Case Blocks in the same way the If blocks are nested. That is, within each Case of a Select Case block, you can code another Select Case block. The nesting can practically go as deep as you would like. (Beware of the problem with clarity though.) As in the case of the If blocks, you should never intertwine a Select Case block with another.

An Example. As an illustration of nesting the Select Case blocks, assume that a university charges tuition based on the student's residence status and the number of hours taken, as shown in the following table.

Hours Taken	In State	Out of State	International
0–5	850	1,250	1,700
6–8	1,000	1,500	2,000
9–11	1,300	2,000	2,700
12–over	1,500	2,300	3,200

You are to design a project to determine the student's tuition when he or she enrolls. How should you proceed?

As usual, you will need to design the visual interface first. The student must declare a residence status among the three categories. These represent mutually exclusive alternatives that will most likely remain unchanged for a long while. Thus, option buttons will be a good choice. The number of hours taken can be entered into a text box. The visual design can appear as in Figure 5.15.

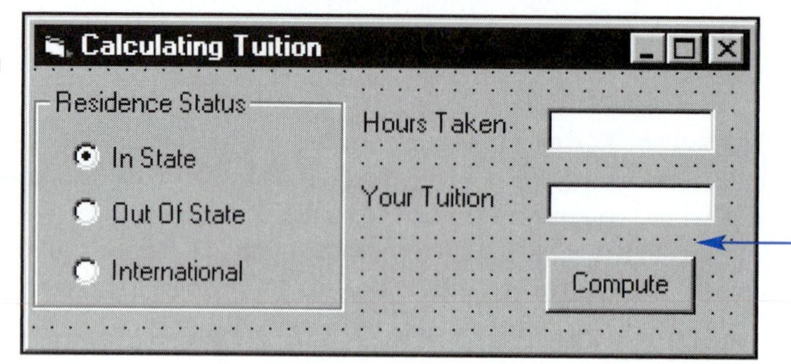

In this application, the user selects the residence status, enters the number of hours taken, then clicks the Compute button. The tuition is displayed in the label named lblTuition.

Figure 5.15
Visual Interface for Tuition Calculation

A list of the properties of the VB controls used in code is given in the following table.

Control	Property	Setting	Remark
Option button	Caption	In State	
	Name	optInState	
	Value	True	As the default option
Option button	Caption	Out Of State	
	Name	optOutOfState	
Option button	Caption	International	
	Name	optInternational	
Text box	Name	txtHoursTaken	To enter hours taken
Label	Name	lblTuition	To display tuition
	BackColor	White	So that the label will look like a text box
	BorderStyle	1-Fxied Single	
Command button	Caption	Compute	To initiate tuition computation
	Name	cmdCompute	

Notice that the Value property of the option button named optInState is set to True so that it will be used as the default status. When the user clicks the Compute command button, your program will show the result in the label named lblTuition.

How can your program determine a student's tuition? There are several different ways to handle this. One possibility is to use the nested Select Case blocks. As you can see from the table, two factors jointly determine the amount of tuition: residence status and hours taken. Either of the factors can be considered the first level of branching. Suppose we use the hours taken as the first level. Then, we can use the following skeleton to code the problem:

```
Private Sub cmdCompute_Click()
Dim Tuition As Currency
    Select Case Val(txtHoursTaken.Text)
    Case 0 to 5
    'For the first bracket
    Case 6 To 8
    'For the second bracket
    Case 9 to 11
    'For the third bracket
    Case Else
    '12 or more hours
```

```
        End Select
        lblTuition.Caption = Tuition 'Display the tuition
    End Sub
```

Within each Case, we can then code the tuition based on the residence status. The question is, Should we also use the Select Case structure? We can, but it takes a bit more analysis. Perhaps, we will begin with the more straightforward If block first. Inspect the table again; under the 0 to 5 hours bracket, you see that a student with an in-state, out-of-state, and international status will pay 850, 1250, 1700, respectively. Thus, the first bracket can be coded as follows:

```
Select Case Val(txtHoursTaken.Text)
Case 0 to 5 'For the first bracket
    If optInState.Value Then
        Tuition = 850
    ElseIf optOutOfState.Value Then
        Tuition = 1250
    Else
        Tuition = 1700
    End If
Case 6 To 8 'For the second bracket
Case 9 to 11 'For the third bracket
Case Else '12 or more hours
End Select
```

The rest of the brackets can be coded in a similar fashion and is left to you as an exercise.

Note that the If block can be conveniently used here to handle the option buttons because the state (value) of each button is a different expression. Using the Select Case structure to handle multiple expressions like this can be a challenge. By syntax, the Select Case structure is more "natural" to branch based on one single expression.

Identifying the Option Button Selected. To "force" the use of Select Case structure to handle option buttons, a commonly used approach is to introduce a form level variable, whose value can then be set in the Click event of each option button. For example, when optInState, optOutOfState, or optInternational is clicked, the variable, ResidenceStatus, can be set to 0, 1, or 2. Then, ResidenceStatus can be used as an expression in the Select Case statement. The following code should set the value of ResidenceStatus properly.

```
Option Explicit
Dim ResidenceStatus As Integer

Private Sub optInState_Click()
    ResidenceStatus = 0
End Sub

Private Sub optOutOfState_Click()
    ResidenceStatus = 1
End Sub

Private Sub optInternational_Click()
    ResidenceStatus = 2
End Sub
```

Once the residence status is determined, you can add the following Select Case block to determine the tuition of the first bracket of hours taken.

```
Select Case ResidenceStatus
Case 0 'In State
    Tuition = 850
Case 1 'Out of State
    Tuition = 1250
Case 2 'International
    Tuition = 1700
End Select
```

The complete code for the command Click event procedure using the nested Select Case blocks can then appear as follows:

```
Private Sub cmdCompute_Click()
Dim Tuition As Currency
    Select Case Val(txtHoursTaken.Text)
    Case 0 To 5 'First bracket
        Select Case ResidenceStatus
        Case 0 'In State
            Tuition = 850
        Case 1 'Out of State
            Tuition = 1250
        Case 2 'International
            Tuition = 1700
        End Select
    Case 6 To 8 'Second bracket
        Select Case ResidenceStatus
        Case 0 'In State
            Tuition = 1000
        Case 1 'Out of State
            Tuition = 1500
        Case 2 'International
            Tuition = 2000
        End Select
    Case 9 To 11 'Third bracket
        Select Case ResidenceStatus
        Case 0 'In State
            Tuition = 1300
        Case 1 'Out of State
            Tuition = 2000
        Case 2 'International
            Tuition = 2700
        End Select
    Case Else '12 hours or more
        Select Case ResidenceStatus
        Case 0 'In State
            Tuition = 1500
        Case 1 'Out of State
            Tuition = 2300
        Case 2 'International
            Tuition = 3200
        End Select
    End Select
    lblTuition.Caption = Tuition 'Display tuition
End Sub
```

The logic in this procedure appears fairly straightforward. Identifying the option button selected, however, takes some analysis. Incidentally, there is a trick that you can use with the Select Case structure to identify fairly easily the option button selected. However, it takes some "inverted" thinking. Rather than explaining its logic here, we present the trick in the Explorer exercise (5-11) for you to explore. We take another look at the issue of identifying the selected option button when we discuss the use of the control array in Chapter 9, "Arrays and Their Uses."

More on the Syntax of Select Case. Because the tuition is jointly determined by the student's residence status and hours taken, can we code the cases as shown here?

```
Select Case ResidenceStatus And HoursTaken
Case 0 And Is <=5
.
.
End Select
```

No. Although "ResidenceStatus And HoursTaken" can be considered as an expression, it means something different to the computer than what a beginner may have in mind. Recall that the expression in the Select Case statement is first evaluated to arrive at a value that will be used to match against the criteria in the Cases. In an attempt to evaluate the expression, the computer will first perform a logical And operation on the variables ResidenceStatus and HoursTaken.

Suppose that ResidenceStatus has a value zero (0). No matter what value HoursTaken may be, the result of the And operation will be a zero. (Recall that the And logical operator requires that the corresponding bits of both operands be 1 to obtain a result 1; otherwise, the result will be a zero.) Thus, the first Case statement that has a zero will be considered the match. Assuming there are no other problems, the result will be both unexpected and unpredictable.

Now, consider this statement:

```
Case 0 And Is <=5
```

"Is <= 5" is an open-range expression. However, on its left is an And operator, which is not expected. Thus, the statement has a syntax error, causing a "compile error" message.

Mixing the Select Case Structure with the If Block. As you may have already noticed in the preceding example, a Select Case structure can have If blocks within its structure. Conversely, an If block can also contain Select Case structures. *There is no restriction as to which structure can enclose the other as long as the nesting constitutes a relationship of the inner and outer blocks,* as discussed in the preceding section.

An Alternative Design. The tuition example can be designed somewhat differently. For example, instead of using the text box to enter hours taken and option buttons for residence status, we can use two combo boxes for both. The first combo box can be used to display the residence status, and the second one can be used for the brackets of hours taken. The visual interface can then appear as in Figure 5.16.

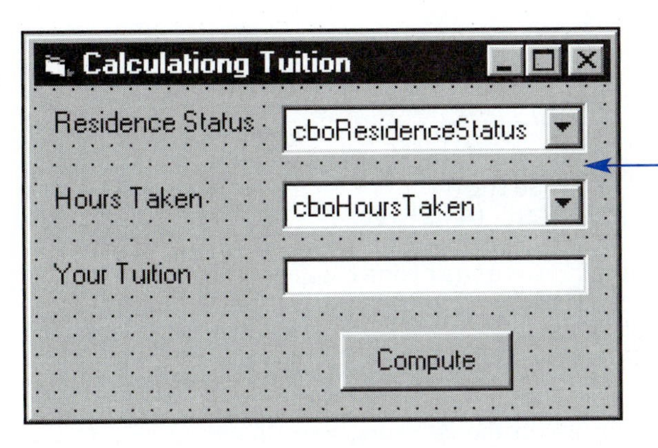

Figure 5.16
Alternative User Interface Design for Tuition Calculation

Here is an alternative design for the preceding tuition problem. The user will select the residence status and the bracket of hours taken from the combo boxes. When he or she clicks the Compute button, the tuition is displayed in the label named lblTuition.

A list of the properties of the controls used in code is given in the following table.

Control	Property	Setting	Remark
Combo box	Name	cboResidenceStatus	
	Style	2-Drop-down list	To disallow user entry
Combo box	Name	cboHoursTaken	
	Style	2-Drop-down list	To disallow user entry
Label	Name	lblTuition	To display tuition
	BackColor	White	So that the label will look like a text box
	BorderStyle	1-Fxied Single	
Command button	Caption	Compute	To initiate tuition computation
	Name	cmdCompute	

In the Form Load event, the two combo boxes can be populated using the AddItem method as follows:

```
Option Explicit
Private Sub Form_Load()
    With cboResidenceStatus
    'Populate combo box with residence status
        .AddItem "In State"
        .AddItem "Out Of State"
        .AddItem "International"
        .ListIndex = 0 'Set default status (In state)
    End With
    With cboHoursTaken
    'Populate combo box with brackets of hours taken
        .AddItem "0 to 5"
        .AddItem "6 to 8"
        .AddItem "9 to 11"
        .AddItem "12 or More"
        .ListIndex = 3 'Set default hours taken (12 or more)
    End With
End Sub
```

Notice that we have also added statements to set the ListIndex properties of both combo boxes. This will make the items corresponding to the ListIndex values appear in the controls' text boxes as the default selections when the program starts.

The Click event procedure for the command button can then be modified with the following code skeleton:

```
Private Sub cmdCompute_Click()
Dim Tuition As Currency
    Select Case cboResidenceStatus.ListIndex
    Case 0 'In state
        Select Case cboHoursTaken.ListIndex
        Case 0 ' 0 to 5 hours
        Case 1 ' 6 to 8 hours
        Case 2 ' 9 to 11 hours
        Case 3 ' 12 or more hours
        End Select
    Case 1 'Out Of state
        'Similar to the Case for In state
    Case 2 'International
        'Similar to the Case for In state
    End Select
    lblTuition.Caption = Tuition
End Sub
```

With the comments in the structure, you should be able to complete the remaining code, which is left to you as an exercise.

Notice that in the procedure, the residence status is used as the first-level Select Case structure. This is done just to show that either of the two factors can be the first level without affecting the result. Indeed, this structure should appear to you logically "more natural" because we typically would check the residence status before asking about the number of hours taken.

Notice also that the Select Case statements now use the combo boxes' ListIndex properties as the expressions. Because the Style properties of both controls are set to 2 (Drop-down List), the user cannot enter any data into the text portion of the combo box. Instead, he or she can select an item from the list. Such an action will set the controls' ListIndex properties.

Which Design Do You Prefer? The original design has the advantage of code clarity. When you review the code, you should be able to have a good feel about what the code is supposed to do. However, it is not flexible. For example, if the hours taken for each bracket change (and the number of brackets remain the same), you will need to change the program to handle the new situation. The second design has the advantage of code brevity. It is also more flexible in handling the changes in data. Although we use the AddItem method to populate the combo boxes, in a real application, the items should be read from a file or database. A change in the hours taken for each bracket will not necessitate a revision in the program as long as the number of brackets remains the same. However, the code is not as clear because the ListIndex itself says very little about the underlying data. In such a case, it is important that you include comments to provide the additional details.

There are actually other alternatives to handle this problem. Another alternative that is even more flexible is considered in an exercise in Chapter 9. We present these alternatives here to illustrate the use of the Select Case structure and the If block to solve a problem. Hopefully, each alternative will stimulate your mind and make you more resourceful in identifying solutions to your next problem.

Summary

This chapter presents coding blocks in VB to handle decision and branching. Becuase logical expressions constitute an integral part of the If block, we have also explained in detail the operations and uses of various relational and logical operators. A clear understanding of how these operators work helps prevent errors in coding mechanics and logic. Indeed, it should also enhance your capability of coming up with efficient and elegant code solutions to various programming problems.

We have studied the structures of If blocks and Select Case blocks. The If block provides a very flexible means to construct code for decisions. However, when various actions to be taken depend on the different results of only one expression, the Select Case block provides a much simpler structure to construct the code for branching. Each of these structures can be nested (with the same or the other structure) for as many levels as you practically need. However, nesting can make your code hard to follow and maintain. Thus, it is sometimes advisable to look for alternatives. Regardless of which structure or approach you use to code, it is always advisable to provide many comments/remarks in the code. These additional explanations can make your code much easier to understand and revise. Also, remember to indent so that each level of the structures can be clearly identified visually.

Visual Basic Explorer

5-1. Use of Logical Operators. Relational operators work on both numeric and string data. Can logical operators do the same? Try the following statements. (*Hint:* To test them, place these lines in the Form Click event procedure with a "Dim A as Integer" statement at the beginning. Then insert a line of code to display the result between the lines below.)

```
A = "34" And "32"
A = "34" Or 32
A = "XY" Or "AB"
```

Why do the first two run, but not the last? (*Answer:* Logical operators work on numeric data only. Data type conversions are performed automatically by VB in the first two cases, making the code executable. It is impossible to convert the strings to numbers in the last case. Thus, the operation fails.)

5-2. The Value Property of the Option Button. Place two option buttons on a new form. Then type in the following code.

```
Option Explicit
Dim A As Integer

Private Sub Option1_Click()
    A = Option1.Value
    MsgBox "A = " & A
End Sub
Private Sub Option2_Click()
    A = Option1.Value
    MsgBox "A = " & A
End Sub
```

Run the project and alternately click the two option buttons. What value of A do you see each time? The numeric value for True is –1 (&HFFFF) and for False is 0 (&H0000).

5-3. The Value Property of the Check Box. Place a check box on the form. Type in the following code.

```
Option Explicit
Dim A As Integer

Private Sub Check1_Click()
    A = Check1.Value
    MsgBox "A = " & A
End Sub
```

What result do you see each time? When the box is checked? And when it is unchecked? Are they the same as the option buttons?

5-4. Assigning "Improper" Values to Option Buttons and Check Boxes. Now you know that the values that an option button can take are –1 (True) or 0 (False), whereas the check box can take 1 (vbChecked) and 0 (vbUnchecked). By code, try to assign a value 1 to the Value property of an option button. Then use MsgBox to display the same property and see what happens. Similarly, try to assign –1 to the Value property of a check box and see what happens. Anything puzzling?

Any numeric value can be converted to True or False, which can be assigned to the Value property of an option button. However, the Value property of a check box can take on only 0, 1, or 2. Assigning any value that cannot be converted to one of these values will cause an error.

5-5. Assigning a Value to the Boolean Variable. Place a text box and a command button on a new form. Name the text box txtNumber and the command button cmdCheck. Set the command button's Caption property to "Check." Type in the following code:

```
Option Explicit
Private Sub cmdCheck_Click()
Dim BoolTest As Boolean
Dim TheNumber as Single
    TheNumber = Val(txtNumber.Text)
    BoolTest = TheNumber
    MsgBox "The resulting Boolean value is " & BoolTest
    If BoolTest = TheNumber Then
        MsgBox "BoolTest and TheNumber are equal."
    Else
        MsgBox "BoolTest and TheNumber are Not equal."
    End If
End Sub
```

Run the program. Enter any number (try at least these numbers: 1000, -30, 0.005, and 0) and click the command button. What does the computer display? What conclusion can you draw from this experiment? What do you also learn? (*Answer:* Any nonzero value will be converted to True for a Boolean variable. Only a value of 0 is interpreted as False. Beware of the potential problem with comparing a Boolean variable with a variable of another data type after assigning the same value to both.)

5-6. Playing with the Truth. Type in the following code:

```
Private Sub Form_Click()
Dim B As Boolean
Dim L As Long
Dim S As String
    B = 3 = 3
    L = 3 = 3
    S = 3 = 3
    MsgBox "B = " & B & ", L = " & L & ", S = " & S
```

```
        MsgBox "Len(B) = " & Len(B) & ",Len(L) = " & Len(L) _
            & ", Len(S) = " & Len(S)
        S = L
        MsgBox "S = " & S & ", Len(S) = " & Len(S)
    End Sub
```

Run the project and click on the form. Does everything turn out to be as expected? Should True have a length of two or four?

5-7. Using the Not Operator. Bring two option buttons and one check box into a new form. Place the following code in the code window:

```
Option Explicit
Private Sub Option1_Click()
Dim B As Boolean
Dim I As Integer
    B = Not Option1.Value
    I = Not Option1.Value
    MsgBox "Not Option1.Value = " & B & ", I = " & I
End Sub

Private Sub Option2_Click()
Dim B As Boolean
Dim I As Integer
    B = Not Option1.Value
    I = Not Option1.Value
    MsgBox "Not Option1.Value = " & B & ", I = " & I
End Sub

Private Sub Check1_Click()
Dim B As Boolean, BB As Boolean
Dim I As Integer
    B = Not Check1.Value
    I = Not Check1.Value
    BB = I
    MsgBox "Not Check1.Value = " & B & ", I = " & I _
        & " BB = " & BB
End Sub
```

Run the project. First, click either of the option buttons. See anything unexpected? (Probably not.) Then click the check box several times. Pay particular attention to the value of I and BB. Anything mysterious? The results, of course, have everything to do with the way the Not logical operator works. You should be able to understand why BB is always True. (Any nonzero value assigned to a Boolean variable is converted to True.) However, if you don't understand why I's value alternates between –2 and 1, recall that logical operators operate on a bit-by-bit basis; that is, every bit in the data is changed when you apply a Not operation on a data field. (*Hint:* Not &H0001 gives &HFFFE. Try to print &HFFFE and see what you get.)

5-8. Using the And Operator on the Same Value. Bring a text box and a command button into a new form. Name the text box txtNumber and clear its text. Name the command button cmdAnd and set its Caption property to "And." Place the following code in the code window:

```
Private Sub cmdAnd_Click()
Dim N As Integer
Dim  R As Integer
    R = Val(txtNumber.Text)
    N = R And R
    MsgBox "The result is " & N
End Sub
```

Run the project. Enter an integer number and then click the And button. Repeat the same experiment with different numbers. What results do you see? (The corresponding bits of the two operands are the same. The result of the And operation should be the same as the operand.)

5-9. Using the Or Operator on the Same Value. (continued from 5-8). Add a command button to the form in 5-8. Name it cmdOr and set its Caption property to "Or." Place the following code in the code window:

```
Private Sub cmdOr_Click()
Dim N As Integer
Dim R As Integer
     R = Val(txtNumber.Text)
     N = R Or R
     MsgBox "The result is " & N
End Sub
```

Run the project. Enter an integer number and then click the Or button. Repeat the same experiment with different numbers. What results do you see? (The corresponding bits of the two operands are the same. The result of the Or operation should be the same as the operand.)

5-10. Use of the Xor Operator on the Same Value. (5-9 continued). Add another command button to the form in 5-9. Name the command button cmdXor and set its Caption property to "Xor." Place the following code in the code window:

```
Private Sub cmdXor_Click()
Dim N As Integer
Dim R As Integer
     R = Val(txtNumber.Text)
     N = R Xor R
     MsgBox "The result is " & N
End Sub
```

Run the project. Enter an integer number and then click the Xor button. Repeat the same experiment with different numbers. What result do you see? (The corresponding bits of the two operands are the same. The result of the Xor operation should give zero.) Can you generalize the results of performing the And, Or, and Xor operations on the same number?

5-11. Inverting the Criterion for the Select Case Block. Typically, the Select Case statement involves a certain expression whose value will vary depending on one or more of the variables or control properties used in the expression. Seldom will you see a single constant used as the expression. However, consider the following code used in the event procedure cmdTest click.

```
Private Sub CmdTest_Click()
     Select Case True
     Case Option1.Value
          MsgBox "Option1 is selected."
     Case Option2.Value
          MsgBox "Option2 is selected."
     Case Option3.Value
          MsgBox "Option3 is selected."
     Case Else
          MsgBox "No option is selected."
     End Select
End Sub
```

Does it mean anything to you? Here, the constant True is used as the expression, whereas the value of each option button is used as the criterion. The "comparison" is inverted.

Test the code by placing on a new form a command button, a frame, and three option buttons inside the frame. Rename the command button to cmdTest. Type in the previous code. Start the program. Click one (or none) of the option buttons. Then click the command button. What do you find? It's a tricky way to test which option button in a group is selected, isn't it?

Exercises

5-12. Sorting Two Random Numbers. Draw a command button on a new form. Name it cmdShow and set its Caption property to "Show."

Provide the code so that when the user clicks the button, your program will display two random numbers in the range of 0 to 1, smaller one first. (*Hint:* Swap the values if the random numbers are "out of order.")

5-13. Sorting Two Random Numbers in a Lottery. Modify the preceding project so that the random numbers are in the range of 1 to 50, representing the first two numbers drawn from a lottery. Again, the smaller number should be shown first. In addition, the two numbers should not be the same.

5-14. Sorting Three Random Numbers in a Lottery. Modify the preceding project so that the program will display three numbers instead of two. (*Hint:* As each number is "drawn," make sure it is not the same as the previous one[s]. Sort the first two numbers in order. Then compare the third number with the smaller one. If the third one is smaller, you have found the order. Otherwise, compare the third one with the larger number.)

5-15. Ordering Names. Write a routine so that it will display two names in alphabetic order regardless the order the names are given. Note that the comparison should not be case sensitive.

Test your routine by drawing two text boxes and a command button on a new form. When your program runs, it will display the names entered in the text boxes in order when the user clicks the command button.

5-16. Testing Divisibility by 4. In the text, you have learned how you can test whether an integer is an odd or even number. The same idea can also be used to test whether a number is divisible by 4 by using the And operator. A number is divisible by 4 when its lowest two bits are zero.

Place a text box and a command button on a new form. Name the text box txtNumber and the command button cmdTest. Then provide the code to test whether the number the user has entered into the text box is divisible by 4. (*Hint:* Use the And operator. A number with the lowest two bits on has a value of 3.)

Use the MsgBox to display the result. Also, use the Mod operator to test the same (place the code in the Form Click event). Compare the results obtained from both approaches.

5-17. Encrypting a Number. A company keeps its employees' salary data in a file in encrypted form. The data-entry screen for the salary data has a masked edit box for the employee number (Social Security number [SSN]) and a text box for the salary amount. When the user clicks the "Save" button, the salary amount is encrypted before being saved. Both the SSN and the salary are internally treated as long integers. The Xor operation is performed on the salary using the SSN as the key. The result is displayed in a label. Then your program displays a message, "Salary saved." (*Note:* Just display the result and the message. Ignore the "Save" operation.)

5-18. Playing with the Flags. You have three check boxes in a general ledger account entry form with the following captions:

```
Is this a control account? (Question 1)
Is this a contra account? (Question 2)
Does this account affect cash flow? (Question 3)
```

You have decided to handle these questions internally with a Flags variable; that is, values in these check boxes will be collectively stored in only one Integer variable named Flags. Bits 0, 1, and 2 will be used to keep track of questions 1, 2, and 3, respectively. When a check box is checked, its corresponding bit will be set on; and when it is unchecked, its corresponding bit will be set off.

Provide the code to handle these flags and display the results (the value of Flags) when a change occurs. (*Hint:* Place the code in the check boxes' Click events. Use the And operator to turn a flag off and the Or operator to turn a flag on. Use a label [name it lblResult] to display the value of Flags at the end of each Click event. When all three flags are on, Flags should have a value of 7.)

5-19. Which Shift Key Has Been Pressed? The KeyDown event has a header:

```
Private Sub Object_KeyDown(KeyCode As Integer, Shift As Integer)
```

Where the *object* can be a form or text box among others and *Shift* refers to the Shift key(s) pressed. The parameter, Shift, is actually a Flags variable, whose lowest (bit 0), second lowest (bit 1), and third lowest (bit 2) bits track the status of the Shift, Ctrl, and Alt keys, respectively. (For example, if the Alt key is pressed, bit 2 will be on and Shift will have a value of 4.) The named constants for these values are vbShiftMask, vbCtrlMask, and vbAltMask.

Set the KeyPreview property of the form to True. Place a few text boxes and masked edit boxes on the form. Then write a routine in the form's KeyDown event procedure to display a message indicating which Shift key has been pressed when one of the three Shift keys is pressed. (*Hint:* Use the And operator. Test for each key separately.)

5-20. Which Mouse Button Is Down? When the mouse button is pressed down on a form, the MouseDown event is raised. The procedure has the following header:

```
Private Sub Form_MouseDown(Button As Integer, _
    Shift As Integer, X As Single, Y As Single)
```

where *Button* is a Flags variable, which tracks the buttons pressed. Its bit 0, 1, and 2 track the left, right, and middle button, respectively.

Write a routine in this event procedure to display a message indicating which mouse button has been pressed when one of the three mouse button is pressed. See the preceding exercise for hints.

5-21. Rotating Background Colors. Write a procedure that rotates the background color of a label, lblSign, in blue, red, green, yellow, and back to blue each time the user clicks a command button named cmdChange, captioned "Change." (*Hint:* Search the online Help file for the names of the colors with the keyword "Color constants." Use a Static long integer variable to keep track of the count. Use the Mod (or And) operator to generate the number sequence 0, 1, 2, 3, 0, 1…and so on, which can then be used in a Select Case block.)

5-22. Rotating Background Colors Automatically. Modify the preceding project so that the colors are rotated automatically every half of a second once your program starts.

5-23. Alternative Solution to the Exploration Problem. The oil exploration investment decision problem presented in this chapter has an alternative solution. Write a line of code (using relational and logical operators) to come up with a correct value for the variable Invest. (*Question:* Which coding alternative executes more efficiently?)

5-24. Random Judgment. When your program starts, it automatically displays one of the three questions on a label, named lblQuestion. (Provide three favorite questions of your own. Use the Rnd function to decide which question to display.) Below the displayed question is a text box, named txtAnswer, for the user to type in the answer. When the user presses the Enter key, your program will display (using MsgBox) either "Yeah! You are right!" or "Nah! You are wrong," depending on the number given by the Rnd function; that is, when the random value is less than 0.5, your program will display the "Yeah!" message; otherwise, it will display the "Nah!" message. (*Hint:* Place your code in the text box's KeyPress event and check for the vbKeyReturn. On the form, use a label to instruct the user to press the Enter key when he or she completes the answser.)

5-25. What Number Is on My Mind? When the user clicks on the command button named cmdPlay and captioned "Play," your program generates a number in the range of 1 to

1000. The user will guess the number by typing a number in a text box, named txtNumber, and then clicking another command button, named cmdCheck and captioned "Check." If the guess is too low, your program will display a message, "Nope. Higher." If it is too high, it will display, "Nah! Lower." When the answer is correct, your program says, "Yes, you've got it. But it takes *n* seconds for you to find out." Where *n* is computed from the time the "Play" button is clicked till the time a correct answer is obtained. (*Hint:* Use the Timer function or Now function to keep track of time.)

5-26. **Port of Entry.** When you come back at the port of entry from a trip to a foreign country, the officer from the Immigration and Naturalization Service (a computer guarding the entrance) displays a check box with a question, "Are you a U.S. citizen?" If you check the box on, the computer displays a text box with the label "Enter U.S. Passport Number." If you check the box off, the computer displays three text boxes with proper labels, "Nationality," "Passport Number," and "Visa Number," respectively. Design the proper visual interface and provide the necessary code. (*Question:* Can you do this one without using the If block?)

5-27. **Long-Term Assets.** A part of a long-term asset entry screen has a check box with the caption "Depreciable Asset?" When the box is checked, a text box with the label "Estimated Life" and a combo box with the label "Depreciation method" are enabled; otherwise, they are disabled. The allowable depreciation methods are straight-line, sum-of-years' digit, ACRE, modified ACRE, and double-declining balance methods. The most often used method is the straight-line method. (Populate the combo box with the AddItem method in the Form Load event.) (*Question:* Can you do this without using the If block? The routine will be shorter if you do it this way.)

5-28. **Broker's Commission.** A broker charges her commission based on the amount of trading involved. If the amount is less than $1,000, the commission rate is 2%. Additional commission on the amount between $1,000 and $5,000 is 1%; between $5,000 and $20,000 is 0.5%; and above $20,000 is 0.025%. There is a minimum charge of $10.

The user interface to compute the commission should allow the user to enter the Date, Ticker Symbol, Price, and Number of Units (shares). When the user clicks the command button captioned "Compute," the computer should display the amount of trade as well as the commission in two labels (with text box appearance), separately.

5-29. **Revisiting the Only-Three Bookstore Problem.** In the Only-Three Bookstore example in the text, the prices (Price1, Price2, and Price3) are assigned in the Form Load event procedure. Actually, the prices are also shown on the captions of the check boxes. A good design should obtain the same data from only one source so that the results are always consistent. Assume that the captions should be the sole source of data. Modify the project so that the Form Load event procedure will assign the prices as given in the captions. (*Hint:* Use the InStr function to obtain the position of the "$" in the caption. Then use the CCur function to convert the string to the Currency type.)

5-30. **The Tuition Problem (I).** In Section 5.3 of this chapter, right after the tuition problem is introduced, we gave a partial solution using an If block as the second-level nesting. Complete the remaining code. For consistency, all the remaining second-level nesting should use the If block.

5-31. **The Tuition Problem (II).** Complete the code for the tuition problem in the text that uses the combo boxes for the residence status and the bracket for hours taken.

5-32. **Year-End Bonus.** A company determines the year-end bonuses for its employees based on rank and performance. The bonus is computed as a percentage of the employee's annual salary as given in the following table.

Rank	Excellent	Good	Mediocre
High	100%	75%	50%
Middle	80%	50%	30%
Low	60%	25%	15%

Your form should provide an interface for the user to specify the employee's rank, performance level, and the employee's annual salary. When the user clicks the "Compute" button, your program will show the amount of bonus for the employee in a label, which should have the appearance of a text box.

Projects

5-33. Computing the FICA Withholding. The FICA tax is computed based on a person's annual income. The formula consists of two parts: the Social Security tax and Medicare tax. A few years ago, the Social Security tax rate was 6.2% and had an upper limit of an annual income of $45,000; that is, there was no Social Security tax on any income above $45,000. The Medicare tax rate was 1.45% with an upper limit on an annual income of $120,000; that is, there was no Medicare tax on any income above $120,000.

For the purpose of your programming practice, assume the same tax rate and bracket. Each time an employee is paid, your company has to withhold Social Security taxes based on his or her current and previous income and withholding. In a real-world situation, the employee's previous income and withholding would have been kept in a file (database) and read in after an employee number was entered. In this project, your program will make the user enter the employee's previous income as well as the current income. Your program will then proceed to compute the previous and current FICA withholding when the user clicks a command button with the caption "Compute." Your program should display the previous and current withholding as well as the total income and withholding including the current amounts. (*Hint:* To compute the current withholding, compute the total withholding based on total income then subtract the previous withholding [based on previous income] from it. This is much easier than if you try to compute the current withholding directly.)

Required: Design a user interface for this purpose. It is suggested that you use three frames: one for previous data, another for current data, and the other for total amounts. Use text boxes for fields that require user input, but use labels for fields that will be computed by your program. Change the BackColor and BorderStyle settings for these labels so that they look like text boxes. You should add two command buttons: one for computation and the other for quitting.

Provide code for the computation and display of results as specified.

The following table can be used to verify the accuracy of your program:

Previous Income (Entered)	Previous Withholding (Computed)	Current Income (Entered)	Current Withholding (Computed)
0	0	10,000	765
40,000	3,060	5,000	382.50
40,000	3,060	10,000	455
40,000	3,060	80,000	1,470
40,000	3,060	100,000	1,470
80,000	3,950	40,000	580
80,000	3,950	80,000	580

5-34. Computing Total for Guest Check. A restaurant offers two kinds of drinks: St. Helen Volcano ($15) and Bloody Mary ($12). They are so strong that diners are allowed to order only one drink per day. Appetizers include cocktail shrimps ($5.95), seasoned mushrooms ($6.45), and hibachi-style crab rangoon ($6.75). Diners can order any combinations (but are restricted to only one from each kind). Main entrees include Boston lobsters ($24.95), New York steak ($21.95), and oriental vegetarians ($28.95). Their portions are so big that no diner should order more than one. Finally, desserts include herb cake ($8.75) and Gin-Sheng ice cream ($8.75). Diners can order either one or both (or none).

Design a user interface that servers of the restaurant can use to enter the order for each diner. (*Note:* Restrict your choice of VB controls to only option buttons and check boxes. Use as many frames as you deem desirable to group items on the form).

Provide necessary code so that when the server clicks the "Compute" command button, the computer will display in a label (named lblTotal) the total charges for a diner. (*Hint:* You may find the code much shorter using formulas as an alternative to If blocks.)

5-35. Computing the Total for a Guest Check: A Variation. Change the code in the preceding project to satisfy the requirement that the restaurant would rather not have the "Compute" button but just for the computer to display the total as soon as the server clicks on any of the available choices on the restaurant menu. Be aware that when a check box is clicked, it can be checked off rather than on.

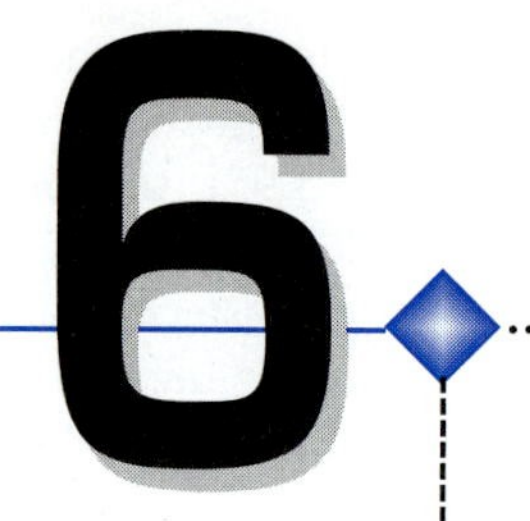

6 Input, Output, and Procedures

This chapter introduces two topics. First, introduction to input and output provides introductory topics to input and output features available in VB. These topics are essential to your understanding of input and output concepts. In addition, some of these features provide a convenient means for you to design sound interactions between your program and the user. Second, the section on procedures discusses the uses of general procedures in structuring VB code. The advantages of using general procedures are too significant to overemphasize and are outlined at the end of that section after you gain a good working knowledge of general procedures. This chapter concludes with an example that represents an attempt to show how all the pieces you learn from this chapter can be put together.

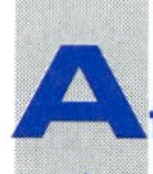

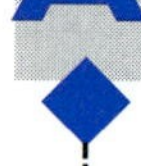

After completing this chapter, you should be able to:

- Use the MsgBox function to ascertain the user's response when your program needs a decision/direction from the user.
- Develop code to handle sequential files for input and output.
- Use the common dialog box to prompt for file paths.
- Understand and use the capability of the Print method for various VB objects.
- Appreciate the need to create and use general procedures.
- Write and use general procedures.
- Differentiate between the situations in which a sub and a function should be written.
- Determine when a parameter is needed for a general procedure.

6.1 Introduction to Input and Output

When your program starts, the variables in the program must be initialized first either with constants or with values provided from external sources, such as users' actions (keystrokes or mouse clicks) or an existing file. The process of obtaining data from a source external to the CPU (central processing unit) is referred to as ***input.***

The data that the variables in your program contain are stored in memory. As soon as your program terminates, all these data will not longer exist in the CPU. Some of the data are temporary in nature and can be discarded without any problem. Others, however, need to be displayed (for the user to view his or her values), printed on a hard copy, or saved in some intermediate storage device (e.g., hard disks) for future uses. The process of sending the data in the CPU to an external device is referred to as ***output***. This section introduces a few possible means that you can use in VB for input and output.

VB provides various ways that your program can obtain input or produce output. Recall in Chapter 3, "Some Visual Basic Controls and Events," you learned that at least six VB controls could be used to obtain input from the user. A text box, for example, can be used for the user to enter data. Indeed, some of those controls can also be used to display output. For example, you can display any data in the same text box. In this section, we explore four additional ways for input and output:

1. The MsgBox function
2. Files
3. The Print Method
4. The Common Dialog box

The MsgBox Function

You have seen MsgBox used to display a pop-up message. When used to display a message (as output), the MsgBox function has the following syntax:

```
MsgBox prompt[, buttons] [, title]
```

where *Prompt* = a text string that is displayed on the message box
Buttons = an optional numeric value specifying the button(s) and icon the pop-up message box is to display; when omitted an OK button is displayed
Title = an optional text string to be displayed as the title of the pop-up message box; when omitted, the name of the project is displayed

The buttons parameter specifies what button(s) and icon the message box is to display. Some of the sample values are listed in the following table.

Named Constant	Value	Display	Type
vbOKOnly	0	OK button only	Button(s)
vbYesNoCancel	3	Yes, No, and Cancel buttons	
vbYesNo	4	Yes and No buttons	
vbRetryCancel	5	Retry and Cancel buttons	
vbCritical	16	Critical Message icon	Icon
vbQuestion	32	Warning Query icon	
vbInformation	64	Information icon	

You can specify one group of buttons and one icon to display at the same time. To display a group of buttons and an icon together, add the values of both as the second parameter. If nothing is specified, the default button, OK, will be displayed. Two examples of the uses of MsgBox follow.

Simple Message. Suppose in your payroll program, you want to display a message informing the user that the maximum allowed number of hours worked per week is 60; you can code the following:

```
MsgBox "Maximum allowed hours worked per week is 60.", _
    vbInformation, "Payroll Entry"
```

The code will display in the message box not only the message but also an Information icon. It will also show "Payroll Entry" as its title. Because nothing is said about the buttons to display, the default button, OK, will be displayed (see Figure 6.1).

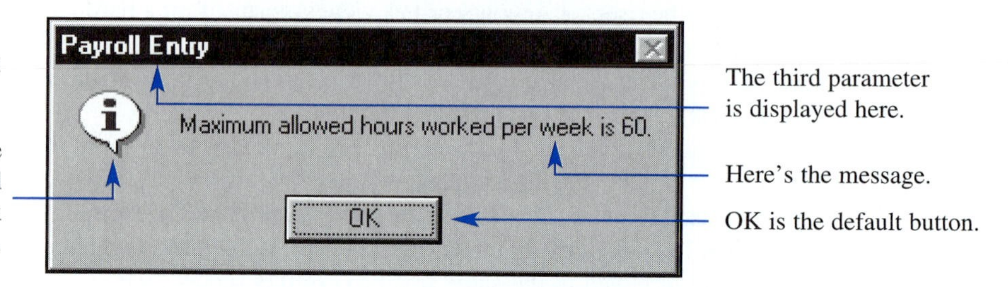

Payroll Entry
Maximum allowed hours worked per week is 60.
OK
The third parameter is displayed here.
Here's the message.
OK is the default button.
vbInformation in the second parameter will make the message box display this icon.

Figure 6.1
A Sample Message Box

Notice again that you can specify an icon along with a group of buttons to display in the message box by adding the icon and buttons values together for the second parameter. For example, you can make it display Yes and No buttons (instead of the default OK button) and the Information icon by coding the following:

```
MsgBox "Maximum allowed hours worked per week is 60.", _
    vbInformation + vbYesNo, "Payroll Entry"
```

The Yes and No buttons, however, do not seem to make any sense in this message. They are usually used when the message box is used to prompt for the user response rather than to display a straight message.

Using MsgBox to Obtain the User Response. The MsgBox function can be used to obtain the response from the user. When used for this purpose, its has the following syntax:

```
Response = MsgBox(prompt[, buttons] [, title])
```

Depending on the button the user clicks on the message box, the MsgBox returns a different value. The following table provides a sample list of the returned values:

Button Clicked	Named Constant	Value
Cancel	vbCancel	2
Abort	vbAbort	3
Yes	vbYes	6
No	vbNo	7

For example, suppose your form has a text box named txtName, which is cleared when data on the form are saved. When the user clicks the close (x) button on the title bar, if the control contains data, it would mean that data have not yet been saved. You would like to warn and ask the user if it is OK to quit. One solution is to place the code in the form's Unload event to handle this situation. The ***Form Unload event*** occurs when the form is being unloaded. It occurs when the user clicks the form's close (x) button or when an Unload statement is executed. The event procedure has the following header:

```
Private Sub Form_Unload(Cancel As Integer)
```

where *Cancel* represents an integer value to indicate whether to cancel the unload operation. A nonzero value will cancel the unload operation.

Using this event procedure, the code can appear as follows:

```
Private Sub Form_Unload(Cancel As Integer)
Dim Response As Integer
    If Len(Trim$(txtName.Text)) > 0 Then
    'The text box contains data.
    'Ask the user whether he or she really means to quit.
        Response = MsgBox("Data not yet saved. Ok to quit?", _
            vbQuestion + vbYesNo, "Testing") 'Display the "?" icon
                                  'as well as yes and no buttons
        If Response = vbYes Then
        ' User clicks the Yes button;
        ' Do nothing (allow program to proceed to unload)
         Else
        ' User clicks the No button, cancel the unload operation
            Cancel = True
        End If
    End If
End Sub
```

In this procedure, the first If statement checks whether the text box, txtName, contains any nonblank text. If so, the message box displays the warning message, the Question mark icon, and the Yes and No buttons (see Figure 6.2). Note that the buttons parameter specifies to display the Question icon as well as the Yes and No buttons. If the user clicks the Yes button, a value vbYes (6) will be returned. The program will proceed normally (unload); otherwise, True is assigned to the Cancel parameter and the unload process will be canceled.

Figure 6.2
Message Box with a Question Icon and Two Buttons

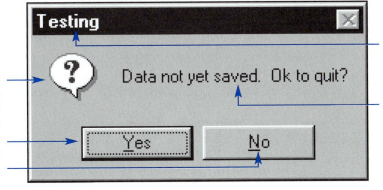

The MsgBox function provides a facility for simple dialogs between your program and the user. It is most appropriate in the following situations:

1. When your program needs to convey a simple message to the user. Examples include messages that do the following:
   - Indicate that a file has been saved
   - Inform the user that an entry is not acceptable
   - Instruct the user to take a certain action, such as inserting a disk in a drive
2. When your program needs a direction (among a few available choices) from the user. Examples include the following:
   - Informing the user of the failure of an operation (e.g., unable to read a specified file) and prompting whether to try again, skip the operation, or quit
   - Warning the user of the possibility of losing data (e.g., when instructed to delete a file) and prompting whether to proceed the operation

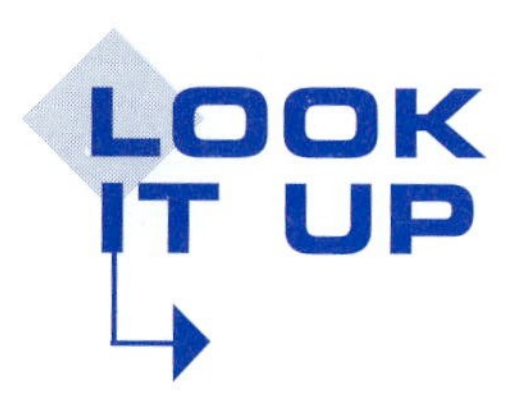

Search the keyword "MsgBox Function" (VB reference) in the Index tab of the online Help file. It explains all the parameters in more detail. It also provides a complete list of button values you can specify for the box to display as well as the values indicating the button clicked.

Files

VB provides three file access types: sequential, random, and binary. As an introduction, we explore only one type—the sequential file. A more complete treatment of file accesses is presented in Appendix A, "Data Management Using Files." When you work with files for input and output, several key steps are involved:

1. Open the file. In this process, your program associates the file number in your program with the physical file residing in the intermediate storage device (e.g., the hard drive or floppy disk).
2. Perform file operations such as reading/writing data from/onto the file. Most of the file activities of your program relate to this aspect.
3. Close the file. This process dissociates your program from the physical file and ensures that all I/O operations are completed by the system.

Opening a File. The syntax to open a sequential file appears as follows:

```
Open FilePath For {Input¦Output¦Append} As [#]FileNumber _
    [Len = Bytes]
```

where *FilePath* = a string specifying the path of the file (e.g., "A:\MyFolder\Phones.txt")

Input = the keyword to specify that the file will be opened for the input mode; the file must exist before it is open

Output = the keyword to specify that the file will be opened for the output mode; if the file specified does not exist, VB creates the file; if the file already exists, all its existing content will be lost

Append = the keyword to specify that the file will be opened for the append mode; if the file specified does not exist, VB creates the file; if the file already exists, all its existing contents are preserved; new data are added (appended) to the end of the file

FileNumber = a number that you assign for the file to be referenced in your program; the # sign prefix for the file number is optional

Len = the number of bytes to be used as the buffer for the file; usually, this parameter is omitted

The following statement will open an existing file named Phones.txt located in the MyFolder folder of Drive A for input.

```
Open "A:\MyFolder\Phones.txt" For Input as #1
```

In this statement, the Len parameter for the buffer size is omitted. The default size of 128 bytes will be used.

About the File Number. The use of a constant literal for the file number in the preceding code should cause your concern for code clarity and the potential problem with file identification. Imagine that you need to open 10 files at the same time. It will be difficult to remember what file number is used for which file. A mistake in your code can cause unthinkable problems. In addition, it would be a challenge for someone, including yourself, to identify the files when reviewing the code in the future.

For this reason, it is a good practice to use a variable, instead of a constant literal, as the file number. You can declare a variable and assign a number to the variable. From then on, the variable can be used in placed of the constant literal. Suppose you want to open the file as soon as your program starts and use the file in several procedures. Using the variable PhoneFile for the file, your code can appear as follows:

```
Option Explicit
Dim PhoneFile As Integer
Private Sub Form_Load()
     PhoneFile = 1
     Open "A:\MyFolder\Phones.txt" For Input as #PhoneFile
End Sub
```

Once the file is opened in Input mode, you are ready to read data from the file sequentially.

Reading Data from a File. Data can be read from a sequential file in several ways. One commonly used statement is the Input statement, which has the following syntax:

```
Input #File Number, Variable List
```

where *File Number* = the file number associated with the input file as explained previously; notice that the "#" in the statement is required, not optional as it is in the case of the Open statement

Variable list = a list of variables to hold the data read from the file

For example, suppose that you have opened the phone file shown in the preceding code example. The file contains your friends' names and phone numbers and appears as follows:

8172223838, John Dole

2145559999, Jane Smith

.

.

Assume your form has a command button named cmdRead. When you click the button, you want to read one line of data into the variables Phone and TheName and display the results. Your code should appear as follows:

```
Private Sub cmdRead_Click()
Dim Phone As Currency
Dim TheName As String
     Input #PhoneFile, Phone, TheName
     MsgBox "Phone is " & Phone & ". Name is " & TheName
End Sub
```

The first time the procedure is executed, the variables Phone and TheName will hold the values of 8172223838 and "John Dole," respectively. The second time the procedure is executed, the variables will have the data on the second line.

Notice that we did not declare Phone as Long because a Long type variable cannot handle a number larger than 2147483647. The Currency type appears to be a good alternative. It has a field width large enough to handle the data. Another alternative is to declare the variable as a String type, which will require more memory.

As a technical side note, at the end of each line in a text file, there is an "end of line" marker that the computer uses to separate one line from the other. The marker consists of two character codes: Return (13; i.e., vbKeyReturn) and Line Feed (10). VB provides the named constant vbCrLf for this marker. Recall that we used this constant in Chapter 3 to display texts on different lines. Although the marker is not visible to us, it is important to be aware of its existence. The awareness helps you understand how the sequential (text) file is handled internally.

The Comma Delimiter for the Input Statement. In the preceding code, the Input statement looks for commas and the end of line markers (vbCrLf) to separate data fields. Because the phone number and name are properly separated by a comma in each line, the Input statement will execute properly. What if each line appears as follows?

8172223838, Dole, John

The value 8172223838 will be correctly assigned to Phone, but TheName will contain only "Dole" instead of "Dole, John." The comma between "Dole" and "John" will lead the Input statement to interpret that they are two separate data fields. What can be done to avoid or correct the problem? A typical way is to create a file with the names enclosed in a pair of double quotes:

8172223838, "Dole, John"

The string enclosed in quotes can then be read and interpreted by the Input statement as a single data field and assigned properly to the variable TheName.

What if for some reason you insist that the file be created without the double quotes? The workaround will take a bit more code. You will use the Line Input statement to read in a line of data and perform your own string parsing.

The Line Input Statement. Unlike the Input statement, the Line Input statement reads one line of data from the file at a time. This statement has the following syntax:

```
Line Input #File Number, Variable
```

where *File Number* = the file number associated with the input file as explained previously; notice that the "#" in the statement is required, not optional as in the case of the Open statement

Variable = a String or Variant variable to hold the line of data read from the file; notice that you can have only one variable in this statement, not a list as in the case of the Input statement

For example, the string variable PhoneName will contain the entire line of data as a result of executing the following statement:

```
Line Input #PhoneFile, PhoneName
```

Note that the Line Input statement does not filter out any characters in the input file. Thus, if the file contains double quotes or commas, these characters will be preserved in the variable. If you need to squeeze out any unneeded characters, you will need to provide the code for that purpose.

To continue our example, assume that the line read in is as follows:

8172223838, Dole, John

And you would like to put the number in Phone and the name in TheName. You can use the code similar to the following to obtain the result:

```
P = InStr(PhoneName, ",")
Phone = Left$(PhoneName, P - 1)
TheName = Mid$(PhoneName, P + 1)
```

In the code, the InStr function is used to find the position of the first comma in PhoneName (the line read in). Then the substring on the left side of the comma is assigned to Phone, and the right side is assigned to TheName.

The Input Function. In addition to the two statements already described to read data from an input file, an ***Input function*** can also be used for similar purposes. The Input function has the following syntax:

```
Input(chars, [#]File Number)
```

where *Chars* = the number of characters to read in

File Number = same as explained previously for the Open statement

To read the first phone number and name in the file in the previous example, you can code the following:

```
Phone = Input(10, #PhoneFile)
TheName = Input(12, #PhoneFile)
```

The Input function does not skip any characters in a file. Thus, the second statement in our code will also include both commas in the input stream; that is, the content of TheName will appear as follows:

, Dole, John

Notice the comma and the space before "Dole, John." In addition, even the "end of line" marker, vbCrLf, will be read into a variable (and counted as two characters) when you use the Input function.

The Relative Advantages of the Input Techniques. At this moment, you probably think that the Input function is of limited use because it requires a lot of additional details, which you may not even be able to supply for the example we have at hand. In the previous example, all phones and names respectively will have to be of equal length to possibly use the Input function.

Actually, there are relative advantages and disadvantages of each type of input technique:

- The ***Input statement*** provides a convenient way to read in data when the file has been created as "comma delimited." However, not all the files are created in this format. Usually, files that are to be exchanged between different software packages are "exported" (created by a software package for another software) in this format. You can then use the Input statement to "import" the data into your application. These files do not look very organized and use much more storage space than files of other formats. Also, it takes much more computer effort to parse the data in this format. Thus, the Input statement is very slow. You should avoid using it for high-volume repetitive data-processing applications.
- The ***Line Input statement*** reads one line of data at a time. If you have files that contain data on a line-by-line basis, this statement can be used conveniently. As the previous example illustrates, it can also be used to parse data to overcome the problem that the Input statement can encounter with improperly delimited files. However, you will then need to provide the code to take care of the details. Thus, the Line Input statement is most often used as a technical supplement for the Input statement.
- The ***Input function*** works the best when the data in a file are structured in a very precise format. It is the fastest technique among the three. Thus, it is the technique most suitable for processing large-volume sequential files. (Note, however, we say, "sequential files." Other file modes can be even faster, but the Input function cannot be used in other file modes.) As you have already seen, when data in a file are not formatted precisely, it will be difficult to use this technique. Some of its uses are illustrated later in this chapter under the headings "LOF Function" and "Reading an Entire File."

The following table summarizes the advantages and disadvantages of the three sequential input techniques.

Input Technique	Feature	Advantages	Disadvantages
Input statement	Reads field by field	Simple, easy to use, good for import and export	Slow; files suitable for this operation require more storage and do not look neat.
Line Input statement	Reads line by line	Faster than Input statement	Additional code is required to parse the string or each field must be of fixed length.
Input function	Reads the number of characters as specified	Fastest among the three techniques	Length of each field must be known before the statement is executed.

The EOF Function. If you continue to execute the Input or the Line Input statement, eventually the file will run out of data. The end of file condition is raised. Further attempt to read the file will result in a runtime "End Of File" (EOF) error. To avoid encountering the EOF error, your code should check for the EOF condition before executing an Input/Line Input statement. The EOF function returns the EOF condition of a file and can be used for this purpose. It has the following syntax:

```
EOF(File Number)
```

If the file specified has run out of data, the function returns a value of True; otherwise, it returns a value of False. In the previous example involving the Input statement, you can modify the code to take into account the EOF condition as follows:

```
Private Sub cmdRead_Click()
Dim Phone As Currency
Dim TheName As String
    If EOF(PhoneFile) Then
        MsgBox "The file has run out of data."
        Exit Sub 'Leave the procedure
    End If
    Input #PhoneFile, Phone, TheName
    MsgBox "Phone is " & Phone & ". Name is " & TheName
End Sub
```

The Exit Sub Statement. Notice that there is an Exit Sub statement after the "Out of data" message is displayed. When this statement is encountered, execution in the procedure will be terminated. No other statement in the procedure will be executed. Additional explanation of this statement is given in the next section.

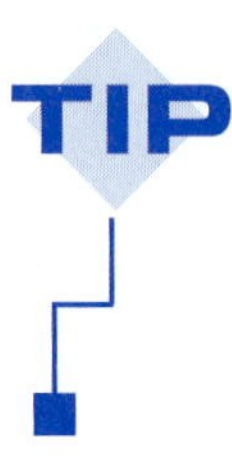

Notice that the number/variable enclosed in the parentheses of EOF has no "#" sign. The EOF function expects numeric data as the parameter. The "#" symbol is not a part of a number or variable name. If you include it in the EOF call, the compiler gives you an error message. On the other hand, it is a good idea to include the "#" character with the file number for all the Input and Output statements. In most I/O statements, the "#" character is required. Without it, the statement may have a compile time error or produce an unexpected result.

The LOF Function. The EOF function works properly for the Input and Line Input statement. However, it does not work for the Input function. Why? This function reads in the number of characters as specified. It makes no attempt to identify the meaning of any characters it reads, which is why it takes the "end of line" marker vbCrLf as a part of the input. For the same reason, it ignores the EOF marker and cannot recognize and generate the EOF condition.

Thus, to identify the EOF condition when using the Input function, you should count the number of characters read and compare the counter with the size of the file, which you can obtain using the LOF function. The ***LOF function*** has the same syntax as the EOF function, but it returns the size of the files. Suppose in the previous phone file that all phone numbers are saved as a 10-character string and names as a 20-character string. In addition, there is no carriage return character in the file. Then, in the routine to read the data (say, the command button cmdRead's Click event), you can code the following:

```
Private Sub cmdRead_Click()
Static CharsRead As Long
Dim Phone As String
Dim TheName As String
    If CharsRead >= LOF(PhoneFile) Then
        MsgBox "All Phones and Names have been read."
        Exit Sub
    End If
```

```
        Phone = Input(10, #PhoneFile)
        TheName = Input(20, #PhoneFile)
        'The above two lines read in a total of 30 characters.
        'Accumulate the number of chars read to compare with
        'the file length
        CharsRead = CharsRead + 30
    End Sub
```

Notice that the variable CharsRead is declared as a Static variable so that its value can be preserved between each event procedure call. It is used to keep track of the number of characters read and is compared with the file size at the beginning of the procedure. If it is greater than or equal to the file size, the entire file has been read. A message is displayed and the procedure is terminated with the Exit Sub statement.

Reading an Entire File. The Input function turns out to be a handy facility when you need to read the entire file in one operation. For example, suppose you would like to read the entire file into a text box named txtDoc from the file number TextFile, which has been opened properly. You can code the following:

```
    txtDoc.Text = Input(LOF(TextFile), #TextFile)
```

This should be a handy way to display the file content in a text box. You can even allow the user to edit the text as in the word processing operations. Of course, to display the text properly, you should set the text box's MultiLine property to True and its Scrollbars property to 2 (Vertical) or 3 (both Vertical and Horizontal).

The FreeFile Function. You have seen that you can designate a file number and use it to open the file. You have also been advised to use a variable for the file number instead of a constant literal in your code. When your program needs to handle many files simultaneously, it can be difficult for you to keep track of which number has been used to open a file. However, all you need is to assign a legitimate number to the variable for each file. It would be nice if the system handles this automatically for you. Is there a way? Yes, the ***FreeFile function*** provides exactly this service. It returns a number that you can safely use to open a file. Instead of designating a number for a file "manually," you should always take advantage of this FreeFile function. The following code from the previous example to open the phone file:

```
    PhoneFile = 1
    Open "A:\MyFolder\Phones.txt" For Input as #PhoneFile
```

should be changed to:

```
    PhoneFile = FreeFile 'Here's the change in code.
    Open "A:\MyFolder\Phones.txt" For Input as #PhoneFile
```

If you have only one file to open, the FreeFile function most likely will return a value of 1, the same number you would have designated. However, if you need to assign a number for another file in a separate part of your project, the use of the FreeFile function will relieve you from the tedious need to check which file number has been used and whether it has been closed.

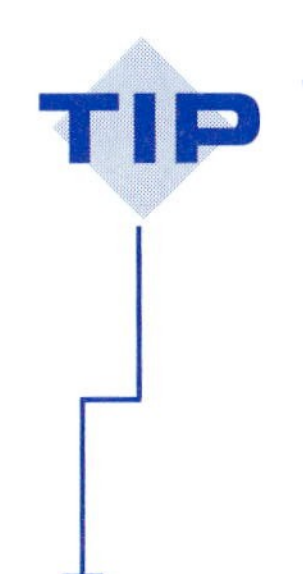

Always use the FreeFile function and the Open statement as a pair in two consecutive statements. Inserting other code between the two lines can make the program harder to read. Furthermore, some errors can sneak in if the FreeFile function is used another time. For example, the following code will result in a ***"File already open" error***.

```
    FileOne = FreeFile
    FileTwo = FreeFile
    Open "A:\MyFileA.txt" for Input As FileOne
    Open "A:\MyFileB.txt" for Input As FileTwo
```

continues

Why? When the FreeFile function is used the second time, FileOne has not yet been open. Thus, the system thinks the number used for FileOne is still available. The same number will be assigned to both FileOne and FileTwo. But the same number cannot be used to open two different files. The ***correct code*** should be:

```
FileOne = FreeFile
Open "A:\MyFileA.txt" for Input As FileOne
FileTwo = FreeFile
Open "A:\MyFileB.txt" for Input As FileTwo
```

The Close Statement. A file left open will be closed when the project ends. However, in many cases, you may need to close the file before the project ends, for example, when you need to open the same file with different mode (e.g., from output mode to input mode). Indeed, it is a good practice to close the file when you are done with it. It eliminates the possibility that your program accidentally performs unexpected operations on the file. It releases the computer resources associated with that file and ensures that all file operations you have performed are actually carried out by the computer. The syntax to close a file is as follows:

```
Close [[#]File Number]
```

To close the phone file in the preceding example, you will write the following:

```
Close #PhoneFile
```

Note that you can simply code:

```
Close
```

In such a case, all open files will be closed.

Output with Files. To output data onto a file, you need to open the file with either the Output or Append mode. If you open a file with an ***Output mode***, any previous content of the file will be erased. In essence, you are creating a brand new file. In most cases, you would probably want to preserve the previous content of the file. In such cases, you should open the file with the ***Append mode***. The previous content will be preserved. The next output operation will be "appended" to the end of the current file content.

The following statements will open the Phone file discussed in the previous example. (Note that the file must be closed if you have previously opened it for other purposes.)

```
Dim PhoneFile As Integer
PhoneFile = FreeFile
Open "A:\MyFolder\Phones.txt" For Append as #PhoneFile
```

You can then use either the Write statement or Print statement to add more phone numbers and names, depending on how you would like to create the data on the file.

The Write Statement. The Write statement will create comma-delimited data and enclose string data in pairs of double quotes. The Write statement has the following syntax:

```
Write #File Number, Variable List
```

where *File Number* = the file number associated with the output; notice that the "#" in the statement is required, not optional as in the case of the Open statement
Variable list = a list of variables to write onto the file

For example, you have a masked edit box named mskPhone and a text box named txtFriend in a form. You would like to save the data entered by the user onto the file just opened. If you use the following statement:

```
Write #PhoneFile, mskPhone.ClipText, txtFriend.Text
```

the line of output data in the file will appear as follows:

"2146668392", "Jones, Allen"

Note that the phone number is also enclosed in a pair of double quotes because the ClipText property is not considered numeric. To avoid the pair of quotes for the phone number, you should code the following:

```
Write #PhoneFile, Val(mskPhone.ClipText), txtFriend.Text
```

Recall that the Input statement explained previously expects this structure of data in the file. Thus, you can think of the Input and Write statements as complementary I/O statements.

The Print Statement. The Print statement does not automatically provide any extra commas or quotes when outputting data. This statement has the following syntax:

```
Print #File Number, Variable List
```

where *File Number* = the file number associated with the output file; notice that the "#" in the statement is required, not optional as in the case of the Open statement
Variable list = a list of variables to output data onto the file

Thus, if you output the data with the following statement:

```
Print #PhoneFile, mskPhone.ClipText, txtFriend.Text
```

the line of data in the file will appear as follows:

2146668392   Jones, Allen

Notice that the phone number and the name are separated with a proper tab position when the variables are separated with a comma (,) in the Print statement. Thus, data output with commas in this statement will appear properly aligned by fields. Note also that you can use semicolons (;) instead of commas in the variable list in the Print statement. That is, the Print statement can appear as follows:

```
Print #PhoneFile, mskPhone.ClipText; txtFriend.Text
```

The output will then appear as follows:

2146668392Jones, Allen

Note that the output produced with the semicolon separator in the variable list will leave no space between the data fields. In addition, you can also conclude a Print statement with a semicolon. That is, you can code the following:

```
Print #PhoneFile, mskPhone.ClipText; txtFriend.Text;
```

In this case, the next output will be placed immediately next to where the current output ends, instead of at the beginning of a new line. The resulting file will appear as follows:

2146668392Jones, Allen8174659333Roberts, Jane . . .

Is there any merit of creating a file using such a format? Files created this way are much more compact. If each field of data is of the same length (fixed length), the data can be retrieved more efficiently (with faster speed) with the Input function or even with other file modes, which are discussed in Appendix A.

Write Versus Print. The differences between the Write statement and the Print statement can be briefly stated as follows:

- The Write statement creates a *comma-delimited* file. The results can be used by other applications. The file can also conveniently be read by using the Input statement. However, the output operation is very slow, just like its input counterpart, the Input statement. The resulting file does not look very neat and therefore is not suitable for reports. In addition, the file takes up more storage space. Thus, you use the Write statement only when the file is intended to be "exported" or when the file size is very small and thus the operational efficiency is not a concern.
- The Print statement can generate files whose columns are neatly aligned. Thus, you can use the Print statement to generate files intended for reports. In addition, you can

also use it to generate files that take up much less storage space than those generated by the Write statement. If each field in a record is created as a fixed-length field, the resulting file can conveniently be read by the Input function. The I/O operations done this way are much more efficient than using the Write or Input statements. However, output from the Print statement generally is not suitable for "export."

We have discussed many statements and functions related to file operations. The following table provides a summary.

Keyword	Statement or Function	Purpose	Code Example
Open	Statement	To associate a file number with a physical file	`Open "PhoneFile.txt" For Output As #PhoneFile`
Close		To close a file	`Close PhoneFile`
Input		To read comma-delimited data from an input file	`Input #PhoneFile, Phone, TheName`
Line Input		To read data line by line	`Line Input #PhoneFile, PhoneName`
Write		To output comma-delimited data	`Write #PhoneFile, Phone, TheName`
Print		To output data without a delimiter	`Print #PhoneFile, Phone, TheName`
Input	Function	To read data with a specified number of characters	`Phone = Input(10, #PhoneFile)`
EOF		Returns a Boolean value indicating whether end of file has been reached	`If EOF(PhoneFile) Then Exit Sub`
LOF		Returns a value giving the size of the file in bytes	`Print LOF(PhoneFile)`
FreeFile		Returns a value that can be used as a file number without causing problems	`PhoneFile = FreeFile`

The Print Method

The ***Print method*** works much like the Print statement. Instead of working with a file, the Print method works with objects, including the form, picture box, Debug, and Printer. The Print method has the following syntax:

```
Object.Print List
```

where *Object* = Form, Picture Box, Debug, or Printer
List = the list to print/display

Items in the list can be separated by commas or semicolons. These separators work exactly the same way as in the Print statement already explained. The output of the Print method is displayed on the object. For example, if the object is a picture box, the output is displayed on the picture box.

The Debug Object. Debug represents the immediate window in the VB's IDE. As the name implies, the Debug object is mainly used by the programmer to output data for the purposes of debugging (tracing the state of program execution to identify the source of errors). As a programmer, you can use it to output anything of interest. In contrast to MsgBox, output to the Debug object does not cause the program to pause for the user's response, making it much easier to work with when you want the program to execute continuously while providing some useful results for debugging clues.

Notice, however, that the immediate window exists only in the IDE. Thus, the user using your program already compiled and running it as an executable will not be able to see that window.

Always bear in mind that the Debug object is meant only for the use of the programmer, not for the user.

The Debug object is referred to as Debug. Thus, to print "Test" in the immediate window, you will code the following:

```
Debug.Print "Test"
```

The Form Object for Print. The form object also has the Print method. Printing output on a form requires careful analysis because the output can be easily cluttered with the VB controls on the form. Therefore, the form is seldom used for regular printed output. Rather, it is used mainly for debugging purposes. The form object is referred to by its name or simply by Me. Thus, to print "Test" on the form, you will code the following:

```
Me.Print "Test"
```

Because the default object of the Print method is the form, you can also code the following:

```
Print "Test"
```

Beware of the fine difference between the following two statements:

```
Print #PhoneFile, mskPhone.ClipText, txtFriend.Text
Print PhoneFile, mskPhone.ClipText, txtFriend.Text
```

The first line uses the Print statement to print the content of the two controls onto the file with the file number PhoneFile. In the second line, the variable PhoneFile is not preceded by a "#" sign; thus, it is interpreted as a part of the list to be printed. The entire line is then taken as a method, not as a Print statement. The method's default object is the form. Thus, the second line will print the file number for PhoneFile as well as the contents of the two controls onto the form. Tricky, isn't it?

The Picture Box for Print. An alternative to printing the output on the form is to use the picture box. Because the picture box is independent of the other VB controls on the form, output to the picture box can easily be isolated from the other controls. Both the form and picture box have the ***CurrentX and CurrentY properties*** whose values you can set or retrieve. The CurrentX property gives the horizontal (print) position of the object, and the CurrentY property gives the vertical (print) position of the object. For example, suppose you want to print the word "Center" at the center of the picture box named picDisplay. You can set the picture box's CurrentX and CurrentY properties to the proper values and then display the text. The following code should accomplish the goal:

```
picDisplay.CurrentX = (picDisplay.ScaleWidth _
     - picDisplay.TextWidth("Center")) / 2
picDisplay.CurrentY = (picDisplay.ScaleHeight _
     - picDisplay.TextHeight("C")) / 2
     picDisplay.Print "Center"
```

In this code, we also use the ScaleWidth and ScaleHeight properties as well as the TextWidth and TextHeight methods. The ***ScaleWidth*** and ***ScaleHeight properties*** refer to the measurements of the interior useable width and height of the picture box (as opposed to the Width and Height properties, which refer to the exterior width and height of the picture box). The ***TextWidth*** and ***TextHeight methods*** return the width and height of the text string in the parameters for the object. Notice that in the preceding code, the picture box is referred to by its name, not by its generic class, PictureBox. This is in contrast to the Debug object, which you refer to as Debug.

All the aforementioned properties and methods are also available for the Printer object (but not for the Debug object) and can be used in exactly the same way. Like the Debug object, you refer to the Printer object as Printer. Thus, to print the string "Center" on the printer (page), you will code the following:

```
Printer.Print "Center"
```

The Common Dialog Box for Files

The files created using the Write or Print statement can be viewed and edited by the use of the Microsoft Notepad program. Files created by Notepad can also be input to your program using the input mode with the Input and Line Input statement or the Input function. Of course, for your program to perform properly, the code and the file structure must match correctly.

Talking about the Notepad, you probably recall that each time you use it to open or save a file, it displays a dialog box for you to specify the file in your computer system. Wouldn't it be nice if we can have the same facility in VB to specify the file? Yes, there is such a facility. It is provided by the common dialog control (see Figure 6.3) with the ShowOpen and ShowSave methods.

The ***common dialog control*** is not a standard (intrinsic) control and needs to be added to the toolbox before you can use it in your form. To add the control to the toolbox:

1. Click the Project menu and select the Components option.
2. Locate and check the "Microsoft Common Dialog Control 6.0" item in the Components dialog box.
3. Click the OK button.

Figure 6.3
Common Dialog Control in the Toolbox and in the Form

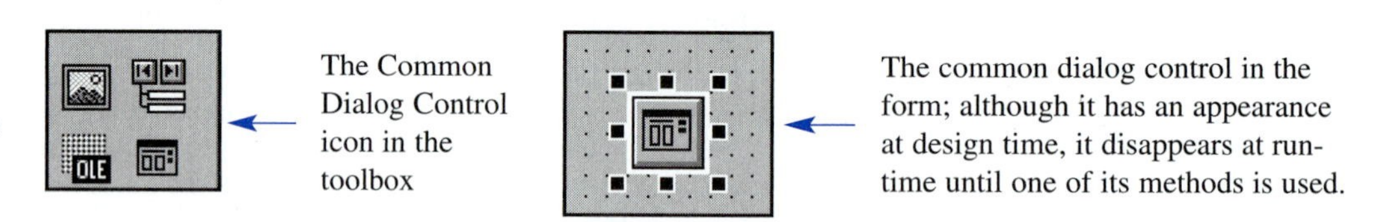

OLE
The Common Dialog Control icon in the toolbox
The common dialog control in the form; although it has an appearance at design time, it disappears at run-time until one of its methods is used.

Once the common dialog control is added to the form, you can set its properties at design time or by code so that it performs the services you need. The following table lists some of its properties that you need to become familiarized with to work with files properly:

Property	Explanation	Example	Effect
Filter	Used to show only the types of file extension in the dialog box.	`.Filter = _ "Text File (*.*) ¦*.txt"`	Only files with the txt extension will be shown in the dialog box.
DialogTitle	A string to be displayed on the title bar of the common dialog box in place of the typical "Open" or "Save as" title.	`.DialogTitle = _ "Where is the File?"`	The title bar will show "Where is the file."
CancelError	When you set it to True and the user clicks the Cancel button, your program generates an error.	`.CancelError = True`	Your program will have an error when the user clicks the Cancel button.
Flags	You can set different values for it to behave differently.	`.Flags = _ cdlOFNFileMustExist`	The common dialog box will insist that the file must exist when the user enters a nonexisting filename.
FileName	This property is set to the user-specified file path after the execution of the ShowOpen or ShowSave method.	`MyFileName = _ .FileName`	MyFileName will have the filename the common dialog box has after the ShowOpen or ShowSave method is executed.

The Filter Property. The Filter property allows you to specify what types of files you would like to be displayed. For each type of files you want to specify, you must give the description and the filter, separated by a "|" symbol. For example, assume that you have named the common dialog cdlFile and that you want it to show only files with the txt extension. You can specify the following:

```
cdlFile.Filter = "Text Files (*.txt)|*.txt"
```

In the preceding code, the string "Text Files (*.txt)" gives the description of the type of files your user will be looking for. The filter "*.txt" (following the "|") specifies that the system will display all files with the txt file extension. The "*" is a wild card specification that indicates to ignore the matching (all names are considered a match).

You can also separate additional filters by additional "|" symbols. The following line will allow either text files or all files to be possible filters, depending on which filter the user chooses.

```
cdlFile.Filter = "Text File (*.txt)|*.txt|All Files (*.*)|*.*"
```

To illustrate how the common dialog box can be used for file specifications, suppose in the previous phone file example that all you know is that there is such a file. The file can be located at any folder with any name in a computer. Thus, you want your user to specify the location for input. Again, assume the control has been named cdlFile. Your code to open the file can appear as follows:

```
'Title on the dialog box
cdlFile.DialogTitle = "Where is the phone file?"
'Display only txt files
cdlFile.Filter = "Text Files (*.txt)|*.txt"
cdlFile.ShowOpen        ' Display the Open dialog box
PhoneFile = FreeFile
' cdlFile.FileName below is obtained from the ShowOpen method
Open cdlFile.FileName For Input As #PhoneFile
```

When the ShowOpen method is executed, the dialog box will appear as in Figure 6.4.

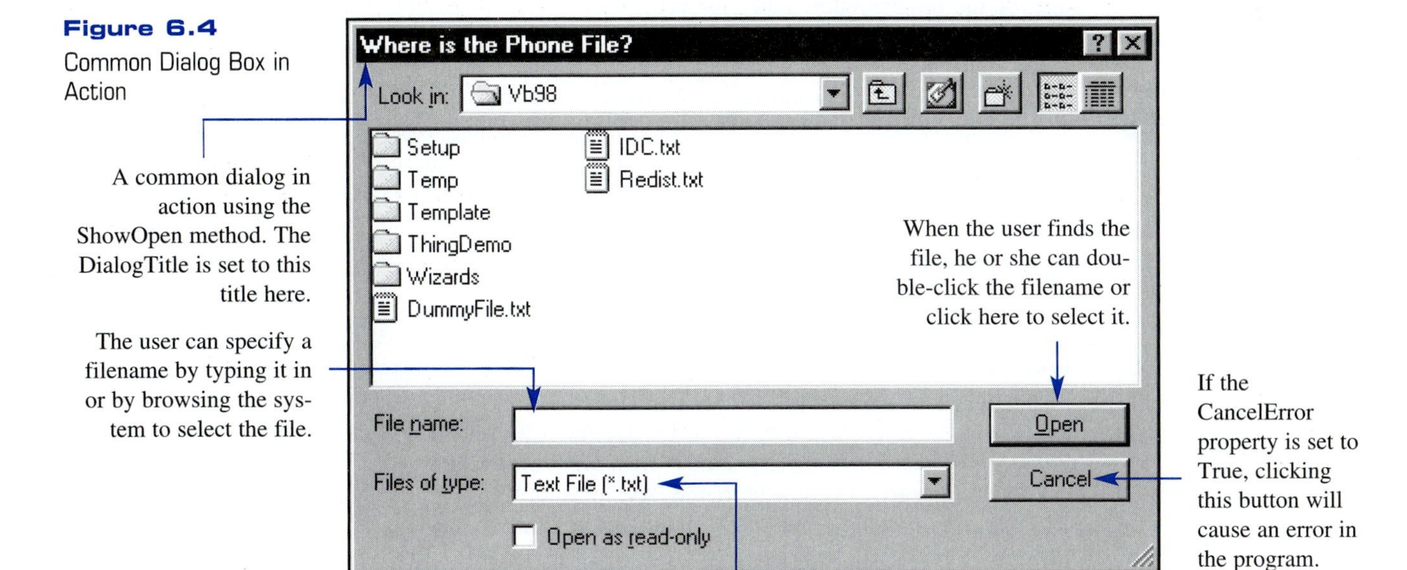
Where is the Phone File?
Look in:
Vb98
Setup
Temp
Template
ThingDemo
Wizards
DummyFile.txt
IDC.txt
Redist.txt
File name:
Files of type:
Text File (*.txt)
Open as read-only
Open
Cancel
A common dialog in action using the ShowOpen method. The DialogTitle is set to this title here.
The user can specify a filename by typing it in or by browsing the system to select the file.
When the user finds the file, he or she can double-click the filename or click here to select it.
If the CancelError property is set to True, clicking this button will cause an error in the program.
The filter description is shown here. The filter is used by the system to select the files to display in the above list. Clicking the drop-down button will show additional filter descriptions.

Figure 6.4
Common Dialog Box in Action

Once the user browses through the computer and selects the proper file, the filename is stored in the control's FileName property, which can then be used as the string for the file specification in the Open statement.

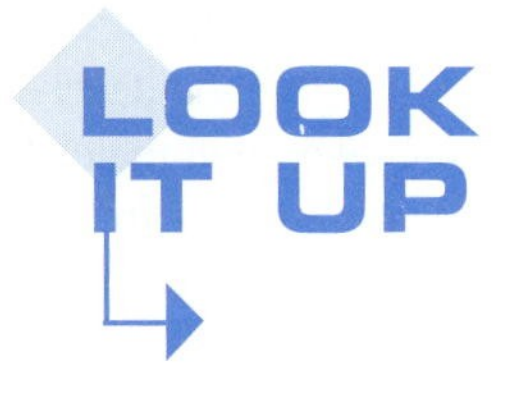

Search for the keyword "CommonDialog constant" in Index tab of the online Help file. You will see how various values (named constants) for the Flags properties can make the common dialog control exhibit additional facilities, such as checking to ensure that a file exists or overwriting an existing file. You can also look up "CommonDialog control" to learn more about its other capabilities, such as Color, Font, and Print dialogs.

Use of the CancelError Property. What if the user clicks the Cancel button instead? The result will be unexpected. To avoid any potential problem, you can set the CancelError property to True and handle the error when it occurs. This will typically mean that the open file operation should be bypassed. Assume you have a command button named cmdOpen with the caption "Open." The following code illustrates how this can be done.

```
Private Sub cmdOpen_Click()
Dim PhoneFile As Integer
    cdlFile.DialogTitle = "Where is the phone file?"
    cdlFile.Filter = "Text Files (*.txt)¦*.txt"
    cdlFile.CancelError = True
    On Error GoTo DoNothing
    cdlFile.ShowOpen
    PhoneFile = FreeFile
    Open cdlFile.filename For Input As #PhoneFile
DoNothing:
End Sub
```

In the preceding code, the common dialog's CancelError property is set to True. Then, the On Error statement, an error-handling statement, is used before the ShowOpen method is invoked. This On Error statement checks whether the execution of any subsequent statements causes an error. When an error condition occurs, the statement (with GoTo) directs the execution control to a statement label named "DoNothing." Thus, if the user clicks the Cancel button, the error will make the execution control jump to the DoNothing label. Because no statement follows the label before the procedure ends, the procedure is done without opening a file.

Recall in Chapter 3, we stressed the importance of following the control naming conventions. It was suggested that a lowercase three-letter prefix be used as the prefix for the name of each control. Use "cdl" as the three-letter prefix to name all common dialog box controls.

About "GoTo" and Statement Label. Notice that you can construct a ***statement label*** (not a label control) with any legitimate name followed by a colon. Usually, a statement label is used as a target of a GoTo statement to which to transfer execution control. In general, it is poor practice to use the GoTo statement to transfer execution control. The execution flow becomes hard to trace, especially when it is transferred "freely" in different directions. The code logic can easily become cluttered. Avoid using "GoTo" in your code by all means and consider the case of "On Error GoTo" statement as a rare exception.

The On Error Statement. As you can see in the previous example, the On Error statement can be used to handle errors that occur during the execution of a program. In general, you want your program to be as error free as possible. However, there are circumstances beyond your control that can cause errors in your program. For example, the user may try to open a file in Drive A without inserting a disk in that drive. Without an error handler in your program, your program gets abruptly terminated and can be perceived by the user as "unfriendly." To the extent possible, you should identify all these potential "troubles" and write code to handle each accordingly. The "On Error GoTo" statement enables your program to branch to a program segment where you can code the "error handler."

There are also cases in which you are sure an error in one statement will not cause any problem in the execution of the subsequent statements. In this situation, you can simply code the following:

```
On Error Resume Next
```

The program will continue to execute without even indicating an error has occurred. Additional discussion of the On Error statement is given in Chapter 10, "Special Topics in Data Entry."

Note that the common dialog control has many other uses. For example, it can also be used to prompt for printers, fonts, as well as colors. You can find additional information by exploring the Index tab of the online Help file using the keyword "CommonDialog control."

6.2 Procedures: Subs and Functions

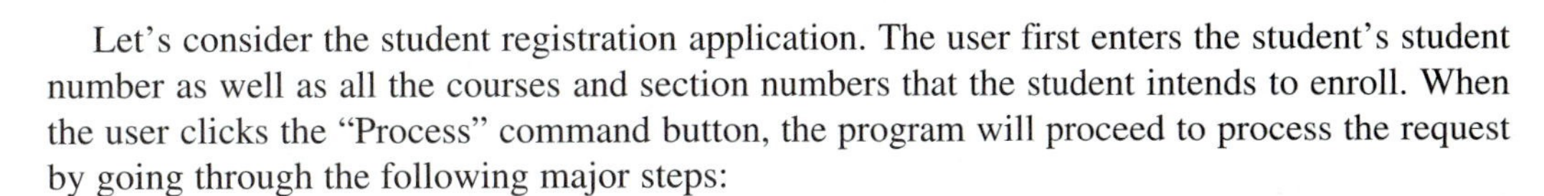

Let's consider the student registration application. The user first enters the student's student number as well as all the courses and section numbers that the student intends to enroll. When the user clicks the "Process" command button, the program will proceed to process the request by going through the following major steps:

1. Verifying that the student number is valid and the student is allowed to enroll
2. Looking for all previous unpaid invoices, campus police tickets, and library fines owed by the student
3. For each course the student requests to enroll:
   3.1 Verifying that the course and the section number are valid
   3.2 Verifying that the class is not yet full
   3.3 Verifying that the student has the prerequisites to take the course
4. Computing the total tuition and previous balance
5. Issuing the invoice
6. Updating the student's record
7. Updating all the class records

The list can go even longer, but the point is simple: in this situation, if you place all the code in the command's Click event procedure, it will be hard to follow the program flow of logic. The program will be too long and difficult to read, understand, debug, change, or maintain. The solution to this problem is to divide the program into several subprograms, each handling a predefined special task (e.g., one of the major steps outlined). The command's Click event procedure will then just provide an "outline" of the steps by calling these subprograms. This arrangement will dramatically reduce the number of lines in the event procedure. Because each subprogram handles a smaller task, it is easier to develop code and to understand when reviewing and debugging.

A partial, conceptual solution to the previous problem will probably be similar to the following:

```
Private Sub cmdProcess_Click()
    If BadStudentID(IDNumber) Then
        MsgBox "Needs a valid student ID number to proceed."
        Exit Sub
    End If
    FindUnPaidRecords IDNumber
      .
      .
End Sub
```

Each procedure referenced inside the event procedure can be written separately as a ***Sub*** or as a ***Function*** procedure. Both types of procedures are different from the event procedure in that the event procedure is typically invoked by the occurrence of an event, whereas the former are invoked by a reference of their names in the code. These procedures are recognized as general (or separate) procedures, as a distinction from the event procedure. The key difference between Sub and Function procedures is that the latter return a value, whereas the former does not. Additional distinctions are explained in the subsection "Additional Notes on General Procedures." For now, we can summarize the classification of procedures as follows.

Procedure Type	How Invoked	Returns a Value?	Remark
Event	Triggered by event	No	
Sub	Referenced by name	No	Collectively recognized as general or separate procedures
Function	Referenced by name	Yes	

Writing a Sub Procedure

So, how do we create a Sub procedure? A ***Sub*** procedure is declared with a Sub keyword with the following syntax structure:

```
[Private¦Public] Sub SubProgramName(Parameter List)
    Statements for the sub program
End Sub
```

where *SubProgramName* = any valid name for a variable
ParameterList = a list of parameters

Note that the parameter list can range from none to many and has the following syntax:

```
Param1 as DataType1, Param2 as DataType2,. . . .
```

The following examples are valid subprogram headers:

```
Private Sub BringData()
Private Sub SearchPreviousInvoice(IDNumber as Long)
Public Sub Enroll(ID As Long, CourseSection As String)
```

The ***Private or Public keyword*** declares the scope of the procedure. A private procedure is recognized only in the current form/module. A public procedure is accessible to all modules in the project; that is, it can be called from another form or module.

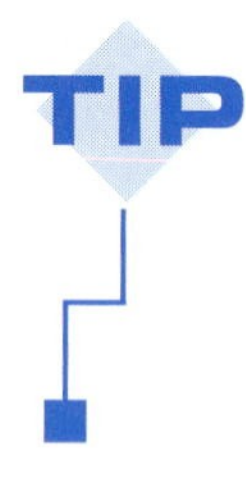

Although the number of parameters for a procedure is determined by the task requirement, it is always difficult to use a procedure with many parameters. Limiting the number to five or fewer appears to be a good rule of thumb. Otherwise, try your best to order the list in a logical way so that you can easily remember the parameters needed one after another. Or, better yet, try to redesign the code structure to see if it is possible to reduce the number of parameters needed.

The statements that are inside the procedure will be executed line by line in sequence when the procedure is invoked. The following Sub procedure computes and displays the area for a circle given its radius:

```
Option Explicit
Const Pi As Double = 3.14159265359

Private Sub ComputeArea(Radius As Double)
' This Sub computes and displays the area of a circle
'given a radius, which is expected to be of the Double type
Dim Area As Double
```

```
        Area = Pi * Radius * Radius
        MsgBox "The area of a circle with a radius of " _
          & Radius & " is " & Area
    End Sub
```

In this example, we declare the procedure to be Private; that is, the procedure will be recognizable and accessible only in this form. The procedure is named ComputeArea. It expects a parameter of the Double type. This parameter will be recognized in this procedure as Radius. Inside the procedure, this parameter is used to compute the area of a circle, and the resulting area is displayed by the MsgBox statement.

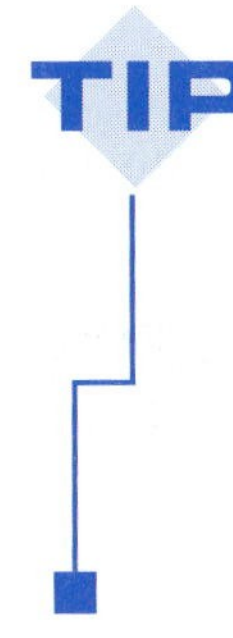
TIP

Recall that a statement declaring variables as follows may not give the data type you expected:

```
Dim One, Two As Integer
```

The variable One will be of the Variant type because no explicit Type declaration is given. The same rule applies to parameters that appear in the header of a procedure. For example, the following header will make the procedure *expect A as a Variant type and B as a Double type* because there is no explicit Type declaration for A.

```
Private Sub AddUp(A, B As Double)
```

Calling a Sub Procedure

You can call (invoke) a Sub procedure by using either of the following syntax:

```
Call SubName(argument list)
```

or

```
SubName Argument list
```

Thus, to call the Sub just written, you can code the following:

```
Call ComputeArea(10)
```

or

```
ComputeArea 10
```

Notice that you do not enclose the argument(s) with a pair of parentheses when you do not use the keyword "Call." However, you have to enclose the argument(s) with a pair of parentheses when you use the keyword "Call" to invoke a Sub procedure. Notice also that you pass an argument with a value 10 to the Sub, ComputeArea, but the argument is recognized in ComputeArea as the parameter Radius. That is, Radius is a symbolic name for any value that the calling procedure passes to the Sub. If you change the value to 8, 8 still will be recognized by the Sub as Radius. The relationship between an argument and a parameter in this context can be depicted as the following diagram:

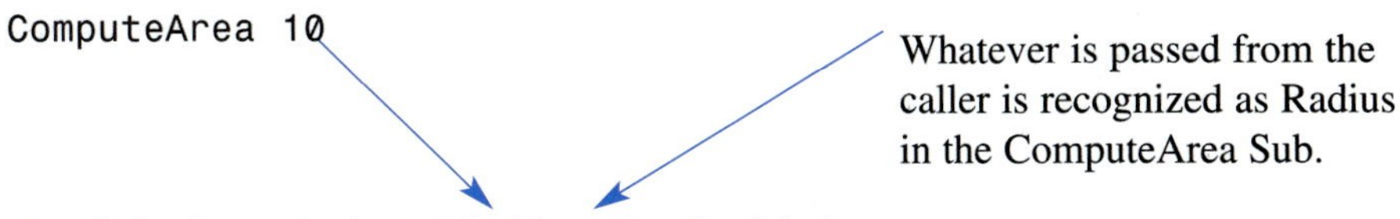
ComputeArea 10
Whatever is passed from the caller is recognized as Radius in the ComputeArea Sub.
Private Sub ComputeArea(Radius As Double)

In addition, you can also use different variables as arguments to call the Sub. For example, assume that you have declared both A and B as Double and assigned proper values to both variables. You can obtain the proper results by using the following statements:

```
ComputeArea A
ComputeArea B
```

To test how it works, draw a new command button on a new form. Name it cmdCompute and set its Caption property to "Compute." Then enter the following code:

```
Private Sub cmdCompute_Click()
Dim A As Double
Dim B As Double
    A = 10
    B = 8
    ComputeArea A
    ComputeArea B
End Sub
```

Run the project and click the command button. The message box should first display the area of the circle for a radius 10; then, for 8.

Code Reusability with the General Procedure. This simple illustration has also demonstrated a powerful use of general procedures. Much like the use of variables to handle different data values, you can use a procedure to even handle different variables that require the same computational formulas or processing steps. You can use the same Sub repetitively anytime you need to handle a similar situation, even when the variables involved are not the same. Thus, *general procedures enhance the reusability of your code.*

To further illustrate this point, consider the program that we wrote in the preceding section to print a text string at the center of a picture box. We can actually rewrite it as a Sub so that it will print any text string at the center of any object that supports the CurrentX and CurrentY properties (e.g., picture boxes, forms, and printers). The Sub can appear as follows:

```
Private Sub PrintAtCenter(Text As String, Obj As Object)
' This Sub prints a string at the center of an object
' The object must have the CurrentX and CurrentY properties
'It must also support the TextWidth and TextHeight methods
    Obj.CurrentX = (Obj.ScaleWidth - Obj.TextWidth(Text)) / 2
    Obj.CurrentY = (Obj.ScaleHeight - Obj.TextHeight(Text)) / 2
    Obj.Print Text
End Sub
```

This Sub takes two parameters. The first parameter is a string, and the second is an object, as indicated in the header. You may recall that *VB objects* is a generic term that refers to a wide spectrum of things, including forms, controls, and printers (and more). Inside the procedure, the position to start printing the string is determined by computing the object's CurrentX and CurrentY properties. The string (a parameter named Text) is then printed using the object's Print method.

If you want to display a text string in the current form, you can call this Sub:

```
PrintAtCenter "At the Center of the Form", Me
```

If you want to print something else on a hard copy, you can use this same Sub:

```
PrintAtCenter "Whatever Text I want to print", Printer
```

If you print onto the printer, your program needs to quit before the document is released (printed). Or, you need to add the following statement to eject a document:

```
Printer.EndDoc
```

Position and Type of Arguments. One very important point you must remember in calling a Sub is that the data or objects you pass as arguments are recognized by their positions, not by their names. With PrintAtCenter's header defined as done previously, if you try to call it with a statement such as the following:

```
PrintAtCenter Me, "At the Center of the Form"
```

you will get a "Type mismatch" error at runtime. Why? The Sub expects that the first parameter to be a string, but Me is a form, not a string. Thus, there is a mismatch in data/object type.

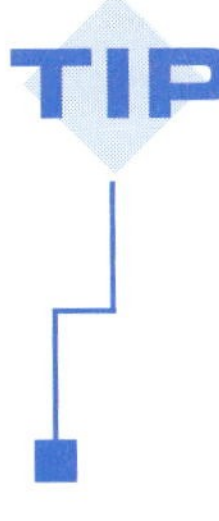

The arguments passed to a procedure are recognized by their position. They must match in data type and purpose (e.g., if the first parameter is expected to be a numerator, you should not pass a number that is meant to be a denominator) with those parameters expected by the procedure.

```
PrintAtCenter "At the Center of the Form", Me

Private Sub PrintAtCenter(Text As String, Obj As Object)
```

You may be wondering why then the statement:

```
ComputeArea 10
```

did not result in a type mismatch error. (Recall that ComputeArea expects a Double type parameter, but the number 10 is an integer.) The explanation is that 10 is a constant literal. Before the compiler constructs the data to pass to the Sub, it converts the constant to a proper data type (Double). If you assign 10 to an integer, for example, then pass the integer variable when calling the Sub, you will definitely get the type mismatch error.

Passing Variables to Sub Procedures

Passing Data By Position. The previous discussion stresses that data passed to the Sub procedure are recognized by position, not by name. This is true even when the data types of the arguments match those parameters expected by the Sub. For example, consider the following Sub:

```
Private Sub MakeTwice(Two As Double, One As Double)
    Two = One + One
End Sub
```

This procedure doubles the value of the second parameter and assigns the result to the first one. Thus, if in another procedure you have two variables, X and Y (both declared to be the Double data type and assigned with proper values), and you use the following statements:

```
MakeTwice Y, X
MsgBox X & Y
```

you should see that Y has a value twice of X. In addition, if you use the statements:

```
MakeTwice X, Y
MsgBox X & Y
```

you should see that X has a value twice of Y.

This holds even if you use the Variables Two and One in the calling procedure. To test, try the following code (be sure to include the MakeTwice Sub):

```
Private Sub Form_Click()
Dim One as Double, Two As Double
    One = 1
    Two = 2
    MakeTwice Two, One
    MsgBox "One = " & One & " Two " & Two
    MakeTwice One, Two
    MsgBox "One = " & One & "Two = " & Two
End Sub
```

Run the project. When you click the form, you should see the first message box display two numbers: 1 and 2 the first time for the variables One and Two. The results are obtained because the arguments are passed to the Sub as shown next (as expected):

```
MakeTwice Two, One

Private Sub MakeTwice(Two As Double, One As Double)
```

However, the second message box will display the numbers 4 and 2 for the variables One and Two. Again, the results are obtained because the arguments are passed as shown next (perhaps, not as expected for some beginners):

```
MakeTwice One, Two

Private Sub MakeTwice(Two As Double, One As Double)
```

Thus, the variable Two in the calling procedure is passed to MakeTwice as One, which is then doubled inside the procedure and assigned to the parameter named Two. However, the corresponding variable in the calling procedure to this parameter is the variable One. Thus, the result in the calling procedure is that One has twice the value of Two.

Passing Data by Name. There is actually a way to pass data by the parameter name. Using this approach, the position of the parameter will no longer be important. The syntax to pass data by name is as follows:

```
SubName Parameter1 := Argument1[, Parameter2 := Argument2] . . .
```

The ":=" symbol is used to indicate that the left side is the parameter name, whereas the right side is the argument. Parameter1 can be a parameter in any position. It does not have to be the first parameter in the parameter list in the Sub procedure's header.

Consider the following statement in previous example again.

```
MakeTwice X, Y
```

Using the named parameter syntax, you can have the same result by coding:

```
MakeTwice Two := X, One := Y
```

or

```
MakeTwice One := Y, Two := X
```

Of course, you can also code the following for the first statement in the above Form Click event procedure:

```
MakeTwice Two := Two, One := One
```

or

```
MakeTwice One := One, Two := Two
```

Again, keep in mind that the name on the left of the ":=" symbol is the parameter name, and the name on the right is the argument to be passed.

ByVal and ByRef. A derived question in the previous discussion is "Why can a procedure change the value of a variable in *another* procedure?" This is because in VB, by default, arguments are passed by their addresses (by reference), rather than by their values. Thus, whatever operations are performed on the parameter are actually performed on the argument. Any change made on the parameter is actually made on the argument.

If you do not want a procedure to accidentally change the value of any variables passed to it, you can use the ***ByVal*** declaration in its header. For example, the header:

```
Private Sub MakeTwice(ByVal Two As Double, ByVal One As Double)
```

will cause only the values of the arguments to be passed to this procedure, not their addresses. That is, a copy of the argument, not the argument itself, is passed to procedure. The effect? Whatever changes made to the parameters inside the Sub procedure will not cause any change in the variables used as arguments in the calling procedure.

In the previous example, the use of ByVal will make no sense because there will be no way to obtain the intended result because ByVal basically nullifies all desired effect of doubling the value of one of the variables. However, not all the Subs are written for the purpose of changing the values of some parameters.

ByVal is used mainly for compatibility with other languages. The Windows application program interface (API) library is developed in C, which by default, passes data by value, not by address. It is also true that in general, passing data ByVal executes faster than ByRef.

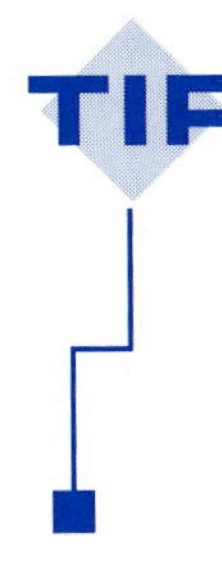

There is another way to have the effect of ByVal if you do not want the variable passed to a procedure gets its value changed. Enclose the variable with a pair of parentheses. For example, you can code the following:

```
MakeTwice (Y), (X)
```

The argument then will be taken as an expression, forcing the compiler to create a dummy variable to pass to the called procedure. Whatever changes are made to the dummy variable are discarded as soon as the called procedure ends.

Terminating a Procedure Before Reaching the End: Exit Sub

In some cases, your program logic in a procedure may be such that when certain conditions arise, there is no need to proceed further to execute the remainder of the code in the Sub. In such cases, you can use the Exit Sub statement to terminate the Sub procedure. The effect will be the same as if the Sub has reached the End Sub statement. For example, assume you have a Sub to save an inventory part in a file. The part number must be greater than 100; otherwise, it is considered invalid. Your Sub may appear as follows:

```
Private Sub SavePart(ID As Integer, PartName As String)
    If ID <= 100 Then
        MsgBox "The ID number is not valid. Part not saved."
        Exit Sub
    End If
' The routine to save the part will continue from here
End Sub
```

Exit Sub Versus End Sub. If both End Sub and Exit Sub statements terminate a procedure, what is the difference between the two? The End Sub statement actually serves two purposes. It not only terminates a Sub procedure when the execution control reaches that point but also physically defines the boundary of a Sub procedure. It tells the compiler that the procedure ends here. No other statements beyond this point should be considered a part of this procedure. On the other hand, the Exit Sub statement terminates only the Sub and returns execution control to the calling procedure. Because no other statements inside the procedure will be executed after the control reaches this statement, the Exit Sub statement is usually included in an If block; that is, you would want to terminate a Sub only when certain conditions occur.

Event Procedures and General Sub Procedures

At this point, you may wonder about the differences between the event procedures and the general Sub procedures. After all, both have the keyword Sub. The two differ in several aspects:

- Event procedures are triggered by events. As you recall, these events are results of something occurring in the systems or the results of the user's actions. There is no explicit call in the code to invoke an event procedure. In contrast, the general Sub procedures must be triggered (invoked) by code. That is, somewhere in the code, the name of the general Sub procedure must be referenced, and only when this line of code is executed will the general Sub be invoked. (Note, however, an event procedure can also be invoked by an explicit call like the way a general Sub is called.)
- A corollary of the preceding difference is that in general, you will find general Subs are called from an event procedure or another general Sub procedure. However, it is rare that a general Sub calls an event procedure even though it is permissible to do so.
- The name of an event procedure must follow a specific syntax structure. The first part of it must be the name of the object with which the event is associated, and the second part must be the name of the event. These two parts are connected with an

underscore. For example, the name of the Form Load event procedure is Form_Load. Form is the name of the object and Load is the event. Between Form and Load, there is the underscore ("_"). Note that the object must exist in the form and the event must be recognized by the object before the event procedure has any effect. In contrast, you can create any name for a general Sub procedure as long as the name can be considered a legitimate variable name.

- The number, order, and data type of parameters for event procedures are predetermined by the system. You cannot change these elements in any event procedure. In contrast, you have complete freedom in deciding these elements in the general procedures that you create.
- In terms of scope, the event procedure must be Private, whereas the Sub procedure can either be Private or Public.

These differences are summarized in the following table.

Difference in	Event Procedure	General Sub Procedure
Trigger	Event (triggered by the occurrence of the event)	Referenced by code (called by another procedure)
Caller	Seldom called from another procedure	Must be called by another procedure, which can be an event or general procedure
Name syntax	Must observe the following structure: *ObjectName_EventName*	Can use any legitimate variable name as the name of a Sub
Parameter list	Predefined by VB	Designed by the programmer
Scope	Private	Public or Private

Function Procedures

Let's consider the previous MakeTwice Sub procedure example again. We use the example to illustrate how arguments passed to a Sub are handled. If we carefully reexamine the design, we should realize that there is a better way to structure the code. Recall that in the Sub, one parameter (One) was used to compute the value of the other (Two), which could then be used by the calling procedure. That is, the Sub procedure was used to generate one result based on the value of another parameter. In such a case, a Function (instead of a Sub) procedure is a better choice. The key difference between a Sub and a Function procedure is that the latter returns a value, whereas the former does not.

The Function Procedure Header. So, how do you create a Function procedure? The Function procedure is declared with the ***Function*** keyword with the following syntax:

```
[Public¦Private] Function Name(parameter list) [As Type]
    Statements (including Exit Function)
    Name = Expression
End Function
```

As you can see in the syntax, the Function procedure header has the scope descriptor (Public or Private) and the parameter list (similar to the Sub procedure). However, the function header accepts a Type declaration, whereas the Sub does not. The Type declaration at the end of the function header specifies the type of data that the function will return. Inside the Function procedure, the function name must appear at least once on the left side of an assignment statement. The value so assigned is the value returned to the caller.

The Differences Between Subs and Functions. There are several differences between Sub and Function procedures.

1. Because the Function procedure is expected to return a value to the calling procedure, you should provide a Type declaration at the end of the header. The type declared here is the data type of the value to be returned by the function. The Sub

procedure is not expected to return a value. A Type declaration in its header is not allowed.

2. Both types of procedures will contain statements that carry out computations. In a Function procedure, however, at least one assignment statement should have the function name on the left side. The execution of this statement will cause the value of the expression on the right side to be returned to the calling procedure. On the other hand, the name of the Sub procedure must not appear in any assignment statement.
3. To call a Sub procedure, you can either use the keyword "Call" or refer to its name. To call a Function procedure, you can only refer to its name but not by the keyword "Call." In addition, because the Function procedure returns a value, it is used as a part of an expression, whereas the Sub procedure is used as a statement (when referenced without the keyword "Call") or a part of a statement (when referenced with the keyword "Call").

Writing a Function Procedure. To illustrate the structure of a function, we can rewrite the MakeTwice Sub into a Function procedure called Twice as follows:

```
Private Function Twice(One As Double) as Double
    Twice = One + One
End Function
```

The function is named Twice and is declared to be a Double type because it is expected to return a value of this type. Inside the procedure, the parameter One is doubled and the result is assigned to Twice, the name of the Function procedure. This statement enables the function to return the value computed. If none of the statements inside a Function procedure assigns a value to the function name (in this case, Twice), the function will return a value of zero (or a zero-length string if the function is expected to return a string).

This function can then be used by other procedures as follows:

```
Two = Twice(10)
```

Or, assuming a proper declaration and assignment of value have been made for A,

```
MsgBox "Twice of " & A & " is " & Twice(A)
```

Note that just like the Sub procedure, the argument passed to the function does not have to be named "One" (the name used for the parameter) but can be any constant, variables, or expressions of the same type.

As another example, the previous Sub to compute the area of a circle can be rewritten as a function as follows:

```
Option Explicit
Const Pi As Double = 3.14159265359

Private Function AreaOfCircle(Radius As Double) As Double
  ' This function computes and returns the area of a circle
'given a radius, which is expected to be of the Double type
    AreaOfCircle = Pi * Radius * Radius
End Function
```

In this function, we only make the function compute and return the area but have omitted the code to display the result. This choice is by design, not by the restriction on a function.

Using a Function Procedure

From the preceding examples, you must have noticed that the way to use/invoke a function is by the reference of the Function procedure's name. Arguments passed to a function must be enclosed in a pair of parentheses. In addition, in contrast to the way to invoke Subs, the keyword "Call" is not used. Because the function is expected to return a value, the name of the function typically appears in an expression. That is, a function can be used exactly like a constant or a variable, in exactly the same way as built-in functions. But a Sub cannot be used in the same manner. Indeed, the only difference between a built-in function and a general function procedure is that the former is predefined (built-in) in the system, whereas you are the one to define the latter whenever you choose to use one.

Additional Notes on General Procedures

Function Versus Sub. Those examples in the discussion of Function procedures may make you wonder when you should create a Sub and when you should create a Function procedure. The key distinction between the two types of general procedures is that one returns a value, and the other does not. Thus, in general, when there is a need for the procedure to return a value, the procedure should be written as a function. This includes the following situations:

- When the value returned from a function will be used like a variable in an expression. Thus, all computational problems that obtain a result based on a list of parameters naturally fall in this category.
- When there is a need to determine whether the computations/actions performed by the procedure are successful. For example, the execution of the procedure may fail because of some external conditions (e.g., required files are missing or not available, an operation is canceled by the user). In such cases, the procedure can be written as a function and then returns an "execution code" (to indicate whether the execution was successful), which can be used by the calling procedure to determine the proper courses of actions.

If the procedure is not required to return any value but just to carry out some activities, it will be more appropriate to create this procedure as a Sub.

Naming the General Procedure. All names (e.g., for constants, variables, and objects) used in a project should be descriptive. Names for procedures are no exception. Because the Sub procedures will be more related to actions, it is advisable to use names that begin with a verb; for example, SaveCustRecord, DisplayAssetItem, and ClearScreen. The names for Function procedures are a bit trickier. Those functions for computational results usually are given the nomenclature of the values they return; for example, AreaOfCircle, CubeRoot, and GrossPay. Those functions used to carry out actions but expected to provide a return code usually are given names that begin with a verb, too. They can be easily confused with Subs. Fortunately, the confusion does not cause coding problems. When you do not need a return value from a function of this kind, you can use it as if it were a Sub by referencing the name without assigning the result to another variable. For example, you have a function CheckDate that returns a value True and displays an error message when a String parameter passed to it is not a valid date. The function appears as follows:

```
Function CheckDate(TheDate As String) As Boolean
'This function checks if a string contains a valid date
'in the mm/dd/yyyy format and
'returns a value True when the date is invalid
    If IsDate(TheDate) Then
        If Val(Left$(TheDate, 2)) <= 12 Then
        'This appears to be a valid date. Do nothing
        Exit Function 'Return to caller
        End If
    End If
    'Execution will reach here only if it fails the above test.
    'Display an error message and set the return code to True
    MsgBox "Must have a valid date to proceed."
    CheckDate = True
End Function
```

But suppose in your code, all you need is to display an error message if the string variable BirthDate is invalid. Its return code will not be used. You can still use the function just like a Sub as follows:

```
CheckDate BirthDate
```

The CheckDate Function. Perhaps some explanation of the code in the CheckDate function is in order. The function takes a string, TheDate, as its only parameter. It assumes that the date is in the mm/dd/yyyy format. In the procedure, it first uses the IsDate function to check whether the string appears to be a valid date. If so, it further checks to see whether the first two characters in the string are not greater than 12. This is necessary because IsDate accepts strings in several different date formats, including the dd/mm/yyyy format. Thus, the string "31/12/1999" will be considered valid, although it should be considered invalid in the CheckDate function. The second If statement in the function ensures that the month portion of the string is not greater than 12.

If a string passes both the IsDate and the second If tests, it should be a valid date. The ***Exit Function statement*** is executed. This statement works in a Function procedure exactly like Exit Sub in the Sub procedure. It will terminate the execution in the function. Execution control will be returned to the caller. No value is assigned to the function. Thus, the function returns a zero or False.

If the string fails either the IsDate or the second If test, it is considered invalid. The MsgBox function is used to display an error message. In addition, the CheckDate function is assigned a value True, indicating the string is not a valid date.

Documenting General Procedures. A procedure typically is written to perform a much more complex task than the examples illustrated previously. Therefore, it is important to document the procedure properly with remarks (comments) when it is being developed. These comments should include at least the following:

- The purposes of the procedure
- What is returned if the procedure is a function
- A description of the required parameters
- Assumptions made
- The algorithm used if the problem is fairly complex

All the examples given previously are coded with this in mind. If you did not notice the comments given at the beginning of each procedure, you may want to take another look now. Of course, additional comments pertinent to any code in the procedure should be added, just as you would typically do for an event procedure.

Recursion. All the VB procedures are recursive; that it, each procedure can call itself. This feature can be a powerful programming tool. A complex programming problem can be solved with an algorithm that recursively (repetitively) divides the problem into a smaller problem of the same nature until the latter is simple enough to solve.

A classical example of the use of recursion is the computation of n factorial (n!). When n is large enough, the computation calls for a fairly long series of computations. However, the problem can be subdivided into a problem of n (n − 1)! That is, if you are able to obtain the result of (n − 1)!, then all you have to do to obtain the result is to multiply n by the factorial of one less. Now, you can solve the problem of (n − 1)! in the same manner; that is, if you think of (n − 1) as n', then n'! can be solved with the same algorithm. Thus, this "divide-and-conquer" method can be continued until the n at hand is a value one (1). Then, there is no need to divide the problem any further. The result is 1. This value can then be returned to the previous level, which can then multiply, obtain the result, and return to yet another previous level. The process repeats until it reaches the original problem level. There the problem is solved.

The following table shows the process of arriving at the solution for 4! based on the description in the preceding paragraph.

Problem-Solving Description	Example	Solution Return Process	Solution
1. Original problem	4! ↓	10. Obtain result and return ↑	24
2. Divide the problem	4 × 3! ↓	9. Obtain result and return ↑	4 × 6

continues

Problem-Solving Description	Example	Solution Return Process	Solution
3. Divide the next problem 3!	3 × 2!	8. Obtain result and return	3 × 2
4. Divide the next problem 2!	2 × 1!	7. Obtain result and return	2 × 1
5. Solve the problem 1!	1	6. Return result to preceding level	1

Column 1 shows the solution process, and column 2 shows the numeric example based on the process. Column 3 shows how the result is obtained at each subsequent step and should be read from bottom to the top with its corresponding numeric results in column 4.

How can this process be implemented in VB? The following code provides the solution:

```
Private Function Factorial(N As Integer) As Long
' This function computes the value of N!
' where N is an integer
' Assumption: N is a number not to exceed 12
' Otherwise, overflow will result
    If N > 1 Then
        Factorial = N * Factorial (N - 1)
    Else
        Factorial = 1
    End If
End Function
```

This function literally implements the algorithm just described. When n is greater than 1, the function calls itself to find the result of the factorial of 1 less than the current n. The result returned from this call is then multiplied and returned to the caller (which can be itself). Only when n reaches a value not greater than 1, does the function consider the problem simple enough to find the solution (1) and return to the previous level.

The following table shows the execution process for an initial parameter value 4.

N	Function Call	Call Return (from Bottom to Top)
Initial call	Factorial (4)	24
4	4 * Factorial(3)	4 * 6
3	3 * Factorial(2)	3 * 2
2	2 * Factorial(1)	2 * 1
1	Return 1	1

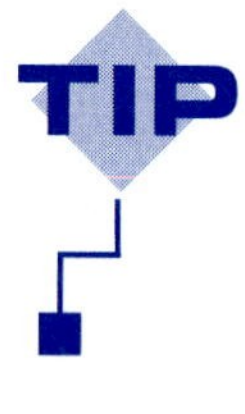

When writing a recursive procedure (Sub or Function), make sure it provides a way to terminate the recursion; that is, there is a way to exit the procedure without calling itself. One of the most commonly encountered problems with the recursive procedure is the "stack out of space" error at runtime. This occurs when the procedure calls itself too many times, causing the computer to run out of memory space used for internal stack.

Cascading an Event Procedure. Even the event procedure is recursive; that is, an event procedure can trigger the same event and invoke itself within itself. In general, recursion for event procedures occurs by "accident," not by design. They are written to handle events. Triggering an event to handle the event itself just does not make much sense. Thus, you should take care not to code an event procedure that causes recursion of itself. As an illustration of event cascading, consider the following code:

```
Private Sub txtNumber_Change()
    txtNumber.Text = 1 + Val(txtNumber.Text)
End Sub
```

The code is placed in the text box's ***Change event***, which occurs when the value of the text box changes. The programmer may think the code will increase the number entered by the user by 1. However, when you run the project and press a numeric key into the text box, you will encounter an "out of stack space" error. Why? Initially, the number entered by the user is increased by 1 and assigned to the Text property of the text box. This action causes a change in the text box and thus triggers another Change event, thus invoking the event procedure itself before the current event procedure ends. This process continues until the computer runs out of stack memory.

Actually, the code was placed in that event procedure because of the misunderstanding of the Change event, which occurs after *each* key is entered or after an assignment of data to the text box. If the intent was to increase the value in the text box by 1 after the field has been properly entered, the code should be placed in either the text box's Validate or LostFocus event when the user leaves the field.

If you encounter "out of stack space" error in your program, look for the possible source of recursion. If you use a recursive procedure, make sure it can exit without calling itself. If the error occurs in an event procedure, examine the code carefully. Look in particular at the left side of the assignment statements for the control name associated with the event. When you find one, check to ensure that the statement does not raise the same event.

Uses of General Procedures

Sometimes, you may wonder why go through all the trouble of creating general procedures. After all, you may end up with more lines of code. In addition, the calls and returns between procedures impose overhead in handling all the housekeeping tasks inside the computer, which can slow down the program. However, these drawbacks must be weighed against the advantages of creating and using these procedures. Here are some of their important advantages:

- They facilitate top-down and modular design. A huge, complex task can be broken down into smaller, manageable tasks, each written as a procedure. When designed this way, the "main" program is much easier to read. Its logic is much easier to trace. The programmer can focus on requirements of the main task at the beginning. He or she can then take care of the details of smaller tasks later. Several programmers can even work together on the same project, each taking care of some of the lower-level procedures. This is the advantage we cited at the beginning of the chapter.
- Problems can be isolated, making the program easier to understand, easier to debug, and easier to revise.
- Procedures can be made reusable. Carefully designed general (public) procedures can be called from any part of the project, eliminating the need to repeat similar code in different parts of the project. This not only reduces the size of the program but also simplifies the coding. Later, if the procedure needs to be revised or corrected, the programmer needs to focus on only one place (the procedure). Any change made to the procedure applies to all parts of the project that call the procedure, making it much easier (and more efficient and effective) to maintain the code.
- Function procedures can make code easier to understand. A function procedure returns a value that can be used just like a constant or variable in a formula. The meaning of the formula can be very clear to the developer and the reader/reviewer. The complexity of the computations is isolated from the main focus of the problem. This design of code will be much easier to review and understand than one that includes complex code to carry out the computations of a value before reaching the point of the formula mentioned previously.
- Recursion simplifies problem solving. Wherever a complex problem can be subdivided into simpler problems using the same algorithm, a recursive procedure can be developed. This makes the program much shorter and easier to code.

6.3 An Application Example

Let's create a project that will use some of the features you have learned in this chapter.

The Project

This program will be used to "maintain" a file that contains your friends' phone numbers and names. This file has been created as a comma-delimited file. Thus, it is easier to handle the file as a sequential file. As you recall, a sequential file can only be opened either for input or for output (or append) mode. This means that you cannot read and write the same file at the same time. Thus, when a sequential file needs to be updated (edit, add, or delete records), you will need to handle it as follows:

- Open (create) a new output file.
- Read the original file and let the user inspect the record one at a time.
  - If a record needs no correction, it can be copied (saved) to the new file "as is."
  - Otherwise, the user can make the change then save the record.
  - If a record needs to be deleted, the user will choose not to save it in the new file.
- To add a new record, the user enters the new data then save it.

For this project, in addition to these maintenance activities, the user can also choose to print a record on either the screen (a picture box) or the printer.

The User Interface

The form should contain the following:

- Data fields for the user to enter the phone number and name
  - These two fields can also be used to display the record read from the existing phone file. The field for the phone number is a masked edit box.
  - The field for the name is a text box.
- Five command buttons for the user to initiate actions to do the following:
  - Read a record from the existing file.
  - Save the record displayed on the fields (these can be either from the file or entered by the user).
  - Erase (clear) the fields so that the user can enter new data.
  - Quit.
  - Print either on the picture box (picOutput) or the printer.
- Two option buttons for the user to choose between the picture box (screen) and the printer when he or she chooses to print a record displayed in the data fields
- A picture box to serve as the area to print on the screen
- A common dialog box (named cdlFile) to prompt for file paths
- Two frames:
  - One to hold the data fields with their proper labels
  - Another to contain the option buttons and the Print button

The resulting visual interface appears as Figure 6.5.

The following table provides a list of controls along with selected properties referenced in the code.

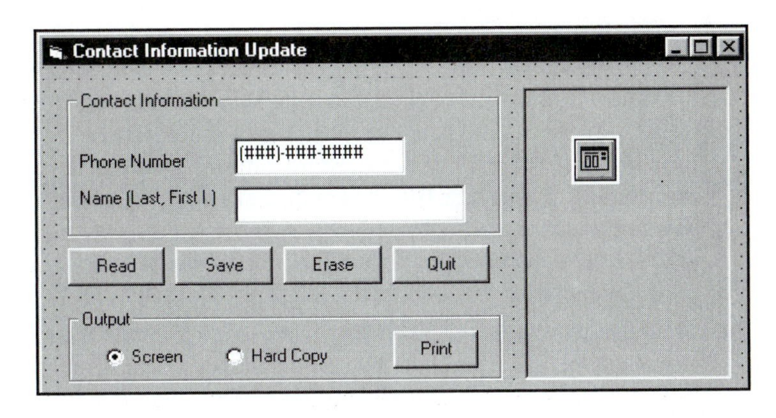

Figure 6.5
Visual Interface for the Phone Project

In this application, existing contact data are read from an old file when the Read button is clicked. Whatever appears on the "Contact Information" frame will be saved onto another file when the Save button is clicked. The user can also print the data by clicking the Print button with proper selection. A common dialog box is used to prompt for the file paths.

Control	Property	Setting	Remark
Common dialog	Name	cdlFile	To prompt for file location
Masked edit Box	Name	mskPhone	Phone field
	Mask	(###)-###-####	
Text box	Name	TxtName	Name field
Picture box	Name	picOutput	To display a record on screen
Command button	Name	cmdRead	To read a record
	Caption	Read	
Command button	Name	cmdSave	To save a record
	Caption	Save	
Command button	Name	cmdErase	To clear the screen
	Caption	Erase	
Command button	Name	cmdPrint	To print data on screen or printer
	Caption	Print	
Command button	Name	cmdQuit	To close file and quit
	Caption	Quit	
Option button	Name	optHardCopy	To select print on printer
Option button	Name	optScreen	To select print on the picture box
	Value	True	To serve as the default choice

The program should behave in the following manner:

- As soon as it starts, it should display a common dialog box to prompt the user for the phone file and again to prompt for the name to save the new file.
- When the user clicks the Read button, it reads a record from the existing file and places the record in the masked edit box and the text box. When the file runs out of records, the program displays a message to such an effect.
- When the user clicks the Save button, the data is saved on the new file, using the Write statement to create another comma-delimited file. After saving the record, the data fields on the screen are cleared.
- When the user clicks the Erase button, the data fields on the screen are cleared.
- When the Print button is clicked, whatever is on the data fields is printed onto the picture box or the printer, depending on which option button is selected.

Designing the Code Structure

If you inspect the program's requirements closely, several points should draw your attention:

- The common dialog box will be used twice to prompt for file paths: once for the input file and another time for the output file. Recall that it takes several lines of code for the dialog box to perform the ShowOpen method properly. However, most of the statements will be the same for both situations. This condition presents itself as a possibility to create a general procedure that can be called to handle both prompts. Should this procedure be a Sub or a function? Recall that the key difference between the two is in whether the procedure returns a value. It seems that requiring the procedure to return the filename will make the procedure more convenient to use. The programmer will not need to remember (or look for) the name of the common dialog box to obtain the result. Thus, the procedure should and will be coded as a function and will be called GetFileName.

- There are two situations in which "clear screen" is called for (when the data is saved and when the Erase command button is clicked). Again, creating a general procedure to handle the clearing will shorten the code. There is no need for the procedure to return a value. Thus, this procedure will be coded as a Sub and will be named ClearScreen.
- When the Print button is clicked, the data will be printed on either the screen (picture box) or the printer. The code will be the same for both. Only the objects to print are different. Here is another situation in which a general procedure can be used. Again, there is no need for the procedure to return a value. Thus, this procedure will be coded as a Sub and will be named PrintData.
- All other requirements can be implemented in the event procedures directly.

Given these considerations, we will create three general procedures and handle all other requirements in the event procedures.

Determining the Parameters for the General Procedures. The preceding discussion suggests that three general procedures should be created: ClearScreen, PrintData, and GetFileName. What parameters, if any, should each procedure have?

Obviously, the action to clear screen will be the same regardless of the situation that triggers the call. Thus, there will be no need for ClearScreen to require any parameters. In the case of printing the data, we know the source of the data will be the same. However, the target (object) to print can be different; it can be either the picture box or the printer. The procedure will need to know the specific object to perform the service properly. Thus, PrintData should require a parameter that allows the calling procedure to specify the object.

Finally, in determining the parameters for the GetFileName function, several factors should be considered:

- Because the common dialog box will be used to prompt for two different files, the user should be properly informed of which file the program is looking for. Recall that the common dialog has the DialogTitle property that can be used to specify the "title." The title can be used to display the prompt. The calling procedure should specify the "title" in order for this procedure to display the proper one. Thus, the "title" should be one of the parameters required by the procedure.
- What types of files should appear in the dialog box? Recall that the common dialog box has a Filter property by which you can specify the type of files to display in the dialog box. For this project, perhaps we can allow only the text file and hard-code the file filter in the procedure. However, if we would like the procedure to be more general, we should also allow different file filters to be specified. This means another required parameters should be the file filter.
- You should also consider the file's existence status. When the program is prompting for the existing phone file for input, it should expect that the file has already existed. On the other hand, when it prompts for the output file, if the file already exists, it should caution the user that the file will be written over. The two situations call for different Flags values. (Recall that the common dialog box has a Flags property that can be used to specify various responses to different conditions.) This should mean that the Flags should also be a parameter to the procedure.

Coding the Project

Based on the preceding discussion, we are now ready to write the code for the project. Let's consider the three general procedures first.

The GetFileName Function. This procedure should:

- Be a function, instead of a Sub.
- Take three parameters: one for the dialog title, another for the file filter, and the other for the flags.
- Thus, the header of the procedure should appear as follows:

```
Private Function GetFileName _
     (Title As String, Filter As String, Flags As Integer) _
       As String
```

Notice that the type of the function is declared to be "As String" because we expect the function to return a filename of the String type. The function is declared as a "Private" procedure because we do not expect it to be called by other forms or modules.

The calling procedure will then supply as its arguments: the dialog title (Title), the file filter (Filter) and the flags (Flags) when calling this function. Inside this function, the Title parameter can then be assigned to the dialog box's DialogTitle property; the Filter parameter, the Filter property; and the Flags parameter, the Flags property. The complete procedure then should appear as follows:

```
Private Function GetFileName _
     (Title As String, Filter As String, Flags As Integer) _
       As String
          On Error GoTo DoNothing
          cdlFile.CancelError = True
          cdlFile.DialogTitle = Title
          cdlFile.Flags = Flags
          cdlFile.Filter = Filter
          cdlFile.ShowOpen
          GetFileName = cdlFile.FileName
          Exit Function
DoNothing:
End Function
```

The detail working of most statements in this procedure has been explained in the first section. The way to use this procedure is further discussed under the heading "Coding the Event Procedures."

Notice the following statement:

```
GetFileName = cdlFile.FileName
```

This statement assigns the filename obtained by the dialog box from the ShowOpen method (the line above this statement) to the function. This statement will make the function return the filename to the calling procedure, as explained in the preceding section.

Note also the statement "Exit Function" below the assignment statement. Recall that the Exit statement will terminate the execution of the procedure. Its presence represents the logical end of this function. In this procedure, there is actually no other executable statements following this one. Therefore, leaving the line out will not affect the result. However, keeping it there will not harm anything either. If in the future some statements will need to be inserted below the statement label "DoNothing" to handle the error, the Exit function statement will be needed. The statement might just save you the potential problem with the "oversight" of failing to include it in the future.

The PrintData Procedure. As already explained, this procedure should take a parameter that specifies the object to print. Because this procedure is not expected to return anything to the caller, it will be written as a Sub. Its header then should appear as follows:

```
Private Sub PrintData(objToPrint As Object)
```

The complete procedure can appear as follows:

```
Sub PrintData(objToPrint As Object)
'This procedure assumes CurrentX and CurrentY of the object
'are pointing at the beginning of the line to print the data
    'Print phone number, stay on the same line
    objToPrint.Print mskPhone.Text;
    'Set print position at 40% of the width
    objToPrint.CurrentX = 0.4 * objToPrint.ScaleWidth
    'Print friend's name
    objToPrint.Print txtName.Text
End Sub
```

Notice the computation of the CurrentX property in the procedure. When the printing starts in an object (the picture box or the printer), the CurrentX and the CurrentY properties are set at the upper-left corner (0,0). As the content of mskPhone is printed, the CurrentX property will be set to the next printable position because the statement concludes with a semicolon (;). Assume that we would like to print the two fields as two columns with the name field starting at the beginning of 40% of the printable area of the object. The ScaleWidth property of the object gives the printable area. Thus, setting the object's CurrentX to 40% of that property will enable the next Print statement to begin at this position. The procedure does not set the CurrentY property. After the content of txtName is printed, the CurrentY property of the object will be pointing to the next line, (while CurrentX will be pointing again to the beginning of the line) ready for another line of new output.

Notice also that the parameter passed to the procedure can be different each time; that is, you can alternate printing between the screen and the printer. The CurrentX and CurrentY properties are associated with each individual object and will not interfere with the values of each other's.

The ClearScreen Procedure. The ClearScreen procedure clears the masked edit box and the text box. The code should be fairly straightforward. It should appear as follows:

```
Sub ClearScreen()
Dim Temp As String
    'See chapter 3 for an explanation of the following code
    'Clear the masked edit box
    Temp = mskPhone.Mask 'Save the mask
    mskPhone.Mask = "" 'Clear the mask
    mskPhone.Text = "" ' Clear the text
    mskPhone.Mask = Temp ' Restore the mask
    ' Clear the text box
    txtName.Text = ""
End Sub
```

Coding the Event Procedures

Recall that as soon as the project starts, the dialog box will prompt the user for the path of the input file and then for that of the output file. In addition, there are five command buttons to allow the user to initiate various activities.

Prompting for the File Paths. Because the program will prompt for the file paths as soon as the project starts, the code should be placed in the Form Load event. The prompt will involve calls to the GetFileName function, which requires three parameters, one of which is the file filter. As discussed, the expected file type should be the text file, whose file extension should be txt. Just in case the user might use a different file extension, we will also allow all other file extensions. The filter string should be just a constant for the purpose of this example. It is suggested that constants be declared at a broader scope so that other procedures can use the same. Thus, we will place the declaration of the filter string in the general declaration area:

```
Option Explicit
Const FileFilter As String = _
    "Text Files (*.txt)|*.txt|All Files (*.*)|*.*"
```

Once the file paths are obtained, the files should be opened. These files should remain open throughout the life of the project because the program will continue to read and write while the project is running. This consideration should also hint that the file numbers associated with the files should be recognized by all the event procedures dealing with the files. Thus, these variables should be declared as the form-level variables. On the other hand, filenames are needed only at the time they are to be opened. Recall that in general, all variables should be declared with a scope as narrow as possible. Thus, we will declare the filenames in the Form Load procedure, while declaring the file numbers in the general declaration area.

In summary, the general declaration area should contain the declaration of two variables and a constant as follows:

```
Option Explicit
Const FileFilter As String = _
    "Text Files (*.txt)¦*txt¦All Files (*.*)¦*.*"
Dim InFileNo As Integer
Dim OutFileNo As Integer
```

The *Form Load procedure* will declare the variables, prompt for the file paths, and open the files. It should appear as follows:

```
Private Sub Form_Load()
Dim InFileName As String
Dim OutFileName As String
    On Error GoTo Bye
'Prompt for the existing input file path
    InFileName = GetFileName("Where is the Phone File?", _
        FileFilter, cdlOFNFileMustExist)
'Prompt for the output file path
    OutFileName = GetFileName("Specify Filename to Save", _
      FileFilter, cdlOFNOverwritePrompt)
    'Open phone file to read
    InFileNo = FreeFile
    Open InFileName For Input As #InFileNo
    ' Open output file
    OutFileNo = FreeFile
    Open OutFileName For Output As #OutFileNo
    Exit Sub
Bye:
    MsgBox Err.Description 'Display the description of the error
    Unload Me
End Sub
```

Using the GetFileName Function. Notice how the GetFileName function is invoked. In the first case, to prompt for the existing input file, the constant literal "Where is the Phone File?" is passed as the Title parameter and the named constant cdlOFNFileMustExist is passed as the Flags parameter. This should make the function display a dialog title to prompt for the phone file. In addition, the Flags parameter should ensure that the user enters an existing filename. (For simplicity, the program assumes the phone file has already existed and takes no steps in creating a new one. Before testing this project, create a comma-delimited file with one phone number and name using Notepad.)

In the second case, to prompt for the output file path, the constant literal "Specify Filename to Save" is passed as the Title parameter so that the dialog box can display it to prompt for the output file. In addition, the named constant cdlOFNOverwritePrompt is passed as the Flags parameter to ensure that the user is cautioned if he or she specifies an output file that already exists because the file will be written over when it is opened.

The two files are then opened as InFileNo and OutFileNo, which are declared as form-level variables to be shared by other event procedures. In this event procedure, a simple error-handling routine is also implemented. Several things can go wrong in this procedure. For example:

- The user may click the Cancel button in response to the prompt for the file path. This will result in a zero-length string being returned as the filename, causing an invalid filename error when the procedure attempts to open the file.
- The user may specify the same filename for both input and output by mistake. This will cause a conflict in an attempt to open the file both for input and output.

The error handler that begins with the statement label Bye includes the following statement:

```
MsgBox Err.Description
```

This statement uses the ***Err object*** that is invoked when an error occurs in the program. The object contains several properties and methods. The Description property gives the description of the error, which you must have seen when an error occurs.

For simplicity, rather than attempting to correct the error, the procedure simply displays the error and quits. This is certainly not a user-friendly design, but our focus here is to illustrate how the various "parts" learned in this chapter can be put together. The perfection aspect is left to you as an exercise.

Reading the Phone File. When the user clicks the Read button, your program should read a record (i.e., the phone number and the name) and display the data on the masked edit and text box controls. If the file runs out of records, a message should be displayed and the execution for the procedure should be terminated with the Exit Sub statement. The code for the event procedure should appear as follows:

```
Private Sub cmdRead_Click()
Dim PhoneNo As String, Name As String
    If EOF(InFileNo) Then
        MsgBox "No more phone records."
        Exit Sub
    End If
    Input #InFileNo, PhoneNo, Name
    mskPhone.Text = Format$(PhoneNo, "(000)-000-0000")
    txtName.Text = Name
End Sub
```

Note that VB controls cannot be used as input fields in the Input statement. Thus, two variables (PhoneNo and Name) are declared and used for that purpose. Once data are read into the variables, they can be assigned to the controls' Text properties, as illustrated in the code.

On the Format String. Notice how the phone number is formatted. The masked edit box has the mask "(###)-###-####," as shown in the visual interface. You can actually use the Mask property as the format string for the phone number. However, if the phone number has fewer digits than the specified format, the resulting string will not fit the mask, producing an error. For example, if the actual number is 2223333, the resulting string will be "()-222-3333." On the other hand, the format string "(000)-000-0000" will force zeros to fill in the leading missing digits, resulting in a string, "(000)-222-3333," which will be acceptable to the masked edit box given the mask.

Saving the Data Fields. When the user clicks the Save button, the program is expected to save the data on screen onto the output file. The data can come from the Read operation either with or without the user's correction and from the user's direct entry into the data fields. A simple Write statement should take care of creating a record that is comma delimited. To be sure that there are data to be saved, the program should also check whether the name field is blank. In addition, after the record is saved, the data fields should be cleared by calling the ClearScreen procedure. The complete code for the event procedure appears as follows:

```
Private Sub cmdSave_Click()
'Create comma-delimited phone file
    If Len(Trim$(txtName.Text)) = 0 Then
        MsgBox "Please enter a valid name."
        Exit Sub
    End If
    Write #OutFileNo, mskPhone.ClipText, txtName.Text
    ClearScreen
End Sub
```

Notice that the masked edit box's ClipText property (not the Text property) is saved. This property strips the mask's literal (parentheses and dashes) from the text string so that only the digits entered by the user are saved.

Erasing the Data Fields. The user can choose to erase the data fields when he or she sees no need to preserve the record. He or she can then proceed to read another record or enter his or her own data. The event procedure can be easily taken care of by a call to the ClearScreen Sub as shown next:

```
Private Sub cmdErase_Click()
    ClearScreen
End Sub
```

Printing Data on Screen or Printer. When the user clicks the Print button in the output frame, the program should determine where the output should be directed: the screen (the picture box) or the printer. You can identify the object to print by testing the value of one of the option buttons. To simplify the testing process, the Value property of one of the option buttons should be set to True at design time (optScreen has been set to True as you can determine from the user interface presented earlier). The complete code of the event procedure is as follows:

```
Private Sub cmdPrint_Click()
     If optHardCopy Then
          PrintData Printer
     Else
          PrintData picOutput
     End If
End Sub
```

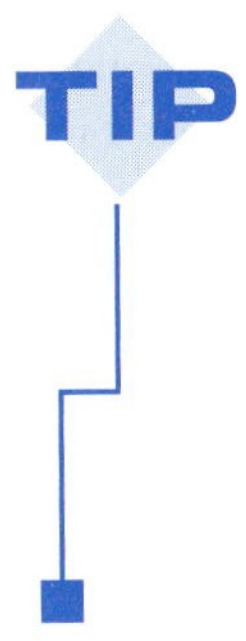

Beware of the syntax difference between the following two statements:

```
PrintData picOutput   'This is correct
PrintData (picOutput) 'This is wrong
```

The first line will execute without any problem. The second line will result in a *type mismatch error.* Why? The extra pair of parentheses enclosing the object makes VB think that it is an expression. Therefore, it attempts to convert picOutput to a value and decides it cannot. The other correct way to call the Sub procedure is as follows:

```
Call PrintData(picOutput) 'Another right way to call
```

Terminating the Program. Finally, terminating the program is a simple procedure that should close all open files and unload the form. A Close statement without specifying the file number(s) will close all open files. Actually, when the project ends, all open files will automatically be closed. However, it is a good practice to explicitly close these files. Thus, the event procedure appears as follows:

```
Private Sub cmdQuit_Click()
     Close
     Unload Me
End Sub
```

Additional Remarks

The preceding procedures should complete the requirements for the project. Before leaving it, keep in mind that this example is presented only for the purpose of illustrating how the various "parts" you have learned in this chapter can be pieced together. Please note the following points in particular:

- This program assumes that the phone file has already existed. Thus, to test the code for this example, you should create a comma-delimited file first, perhaps with

Notepad. The phone number should be the first field; and the name (enclosed in double quotes), the second field of each record (line).

- When you work with the program as the user, you should feel very nervous about the accuracy of the results. For example, if you repetitively click the Read button, the program will continue to read the records from the existing file. There is no warning that the previous record has not yet been saved. Also, the records in the old file that have not been read before the program quits will not be saved. All these situations can certainly cause the new file to miss records that should have been kept. The needed refinements to guard against potential losses of data are left to you as an exercise.
- In general, we would rather have a way to update/edit a record "randomly"; that is, we would rather have the ability to recall a record for edit at our random choice instead of having the program dictate the sequence in which records are retrieved. The approach used in the example will take too long and cost a lot of unnecessary effort and attention (plus potential errors) of the user. A better approach would be to structure the file so that it is capable of being randomly accessed or to save the records in a database table. In either case, a record can be retrieved and updated directly. New records can also be added to the file (database table) without any need to deal with the existing records. Databases are discussed in Chapter 10. The use of random files is discussed in Appendix A.
- Despite the shortcomings of the example project just noted, you should be able to appreciate the reasons for creating those general (separate) procedures and the design for the parameter(s) called for by each procedure. In addition, you should also notice the contexts in which various statements such as Exit Sub can be used.

Summary

This chapter introduces you to input, output, and general procedures. Sequential files are discussed among MsgBox, common dialog control, and the Print method for various VB objects. Then, the need and desirability for general procedures are presented. Various issues such as passing data among procedures and naming procedures are explored. Finally, an example is provided to illustrate how the various VB features you have learned in this chapter can be used in a project. We note that the design presented in the example has several shortcomings. However, you should note that the reasons for the creation of general procedures and design for their parameters are sound, and you should study the topics carefully.

Although the example does not show the usefulness of sequential files, it does not follow that sequential files are not useful. Text files that abound in all computer systems generally are handled as sequential files. In addition, text (sequential) files are also used as a means of exchanging data between different software systems using the importing or exporting protocol. Usually, these files are created as comma-delimited files. Finally, studying sequential files lays a good foundation for an understanding of other file modes as well as databases.

Visual Basic Explorer

6-1. Default Button for the MsgBox Function. Enter the following code in a new project:

```
Private Sub Form_Click()
Dim Answer As Integer
    Answer = MsgBox("Cannot find the file. Proceed?", _
        vbYesNoCancel + vbQuestion)
    Debug.Print Answer
End Sub
```

Run the project and click the form. What do you see the message box display as the default button? Press the spacebar. What value do you see in the immediate window?

Revise the MsgBox statement as follows:

```
Answer = MsgBox("Cannot find the file. Proceed?", _
    vbYesNoCancel + vbQuestion + vbDefaultButton2)
```

Run the project again and click the form. What do you see the message box display as the default button? Press the spacebar. What value do you see in the immediate window this time?

6-2. Help Button for the MsgBox Function. Add another value to the second parameter in the preceding exercise such that the message box will display a Help button. (*Hint:* Find the named constant from the online Help file using "MsgBox Function" as the search keyword in the Index tab.)

6-3. What is App.Path? VB provides an object App that contains several properties and methods for your application (project). One of its properties is Path. Try the following code:

```
Private Sub Form_Click()
    Debug.Print App.Path
    Debug.Print CurDir
End Sub
```

Run the project and click the form. What do you see in the immediate window? App.Path is the folder where your project file (vbp) (or your compiled program) is located, and CurDir is the current folder that the system is pointing to. To set the App.Path as your current directory, you can use the following command:

```
ChDir App.Path
```

6-4. Append Versus Output Mode. Draw two command buttons on a new form. Name the first one cmdAppend and set its Caption property to "Append." Name the second one cmdOutput and set its Caption property to "Output."

```
Option Explicit

Private Sub cmdAppend_Click()
Dim TestFile As Integer
     TestFile = FreeFile
     Open "C:\Temp\TestFile.txt" For Append As #TestFile
     Print #TestFile, "ABCD"
     Close TestFile
End Sub

Private Sub cmdOutput_Click()
Dim TestFile As Integer
     TestFile = FreeFile
     Open "C:\Temp\TestFile.txt" For Output As #TestFile
     Print #TestFile, "ABCD"
     Close TestFile
End Sub
```

Note that the only difference between the two procedures is the mode for the file (Append versus Output). Note also that to test this project, you need to have a Temp folder in Drive C. Change the path to some other folder if you do not wish to create a Temp folder.

Run the project. Click the Append button. Then use Notepad to inspect the file. Each time you click the Append button, you should see one more line of "ABCD" when you reopen the file from Notepad.

Click the Output button. Then inspect the file again. What do you see? Click as many times as you wish. You should always see only one line of "ABCD" in the file. The Output mode erases the previous content of the file, whereas the Append mode appends data at the end of the existing file.

6-5. Printing Text in the Picture Box. Draw a picture box in a new form. Make the picture box's size and shape look like a check. Name it picCheck. Set its Picture property to Check.wmf. The file is available in the following folder:

Microsoft Visual Studio\Common\Graphics\Metafile\Business

Also set the picture box's font size to 18 and font style to Italic. Then enter the following code:

```
Private Sub picCheck_Click()
    picCheck.CurrentX = (picCheck.Width - _
      picCheck.TextWidth("Cancelled!")) / 2
    picCheck.CurrentY = _
      (picCheck.Height - picCheck.TextHeight("C")) / 2
    picCheck.Print "Cancelled!"
End Sub
```

Run the project and click the check. Can you print any text on a picture? What do you conclude?

6-6. The ShowPrinter Method of the Common Dialog Box. The common dialog box has several methods. One of these is the ShowPrinter method. To see how it works, add a common dialog control to a new project and then draw it on the form. Name it cdlPrint. Also draw a command button on the form. Set its Caption property to "Print" and name it cmdPrint. Type in the following code:

```
Private Sub cmdPrint_Click()
    cdlPrint.ShowPrinter
    Printer.Print "Test"
    Printer.EndDoc
End Sub
```

Run the project and click the button. Set the number of copies in the dialog box to 2 and then click the OK button. How many pages of hard copies do you get? This control makes your job in programming the printer easy, doesn't it?

6-7. The InputBox Function. Draw a text box onto a new form. Enter the following code:

```
Private Sub Form_Click()
    Text1.Text = InputBox("What is your name?", _
      "Name Prompt", "Debbra Solomon")
End Sub
```

Run the project. Click the form and inspect carefully the dialog box that shows up on the screen. Can you associate the code with the text in the dialog box? After you click the form, do the following (one each time) and inspect the result in the text box:

A. Click the OK button.

B. Press the Enter key.

C. Click the Cancel button.

D. Enter your name in the box then click the OK button.

E. Enter your name in the box then click the Cancel button.

Have you got a good feel about how the InputBox function behaves? This function allows the program to obtain data from the user "on the fly" and can be used conveniently to test your program logic under certain circumstances. However, it cannot be used in a serious data-entry application because it pops up only when called and input from the function can be verified only afterward (not while the data is being typed in). Therefore, it is not further discussed in the text.

6-8. Relationship of Argument and Parameter. Use two command buttons. Name One cmdTestA and the other cmdTestB. Set their Caption properties to "Test A" and "Test B," respectively. Enter the code that follows. Run the program. Click each command button. What message do you see? You should see that there are two different syntactical expressions to call a Sub procedure. Also, how are A and B related to C in this illustration?

```
Sub Messenger(C As Integer)
    MsgBox "I get a value " & C
End Sub

Private Sub cmdTestA_Click()
Dim A As Integer
```

```
    A = 100
    Call Messenger(A)
End Sub
Private Sub cmdTestB_Click()
Dim B As Integer
    B = 120
    Messenger B
End Sub
```

6-9. Positions of Arguments and Parameters. Use a command button. Name it cmdTest. Set its Caption property to "Test." In its Click event procedure and a separate Sub procedure named Divider, give the code as follows:

```
Option Explicit
Sub Divider(A As Single, B As Single)
    MsgBox "The quotient is " & A / B
End Sub
Private Sub cmdTest_Click()
Dim A As Single
Dim B As Single
    A = 4
    B = 2
    Divider B, A
End Sub
```

Click the command button. Is there anything puzzling to you? Recall that arguments passed to a Sub procedure are recognized by their positions, not by their names. What is recognized in the event procedure as A is recognized as B in Divider. It's the position, not the name, of the variable in the argument list that matters.

6-10. Passing by Name. (continued from 6-9). If you pass the arguments without referencing the names of the parameters, they are recognized by position, as shown in the preceding exercise. However, as explained in the text, there is a way you can pass the arguments by the parameter names. For example, without any change to the Divider Sub in the preceding exercise, you can rewrite the Test command Click event procedure as follows:

```
Private Sub cmdTest_Click()
Dim A As Single
Dim B As Single
    A = 4
    B = 2
    Divider B := B, A := A
End Sub
```

Run the program and click the command button. Do you see the correct result? Inspect the syntax carefully. The ":=" symbol is used to indicate the parameter assignment. The name on the left side of the ":=" symbol is the parameter name. The name on its right is the argument.

Replace the line in the event procedure to call Divider as follows:

```
    Divider B := 2, A := 4
```

Run the project again. Do you still obtain the correct result?

When you use this syntax, the positions of the parameters no long matter. They are recognized by name. Can you think of situations in which the use of named parameters is more convenient?

6-11. Optional Parameters. VB provides a way to write procedures that require optional parameters. For example, suppose you are interested in a function that will return the largest value from a list of two or three arguments. You can code the function as follows:

```
Function Biggest(X1 As Variant, X2 As Variant, _
Optional X3 As Variant) As Variant
```

```
Dim X As Variant
    If X1 >= X2 Then
        X = X1
    Else
        X = X2
    End If
    If IsMissing(X3) Then
    ElseIf X3 > X Then
        X = X3
    End If
    Biggest = X
End Function
```

Note that the third parameter starts with the keyword "Optional," which denotes that the parameter can be omitted. To check whether it is present (passed from the calling procedure), you use the ***IsMissing function***, which returns True if the parameter is missing; otherwise, False.

Try the preceding code with the following event procedure:

```
Private Sub Form_Click()
    Print Biggest(12, 34, 53)
    Print Biggest("A", "c")
End Sub
```

Are there other situations in which optional parameters can be useful?

6-12. Effect of ByVal and ByRef. Draw a command button on a new form. Name it cmdTest. Set its Caption property to "Test." In its Click event procedure and a separate Sub procedure named Setter, give the following code.

```
Option Explicit

Sub Setter(ByVal C As Integer, ByRef D As Integer)
    C = 10
    D = 10
End Sub

Private Sub cmdTest_Click()
Dim A As Integer
Dim B As Integer
    Setter A, B
    MsgBox "After setting the values, A = " & A _
      & "and B = " & B
End Sub
```

Click the command button. Why don't you get the same result for A and B? Recall that a ByVal parameter uses a copy of the value of the argument. Any change to that parameter will not cause a corresponding change to the argument passed to the Sub procedure.

6-13. Expressions as Arguments. (Continued from 6-12). Suppose the previous Setter procedure is revised as follows:

```
Option Explicit

Sub Setter(ByRef C As Integer, ByRef D As Integer)
    C = 10
    D = 10
End Sub
```

Thus, the parameters will be passed by reference, by default. However, you code the calling event procedure as follows:

```
Private Sub cmdTest_Click()
Dim A As Integer
Dim B As Integer
    Setter (A), (B)
    MsgBox "After setting the values, A = " & A & _
      "and B = " & B
End Sub
```

What results do you obtain when you test the program? Why are A and B's values not set to 10? The pairs of parentheses enclosing the variables make each argument an expression, not the original variable. Expressions are passed to procedures by value, not by reference, no matter how the parameters are declared in the header of the procedure.

Exercises

6-14. **Using the MsgBox Function.** Add the masked edit box control to your project. Draw a masked edit box and a command button on the form. Name the masked edit box mskPhone and set its Mask property to "(###)-###-####." Also set its Prompt Character property to a blank space. Set the command button's Caption property to "Save" and name it cmdSave.

Provide code so that when the button is clicked, your program will check whether the user has entered a 10-digit number. If not, your program should display a message (use the MsgBox function) indicating that the phone number field is incomplete and ask the user whether it is okay to save. If the user clicks the No button, the Save procedure is exited, returning the focus to the masked edit box. When the masked edit box has a legitimate number or when the user indicates that it is okay to save, the program displays a message stating that the record has been saved. (Do not provide code to actually save the record.)

6-15. **Avoiding Errors in Opening Files.** Refer to the Form Load event procedure in the PhoneBook example in Section 6.3. Modify the procedure so that the errors are handled as follows:

A. When the user clicks the Cancel button when prompted for a filename either for input or for output, your code should indicate no filename has been specified and ask the user to specify the filename again. If no filename is specified, your program will quit.

B. When the user specifies the same filename for output as for input, your code should ask the user to specify another filename. If the user specifies the same filename again, your program will display a message and quit.

6-16. **Ensuring Data Are Saved.** (continued from 6-15). Add code to the PhoneBook example in Section 6.3 so that when the Read button is clicked, your program will check whether the name field has any data. If so, your program will display a message box asking the user whether to save the data before reading another record. The message box should display three buttons: Yes, No, and Cancel. If the user clicks the Yes button, your program should save the data fields before reading in another record. If the user clicks the No button, your program should proceed to read another record. If the Cancel button is clicked, your program should neither save the record nor read another record.

6-17. **Ensuring Data Are Saved** (continued from 6-16). Refer to the PhoneBook example in Section 6.3 again. Add code to the project so that the remaining records in the original file can be saved when the user wants to quit. The additional code should work as follows:

A. When the user clicks either the Quit button or the close (x) button, the program checks to see whether the original file contains any unread data. If not, the program quits; otherwise, the program proceeds to step B.

B. Displays a message (use the MsgBox function) warning the user of the unread/unsaved data and asks the user whether the data should be copied into the new file. The MsgBox function should display a Question icon with three buttons: Yes, No, and Cancel.

C. If the Yes button is clicked, your code will copy the remaining records in the old file to the new one and quit. If the No button is clicked, your program quits. If the Cancel button is clicked, your program does not quit. (*Hint:* Place your code in the Form Unload event.)

6-18. Print/Display a Number in an Object for a Specified Length. Write a Sub procedure with the following header to print or display a number in the specified object:

```
Private Sub PrintNumber(Number As Variant, _
    Obj As Object, Length as Integer)
```

Where *Number* can be any numeric type; *Obj* is the object in which the number is to be printed; and *Length* is the width (in number of characters) the number should be printed (right-justified). Use the standard numeric format for the output. Can you enumerate the situations in which such a routine can be useful? (Note that the function as specified works well only with monospace fonts.)

6-19. Print/Display a Centered Heading in an Object. Write a Sub procedure to print a string at the centered position on the current line in an object. The Sub should have the following header:

```
Sub PrintCentered(Text As String, Obj As Object)
```

Can you enumerate the situations in which such a routine can be useful?

6-20. Print/Display a String in a Specific Column. Write a Sub with the following header:

```
Sub PrintInCol(Text As String, Obj As Object, _
    Col As Integer, Cols As Integer)
```

Where *Text* is the string to be printed; *Obj* is the object in which the text should be printed; *Cols* is number of equal width columns the object should print; *Col* is the specific column the string should be printed (0 = the first column). Can you enumerate the situations in which such a routine can be useful?

6-21. Save a Record (Screen). Suppose that a form has a masked edit box and two text boxes. They are named mskSSN, txtLastName, and txtFirstName, respectively. You would like for the data entered to be saved as a record in fixed-length format (one record per line); that is, data in each field are to have the same length (pad with blank spaces if necessary). The lengths for the fields should be 9, 12, and 12, respectively. Write a Sub to save data entered. Use the Print statement to save the data in a file named Employees.

From what event procedure should the Save Record procedure be called? Is there a reason why the Save routine should be written as a separate procedure?

6-22. Read and Display a Record. Write a general Sub procedure to read the data saved in the preceding exercise and display the results in the three VB controls.

From what event procedure should the Read Record procedure be called? Is there a reason why the Read routine should be written as a separate procedure?

6-23. The Missing Data Function. Write a function to return a Boolean value True if the text string passed to this function contains only blank spaces or zero length. (Otherwise, the function returns False.) Name the function Missing. Its header should appear as follows:

```
Function Missing(Text As String) As Boolean
```

6-24. Write a Function That Will Return a Random Uppercase Letter. Test the function as follows:

1. Draw a text box (with proper label) and command button on a new form.
2. Name the command button cmdGenerate.
3. Provide the code so that when the user clicks the button, the function is called and the letter it generates is displayed in the text box.

6-25. The Month End Function. Write a Function that will take the month and year as its parameter and will return a string that represents the last day of that month; for example,

MonthEnd(2, 1996) will return the string "02/29/1996." (*Hint:* Use the DateAdd function. Keep in mind that the last day of January is always 31. Add the proper number of months to that date. Or, use the DateSerial function. The last day of a month is 1 day before the first day of the next month.)

6-26. The Julian Date Function. Write a function that will return a Julian date given a valid date string such as "01/01/1999." A Julian date is a date represented by a five-digit number whose first two digits represent the year and the last three digits give the sequence number of the day in the year. For example, the Julian date for "01/01/1999" is 99001. (*Note:* Given the problem with Y2K, do you expect the Julian date to be very popular?)

6-27. The GetFileName Function. Assume your form has a common dialog control named cdlFile. Write a function that will use this control to prompt the user for the filename. The function should have the following header:

```
Function GetFileName(ForWhat As String, Filter As String) _
    As String
```

The parameter ForWhat expects an "O" (for ShowOpen) or "S" (for ShowSave). The parameter Filter expects a string specifying the file filter, as explained in the chapter. Set the Flags in the function such that when "O" is specified, the dialog box will insist that the file must exist; and when "S" is specified, the user will be warned if the file already exists.

The function will return the filename (a string) specified by the user in the dialog box. If the user clicks the Cancel button in the common dialog box, the function should return a zero-length string.

6-28. The Grade Function. Write a function that will return a letter grade. The function expects an integer parameter that represents the score. The grading system is based on the typical 90, 80, 70, etc., cut-off criteria.

6-29. The Present Value of an Annuity Function. The present value of the annuity of one dollar ($1), P, can be computed by the following formula:

$$P = (1 - (1 + R)^{-n}) / R$$

Where *R* is the rate of interest per period and *N* is the number of periods.

Write a function with the following header to perform the computation:

```
Function PresentValue(R As Double, N As Integer) As Double
```

Compare the results obtained from this function with the results from using the built-in NPV function. (Use the keyword "NPV function" to search the Index tab of the online Help file for additional information on how to use the function.)

6-30. Recursive Function. Write a recursive function to compute the following series:

$$S = 1 + 2 + 3 + \ldots + N$$

The function should have the following header:

```
Function Series(N As Integer) As Long
```

(*Hint:* Rewrite the formula as follows:

$$S = N + (N - 1) + (N - 2) + \ldots + 2 + 1)$$

6-31. Recursive Function. Write a recursive function to approximate the following infinite series:

$$S = B + B / D + B / D^2 + B / D^3 + \ldots$$

Where *D* is greater than 1.

The function should have the following header:

```
Function Series(B As Double, D As Double) As Double
```

(*Hint:* Rewrite the formula as follows:

$S = B + (B + (B / D + (B / D^2 + . . .))) / D$

That is, the series can be evaluated by the beginning value (B) plus the series that begins with the current beginning value divided by D. Terminate the function when B/D is very small (say, .1E-10).

Projects

6-32. Revisiting the FICA Computation Project. Refer to 5-33. Modify the FICA withholding computation project so that the previous data come from an existing file and the resulting year-to-date (y-t-d) data are saved onto a new file.

The existing file contains the y-t-d data on all employees who have been paid previously. Each record consists of employee Social Security number (SSN), employee name, y-t-d pay, and FICA withholding. A sample record from the data file appears as follows:

"111-11-1111", "John Smith", 10000, 465

Your program should have command buttons to Read, Compute, Save, and Quit. These buttons should align across the top of the form. You should add controls to display the employee SSN and name in the form, while all other data fields in your visual interface remain the same.

Your project should behave in the following manner:

A. When the project starts, it should prompt for the existing (y-t-d) file and the file to which updated data will be saved. To simplify your code, create an empty y-t-d file using Notepad for the first round before testing your program.

B. When the user clicks the Read button, your program will read a record from the existing file. (If the file runs out of records, your program should display a message to that effect.) The pay data will be displayed in the frame for the previous period, and the employee SSN and name should be displayed in the proper controls. Before your program proceeds to read, it should check to see whether the data in the current screen have been saved. If not, it should prompt the user whether to save and should save the data if so instructed. (See D for instruction on what to save.)

C. The user should enter current pay in the frame for current data then click the Compute button. Your program will then display the results in the proper fields as described in 5-33.

D. When the user clicks the Save button, the data in the frame for cumulative total should be saved in the same format as the previous sample record. All fields on the form should then be cleared.

E. Data on new employees can be entered when all the fields are cleared. The user should enter the employee SSN, name, and current pay; click the Compute button; and then click the Save button. (This is what you should do to create an existing y-t-d file for the first round.)

F. When the user clicks the Quit button or the Close button on the title bar, your program should check whether the existing file has any unread data. If so, it should copy all these records to the new file and display a message informing the user of this action.

(*Note:* This project emulates a sequential file processing system although it is very much simplified.)

6-33. A Mini Word Processor. Develop a project that will provide the following word processing capabilities: opening a file; allowing the user to edit, search, and replace text; and saving text onto a file. The user interface should have command buttons for Open, Search, Save, and Quit across the top of the form; a text box for text editing and processing at the center of the form; and a frame for search and replace. The frame should be placed below the text box and should contain a text box for search text, another text box for replace text, a command button with a "Find Next" caption, another with a "Replace" caption, and the other with an "OK" caption. The text boxes in the search frame should be accompanied with proper labels.

The application should behave as follows:

1. When the project starts, all the buttons across the top of the form and the text box (txtDoc) for word processing should appear. The form should have space enough to show all these controls. (The aforementioned frame is not visible. In addition, there is no space in the form to hint its existence.) The user can start entering and editing text, or he or she can click the Open button to bring text from an existing file. (*Hint:* Set the frame's Visible property to False. Compute the Form's Height property using the Top and Height properties of txtDoc.)
2. When the user clicks the Open button, a common dialog box should appear to prompt for an existing file. (*Hint:* Use the proper Flags property.) Then the data should be retrieved and displayed in the text box. Note that before your program retrieves data from an existing file, if the text box contains text and has been changed, your program should prompt the user whether to save the change. (*Hint:* Use a form-level variable to keep track of the change. Set it to False when the file is first open or when the text is saved. Then set it to True when the text changes.)
3. When the user clicks the Save button or when the user indicates to save in requirement 2, your program should prompt for an output file path. The text will then be saved in the specified file path.
4. When the user clicks the Search button, the frame for Search and Replace will appear below txtDoc. (*Hint:* Compute the form's Height property using the Frame's Top and Height property.) Once the frame appears:
   A. When the user clicks the Find Next button, your program will search the text in txtDoc for the text specified in the Search text box. If a match is found, it will be highlighted; otherwise, the program displays an error message.
   B. When the user clicks the Replace button, whatever appears in the Replace text box will replace the highlighted text in txtDoc. (*Hint:* See 4-10 for hint for replacing text.)
   C. When the user clicks the OK button, the frame disappears and the form goes back to its previous size.
   D. When the user clicks the Quit button, the program should check to ensure that the changes in the text have been saved. If not, it should prompt the user whether to save. If so, handle the saving operation as specified in requirement 3.

7 Repetition

One of the most powerful features of the computer is its ability to execute a group of instructions repetitively while the data handled by these instructions change. With this capability, many tasks that are repetitive in nature can be handled with much shorter code and a lot of flexibility. Imagine a payroll routine that computes for each employee the gross pay, various deductions, and the net pay. The steps to handle each employee's pay are basically the same. Only the data (the employee and the pay) in question change. Without the capability to execute the group of instructions repetitively, the same code will have to be "repeated" for each employee. The length of code will be sizable to say the least. Worse yet, the number of repetitions in code (which vary with the number of employees to be paid) will have to be known beforehand. Each time the number of employees changes, the program will have to be modified, an extremely tedious task.

Many of the problems (much more than we can imagine) handled by the computer are repetitive in nature. Just to list a few, populating a list box or combo box, reversing a string, computing the square root of a number (indeed searching for the root of any function in general), and listing the content of a file (e.g., customers), all require repeating a selected group of instructions.

In VB, there are two structures by which you can construct code for repetition: the Do...Loop structure and the For...Next structure. In each of these structures, the repetition starts with a keyword (Do or For) in an opening statement and ends with another keyword (Loop or Next) in the closing statement. Statements enclosed physically inside the two statements are repeated until a certain condition is satisfied. Because the execution of the group of statements starts from the opening statement top down, ends at the closing statement, and starts over again from the opening statement, the repetition looks like a loop and is commonly so referenced. This chapter provides detailed discussions of these two loop structures.

After completing this chapter, you should be able to:

- Understand all variations of the Do...Loop structure.
- Develop code that calls for the use of the Do...Loop structure with all variations.
- Understand the For...Next structure with different values and signs of the increment parameter.
- Develop code that requires the use of the For...Next structure.
- Understand and develop code that calls for the use of nested loop structures.

7.1 The Do...Loop Structure

You can construct the Do...Loop structure with either of the following syntax:

```
Do [{While¦Until} condition]
     Statements to be repeated
Loop
```

or

```
Do
     Statements to be repeated
Loop [{While¦Until} condition]
```

where *condition* = any expression that can be evaluated to True or False; any expression that can be used in an If statement can be used here

While = the keyword that will make the loop continue as long as the condition is true

Until = the keyword that will make the loop continue as long as the condition is false

When the loop ends, the execution continues to the line below the Loop statement. The following examples illustrate how the various variations of the Do...Loop structure work.

Example 1. Showing a Sequence of Numbers

You would like to know the sequence of numbers in the range of 1 and 1,000, which are successively doubled beginning with 1. To solve the problem, you can do the following:

1. Create a variable (e.g., N) and assign it with a value 1.
2. Print N.
3. Double N.
4. Compare N with 1,000. If N is less then 1,000, repeat steps 2 and 3; Otherwise, end the process.

A flowchart that depicts the process is presented in Figure 7.1.

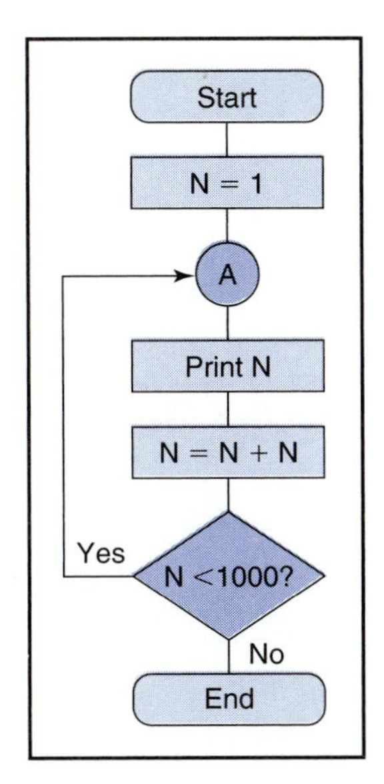

Figure 7.1
A Flowchart to Print a Sequence of Numbers

The flowchart gives a visual hint that the connector (A) and the decision (N <1,000) form a loop. Thus, the routine can look like the following:

```
Private Sub Form_Click()
Dim N As Integer
```

```
        N = 1
        Do
            Print N
            N = N + N
        Loop while N < 1000
    End Sub
```

Before the loop is executed, N is set to 1. Within the loop, the value N is printed (on the form). Then N is added by itself, doubling its value in effect. When the loop reaches the end (the Loop statement), N is compared with 1,000. The While condition states that if N is less than 1,000, the repetition continues. The execution transfers back to the beginning of the loop (the Do statement). The two statements inside the loop will be executed again. This cycle continues until N is greater than or equal to 1,000, then the While condition is no longer true. Thus, the execution control goes to the statement immediately below the Loop statement. In this case, the End Sub statement is reached and the Form Click event procedure ends.

The process can be depicted with the following execution table.

Iteration No.	N (Printed)	N (After doubling)
1	1	2
2	2	4
3	4	8
4	8	16
.	.	.
10	512	1024

Notice that the Loop While statement can be rewritten with the Until keyword as follows:

```
Loop Until N >= 1000
```

Replacing this statement for the preceding Loop While line will have exactly the same result as the original routine. (Try both ways. The last number you should see on the form is 512.)

Example 2. Reading a Name List and Populating a List Box

Suppose you have created a list of names (one name per line) and kept it in a file located at "c:\friends\namelist.txt." The content of the file appears as follows:

Andrea Aaron

Ben Bennett

.

.

Zeff Zenor

You would like to populate the list box (named lstNames) with these names as soon as your program starts. To do this, you must open the file first. Then your program should do the following:

1. Read a name from the file.
2. Add the name to the list box using the AddItem method.
3. Repeat steps 1 and 2 until the file runs out of names (reaches the end of file).

Assume the file number is NameFile and the list box name is lstNames. Then, the "first approximation" of the repetition should appear as follows:

```
Do
    Line Input #NameFile, TheName 'Read a name
    lstNames.AddItem TheName 'Add the name to the list box
Loop Until EOF(NameFile)
```

In this structure, when the loop is executed, the computer will read the name from the file and add it to the list box before the execution reaches the Loop statement, where the EOF condition is tested. Recall that when reading a sequential file, the EOF function returns a value of True when the end of the file is reached; otherwise, it returns a value of False. Because the Loop statement uses the keyword "Until," the loop will continue when the EOF condition is False.

Dealing with an Empty File. As long as there is at least one name in the file, the preceding code structure will perform properly without any error. However, if the file happens to be empty, this structure will have a problem. When it attempts to read the name the first time, the EOF condition is encountered and an error occurs. The program will fail.

To guard against this possibility, the EOF condition should be tested at the beginning of the loop; that is, the condition should be placed in the Do statement. If the file is empty, no statements inside of the loop will be executed. The loop should appear as follows:

```
Do Until EOF(NameFile)
    ' Read a name from NameFile
    Line Input #NameFile, TheName
    ' Add the name to the list box
    lstNames.AddItem TheName
Loop
```

The Complete Procedure. Because you want to populate the list box as soon as the program starts, you should place the code in the Form Load event procedure as shown here:

```
Private Sub Form_Load()
Dim NameFile as Integer
Dim TheName as String
    NameFile = FreeFile
    Open "C:\Friends\NameList.txt" for Input as #NameFile
    Do Until EOF(NameFile)
        Line Input #NameFile, TheName
        lstNames.AddItem TheName
    Loop
End Sub
```

In the procedure, the variable NameFile is assigned with a file number returned by the FreeFile function. Then the NameList file is opened and associated with the file number NameFile. Once the file is open, the Do...Loop structure will perform the required repetition until it exhausts the records in the file.

Difference in Effect Between the Two Structures. The preceding discussion indicates that the key difference in effect between the two structures of placing the condition is whether the statements inside the loop will be executed at least once. Placing the condition with the Do statement can prevent those statements from being executed, whereas placing the condition with the Loop statement ensures that those statements will be executed at least once.

Thus, if the execution of those statements strictly depends on the condition, you should place the condition in the Do statement. On the other hand, if those statements must be executed at least once or if it is inconsequential whether the condition is checked before entering the loop, you should (may) place the condition in the Loop statement. For example, the code given in Example 1 can be changed to the following without affecting the result or exposing to any potential possibility for errors:

```
Private Sub Form_Click()
Dim N As Integer
    N = 1
    Do While N < 1000
        Print N
        N = N + N
    Loop
End Sub
```

Why? We know for certain that the first time the loop is executed the value of N will be 1 and thus is less than 1,000. When the loop is executed enough times such that N is at least 1,000, the loop will end regardless of where the checking is performed (with Do or with Loop).

Handling the Endless Loop

Notice that in the previous structures, some of the statements inside the loop must cause the condition to be False (in conjunction with the keyword "While") or True (in conjunction with the keyword "Until"). Otherwise, the loop will execute endlessly, resulting in an undesirable trap. When testing your programs, if you happen to encounter such a situation, you will notice that you cannot click the form's close (x) button or the End button in the menu bar to terminate the program. In such a case, you should press Ctrl+Break first. You can then end the program in the typical way (e.g., click the End button).

Do Loop Without a Condition on Either Statement

If you inspect the syntax of the Do...Loop structure again, you may discover that the While/Until condition is optional; that is, the entire structure can do without any While/Until condition. For example, it is perfectly legitimate to have a Do...Loop structure as follows:

```
Do
    'Statements to be executed
Loop
```

Like the preceding structures, there must be some condition(s) (plus some statements) inside the loop that can terminate the loop; otherwise, the loop will repeat endlessly. Typically, this structure is used when the condition to be checked is neither at the beginning nor at the end of the group of statements to be executed. The following example illustrates this situation.

Example 3. Computing the Value of an Infinite Series

Consider the following series:

$S = 1 + 1/2 + (1/2)^2 + (1/2)^3 + ...$

Is there a way to approximate the value of the series numerically? The series starts with a value of 1. Each subsequent value to be added is half of the previous value. Although the addition is supposed to be carried out "infinitely," our intuition is that at a certain point, the number in the series will be so small that any further addition will not alter the "tangible" value of the result. We can certainly stop the addition (get out of the loop) at that time. For practical purposes, we can consider 0.1E-07 (10^{-8}) "very small."

Let *S* = the variable to accumulate the value for the series
V = the variable to represent the value at each point of the series

Then, the algorithm to compute the series can be described as follows:

1. Set both V and S to 1.
2. Divide V by 2; that is, V = V/2.
3. Compare V with the "very small" number. If V is less than that number, terminate the computation; otherwise, proceed to step 4.
4. Add V to S; that is, S = S + V.
5. Go to step 2 (repeat the process).

With this algorithm, the following code can be written to approximate the result:

```
Dim S as Single, V as Single
V = 1
S = 1
Do
    V = V / 2
    If V < .1E-07 Then Exit Do
    S = S + V
Loop
Print "The value of the series is " & S
```

The following execution table shows the value of S and V at various stages.

Iteration No.	Value of V	Value of S
0	1	1
1	1/2	1 + 1/2
2	$(1/2)^2$	$1 + (1/2) + (1/2)^2$
3	$(1/2)^3$	$1 + (1/2) + (1/2)^2 + (1/2)^3$
.	.	.
.	.	.
.	.	.
N	$(1/2)^n$	$1 + (1/2) + (1/2)^2 + \ldots + (1/2)^n$

The Exit Do Statement. Notice how the loop is ended in the previous routine. We place an If statement among the group of statements inside the loop. Each time the statement is reached (after V has been divided by 2), it checks whether V is "very small" (when V < 0.1E-07). If the value is not "very small," execution will drop down to the next statement and V will be added to S. When V is "very small," the ***Exit Do statement*** will be executed, terminating the loop. When this statement is executed, the execution control is transferred to the statement immediately following the Loop statement (i.e., the Print statement), exactly like the situation in which the condition with the Until/While keyword is True.

Place the preceding code in an event procedure and test the result. (*Note:* VB will automatically convert the number 0.1E-07 to 0.00000001.) It should print 2 as the result.

Example 4. Finding the Solution of an Equation Numerically

Now you have learned how to perform computations repetitively using the Do...Loop structure. Repetition is a powerful feature that you can use to solve various mathematically problems. To illustrate, let's consider the following equation:

$a\ x^c = 4{,}000$

where $a = 100$

$c = 1 + \log(.8)/\log(2)$

You are to write a VB program to find the solution (the value of x that makes the equation true). One possible way, of course, is to perform some analysis so that you can express x in terms of all the other values. You can then just code the formula into your program. In this case, it should work.

However, sometimes the equation is so complex that it defies any analysis. It will then be impossible to solve the problem "analytically." In such a case, you may still be able to use the computer to find the solution "numerically." Let's pretend that this problem is complex enough that you would rather solve it numerically.

Where do we start? First, let's examine the left side and let y be the function; that is:

Let $y = a\ x^c$

We can then plot the function as shown in Figure 7.2.

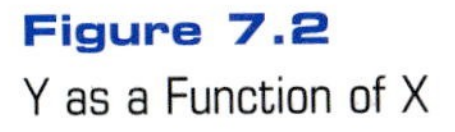

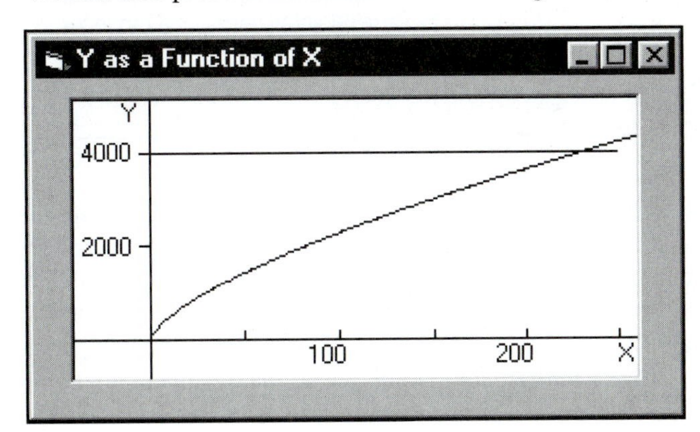

Figure 7.2
Y as a Function of X

Notice that the x value at which the y value is equal to 4,000 is the solution. As you can see, the function increases monotonically with respect to x. In such a case, there is a fairly simple but efficient way to find the solution.

An Algorithm for the Numerical Solution. Inspect the chart again. Notice that for any x value beyond the solution, y is greater than 4,000 and below the solution y is less than 4,000. Now, suppose you know that x must fall in a certain range. Then you can do the following:

1. Compute the midpoint of the range of x.
2. Find the new y for the midpoint of x.
3. Compare the resulting y with 4,000.
   3.1 If y is less than 4,000, this x value is too small. We can then change the lower bound of the range to this midpoint.
   3.2 On the other hand, if y is greater than 4,000, this x value is too large. We can change the upper bound of the range to this midpoint.

In either case, we have narrowed the possible range of the solution by half of the current range. The revised range can again be used to compute a new midpoint, which will give a clue to revising the range of the solution.

When this trial-and-error method is repeated a sufficient number of times, you will find the range is so small that any value within it can be considered a good approximation to the solution. This method of finding a solution of an equation numerically is recognized as the ***half interval method***. Figure 7.3 illustrates graphically how this trial-and-error method is carried out.

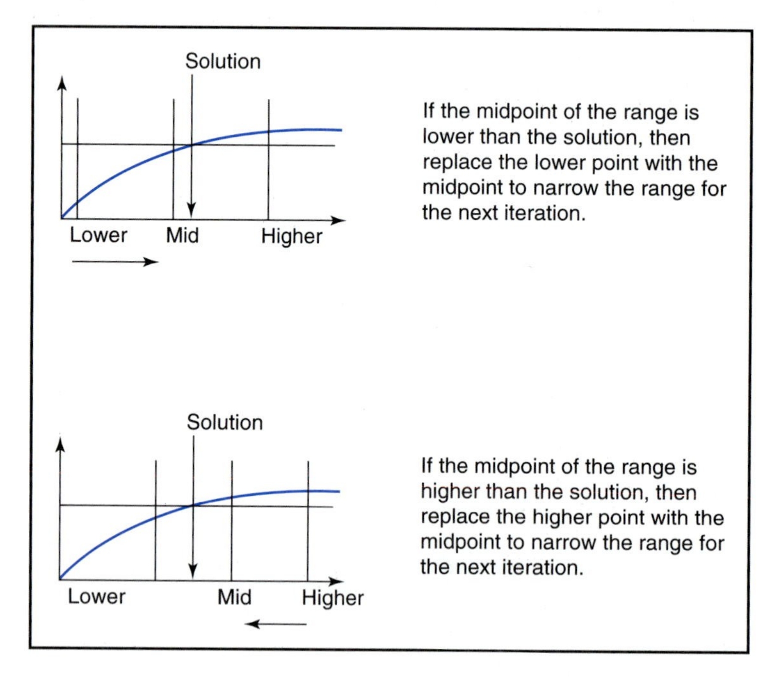

Figure 7.3
The Half Interval Method at Work

Searching for the Initial Range. How do you set the initial range to search for the solution? In our case, it is obvious that the lower bound cannot be anything less than 0. The upper bound can be identified by a "reverse" half interval method. Suppose you try a value for x at 1. You should find the function gives a y value that is smaller than 4,000. So, we can double this value of x and try again. If it is still smaller than 4,000, you can double x again. You can repeat this process until you obtain a x value that results in a y value greater than 4,000. This x value can then be used as the upper bound.

In sum, the procedure to find the numerical solution can be stated by the pseudo-code as follows:

1. Finding an appropriate upper bound:
   1.1 Let x = 1.
   1.2 Double x.
   1.3 Compute y for the given x.
   1.4 If y is less than 4,000, repeat 1.2 through 1.3; otherwise, proceed to step 2.
2. Find the numerical approximation (solution) using the half interval method:
   2.1 Let Low = 0; and High = X, which is obtained in step 1. (Low and High represent the lower and upper bounds of the range to search for the solution.)
   2.2 Compute x = (Low + High)/2.
   2.3 Compute y.
   2.4 If y is less than 4,000, let Low = X (i.e., adjust the lower bound); otherwise, let High = X (i.e., adjust the upper bound).
   2.5 If (High – Low) is still not small enough, repeat steps 2.2 through 2.4; otherwise, terminate the search. X is a good approximation to the solution.

Suppose the user will click a command button named cmdSolve to initiate the computation. Then, the complete procedure using this algorithm can be coded in VB as follows:

```
Private Sub cmdSolve_Click()
Dim R As Double
Dim C As Double
Dim A As Double
Dim Y As Double
Dim T As Double
Dim Low As Double
Dim High As Double
Dim X As Double
    R = 0.8
    A = 100
    T = 4000
    C = 1 + Log(R) / Log(2)
    ' Search for a point that Y(X) > T
    X = 1
    Do
        X = X + X
        Y = A * X ^ C
    Loop Until Y >= T
    ' Search for X using the half interval method
    Low = 0
    High = X
    Do
        X = (High + Low) / 2
        Y = A * X ^ C
        If Y < T Then
        ' Too low; adjust lower bound
            Low = X
        Else
        ' Too high; adjust upper bound
            High = X
        End If
    Loop Until (High - Low) / X < 0.000001
    MsgBox "X = " & X
End Sub
```

Notice that we have assigned 0.8 to a variable R, 100 to A, and 4,000 to T. You can redesign the project so that the values of these variables can be obtained from data entered through text boxes. The modification is left to you as an exercise.

The Termination Criterion. Also notice that we use the formula (High – Low)/X to determine whether the range of the "true" solution is small enough. The criterion is based on a precision "relative" to the value of the solution. In contrast, you can also use "absolute" precision as the criterion by comparing the difference between High and Low with a "very small" value without dividing by X. In general, the relative precision is better, especially when X is relatively large. When X is near zero, however, you may encounter an overflow problem with the computation of the relative precision.

The Practical Meaning of the Example. Is there a practical meaning of the preceding example? Yes. You have just solved a learning curve problem, which asks, "If the first product unit takes 100 hours (A) to complete, how many units can we produce if we have 4,000 hours (T), assuming our factory has a 0.8 learning rate (R)?" The learning curve model asserts that because of the task complexity, the initial time (A) to complete a unit of product takes longer. As the experience (production) doubles, the average time required to perform the same task decreases by a constant percentage, R. The formula you see at the beginning of this example is the one to compute the total hours required to produce X units. The solution to the problem is approximately 230.5 units. This should intrigue you. If every unit takes 100 hours to produce (the initial time), then you can produce only 40 units with 4,000 hours available!

Perhaps, you have also learned a "moral." When you first attempted to solve the problem, you were unaware of the problem's practical meaning. As long as you know how the function behaves, your knowledge (or the lack) of the "practical meaning" of the problem should not affect your ability to solve the programming problem.

You may encounter a situation to code a loop that will continue until the user clicks a command button (e.g., cmdStop). Apparently, the loop cannot include the Click event procedure that is triggered when the button is clicked. How can you then terminate the loop when the event is fired? Here is a possible solution. Declare a form-level Boolean variable (e.g., GoodBye). Set the variable to True in the button's Click event procedure; that is, code the following:

```
Private Sub cmdStop_Click()
    GoodBye = True
End Sub
```

Then assume that the Do...Loop has no other termination conditions in the opening or closing statement. The loop can be structured as follows:

```
Do Until GoodBye
    ' Place all other statements for the loop here.
    DoEvents ' Release execution control to the system
Loop
```

Notice that there is a DoEvents statement inside the loop. The statement releases execution control to the system for it to perform system-level activities, including checking for the button's Click event so that the Boolean variable GoodBye can be set properly. Without the DoEvents statement, the loop will never terminate.

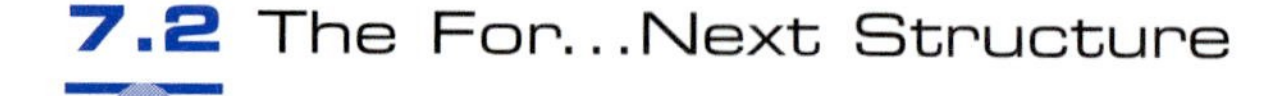

7.2 The For...Next Structure

The For...Next structure has the following syntax:

```
For Counter = Starting Value To Ending Value [Step Increment]
    Statements to be executed
Next [Counter]
```

where *Counter* = a variable to serve as the counter in the repetition

Starting Value = an expression that can be evaluated to a numeric value, which will be assigned to *Counter* when the loop starts

Ending Value = an expression that can be evaluated to a numeric value, which will be compared with *Counter* after adding *Increment* for each iteration

Increment = an optional parameter that will be added to *Counter* for each iteration; *Increment* can be either a positive or a negative value; if this parameter is omitted, 1 is the default value.

As the syntax shows, The For...Next structure starts a loop with the For statement and ends with the Next statement. The counter in the Next statement is optional. However, you are strongly urged to include the counter name in the statement for code clarity.

When the loop starts, the counter is set to the starting value for the first iteration. The increment is then added to the counter for each of the subsequent iterations. At the beginning of each iteration, the counter value for the upcoming iteration is first compared with the ending value. Either the statements inside the loop will be executed or the loop will terminate, depending on the sign of the increment and the result of comparison.

The Increment Can Be Either Positive or Negative. If the increment is positive, the loop will end as soon as the counter is greater than the ending value. Thus, if the starting value is greater than the ending value, the loop will terminate immediately and the statements inside the loop will never be executed.

On the other hand, if the increment is negative, the loop will end as soon as the counter is less than the ending value. Thus, in this case, if the starting value is less than the ending value, statements inside the loop will never be executed. The two flowchart fragments in Figure 7.4 show how the For...Next loop works with positive and negative increment.

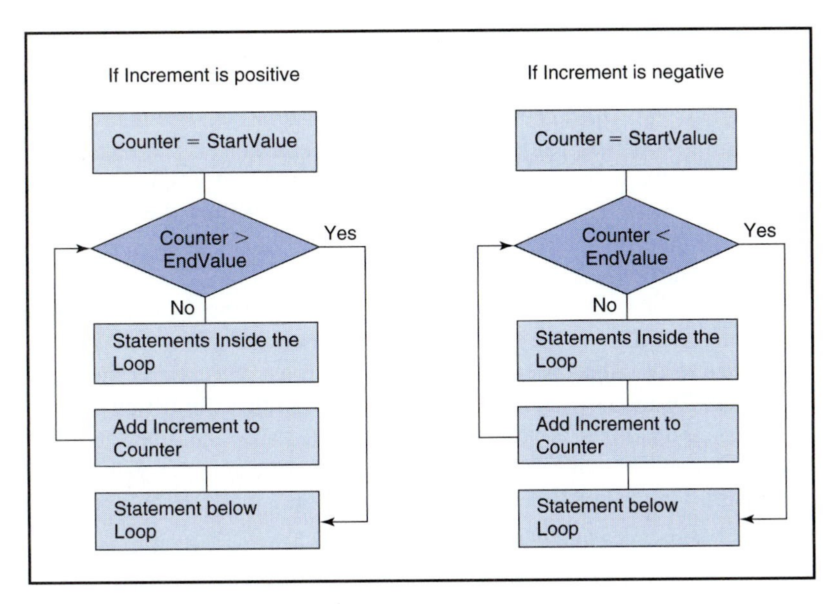

Figure 7.4
For Loops with a Positive and Negative Increment

Notice that when the increment is negative, adding it to the counter will decrease the value of the counter. The following examples illustrate how the For...Next loop can be used.

Example 5. Printing a Sequence of Numbers

Suppose you would like to print the numbers 1 through 10 on the form on the same line. What would be the easiest to do? You can use the For...Next loop, setting the starting value to one (1) and ending value to 10 with an increment of 1. You can then print the value of the counter inside the loop. The code should appear as follows:

```
Dim Counter As Integer
For Counter = 1 To 10
    Print Counter;
Next Counter
Print
```

You should be able to see the following output on your form:

1 2 3 4 5 6 7 8 9 10

Recall that in the For statement, if the Step optional parameter is omitted, the increment defaults to 1. In the preceding code, when the loop starts, the starting value 1 is assigned to the variable Counter. Then the Print statement inside the loop is executed. (Note that the semicolon [;] at the end of the Print statement instructs the computer to stay at the next printable position [not to move to the next line] after printing.)

In the next iteration, the default increment 1 is added to Counter, resulting in 2, which is compared with the ending value 10. Because 2 is not greater than 10, the statement inside the loop is executed. The iteration continues until Counter has a value of 11, which is greater than the ending value 10. The loop is then terminated. The execution control is transferred to the Print statement immediately below the Next statement. That Print statement instructs the computer to move to the next line in the form because it does not end with a semicolon. As a result, the loop prints the numbers 1 through 10. (Try the routine in a form Click event. Click the form a few times and inspect the results.)

Example 6. Listing Who's Invited

In Example 2, you saw how the list box named lstNames was populated with the list of your friends' names in a file. Suppose the list box's Style property has been set to 1 (Checkbox). You can check each of the names in the list box on or off. When you click a command button named cmdInvite with a caption "Invite," you would like the computer to print on the form the list of friends whom you plan to invite to your birthday party (see Figure 7.5 for a sample result). How can we do that? (Eventually, you want to modify the program so that the computer will print a personal invitation to each of the friends invited.)

Recall that the list box has a Selected property and a List property for each individual item. These properties are indexed. Selected(0) indicates whether the first item is checked, whereas List(0) gives the content of the first item (name). Notice that the index of either property in the pair of parentheses does not have to be a constant. It can be a variable. Thus, if we use a variable for the index and have a way to change this variable such that it will go 0, 1, 2, . . . until the end of the list, we would be able to test the Selected property for each value of the index. If the Selected property for a given value of the index is True, we will print the List property with the corresponding index value.

Now, if we set up a For loop with a beginning number 0 and an increment 1, the loop's counter will go 0, 1, 2 . . . , exactly the same values we would like for the index of the two properties to be. Thus, the Counter of the loop can be used as the index. What is the value of the index for the last item in the list box? Recall that the list box has a ListCount property, which gives the number of items in the control. Because the index starts with a value of 0 for the first item in the list, the last item in the list must have an index value of ListCount – 1. Thus, the code to print the list of friends to be invited should appear as follows:

```
Private Sub cmdInvite_Click()
Dim I as Integer
     Print "The following friends will be invited to" & _
       " my birthday party:"
     For I = 0 To lstNames.ListCount - 1
          If lstNames.Selected(I) Then
               Print lstNames.List(I)
          End If
     Next I
End Sub
```

In the procedure, the first Print statement is placed before the loop starts because you want the line to be printed only once and before any of your friends' names appear. The For statement sets the starting value for the counter, I to 0 and the ending value to the number of items (ListCount) minus one. Inside the loop, the If statement tests whether the item with an index value of I is selected (True if checked on). If it is, the name with the same index is printed. Figure 7.5 shows the results of a sample run. The following execution table depicts the process of executing the For loop when the list box contains five names.

Iteration	I	Selected(I)	Value of Selected(I)	List(I)	Value of List(I)	Action
1	0	Selected(0)	True	List(0)	Andrea Aaron	(Printed)
2	1	Selected(1)	False	List(1)	Ben Bennett	(None)
3	2	Selected(2)	True	List(2)	George Gunther	(Printed)
4	3	Selected(3)	True	List(3)	Lisa Latimer	(Printed)
5	4	Selected(4)	False	List(4)	Zeff Zener	(None)

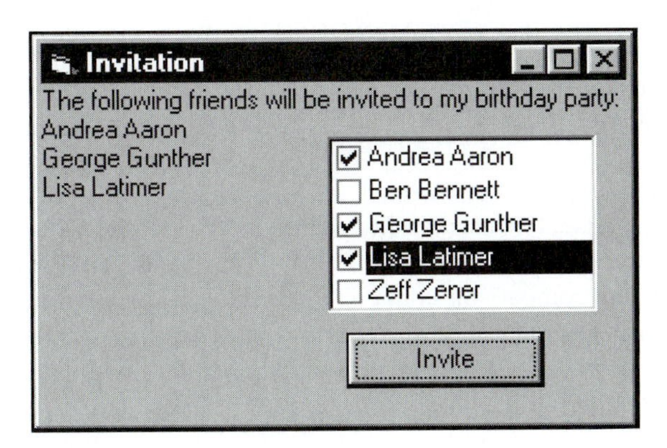

Figure 7.5
Printing Names Selected from a List Box

Example 7. Every Other Day

You have made a decision to run every other day in the month of October beginning on October 1. You would like to print all the days you should run as a reminder. How can you do this? You can still use the counter in a loop to represent the days that you are supposed to run. The only difference in this problem from Example 5 is that the increment is no longer one (1) but two (2). Thus, the routine can appear as follows:

```
Dim Counter As Integer
Print "I am determined to run on the following days of October:"
For Counter = 1 to 31 Step 2
    Print Counter,
Next Counter
Print
```

In this example, the Step parameter is specified explicitly as 2. Thus, Counter will begin with the starting value of 1. After the first iteration, it is increased by 2, resulting in 3 being printed. The numbers printed should appear as follows:

1 3 5 7 9 11 13 15 17 19 21 23 25 27 29 31

Notice that the Print statement inside the loop ends with a comma (,), which instructs the computer to move to the next tab position before the next data element is printed. This should make the numbers more clearly separated apart on the form.

In some languages, there is a restriction that the counter as well as the increment for the For loop must be Integer (or Long) variables. There is no such restriction in VB. However, it is advisable that both the counter and the increment are of the same data type. In addition, fractional increments should be avoided to guard against unexpected rounding problems, some of which are illustrated in the Visual Basic Explorer exercises at the end of this chapter.

Example 8. Printing a String on Two Lines

Suppose you have a text string, Text, that is longer than 80 characters but shorter than 140. You would like to print it on a form in two lines and you don't want the first line to be longer than 80 characters. How can this be done?

Assume your text string has embedded spaces between positions 1 and 80. One way to handle this is to search the string backward for a blank space starting from the 80th position. This space position can then be used as the split point; everything on the left can be printed on the first line, and the remainder on the second.

To search for the space backward, you can compare each character in the string with the space character beginning with the 80th position and going backward until the comparison is true. Recall that you can use the Mid$ function to extract a character from a string. Thus, the code to search for a blank space for this purpose should appear as follows:

```
Dim P As Integer
For P = 80 to 1 Step -1
    If Mid$(Text, P, 1) = " " Then
        Exit For
    End If
Next P
```

In the preceding code, P is used as the counter with a starting value of 80. Inside the loop, the Mid$ function extracts a character at position P. This character is then compared with the space character (" "). If the comparison is not True, nothing is done within the If block. The Next P statement transfers execution control to the For statement. In the next iteration, a value −1 is added to P. As long as P is greater than or equal to 1, the loop will continue. When at certain position P of the text string the character is a space, the comparison will be True. The statement inside the If block will then be executed. The ***Exit For statement*** will immediately terminate the loop and transfer the execution control to the statement immediately following the Next P statement (much like the Exit Do statement for the Do...Loop structure).

For example, assume the two words near position 80 are "getting excited" and are positioned as follows:

Position	69	70	71	72	73	74	75	76	77	78	79	80	81	82	83
Character	g	e	t	t	i	n	g		e	x	c	i	t	e	d

The following execution table depicts how the For loop is executed.

Iteration	P	Mid$(Text, P, 1)	= " "	Action
1	80	i	False	(Next P)
2	79	c	False	(Next P)
3	78	x	False	(Next P)
4	77	e	False	(Next P)
5	76	(space)	True	Exit For

Thus, when the loop terminates, P should have a value of 76. Once the position for the space is found, you can print the string in two separate lines as follows:

```
Print Left$(Text, P - 1)
Print Mid$(Text, P + 1)
```

Partial results from the preceding example may appear as follows:

. . . getting

excited . . .

To test the preceding code, let's convert the problem into a project. Here are the steps to create the visual interface:

1. Draw a text box on a new form. Name it txtInput. This text box will be used to input the text string, which will be approximately 140 characters long.
2. Draw a label above the text box. Use "Enter the text here:" as its caption.
3. Add a command button to the form. Name it cmdPrint. The resulting visual interface should be similar to that shown in Figure 7.6.

After the user enters the text string in txtInput, he or she will click the button to initiate printing the text string in two lines.

With this modification, your code should be placed in the cmdPrint Click event. The complete code for the procedure should appear as follows:

```
Private Sub cmdPrint_Click()
Dim P As Integer
Dim Text As String
    Text = txtInput.Text
    For P = 80 to 1 Step -1
        If Mid$(Text, P, 1) = " " Then
            Exit For
        End If
    Next P
    Print Left$(Text, P - 1)
    Print Mid$(Text, P + 1)
End Sub
```

Notice that we have added the declaration for the variable Text. Because the source of the text string is the text box txtInput, Text is assigned with the Text property of that control. If everything goes well, the program should print the text you have entered in the text box in two lines when you click the command button. A sample output from the project is shown in Figure 7.6.

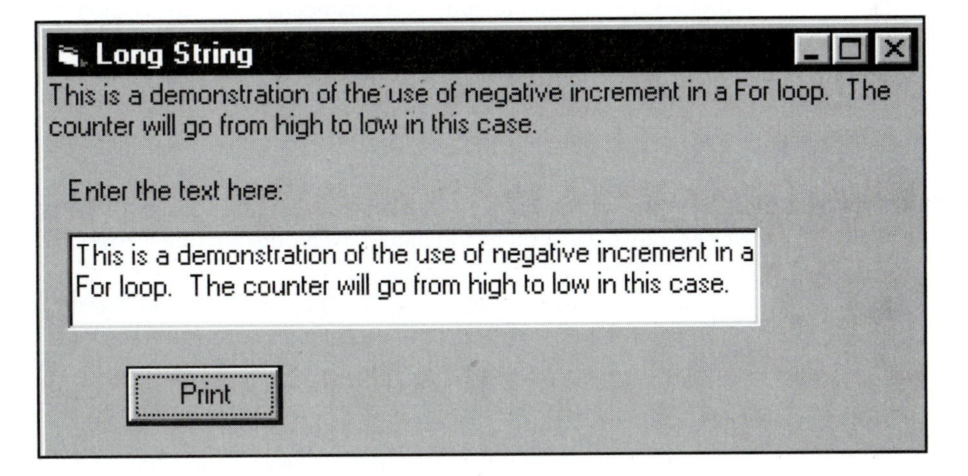

Figure 7.6
Printing a Long String in Two Lines

The code does not test whether the string is actually longer than 80 characters. If the string is not, the code will fail because the Mid$ function begins with testing the character at the 80th position. The additional code to safeguard against this error is left to you as an exercise.

Note that the preceding For loop was one way to find the position of a character in a string backward before VB6 was available. As you may recall, there is a string function, InStrRev (introduced in VB6 as discussed in Chapter 4, "Data, Operations, and Built-In Functions") that can perform the same computation much more effectively. A statement such as the following:

```
P = InStrRev(Text, " ", 80)
```

will give the same result as the For loop. Thus, practically, you should use the For loop for this purpose only if you are using an older version of VB. Even so, the preceding example should give you a fairly good idea about how a For loop works with a negative increment.

Nesting the Loops

Like the If blocks, the loop structures (both the Do and For structures) can be nested; that is, a Do...Loop structure can contain several Do...Loop structures inside itself. Similarly, a For...Next structure can contain several For...Next structures inside itself. In addition, a

Do...Loop structure can also contain For...Next structures and vice versa. The nesting can go practically any levels deep. The nested structure can appear as follows:

```
Level 1 / Level 2 / Level 3
For I = 1 To 20
    Statements to be executed (Level 1)
    For J= I to 40
        Statements to be executed (Level 2)
        For K = J to 1 Step -1
            Statements to be executed (Level 3)
        Next K
        Statements to be executed (Level 2)
    Next J
    Statements to be executed (Level 1)
Next I
```

Notice that the loops cannot be interposed; that is, one loop can contain another, and the inner loop must be complete before the end of the outer loop. In addition, you should not use the same counter variable for more than one loop. Example 9 illustrates the use of a nested loop structure.

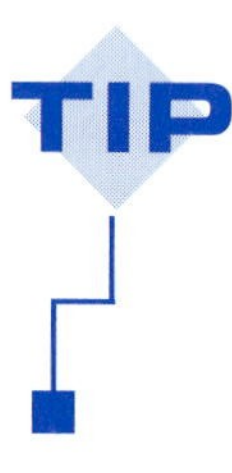

Always attach the counter to the Next statement (e.g., Next I, instead of just Next), as shown previously. Coding this way enables you to trace your own programming logic much more easily, especially when you have nested loops. You can see clearly where in your code you mean to conclude a particular For loop. Without the counter, it can create uncertainty in your mind as to which loop you mean to conclude. You can even lose track of the level of nesting while developing your code.

Example 9. Matching Up Teams in a League

Suppose there are eight teams in a sport league. In a season, each team is to play with all other teams exactly once. You would like to list all the possible games showing which team is to play against the other team. How can this be done?

Consider the situation for Team 1. They will play all the other teams, that is, Teams 2, 3, . . . , and 8. Thus, we can list all these "other" teams they will play against. How about Team 2? They will also play against all other 7 teams. But we should notice that the game Team 2 against Team 1 is the same game as Team 1 against Team 2. This game has already been listed for Team 1. There is no need to list this one again. So, for Team 2, we only need to list Teams 3, 4, . . . , and 8. Thus, to avoid listing the same games, the general rule is to list as the opponents only those teams whose numbers are higher than the current team we are considering. This analysis gives the following table.

Pivotal Team	Opponents to List
1	2, 3, . . . 7, and 8
2	3, 4, . . . 7, and 8
3	4, 5, . . . 7, and 8
.	
.	
6	7 and 8
7	8

Notice that Team 8 is not listed as a pivotal team because it has been listed as the opponent to *all* other teams already.

Let *Team* = the focal team

Other = the other team that Team will play against

Then the following code should print all the games for the league during a season.

```
For Team = 1 To 7
    For Other = Team + 1 to 8
        Print "Team " & Team & " against Team " & Other
    Next Other
Next Team
```

The inner For loop actually prints the other teams that Team will be playing against. The counter Other starts with a value Team +1. As explained, all games against teams with a team number smaller than this team have already been printed. The following table shows the results at different states of the two loops.

Team	Other	Game
1		
	2	Team 1 against Team 2
	3	Team 1 against Team 3
	.	
	.	
	7	Team 1 against Team 7
	8	Team 1 against Team 8
2		
	3	Team 2 against Team 3
	4	Team 2 against Team 4
	.	
	8	Team 2 against Team 8
.	.	
	.	
7		
	8	Team 7 against Team 8

Note that the inner loop with the counter Other repeats seven times. Each time, Other starts with a different value. When Team is 1, Other starts with 2; when Team is 2, Other starts with 3. The inner loop always ends after Other reaches 8. A total of 28 lines should be printed when the entire routine ends.

Example 10. What Is Your Chance?

Nested loops are often used to solve complex computational problems. It is therefore important for you to become familiar and comfortable with their working. Here is another illustrative problem that calls for the use of nested loops: The probability for a gambler to win a hand of blackjack against the house is 49%. What is the chance to win at least 60 hands out of 100?

To solve this problem *analytically*, you will need to find the formulas to compute the probability to win 60, 61, 62, . . . and 100 out of 100 hands and then sum the results. You can imagine how long the formula may look.

An alternative is to solve the problem *numerically by simulation*. You can use the random numbers generated by the computer to simulate the event and outcome. The resulting experience can then be used as an approximation to the probability of interest.

For example, the probability to win a hand is 49%, so you can draw a random number and examine its value. If it is less than or equal to 0.49, you can consider that you have won a hand; otherwise, you have lost. Given sufficient repetition, the probability of "winning" will be approximately 49%, using this simulation scheme. Thus, to simulate playing a hand, you will draw a random number and examine whether it is less than or equal to 0.49.

In the original problem, the question is the chance of winning 60 hands out of 100. You can simulate playing 100 hands. As each hand is played, you can determine whether you win or lose and accumulate the number of hands won. At the end of this "experiment," you can check to see how many hands you have won. If you have won at least 60 hands, you can claim it a success by the definition of the problem.

Let *R* = the random number

Wins = the number of hands won

Then the previous discussion can be translated into the following pseudo-code:

1. Let Wins = 0.
2. Repeat steps 2.1 and 2.2 100 times.
   2.1 Draw a random number, R.
   2.2 If R is less than or equal to 0.49, add 1 to Wins.
3. If Wins is greater than or equal to 60, you have succeeded in winning 60 hands out of 100.

The code to implement the algorithm can appear as follows:

```
Wins = 0
For I = 1 To 100
     R = Rnd
     If R <= 0.49 Then
          Wins = Wins + 1
     End If
Next I
If Wins >= 60 Then
' Claim that you have succeeded
End If
```

Notice that a For...Next loop has been used to "play 100 hands." Inside the loop, a hand is played by drawing a random number, and the outcome (win or loss) is determined by comparing the random number with 0.49.

The preceding code gives the result of one experiment. That is, you experiment by playing 100 hands and see whether you succeed. To approximate the probability of success, you will need to experiment many times, some successful, others unsuccessful. The probability of success can then be approximated by the relative frequency by dividing the number of successes by the total number of experiments. Assume you experiment 1,000 times. The algorithm can be described as follows:

1. Repeat steps 1.1 and 1.2 1,000 times.
   1.1 Experiment 100 hands and count the number of wins (W).
   1.2 If Wins is greater than or equal to 60, add 1 to Successes.
2. The probability of success = Successes/1,000.

The code to implement the algorithm should appear as follows:

```
For J = 1 To 1000
     ' Include the experiment to play 100 hands here
     If Wins >= 60 Then
     ' Claim that you have succeeded
          Successes = Successes + 1
     End If
Next J
ProbOfSuccess = Successes / 1000
```

The Complete Simulation Procedure. Assuming the computation will be initiated by a click of a command button named cmdSimulate, the complete procedure can appear as follows:

```
Option Explicit

Private Sub cmdSimulate_Click()
Dim R As Single
Dim Wins As Single
Dim Successes As Single
Dim I As Integer
Dim J As Integer
```

```
Dim ProbOfSuccess As Single
    Randomize
    For J = 1 To 1000
        Wins = 0
        For I = 1 To 100
            R = Rnd
            If R <= 0.49 Then
                Wins = Wins + 1
            End If
        Next I
        If Wins >= 60 Then
        ' Claim that you have succeeded
            Successes = Successes + 1
        End If
    Next J
    ProbOfSuccess = Successes / 1000
    MsgBox "Probability of winning 60 hands out of 100 is " & _
      ProbOfSuccess
End Sub
```

Notice that the Randomize statement has been inserted at the beginning of the program so that a different series of random numbers will be generated each time the simulation is performed. Test the program. You will see that the result oscillates around 2%. Does it surprise you?

Additional Remarks. The accuracy of the program depends primarily on the quality of the random number generator. If the random numbers are truly random, the results can be very accurate when the number of experiments is large.

Of course, you can modify the program so that it can be used to simulate a broad number of intriguing probability problems. For instance, in the previous example, the probability of winning a hand, the number of hands played, and the number of experiments are fixed at 0.49, 100, and 1,000, respectively. You can replace these simulation parameters with variables and allow the user to specify their values. The program can then be used to answer a question such as "If the probability for a particular baseball player to hit a home run each time he is at bat is 10%, what is the probability that he hits two or more home runs in a game when he is at bat 5 times?" The desired revision is left to you as an exercise.

The For Each...Next Structure

A variation of the For... Next structure is the For Each...Next structure, which has the following syntax:

```
For Each Object In Collection
    Statements to be Executed
Next [Object]
```

where *Object* = an object variable that represents an object such as a text box

Collection = a variable or predefined term that represents a set of object items; for example, the term ***Controls*** represents all the VB controls in a form and is recognized by VB.

It is probably easier to show you how the For Each structure works by example than by the explanation of concept. The following code will count the number of text boxes in a form:

```
Dim Ctrl As Control
Dim Count As Integer
For Each Ctrl In Controls
    If TypeName(Ctrl) = "TextBox" Then
        Count = Count + 1
    End If
Next Ctrl
```

As you can see in the code, the variable Ctrl is declared to be of a Control type and Count is declared to be an integer. Count is used to count the number of text boxes. In the For Each statement, the variable Ctrl is set to a control in the form (all these controls are collectively recognized by VB as Controls). Inside the loop, the ***TypeName function*** returns a string representing the type name of the control. For example, if the control is a TextBox, the function returns a string "TextBox." The string is compared with "TextBox," and if the two are equal, Count is increased by 1. In the next iteration, Ctrl is set to the next control in the Controls collection. The loop continues until the Controls collection runs out of the control object; that is, until all controls in the form have been enumerated.

Clearing Text Boxes and Masked Edit Boxes in a Form. With this understanding, you should be able to explain why the following code clears all the text boxes and masked edit boxes in the form:

```
Dim Ctrl As Control
Dim Temp As String
    For Each Ctrl In Controls 'Enumerate controls in the form
        Select Case TypeName(Ctrl)
        Case "TextBox"
        ' If the control is a text box
            Ctrl.Text = "" 'Clear the text box
        Case "MaskEdBox"
        ' If the control is a Masked Edit box
            Temp = Ctrl.Mask 'Save the mask
            Ctrl.Mask = "" 'Clear the mask
            Ctrl.Text = "" 'Clear the text box
            Ctrl.Mask = Temp 'Restore the mask
        End Select
    Next Ctrl
```

The routine uses the For Each...Next loop to enumerate through all the controls in the form. If a control is a text box, a zero-length string is assigned to its Text property to clear the text box. If a control is a masked edit box, its Mask property is saved before the Mask is cleared. Its text box is then cleared, and the Mask property is restored. This method to clear the text box of the masked edit box was explained in Chapter 3, "Some Visual Basic Controls and Events."

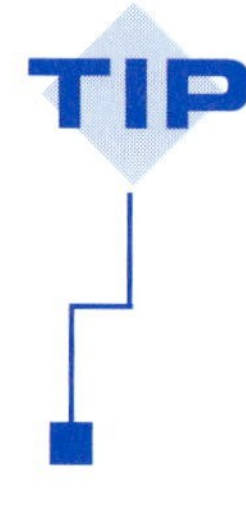

The online Help file does not appear complete in documenting the TypeName function. It only provides a list of data types returned by the function, but not any of the specific object types. You can find the type of the control by looking into the Properties window. The object box at its top contains a list of the objects in your form. Click on one of the objects of interest in the drop-down list. The name of the object and its type will appear in the object box. The type name that appears in this box is exactly the same string as returned by the TypeName function for the same object (see Figure 7.7).

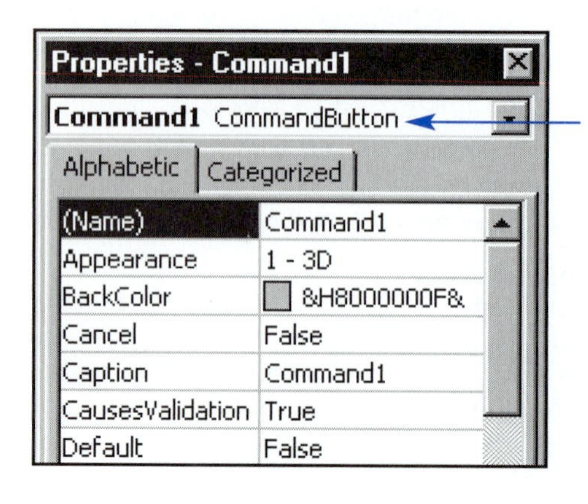

Figure 7.7
Properties Window

The Advantages of Generality. You may be wondering whether you would need a routine like this one at all. After all, when you develop a project and design the visual interface, you certainly know all the text boxes and the mask edit boxes in the form. Will it not be equally convenient to just code like the following?

```
txtName.Text = ""
```

The answer is that the loop approach is better in most cases, especially for an application with many controls on a form. You do not need to know the names of the controls to make the code work properly. In addition, one statement (or a group of statements) such as:

```
Ctrl.Text = ""
```

will take care of clearing all controls of the same type.

Furthermore, when the visual interface is changed (e.g., addition or deletion of some controls), you do not have to worry about revising the code. It is generalized and will work properly for all text boxes and masked edit boxes.

7.3 Additional Notes on Coding Repetition

You have seen all the structures to construct code for repetition. Have you wondered under what situations you should use which structure (a question of *suitability*)? In addition, recall that statements within the loop will be repeated "many" times. Thus, any performance efficiency/inefficiency associated with these statements can be magnified dramatically (a question of *speed* or efficiency). Are there tips that can enhance the efficiency of code for loops? Here are some notes in these regards.

Do Versus For

Suitability. The Do...Loop structure has no counter, whereas the For...Next structure does. In nearly all cases, one structure can be used in place of the other. However, one structure will appear to be more suitable than the other for a given situation. Basically, the For...Next structure is clearly intended for a situation in which the lower and the upper limit as well as the increment are known, whereas the Do...Loop structure is designed for the situation in which such parameters are undeterminable.

For example, when reading an entire sequential file record by record, it will be difficult for the program to determine ahead of time how many records there are in the file. In such a situation, it will be more appropriate to use the Do...Loop structure and check for the EOF condition to terminate the loop. Even if there is a need to use a counter while the input process is in progress (e.g., displaying the record number being read), a variable can be used to perform the count in the Do loop. You will be still better off not to use the For...Next structure by assuming an arbitrary upper limit then check for the EOF condition inside the loop. Such an approach leaves open the possibility that in the future the arbitrary upper limit might be unexpectedly exceeded when the file grows too large.

On the other hand, the For...Next structure will be more appropriate when its parameter values are known. Take the computation of the series of 1, 2, 3, . . . to n for example. At the time of computation, the value of n is certainly known, as are the starting value and the increment. Therefore, it is natural that the For...Next structure is used. Although you can still accomplish the requirement by using the Do...Loop structure, you will find that more lines of code are needed. The code will not be as concise and easy to understand.

Speed. How does the For...Next structure compare with the Do...Loop structure in terms of speed? In general, the difference is negligible. In fact, the performance difference of the two structures depends more on the way the condition in the Do loop is coded and on the data types of the parameters in the For loop than on the structures themselves.

For example, just like the "condition" in the If statement, a complex logical expression such as A >= B And C = D Or Not (X = Y And W < V) in the Do or Loop statement will be much slower than a simple expression such as A <> B. In the case of For loops, using variables of

Currency or Double type to serve as counter will certainly take more time to execute than using variables of the Integer or Long type. Because loops are to be executed many times, their performance difference will be magnified and more noticeable. One of the Visual Basic Explorer exercises at the end of this chapter illustrates the difference in speed between the Long counter and the Currency counter for the For...Next loop.

For Versus For Each

The For Each...Next structure is a convenient way to enumerate objects (especially of different types) in a collection, as you have seen in the example of enumerating all controls in a form. When you learn more about multiple form applications and databases in later chapters, you will find more opportunities to use this structure.

Note, however, that in many cases, the objects in a collection are of the same type. Usually, in such cases, the For...Next (with a counter, instead of with the keyword "Each") can also be used. When this is the case, the For...Next structure is usually more efficient than the For Each ...Next structure.

Tips for Efficiency

To repeat the point, because loops are to be executed many times, the efficiency or inefficiency of the group of statements in the loops is magnified. Thus, it is far more important to examine the code in the loops (especially the inner-most loops) very closely. Here are a few tips to improve the efficiency in coding the loops:

- *Move all constant assignments/operations out of the loop.* For example, consider the following loop:

```
For I = 1 To 20000
    A = 10 + B
    ' Other statements
Next I
```

Where none of the other statements inside the loop change the value of A or B. The code will be more efficient if it is rearranged as follows:

```
A = 10 + B
For I = 1 To 20000
    ' Other statements
Next I
```

- *Replace complex mathematical operations with simpler ones.* For example, the present value of an ordinary annuity of $1 for n years can be computed by the following formula:

$P = (1 + r)^{-1} + (1 + r)^{-2} + ... + (1 + r)^{-n}$

Assuming the proper values for R and N have been obtained, a straightforward way to implement the formula will be to code the following:

```
Dim PresentValue As Double
Dim I As Integer
    PresentValue = 0
    For I = 1 To N
        PresentValue = PresentValue + (1 + R) ^ (-I)
    Next I
```

However, the preceding code is not efficient for two reasons. First, the value of (1 + R) will never change inside the loop. It will be more efficient to perform the computation before the loop. Second, the ^ operator takes much more time than a simple multiplication. The following code can accomplish the same and would be much more efficient:

```
Dim PresentValue As Double
Dim Factor1 As Double
Dim FactorN As Double
Dim I As Integer
PresentValue = 0
FactorN = 1    ' The present value of a dollar for n years
```

```
Factor1 = 1 / (1 + R) 'The inverse factor, i.e., (1 + r)-1
For I = 1 To N
    FactorN = FactorN * Factor1 'Compute V = V ^ I
    PresentValue = PresentValue + FactorN
Next I
```

The following execution table shows the state of each iteration.

I	FactorN	PresentValue
1	$(1 + r)^{-1}$	$(1 + r)^{-1}$
2	$(1 + r)^{-2}$	$(1 + r)^{-1} + (1 + r)^{-2}$
.		
N	$(1 + r)^{-n}$	$(1 + r)^{-1} + (1 + r)^{-2} + \ldots + (1 + r)^{-n}$

- *Avoid data type conversions inside the loop.* In the previous example, some might not see a need for the variable Factor1 or FactorN to be of the Double type. However, as long as PresentValue is of the Double type, making either Factor1 or FactorN (or both) as a Single type variable will force data type conversion inside the loop, creating additional work for the computer.
- *Avoid using the concatenation operator for string operations.* The concatenation operation is very slow. If you can find a way to avoid using it, you should. For example, suppose you need to generate the string "ABCD...Z." One way to do it is to code the following:

```
Dim Alphabet As String
For I = vbKeyA To vbKeyZ
    Alphabet = Alphabet & Chr$(I)
Next I
```

However, the following code is much faster because it does not involve the concatenation operation.

```
Dim Alphabets As String
Dim I As Integer
Alphabet = Space$(26) ' Generate a string with 26 spaces
For I = 1 To 26
    Mid$(Alphabet, I, 1) = Chr$(I + 64) ' Note that vbKeyA = 65
Next I
```

- *Replace reference to a control's property by a variable.* It takes longer to refer to a control's property than to a variable. Thus, for repetitive references in a loop, a variable should be used. For example, consider the following code:

```
For I = 1 To Len(txtName.Text)
    Ch = Mid$(txtName.Text, I , 1)
    ' Other statements
Next I
```

The code will be more efficient if it is rearranged as follows (assuming Text has been declared as a String variable):

```
Text = txtName.Text
For I = 1 To Len(Text)
    Ch = Mid$(Text, I, 1)
    ' Other statements
Next I
```

7.4 An Application Example

Loops are used extensively in programs but are pretty hard for the beginner. To illustrate how they can be used in a practical problem, let's consider a simplified aspect of a payroll system.

When a new employee is hired, the payroll department needs to establish an employee record for the employee so that proper payroll withholdings can be handled. An aspect of this involves the completion of a W-4 form, which requires the employee to fill out information concerning employee's tax status, such as the marital status and number of dependents. Our simplified example focuses on the programming steps, rather than the information required.

The Project

The project involves the entry of the employee W-4 form. We will assume one or more new employees will be entered into the W-4 file each time the program runs. We will also assume that the company has fewer than 100 employees. The program will require the entry of the following data:

Employee Social Security number

Name (last, first)

Sex

Number of dependents

The data will be saved in a file called W-4Info.txt as a fixed-length file (the length of each field remains constant), one line per record. Pretty simple? The following lists additional specifications.

Design Considerations

One important consideration of the project is that there should be no duplicate employee records. To handle this, we will populate the existing employee records in a list box. As each new employee is to be saved, the list box will be searched for the "new" Social Security number. If found, an error message will be displayed and the record will not be saved. Otherwise, the record will be saved. In addition, it will be added to the list box so that any duplicate entry later can be identified.

The Visual Interface

We will use the following controls to handle the data fields:

Data Field	Control
Employee Social Security number	Masked edit box
Name (last, first)	Text box
Sex	Option buttons
Number of dependents	Text box

To make the form appear uncluttered, we will use a frame to group all these fields. In addition to the VB controls for these data fields, we will add a list box to list the existing employees, as mentioned previously. Furthermore, we should also have two command buttons: one to save the data and another to end the program.

The properties for these controls should be set to proper values. Some selected ones are as listed in the following table.

Control (Field)	Property	Setting
Masked edit box (S-S-N)	Name	mskSSN
	Mask	"###-##-####"
Text box (Employ Name)	Name	txtName
	MaxLength	24
Option button (for male)	Name	optMale
	Caption	Male
	Value	True
Option button (for female)	Name	optFemale
	Caption	Female
Text box (No. of dependents)	Name	txtNoOfDependents
	MaxLength	3

Control (Field)	Property	Setting
List box (to list employees)	Name	lstEmployees
Command button	Name	cmdSave
	Caption	Save
Command button	Name	cmdQuit
	Caption	Quit

The visual interface appears as in Figure 7.8.

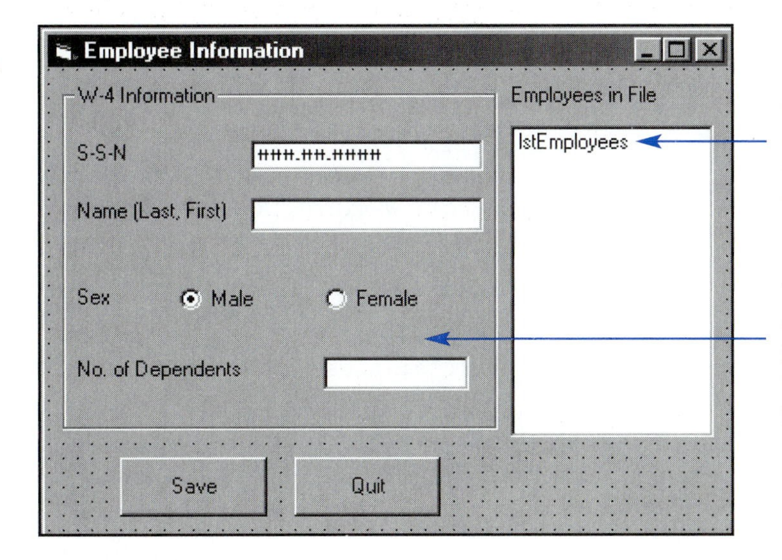
Employee Information
W-4 Information
S-S-N
###-##-####
Name (Last, First)
Sex
Male
Female
No. of Dependents
Employees in File
lstEmployees
Save
Quit
This list box allows the user to view existing employees and the program to verify whether a newly entered employee already exists.
The W-4 information to be entered here is highly simplified. However, all additional data elements will be processed through the same steps as discussed in this example.

Figure 7.8
Visual Interface for W-4 Form Entry

Coding the Project

The code needs to handle the following situations:

- As soon as the program starts, the list box should be populated with employee records in the W-4 info file. This will involve opening the file with the Input mode, reading the records one at a time in a loop and adding each to the list box as it reads. The file needs to be closed and reopened with the Append mode so that data for additional employees can be saved during the remaining duration of the program.
- When the user clicks the Save command button, several major steps should be carried out:
  - There should be an input error-checking routine to ensure that data entered are legitimate. For simplicity, we will check only the employee's Social Security number to ensure that duplicate records for the same employee will not be allowed.
  - The data should be saved in the W-4 Info file. In addition, the same record should appear in the list box.
  - The screen should be cleared to facilitate the entry of the next record.
- When the user clicks the Quit button, the program should end.

Populating the List Box. The list box will be populated with all existing employee records. Assuming the file (with the variable named W4File) has been open, how can this be accomplished? For simplicity, we will assume all fields in the record will be kept in the list box. We can set up a loop and read the file one record (line) at a time (in each iteration). As the record (named EmpRec) is read, it is added to the list box. The code in Example 2 can be easily modified to handle this:

```
Do Until EOF(W4File)
     Line Input #W4File, EmpRec
     lstEmployees.AddItem EmpRec
Loop
```

As already stated, this should be done as soon as the program starts. Thus, it should be placed in the Form Load event. This event procedure should also do the following:

1. Open the file for input.
2. Close the file after all records have been read.
3. Reopen the file for Append (because we will be adding new records for the remaining duration of the program).

The complete code for the Form Load event procedure appears as follows:

```
Option Explicit
Dim W4File As Integer

Private Sub Form_Load()
Dim EmpRec As String
     ' Open W-4 Info file
     W4File = FreeFile
     Open "A:\Payroll\w-4info.txt" For Input As #W4File
     ' Read employee w-4 info file and populate the list box
     Do Until EOF(W4File)
          Line Input #W4File, EmpRec
          lstEmployees.AddItem EmpRec
     Loop
     ' Input complete; close the file
     Close W4File
     ' Reopen the file for Append
     Open "A:\Payroll\w-4info.txt" For Append As #W4File
End Sub
```

Note that the variable W4File is declared in the general declaration area at the form (module) level. This is necessary because the file will also be used in another event procedure in which the employee W-4 records are saved. *Note also that this routine will not run when it attempts to open the W-4 Info file for Input if it does not exist. You should create an empty file with Notepad before testing this program.*

Handling the Save Command. As indicated previously, when the user clicks the Save command button, the program should do the following:

1. Ensure that the current entry is not a duplicate of an existing record.
2. Save the record if it is a new one.
3. Clear the screen.

These steps can be coded in the cmdSave click event procedure as follows:

```
Private Sub cmdSave_Click()
' Make sure s-s-n does not already exist
' Don't save the record if it does exist
   If SSNExists Then Exit Sub
' Save the employee record
' Also add the record to the list box
   SaveRec
' Clear screen and reset the default option button
   ClearScreen
' Set focus on the first control for the convenience of the user
   mskSSN.SetFocus
End Sub
```

Our coding design takes advantage of using general procedures for the top-down design. Each major step is coded either as a function or as a Sub and is invoked from this procedure. The code should be self-explanatory.

The first step is to make sure the Social Security number entered does not already exist in file. This is done by calling a function SSNExists, which is expected to return True or False, depending on whether the Social Security number actually exists. How does the function carry out the checking? To understand how it is done, we need to understand the format of the records saved first. Thus, we will take a look at the SaveRec Sub now.

Saving a W-4 Record. As mentioned, the file is created as a fixed-length file; that is, each field in the file remains constant. We will assume the lengths for S-S-N, name, sex, and number of dependents are 9, 24, 1, and 3, respectively. The lengths for S-S-N and sex should pose no problem because their field lengths appear fixed. For ease of browsing the file, we will also pad a blank space between each field.

How do we handle the length for Name? Note that the actual length of names can vary. We can solve this problem by assigning the data to a fixed-length string variable first. This type of variables ensure that the length of the string is always the same as declared by either padding with blank spaces or truncating extra characters. Once assigned to it, the content of this variable can be saved into the file. The following declaration will ensure that the variable TheName will always be 24 characters long:

```
Dim TheName As String * 24
```

How do we ensure that the number of dependents will be always three characters long? This can be accomplished by using the format function. Recall the format character "@" is a space-holder for string data and will right-align the data being formatted. This fits our needs exactly. The following expression should ensure that the number of dependents will be three characters long:

```
Format$(txtNoOfDependents,"@@@")
```

The following code for Sub SaveRec should save the employee record in the format we want.

```
Sub SaveRec()
' This Sub saves an employee w-4 record
' It also adds the same to the list box
Dim TheName As String * 24
Dim Sex As String
Dim EmpRec As String
     TheName = txtName.Text
     If optMale.Value Then
          Sex = "M"
     Else
          Sex = "F"
     End If
     EmpRec = mskSSN.ClipText & " " & TheName & " " & Sex & " " _
       & Format$(txtNoOfDependents.Text, "@@@")
     Print #W4File, EmpRec
     ' Also add to the list box
     lstEmployees.AddItem EmpRec
     ' Tell the user what has been done
     MsgBox "Employee data for " & Trim$(TheName) & " Saved"
End Sub
```

Notice that in the code we also "convert" what the user specifies as the employee's sex by the option buttons (optMale and optFemale) to a string variable, Sex, which is assigned a value "M" or "F" depending on which option button is clicked. Notice also that the variable EmpRec is used to prepare the employee W-4 record to be saved. In addition, the ClipText (not the Text) property of the masked edit box for S-S-N is used. Thus, there will be no embedded dash (-) in the saved S-S-N. Once the W-4 Info record is assembled, it is printed to the file. The same record is also added to the list box for content consistency and to facilitate the prevention of duplicate employee records.

Checking for Existence of an S-S-N. Now we know the Social Security number is the first field in the file and the list box. Thus, searching for the S-S-N involves the comparison of the data entered in the masked edit box with the first field of each item in the list box until a match is found or the list box runs out of items. To speed up the operation, a string variable SSN can be used to store the data extracted from the masked edit box. (Recall that data stored in variables can be accessed much faster than those properties in controls.) The pseudo-code to search for the SSN can appear as follows:

1. Let SSN = the number extracted from the masked edit box.
2. For each I = 0, 1, 2... for all items in the list box, perform the following:
   2.1 Compare SSN with the S-S-N in the Ith item in the list box. If the two are equal, conclude that SSN exists and exit the function; otherwise, proceed to next I.
3. When all items are compared, exit the function.

How do you extract data in the first field (S-S-N) of a list item? Each item (record) in the list box can be accessed by the list box's List(I) property. To extract the first substring from a string, you can use the Left$ function. Because the S-S-N field has a length of 9, the expression Left$(lstEmployees.List(I), 9) should return the S-S-N of the Ith (0th being the first) employee.

How do we set the value for I? The value can vary in the range of 0 through ListCount –1. This range can be used to set up the counter of a For loop. The following code tests the existence for a given S-S-N and returns a value True when the S-S-N is found:

```
Function SSNExists() As Boolean
' This function checks if the SSN in the masked edit box
' already exists; if so, it displays an error message
' Returns True; otherwise, it returns False
Dim SSN As String
Dim I As Integer
    SSN = mskSSN.ClipText
    For I = 0 To lstEmployees.ListCount - 1
        If SSN = Left$(lstEmployees.List(I), 9) Then
            MsgBox "S-S-N already in file", vbInformation
            SSNExists = True
            Exit Function
        End If
    Next I
End Function
```

In the loop, when SSN (the entered S-S-N) is found to be equal to one of the S-S-Ns in the list box, a message is displayed, True is assigned to the function, and the function ends (with the Exit Function statement). Otherwise, the search continues until the end of the loop. Because in this case no value is assigned to the function, it returns a value of False.

Clearing the Screen. The third major step in the Save event procedure is to clear to screen. The previous code example to clear the text boxes and masked edit boxes on the screen (form) can be literally copied and used here. Notice that the routine is capable of clearing all text boxes and masked edit boxes in a form.

This W-4 info screen also has option buttons. What we would like to accomplish is to reset the default button (i.e., set optMale on). To do this in the For Each loop appears to be a bit trickier. Thus, we will take the direct approach of setting the value property of optMale to True. The complete code for this Sub appears as follows:

```
Sub ClearScreen()
' This Sub clears all the text boxes and
' masked edit boxes in a form
' it also sets optMale.Value to True
Dim Ctrl As Control
Dim Temp As String
    For Each Ctrl In Controls
        Select Case UCase$(TypeName(Ctrl))
        Case "TEXTBOX"
            Ctrl.Text = ""
        Case "MASKEDBOX"
            Temp = Ctrl.Mask
            Ctrl.Mask = ""
            Ctrl.Text = ""
            Ctrl.Mask = Temp
        End Select
```

```
        Next Ctrl
        optMale.Value = True
    End Sub
```

Finally, when the user clicks the Quit button, the program should end. This is left to you as an exercise. This completes the code for the application example.

Testing the Program. Run the program. You should be able to observe the following:

- As soon as the program starts, you should be able to see the existing employees in the list box. (If you do not see all fields for the employee appear in the list box, stop the program and make the list box wider.)
- After you have entered data for an employee and click the Save button:
  - If the SSN already exists, the program should display a message box and wait for your additional action.
  - If the SSN is new, the data will be saved and the screen will be cleared. In addition, the computer will display a message indicating that the data have been saved.
- When you click the Quit button, the program terminates (assuming you have entered the proper code).

Additional Remarks. We have made this application example as simple as we can. As simple as it is, however, it illustrates how useful and widely used loops are. You have seen that all the following activities involve the use of loops:

- Populating the list box
- Reading records from a file
- Looking for certain data in a list (list box is just an example)
- Clearing edit boxes in a form

You may have also noticed that each situation calls for a different loop structure. The implication is that you should not rely exclusively on only one structure. Become well acquainted with all of them, and you will become more proficient in programming in VB.

If you compare this example with the one at the end of the preceding chapter for the phone file update, you may find some differences in design. For example, the current example involves only one file. Recall that a case was made in the preceding chapter that updating a sequential file calls for the use of two files (one for input and one for output). The current example imposes additional restrictions. Records can only be added to the file. No record can be recalled for editing, nor can a record be deleted from the file. In addition, the entire file is read into a list box. This is feasible only when the file is fairly small.

Summary

This chapter introduces you to the coding structures for repetition. You have seen and worked with the Do...Loop structure, For...Next structure, and For Each...Next structure. They constitute a powerful group of statements that can be used to solve very complex problems. Typically, the data manipulated within the loop will change from iteration to iteration.

Both the Do and For structures have variations in the parameters. These variations provide additional flexibility that you may need in designing the solutions to handle different problem situations. The exercises at the end of this chapter should further impress you with the power of the repetition structures. Indeed, you should consider these exercises an integral (inseparable) part of the chapter and complete all of them.

You have also learned that using the capability of repetition, many complex problems that may defy analytical solutions can be approximated numerically as illustrated in Examples 4 and 10. Although the discussion of numerical methods is beyond the scope of this book, you should be aware of this general approach to fully use the power of the computer.

This chapter further discusses the different situations in which different loop structures might be most appropriate. In addition, tips on how to structure code for efficiency have been explored. Because loops repeat execution of statements, code efficiency is amplified and can become highly noticeable. Therefore, it pays to examine the code inside the loops very carefully. This is particularly important for those statements in the inner-most loops.

Coding for repetition is one of the most difficult subjects in programming to the beginner, especially when the situation calls for nested loops. There is no shortcut in gaining proficiency in this respect. It takes a lot of practice, a lot of mental focus, and even a lot of patience for the beginner just to become "comfortable" with the code structure. When the problem appears to be very complex, draw an execution table (similar to the ones illustrated in Examples 1, 3, 6, 8, and 9). It can help you track the steps of the execution and understand the process more clearly.

Visual Basic Explorer

7-1. Conditions with Both the Do and Loop Statements. Test the following code:

```
Option Explicit
Private Sub Form_Click()
Dim I As Integer
Dim C As Integer
     I = -10
     Do Until I > 0
          I = I + 1
          C = I - 1
     Loop While C < 0
End Sub
```

After you click the form, what does the compiler say? (Although the compiler's message does not seem to make much sense, the point is that VB does not allow both the Do and Loop statements to include conditions at the same time.)

7-2. Changing the Parameters of a For Block. Enter the following code:

```
Option Explicit
Private Sub Form_Click()
Dim I As Integer
Dim K As Integer
Dim Z As Integer
Dim Total As Integer
     K = 1
     Z = 10
     For I = K To Z
          Total = Total + I
          K = 10
     Next I
     Print Total
End Sub
```

Run the project and click the form. What is the value of Total? Does the change in value for K inside the loop affect the loop?

7-3. Changing the Parameters of a For Block. (continued from 7-2). Test the following code:

```
Option Explicit
Private Sub Form_Click()
Dim I As Integer
Dim K As Integer
Dim Z As Integer
Dim Total As Integer
     K = 1
     Z = 10
```

```
        For I = K To Z
            Total = Total + I
            Z = 1
        Next I
        Print Total
    End Sub
```

What is the value of Total? Does the change in value for Z inside the loop affect the loop?

7-4. Changing the Parameters of a For Block. (continued from 7-3). Test the following code:

```
    Option Explicit
    Private Sub Form_Click()
    Dim I As Integer
    Dim K As Integer
    Dim Z As Integer
    Dim Total As Integer
    Dim S As Integer
        K = 1
        Z = 10
        S = 1
        For I = K To Z Step S
            Total = Total + I
            S = 2
        Next I
        Print Total
    End Sub
```

What is the value of Total? Does the change in the value of S inside the loop affect the initial setting? What is your conclusion concerning the effect of changing the parameter values of the For loop?

7-5. Changing the Counter of a For Block. Test the following code:

```
    Option Explicit
    Private Sub Form_Click()
    Dim I As Integer
    Dim K As Integer
    Dim Z As Integer
    Dim Total As Integer
    Dim S As Integer
        K = 1
        Z = 10
        S = 1
        For I = K To Z Step S
            Total = Total + I
            I = 10
        Next I
        Print Total
    End Sub
```

What is the value of Total? Why is the result different from that of previous situations? (The parameters for the loop are set the first time the loop is executed and remain the same. The counter value (which is allowed to be changed inside the loop) is always compared with the ending value each time the For statement is executed.) (*Note:* Changing the counter value inside the loop can make the code logic difficult to trace. Avoid such a coding practice.)

7-6. Fractional Progression. Test the following code and observe the result:

```
    Option Explicit
    Private Sub Form_Click()
    Dim I As Single
    Dim C As Integer
        For I = 1 To 100 Step 0.1
            C = C + 1
        Next I
```

```
        Print " C = " & C
    End Sub
```

Is the result what you expected? How do you explain it?

7-7. Fractional Progression. (continued from 7-6). Test the following code and observe the result (notice that I is declared as Integer this time):

```
Option Explicit
Private Sub Form_Click()
Dim I As Integer
Dim C As Integer
    For I = 1 To 100 Step 0.1
        C = C + 1
    Next I
    Print " C = " & C
End Sub
```

Why does the program result in an overflow for C? (The loop turns out to be an endless one. I is an integer. After I is added by 0.1, it is truncated to be 1. Thus, the counter never increases, regardless of how many iterations the loop executes.)

7-8. Counter Value After Exit For. Consider the following code:

```
Dim I as Integer
For I = 10 To 1 Step -1
    If I = 5 Then Exit For
Next I
Print I
For I = 10 To 1 Step -1
Next I
Print I
```

Place the code in an event procedure (e.g., a Command Click or Form Click event) and test it. What results do you obtain? When the loop is terminated by Exit For, the value of the counter is exactly what it is within the loop. When the loop is terminated from the For statement (by comparing the counter value with the ending value), the counter value should be one increment value (as specified by Step) away from the ending value.

7-9. The Puzzling Fractional Increment. Test the following code:

```
Private Sub Form_Click()
Dim S As Single
    For S = 0 To 2 Step 0.2
        Print S
    Next S
End Sub
```

What is the last number printed? Is it 2, which is what we should expect? Now, insert the following three lines between Next S and End Sub:

```
Print S
Print S = 2
Print S > 2
```

Run the program again. What do you see? Although S is printed to be 2, the result of comparing S = 2 is False and S > 2 is True! As explained in Chapter 4, Single type variables have a precision of approximately seven significant digits. Some numbers are very hard for this type of variables to represent exactly. Repetitively adding 0.2 to S causes the variable minutely off its "True" value. See the potential problem with using the Single type variable (especially as a counter)? (Contributed by Wen-Hao Chuang via Ben Wu, both of Indiana University.)

7-10. Use of the For Each...Next Structure and the Variant Type. Draw a few different types of controls on a form. Give each a name of your favorite. Then test the following code:

```
Option Explicit
Private Sub Form_Click()
Dim V As Variant
    For Each V In Controls
        Print V.Name; " "; TypeName(V)
    Next V
End Sub
```

Does it work properly? See the power and flexibility of the Variant type variable? It can even be used as an object variable.

7-11. Does It Really Matter What Data Type the Counter Is? Draw two command buttons on a new form. Name one cmdLong and set its Caption property to "Long." Name the other cmdCurrency and set its Caption property to "Currency." Then enter the following code:

```
Private Sub cmdCurrency_Click()
Dim I As Currency
Dim J As Currency
Dim T As Single
    T = Timer
    For I = 1 To 10000
        For J = 1 To 10000
        Next J
    Next I
    Debug.Print Timer - T
End Sub
Private Sub cmdLong_Click()
Dim I As Long
Dim J As Long
Dim T As Single
    T = Timer
    For I = 1 To 10000
        For J = 1 To 10000
        Next J
    Next I
    Debug.Print Timer - T
End Sub
```

Notice that the only difference between the two procedures is the type of data declared for the counters. Click the Long button. Observe the time displayed in the immediate window. Do the same with the Currency button. Do you see a difference in the time it takes to execute each procedure? Currency counters use approximately one-third more time than Long counters in getting an empty loop executed.

Exercises

7-12. Series. Write a routine to compute the total of 1 + 2 + 3 +. . . + n, where n is taken from a text box. The result is displayed in the caption of a label, called lblSeries, when the user clicks a command button, named cmdCompute.

7-13. Factorial. Write a routine to compute the product of $1 \times 2 \times 3 \times \ldots \times n$, where n is taken from a text box. The result is displayed in the caption of a label, called lblFactorial, when the user clicks a command button, named cmdCompute. Use the Double data type for the result. (*Remarks:* Recall that this problem was solved by the use of recursive procedures. Most problems that can be solved by recursion can also be solved by iteration. Iteration can be "easier" for the computer, but recursion is easier for human beings to solve a complex problem.)

7-14. Setting the ListIndex Property of Combo Boxes in a Form. Write a Sub procedure (call it ComboSetter) to set to zero the ListIndex property of all combo boxes in your form when the user clicks the command button with a caption "Set Default." Your procedure should not explicitly refer to the names of the combo boxes. Test the program using a form that contains combo boxes mixed with other controls. The Sub should be invoked by a call from a command button's Click event procedure. (*Hint:* Use the For Each loop to identify the combo boxes in the form.)

7-15. Are All Text Boxes Blank? Write a routine to check whether all text boxes in a form are blank. When the user clicks the command button with the caption "All Blank?" your code will display either the message, "Yes. All text boxes are blank," or the message, "No. Some text boxes contain data," depending on the state of the text boxes. (*Hint:* Use the For Each loop to identify the text boxes in the form. *Note:* Write the routine as a function. Then use this function from the Click event procedure.)

7-16. Reversing a String. Develop the code to reverse a string; that is, given a string "abcde," your code will produce "edcba" as a result. Test your code by taking the string from a text box (named txtOriginal) into which the user enters the data and displaying the result in the caption of a label named lblReversed. (*Note:* VB6 has a reverse string function, StrReverse, to handle this. However, the purpose of this assignment is for you to practice using the loop. So, don't allow yourself to use that built-in function.)

7-17. Encrypting a String. Write code to encrypt a string in a text box named txtUserName using another string (named txtPassWord) as the key. The result is displayed in the same text box, txtUserName, when the user clicks the command button named cmdEncrypt with the caption "Encrypt/Decrypt." Use the Xor logical operator to perform the encryption. You should be able to see the "toggle effect"; that is, without changing either of the text boxes, the username will be encrypted and decrypted alternately when you click the command button repetitively. Each character in the username should be Xored with the corresponding character in the key. If the username is shorter than the key, the remaining portion of the key is ignored. If the username is longer than the key, the key will be used repetitively until the entire string of the username is encrypted; that is, as soon as the key runs out of characters, it will start over from the first character again. (*Hint:* Use the length of the name as the upper limit of the loop. Use the Mid$ function to extract a character from the name to encrypt. Use the Mod operator on the counter to compute the position of the password from which to obtain the character as the encryption key. Convert both the characters from the name and the encryption key to ASCII values to perform the Xor operation. (*Note:* For some technical reasons, mask off the upper 4 bits of each password character before performing the Xor operations.) Then covert the result back to a character using the Chr$ function.)

7-18. Finding the Last Comma in a String. Write a function that will find the position of the last comma in a string that is passed as the function's parameter. (*Hint:* One easy way to do this is to compare the string character by character backward with "," using the Mid$ function to extract a character from the string. A more efficient approach is to use the Instr function and search forward for "," in the string starting one position to the right of the previously found "," until there's no more ",". *Note:* There is a string function in VB6, InStrRev, that can handle this. However, the purpose of this assignment is for you to practice using loop. Do not use that built-in function exclusively for this assignment, although you may want to verify the solution by comparing the results from both.)

7-19. Counting the Number of Periods in a Paragraph. Write a function to count the number of periods (.) in a text string (paragraph), which is passed to the function as a parameter. Test the function by calling it from an event procedure. (*Hint:* Use the InStr function in a Do loop. Make sure its first [optional] parameter is used.)

7-20. Counting the Number of Option buttons in a Form. Write a routine to count the number of option buttons in a form by using the For Each...Next structure. Test your code by drawing five option buttons on a form in addition to one text box, one picture box, one list box, and one command button. The command button should have a name cmdCount with the caption

"Count." When you click the Count button, your routine should display the message, "There are 5 option buttons on the form."

7-21. Adding an Item to the Combo Box. Set up a new form such that it will contain the following fields for data entry:

Field	Control	Control Name
Name	Text box	txtName
Address	Text box	txtAddress
Zip code	Combo box	cboZipCode

Also, there should be two command buttons: one with the caption "Save" and the other with the caption "Quit."

When the user clicks the Save button, your program checks whether the zip code entered in the combo box (cboZipCode.Text) already exists in its list. If not, this new zip code is added to the list.

7-22. Populating and Saving the Content of a Combo Box. Modify the preceding exercise in the following manner:

- When the program starts, the combo box will be populated with a list of zip codes in a file called ZipCodeList.txt. (Open the file for Input.)
- When the user clicks the Save button, if the zip code is new, it is added to the combo box's list and saved in the file. (*Hint:* In the Form Load event, after the combo box is populated, close the file. Then reopen it for Append. Close this file in the form's Unload event. Be consistent in saving your data; that is, if your previous data were saved with a Write [Print] statement, you should use the same statement this time.)

7-23. Generalized Routine for Series Computation. Write a function to compute the value of an infinite series of the form:

$$S = a + a\,(1/d) + a\,(1/d)^2 + a\,(1/d)^3 + \ldots + a\,(1/d)^n$$

where $d > 1$

The function should have the following header:

```
Function Series(A As Double, D as Double) As Double
```

Test your routine by calling it from a command button Click event. The values of a and d should be taken from two text boxes whose values are entered by the user.

7-24. Computing the Present Value of an Annuity. The present value of an annuity can be computed with the following formula:

$$P = a\,(1 + r)^{-1} + a\,(1 + r)^{-2} + a\,(1 + r)^{-3} + \ldots + a\,(1 + r)^{-n}$$

where a = the amount of payment per period
r = the interest rate per period
n = the number of periods
p = the present value of the annuity

Write a routine to compute p and display the result when the user clicks the command button captioned "Compute." The values of a, r, and n are to be taken from the text boxes named txtAmount, txtRate, and txtPeriod. (*Note:* Do not use the PV built-in function for this purpose. Instead, set up a For loop to perform the computation.)

7-25. The Present Value of a Bond. A coupon bond pays an interest semiannually at the stated rate of its coupon (e.g., 6%). On the date of maturity, it pays its face value ($1,000 per unit) in addition to its interest coupon. Because the coupon rate can never be the same as the market rate (which fluctuates daily), the price (present value) of the bond is seldom the same as its face value. The formula to compute the present value (price) of a coupon bond is as follows:

$$P = c\,(1 + r)^{-1} + c\,(1 + r)^{-2} + c\,(1 + r)^{-3} + \ldots + c\,(1 + r)^{-2n} + f\,(1 + r)^{-2n}$$

where P = the present value (price) of the bond
C = coupon rate × Face value/2
R = market rate/2
N = number of years to maturity
F = face value (usually $1,000)

Write a function to compute the price of a bond given the coupon rate, market rate, years to maturity, and face value (set all these as the function's parameters).

Your visual interface should include three text boxes for the user to enter the coupon rate, the market rate, and years to maturity. You can assume that the face value is $1,000. You should also have a box (a label with an appearance similar to a text box) to display the result of computation (price). There should also be two command buttons: one to initiate the computation and the other to end the program. Invoke the function from the Click event of the button to initiate computation and display the result.

7-26. Computing the Square Root of a Number. The square root of a number can be computed by a set of iterative formulas:

$$D = (X_n^{\,2} - A)/(2\,X_n)$$
$$X_{n+1} = X_n - D$$

where A = the number for which to compute the square root
X = the square root of A
N = the subscript of X, denoting the number of iterations

The formulas state that you can start with any positive number for X as an approximation for the square root of A. (You can just start with A except when it is zero. In the case of zero, there no need to compute. The root is zero.) Then, a better approximation can be computed by subtracting from the current approximation (X_n) a value D, which is computed by the formula just given.

Each approximation will move closer to the true square root of A. When D (the amount of adjustment/correction) is sufficiently small, the new X can be considered a good approximation to the root. You can then stop the iteration (repetition). You can consider D "sufficiently small" when Abs(D/X) < 0.0000001.

Write a function (call it SqRt) to compute the square root of any positive number using this method. Test your program by taking a number from a text box entered by the user and displaying the result in the caption of a label. Compare your result with the result given by the Sqr built-in function.

7-27. Computing the Cube Root of a Number. Refer to the preceding exercise. In a similar fashion, the cube root of a number can be computed by a set of iterative formulas:

$$D = (X_n - A/X_n^{\,2})/3$$
$$X_{n+1} = X_n - D$$

Write a function to compute the cube root of any positive number using the same iterative method. Test your results with the following numbers: 1, 8, 27, 64, and 125. The solution should be 1, 2, 3, 4, and 5.

7-28. Computing the Economic Order Quantity (EOQ): The Sequential Method. The relevant cost of an inventory replenishment policy has an optimum point with respect to the quantity reordered each time. The total inventory cost for such a purpose is given as follows:

TCC = CC x (Q / 2)

TOC = PC x (D / Q)

TIC = TCC + TOC

where Q = the quantity to order each time
CC = the cost to carry an item per period
PC = the cost to place an order
D = the total demand per period for the product
TCC = total carrying costs
TOC = total ordering costs
TIC = total relevant inventory cost

You can compute the total relevant inventory cost beginning with Q = 1. Then perform the cost computation when Q is increased by 1 each time. Initially, you will find the cost decreases as Q increases. Eventually, you will find the total cost increases as Q increases. The EOQ is the quantity at which the total cost is the lowest (before it starts to increase as Q increases).

Write a routine to compute the Q at which the total inventory cost is the lowest, using this method. Your visual interface should include three text boxes for the user to enter the total demand per period, the carrying cost per unit per period, and the cost to place an order. You should also have a box (a label with an appearance like a text box) to display the result (EOQ). In addition, you should have two command buttons: one to initiate the computation and one to end the program.

7-29. Computing the EOQ with the Half Interval Method. The preceding problem can be solved using another (more efficient) algorithm. If you draw a graph depicting the cost behavior of the total carrying costs and the total order costs, you will notice that a Q below the optimum EOQ, the total ordering costs, are higher than the total carrying costs. However, a Q above the EOQ has higher total carrying costs than the total ordering costs. You can start by setting a very low quantity (e.g., 1 and call it Low) and a very high quantity (e.g., 10 times the demand and call it High) such that you are ensured that the EOQ is in between the two quantities.

You can approximate the EOQ by finding the half point of the Low and High (i.e., Q = (High + Low)/2). Then compute the total carrying costs and the total ordering costs. If the total carrying costs are higher than the total ordering costs, the Q is too high (higher than the EOQ according to the previous explanation). You should then adjust the high bound; that is, set High = Q. Otherwise, you should adjust the low bound. You can then repeat this computational process until High and Low are very close to each other (e.g., a difference less than 0.1). There you have the solution. (This method of arriving at a numerical solution is recognized as the half interval method as explained in this chapter.)

Write a routine to compute the EOQ using this method. The visual interface should be the same as the preceding exercise.

7-30. Searching for a Town by Zip Code. You can download a complete U.S. zip code list from the following Internet URL:

http://www.qrs.com/files/misc/zipcodes.txt

Save the file in your favorite folder. Each line in the file contains a zip code followed by a comma, a blank space, then by the township, county, and state code, as the following lines show:

10081, New York, New York, NY

10087, New York, New York, NY

The file is arranged in ascending order by zip code.

Design a VB project to facilitate the search for a township/city or zip code. The form should contain a combo box and a list box. Set the combo box's Style property to Dropdown list.

When your program starts, it will populate the combo box with the zip codes and the list box with the corresponding township/city names. The file is too large for the combo box to handle. So, load both controls only up to the zip code number 60000.

When the user selects a zip code from the combo box, the list box will highlight the corresponding city/township name. When the user selects a city/township in the list box, the combo box will show the corresponding zip code. (*Hint:* when populating the two controls, use the Line Input statement to read a line from the zip code file. Then use the Left$ and Mid$ functions to obtain the zip code and city name. Use the AddItem method to add these items to their proper controls. *Note:* We will visit this zip code problem again in Chapter 9, "Arrays and Their Uses.")

7-31. Listing All Available Lottery Numbers. Assume that a lottery involves the random selection (without replacement) of three balls from a box. The box contains 25 numbers labeled from 1 to 25. Write a routine that will list *all possible combinations* of numbers for the lottery. Place the results in a list box.

7-32. Clearing Selections of a List Box. Write a Sub procedure that will take a list box as its parameter and clear all selections in the list box. (*Note:* Just deselect; do not remove the item[s].) Note that if the MultiSelect is set to 0 (none) and the Style is also 0 (standard), all you have to do is to set the ListIndex to −1; otherwise, you will also need to deselect all selected items.

7-33. Write a Sub procedure that will clear all controls in a form that are used to accept the user input. These controls should include text boxes, masked edit boxes, option buttons, check boxes, combo boxes, and list boxes. Deselect items selected in combo boxes and list boxes but do not clear the items from these controls. Refer to the preceding exercise (7-32) for the fine points concerning deselecting items in the list box.

7-34. Generalizing the Simulation Example. Modify the blackjack simulation program so that it can be used for a general class of problems. Your project should allow the user to specify the following:

1. The probability of success per trial (winning a hand)
2. The minimum desired number of successes per 100 trials (e.g., winning at least 60 out of 100 hands)
3. The number of experiment (this was assumed to be 1,000 in the example)

Test your project by answering the following question: "Assume the probability that Mark McGwire hits a home run each time that he is at bat is 10%. He is at bat five times per game. What is the probability that he hits 70 home runs in a season of 162 games?"

Without revising the program, can you use it to answer the question, "In order for Mark McGwire to have a 50% probability to hit 70 home runs in a season, at what rate (probability) he must be able to hit a home run each time he is at bat?" (*Hint:* Try different values of the probability to win per trial until the probability of success is around 50%. You can minimize your trials by mimicking the "half interval method.")

Projects

7-35. Finding the Effective Rate of a Bond. Refer to exercise 7-25 for the computation of the bond price (present value). In the financial market, the bond price is found through the bid and ask process (quote). Thus, when you are buying or selling a bond, you know the price first.

As an investor, you, of course, would want to know the effective (market) interest rate of the bond given the price. You are to develop a project for such a purpose.

Input: The user will enter the coupon rate, the years to maturity, and the price of the bond. (The price is quoted as if the face value were 100. Thus, a quote of 101 actually means 101% of the face value.)

Output: The computed market rate should be displayed in a label's caption, which should look like a text box and be accompanied by another label with a proper caption.

Computation: The bond price changes inversely with the market rate of interest. The higher the market rate, the lower the bond price. You should first write a function to compute the bond price (present value) given the market rate, coupon rate, and years to maturity as the parameters (call this function BondPrice). (Refer to the formula in Exercise 7-25.) The rate that makes the present value of the bond equal to the current bond price is the market (effective) rate on the bond. You can approximate the market rate by using the half interval method. For any practical problem, you can assume the market rate will be between 0% and 100%. Your algorithm to find the market rate will be as follows:

1. Set the lower rate to 0 and the higher rate to 1.
2. Compute the midpoint of the lower rate and higher rate.
3. Use the midpoint rate to compute the bond price, using the BondPrice function.
4. Compare the computed bond price with the bond price given by the user.
   A. If the computed price is higher than the one given, the current midpoint rate is lower than the true market rate. Adjust the lower rate by setting the lower rate to the current midpoint rate.
   B. Otherwise, adjust the higher rate by setting the higher rate to the current midpoint rate.
5. Repeat steps 2 through 4 until the lower rate and the higher rate are "very close" to each other. We will consider the two rates "very close" when the difference between the two rates is less than 0.1E-06.

7-36. Updating the Accounts Receivable File: Sequential File Processing. Develop a project that will update customer balances in an accounts receivable master file, using a customer transaction file. Each record in the accounts receivable master file consists of two data fields and are structured as follows:

Field	Length	Description
Account number	5 digits	xxxxx
Account balance	10 digits	xxxxxxx.xx; begins at position 7

Sample records of the file appear as follows:

10001 8000.00

10002 10000.00

.

.

Each record in the transaction file consists of four data fields and is structured as follows:

Field	Length	Description
Date	10 characters	mm/dd/yyyy
Account number	5 digits xxxxx;	begins at position12

Field	Length	Description
Charge or credit	1 character	C or D; in position 18; C = Credit; D = Charge
Amount	9 digits	xxxxxx.xx; begins at position 20

Sample records of the file appear as follows:

01/10/1999 10002 D 7000.00

01/05/1999 10002 C 5000.00

.

.

Both files are text files created with the Print statement (one record per line) and have been sorted in ascending order by the account number.

To update the account balances, your program needs to read both files and use the data to create a new account receivable (customer balance) file. Note that the customer master file contains all valid accounts. Thus, an account number in the transaction file that fails to match one in the master file represents an invalid number. The transaction record should be logged in an error log file and discarded.

Hints:

1. You need to open and use four files for the duration of your program. These are the "old" (existing) account receivable master file (for Input), the transaction file (for Input), the "new" (updated) account receivable file (for Output), and the error log file. Note that the new master file should have the same format as the existing one.
2. Use a command's Click event to initiate the update process.
3. The major steps involved in the update are as follows:

   3.1 Read transaction records for an account (TFAcctNo) until a different account or EOF is encountered. For each record for the same account, accumulate the transaction amount. (Note that you have an unprocessed transaction record here.)

   3.2 Read a customer master record. If the account number (MFAcctNo) is smaller than the one from the transaction file (TFAcctNo), this master record has no current transactions. Just output the record onto the new account receivable master file and repeat step 3.2. If MFAcctNo equals TFAcctNo, update the balance with the amount accumulated from step 3.1 and output the result onto the new master file. If MFAcctNo is greater than TFAcctNo, TFAcctNo is invalid; print an error log (message) in the error log file.

   3.3 If it is not the EOF of the transaction file, set the TFAcctNo and the accumulated transaction amount to the last record read in step 3.1 and repeat steps 3.1 and 3.2; otherwise, copy all the remaining records in the old master file to the new master file and then quit.

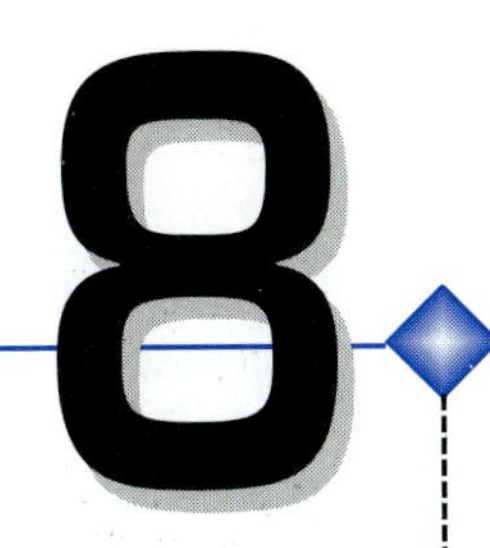

8 Database and the ActiveX Data Objects

All organizations must keep records of their activities (financial or nonfinancial) to satisfy their own information needs and to meet legal requirements. The activities required to create, store, and retrieve these data are recognized as data management. There are two general approaches to data management: the file-oriented approach and the database approach. The former approach focuses on individual application system's needs. Each application system develops and handles its own files. The database approach takes an enterprise view on the data. When more than one application system uses the same set of data, the set of data will be shared by these applications. The management of data under shared ownership can become very complex and thus calls for pecialized software, which is recognized as the database management system (DBMS).

This chapter presents topics related to the database, including the ActiveX Data Objects (ADO) provided by VB6 to interface with the database.

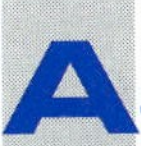

After completing this chapter, you should be able to:

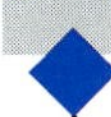

- Understand the concept of relational database.
- Know how to construct SQL statements.
- Use the ADO data control with bound controls.
- Write code to use the ADO data control without using bound controls.
- Use the ADO by code only (without the use of ADO data control).
- Understand data shaping and create code to construct hierarchical recordsets.
- Use the Data Environment Designer to create data environment objects for data access.

8.1 Introduction to Database

A *database* is defined as a collection of stored data that are managed by the database management system (DBMS). There are several conceptual models for the database. One of these is the relational database model. Under this model, a database is a collection of tables, each consisting of rows and columns. Each row represents a record, and a column represents a field. (A *field* is the smallest data element that has practical meaning. Examples of a field include the transaction date, Social Security number, and employee name.) Because this model is easy to understand, it is very popular. Almost all the current commercial database software packages for personal computers are built under this model. The Microsoft Access, SQL Server, FoxPro, Dbase, and Btrieve are all relational database software.

Table Definitions and Recordsets

Two distinct types of activities are required to create a database. Before a database comes into existence, you need to define tables and fields for the database. For example, if you are designing a payroll database, you will include at least an Employees table to keep data pertaining to all employees and a Paychecks table to record all paychecks paid to employees. For each table in the database, you will further specify what fields and their data types are in the table. For example, the Employees table will probably have at least the following fields:

Field Name	Data Type	Length
Employee Number	Long Integer	
Last Name	String	15 characters
First Name	String	15 characters
Middle Initial	String	1 character
Sex	String (M or F)	1 character
.		
.		

Once the tables and fields in a database are defined in the "table definition" phase, the user will be able to *store and retrieve data from the tables*. In many applications, the VB program is used to serve as the "front-end" interface, while the database "engine" is used as the "backbone" to handle the actual storage and retrieval of the data. A set of data records constructed by the database software and presented to VB is recognized as a recordset. In other words, a ***recordset*** is a "virtual" table that can be an actual table of the database, a subset of this table, or a subset of data extracted from various tables.

DDL and DML. Perhaps we should also mention a few technical terms. In the previous discussion, the language that is used to "define tables" is referred to as the ***data definition language (DDL)***. The result of using the language that defines an overall view of the structure of the database is referred to as the ***schema*** of the database. Some software allows the user to further define his or her own partial views of the database. These definitions are recognized as ***subschemata***.

The language that allows the user to "manipulate" the data is recognized as the ***data manipulation language (DML)***. Examples of the types of data manipulation that can be performed include updating, editing, adding, and deleting records.

Indexes, the Primary Key, and the Foreign Key

In many applications, you will need to search the table for needed data. To facilitate the search, you can create indexes to the table. An index allows the computer to find the location of a record given a field value. For example, assume the employee whose employee number is 1001 is the 50th record in the table. If the table has the employee number as one of its indexes, when you specify the employee number 1001 using the index, the computer will be able to identify that the record is located at the 50th position and thus retrieve it quickly. An index can be built on one field or several fields. For example, an index can be built on the Employee Number field. Another index can be built on the fields Last Name, First Name, and Middle Initial.

Index Uniqueness. When you create an index, you need to indicate whether it should be unique. A ***unique index*** will not allow a new record with the same index value as an existing one to be added. Some indexes by nature should be unique. For example, in the Employees table, the Employee Number index should be unique; otherwise, you will encounter difficulty in identifying an employee given an employee number. In the Paychecks table, the Check Number index should be unique as well. (You won't write two checks with the same check number, will you?) On the other hand, some indexes by nature will never be unique. For example, in the Employees table, if you decide to build an index on Sex, the index will have approximately half of the records with the same field value!

A ***primary key*** is an index of which each value is uniquely identified with a record. Thus, by definition, a primary key *must* be a unique index, although not all unique indexes are primary keys. In a way, this distinction is more conceptual than technical. There can be only one primary key in a table. We are willing to call a unique index the primary key of a table only if it is "identified" with the record. The employee number should be the primary key of the Employee table, whereas the check number should be the primary key of the Paychecks table.

The primary key of a table is often also used in another table to establish a relation/reference to the record in that table. For example, there should be an Employee Number field in the Paychecks table to indicate to whom the check is paid. The Employee Number in the Paychecks table can be considered the ***foreign key*** to the Employees table.

Introduction to the SQL

There are basically two different approaches to access data in the relational database. The ***navigational approach*** uses the Move and Find methods to locate and retrieve the records in data tables. The ***structured query language (SQL) approach*** uses the special query-handling features provided by the relational database software to handle the data. The SQL is a standard database query language supported by all relational database software. VB provides ways to interact with the database software that will interpret and act on the SQL. A good understanding of the SQL will enable you to code in VB programs that can interact with the database software smoothly. The following discussion covers some basics of the SQL that pertain to the MS Jet data engine (for MS Access). Different software can have its own "dialect." If you use different software (server) for your database, you should consult the particular software manual for the specific vocabulary, which can be slightly different from what's presented here.

The Basic Syntax. The SQL to construct a recordset has the following basic syntax:

```
Select Field1[, field2][, . . .] From Table [Where Criteria] _
        [Order by fields to sort];
```

where *fields to select* = the list of fields in the table to be included in the results
Table = the name of the table to be queried
Criteria = the criteria to include records; only records satisfying the criteria will be included in the resulting recordset
Fields to sort = records included will be sorted by the fields specified here

The statement should be concluded with a semicolon (;) although in most cases, its absence will not cause any problem.

Notice that the selection and sort criteria are optional. Thus, a very simple SQL statement can appear as follows:

```
Select EmployeeNumber From Employees;
```

The preceding statement will result in a recordset that contains a column of all the employee numbers from the Employees table. Note that the field name, EmployeeNumber, is one word. MS Access allows a field name to be created with embedded spaces. In such a case, you will need to enclose the name in a pair of brackets to avoid confusing the database engine (server) in interpreting the code. Thus, if the field name in the database table is "Employee Number," the preceding SQL code will have to be changed to the following:

```
Select [Employee Number] From Employees;
```

Note, however, you should avoid creating table or field names with embedded spaces. Most DBMS do not allow names of this structure. The following discussion assumes that field and table names are not created with embedded spaces.

More Than One Field. To select more than one field, you will list the fields, separated by commas. To select both the Employee Number and Name, you will code the following:

```
Select EmployeeNumber, LastName, FirstName From Employees;
```

Note that commas are used to separate the field names.

Sorting the Recordset. You may want the previous results sorted by last name and then by first name. You can use the "***Order By***" clause to handle this:

```
Select EmployeeNumber, LastName, FirstName From _
    Employees Order by LastName, FirstName;
```

You can also specify whether the sort is in ascending or descending order by adding the ***Asc*** or ***Desc*** keyword after the sort field in the Order clause. For example, the following code will sort the last name in descending order and first name in ascending order:

```
Select EmployeeNumber, LastName, FirstName From _
    Employees Order by LastName Desc, FirstName Asc;
```

You may encounter the field name Desc for "Description." When you need to refer to this field name in an SQL, be sure to enclose it with a pair of brackets to avoid confusion. That is, in an SQL, you should code the field name Desc as [Desc].

All Fields in the Record. Rather than selecting only a few specific fields, what if you would like to select all fields in the Employees table, while sorting the same way as done previously? You can use the wildcard "*" character to indicate all fields in the table:

```
Select * From Employees _
    Order by LastName, FirstName;
```

A Specific Record. What if you want only the record for employee number 1001? You can specify this criterion by using the "Where" clause with the "=" operator:

```
Select * From Employees _
    Where EmployeeNumber = 1001;
```

A Range. Note that the comparison criterion described can also be other "relational" operators, which were presented in Chapter 5, "Decision." For example, if you want all the records for employee numbers in the range of 1,000 and 2,000, you can code the following:

```
Select * From Employees _
    Where (EmployeeNumber >= 1000) And (EmployeeNumber <= 2000);
```

Notice the use of the logical operator And. Specifying the criteria for the SQL is similar to specifying the conditions for an If statement in VB. Or and Not are also recognized logical operators in the SQL. Also, the two pairs of parentheses are used to enhanced code clarity; they are not required.

Matching a Name. When the query involves a text string, the string should be enclosed in a pair of either single or double quotes. Because it is easier to handle the single quotes than double quotes in VB code, you should use the single quotes. For example, suppose you would like the record for the employee named Charles Smith. The SQL statement should appear as follows:

```
Select * From Employees _
    Where (LastName = 'Smith') And (FirstName = 'Charles');
```

Note that the MS Access string comparisons are not case sensitive; that is, the preceding query will produce all records that contain the name "Charles Smith," whether they are uppercased, lowercased, or any combination thereof.

Matching a Partial Text. If your search requires a partial match of a text string such as all last names that begin with "Sm," you should use the Like operator instead of the relational (comparison) operator(s). For example, the following SQL will select all employees with a last name that begins with "Sm," such as Smart, Smiley, and Smith:

```
Select * From Employees _
    Where LastName Like 'Sm%';
```

What if you want to limit the records to those last names with only five characters (thus excluding Smiley in the previous example)? You will still use the Like operator. However, instead of using the "%" wildcard specification, you can use the "?" character, which represents a positional parameter that does not require a match. Thus, you can code the following:

```
Select * From Employees _
    Where LastName Like 'Sm???'
```

The three "?"s ensure that only those last names with five characters are selected for comparison. Then as long as the first two characters are "Sm," the record is considered to have satisfied the search criterion. (Note again that MS Access string comparisons are not case sensitive.)

Here is a "clarification." The wildcard character for MS Access in the Like criterion is actually "*." However, depending on the tool you use in VB to interface with Access, you will need to choose between "%" and "*" in order for your specification to work properly. The ADO requires "%," but the intrinsic data control and DAO require "*." These new terms, ADO, data control, and DAO, are explained later in this chapter.

The Inner Join and Outer Join. Suppose in the previous payroll application that you would like to retrieve all fields of all checks. In addition, you would like to include the names of employees to whom each check is paid. The Paychecks table should have an Employee Number field to identify the employee being paid. However, it should not have the Employee Name fields because they are already available in the Employees table. Thus, the query involves fields that are in two tables: all fields in the Paychecks table and the Employee Name fields in the Employees table. These records should be matched by the Employee Number in the two tables.

Inner Join. You can use the Inner Join clause to join the two tables and obtain the desired results:

```
Select Employees.LastName, Employees.FirstName, Paychecks.* _
  From Paychecks Inner Join Employees _
  On Paychecks.EmployeeNumber = Employees.EmployeeNumber;
```

Notice how the fields are listed. Because the selection involves two tables, the field names should be qualified with the table names. Thus, because the Last Name and First Name fields are in the Employees table, they are coded as follows:

```
Employees.LastName, Employees.FirstName
```

In addition, to indicate all fields in the Paychecks table, you code the following:

```
Paychecks.*
```

If a field name exists in only one table, you can omit the table name. Because LastName and FirstName appear only in the Employees table, you can also code the SQL as follows:

```
Select LastName, FirstName, Paychecks.* _
  From Paychecks Inner Join Employees _
  On Paychecks.EmployeeNumber = Employees.EmployeeNumber;
```

For code clarity, it is preferable to qualify the field name with the table name.

The Inner Join operation will return only those records that have the matching fields specified by the "On" criterion. In our example, only those checks with matching employee numbers in the Employees table will be included in the resulting recordset. Neither employees who have no paychecks nor paychecks without matching employee numbers in the Employees table will be included. If you want either of these types of records, you should use the Left or Right (outer) Join clause.

Outer Join. The Left (Right) Join clause will include all records in the first (second) table regardless of whether they have a match on the second (first) table. For example, if you are interested in *all* checks paid, regardless of whether they have matching employee numbers in the Employees table, you can code the following:

```
Select Employees.LastName, Employees.FirstName, Paychecks.* _
  From Paychecks Left Join Employees _
  On Paychecks.EmployeeNumber = Employees.EmployeeNumber;
```

This statement will return all checks paid. (Paychecks is the first [left] table used in the SQL.) If the check has a matching employee number, the name will be included; otherwise, there will be no name.

As a side note, you will hope your company never has this type of paycheck. Indeed, in a well-designed database, there should be a primary key–foreign key relation for the employee number between the two tables. You can then impose the "***referential integrity***" rule, which stipulates that a foreign key cannot be entered without the existence of the primary key. That is, in our case, the employee number in a paycheck must have a corresponding employee number in the Employees table. Otherwise, the paycheck cannot be saved into the Paychecks table.

The previous SQL will not list employees who are not paid. If you are interested in retrieving *all* employees, whether they are paid or not, you will use the Right Join clause; that is, you will code the following:

```
Select Employees.LastName, Employees.FirstName, Paychecks.*
  From Paychecks Right Join Employees _
  On Paychecks.EmployeeNumber = Employees.EmployeeNumber;
```

If you need to include the Where or Order clause while using the Inner/Outer Join clause, you will place it after the preceding lines. For example, if you are interested in only those checks with an amount greater than $10 and would like to sort the result by name, you can code the following:

```
Select Employees.LastName, Employees.FirstName, Paychecks.* _
  From Paychecks Inner Join Employees _
  On Paychecks.EmployeeNumber     = Employees.EmployeeNumber _
  Where (Paychecks.Amount > 10) _
  Order By Employees.LastName, Employees.FirstName;
```

The Create Table Statement. The Select statement introduced provides you with the capability to construct recordsets for various requirements. The SQL can also be used to define tables (schema) in a database; that is, the SQL also has the DDL capability. For example, you can use the ***Create Table statement*** to create a new table. The syntax appears as follows:

```
Create Table TableName (Field1 Type[(Length)] _
    [, Field2 Type[(Length)]. . .);
```

where *TableName* = name of the new table to be created

Field1, Field2 . . . = name of the nth field in the new table

Type = data type (as recognized in the database, not necessarily the same as in VB); for example, Text (for String in VB) and Integer (for Integer in VB)

Length = length of the (Text) field

The following code will create a new table for a phone directory that contains two fields, Phone and Name:

```
Create Table PhoneDirectory (Phone Text(10), Name Text(50));
```

A thorough discussion of the SQL requires an entire book and is beyond the scope of this chapter. Consult a book on database programming for a complete treatment of the subject.

8.2 Using the ADO Data Control

Data Control, DAO, and ADO

VB provides several tools for the programmer to work with the database. Prior to VB6, the data control and the data access objects (***DAO***) were the primary tools. The ***data control*** is one of the intrinsic VB controls available in the toolbox. It provides various properties, methods, and events that enable you to work with a recordset constructed from a database. The DAO has no visible element (thus, it is not called a *control* but rather an *object*) but offers a more complete set of properties and methods that you can use to work with not only recordsets but also table definitions.

VB6 introduces yet another technology, the ***ActiveX data objects*** (***ADO***) that can be used to handle not only the database (whether local or remote) but also various data "stores" (data that are stored in any form, not just the database format). These objects provide a standard programming interface for you to develop the code in handling data. Thus, "theoretically," once you learn the ADO, you should have no need to learn other technology to access any kind of data from your VB program, such as Excel files and email messages, a technology still under development.

As you can imagine, different kinds of databases require different database servers to manage. For example, the MS Access database is driven by the ***MS Data Jet Engine***. However, Oracle has its own database server for the Oracle database. Many of these servers are ***ODBC*** (open database connectivity) ***compliant***, meaning they provide a cross-platform database-independent interface to access the database. So, where does the ADO stand in this context? The ADO is based on a data access technology recognized as ***OLE-DB*** that defines a set of low-level services to access the database. Perhaps the diagram in Figure 8.1 can help illustrate the relationship among these terms (software).

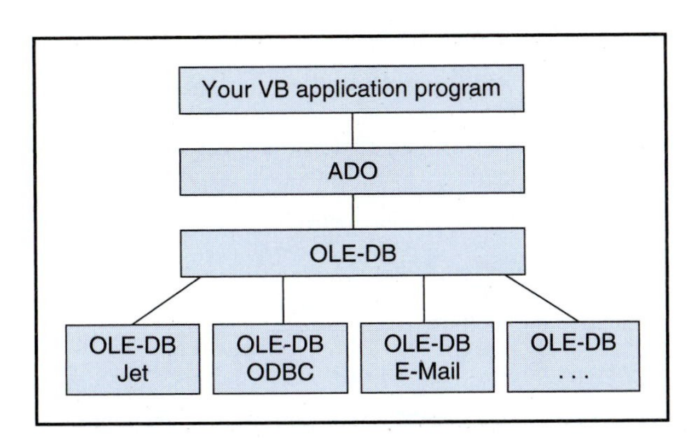

Figure 8.1
A Sketch of the Relationship of ADO to OLE-DB

From your point of view, you learn to work with the ADO so that you can get access to the underlying data that your program needs to handle. The ADO provides a uniform set of interfaces (properties, events, and methods) that you can use to handle all kinds of data, thus alleviating the need to learn different interfaces/code for different kinds of data. This chapter focuses only on the use of ADO to handle the MS Access database as an introduction to database and to the ADO technology.

From your VB program, you can use the ADO to access the database via the ADO data control or by code directly. VB6 also provides data tools such as the ***Data Environment Designer*** that creates data environment objects, enables you to design your data access at design time, and generates necessary code to access the data at runtime. The remainder of this chapter introduces each of these features.

Working with the ADO Data Control

The ADO data control (ADODC) provides features that enable you to interact with the underlying database with bound controls and code. A VB control can be bound to data through the ADODC if that control has the DataSource property. Many of the VB controls, such as the text box and label controls, have this property.

To illustrate how to work with the ADODC, let's consider a simple project that involves the Biblio database, which comes with VB. (If you follow the standard installation procedure, the database should be located under the "C:\Program Files\Microsoft Video Studio\VB98" folder.) The database contains several tables, one of which is the Authors table. The following discussion shows the steps to connect an ADODC data control to this table. These steps are as follows:

1. Add the control to your project.
2. Set the ConnectionString Property.
3. Set the RecordSource Property.

Adding the ADO Control. The ADODC is not an intrinsic VB control. Thus, you will need to add the control to the toolbox first. Adding this control to the toolbox takes exactly the same steps as adding all other nonstandard controls (e.g., the masked edit). That is, to add the ADODC to the toolbox, do the following:

1. Click the Project drop-down menu.
2. Click the Components option. The Components dialog box should appear.
3. Look for "Microsoft ADO Data Control 6.0 (OLEDB)" in the list box in the Controls tab and check the item.
4. Click the OK button.

Once it appears in the toolbox, you can do the following:

1. Draw it on your form just like all other controls. (See Figure 8.2 for its icon and appearance.)
2. Set its Name property to adcAuthors because this control will be used to work with the Authors table.

Figure 8.2
ADO Data Control: Icon and Appearance

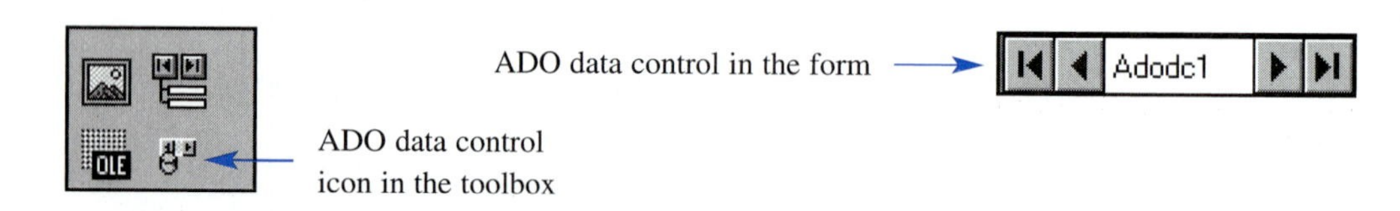

Setting Up the Connection String Property. The ***ConnectionString property*** is used to specify the provider, data source, and other parameters concerning a "connection" to the data source. The provider refers to the driver (server) that provides the data access services. The data source refers to the database to access.

To set the ConnectionString property for the control:

1. Double-click that property of this control in the Properties window. A Property Pages dialog box should appear as in Figure 8.3.

2. Select the "Use Connection String" option and then click the Build button. The Data Link Properties dialog box will appear (Figure 8.4).
3. Select "Microsoft Jet 4.0 OLE DB Provider." (*Note:* If you do not see Jet 4.0, select Jet 3.51.)
4. Click the Next button as shown in Figure 8.4. This button moves the same dialog box to the next tab, Connection.
5. Click the ellipsis (. . .) button in the Connection tab to browse the system and locate the database (Biblio.mdb) as the data source.
6. Test the connection by clicking the "Test Connection" button to ensure all parameters are specified correctly.
7. Click the OK button to return to the Property Pages dialog box.
8. Click the Apply button to set the ConnectionString so built. You should see more tabs appear on the same dialog box as shown in Figure 8.5.

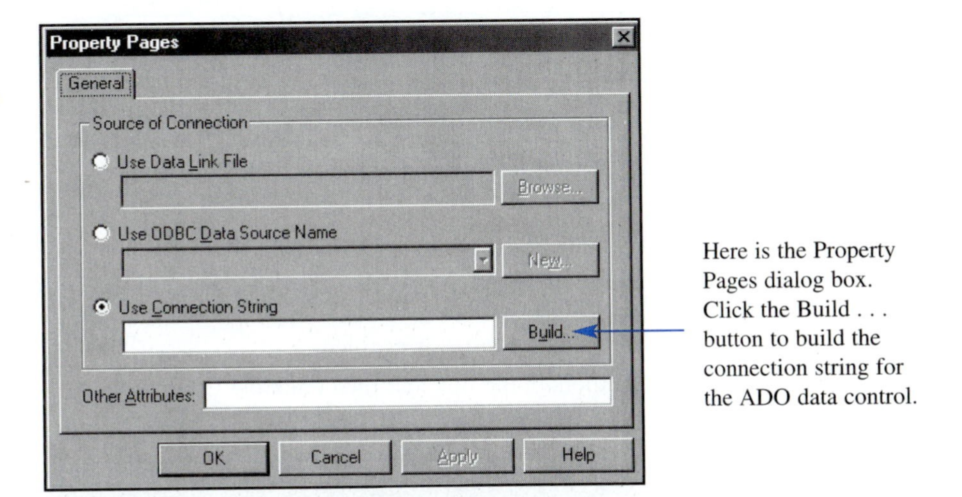

Figure 8.3
Property Pages Dialog Box for ADO Connection

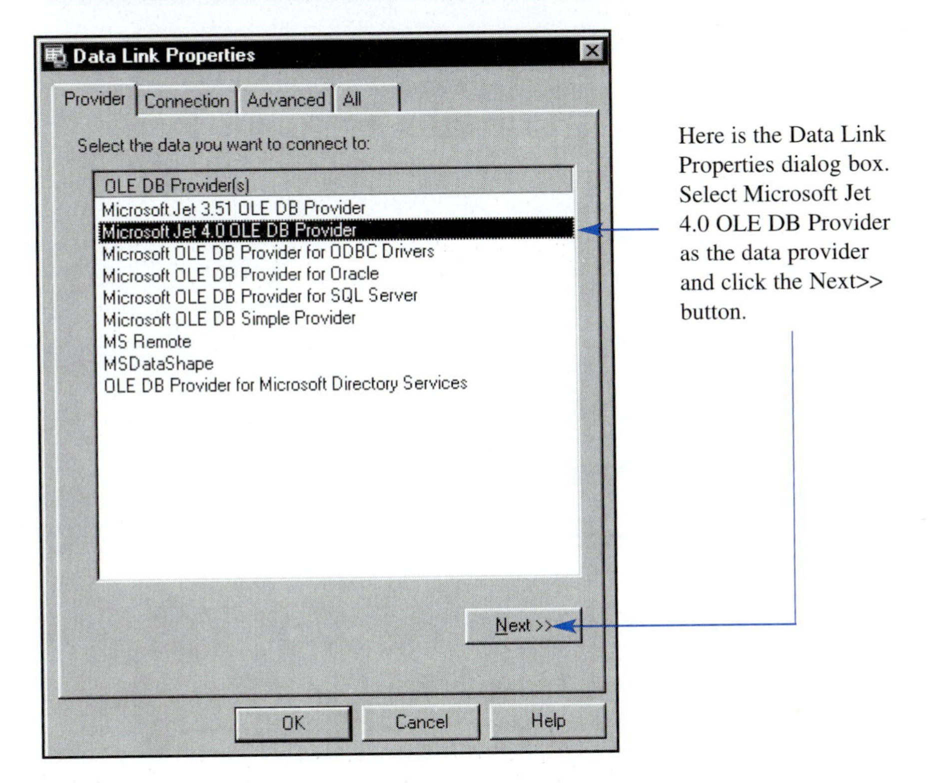

Figure 8.4
Data Link Properties Dialog Box

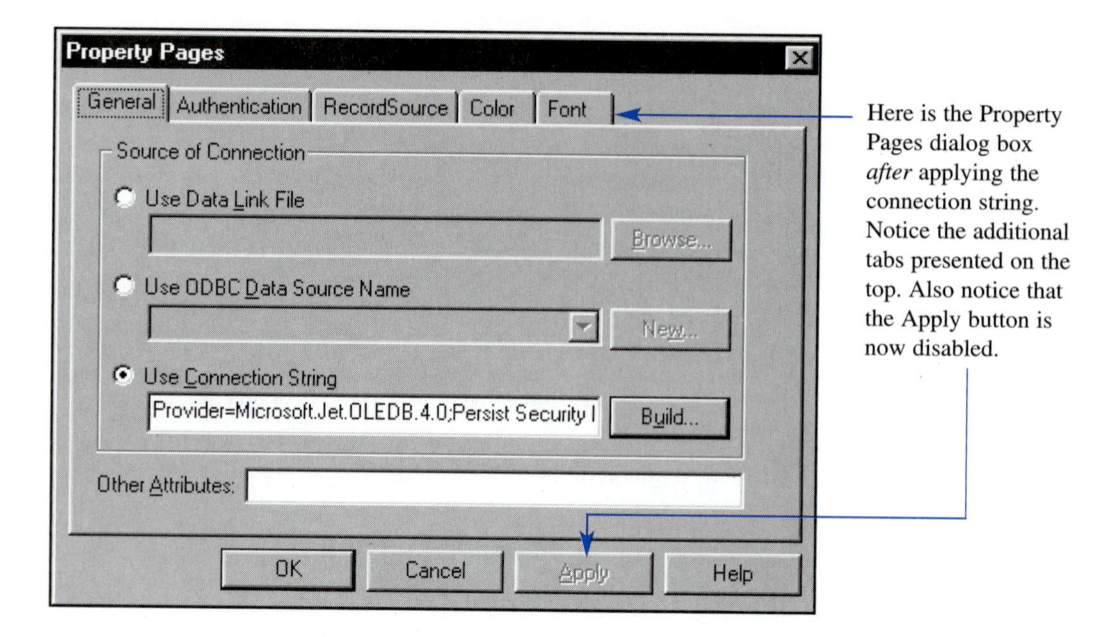

Figure 8.5
Property Pages After Setting the Connection String

Setting the RecordSource Property. You are now ready to specify the record source. Follow these steps:

1. Click the RecordSource tab. The tab appears as in Figure 8.6.
2. In the Command Type combo box, select 2-adCmdTable, which means that you are specifying to use a database table. You should see that the combo box for "Table or Stored Procedure Name" is enabled.
3. Select Authors in the box and then click the OK button.

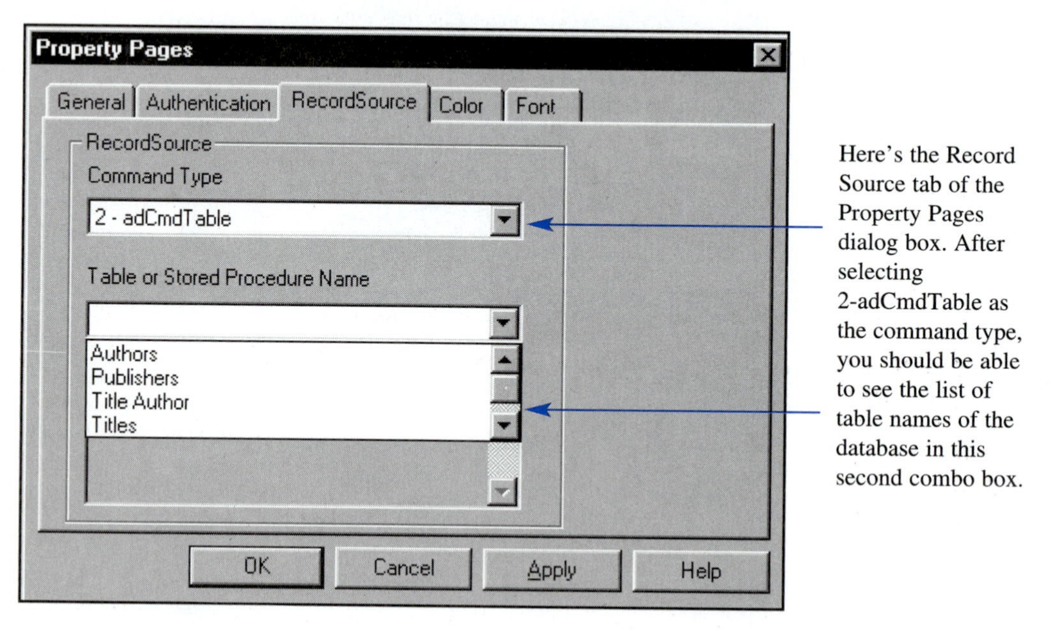

Figure 8.6
The RecordSource Tab on the Property Pages

Verifying the Settings. You have completed the specification for the ConnectionString and the RecordSource Property. To verify, you can check the Properties window and examine the content of both properties. The ConnectionString property box should contain a long text string; and the RecordSource property should show "Authors." If the RecordSource property is somehow not specified correctly, you can double-click this property box in the Properties window and work on the RecordSource tab of the Property Pages dialog box again.

After you complete setting these two properties and start the project, the ADODC will generate a recordset when you run the project. In this case, the underlying data is the Authors table of the Biblio database.

Binding Text Box Controls to the ADO Data Control

As mentioned previously, various VB controls can be bound to a recordset via the ADODC to perform input/output (I/O) operations. When controls are bound, many of the I/O operations are carried out automatically. Thus, only a minimum amount of code is required.

To illustrate the use of bound controls, let's continue the previous example. The Authors table has three fields: Au_ID, Author, and Year Born. Suppose we would like to browse through the table one record at a time. We can bind three text boxes to these fields at design time and then use the arrow buttons in the ADODC to navigate through the table at runtime. (As mentioned, text boxes are data-bound controls.)

Let's begin with the visual interface. If you have followed the steps discussed previously, the ADODC should be already on your form and named adcAuthors. You can then do the following:

1. Align the control at the bottom of the form by setting its Align property to 2-vbAlignBottom.
2. Draw three labels and three text boxes on the form.
3. Set the Caption property of the labels to Author ID, Author Name, and Year Born, respectively.
4. Name the three text boxes txtAu_ID, txtAuthor, and txtYearBorn to correspond to the field names in the database table. Also, clear their Text properties.

The completed interface should appear as in Figure 8.7.

Figure 8.7
Visual Interface for the Authors Table

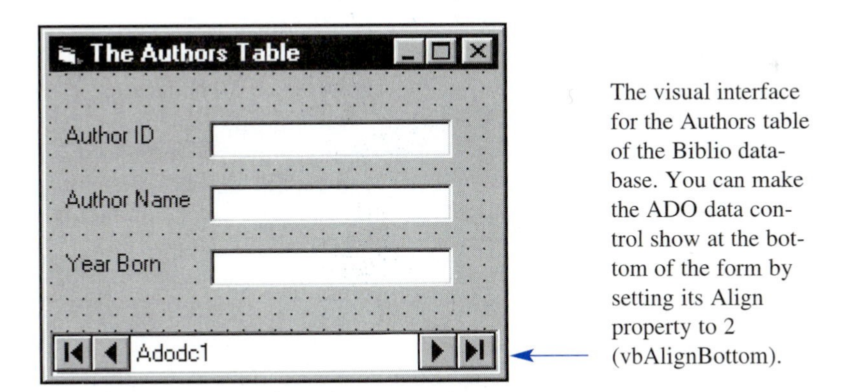

The visual interface for the Authors table of the Biblio database. You can make the ADO data control show at the bottom of the form by setting its Align property to 2 (vbAlignBottom).

Setting DataSource and DataField Properties for Bound Controls. You can bind the text box controls to the recordset for the Authors table via the ADODC by specifying the ***DataSource*** and ***DataField properties*** for each control. For example, to bind txtAu_ID to the table:

1. Click txtAu_ID; then click the Properties window.
2. Look for the DataSource property in the Properties window. Click the box for this property. You should see (only) adcAuthors in the drop-down list.
3. Click this item. adcAuthors should appear in the box for DataSource property.
4. Look for the DataField property in the Properties window. Click the box for this property. You should see all fields of the Authors table in the drop-down list.
5. Click Au_ID. It should appear in the property box.

You can follow the same steps to have txtAuthor and txtYearBorn bound to the database table.

You are now ready to see how the bound controls work. Start the project. The form should appear as in Figure 8.8.

Figure 8.8
Data Bound Controls in Action

The Authors Table

Author ID 1

Author Name Jacobs, Russell

Year Born

Adodc1

The MovePrevious button

The MoveFirst button

The MoveNext button

The MoveLast button

Data bound controls in action; when the project starts, the first record in the Authors table appears. The user can click the buttons on the ADODC to move around the recordset. Click the Move first (Last) button and the first (last) record will appear in the bound controls. Click the Move Next (Previous) button and the next (previous) record will appear.

As you can see, the first record in the Authors table automatically appears. Click the arrow buttons on the ADODC. You should be able to observe the following:

- The MoveNext button makes the next record appears on the text boxes.
- The MovePrevious button makes the record before the current one appear.
- The MoveFirst (MoveLast) button moves to the first (last) record of the recordset.

Behavior of the Bound Controls. Bound controls allow the user to move around a database table without any code. In addition, the user can also update the records without any code; that is, *if the user changes the data in the text boxes in the form and moves away from the record, the record is updated automatically*. This can be very convenient for the development of an application that requires no data validation.

Although you can perform data validation with bound controls, various restrictions can limit the flexibility your program may need to handle the data. Thus, if your application requires serious data validation and maximal flexibility in moving around the data table (as in the case of most serious business applications), you should stay away from binding the controls. Later in this chapter, we show how to perform input and output without binding the controls.

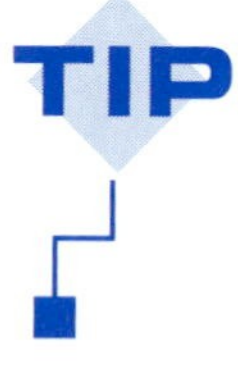

If you bind the text box controls only to browse a data table, you should set the Locked properties of the bound text boxes to True to prevent accidental changes to the data. Another alternative is to bind the labels, instead of the text boxes, to the database table. The properties and steps involved to bind the labels are exactly the same as those for the text boxes.

The DataGrid

Binding text boxes and labels to a recordset as shown previously allows you to browse/update the table one record at a time. In many instances, you may find it much easier for the user to see the entire table when browsing or even updating the records. The ***DataGrid control*** is designed exactly for this purpose. When bound to a data table, this control shows the entire recordset in a tabular form in a manner similar to the familiar electronic spreadsheet. The first row shows the heading of each column, which is the name of the field, and the remaining rows show all the records in the table. A DataGrid bound to the Authors table of the Biblio database is shown in Figure 8.9.

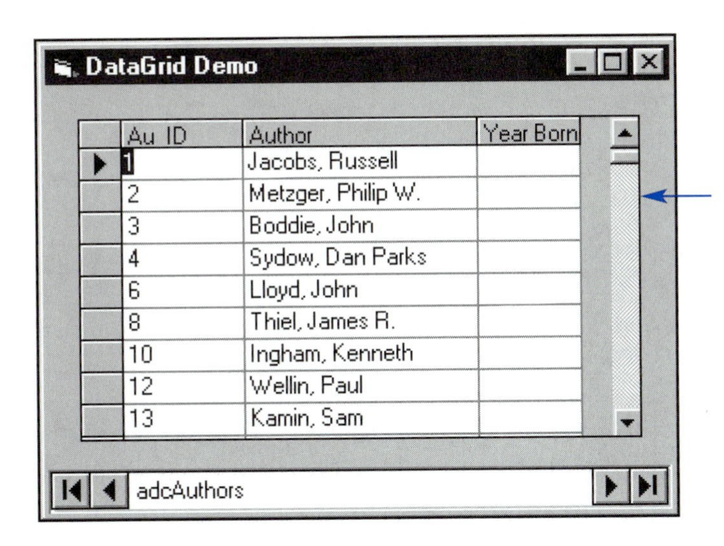

Figure 8.9
DataGrid in Action

The DataGrid displays the data automatically in the database table to which the grid is bound. The grid also automatically adjusts its column width to accommodate the field sizes. The user can also change the column width and row height by using the mouse to drag the grid line in the fixed cell.

As you can see, the grid consists of rows and columns. The first row and first column are set to "fixed" by default. A fixed row (column) appears in gray and behaves differently in that it does not move when the user scrolls around the data in the grid. Each intersection of a row and a column is called a cell. The row and column count from 0. Thus, the first cell in the grid is located at row 0 and column 0.

The user can set focus on a cell by clicking the mouse or using the navigational arrow keys. When a cell on the fixed column (on the left) is clicked, the entire row is highlighted (selected). When the height of the grid is not sufficient to present the entire recordset, the vertical scrollbar is automatically shown so that the user can scroll up and down to browse the records (much like the list box control). Similarly, when its width is not sufficient to show all fields in the data table, the horizontal scrollbar is added.

Adding the DataGrid to a Project. How do you bring a DataGrid control to a form and bind it to a recordset? This control is not a standard control and can be added to the toolbox by following the same steps used to add any nonstandard controls (as described previously). That is, to use the DataGrid:

1. Click the Project menu and select the Components option.
2. Locate "Microsoft DataGrid Control 6.0 (OLEDB)" in the list box and check it.
3. Click the OK button. You should see the DataGrid icon in the toolbox.
4. Draw the DataGrid on the form and adjust its size and location (see Figure 8.10).

Watch what you are adding to your project. In the Components dialog box, you will also see a control named "Microsoft Data Bound Grid Control," which is designed to work with the intrinsic data control, not the ADODC. The control you should add to your project is the "Microsoft DataGrid Control 6.0 (OLEDB)." Notice the slight difference in the names.

Figure 8.10
The DataGrid Control: Icon and Appearance

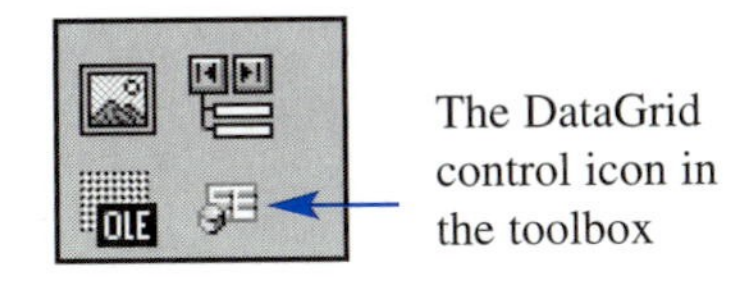

The DataGrid control icon in the toolbox

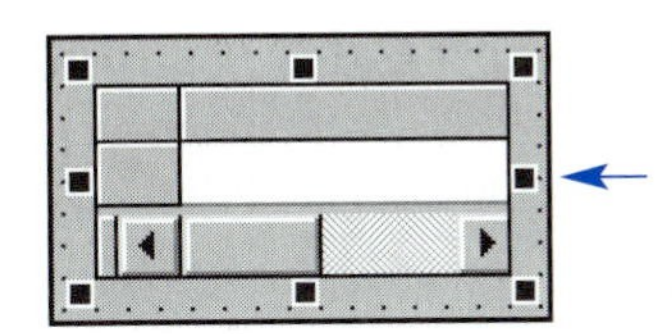

The DataGrid in a form when you double-click its icon in the toolbox. Just like most other controls, you can change its size by dragging its sizing handles.

Binding the DataGrid to a Recordset. To bind the grid to a recordset, you will need an ADODC on the form. Once the ADODC is connected to a recordset, you can set the grid's DataSource property to the ADODC. That is all it takes for the grid to become "functional" and to behave as described previously.

As a practice, start a new project and complete the following steps to bind the DataGrid control to the Authors table of the Biblio database:

1. Add the ADODC and DataGrid control to the toolbox using the Components option of the Project menu as described previously.
2. Draw an ADODC on the form. To make the control show at the bottom of the form, set its Align property to 2 (vbAlignBottom).
3. Set its Name property to adcAuthors. Then set up its ConnectionString and RecordSource in exactly the same way as described in the preceding example.
4. Draw a DataGrid on the form and adjust its position and size.
5. Set the Name property of the DataGrid control to dtgAuthors and its DataSource property to adcAuthors. (Unlike the text box, this control has no DataField property.)

Run the project. You should be able to verify that all the records in the Authors table are loaded into the grid.

DataGrid Properties. The DataGrid control has several properties that deal with the recordset. If the ***AllowUpdate property*** is set to True (default), any change made to a cell will cause a corresponding change in the underlying data. Thus, you should set this property to False if you intend for the user only to browse the data. If set to True, the ***AllowAddNew property*** will cause the grid to show a blank row at the bottom for the user to add new records. (The default setting is False.) The ***AllowDelete property***, if set to True (the default is False), will allow the user to delete a row by highlighting the row and pressing the Delete key.

The Hierarchical FlexGrid

When you want to show the content of an entire recordset in a grid but you intend for the user only to browse and not to update, delete, or add new records, you have another alternative. You can use the ***Microsoft Hierarchical FlexGrid*** (HFG), instead of the DataGrid. The HFG does not allow the user to directly manipulate any data in the grid but provides several interesting features that the DataGrid does not have. The HFG control can be added to the toolbox by following the same steps as the DataGrid control:

1. Click the Project menu and select the Components option.
2. Locate "Microsoft Hierarchical FlexGrid control 6.0" in the list box of the Controls tab.
3. Click the OK button.

Figure 8.11 shows the icon and appearance of the HFG.

Figure 8.11
Microsoft Hierarchical FlexGrid Control: Icon and Appearance

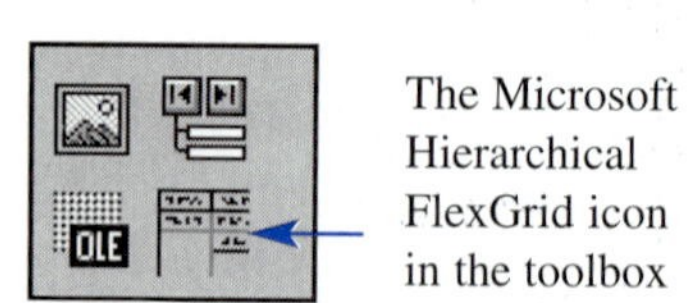

The Microsoft Hierarchical FlexGrid icon in the toolbox

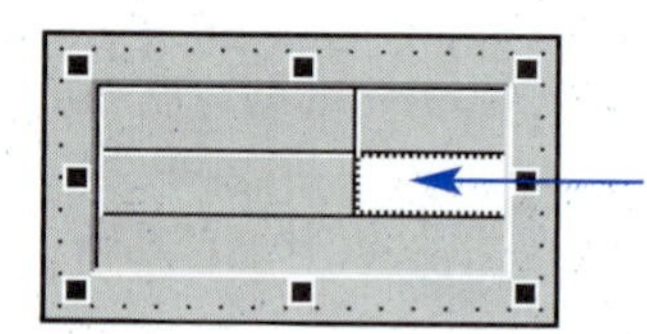

The Microsoft Hierarchical FlexGrid appears in the form after you double-click its icon in the toolbox.

Again, watch what control you are adding to your project. There is also a "Microsoft FlexGrid control," which works with the intrinsic data control. The name of the control you should add to your project is the "Microsoft Hierarchical FlexGrid control 6.0 (OLEDB)."

You can bind this control to a recordset in exactly the same manner as the DataGrid. However, this control behaves differently in several respects when you run the project.

Properties of the HFG. The HFG does not have the AllowAddNew, AllowUpdate, or AllowDelete properties. Thus, there is no way you can allow the user to add, update, or delete any record in the recordset, as already mentioned. Also, the control does not automatically adjust its column or row size to the data field, unlike the DataGrid. Whereas the DataGrid automatically allows the user to adjust the row and column size by dragging the grid line in the fixed column or row area, the HFG allows the user to do the same only when its ***AllowUserResizing property*** is set "properly." This property can be set to one of the four different settings, as listed in the following table.

Setting	Constant Name	Explanation
0	flexReSizeNone	Default; no resizing is allowed.
1	flexResizeColumns	The user can resize the columns.
2	flexResizeRows	The user can resize the rows.
3	flexResizeBoth	The user can resize both the columns and rows.

Binding the HFG. For practice, start a new project and complete the following steps to create a HFG bound to the Authors table of the Biblio database.

1. Add the ADODC and the HFG to the toolbox using the Components option of the Project menu.
2. Draw an ADODC on the form. Name the ADODC adcAuthors.
3. Set up the ADODC's ConnectionString and RecordSource properties. Connect the control to the Biblio database and set its RecordSource property to the Authors table.
4. Draw an HFG on the form. Adjust its location and size.
5. Name the HFG grdAuthors. Set its AllowUserResizing property to 1 (flexResizeColumns).
6. Set the HFG's DataSource property to adcAuthors.

Run the project. The result should appear as in Figure 8.12.

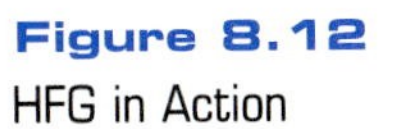
Figure 8.12
HFG in Action

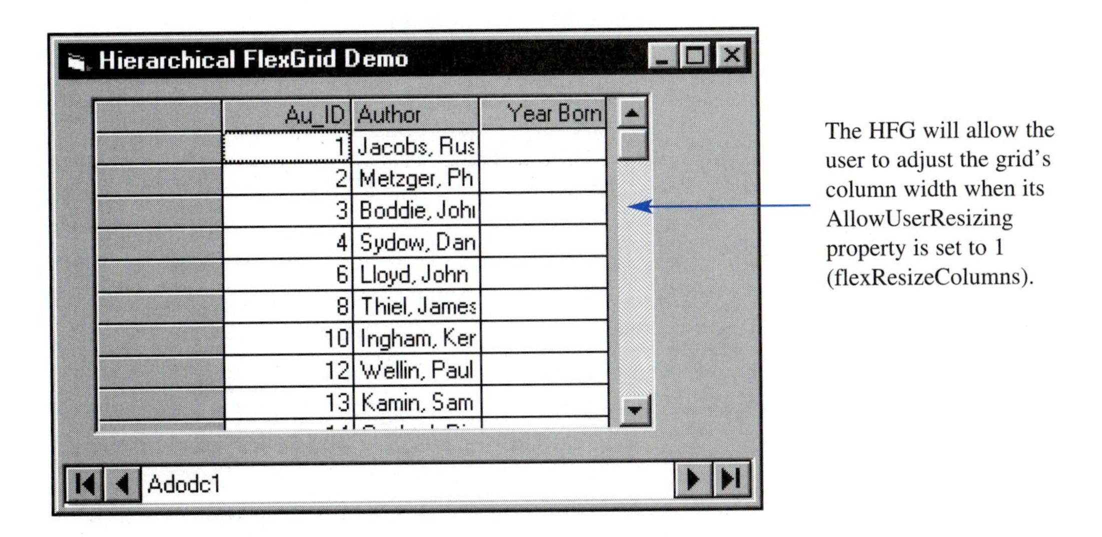

The HFG has many additional features and can be conveniently used to display reports and tables. Some of these additional features are further explored in Chapter 13, "Selected Topics in Input and Output."

Always use a three-letter prefix to name a VB control. The text uses "adc," "dtg," and "grd" as the name prefix for ADODC, DataGrid, and HFG, respectively.

Using the SQL with the ADO Data Control

Our preceding discussion focused on binding VB controls to an existing database table. The ADODC can also be used to handle the SQL. Several properties will have to be set differently:

- The ADODC's ***CommandType*** property has to be changed to adCmdText (for SQL), instead of adCmdTable (for an underlying table). You can do this at design time using the Properties window (select 2 in the CommandType property) or at runtime by coding the following:

  ```
  AdcAuthors.CommandType = adCmdText
  ```

- The ADODC's RecordSource property should be set to the SQL statement either at design time or runtime. If it is set at runtime, the control's refresh method should be executed to bring about the results.
- The HFG's DataSource property should be set at runtime because the resulting recordset to which this control is bound is not available until the execution of the SQL statement.

As an example, suppose you would like to display all authors with the last name "Smith." You can follow these steps to create the project:

1. Add the ADODC and HFG to the toolbox using the Components option of the Project menu.
2. Draw an ADODC on the form. Name it adcAuthors.
3. Set up the ConnectionString property for the ADODC. Do not set its RecordSource property.
4. Draw an HFG on the form. Name it grdAuthors. You may also want to set its AllowUserResizing property to 1 (flexResizeColumns).
5. Add the following code in the Form Load event:

   ```
   Private Sub Form_Load()
   Dim SQL As String
       SQL = "Select * From Authors Where Author Like 'Smith%'"
       adcAuthors.CommandType = adCmdText
       adcAuthors.RecordSource = SQL
       adcAuthors.Refresh
       Set grdAuthors.DataSource = adcAuthors
   End Sub
   ```

Several points in the preceding code are worth your attention.

- The SQL to be passed to the ADO should be enclosed in a pair of double quotes as a string, which is assigned to the RecordSource property of the ADODC.
- The Author field in the Authors table is of the String type. Thus, the search criterion in the SQL, "Smith%," should be enclosed in a pair of single quotes.
- The ADODC's Refresh method is used to activate SQL query to generate the resulting recordset. The method is analogous to an Open statement in a file operation.
- The grid's DataSource property is set to adcAuthors by a Set statement. adcAuthors is an object (a control), which cannot be assigned with an assignment statement to a variable/property directly. The Set statement associates the DataSource property (of the HFG) with the ADODC.

As explained previously, the HFG's DataSource property should not be set at design time because the recordset is not ready until the execution of the ADODC's Refresh method. Notice also that the

ADODC's ***CommandType*** property is set by code to adCmdText indicating that the RecordSource is a SQL statement. This can actually be done at design time using the Properties window.

Using the DataGrid with SQL. Of course, the same process can also be done with a DataGrid. Note also that the SQL query does not have to be limited to one data table. For example, the following code will make the grid (named dtgAuthors) display all authors with a name beginning with "Smith" along with the author's book(s). The query result will be sorted by the authors' ID number.

```
Private Sub Form_Load()
Dim SQL As String
    SQL = "Select Author, Title From Authors " _
      & " Inner Join ([Title Author] Inner Join" _
      & " Titles on Titles.ISBN = [Title author].ISBN) " _
      & " on Authors.Au_ID = [Title Author].Au_ID " _
      & " Where Author Like 'Smith%'" _
      & " Order by Authors.Au_ID"
    adcAuthors.CommandType = adCmdText
    adcAuthors.RecordSource = SQL
    adcAuthors.Refresh
    Set dtgAuthors.DataSource = adcAuthors
End Sub
```

The SQL in the code involves three data tables, although only two fields are selected. Our objective is to find the books written by all the Smiths. However, there is no field in the Titles table that indicates the author of a book. This table does have a field ISBN, which also appears in the Title Author table, which has an AU_ID field. The AU_ID field also appears in the Authors table. Thus, our query begins with an Inner Join of the Title Author and Titles tables (in the pair of parentheses) matched on the ISBN so that the author's ID (AU_ID) and the title of the book appear in the same record. This result is then inner-joined with the Authors table matched on the Author's ID, thus resulting in AU_ID, author, and title in the same record. Figure 8.13 illustrates the SQL steps. Figure 8.14 shows the query result.

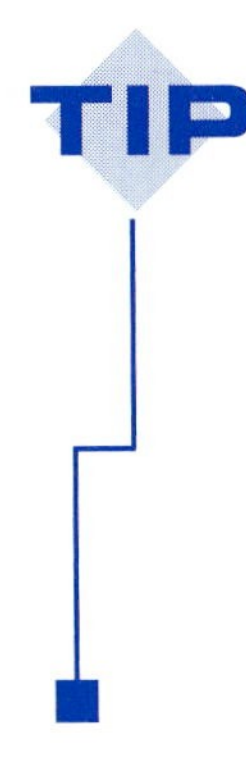

One of the most commonly found errors in coding an SQL statement is the missing spaces between clauses. This error is often made when the string is broken into several lines. Consider the following code:

```
SQL = "Select * From Authors" _
    "Where Author Like 'Smith%'"
```

There is no space within the pair of double quotes either immediately after "Authors" or before "Where." Thus, the two words will actually turn out to be "AuthorsWhere" when the VB compiler parses the string and passes to the SQL processor. An error message from the SQL will ensue at runtime. In such cases, always make sure that there is at least one space either after "Authors" (i.e., "Authors ") or before "Where" (i.e., " Where").

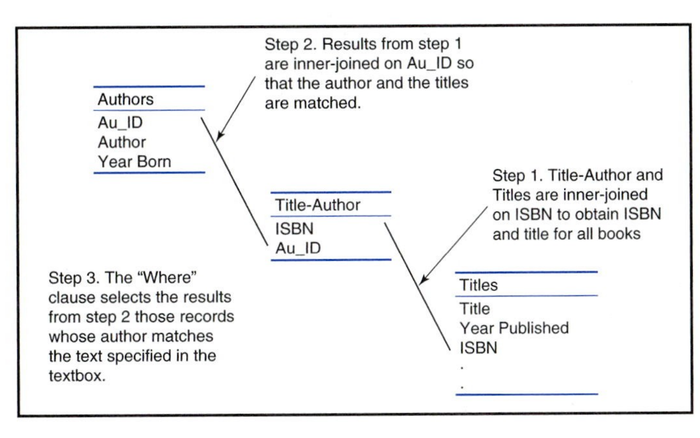

Figure 8.13
Steps in Extracting the Author and Title Fields for an Author

Figure 8.14
Sample SQL Result

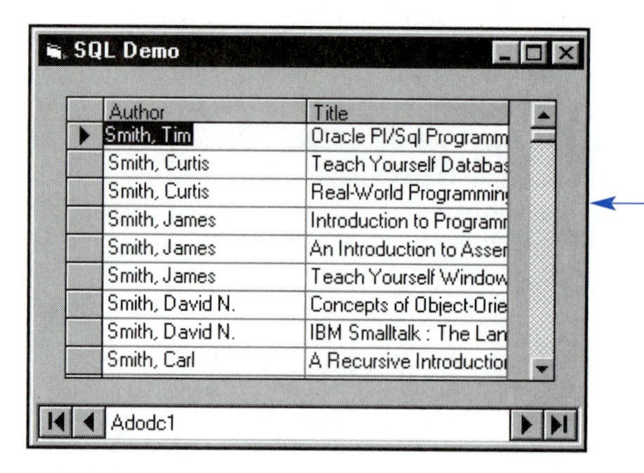

The ADODC and DataGrid can be used to display the results of an SQL query. This demo shows the result of querying the Biblio database for all the Smiths and the books they authored.

Populating an Unbound Control

As mentioned, you may not always want to bind a VB control to a recordset because of the need for flexibility. To illustrate how an unbound control can be populated, assume a form contains a text box (named txtName) for the user to enter a portion of the author's name. When the user clicks the Search command button (named cmdSearch), your program will show in a list box (named lstAuthors) all authors in the Authors table of the Biblio database with the names matching the string in the text box. How can this be done?

The first few steps should be the same as before:

1. Add an ADODC in the form and name it adcAuthors.
2. Set the adcAuthor's ConnectionString property. The Provider is Microsoft.Jet.OLEDB.4.0 (use 3.51 if your computer does not have 4.0) and the Data Source to the path for the Biblio database.

In code, you will need to construct an SQL statement to find all the authors with names matching the search string and assign this SQL to the ADODC as its record source. This step is similar to that in a previous example. The only difference is that the search string comes from the text box. The code should appear as follows:

```
Dim SQL As String
SQL = "Select Author From Authors " _
     & " Where Author Like '" & txtName.Text & "%'"
adcAuthors.CommandType = adCmdText
adcAuthors.RecordSource = SQL
adcAuthors.Refresh 'Build/Rebuild the record set
```

Notice how the "Where" clause of the SQL is coded. There is a space followed by a single quote (') after the "Like" operator. This string is then concatenated with the search string contained in the text box, which is then concatenated with a "%" (wild card character) followed by another single quote. If the text box contains "Smith," the "Where" portion of the SQL string will appear as follows:

```
Where Author Like 'Smith%'
```

The following SQL (constructed by a student of mine) fails to bring the desired results. Can you see why?

```
SQL = "Select Author From Authors "  & _
    " Where Author Like ' " & _
      Trim$(txtName.Text) & "%'"
```

Answer: Notice the extra space between the first single quote and the closing double quote in the Where line? That makes the actual SQL of the Where clause appear as follows:

```
Where Author Like ' Smith%'
```

The extra space causes the failure to recognize "Smith" as a match even when the student was so keen on avoiding extra spaces by using the Trim$ function. A brain teaser, isn't it?

After the SQL is assigned to the RecordSource property of the ADODC, the control's Refresh method is used to build the recordset based on the SQL string.

You can use one of the several Move methods to move around the recordset and thus access to the records. The following table lists these methods.

Method	Effect
MoveFirst	Sets the record pointer to the first record of the recordset
MoveNext	Sets the record pointer to the record next to the current one
MovePrevious	Sets the record pointer to the preceding record
MoveLast	Sets the record pointer to the last record of the recordset

Once the record pointer is set to a record, you can retrieve its content by code using various syntax structures. For example, all the following refer to the same data field from the previous query (for Author):

```
adcAuthors.Recordset.Fields(0) 'The first field in the record set
adcAuthors.Recordset.Fields("Author") 'The field named "Author"
adcAuthors.Recordset.Fields!Author 'Another way to refer to '"Author"
```

Fields is the default property of Recordset. Thus, the following lines are also equivalent:

```
adcAuthors.Recordset(0) 'The first field of the record set
adcAuthors.Recordset("Author") 'The field named "Author"
adcAuthors.Recordset!Author 'Another way to refer to "Author"
```

To populate the list box with the authors from a query, you can do the following:

1. Set the record pointer to the first record using the ADODC's MoveFirst method.
2. Use the list box's AddItem method to add the author in the record to the list box.
3. Move the pointer to the next record.
4. Repeat steps 2 and 3 until the entire recordset is exhausted. At that point, the recordset's EOF property will be True.

The code should then appear as follows:

```
adcAuthors.Recordset.MoveFirst 'Move to the first record
' Quit the loop when records are exhausted
Do Until adcAuthors.Recordset.EOF
     ' Add the author of current record to the list box
     lstAuthors.AddItem adcAuthors.Recordset!Author
     ' Move to next record
     adcAuthors.Recordset.MoveNext
Loop
```

Because not all queries will be successful in finding matching records (i.e., some queries can result in an empty recordset), we should add code to check the existence of records in the recordset. If the record set is empty, the preceding routine should not be executed. If the recordset is empty, both the *BOF* (beginning of file) and *EOF* (end of file) properties will be True. Thus, we can add the following line:

```
If adcAuthors.Recordset.BOF And adcAuthors.Recordset.EOF _
        Then Exit Sub
```

Also, the list box should be cleared before it is populated with the query results. Therefore, the following line should also be inserted before the loop:

```
lstAuthors.Clear
```

The Complete Procedure. The previous routine should be placed in the cmdSearch_Click event procedure because we want to populate the list box when the user clicks the Search button. The complete code should appear as follows:

```
Private Sub cmdSearch_Click()
Dim SQL As String
```

```
        ' Set up the record set with the following SQL
        SQL = "Select Author From Authors " _
          & " Where Author Like '" & txtName.Text & "%'"
        adcAuthors.RecordSource = SQL
        adcAuthors.CommandType = adCmdText
        adcAuthors.Refresh 'Construct the record set
        ' Clear the content of the list box
        lstAuthors.Clear
        ' If the query is empty, then do nothing
        If adcAuthors.Recordset.BOF and adcAuthors.Recordset.EOF _
          Then Exit Sub
        ' The following lines will populate the list box
        adcAuthors.Recordset.MoveFirst 'Move to the first record
        ' Terminate the loop when there is no more record
        Do Until adcAuthors.Recordset.EOF
            ' Add the author of current record to the list box
            lstAuthors.AddItem adcAuthors.Recordset!Author
            ' Move to next record
            adcAuthors.Recordset.MoveNext
        Loop
    End Sub
```

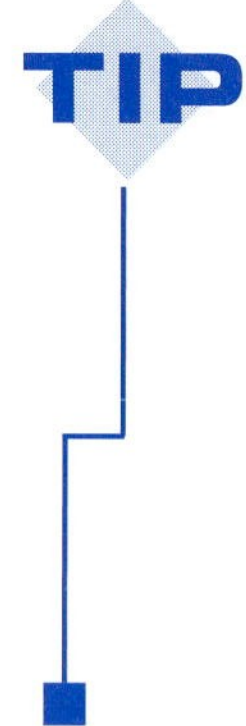

When your code refers to an object several times, you can minimize your coding effort and improve the code efficiency by the use of the With *Object*...End With coding structure. This structure allows you to omit the reference of the object within the structure when the object precedes a dot (.) or a bang (!). Thus, the routine to populate the list box can be coded as follows:

```
With adcAuthors.Recordset 'adcAuthors.Recordset is an object
    .MoveFirst
    Do Until .EOF
        lstAuthors.AddItem !Author
        .MoveNext
    Loop
End With
```

Using Unbound Controls for Input and Output

As mentioned in the first example, the bound text controls will automatically perform input and output on the underlying database table without code. When controls are not bound, you can still perform input and output on the data table by code. You will first associate an ADODC with the database table by setting the proper ConnectingString and RecordSource properties. To perform any I/O with the recordset, you will need to open it with the Refresh method first.

For example, suppose you would like to perform I/O on a Phones table in the Directory database:

1. Connect an ADODC (adcPhones) to the data table, specifying the provider as Microsoft.Jet.OLEDB.4.0 (or 3.51 if your computer does not have 4.0), the file path for the Directory as the DataSource, and the Phones table as the RecordSource.
2. Open the recordset as soon the project starts (because the I/O operations will be performed throughout the duration of the project).

So, you will place the statement to open the recordset in the Form Load event as follows:

```
Private Sub Form_Load()
    adcPhones.Refresh
End Sub
```

Once the recordset is open, you will be able to perform the desired input and output. The following discussion illustrates how to do the following:

- Display a record retrieved from the recordset.

- Update an existing record.
- Add a new record.
- Search for and update a specified record.

Displaying a Record. To show a record in the database table on an unbound control:

1. Point (move) to the record in the recordset.
2. Move the data in the record to the unbound controls.

To continue this example, assume the Phones table has two fields: Phone and Name. The Phone field is the primary key and is a 10-character text field with no embedded dashes (-). The Name field is a variable-length text field. Data in a record will be displayed in a masked edit box and a text box (mskPhone and txtName). Suppose you would like to show the first record when the user clicks the Show button. Your code will appear as follows:

```
Private Sub cmdShow_Click()
    adcPhones.Recordset.MoveFirst 'Move to the first record
    ' Move Phone Number to mskPhone with proper Format
    mskPhone.Text = _
      Format$(adcPhones.Recordset("Phone"), "(000)-000-0000")
    ' Move Name in record to txtName
    txtName.Text = adcPhones.Recordset("Name")
End Sub
```

Beware! Our discussion in this subsection involves *unbound* controls. When testing the code, be sure that the text boxes are *not* bound to the underlying table; that is, the masked edit box and the text box's DataSource and DataField properties must be cleared.

Updating an Existing Record. To update a record that has been just accessed:

1. Move the updated data to the recordset's data field.
2. Complete the operation with the Update method.

For example, assume that you would like to update the Name field just retrieved after the user corrects the name in the text box and clicks the Update button. You can code the following:

```
Private Sub cmdUpdate_Click()
    ' Note: This routine updates only the name field, phone
    ' number should be unchanged; that is,
    ' You can't change the primary key when updating.
    ' Move the corrected data to the field to be updated
    adcPhones.Recordset("Name") = txtName.Text
    ' Perform update
    adcPhones.Recordset.Update
End Sub
```

Adding New Records. What if instead of updating a record, you want to add a new record to the recordset? Then, you will need to use the recordset's AddNew method to prepare the record first. Suppose you want to add a new phone record to the Phones table when the user clicks the Add button. Your code will appear as follows:

```
Private Sub cmdAdd_Click()
    ' Use the AddNew method to prepare a new record
    ' You must do this before moving any data to the record
    adcPhones.Recordset.AddNew
    ' Move the phone # to the Phone field in recordset
    adcPhones.Recordset("Phone") = mskPhone.ClipText
```

```
        ' Move name to the name field in recordset
            adcPhones.Recordset("Name") = txtName.Text
            ' Then perform update
            adcPhones.Recordset.Update
End Sub
```

Notice that when you are adding a new record to the table (recordset), you must provide values to all fields that are expected to contain values. Otherwise, the field(s) will have a Null value. However, when you are updating a record, you only need to provide values to the fields that you want to update. All other fields will be left unchanged when your code performs the recordset's Update method. In addition, you must first set the record position properly (i.e., you must move to [or find] that record first) before any code to edit the fields is executed.

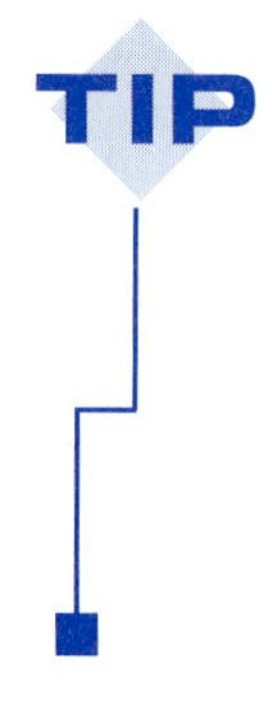

You can improve the efficiency of the preceding code by using the With...End With structure:

```
Private Sub cmdAdd_Click()
    With adcPhones.Recordset
        .AddNew
        !Phone = mskPhone.ClipText
        !Name = txtName.Text
        .Update
    End With
End Sub
```

Modifying Program Requirements. Let's modify the preceding program requirements slightly. Suppose we will allow the user to enter the phone number and name. Then when he or she clicks a button captioned "Save" (named cmdSave), the program will check to see whether the record exists in the Phones table. If it does, the record will be updated. Otherwise, the record will be saved as a new record. Thus, the process starts with determining whether the record exists in the table.

The Find Method. It is apparent that the record (if it exists) may lie anywhere in the recordset. It would not be efficient to search through the entire recordset for that record one by one using the MoveNext method. Rather, you should use the ***Find method*** to locate the record. The Find method has the following syntax:

```
Recordset.Find criteria, SkipRecords, searchDirection, start
```

where *Recordset* = the recordset in which the Find method is to perform the search

Criteria = a string expression similar to the Where clause in the SQL statement as the search criteria; for example, to find a match for an author whose name is Smith, you will code the following:

```
Author Like 'Smith%'
```

Skip Records = a Long integer indicating the number of records to skip before starting the search from the current record (zero is the default)

Search Direction = a value indicating whether the search is forward (default) or backward; the named constants are adSearchForward and adSearchBackward

Start = a bookmark specifying the position to start the search

The Start (the fourth) parameter requires a "***bookmark***," which is a variant variable representing the position of a record in the recordset. For example, the following code will keep the bookmark for the first record in the variable, FirstRec:

```
Dim FirstRec As Variant
adcPhones.Recordset.MoveFirst
FirstRec = adcPhones.Recordset.BookMark
```

After you use other Move methods to move away from the first record, you can set the bookmark of the recordset to the first record by coding the following:

```
adcPhones.Recordset.BookMark = FirstRec
```

This statement will make the recordset move back to the first record.

To go back to the example, you can use the Find method to locate the record by coding the following:

```
AdcPhones.Recordset.Find "Phone = '" & mskPhone.ClipText & "'"
```

Note again that because the Phone field is a text field, the phone number is enclosed with a pair of single quotes.

There are more restrictions in specifying the search criteria in the parameter for the Find method than those in a SQL statement. You can use a complex expression with logical operators (e.g., And, Or) in a SQL statement, such as follows:

```
Select * From PayChecks Where
(PayDate >= #01/01/2000#) And (PayDate <= #03/31/2000#;
```

However, you can use only the simple comparison expression in the criteria parameter for the Find method (with no logical operator). That is, you can only code the following:

```
rsPayChecks.Find "PayDate >= #01/01/2000#"
```

Then, you can use the If statement to filter out those records beyond March 31, 2000. Notice that to specify a date for comparison, you must enclose it in a pair of "#" signs.

Searching from a Specified Position. The preceding code will start the search from the *current record*, which may not be the first record. If the record you are searching for is located before this current record, the search will not be successful. To ensure that the record will be found, the search should start from the beginning. Assume the bookmark value for the first record has been assigned to the variable FirstRec. To search from the first record, the statement should be changed as follows:

```
adcPhones.Recordset.Find "Phone = '" & mskPhone.ClipText & "'" _
    ,,,FirstRec
```

In this line, the parameter values for "skip records" and "search direction" are left unspecified. Thus, their default values (skip 0 and search forward) will be used.

The EOF Property. When searching forward after the execution of the Find method, the Recordset's EOF property will be set to True if no match is found. Thus, if the Phones table has no phone number that matches the number in mskPhone, the EOF property will be set to True. You can use this indicator to take proper action. That is, if no match is found, you can use the AddNew method to add the data as a new record; otherwise, you will have the record ready for update. Thus, the code will appear as follows:

```
If adcPhones.Recordset.EOF Then
' No match found; prepare the recordset for a new record
    adcPhones.Recordset.AddNew
Else
' the record is ready; do nothing
End If
```

Once the way to treat the record is decided, the remaining code will be almost the same whether it is a new record or an update. The "complete" code appears as follows:

```
Private Sub cmdSave_Click()
' The routine update/add a record to recordset
```

```
         ' Find the matching record
         adcPhones.Recordset.Find "Phone = " & mskPhone.ClipText _
           ,,,FirstRec
             ' Is a match found?
           If adcPhones.Recordset.EOF Then
               ' No match found; prepare the recordset for a new record
                 adcPhones.Recordset.AddNew
                 ' Also move the phone number to the field in recordset
                 adcPhones.Recordset("Phone") = mskPhone.ClipText
           Else
                 ' A match is found; ready to update the record
           End If
           ' move name to the name field in recordset
           adcPhones.Recordset("Name") = txtName.Text
           adcPhones.Recordset.Update ' Then perform update
End Sub
```

Note that in the preceding code, the phone number is moved to the Phone field only when it is a new record. There is no need to do anything about the number if it is already the same, which is the case when the record is being updated.

Recall that you can perform I/O on the recordset only after the ADODC has been "refreshed" (opened). This should be done in the Form Load event. The variable for the bookmark FirstRec can also be set in this procedure. Thus, the code will appear as follows:

```
Option Explicit
Dim FirstRec As Variant

Private Sub Form_Load()
     adcPhones.Refresh
     adcPhones.Recordset.MoveFirst
     FirstRec = adcPhones.Recordset.BookMark
End Sub
```

A Note on Flexibility. Perhaps you should also notice the "flexibility" provided in the previous example by using the unbound controls. The masked edit control does not automatically handle its Mask property when bound. Thus, it is difficult to work with a bound masked edit box with a desired mask. Using the unbound controls, your code can take care of the formatting and clipping (using the ClipText property) in a usual manner.

8.3 Using the ADO Without the ADODC

The ADODC introduced in the preceding section has the capability to work with recordsets. It provides various means to manipulate the data, such as adding, updating, and deleting records. However, the ADODC is pretty "expensive" in terms of its resource consumption. You can actually use the ADO capabilities without having the ADODC; that is, *you can access data with the ADO just by code*. To do so, you will need to add the ActiveX Data Objects Library 2.1 (or 2.0 if your computer does not have version 2.1) to your project. Using the library, you can do the following:

- Perform input and output on database tables.
- Execute SQL statements that construct or perform operations on recordsets.
- Bind VB controls to recordsets by code.
- Bind VB controls to recordsets by the use of the data environment object, which is explained later.
- Execute SQL statements that perform DDL functions, such as creating tables in a database.
- Browse the database for table definitions (schema).

As you can see, the first four capabilities are those that the ADODC is able to perform. However, the last two capabilities are not provided by the ADODC. In fact, you will have more flexibility and capabilities by code without involving the control.

Adding the ADO Object Library to Your Project

As mentioned, to use the ADO capabilities by code only, you will need to add the ADO Objects Library to your project. Here are the steps to include the ADO Library in your project from the VB IDE:

1. Click the Project menu.
2. Click the References option (the one above the familiar Components option). The References dialog box should appear.
3. Locate "Microsoft ActiveX Data Objects 2.1 Library" in the list box and check the item. (See Figure 8.15. If your computer does not have version 2.1, then select 2.0.)
4. Click the OK button in the References dialog box.

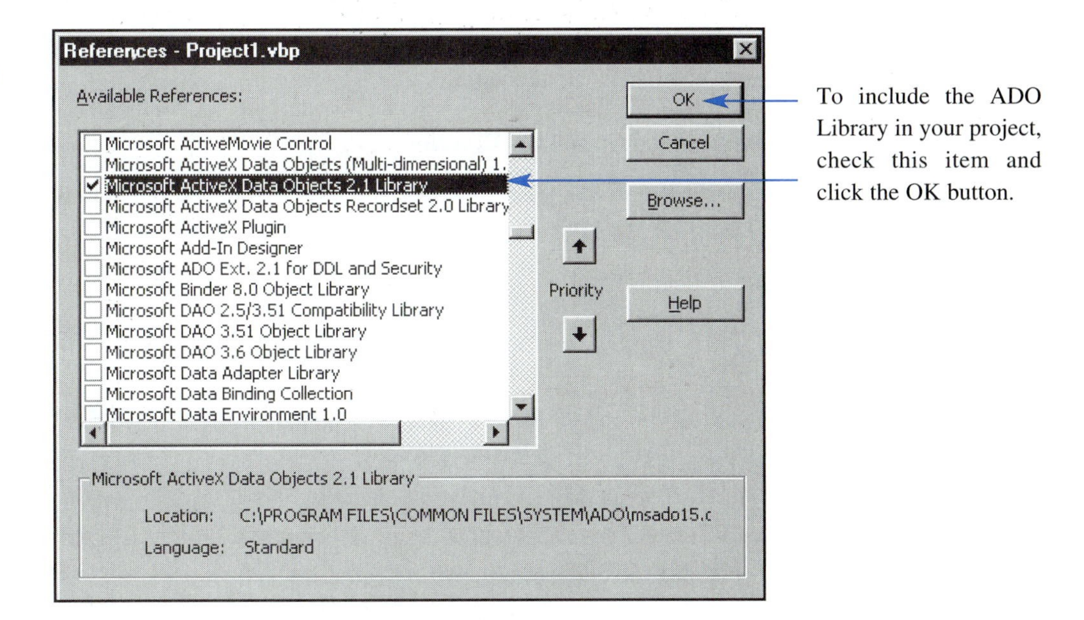

Figure 8.15
The References Dialog Box

After you add the reference, nothing will appear in the toolbox. Thus, you will not notice any difference on appearance. However, without adding the ADO Library and without an ADODC in a form, you will notice that none of the "vocabulary" related to the ADO are recognized by the VB IDE.

Objects and Object Variables

Before we proceed further, it is desirable to differentiate between two terms: the *object* and *object variable*. An *object* consists of code and data that work together as a unit. You have seen many objects that are visible at design time. All VB controls, including the ADODC, belong to this group. Some objects have no visible element at design time. The ADO objects are this type.

You can create a VB control and set its Name property at design time. Thus, in your code, you can readily reference the control by its name. At design time, however, you cannot create an object that has no visible element or set its name. You have to resort to code to accomplish both. In this case, you need to declare an ***object variable*** and then associate it with the object created by your code. It will be difficult to reference an object that has no name. Conversely, an object variable without being associated with an object has Nothing.

You can declare a generic object variable as follows:

```
Dim MyObject As Object
```

You can then associate the variable with any object by using the Set statement. For example, you can associate it with the adcAuthors' recordset that you used in the preceding example by coding the following:

```
Set MyObject = adcAuthors.Recordset
```

Then instead of coding:

```
adcAuthors.Recordset.MoveNext
```

you can just code:

```
MyObject.MoveNext
```

In general, your code will be more efficient when the object variable is declared as specific to its type as possible. In addition, you should always use a meaningful name for the variable. Thus, in actual practice, the preceding code should appear as follows:

```
' Declare a recordset object variable
Dim rsPhones As ADODB.Recordset
' Associate the object variable with the ADODC (object)
Set rsPhones = adcAuthors.Recordset
rsPhones.MoveNext 'Move to the next record
```

With this understanding of how to use the object variable, you are now ready to work with the ADO objects with code only.

Working with Recordsets by Code

To work with a recordset by code, you must create and open a recordset. A recordset can be opened in two ways:

- Use a connection's Execute method. To use this approach, you must create and open a connection object first.
- Use the recordset's Open method.

Creating and Opening a Connection Object. Let's look at the first approach first. Using this approach, you will do the following:

1. Declare an ADO connection object variable.
2. Create a connection object and associate it with the variable declared in step 1.
3. Open the connection.

To declare an ADO connection object variable, use the following syntax:

```
Dim Connection Name As ADODB.Connection
```

For example, to declare a connection variable for the Directory database, you can code the following:

```
Dim cnnDirectory As ADODB.Connection
```

To create a new connection object and associate it with an object variable, you use the Set statement with the New keyword. For example, you can code the following:

```
Set cnnDirectory = New ADODB.Connection
```

The expression on the right with the New keyword creates an ADO Connection object. The Set statement associates the variable cnnDirectory with this newly created object.

Finally, the syntax to open a connection appears as follows:

```
Connection.Open Connection String[, User ID][, Password][, Options]
```

where *Connection* = an object variable of the ADO connection type

Connection String = a text string that specifies the provider and the data source and is the same as you would specify for an ADODC

User ID = a string containing the username to use if the database requires one

Password = a string containing the password to use if the database requires one

Options = optional; can be used for remote connection if adConnectAsync is specified

The following code will declare an ADO Connection variable, associate it with a newly created Connection object, and open the connection:

```
' Declare an ADO Connection object variable
Dim cnnDirectory As ADODB.Connection
' Create a new connection object and associate it with
' cnnDirectory
Set cnnDirectory = New ADODB.Connection
' Open the connection with a connection string
cnnDirectory.Open "Provider=Microsoft.Jet.OLEDB.4.0;" & _
     "Data Source=C:\Directory\Directory.mdb"
```

Notice that the connection string used is the same as that required for the ADODC.

The Execute Method of the Connection Object. Once a connection is open, you can create a recordset by using the connection's Execute method, which has the following syntax:

```
Connection.Execute(Command Text[, Records Affected][, Options])
```

where *Connection* = a connection object variable

Command Text = a text string that contains an SQL statement, table name, or provider specific statement

Records Affected = a Long type variable returned by the provider indicating the number of records affected

Options = a Long type value that specifies how the provider should evaluate the command text (For example, adCmdTable specifies that the command text represents a table name. This is the same parameter that is used in specifying the CommandType property for the ADODC.)

For example, the following expression will open the Phones table as a recordset under the connection cnnDirectory.

```
cnnDirectory.Execute("Phones",,adCmdTable)
```

Associating a Recordset with a Variable. To refer to a recordset, you need to declare an ADO Recordset object variable first. To declare a Recordset variable for the Phones table, you code the following:

```
Dim rsPhones As ADODB.Recordset
```

You can then open the Recordset and associate it with this variable by coding the following:

```
Set rsPhones = cnnDirectory.Execute("Phones",,adCmdTable)
```

You may recall that there is a Set statement with the New keyword previously when we were creating the Connection object. No equivalent statement is used here. Why? A new recordset object is created by the connection's Execute method. There is no need to create another "new" object when the object variable rsPhones is being associated with the recordset object by the Set statement.

Using the Recordset's Open Method. Recall that you can also use the recordset's Open method to open a recordset instead of using the connection's Execute method. The recordset's Open method has the following syntax:

```
Recordset.Open Source, Active Connection, Cursor Type, _
     Lock Type, Options
```

where *Source* = a string that represents the name of the table or an SQL query

Active Connection = a connection object or a connection string to open a connection

Cursor Type = the type of "cursor" that the provider should use; refers to the manner in which the recordset can be accessed

Lock Type = the type of locks placed on records during editing

Options = a Long integer indicating how the string in the Source parameter is to be interpreted; for example, adCmdTable will indicate that the string is a table name, whereas adCmdText will indicate that the string is a SQL statement

The following table summarizes the four different cursor types.

Curser Type	Explanation
adOpenForwardOnly	The recordset can only move forward (the MovePrevious method will not be allowed).
adOpenKeySet	The recordset can be accessed in any direction or randomly. Changes made to records by other users are visible. Records deleted by other users are not accessible. In addition, records added by other users are not visible.
adOpenDynamic	The recordset can be accessed in any direction or randomly. Changes, additions, and deletions by other users are visible.
adOpenStatic	The recordset can be accessed in any direction or randomly. However, changes, additions, and deletions by other users are not visible.

Why different types of cursors? These cursors have *performance implications*. The forward-only cursor is the fastest, but it has many access restrictions. It will be most suitable when you need to read the recordset only once. The static cursor type will be most suitable for constructing reports or for applications in a single-user setting. The dynamic cursor is the slowest, but it reflects the current status of the recordset most accurately. It will be most suitable for applications in which the recordset must remain up-to-date all the time (e.g., airline reservation systems).

The four types of locks are listed in the following table.

Lock Type	Explanation
adLockReadOnly	Records cannot be edited.
adLockPessimistic	Lock the data source as soon as the record is being edited. Apply the most restrictive rule to ensure successful editing.
adLockOptimistic	Lock the data source only when the Update method is called.
adLockBatchOptimistic	Used in batch update mode with the optimistic lock.

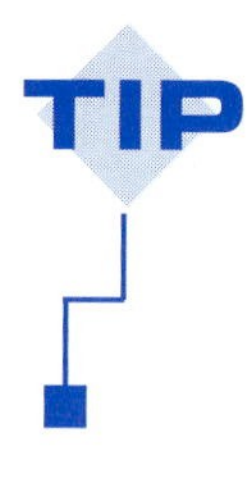

The default cursor type and lock type for the ADODC are adOpenStatic and adLockOptimistic. However, the default cursor type and lock type for ADO objects opened by code are adOpenForwardOnly and adLockReadOnly. The latter places emphasis on performance efficiency. Thus, when you use the ADO with code only, if you need to update data, you have to explicitly use the appropriate cursor type and lock type. For the single-user setting, adOpenStatic and adLockOptimistic will be the best choices.

When the cnnDirectory is already open, you can code the following to open the rsPhones recordset:

```
Dim rsPhones As ADODB.Recordset
Set rsPhones = New ADODB.Recordset
rsPhones.Open "Phones", cnnDirectory, adOpenStatic, _
    adLockOptimistic
```

Note that you will need to create a new ADO recordset and associate it with the ADO recordset variable (rsPhones) before you can use the variable to open the recordset. An object must exist before you can make it to perform it methods.

Using the Open method, you have a choice not to even open a connection explicitly. If you so choose, the code can appear as follows:

```
Dim rsPhones As ADODB.Recordset
Dim ConnStr As String
ConnStr = "Provider=Microsoft.Jet.OLEDB.4.0;" & _
    " Data Source=C:\Directory\Directory.mdb"
Set rsPhones = New ADODB.Recordset
rsPhones.Open "Phones", ConnStr, adOpenStatic, _
    adLockOptimistic
```

Why Open a Connection? It would appear that opening a recordset without having to open a connection is more direct. You would therefore be tempted to do so. However, when you do so, each recordset implicitly opens a connection. Thus, the number of open connections will be the same as the number of open recordsets. On the other hand, as shown previously, if you open a connection first, you can open a recordset either by the recordset's Open method or by the connection's Execute method. *You can open many recordsets under the same connection*. Apparently, if you have multiple recordsets that can be opened with the same connection, this approach will be much more efficient in terms of resource consumption. Incidentally, each ADODC requires two connections. This is why it is considered "expensive" to use.

There is a way that you can have several recordsets share the same connection even if a recordset is opened directly with a connection string. The recordset has an ***ActiveConnection property***, which represents the recordset's current connection. Assume rsOne and rsTwo are recordset variables, ConnStr is a connection string, and SQL1 and SQL2 are SQL strings. All these strings have been assigned with proper values. Then the following code will allow rsOne and rsTwo to share the same connection:

```
Set rsOne = New ADODB.Recordset
rsOne.Open SQL1, ConnStr
Set rsTwo = New ADODB.Recordset
rsTwo.Open SQL2, rsOne.ActiveConnection
```

Of course, you can also set the ActiveConnection to a connection variable. For example, assume cnnOne has been properly declared. You can code the following:

```
Set cnnOne = rsOne.ActiveConnection
```

Input and Output with ADO Code. To continue the Phone example, suppose the data-entry form that has the masked edit box (mskPhone) and the text box (txtName) also has a command button named cmdAdd. When the user clicks this button, the data on the screen will be saved. The code to save the record will be as follows:

```
Private Sub cmdAdd_Click()
    rsPhones.AddNew
    rsPhones("Phone") = mskPhone.ClipText
    rsPhones("Name") = txtName.Text
    rsPhones.Update
End Sub
```

You may recall that code and coding efficiency can be improved by using the With...End With structure for objects repetitively referenced in a procedure. Recall also that the following two different kinds of code syntax refer to the same field:

```
Recordset("FieldName")
Recordset!FieldName
```

Adopting the With...End With structure, we can code the above procedure as follows:

```
Private Sub cmdAdd_Click()
```

```
        With rsPhones
            .AddNew
            !Phone = mskPhone.ClipText
            !Name = txtName.Text
            .Update
        End With
    End Sub
```

The code structured this way is more efficient and should be considered "preferred" coding structure.

Reworking the Phone Project

You have learned quite a lot in this chapter. Perhaps it will help if we rework the Phone project to piece everything together. Rather than repeating the same previous requirements, we will modify the project slightly. The "new" project will be as follows:

- The visual interface will appear as in Figure 8.16, which contains a masked edit box (with label), a text box (with label), three command buttons (Save, Delete, and Quit), and a list box.
- The ADODC will not be used. All the requirements will be done by code.
- When the project starts, the list box will be populated with existing names and phones in the Phones table.
- When the user double-clicks a name on the list box, the corresponding record will be displayed in the two data fields.
- When the Save button is clicked, the program checks whether the phone number exists in the Phones table. If it does, the record is updated; otherwise, a new record is added.
- When the Delete button is clicked, the program checks whether the record exists in the table. If it does, the record is deleted; otherwise, a message indicating the nonexistence of the record is displayed.
- When the Quit button is clicked, the program quits.

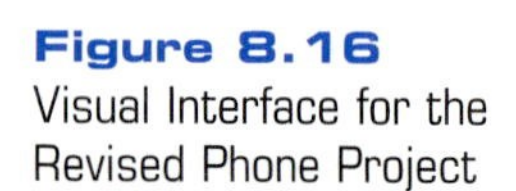

Figure 8.16
Visual Interface for the Revised Phone Project

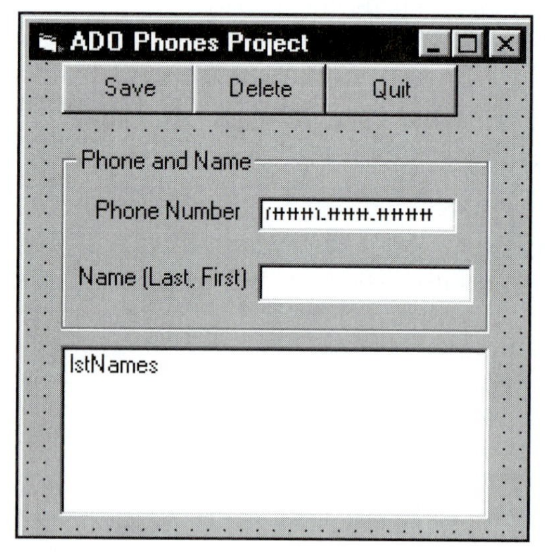

When the project starts, the list box will be populated with existing records. When the user double-clicks an item in it, the record will appear in the phone/name frame. The user can save or delete a record by clicking the proper command button.

Major Steps. Here are the key steps in developing the project:

1. Prepare the database and the Phones table. If the Directory database does not exist, you can create one using MS Access.
2. Add the Microsoft ActiveX Data Objects Library 2.1 (if it is not available, use 2.0) to your project from the References option of the Project menu. The steps have been described previously.

3. Design the visual interface. After all the needed controls as shown in Figure 8.16 are in place, set their properties as shown in the following table.

Control	Property	Setting	Remarks
Masked edit box	Name	mskPhone	For the Phone field
	Mask	(###)-###-####	
Text box	Name	txtname	For the Name field
List box	Name	lstNames	To display names
Command button	Name	cmdSave	To initiate the save routine
	Caption	Save	
Command button	Name	cmdDelete	To initiate the delete routine
	Caption	Delete	
Command button	Name	cmdQuit	To end the project
	Caption	Quit	

Code the project. The following discussion focuses on this aspect.

Declaring the Connection and Recordset Variables. Although we can elect to open a recordset without explicitly referencing a connection, we will use one here for practicing and building a habit for efficiency. The recordset variable will be referenced in different event procedures; therefore, it should be declared in the general declaration section. The connection variable will be used only once in this project. The reason for the use of a connection variable is that it can be used several times in a project. It will then appear more logical to place its declaration in the general declaration area. Finally, we will also declare a variable for bookmark. Its use should be obvious from the previous discussion. The declaration of these variables appears as follows:

```
Option Explicit
Dim cnnDirectory As ADODB.Connection
Dim rsPhones As ADODB.Recordset
Dim FirstRec As Variant 'For bookmark for the first record
```

Opening the Recordset. The recordset will be accessed in various procedures. It should remain open throughout the life of the project and should be opened as soon as the project starts. Thus, the code to open the recordset should be placed in the Form Load event as follows:

```
Private Sub Form_Load()
Dim ConnStr As Variant
    ' Construct connection string
    ConnStr = "Provider=Microsoft.Jet.OLEDB.4.0;" & _
      "Data Source=C:\vbsource\ado\directory\Directory.mdb"
    ' Create a connection object and associate it with cnnDirectory
    Set cnnDirectory = New ADODB.Connection
    ' Open the connection using the connection string
    cnnDirectory.Open ConnStr
    ' Open the Phones recordset through the connection
    Set rsPhones = New ADODB.Recordset
    rsPhones.Open "Phones", cnnDirectory, _
      adOpenStatic, adLockOptimistic, adCmdTable
End Sub
```

A Note on Creating the Recordset. In the code, the connection is open first. (Note that you may need to modify the connection string for the path to the Directory database.) The recordset is then opened using its Open method, rather than using the connection's Execute method. Recordsets *opened through the connection's Execute method assume several default settings*, which are not appropriate for recordsets to be used for updating operations. For example, the defaults for the cursor type and lock type properties are adOpenForwardOnly and adLockReadOnly, respectively. Furthermore, *bound grids cannot display properly recordsets created with these defaults.*

The recordset's Open method allows you to specify the cursor type as well as the lock type. As you can see, the recordset is opened with the adOpenStatic cursor type and adLockOptimistic lock type. These settings allow you to properly update the underlying database table under the single-user environment.

Populating the List Box. As soon as the recordset is open, the list box should be populated because we want the list box to show all records when the program starts. The following code can be inserted to the previous procedure:

```
' If there is no record in the recordset, then don't try to
'populate the list box.
    If rsPhones.BOF And rsPhones.EOF Then Exit Sub
    With rsPhones
        .MoveFirst 'point to the first record
        FirstRec = .Bookmark ' Keep the bookmark for future use
        Do Until .EOF
            ' Populate list box with phones and names
            lstNames.AddItem !Phone & vbTab & !Name
            .MoveNext
        Loop
    End With
```

Responding to the DblClick (Double-Click) Event on the List Box. When the user double-clicks an item in the list box, your program should show the corresponding record. The following code should accomplish this:

```
Private Sub lstNames_DblClick()
Dim Phone As String
    Phone = Left$(lstNames.Text, 10)
    With rsPhones
        .Bookmark = FirstRec
        .Find "Phone = '" & Phone & "'"
        mskPhone.Text = Format$(!Phone, "(000)-000-0000")
        txtName.Text = !Name
    End With
End Sub
```

In the code, the recordset's Bookmark is first assigned with the value of FirstRec, which has been assigned with the Bookmark setting in the Form Load event. This in effect makes the recordset point to its first record. Then, the recordset's Find method is used to search for the record with the matching phone number as extracted from the Text property of the list box. You may recall that previously, FirsRec was placed as the fourth argument in the Find method to perform the search. Why do it differently here? We have found that when the recordset's EOF property is True, the Find method does not perform as expected with the fourth argument. The current code ensures the correct result.

Notice that the Phone field is a text (string) field. Therefore the phone number is enclosed in a pair of single quotes as a part of the first parameter for the Find method. If the phone number is 1234567890, the statement with "Find" will appear as follows:

```
.Find "Phone = '1234567890'
```

A Note on a Design Issue. You may be wondering, "If all the data fields are already stored in the list box, why search the database table for the same thing?" After all, data in the list box are readily available. You have raised a perfect design question.

Our example is simplified to illustrate how a record in a recordset can be searched for and displayed in the controls on the form. The actual table that you would use to keep track of contact information of your friends probably will include many more fields such as Address, Email, and other remarks. In such a case, the list box will still hold a few selected fields as we have, whereas all other fields are retrieved from the recordset and updated when needed. The code illustrated here can be conveniently expanded to handle the additional fields.

Handling the Save Event. When the Save button is clicked, your code needs to decide whether the data in the controls represent a new record or an update of an existing record. Using the recordset's Find method, you can search for the phone number to see whether it exists. The code should be similar to that illustrated previously in the cmdSave Click event:

```
Private Sub cmdSave_Click()
Dim Phone As String
    Phone = mskPhone.ClipText
    With rsPhones
        If .BOF And .EOF Then
        ' The recordset is empty. There's no need to search.
        Else
        ' Look for the record as specified in the masked edit box.
            .Bookmark = FirstRec
            .Find "Phone = '" & Phone & "'"
        End If
        If .EOF Then
        ' Empty recordset or rec not found; prepare a new record
            .AddNew
            !Phone = mskPhone.ClipText 'move phone # to field
            ' Also add the new record to the list box
            lstNames.AddItem mskPhone.ClipText & vbTab & _
              txtName.Text
        Else
        ' Found the existing record; everything is ready
        End If
        ' Move name to name field
        !Name = txtName.Text
        ' Write the record using the update method
        .Update
    End With
End Sub
```

The first few lines of code involving the Find method may need additional explanation. This method can result in an error when the recordset is empty. Thus, we check the recordset's BOF and EOF properties. If both are True, the recordset has no record and there is no need to perform the search. Otherwise, the search will be done by the Find method. Before the Find method is used, the recordset's Bookmark is set to FirstRec so that the recordset will point to the first record. The need for this statement has been explained in the discussion of the list box DblClick event (p. 304).

Deleting a Record. When the Delete button is clicked, the record that is displayed on the screen (controls) should be deleted. In addition, the same name and phone in the list box should be removed for consistency.

To delete a record from a recordset, you can use the recordset's Delete method. For example, the following statement will delete the current record from the recordset, rsPhones:

```
rsPhones.Delete
```

When the user clicks the Delete command button, your code needs to take care of several details:

1. The "current" record must be set. The masked edit box mskPhone contains the phone number to be deleted. Therefore, you can use the recordset's Find method to search for the record that contains this number.
2. If the record is not found, it does not even exist. There will be no need to proceed further. However, a message should be displayed.
3. If the record is found:
    3.1 The record should be deleted from the recordset.
    3.2 The same item should be removed from the list box. To identify the item to remove, you can set up a For loop to check through the list box. The InStr

function can be used to check whether an item in the list box contains the phone number. The statement can appear as follows:

```
If Instr(lstNames.List(I), Phone) > 0 Then
```

The item that satisfies this condition is the one to remove. Once the item is removed the loop can be terminated.

The *complete code* for the Delete button's Click event appears as follows:

```
Private Sub cmdDelete_Click()
Dim Phone As String
Dim I As Integer
    Phone = mskPhone.ClipText
' Find the record and delete it from the recordset
    With rsPhones
        .Bookmark = FirstRec
        .Find "Phone = '" & Phone & "'"
        If .EOF Then
            MsgBox "Not an existing record."
            Exit Sub
        End If
        .Delete
    ' If the first record is deleted, we will need to reset bookmark
        .MoveFirst
        FirstRec = .Bookmark 'Reset the bookmark
    End With
    ' Find and remove the same from the list box
    With lstNames
        For I = 0 To .ListCount - 1
            If InStr(.List(I), Phone) > 0 Then
                .RemoveItem I
                Exit For
            End If
        Next I
    End With
    MsgBox "Phone no. " & mskPhone.Text & " deleted"
End Sub
```

The two statements immediately below the Delete method may require additional explanation. The MoveFirst method is executed, and the bookmark (FirstRec) to the first record is reassigned. These two statements are needed just in case the deleted record is the first record in the recordset. When this happens, the bookmark to the original first record will no longer be valid. These two statements ensure that FirstRec will point to the valid first record in the recordset.

A Finishing Touch. Objects created in a program are automatically destroyed when they go "out of scope." For example, if you declare and create a recordset in an event procedure, the recordset along with all the local variables in that procedure will be out of scope when the event procedure terminates. By the same token, form-level (module-level) objects are out of their scope when the form is destroyed.

There are situations in which the objects created should be destroyed before they are out of scope. In such cases, you should provide proper code. The following code will destroy the rsPhones recordset:

```
rsPhones.Close
Set rsPhones = Nothing
```

The Close method closes the object. The ***Nothing*** keyword in the Set statement dissociates the object variable rsPhones from the recordset object, allowing the object to be destroyed and releasing the resources used by both.

In our example project, the connection and recordset objects are needed for the duration of the project. They should go out of scope with the form. It is not necessary to provide code to destroy them. However, some writers maintain that it is a good practice to explicitly destroy the objects created in a program. The code provides a visual clue as to the exact timing that the objects are expected to terminate.

If we follow this practice, we should explicitly destroy the connection and recordset objects when the form unloads. Thus, we should add the following code:

```
Private Sub Form_Unload()
    rsPhones.Close
    Set rsPhones = Nothing
    cnnDirectory.Close
    Set cnnDirectory = Nothing
End Sub
```

Additional Remarks. The previous example, of course, has been simplified in several respects. For example, after the record is saved or deleted, the screen should be cleared. Similarly, a button to allow the user to clear the screen can be added. In addition, before a record is actually deleted, the program should confirm with the user about his or her true intention to prevent accidental deletion. There should also be code for data validation. Furthermore, as mentioned, a realistic database table should include more fields. All of these desirable enhancements are left to you as an exercise.

Coding the ADO with SQL

Recall the syntax to open a recordset using the connection's Execute method is as follows:

```
Connection.Execute(Command Text[, Records Affected][, Options])
```

The syntax for the recordset's Open method is as follows:

```
Recordset.Open Source, Active Connection, Cursor Type, _
    Lock Type, Options
```

In both cases, the first parameter can be either a table name or an SQL statement. Thus, to open a recordset with a SQL statement, you can use either of the two forms. (Recall, however, you can only open an adOpenForwardOnly, adLockReadOnly recordset with the connection's Execute method.)

Modifying the Author Title Project. As an illustration, consider the previous example to display all authors with the last name "Smith" and their books in a DataGrid. Suppose you want to display the same results without the ADODC. You can do the following:

1. Draw an HFG in the form, instead of the DataGrid. (The latter works only with ADODC.) Name the HFG grdAuthors.
2. Add the ADO library reference to your project.
3. Use the Recordset's Open method to generate the recordset.
4. Set the HFG's DataSource property to the recordset.

The following code shows how the recordset is created and the grid is bound to it.

```
Private Sub Form_Load()
Dim cnnBiblio As ADODB.Connection
Dim rsAuthors As ADODB.Recordset
Dim ConnStr As String
Dim SQL As String
    SQL = "Select Author, Title From Authors " _
      & " Inner Join ([Title Author] Inner Join" _
      & " Titles on Titles.ISBN = [Title author].ISBN) " _
      & " on Authors.Au_ID = [Title Author].Au_ID " _
      & " Where Author Like 'Smith%'" _
      & " Order by Authors.Au_ID"
    ConnStr = "Provider=Microsoft.Jet.OLEDB.4.0;Data Source=" & _
      "C:\Program Files\Microsoft Visual Studio\Vb98\Biblio.mdb"
    Set cnnBiblio = New ADODB.Connection
    cnnBiblio.Open ConnStr
    Set rsAuthors = New ADODB.Recordset
    rsAuthors.Open SQL, cnnBiblio, adOpenStatic, _
      adLockReadOnly, adCmdText
    Set grdAuthors.DataSource = rsAuthors
End Sub
```

As you can see from the code, the steps to open a recordset with SQL are exactly the same as those used to open a database table. The only difference is that the SQL statement is used in place of the table name in the first parameter of the recordset's Open method.

Other SQL Capabilities

The previous discussion focuses on the ADO's capabilities to handle the recordset. Actually, all SQL statements can be executed on the database using the connection's Execute method. These include the creation/dropping of tables and columns. For example, the following code will create a database table, JrnlHead, in the GL database. The table will have three fields: a Long type EntryID field, a Date/Time type TrnsDate field, and a String type Description field that is 50 characters long.

```
Dim cnnGL As New ADODB.Connection
Dim CreateJournal As String
    CreateJournal = "Create Table JrnlHead" & _
       " (EntryID Long, TrnsDate Date, Description Text(50))"
    cnnGL.Open "Provider=Microsoft.Jet.OLEDB.4.0;" & _
       "Data Source=C:\gl\gl.mdb"
    cnnGL.Execute CreateJournal
```

Note the last line in the code. Because the Execute method is not expected to return a recordset in this case, it is not set to any recordset variable.

Notice also that in the first line, the Dim statement declares cnnGL with the New keyword. When declared this way, cnnGL is a variable that is associated with a newly created connection object. This is another way to create a new object. You will then no longer need to use a Set statement to associate the variable with a connection object.

In terms of coding, this would seem more convenient. However, a potential pitfall with this approach is that after you destroy the object by setting the object variable to Nothing, if you accidentally reference the object or its property, the object will come to exist again. This situation can create "mysterious" problems for your code. For this reason, it is advisable to avoid using this way of declaring an object. In other words, the previous approach of declaring an object variable and then using the Set statement with the New keyword is still the preferred method.

As stated, a complete treatment of the SQL is beyond the scope of this book. Consult with an SQL book for information on additional SQL capabilities.

Browsing Database Table Definitions (Schema)

From time to time, you will have a need to browse through the database to verify the existence of certain tables or columns. The ADO connection provides such a capability with the OpenSchema method, which has the following syntax:

Connection.OpenSchema(*QueryType*[, *Criteria*][, *SchemaID*])

where *Connection* = the connection to perform the schema query

Query Type = a value specifying the type of schema query; for example, adSchemaTables specifies a query for the table names, and adSchemaColumns specifies a query for the column names in the database

Criteria = a Variant type array specifying the criteria for the query; different query type will require different array parameters (The online Help file provides a complete listing.)

Schema ID = a provider-specific parameter, not used by MS Access

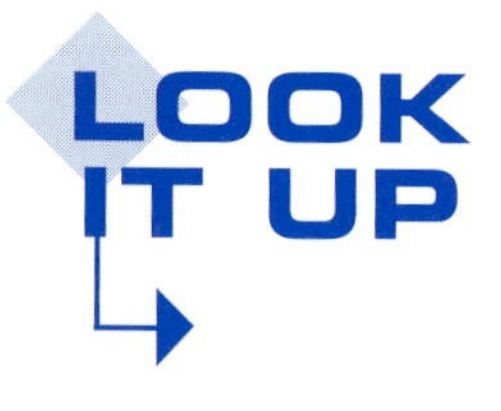

Use the keyword "OpenSchema Method" to search the Index tab of the online Help file. The page shows all available query types. In addition, it shows the available criteria under each query. The number of criteria varies from one to as many as seven, depending on the query type. These criteria are recognized by their positions in the array specified in the second parameter. For example, the query adSchemaColumns provides four criteria: TABLE_CATALOG, TABLE_SCHEMA, TABLE_NAME, and COLUMN_NAME. If you are looking for the columns for the Authors table, you will specify the array as Array(Empty, Empty, "Authors") because Table_Name is the third criterion in the parameter.

To illustrate the use of this method, let's consider a project. Suppose we would like to show all the tables of the Biblio database in a list box (named lstTables) as soon as the project starts. Then when the user clicks a particular table name in this list box, the field names of this table will show in yet another list box, named lstFields. Where do we begin?

As usual, we will begin with designing the visual interface:

1. Draw two list boxes on a new form.
2. Name the first list box lstTables and the second lstFields.
3. Draw an MS HFlexGrid onto the form. (You will need to add the control to the toolbox first.) Name this control grdSchema. Also set its AllowUserResizing property to 1 (flexResizeColumns) and the FixedCols property to 0 (this will allow all columns to contain data from the recordset). This control is not required in the project description. However, we will use it to show the results of some schema query. It is easier for you to understand the operation when you see the actual results.

Figure 8.17 shows the visual interface at runtime. Let's now consider the code.

Figure 8.17
Visual Interface for Querying the Table Definitions

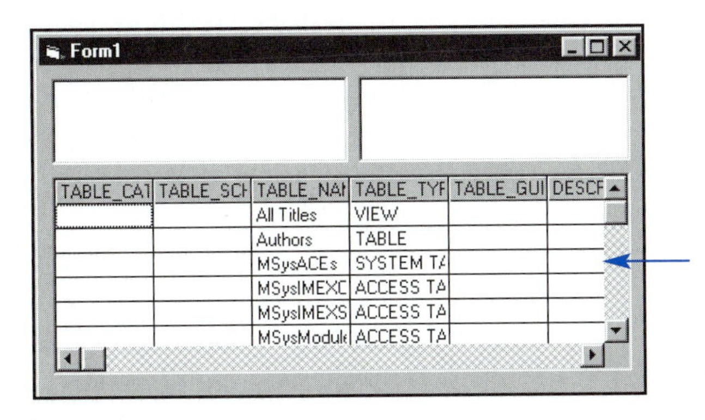

By binding the resulting recordset to an HFG from the OpenSchema query, you are able to see what the query can bring. The two list boxes above the grid will be used to display the tables and fields as specified in the project description.

Querying the Biblio Table Definitions. We will begin with opening the connection and will then use the OpenSchema method, specifying adSchemaTables as the query type. We will declare the connection variable in the general declaration area and open the connection in the Form Load event procedure:

```
Option Explicit
Dim cnnBiblio As ADODB.Connection

Private Sub Form_Load()
Dim rsTables As ADODB.Recordset
Dim ConnStr As String
    Set cnnBiblio = New ADODB.Connection
    cnnBiblio.Open "Provider=Microsoft.Jet.OLEDB.4.0;" & _
      "Data Source =" & _
      "C:\Program Files\Microsoft Visual Studio\VB98\Biblio.mdb"
End Sub
```

In the preceding code, we have also declared a recordset variable rsTables for the table query. We can then code our "first approximation" to query the "schema" (table definitions):

```
Set rsTables = cnnBiblio.OpenSchema(adSchemaTables)
```

What do you get with this line of code? To see the results, you can bind the HFG to this recordset:

```
Set grdSchema.DataSource = rsTables
```

The DataGrid can work only with the recordset generated with an ADODC. Thus, HFG is your only choice if you want to bind the returned recordset from the OpenSchema method to a grid.

Insert the preceding two lines of code in the Form Load event procedure and run the project. You should see that the HFG contains nine columns and many records. The columns include TABLE_NAME and TABLE_TYPE. Examine the TABLE_NAME column. You should see many unfamiliar names, whose corresponding TABLE_TYPE is SYSTEM TABLE (see Figure 8.17). Apparently, these are not user-created tables and should be filtered out.

Specifying the "Table" Criterion. To make the recordset return only the "Table" type, you will need to specify the criteria, which is the second parameter of the OpenSchema method. The following line of code should accomplish this (modify the preceding OpenSchema line as follows):

```
Set rsTables = cnnBiblio.OpenSchema _
    (adSchemaTables, Array(Empty, Empty, Empty, "Table"))
```

The second parameter in the OpenSchema method varies with the first parameter. When the first parameter is adSchemaTables, this second parameter expects an array that specifies four criteria: TABLE_CATALOG, TABLE_SCHEMA, TABLE_NAME, and TABLE_TYPE. Notice that the fourth criterion deals with the type of tables and is what we are interested in.

In the code, these criteria are specified with the ***Array function***, which returns an array of the given elements enclosed in the pair of parentheses. Because we are interested in only the fourth criterion, the first three are left ***Empty***, which is a special value indicating the absence of a value for an element of an array. The resulting parameter specifies that only the "Table" type tables are to be returned.

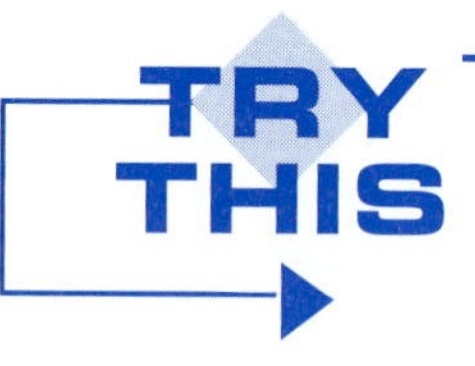

Want to know the names of the columns (fields) returned from the adSchemaTables query? Because the result of the query is a recordset (rsTables in our example), you can use the following code to identify the field names of the recordset:

```
For I = 0 To rsTables.Fields.Count - 1
    Debug.Print rsTables(I).Name
Next I
```

Even with the "Table" criterion, the resulting recordset still includes some table names that are system created, not user created. The names of all system-created tables begin with "Msys." Therefore, you can easily filter them out before showing the table names in the list box lstTables. The following code should accomplish this:

```
Dim TableName As String
rsTables.MoveFirst
Do Until rsTables.EOF
    TableName = rsTables("Table_Name")
    If Left$(TableName, 4) <> "MSys" Then
        lstTables.AddItem TableName
    End If
    rsTables.MoveNext
Loop
```

Again, the preceding code should be included in the Form Load event.

Querying for the Column Names of a Table. When an item (a table name in the database) in the list box lstTables is clicked, the field names in that table should appear in another list box, lstFields. Again, the OpenSchema method can be used to obtain the column (field) names. Because this method returns a recordset, a recordset variable (e.g., rsFields) should be declared. The statement to use the method should be as follows:

```
Set rsFields = cnnBiblio.OpenSchema(adSchemaColumns, _
    Array(Empty, Empty, lstTables.Text))
```

The first parameter (adSchemaColumns) specifies the query type to be "schema columns" (data fields). As mentioned previously, the second parameter varies with the first. Under adSchemaColumns, the second parameter specifies four criteria: TABLE_CATALOG, TABLE_SCHEMA, TABLE_NAME, and COLUMN_NAME. Notice that the third criterion relates to the table name. Because we are interested in only those columns of a particular table, the table name is specified as the third element of the second parameter. Note that you can omit the criteria after the criterion you need to specify. Thus, the Array function in the second parameter specifies only three criteria instead of four.

The code to populate the list box with the field names of the table selected by the user (by clicking the item) is given as follows:

```
Private Sub lstTables_Click()
Dim rsFields As ADODB.Recordset
    lstFields.Clear 'Clear the list box
    Set rsFields = cnnBiblio.OpenSchema(adSchemaColumns, _
      Array(Empty, Empty, lstTables.Text))
    Do Until rsFields.EOF
        lstFields.AddItem rsFields("Column_Name")
        rsFields.MoveNext
    Loop
End Sub
```

The returned recordset has a field containing the field names. The field name for this field is Column_Name. Thus, the expression rsFields("Column_Name") should give the field names in the database table.

You can easily modify this project to show the table definitions of any database. All you have to do is to change the database path specified in the connection string. Indeed, you can have the user specify the database path. Then the database path can be concatenated to the connection string to open the connection. Such an enhancement is left to you as an exercise.

8.4 Data Shaping: Hierarchical Recordsets

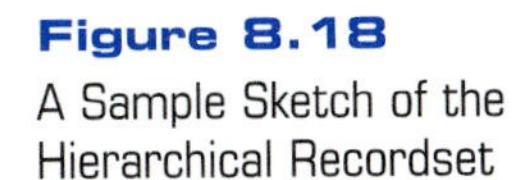

Imagine a sales database contains a Customers table and an Orders table. Each customer can place many orders. There is a one-to-many (parent-child) relationship between the records in the two tables. In a query of orders by the customer, it is traditionally done by an inner join operation with a Select statement.

The resulting recordset will have a customer for each order. Thus, the customer data are repeated when there is more than one order from the customer. The ADO 2.x provides a new way, called data shaping, to handle this situation differently. Data shaping allows you to retain the one-to-many (parent-child) relationship by creating a ***hierarchical recordset*** in which a parent record can contain a child recordset. This relationship can be depicted as in Figure 8.18:

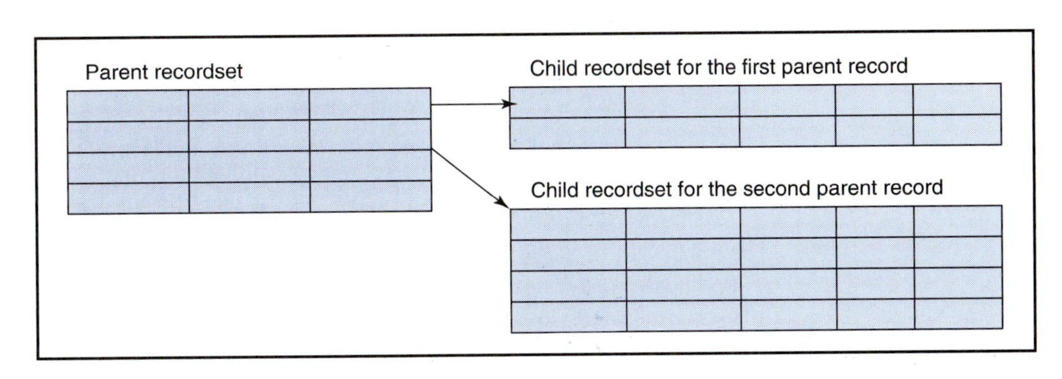

Figure 8.18
A Sample Sketch of the Hierarchical Recordset

Syntax

Data shaping requires a slightly different syntax to construct a "hierarchical" recordset:

```
Shape {Select ...} As ParentName
    Append ({Select....} As ChildName
    Relate ParentFieldName = ChildFieldName) As ChildName
```

Notice the pairs of braces ({ }) that enclose the Select clauses and parentheses that enclose the construct for the child recordset. They are required in constructing the statement. The ***Shape*** clause constructs a parent recordset. The ***Append*** clause creates child recordsets using the fields specified in the ***Relate*** clause to organize the relationship. For example, the following code will create a hierarchical recordset for the Customers and Orders:

```
Shape {Select * From Customers} As Customers
    Append ({Select * From Orders} As Orders
    Relate CustomerID = CustomerID) As Orders
```

The Authors-Titles Hierarchical Recordset. The same concept can also be applied to the Authors-Titles relationship; that is, an author can have several books. There is a one-to-many relationship that can be presented as a parent-child recordset relationship. For example, suppose we would like to show all authors and their respective book titles in the Biblio database. We can construct a query to generate a hierarchical recordset with the following statement:

```
ShapeStr = "Shape {Select Au_ID, Author From Authors}" & _
    " As Authors" & _
    " Append ({Select Title, Au_ID From Titles Inner Join " & _
    "[Title Author]  On Titles.ISBN =[Title Author].ISBN} " & _
    " As Titles " & _
    "Relate Au_ID To Au_ID) As Titles"
```

Note again that this query involves three tables. However, the relationship between the Titles and Title Author tables is a one-to-one relationship, whereas the relationship between Authors and Titles is a one-to-many (parent-child) relationship. Thus, we structure the Authors table as the parent recordset, while joining the Titles and Title Author tables together as a child recordset.

The Provider and the Connection String

The data shaping feature is handled by the MSDataShape provider. Thus, to construct a hierarchical recordset, you need to specify the provider by the following statement:

```
cnnShapeBiblio.Provider = "MsDataShape"
```

In addition, when opening the connection, the "Provider" specification in the connection string should also be changed to "Data provider," as illustrated here.

```
cnnShapeBiblio.Open " Data Provider=Microsoft.Jet.OLEDB.4.0;" & _
    "Data Source=" & _
    "C:\Program Files\Micorsoft Visual Studio\Vb98\Biblio.mdb"
```

Then you can open the recordset with the following statement:

```
rsAuthors.Open ShapeStr, cnnShapeBiblio
```

The Hierarchical FlexGrid, Again. The resulting hierarchical recordset can be bound to an HFG by associating the HFG's Data Source (or recordset) property with the hierarchical recordset. For example, assume you have an HFG in your form with the name grdAuthors. The entire recordset constructed previously can be displayed in the HFG with the following statement (to test the code, use the "complete" procedure given on page 314):

```
Set grdAuthors.DataSource = rsAuthors
```

The upper half of the form in Figure 8.19 shows the HFG containing the results.

Perhaps you have been wondering why the grid is called a "Hierarchical" FlexGrid. After all, a "FlexGrid" was also introduced in VB5 and is still available in VB6. The HFG is meant to be a replacement for the FlexGrid and is introduced to work with the "hierarchical" recordset.

Therefore, it gets this name for this extra capability. (Note also that the "old" FlexGrid is not compatible with the ADO and cannot be bound to an ADO recordset.)

Referencing the Hierarchical Recordset

How do you refer to a hierarchical recordset? The parent recordset can be referenced in exactly the same manner as a typical recordset. Thus, the Author column in the rsAuthors recordset can be referenced as follows:

```
rsAuthors!Author
```

The child recordset is referenced as a column in the parent recordset. For example, the Titles recordset (call it rsTitles) can be set with the following statement:

```
Set rsTitles = rsAuthors("Titles").Value
```

Notice how "Titles" is referenced in this statement and in the Shape statement in the preceding subsection. The "Titles" field here is the child recordset name in the preceding Shape statement.

To illustrate how the hierarchical recordset is referenced, let's continue the Authors-Titles example. Suppose we would like to display the authors (along with the ID) in a list box (named lstAuthors). Then when the user clicks an item (author name) in the list box, the books written by this author will appear on another list box, named lstTitles. The lower half of the form in Figure 8.19 shows lstAuthors on the left and lstTitles on the right. The routine to populate lstAuthors will appear as follows:

```
With rsAuthors
     .MoveFirst
     Do Until .EOF
          lstAuthors.AddItem !Author & vbTab & !Au_ID
          .MoveNext
     Loop
End With
```

Populating the List Box with a Child Recordset. As stated, when the user clicks an item in the Authors list box, the program will display all the titles of this author. The procedure to display the titles (records in the child recordset) given an author will appear as follows:

```
Private Sub lstAuthors_Click()
Dim Au_ID As Long
Dim P As Integer
     lstTitles.Clear 'Clear the list box
     P = InStr(lstAuthors.Text, vbTab)
     Au_ID = Val(Mid$(lstAuthors.Text, P + 1)) 'Obtain the ID
     ' Find the author record in the parent recordset
     rsAuthors.MoveFirst 'Start the search from the first record
     rsAuthors.Find "Au_ID=" & Au_ID
' Associate the child recordset with a recordset variable
     Set rsTitles = rsAuthors("Titles").Value
     With rsTitles
          Do Until .EOF
               lstTitles.AddItem !Title
               .MoveNext
          Loop
     End With
End Sub
```

As you can see in the code, the author's record is found by using the recordset's Find method, using Au_ID as the search key. Once the record is found, its "Titles" column (representing the child recordset) is associated with the recordset variable rsTitles by the Set statement. Then the loop to populate the list box with Titles by the author is just a typical routine.

The "Complete" Code for the Authors-Titles Example

The "complete" code to handle the Authors-Titles hierarchical recordset follows. The procedure to populate the Titles is omitted because it is already complete as shown immediately before this section.

```
Option Explicit
Dim cnnShapeBiblio As ADODB.Connection
Dim rsAuthors As New ADODB.Recordset
Dim rsTitles As ADODB.Recordset
Private Sub cmdOpen_Click()
Dim ShapeStr As String
Dim ConnStr As String
    Set cnnShapeBiblio = New ADODB.Connection
    cnnShapeBiblio.Provider = "MsDataShape"
    cnnShapeBiblio.Open _
      "Data Provider=Microsoft.Jet.OLEDB.4.0;Data Source=" & _
      "C:\Program files\Microsoft Visual Studio\Vb98\Biblio.mdb"
    ShapeStr = "Shape {Select Au_ID, Author From Authors}" & _
      " as Authors" & _
      " Append ({Select Title, Au_ID From titles Inner Join " & _
      "[Title Author]" & _
      " On Titles.ISBN =[title Author].ISBN} as Titles " & _
      "Relate Au_ID To Au_ID) As Titles"
    rsAuthors.Open ShapeStr, cnnShapeBiblio
    Set grdAuthors.DataSource = rsAuthors 'Bind the HFG to the
                                          'recordset
    ' Populate the list box with authors
    With rsAuthors
    .MoveFirst
    Do Until .EOF
        lstAuthors.AddItem !Author & vbTab & !Au_ID
        .MoveNext
    Loop
    End With
End Sub
```

You can see the complete results of running this procedure in Figure 8.19.

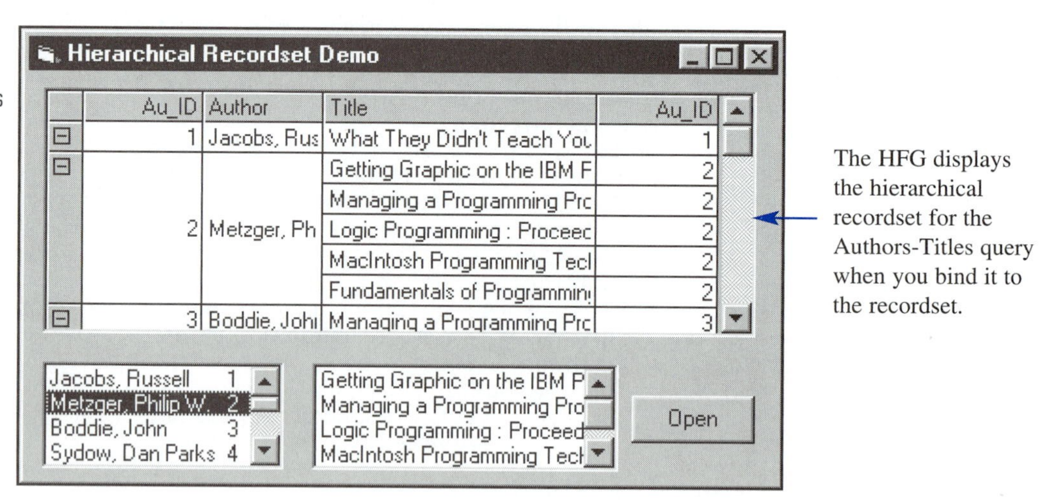

Figure 8.19 Sample Results of Hierarchical Authors-Titles Recordset

These two unbound list boxes display the results of the hierarchical Authors-Titles recordset. When the user clicks the author in the list box on the left, all books authored by him or her are displayed in the list box on the right.

The HFG displays the hierarchical recordset for the Authors-Titles query when you bind it to the recordset.

More on Data Shaping

Data shaping can also generate multiple child recordsets and multiple hierarchies resulting in a parent-child-grandchild recordset relationship. The following syntax illustrates how these can be done.

To generate multiple child recordsets:

```
Shape {Select...} As ParentName
    Append ({Select...} As ChildName1
        Relate ParentField1=Child1Field1) As ChildName1,
        ({Select...} As ChildName2
        Relate ParentField2=Child2Field2) As ChildName2
```

To generate hierarchies of child recordsets:

```
Shape {Select ...} As ParentName
    Append ({Select...} As ChildName
        Append ({Select...} As GrandChildName
            Relate ChildField1=GrandChildField) As GrandChildName
            Relate ParentField = ChildField2) As ChildName
```

As implied at the beginning of this section, data shaping is more efficient in terms of memory usage because only the pointers to the child recordset are kept in the parent records. However, this does not necessarily mean that it will perform faster in all cases. All records in the child recordset will have to be retrieved at one time. In a remote access situation, this can take quite a long time. Thus, the performance can vary from situation to situation. Coding for data shaping can become fairly complex and difficult. VB6 provides the Data Environment Designer that can aid the construction of code for this purpose. The next section provides a brief description of how to use the Data Environment Designer.

8.5 Using the Data Environment Designer

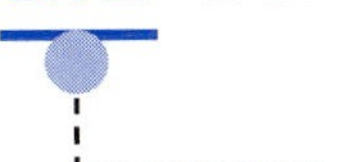

The Data Environment Designer comes with VB6. You can use it at design time to create "data environment" (DE) objects that can contain multiple connections with commands (which are just yet another type of ADO objects that can create recordsets and execute procedures). The DE Designer provides the capability to build SQL statements by drag and drop and point and click at design time. An interesting capability that DE objects have is to bind controls to recordsets without involving the ADODC. You can explore the online Help file for its full capability. The following walk-through examples introduce you to some of its uses. The instructions will make sense only if you actually work with the examples, step by step.

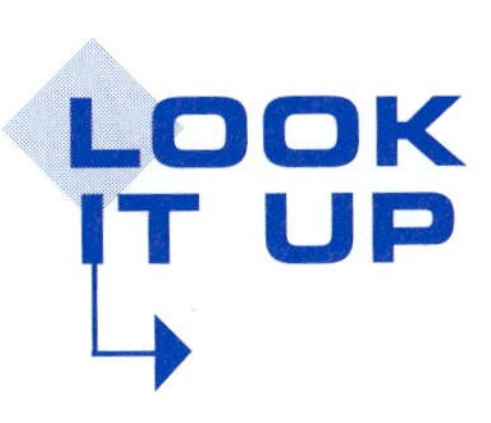

The data access guide has a tutorial about the Data Environment Designer. Go over the tutorial. You should be able to learn more about the capabilities of the Designer. One way to get to the tutorial is to start from the center of the online Help file and click Visual Basic. Then in the Visual Basic page, click the third item, Data Access Guide. The fifth chapter is titled "Tutorial: Interacting with Data in a Microsoft Jet/Microsoft Access Database." Follow the instructions in that chapter to gain familiarity with the Designer and to learn about its potential uses.

Example 1. Accessing the Authors Table and Binding a Hierarchical FlexGrid

In this example, we create a recordset built from the Publishers table in the familiar Biblio database. Here are the steps:

1. Start a new project.
2. Add a DE object to your project. Click the Project menu and select the "Add Data Environment" option. The DE Designer should come to action displaying the DE Design dialog box (form).
3. Change the name of the DE object from DataEnvironment1 to deBiblio. This should be very similar to the way you change the name of a control. First, click the DE object icon (which should have the name DataEnviroment1). Then click the Name property in the Properties window and enter "deBiblio."
4. Change the name of the connection object from Connection1 to cnnBiblio. The steps should be similar to those in step 3.

5. Set the properties for cnnBiblio.
   5.1 Right-click the connection's icon. A context menu should appear.
   5.2 Select the Properties option. The Data Links Properties dialog box will appear.
   5.3 Select Microsoft Jet 4.0 OLE DB Provider and then click the Next button. (*Note:* If you do not see MS Jet 4.0, use MS Jet 3.51.)
   5.4 In the Connection tab, click the "..." button to browse through your system to find and select the Biblio.mdb database.
   5.5 Click the OK button. (These steps are the same as those to set up the connection string for the ADODC.)
6. Add a command under cnnBiblio. Right-click the connection object. The context menu you saw before should appear. This time, click the Add Command option. You should see Command1 with its icon appear below cnnBiblio.
7. Change the command name to cmdPublishers.
8. Set the properties for cmdPublishers.
   8.1 Right-click the command icon. A context menu should appear. Select the Properties option and the Properties dialog box should appear.
   8.2 Click the drop-down button of the Database Object box and select the item Table.
   8.3 Click the drop-down button of the Object Name box and select the item Publishers.
   8.4 Click the Apply button.
   8.5 Click the OK button.
9. Drag the command cmdPublishers to your form.
   9.1 Click the Window menu of the VB IDE and select the "Tile Horizontally" option. You should see both your standard form and the DE designer form (dialog box).
   9.2 Use the *right* mouse button to drag cmdPublishers to your form. As you let go of the mouse, you should see a context menu, listing various controls to use.
   9.3 Select the Hierarchical FlexGrid.
10. Adjust the appearance of the grid.
    10.1 Click the Close button of the DE designer dialog box.
    10.2 Click the Window menu of the VB IDE and click the "Tile Horizontally" option again. Now, only your form should appear in the center of the VB IDE.
    10.3 Resize the grid to fit your form or resize the form to accommodate the grid.
11. Run the project. You should see the grid display the Publishers table.

Once you are familiar with the navigation steps around the DE designer, you will be able to see how easy it is to create bound control applications using the designer without involving the ADODC.

Example 2. Creating a Hierarchical Recordset

This example can be considered a continuation of the preceding example and will create a hierarchical recordset that contains the Publishers as the parent recordset and the Titles as the child recordset. Here are the steps:

1. Perform the steps listed in the preceding example from step 1 through step 8 so that you have the cnnBiblio and cmdPublishers created. Do not drag or drop any command to your form yet. A shortcut for this step will be to delete the HFG from the previous form and double-click the deBiblio object in the Object Explorer window to make the Data Designer form (dialog box) appear.

2. Create a child command for cmdPublishers.
   2.1 Right-click the cmdPublishers icon. A context menu should appear.
   2.2 Select the Add Child Command option. The command icon with the name Command1 should appear at the bottom of the list under cmdPublishers.
3. Change the name of the child command from Command1 to cmdTitles.
4. Build SQL for cmdTitles.
   4.1 Right-click the cmdTitles Icon. A context menu should appear.
   4.2 Select the Properties option. A Properties dialog box should appear.
   4.3 Select the SQL Statement option and then click the SQL Builder button. The SQL Design dialog box and the Data View window should appear.
   4.4 Drag the Titles table from the Data View window to the SQL Design dialog box. You can find the Titles table in the Tables folder under the cnnBiblio object in that window. If the folder is not open, double-click it and then look for "Titles" under it.
   4.5 Select the Title, Year Published, and PubID fields from the Titles list box, which becomes visible in the SQL Design dialog box after you drag the Titles tables here.
   4.6 Close the SQL Design dialog box by clicking its close button. You will be asked whether to save changes to query cmdTitles. Click the Yes button to save.
5. Add Relation.
   5.1 Right-click the cmdTitles icon. Select Properties from the context menu.
   5.2 Select the Relation tab in the Properties dialog box.
   5.3 Make sure that in the Relation Definition frame both the combo box for parent fields and the combo box for child fields show PubID as the selected field.
   5.4 Click the Add button.
   5.5 Click the Apply button.
   5.6 Click the OK button.
6. Drag cmdPublishers to your form from the DE Designer dialog box. Follow the same steps as outline in step 9 of the preceding example to drag this object.
7. Adjust the appearance of the HFG on your form. The steps should be the same as outlined in step 10 of the preceding example.
8. Run your project to see how the HFG looks.

The recordset created in this example is a hierarchical recordset, as you may be able to tell from the appearance of the HFlexGrid when you run the project. You can indeed inspect the Shape statement that this example creates. At design time (if you do not see the DE designer form [dialog box], double-click the deBiblio object in the Project Explorer window), right-click the cmdPublishers icon and select the Hierarchy Info option. You should be able to see the Shape statement in a window.

As you can see from the previous examples, the DE Designer makes it easy to develop code and objects to access databases. You can also use it to learn to write SQL statements. However, it is important that you understand the basic concepts of database. A good knowledge in database will enable you to use the DE Designer more effectively. In many cases, you will have to modify or add to the code generated by the Designer to satisfy the requirements of your applications.

Summary

This chapter focuses on working with the database. It begins with an introduction to the SQL. Then, the ADODC is introduced. The ADODC can be used to query or perform I/O on the database either with or without VB controls bound to the database. The use of bound controls minimizes the need for code in providing data access functionality. However, you will have much more flexibility in handling the data when the controls are not bound. In either case, the use of the ADODC consumes many more resources than using ADO with code only.

By using the ADO library, you can write code that not only can handle the recordset but also can perform DDL functions such as adding or deleting tables or columns. Such capabilities are carried out through the use of SQL statements. Thus, you will need to consult SQL books to enhance your ability to use the ADO. You have also been introduced to the concept of data shaping and hierarchical recordsets. Data shaping is a rather new technology. In many cases, it is more advantageous to use hierarchical recordsets than typical recordsets built by the use of the Join clause.

We conclude the chapter with two walk-through examples of using the DE Designer. Once you become familiar with it, you can easily use it to create command objects to construct recordsets, including hierarchical recordsets. These recordsets can be bound to VB controls without the ADODC. Thus, the DE Designer can be a helpful rapid application development (RAD) tool. However, you still need to know the fundamentals of coding with the ADO and SQL. This chapter covers many important concepts and topics. However, they only scratch the surface of data access and ADO. It is hoped that the chapter provides you with sufficient background for you to explore your knowledge in these areas.

Visual Basic Explorer

8-1. Default Cursor Type and Lock Type of the ADODC. Draw an ADODC on a new form.

Then, with the ADODC selected, look for the CursorType and LockType properties in the Properties window. What setting for each property do you see? (You should see adOpenStatic and adLockOptiministic, respectively, as the default setting for each.)

8-2. Binding Controls by Code with ADODCs. (continued from 8-1). Name the ADODC adcAuthors. Then, add three text boxes to the form. Name them txtAu_ID, txtAuthor, and txtYearBorn. Run the project. Click the arrow buttons in the ADODC. Did anything happening?

Then in the Form Load event, enter the following code:

```
Private Sub Form_Load()
    Set txtAu_ID.DataSource = adcAuthors
    txtAu_ID.DataField = "Au_ID"
    Set txtAuthor.DataSource = adcAuthors
    txtAuthor.DataField = "Author"
    Set txtYearBorn.DataSource = adcAuthors
    txtYearBorn.DataField = "Year Born"
End Sub
```

Run the project again. What do you see this time? Click the arrow buttons in the ADODC. Did anything happening? Although you did not set the properties in the text boxes to bind them to the recordset, the code in the preceding procedure accomplishes that. This approach provides you with some flexibility in binding and unbinding controls to recordsets. As discussed in the text, you have even more flexibility by not binding controls to the recordset. However, you do need to provide the code to perform whatever operations your applications call for.

8-3. Default Cursor Type and Lock Type of the ADO with Code Only. Start a new project. Add the ADO Library reference to the project. Try the following code:

```
Private Sub Form_Load()
Dim rsAuthors As ADODB.Recordset
Dim ConnStr As String
    ConnStr = "Provider=Microsoft.Jet.OLEDB.4.0;" & _
      "Data Source=" & _
      "C:\Program Files\Microsoft Visual Studio" & _
      "\VB98\Biblio.mdb"
```

```
        Set rsAuthors = New ADODB.Recordset
        rsAuthors.Open "Authors", ConnStr
        Debug.Print rsAuthors.CursorType; rsAuthors.LockType
        Debug.Print rsAuthors.CursorType = adOpenForwardOnly; _
          rsAuthors.LockType = adLockReadOnly
    End Sub
```

Verify that the data source parameter in the connection string is correct for your system. Run the project. What results do you see? Compare the results with those in Visual Basic Explorer Exercise 8-1. Do you see the same results?

8-4. Binding a Hierarchical FlexGrid by Code Only? (continued from 8-3). Draw an HFG on the form you have created for the preceding exercise. Name the grid grdAuthors. Add the following statement to the previous procedure:

```
    Set grdAuthors.DataSource = rsAuthors
```

Run the project. What do you see? Change the statement to open the recordset as follows:

```
    rsAuthors.Open "Authors", ConnStr, adOpenStatic
```

Run the project again. What do you see this time? You can bind the HFG to a recordset by code if the cursor type is not adOpenForwardOnly.

8-5. Can DataGrid Automatically Display a Hierarchical Recordset? The Authors-Titles hierarchical recordset example in this chapter demonstrates that an HFG can automatically display a hierarchical recordset when the HFG's record source is set to point to the recordset. Design a project to test whether the DataGrid can perform the same by using the same code example. (*Answer:* No.)

Exercises

Note: The Biblio and NWInd databases from Microsoft referenced in many of the following exercises are available in the VB98 folder of Microsoft Visual Basic 6 installed on your computer. If you are not familiar with the SQL but are familiar with MS Access, there is a way for you to learn the SQL. Make your query with MS Access first. Then, while in query design, you can view the SQL constructed by Access by clicking the SQL view option in the View drop-down menu. You can also use the DE Designer to build SQL statements as discussed in the last section of this chapter.

8-6. Browsing a Database Table with Bound Text Boxes. Add the ADODC to your project. Draw an ADODC, five labels, and five text boxes on a form. Align the data control at the bottom of the form. Align the labels vertically. Place the text boxes on the right side of the labels and align them vertically, too.

Name the ADODC adcCustomers. Set its Connection String property so that Microsoft Jet OLEDB 4.0 (or 3.51) is the provider and the NWInd database mentioned previously is the data source. Also, set the RecordSource property to the Customers table.

Set the DataSource property of the first text box to adcCustomers (the only one available in the drop-down list of this property). Then set its DataField property to the first field in the drop-down list of this property (CustomerID). Name this text control txtCustomerID.

In a similar fashion, set the DataSource property of all the remaining text boxes to adcCustomers. Then set their DataField properties to the second, third, fourth, and fifth fields available in the drop-down list of the respective DataField property. (The field names should be CompanyName, ContactName, ContactTitle, and Address). Name these text boxes the same names as the field names but with the "txt" prefix.

Start the program. Click the MoveNext button on the data control several times. Each time you click the button, you should see a different record. Click the MoveLast button to move to the last record. Click the MovePrevious button and you will be browsing the table backward. Click the MoveFirst button to go back to the first record.

As you are browsing the table, be careful not to accidentally change the content in the text boxes. This can change the corresponding record in the database table. To prevent this type of accidental updating, you can (and should) set the Locked property of each text box to True, ensuring that the text box is read-only.

8-7. Browsing a Database Table with Bound Label Controls. Replicate what you did in the preceding exercise on a new form with the following two changes:

1. Use the Authors table in the Biblio database instead of the Customers table in NWInd.
2. Replace the text boxes with the label controls. Make these labels look like text boxes by setting their properties properly.

Observe good naming practice; that is, give these labels the field names they are bound to but begin with the "lbl" prefix.

8-8. Browsing a Database Table with the DataGrid Control. Add the Microsoft DataGrid control and the ADODC to the toolbox of a new project. Draw an ADODC and a DataGrid control on the new form. Align the ADODC at the bottom of the form. Make the DataGrid cover nearly all the available space of the form. Name the ADODC adcOrders and the data bound control dtgOrders.

Set the Connection String property of the ADODC so that the provider is Microsoft Jet OLEDB 4.0 and the data source is the NWInd database. Also, set the ADODC's RecordSource property to Orders. Then set the DataSource property of the DataGrid control to adcOrders (the only choice in the drop-down list for this property.) To avoid accidental updating, set the DataGrid's Allow-Update property to False.

Run the project. Browse the table by clicking on the scrollbars (vertical and horizontal) on the DataGrid.

8-9. Browsing a Database Table with the MS Hierarchical FlexGrid. Replicate what you did in the preceding exercise in a new form with the following changes:

1. Replace the DataGrid with an HFG.
2. Name the ADODC adcAuthors and the HFG grdAuthors.
3. Delay setting the Connection String and Record Source properties for the ADODC until runtime:
   - 3.1 Use a common dialog box and provide code (in the Form Load event) for the user to specify the location of the database Biblio. Assign the filename obtained at runtime to the connection string. (You may want to create a Function procedure [name it GetFileName] for the code to prompt for the file path and invoke this function from the Form Load event. This function can be useful for many of your assignments as well as any actual work.)
   - 3.2 The table to be browsed is Authors.
4. Run your project. If you do not see any result, add the following line after the assignment of the Connection String and setting of the Data Source properties by code:

   ```
   adcAuthors.Refresh
   ```
5. Also, set the AllowUserResize property of the HFG to flexResizeColumns (1) so that the user can change the size of any column to fit its content.

8-10. Browsing a Database Table with the DataGrid Control (SQL). Modify your solution to 8-8 such that only the orders from Brazil are displayed. (The field to search on is ShipCountry. Note that at design time, you should clear the RecordSource property of the ADODC.)

8-11. Browsing a Database Table with the MS HFlexGrid Control (SQL). Modify your solution to 8-9 so that the user can specify a portion of the author's last name in a text box and when he or she clicks the search button, all authors with the specified last name will be displayed. Note that you should clear the RecordSource property of the ADODC at design time. The field name to search on is Author.

8-12. Browsing Database Tables with the DataGrid Control (SQL). Draw a DataGrid, an ADODC, and a command button on a new form. Connect the ADODC to the Biblio database. Provide the code to extract all the books published since 1995 with the following fields when the user clicks the command button.

Title (Book title)
Year published
Description
Name (Publisher name)

Display the results in the DataGrid. (Note that the SQL should involve two tables: Title Author and Publishers. Note also that the table Title Author should be coded as [title author] in the SQL.)

8-13. Populating an Unbound Combo Box with Data in Database Tables (SQL). Develop a project that will perform the following, using the Biblio database:

1. When the user clicks the Search command button after he or she enters a portion of the author's name in a text box, your code will construct a SQL statement to identify all the authors matching the search string, along with all the books each of these authors have published. The results should be sorted by author. (Use the SQL to perform the sorting.)
2. The search results should be populated by code in a combo box with the author's name on the left and the book title on the right. The combo box's Style property should be set to Dropdown List.

8-14. Populating an Unbound List Box with Data in Database Tables (SQL). Using the Biblio database, develop a project that will perform the following:

1. The user interface will let the user specify in two text boxes the range of years the books are published.
2. When the user clicks the Search command button, your code will construct a SQL statement to identify all books published during these years. The fields to retrieve should include year published, title of the book, and name of the author, sorted by year and book title.
3. The search results should be populated by code in a list box showing all three fields selected. Use vbTab to separate the fields.

8-15. Retrieving Data with Items Selected from a List Box. Use MS Access to create a database called Friends with a table named Directory, which has the following fields:

Field Name	Name	Description
Name	Name (Last, First Init)	Text field; make this an index field allowing duplicates
Phone	Phone Number	Text field (no embedded special characters such as parentheses or -); make this the primary key

Field Name	Name	Description
Address	Street Address	Text field
City	City	Text field
State	State Code	Text field
ZipCode	Zip Code	Text field

You can use this exercise and those following to create your personal directory. So, feel free to add more fields in this table.

Enter five records in the table directly from Access. Then develop a project that satisfies the following requirements:

1. Design a user interface that has all the aforementioned fields in a form. In addition, there should be a list box on the right side of the form to show the names and phone numbers in the table. None of these VB controls should be bound to the ADODC that is connected to the database table.
2. As soon as your project runs, the list box will be populated with the names along with their phone numbers in the table.
3. When the user double-clicks a name in the list box, your code will retrieve the record from the table and show the content in the user interface.

8-16. Saving Data Entered in Unbound VB Controls to a Database Table. (continued from 8-15). Add a Save command button to the interface you created for 8-15. Provide code to save a new record when the user clicks the Save button. You may also want to provide code for certain error checking. The minimum should include ensuring that the name and the phone number have been entered properly. After the record is saved, the screen should be cleared. Your code should display a "Record saved." message.

Note that the user can double-click the list box any time to retrieve an existing record. Thus, you should provide code to prevent an accidental loss of entered data. That is, if the user has already entered something in the form, your code should confirm with the user that it is okay to overwrite the data on the screen.

8-17. Adding and Updating Data Entered in Unbound VB Controls to a Database Table. (continued from 8-16). Modified the code in the preceding exercise such that at the time of saving the record, if the phone number is found to be already in the table, your code will verify with the user that this is an update of an existing record. If the user affirms, your program proceeds to update the record. Otherwise, your program will inform the user that no two records should have the same phone number (primary key).

Of course, if the phone number is not found in the table, your program should proceed to save the screen as a new record.

8-18. Replicating Exercises 8-15 Through 8-17 with Different Application Context (Inventory). Replicate what you did in Exercises 8-15 through 8-17 with the Products table of the Inventory database described as follows:

Field Name	Description	Remarks
ProductID	Product ID	Has a pattern aaa-nn where *a* = letter; *n* = number. Make this field the primary key
Name	Product Name	Text string; make this field an index with no duplicate
Description	Description	Text string

Field Name	Description	Remarks
Quantity	Quantity on hand	Maximum is 50,000; no fractional unit
Price	Unit cost	Ranges between 20 and 100 with decimal point

8-19. Logging Phone Calls to Your Friends (Expanding on the Friend's Directory Exercises). By working on Exercises 8-15 through 8-17, you have created a database table to keep track of the directory of your friends. Now, you would like to log all the phone calls you make to your friends. To do this, you will create another table, PhoneLog, in your Friends database. The table has the following fields:

Field Name	Description
RecordID	An auto number field for record identification; make this field the primary key
Date	Date phone call is made; date/time
Phone	The phone number you call (this enables you to identify whom you call)
Duration	Time length of the call
Description	A description of the content of the conversation

Develop a project that will satisfy the following requirements:

1. Design a user interface for the user to enter the logs. Note that the record Id need not be entered (or even shown). Note also that all phone numbers entered here must have already been in the Directory table. You may want to use a list box (similar to the one in 8-15) to show the names and phone numbers.
2. Provide the code to save the logs. Note that a future date would suggest a user error. Also remember to check the existence of the phone number in the directory.

8-20. Purchase Orders. (continued from 8-18). (*Note:* This project involves multiple forms and may be more suitable after you have learned to work with multiple forms.) After completing the requirements for 8-18, you would like to create an additional database table to keep track of the purchase orders for the same company. This table should have the following fields:

Field Name	Description
Order Number	Purchase order number; a seven-digit numeric field; primary key of the table
Date	Date of purchase order
Vendor ID	A six-digit numeric field
ProductID	The product ordered
Quantity	Quantity ordered
Price	Negotiated purchase price

Develop a project that will satisfy the following requirements:

1. Design a user interface for the purpose of performing the purchase order entry. Next to the product ID field, there should be a command button that allows the user to invoke a dialog box to search for the product ID. (We assume that there are many products and therefore it is not practical to use a list box in the same form for the purpose of search.)
2. Design a dialog box (another form) that will allow the user to search for the product ID. The user will enter a portion of the product name into a text box and then click a Search command button. There should be another command button for the user to signal that the search is complete. Use a HFG to display the search results.

3. Provide the code to save the data entered in the purchase order entry screen. The code should include error-checking routines. Note that the product ID must exist in the Products table. Also, the new purchase price will be considered "unusual" if it is 10% higher or lower than that in the Products table.
4. Provide the code to invoke the product search dialog box. Note that the procedure to invoke the search dialog box should wait until the search is complete before it proceeds to execute the remainder of the code in the procedure. The code should place the search result in the VB control for the product ID field. (Hint: To invoke the dialog box, use the following syntax:

```
FormName.Show vbModal
```

where *Form Name* is the name of the dialog box (form).

5. Provide the code in the dialog box to perform the search for the product. When the user clicks the Search button (after entering the search string), your code will display the search results in the HFG. When the user double-clicks an item in the HFG the item is "selected." The dialog box will disappear. The selected item is "picked up" by the code in the purchase order entry form as described in step 4. (*Hint:* When the user clicks a nonfixed cell of an HFG, its three properties are set to that cell: Row, Col, and Text.)

8-21. What Tables Are in a Database? Draw a command button and a list box on a new form. Name the command button cmdBrowse and set its Caption property to "Browse." Name the list box lstTables. Using the ActiveX Data Objects Library 2.1 (or 2.0), provide the code to obtain all the user-defined table names from the NWInd database and to place these names in the list box when the user clicks the Browse button. Note also that you need to add the ADO library to the project.

8-22. What Fields Are in a Database Table? (continued from 8-21). Add one more list box to the form designed in 8-21. Name this control lstFields. Now, add this additional feature to your project: When the user double-clicks on a table name in the lstTables list box, your code will show all the fields of this table in the list box lstFields.

8-23. A Generalized Database Table Definition (Schema) Browser. (continued from 8-22). Modify the interface and your code in 8-21 and 8-22 in the following manner:

1. Change the caption of the command button to "Browse a DB" and the name to cmdGetDBName.
2. Add a common dialog box to your form. Name it cdlFile.
3. When the user clicks the "Browse a DB" button, your code will prompt the user for a database to browse, using the common dialog box. The filename so obtained should be the data source specified in the connection string. Your code will then display all the user-defined tables in the lstTables list box.
4. When the user double-clicks a table name in the lstTables list box, your code will display all the fields of this table in the lstFields list box.

8-24. Creating DB Tables with ADO. Using the ADO, provide code to create the following two tables for a clinic:

Accounts table

Field Name	Description
Account Number	Numeric; Long integer
Name	Account holder name (Last First, Init); text
Insurance ID	Text

Patients table

Field Name	Description
Account Number	Numeric; Long integer
Patient Sequence Number	Numeric; integer 0 for the account holder
Name	Patient name
Sex	M or F

(*Note:* ADO cannot create a database. Use MS Access or VB's Visual Data manager to create one before attempting to add tables to it.)

8-25. Creating a Hierarchical Recordset. The NWInd database has a Customers table and an Orders table. Construct a hierarchical recordset that contains all customer orders in 1995. The parent recordset should contain CustomerID, CompanyName, and ContactName fields. The child recordset should contain OrderDate, ShippedDate, and CustomerID fields. The two recordsets are related by CustomerID. Display the results in a HFG.

8-26. Referencing a Hierarchical Recordset. (continued from 8-25) Add two list boxes to the preceding exercise. Name them lstCustomers and lstOrders. Populate lstCustomers with all the records in the parent recordset. When the user double-clicks a customer in lstCustomers, all orders by that customer will be displayed in lstOrders.

8-27. Adding and Updating Records with ADO by Code. Replicate Exercises 8-15 through 8-17 using the ADO by code only (without the ADODC). Note that now you can (and should) create the Directory table by the ADO using SQL statements instead of relying on MS Access.

8-28. Adding and Updating Records with ADO. Replicate Exercise 8-18 using the ADO by code only. Note that now you can (and should) create the Products table by the ADO using the SQL instead of relying on MS Access.

8-29. Using the Data Environment Designer. Use the DE Designer to develop a project to display (in a DataGrid) CompanyName, ContactName, and ContactTitle of all Suppliers (from the Suppliers Table of the NWInd database).

8-30. Using the Data Environment Designer to Create Hierarchical Recordset. The NWInd database has an Orders table and an Order Details table. Use the DE Designer to create a hierarchical recordset that retrieves Orders (OrderID, CustomerID, and RequiredDate) as the parent recordset and Order Details (all fields) as the child recordset. The two should be related by OrderID. Only the orders between 10301 and 10500 should be retrieved and displayed in an HFG.

Projects

Note: Many of the exercises that are related to each other in this chapter (e.g., 8-15 through 8-17 plus 8-19) are of the magnitude of a project.

8-31. Circle of Luck. Design a project that will play the Circle of Luck by two players. The visual interface appears in Figure 8.20. (The solution to the puzzle is "Dress for Success." Notice that the cells not expecting a letter are set to gray. You can accomplish this by setting the individual cells' CellBackColor property to vbGrayText.)

At the start of the game, the grid (HFG) at the upper-left corner displays the blanks where the puzzle phrase should appear. (Name the HFG grdPuzzle.) Cells expecting blank spaces should display a different color. The grid has 36 cells (3 rows and 12 columns). Below the grid, a label should show the category (e.g., movie star, idiom, history) of the puzzle. Another label should show who the current player is. (Name this label lblPlayer.) At the bottom of the form, there is another grid displaying the 26 letters of the alphabet. (Name this HFG grdAlphabet.) The label with the caption "Enter your guess" (name it lblGuess) and the text box (name it txtGuess) below it should be invisible.

The scores represent the amount each player has earned in the current game. The winner of a game gets the score added to the prize, which continues to accumulate until the program ends.

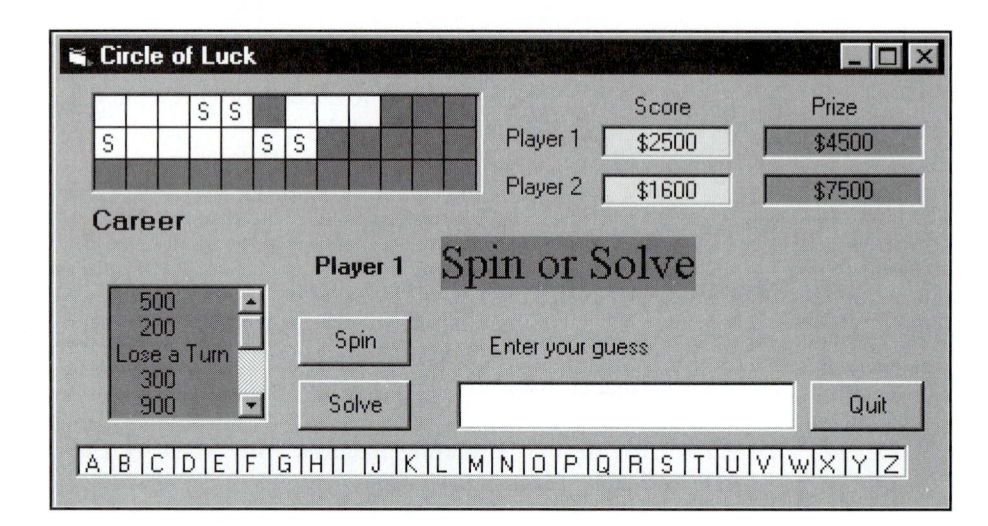

Figure 8.20
Circle of Luck

The label at the center of the form (name lblInstruct) displays different instructions to the player depending on the stage of the game:

A. When the games starts, it will display "Spin or Solve."

B. If the player clicks the Spin button and ends with an amount in the circle (list box), it displays "Pick a letter." The player is expected to click a letter in the grid at the bottom of the form.

- If the letter the player picks is found in the puzzle, the score is increased by the amount in the circle times the number of letters in the puzzle.
- If the letter is not in the puzzle, the next player gets his or her turn. (lblPlayer should display a different player.)
- Regardless of the outcome, lblInstruct will display "Spin or Solve" again.

C. If the player clicks the Spin button and ends with "Lose a Turn," the next player gets to play. Nothing else changes. (LblInstruct continues to display "Spin or Solve.")

D. If the player clicks the Spin button and ends with "Bankrupt," the player loses a turn. In addition, the player's score goes to zero. (LblInstruct continues to display "Spin or Solve.")

E. When the player clicks the Solve button, lblInstruct displays "Guess." In addition, both lblGuess and txtGuess will appear, waiting for the player to enter the solution. The player will press the Enter key to signal completion.

- If the solution is correct, the player's score is added to the prize. Both players' scores are cleared. A new game is automatically set up. (See the following for details.)
- If the solution is incorrect, the text box is cleared. The other player gets his or her turn.

Spinning the Circle. A random number will be drawn to determine how many positions the circle (represented by a list box) will spin. (Make the maximum possible advances three turns of the circle.) The end position determines the "luck" of the player as described previously.

You can make the list box emulate the spinning by assigning consecutive numbers to the control's list index in a loop. Try the following code fragment to get a feel:

```
For I = 0 To lstCircle.ListCount - 1
    lstCircle.ListIndex = I
    DoEvents
Next I
```

As the wheel advances, if the value to be assigned to the ListIndex reaches the upper limit (ListCount − 1), set that value to 0 and continue.

Source of Puzzle Phrases. Create a database with a table consisting of three fields: Record Number, Category, and Phrase. Enter at least 20 phrases (records). At the beginning of a game, use a random number to select the record number. Use the ADO recordset's Find method to retrieve the record. Display the category in the appropriate label. And use the phrase as the puzzle.

Hints:

- Use the Custom dialog box in the Properties window to set the HFG's rows and columns. Also set its FixedRows and FixedCols to 0. (Click the HFG in the form. Then double-click (Custom) in the Properties window to start the dialog box.)
- The following HFG properties are pertinent to programming this game. Check the online Help file for their proper uses:

  Col, Row, ColWidth, TextMatrix, CellForeColor, CellBackColor
- You can hide the letters in the grid by setting the CellForeColor property to the same as CellBackColor. To set these properties for a cell, set the Col and Row property to point to the cell first.
- Disable the controls so that the current "state" does not expect them to respond when the player clicks on them. For example, when the instruction is "Pick a Letter," the Spin or Solve button should not be active and should be disabled.

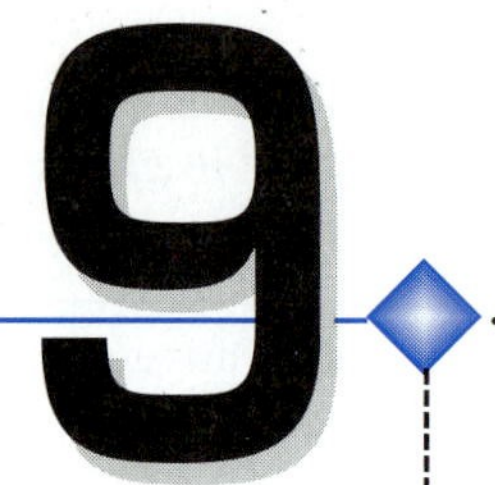

9 Arrays and Their Uses

So far, the variables we have used have been scalar variables. That is, each of these variables holds one value, a number or a string. Sometimes, you may encounter a situation in which your program needs to handle a large group of homogeneous data and it needs to access these data back and forth. In this case, using array variables will be more elegant and/or efficient. An array is a collection of more than one element of data and is collectively recognized by the same variable name. Each element in the array is indexed with the variable's subscript(s). You can refer to these elements by their indexes.

Although the concept of arrays appears simple, their applications can be fascinating. Their uses can make many complex problems much easier to solve. One interesting problem is sorting, which involves arranging data in order. The goal is simple and well defined, but the algorithms to solving the problem are diverse and fascinating.

Arrays are not limited to numeric or string data. You can also create arrays for controls. In many cases, control arrays can simplify your code.

An array can have one or more subscripts. The number of subscripts of an array is also referred to as the number of dimensions. Thus, an array with two subscripts is recognized as a two-dimensional array. Although most of this chapter is devoted to discussing uses of one-dimensional arrays, the last section deals with two-dimensional arrays.

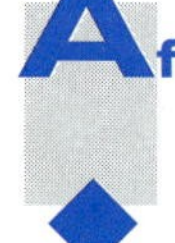

After completing this chapter, you should be able to:

- Create and use one-dimensional arrays.
- Understand some practical applications of one-dimensional arrays.
- Appreciate and implement several sorting algorithms.
- Know the different ways to create control arrays.
- Use control arrays properly and effectively.
- Create and use two-dimensional arrays.

9.1 One-Dimensional Arrays

Creating One-Dimensional Arrays

To declare a one-dimensional array, you use the Dim statement with the following syntax:

```
Dim Name([Lower bound To] Upper bound) As Type
```

where *Name* = any unique name that is legitimate as a variable name

Lower bound = lower value of the subscript; if not specified it *defaults to zero*

Upper bound = upper value of the subscript

Type = any data type, such as Integer, Long, and so on

Scope of Array Variables. Just like the declaration of scalar variables, the declaration of array variables can be placed in the general declaration area or in a procedure. Array variables declared in the general declaration area are form-level (module-level) variables and are recognized by all procedures in the form. Array variables declared in a procedure are local (procedure-level) variables.

Declaration Examples. Here are some examples of valid array declarations:

```
Dim A(5) As Double
Dim Student(1 To 50) As String
Dim Balance(1001 To 2000) As Currency
```

The first Dim statement declares A to be a variable containing six elements of the Double type with a subscript range of 0 to 5, as shown here:

A(0) A(1) A(2) A(3) A(4) A(5)

The second Dim statement declares a string variable, Student, to contain 50 elements with a subscript range of 1 to 50, as shown next:

Student(1) Student(2) ... Student(49) Student(50)

The third statement declares a Currency variable, Balance, to contain 1,000 elements with a subscript range of 1,001 to 2,000:

Balance(1001) Balance(1002) ... Balance(1999) Balance(2000)

Addressing Elements in an Array. Once the array has been declared, we can refer to individual elements in the array by the use of an index (subscript). For example, Student(1) refers to the first element in the Student array. Thus, you can code the following:

```
Student(1) = "Angela Allen"
```

This statement will assign the text string (name) "Angela Allen" to the first element of the Student array. You can then use the element just as you would any scalar variable. For example, to display the name, you can code the following:

```
MsgBox "The first student in the array is " & Student(1)
```

Similarly, A(5) refers to the sixth element in A. Notice that A's smallest subscript value is 0.

Using Variables as the Index. The index in the pair of parentheses does not have to be a constant. It can also be a variable or any expression that results in a numeric value. Thus, you can code the following:

```
Balance(N) = 10000
```

Depending on the value of N, 10,000 will be assigned to the corresponding element. That is, if N is 2,000, Balance(2000) will be assigned with a value 10,000. The ability to handle an expression as the index greatly enhances the flexibility and power of arrays, as we will see in the examples in the next section. Here are some simple uses of this capability:

Example 1. The following code lists all the names of students (assuming that the array has been properly populated with the names):

```
' List Student(1) Through Student(50)
For I = 1 to 50
    Print Student(I)
Next I
```

Recall that in the For loop, the counter I will vary from the starting value (1) to the ending value (50) with the specified increment. Because the increment is not specified, its default is 1. Thus, the loop will execute 50 times, with I taking on 1, 2, 3, ... 49, 50. The following execution table shows the process:

Iteration	I	Element of Student(I) Referenced	Example Result
1	1	Student(1)	Angela Allen
2	2	Student(2)	Bob Bunker
.	.	.	.
.	.	.	.
50	50	Student(50)	Zeff Ziegler

Example 2. The following code increases each element in Scores() (again, assuming that the array has been properly declared and populated with values) by 5.

```
' Add 5 points to Scores(1) through Scores(50)
For I = 1 To 50
    Scores (I) = Scores (I) + 5
Next I
```

Variable Size Arrays

When the size of an array cannot be determined until runtime, you can use the ReDim statement to size or resize the array when the information on its size is available. The syntax for the ***ReDim statement*** is as follows:

```
ReDim Name([LowerBoundExpression To] UpperBoundExpression) [As Type]
```

The ReDim statement can be placed only within procedures; that is, you are not allowed to use the ReDim statement in the general declaration section. The following are examples of valid uses of the ReDim statement.

```
ReDim A(10) As Long
ReDim Employees(1 To EmployeeCount) As String
ReDim Holder(3 * N)
```

If you use a variable as a part of an expression to compute the subscript of an array, the variable must have its proper value before the ReDim statement is executed. In the preceding examples, we assume proper values have been assigned to the variables EmployeeCount and N in lines 2 and 3.

Scope of ReDimed Variables. If the ReDim statement can be used only within procedures, does it mean that all variables sized with the ReDim statement are procedure-level (local) variables? Not necessarily. If the variable is "declared" only in a procedure with the ReDim statement (and nowhere else), it is a local variable. However, you can declare a form-level dynamic array variable by placing a Dim statement for that variable in the general declaration section with nothing inside the pair of parentheses for the subscript, as shown here:

```
Option Explicit
Dim Employees() As String
```

Then in a procedure, you can declare its actual size:

```
Private Sub Form_Load()
Dim N As Integer
```

```
' various statements, including one that sets the value of N
    ReDim Employees(N)
' other statements
End Sub
```

Note that in the preceding ReDim statement, the variable's data type does not need to be declared again (it has been declared as the String type in the general declaration section). If you do include the type declaration, be sure it is the same as in the original declaration; otherwise, an error will result.

Passing Arrays to Procedures. Sometimes, an entire array needs to be passed to another procedure for computation or data manipulation. To pass an array to a procedure, the called procedure must be written to expect an array as its parameter. The array argument to be passed should have the variable name followed by a pair of parentheses with nothing in between. The header of the procedure being called should be written in a similar manner. The following example illustrates the syntax:

```
Function Sum(A() As Double) As Double
'  statements
End Function
```

To pass an array (e.g., Salary) in another procedure to the Sum function, you can code the following:

```
Total = Sum(Salary())
```

Here we assume that the variable Salary has been properly declared as an array of the Double type.

There are additional fine points and interesting variations. They are further explored in the Visual Basic Explorer assignments at the end of this chapter. In general, it is advisable to observe the rules explained here for the robustness of your program.

Determining the Boundary of an Array. If you inspect the Sum function in the preceding example again, you may notice that any Double array can be passed to it. The array parameter passed each time may not have the same size. How does the function know the starting and ending subscript values to perform the summation? There are two built-in functions that can be used to solve this problem. The ***LBound*** and ***UBound functions*** give the lower and upper boundaries of an array. For example, LBound(A) will return the smallest subscript of the array A. Similarly, UBound(A) will return the largest subscript of A. Thus, the preceding Sum function can be written as follows:

```
Function Sum(A() As Double) As Double
' This function returns the total of a Double type array, A()
Dim Total As Double
Dim I as Long
     For I = LBound(A) To UBound(A)
          Total = Total + A(I)
     Next I
     Sum = Total 'Return total to the caller
End Function
```

Then, suppose in the Form Click event procedure, you code the following:

```
Private Sub Form_Click()
Dim Salary(101 To 103) as Double
Dim CashNeeded As Double
' Populate the Salary array with pay data
' In real operations, data will be read from a file
    Salary(101)=40000
    Salary(102)=80000
    Salary(103)=55000
' Compute total salary to arrive at cash needed for payroll
    CashNeeded = Sum(Salary())
    MsgBox "We need " & CashNeeded & " dollars."
```

```
    ' additional statements follow
End Sub
```

When the Sum function is invoked, the lower and upper bounds of the array parameter A will be exactly 101 and 103, respectively (because Salary's subscript has 103 and 105 as its lower and upper bounds, respectively). Thus, the For loop in the Sum function will be set up equivalently to the following:

```
For I = 101 To 103
```

All elements in Salary will be involved in the computation. The result should be correct. Test the preceding procedures. You should see the total cash needed is 175,000.

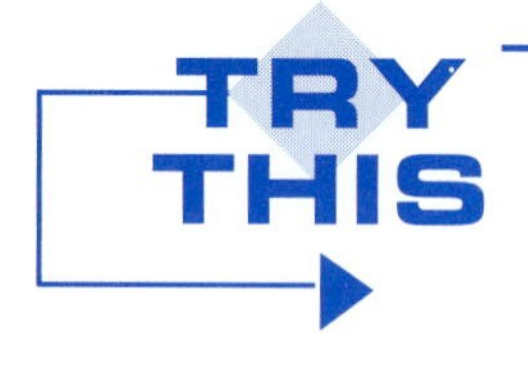

Enter the following code in a new form:

```
Option Explicit
Dim A() As Long
Private Sub Form_Load()
    ReDim A(100)
End Sub
Private Sub Form_Click()
    Debug.Print UBound(A); TypeName(A)
End Sub
```

Run the project and click the form. You should see the following in the immediate window:

100 Long()

This should indicate that A() is a form-level array variable with an upper bound of 100. In addition, it is of the Long type as initially declared. *The ReDim statement in the Form Load event does not (cannot) change its data type.*

9.2 Sample Uses of Arrays

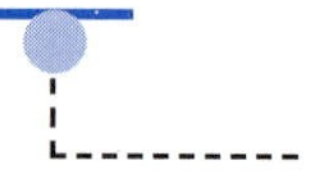

In addition to their uses in simplifying repetitive operations (as illustrated in the preceding examples), arrays can be used to solve various programming problems. It is difficult to exhaust the list of their uses. The following examples represent a small sample.

Simplified Selection

What is considered your normal weight? This depends on your sex, height, and frame size. For simplicity, let's consider only the case of males with a medium frame. The following table gives an abbreviated list.

Height (In Shoes)	Normal Weight
5'2"	118-129
5'3"	121–133
5'4"	124–136
.	
.	
6'3"	167-185
6'4"	172-190

Suppose your program is expected to give an answer when the user enters the height and clicks the Show command button. How can this be handled in code? (Assume the height is given in two text boxes: txtFeet and txtInches.)

When the program starts, we can populate the normal weight in an array. The array subscript can be declared in such a way that the subscript range corresponds to the height in inches. Then in response to repetitive queries, the height entered in the text boxes can be converted to inches, which can then be used as the index to obtain the weight stored in the Weight array. Thus, the Form Load event procedure may appear as follows:

```
Option Explicit
' Declare an array to hold weights for heights from 5'2" to 6'4"
Dim Weights(62 To 76) As String
Private Sub Form_Load()
' populate the weight array with data
' In real application, data will be read from a file
    Weights(62) = "118-129"
    Weights(63) = "121-133"
    .
    .
    Weights(76) = "172-190"
End Sub
```

The preceding code appears tedious. In real situations, the data should be stored in a file. Thus, the data will be read and assigned to each element one at a time with a loop. (See the next example for an illustration.)

How can the stored data be used when the user enters the height and clicks the Show command button? As explained, the entered height will first be converted to inches. This value can then be used as the index to obtain the weight data as illustrated in the following code:

```
Private Sub cmdShow_Click()
Dim Inches As Integer
' Convert height to inches
    Inches = Val(txtFeet.Text) * 12 + Val(txtInches.Text)
' Display the weight
    MsgBox "Your normal weight should be " & Weights(Inches) _
      & " lbs."
End Sub
```

The following table shows by example how the procedure works.

(User Entered) txtFeet	(User Entered) txtInches	Inches (Computed)	Weight(Inches)	Value of Weight(Inches)
5	2	62	Weight (62)	"118-129"
5	3	63	Weight (63)	"121-133"
6	4	76	Weight (76)	"172-190"

Suppose a person's height is 5'3". This height measurement will be converted to 63 inches by executing the line to convert the height. Thus, Weights(Inches) refers to Weights(63), which contains the string "121-133." The message box will display the following:

Your normal weight should be 121-133 lbs.

Note that the last line of code can also be done by the use of the Select Case structure as follows:

```
Select Case Inches
Case 62
    Weight  = "118-129"
Case 63
    Weight = "121-133"
Case 64
    .
    .
Case 76
    Weight = "172-190"
End Select
MsgBox "Your normal weight should be " & Weight & " lbs."
```

The code using this structure not only is much longer but also will have to be revised when the data change (over the years the height and weight can change). However, when you use the array and the data are stored in the file, the data can be revised without the need to revise the program.

Table Look Up

Imagine the information service desk of a midsize company. When a customer calls in to ask for the phone number of a particular employee, the clerk will use your program to find the needed information in response. How should you code this program?

Looking Up the Array. There are, of course, several ways to accomplish this. One possibility is to keep all the employees' names and phone numbers in two separate arrays; for example, (Employees() and Phones()). These arrays can be populated as soon as the program starts. When the clerk enters a name in a text box (e.g., txtName) and clicks a command button (e.g., Search), your program can search through the Employees array, find the match, and give the corresponding phone number. If the arrays have been populated properly, the following code should accomplish the search:

```
Private Sub cmdSearch_Click()
Dim TheName As String, I As Integer
    TheName = txtName.Text 'Get the name entered by the user
    For I = 0 To EmployeeCount -1
        If TheName = Employees(I) then
        ' The ith employee the name searched for.
        ' Give the ith phone number along with the name.
            MsgBox "The phone number for " & Name _
              & " is " & Format$(Phones(I), "(000)-000-0000")
            Exit Sub
        End If
    Next I
    MsgBox "Employee name " & Name & " not found."
End Sub
```

In this procedure, the name of the employee to look up from the Employees array is taken from the text box txtName. A For loop is then used to compare TheName with each element (name) in the Employees array. The loop counter, I, will vary from 0 to EmployeeCount – 1 (where *EmployeeCount* is a form-level variable used to represent the number of employees). When I is 0, TheName will be compared with Employees(0), the first employee name in the list. When I is 1, TheName will be compared with Employee(1), and so on. If a match is found, a message box will display the employee's name and phone number, which is presented with the proper format. The procedure is then terminated with the Exit Sub statement. If no match is found, the loop will continue until all employees in the list are compared. When the loop ends, the list of employees has been exhausted without a match. A message indicating the employee name is not found is thus displayed.

Populating the Array. In the previous procedure, we also assume that the value of the variable EmployeeCount has been set properly. How is the value of this variable set and how are the two arrays populated? Assume that the employee phone file has been properly created for "Input" operations (i.e., it has been created with the Write statement) and the phone number precedes the employee name in each record. The following code should accomplish populating the arrays and setting the value for EmployeeCount:

```
Option Explicit
Dim Phones(500) As Double
Dim Employees(500) As String
Dim EmployeeCount As Long

Private Sub Form_Load()
' When the project starts, this routine populates the Phones()
' and Employees() arrays
Dim PhoneNumber As Double
Dim TheName As String
Dim PhoneFile As Integer
' First, Open the file
    PhoneFile = FreeFile
    Open "C:\Employees\Phones.txt" For Input As #PhoneFile
```

```
' Populate the arrays
    Do Until EOF(PhoneFile)
        Input #PhoneFile, PhoneNumber, TheName
        Phones(EmployeeCount) = PhoneNumber
        Employees(EmployeeCount) = TheName
        EmployeeCount = EmployeeCount +1
    Loop
' Close the file
    Close PhoneFile
End Sub
```

You may have noticed that populating an array from a file is basically the same as populating a list box or combo box. You are exactly right. The steps are identical. Only the "objects" that you are populating are different. Also, you use the AddItem method to add items (elements) to the controls, but you use the assignment statement to add elements to arrays.

Tracking Random Occurrences

Arrays can conveniently be used to keep track of the occurrence of "random" events; for example, the number of times each customer called during a period, the number of purchase orders issued for each parts inventory, and the number of times each depositor made deposits in a month. All of these involve frequency counting.

Frequency Count. As an illustration of how arrays can simplify frequency count, consider this simple problem. You would like to know that given 1,000 random numbers in the range of 0 to 9, how many times each number appears. The first reaction is probably to code the count routine as follows:

```
For I = 1 to 1000
    Number = Int(Rnd * 10) ' generate a random # in range 0 - 9
    If Number = 0 Then Freq0 = Freq0 + 1
    If Number = 1 Then Freq1 = Freq1 + 1
         .
         .
    If Number = 9 Then Freq9 = Freq9 + 1
Next I
```

Notice the variables Freq0 through Freq9. Each is serving a similar purpose. Why not use an array, such as Freq() instead? If you declare the variable Freq() as follows:

```
Dim Freq(9) As Integer
```

you can use it in the following manner:

```
If Number = 0 Then Freq(0) = Freq(0) + 1
If Number = 1 Then Freq(1) = Freq(1) + 1
.
.
```

Now, inspect this line carefully:

```
If Number = 0 Then Freq(0) = Freq(0) + 1
```

The If condition tests whether Number is equal to zero. If so, Freq(0) is increased by 1. Note that if Number is zero, Freq(Number) and Freq(0) both refer to the same element. Thus, when Number is zero, you can code the following:

```
Freq(Number) = Freq(Number) + 1
```

That is, you do not need the If condition to accumulate total count for zero. It turns out that all the lines below this one are the same way. There is no need to test the value of Number! All you have to code to count the frequency is the following:

```
Freq(Number) = Freq(Number) + 1
```

This statement has the effect that when Number is zero, Freq(0) is increased by 1, and when Number is 1, Freq(1) is increased by 1, and so on as shown in the following table.

When Number Is	Freq(Number) Refers to	Effect of Freq(Number) = Freq (Number) + 1
0	Freq(0)	Freq(0) is increased by 1.
1	Freq(1)	Freq(1) is increased by 1.
.		
.		
9	Freq(9)	Freq(9) is increased by 1.

Thus, the statement can be used to replace *all* the 10 statements in the previous loop! The previous routine can now be rewritten as follows:

```
Dim Number As Integer
Dim Freq(9) As Integer
For I = 1 To 1000
     Number = Int(Rnd * 10)
     Freq(Number) = Freq(Number) + 1
Next I
```

To see the results after the count, you can code the following:

```
For I = 0 to 9
     Print I; Freq(I)
Next I
```

You can test the program by placing the preceding two loops in the Form Click event. Inspect the results. The total of frequency counts for all numbers should be 1,000. Note that the use of the array simplifies the code not only for counting but also for output.

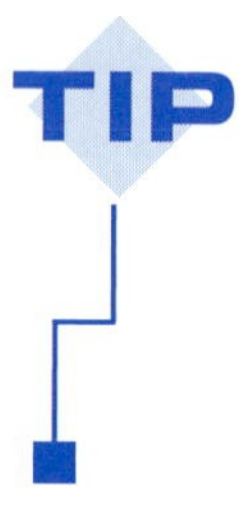

Beginners tend to associate the range of the loop counter with the size of the array involved in the loop. Beware of this general tendency (and misconception). The two are not necessarily related. If you inspect the second loop in the preceding example, the counter and the size of the variable Freq do correspond to each other because the counter is used to retrieve the content of each element in the array. However, in the first loop, the counter goes from 1 to 1,000, not from 0 to 9 (subscript of the array). They are completely independent of each other.

Counting Letters. How would you like to know how often each letter of the alphabet is used in our daily life? Let's assume you have a text box named txtText for the user to enter a long text string. Then when the user is ready, he or she clicks the command button "Count."

How should your program proceed to count? Recall that the ASCII value for "A" and "Z" are 65 (vbKeyA) and 90 (vbKeyZ), respectively. Before any letter is counted, it can be converted to uppercase. Then its ASCII value will have to fall in the range of vbKeyA (65) through vbKeyZ (90). Thus, if we declare an array variable LetterCount as follows:

```
Dim LetterCount(vbKeyA To vbKeyZ)
```

we will be able to use it to count the frequency of each letter in a fashion similar to the previous example. The following code represents a sample solution:

```
Dim LetterCount(vbKeyA To vbKeyZ) As Long
Dim I As Long
Dim Text As String
Dim Ascii As Integer

Text = txtText.Text 'Get the entered text
For I = 1 to Len(Text)
     ' Obtain the ASCII value of the character being inspected
     'Ensure the letter is uppercased
     Ascii =Asc(Ucase$(Mid$(Text, I, 1)))
```

```
        Select Case Ascii
        Case vbKeyA To vbKeyZ
        ' alphabet, count its frequency
            LetterCount(Ascii) = LetterCount(Ascii) + 1
        Case Else
        ' non-alphabetic characters, ignore
        End Select
    Next I
```

Notice that the subscript of LetterCount is declared with named constants as its range. This is certainly permissible (and more readable). To VB, the literal constants and their corresponding named constants have exactly the same values. The For...Next loop is used to inspect each character in the text string (from the first through the last character) one at a time using the Mid$ function. The character extracted is first converted to uppercase. Its ASCII value is then obtained using the Asc function. The ASCII value is used in the frequency count if it falls within the range of alphabet values, in a similar fashion to the frequency count for random numbers. If the ASCII value falls out of the range of the alphabet, it is ignored.

Want to inspect the results? The following code will display the results in a list box named lstResults:

```
' Output the results into a list box
For I = vbKeyA To VbKeyZ
    lstResults.AddItem Chr$(I) & vbTab & LetterCount(I)
Next I
```

You can test the preceding code by placing both loops in the cmdCount Click event (assuming the "Count" command button mentioned previously is named cmdCount).

The two frequency counting examples can easily be modified to count the frequency of scores and letter grades for a class when data are available in a file or database table. Indeed, they can be generalized to handle all the problems mentioned at the beginning of this subsection. Such an enhancement is left to you as an exercise.

Simulation

Because of their capability to accumulate frequency count easily, arrays can also be used conveniently to simulate/approximate probabilities in conjunction with the use of random numbers. As an illustration, assume the product spoilage rate in a production process is 2% (i.e., 98% of the product going through the process will turn out to be good). What is the probability that you will obtain 100, 101, . . . or more good units, when you put 105 raw units in a batch through the process? You can, of course, solve this problem analytically. However, it will take a long time to get the formula right (assuming you have average math skills) and obtain the correct computation thereof.

With the computer, you can use an alternative approach, which involves using random numbers to simulate the event and accumulate the "experiences." (This kind of simulation is recognized as the Monte Carlo simulation.) You can simulate whether a unit from the process is good or bad by "drawing" a random number. Because the probability of getting a spoiled unit is 2%, if the random number is higher than .02, you can claim that it is a good unit; otherwise, it is spoiled. If you simulate this inspection of good/bad output units 105 times, you should be able to find how many units turn out to be good. This "experiment" is equivalent to running 105 raw units through the process and counting the number of good units. Thus, if you run the experiment 1,000 (or even 10,000) times, you should be able to count the number of times good output units equal 100, 101, . . . or more units.

Let's code this simulation process step by step. Assume that the variable GoodUnits is used to accumulate the number of good units in each experiment. When you inspect a unit of output and find it to be good, you add 1 to GoodUnits. (A random number greater than or equal to .02 represents the event of obtaining a good unit.) The code appears as follows:

```
If Rnd >=.02 Then
    GoodUnits = GoodUnits + 1
End If
```

However, each batch consists of 105 units. Thus, we need to inspect 105 times:

```
GoodUnits = 0 'Before the process, there is no good unit.
For I = 1 to 105
    If Rnd >=.02 Then
        GoodUnits = GoodUnits + 1
    End If
Next I
```

After the "inspection," the value of GoodUnits represents the number of good units produced from this batch. This "experience" can be accumulated by a frequency count. Assume that the array variable GoodUnitCount is declared with a proper range of its subscript. We can place the following line immediately below the loop:

```
GoodUnitCount(GoodUnits) = GoodUnitCount(GoodUnits) + 1
```

We have just finished simulating one batch of production. To arrive at a probability distribution, we need to repeat the "experiment" many times. For the interest of fairly accurate approximation, let's repeat the experiment 1,000 times. In addition, to make the code complete, we also show the proper declaration for all the variables used:

```
Dim I As Integer
Dim J as Integer
Dim GoodUnits As Integer
Dim GoodUnitCount(105) As Integer
    ' Randomize to get a different sequence of random numbers
    ' each time
    Randomize
    For J = 1 to 1000
        ' Set good units to 0 at start of each production run
        GoodUnits = 0
        'Inspect a batch and count the number of good units
        For I = 1 to 105
            If Rnd >=.02 Then
                GoodUnits = GoodUnits + 1
            End If
        Next I
        ' Accumulate the frequency for good units
        GoodUnitCount(GoodUnits) = GoodUnitCount(GoodUnits) + 1
    Next J
```

Notice that GoodUnitCount is declared with an upper bound of the subscript of 105 and with a default lower bound of 0. We allow the possibilities that in a production run, the entire batch can be either all bad or all good. Notice also that before the "inspection" of a batch, the variable GoodUnits is assigned a value of 0. This must be done; otherwise, the count from the previous batch will be carried over, resulting in an extremely unreasonable large number (much greater than 105 units). Note also that we place the Randomize statement before the simulation starts so that the random number sequence will be different each time the program is run.

Interested in the results of the simulation? If you print the results as a table in a form, there will be too many lines. Instead, you can place the results in a list box named lstResults:

```
For I = 0 To 105
    lstResults.AddItem I & vbTab & GoodUnitCount(I)
Next I
```

You can place these lines along with the preceding code in a Command (e.g., Simulate) Click event. Alternatively, you can place them in a Sub procedure and call the procedure from a Command Click event. The following table is a sample result from one simulation.

Number of Good Units	Frequency
98	3
99	14
100	33
101	97
102	194

Number of Good Units	Frequency
103	278
104	262
105	119

Because the random number sequences will differ in each simulation, the results will vary slightly. However, the results should give a pretty good approximation of the probability of obtaining a specified number of good units. (The preceding results show that there is approximately a 98.3% probability that you will get 100 or more good units if you place a batch of 105 raw units into production, given a spoilage rate of 2%.) If you are interested in more stable (accurate) results, you can increase the number of experiments. Of course, it will then take longer to compute the results.

Random Sampling Without Replacement

Consider the drawing of a lottery. There are 50 balls, numbered from 1 to 50. Six balls will be drawn. None of the drawn balls will be placed back in the bin. Thus, none of the six numbers will be repeated. (This type of problem is recognized as random sampling without replacement.) You want your program to emulate the drawing; that is, your program will display six random numbers in the range of 1 to 50, without repetition, when the user clicks the Draw command button. How do you proceed?

Drawing a Ball. Drawing a random number in the range of 1 to 50 can be done with the following statement:

```
BallNumber = 1 + Int(Rnd * 50)
```

Recall that the Rnd function generates a random number between 0 and 1 (but can equal 0). When this value is multiplied by 50, the result will be between 0 and 50 (but less than 50). The Int function truncates the fractional number and should return a number in the range of 0 to 49. When 1 is added to this value, the resulting BallNumber should be in the range of 1 to 50.

Avoiding Repetition. The preceding statement does not guarantee that some of the six numbers drawn will not be the same. We need to find a way to verify that a new number has not already been "drawn."

There are two possible ways to accomplish this. Let's consider an *intuitive approach* first. As soon as we draw a number, we can compare it with all those numbers previously drawn. If a match is found, we should draw another number (discarding the current number) and compare again until the new number has no match with the previously drawn numbers. This number is then included in the numbers already drawn. When the total number of numbers drawn is equal to six, your program has done the job and can display the results and quit.

You can use a variable, for example, NumbersDrawn, to count the number of numbers drawn. To keep track of the numbers drawn, you can set up an array, for example, Ball(1 To 6). Each time a number is drawn, you can use a For loop, varying the counter from 1 to NumbersDrawn, to compare this new number with the ones drawn to determine whether the number is already drawn. So that at the end of the loop you can easily determine whether a match is found, you can use another variable (e.g., NotFound). Before the loop, you can assume the new number has no match, thus set NotFound to True. Within the loop, if a match is found, the variable is set to False and the loop is terminated.

The description can be translated into the following code:

```
BallNumber = 1 + Int(Rnd * 50) 'Draw a random number
NotFound = True 'Assume this number is not already drawn
For I = 1 To NumbersDrawn
    If BallNumber = Balls(I) Then
    'A match is found; so NotFound is false
        NotFound = False
        Exit For 'and terminate the search
    End If
```

```
Next I
If NotFound Then
' The current ball number is indeed new
    NumbersDrawn = NumbersDrawn + 1 'Increase the number count
    Balls(NumbersDrawn) = BallNumber 'Keep the ball number
End If
```

Notice how a new number is added to the "already drawn" list. First, the count (NumbersDrawn) is increased by 1. The value is then used as the subscript to identify the position in the array Balls where the ball number is stored.

The routine should be repeated as long as NumbersDrawn is less than six. You should enclose the preceding code within a Do loop as follows:

```
Do
' Place all the above statement here
Loop While NumbersDrawn < 6
```

Complete Code for the Intuitive Approach. Assume the routine will be triggered by the user's click on a command button named cmdDraw. The complete procedure can appear as follows:

```
Option Explicit

Private Sub cmdDraw_Click()
Dim I As Integer
Dim NumbersDrawn As Integer
Dim BallNumber As Integer
Dim Balls(1 To 6) As Integer
Dim NotFound As Boolean
    Randomize 'Use a new random number sequence
    Do
        BallNumber = 1 + Int(Rnd * 50)
        NotFound = True
        For I = 1 To NumbersDrawn
            If BallNumber = Balls(I) Then
                NotFound = False
                Exit For
            End If
        Next I
        If NotFound Then
            NumbersDrawn = NumbersDrawn + 1
            Balls(NumbersDrawn) = BallNumber
        End If
    Loop While NumbersDrawn < 6
    Me.Cls 'Clear the form
    ' Print results
    For I = 1 To 6
        Print Balls(I)
    Next I
End Sub
```

Notice that in this code we have included proper declarations for all variables used in the procedure. A For... Next loop is also used at the end to display the results. There is a ***Me.Cls*** statement before the loop. The statement uses the Form's ***Cls method*** to clear all the text previously printed on the form. The CurrentX and CurrentY property of the form will also reset to zero after the execution of the method.

Another Approach. The preceding routine keeps track of which numbers have been drawn. Alternatively, you can focus on each number in the entire range. That is, when a number is drawn, you can ask whether the ball has been drawn not by comparing the numbers that have been drawn but by checking a "marker" for the particular number. If the marker is not turned on, the ball has not yet been drawn and you can display the number and turn its marker on; otherwise, it has been drawn and the number should be discarded.

If you want to set up a marker for each ball, you will need 50 markers because there are 50 balls. Thus, the marker should be an array with 50 elements. Let the array name be AlreadyPicked. Then you can declare it as follows:

```
Dim AlreadyPicked(1 to 50) As Boolean
```

Now, imagine you have drawn the number 3. You can test the value of AlreadyPicked(3) to determine whether it has already been drawn. If AlreadyPicked(3) is False, you can set it to True and display 3; otherwise, you can ignore the number and repeat the drawing. Notice that 3 is just a particular number. Any number you draw (BallNumber) should work the same way. Thus, the routine to obtain a legitimate (nonrepeated) ball number can be coded as follows:

```
Do
    BallNumber = 1 + Int(Rnd * 50) 'Draw a number
' If the number has been drawn, repeat the drawing.
Loop While AlreadyPicked(BallNumber)
AlreadyPicked(BallNumber) = True
Print BallNumber 'display the number currently drawn
```

You need six numbers. Thus, the routine should be repeated six times. You can accomplish this by enclosing the preceding routine in a For...Next loop as follows:

```
For I = 1 to 6
' Place the above drawing routine here
Next I
```

Complete Code for the Second Approach. To test this approach, you can draw another command button on the same form. Name it cmdDrawAlt and set its Caption property to "Draw, Alternative Way." The complete code should appear as follows:

```
Private Sub cmdDrawAlt_Click()
Dim AlreadyPicked(1 To 50) As Boolean
Dim BallNumber As Integer
Dim I As Integer
    Randomize 'Start a new random number sequence
    Me.Cls 'Erase previous output
    For I = 1 To 6
        Do
            BallNumber = 1 + Int(Rnd * 50) 'Draw a ball
        ' If it is already picked, then repeat the drawing
        Loop While AlreadyPicked(BallNumber)
        AlreadyPicked(BallNumber) = True 'Mark the ball drawn
        Print BallNumber 'Display the number
    Next I
End Sub
```

When you run the project, you should be able to verify that each time you click the command button, six unique numbers in the range of 1 to 50 are displayed in the form. These numbers should vary randomly from one round to the next.

Notice that with this approach, there is no need to have another array, Balls(), which keeps track of all the ball numbers drawn. Each number is displayed when it is determined to be legitimate. These numbers are also implicitly kept in the AlreadyPicked array. The position of the element that has been set to True represents the ball number that has been drawn; that is, if AlreadyPicked(5) is True, 5 is a number that has been drawn. Thus, the following loop should also give the numbers that have been drawn:

```
For I = 1 To 50
    If AlreadyPicked(I) Then
    ' I has been picked
        Print I 'Print the ball number
    End If
Next I
```

Comparing the Two Approaches. When you inspect the two procedures, you should notice that the first approach requires longer code but takes a smaller array, whereas the second approach requires shorter code but takes a longer array. The second approach should be faster because the loop to determine whether a ball (number) has been drawn requires a test on one element of the array; that is, AlreadyPicked(BallNumber). In contrast, the first approach requires the execution of a loop. Only after the loop is completely executed can the routine conclude that the number has not been drawn. Thus, there is a trade-off between speed and space (storage) used.

You will encounter many problems of similar nature and therefore be faced with the same design issue as to which approach to use given a situation. If speed of execution is the most important consideration, you should use the second approach. Indeed, you should use the first approach only when the number of elements to keep track of (balls to draw) is relatively small. When this number approaches the total potential number (50 in this example), you will always be better off using the second approach.

9.3 Sorting and Searching

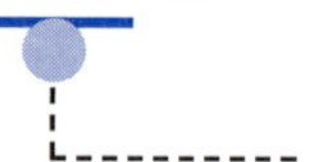

The main advantage of keeping data in an array is that the array allows you to conveniently handle the data in it randomly without any restriction. One of the uses of arrays is sorting: data in the array can be arranged in either ascending or descending order. The sorted data can then be output or further processed.

Humans prefer sorted data. Sorted data are easier to browse and facilitate lookup. Sorted data are also "helpful" to the computer. More efficient search/processing algorithms can be used with sorted data. Thus, if an array is to be searched repetitively for different search values, it pays to sort the array first. In batch processing (where transactions are collected into a "batch" and all are processed at one time), transactions sorted in the same order as their master records (e.g., customer accounts) eliminate the need to search the master file back and forth to update the affected master records. In this case, sorting is a necessity for efficient processing.

Selected Algorithms for Sorting

You may be amazed that as simple as the goal of sorting is, virtually countless algorithms to sort data exist. In this section, we discuss the following four algorithms:

1. Bubble sort
2. Insertion sort
3. Shell sort
4. Quick sort

A careful study of the sorting algorithms allows you to appreciate the performance differences as well as helps you develop the capability to design elegant solutions to new programming problems.

A study of sorting algorithms is both important and interesting. About 25 years ago, Knuth asserted that nearly 20% of the computer resources at that time were used to perform sorting, according to a survey. This would suggest several alternative explanations: (1) Sorting is very important and indispensable in computer applications, (2) sorting is not conducted efficiently, or (3) sorting has been used unnecessarily. A careful study of sorting algorithms could help improve all these situations.

Bubble Sort

In bubble sort, each element in the array is compared with the next element. If these elements are out of order, they are swapped. When one round of comparisons (and the resulting swaps) is done, the largest value in the array will be placed at the right-most position as a result. Thus, in the next round, one fewer element needs to be compared. This process continues until the last round in which only two elements need to be compared.

The process is illustrated in the following example.

Position	1	2	3	4	5
Value	38	51	23	56	34

The comparisons start from left to right, element by element. The first element, 38, is compared with the second element, 51. Because they are in order, nothing is performed. Then, the second element, 51, is compared with the third element, 23. Because they are out of order, the two elements are swapped. The result appears as follows:

Position	1	2	3	4	5
Value	38	23	51	56	34

The third element, now 51, is compared with the fourth element, 56. Then 56 is compared with 34, resulting in another swap. After the first round of comparison, the array will appear as follows:

Position	1	2	3	4	5
Value	38	23	51	34	56

Notice that the largest element in the array is now at the right-most position.

The same process of comparisons for the second round will start from position 1 again but will stop at position 4, resulting in the second largest element being moved into this position. This process is repeated until all elements are placed in their proper position.

Comparing and Swapping. How do we implement such an algorithm? Assume X() is the array to be sorted and the Ith element is to be compared with the next element. Then, the following statements should accomplish the comparison and swap:

```
If X(I) > X(I+1) Then
' out of order; swap
    Temp = X(I)
    X(I) = X(I+1)
    X(I+1) = Temp
End If
```

The Number of Elements to Compare. What range of I should the preceding code execute? I should always start with the lower bound of the array. In the first round, it should go until I + 1 is the last element of the array; that is, I should be one less than the upper bound of the array. In the second round, this number should be one less than the preceding round; the next round, one further less, and so on. Before we have a formula to compute this value, let's just name a variable, H, to represent the value. The loop to complete a round of comparisons can then appear as follows:

```
For I = LBound(X) To H
    If X(I) > X(I+1) Then
        ' out of order; swap
        Temp = X(I)
        X(I) = X(I+1)
        X(I+1) = Temp
    End If
Next I
```

The Number of Rounds of Comparisons. Because one round of comparisons will move only one element (the largest in range considered) to its proper position, if the array X has n elements, it will take n – 1 rounds of comparisons to complete the sort (n –1, not n rounds because the smallest will automatically be placed in its position when the second smallest element is moved to its proper position). This means the preceding For loop should be executed n –1 times. In other words, the loop should be enclosed by another loop that will execute n –1 times:

```
For J = LBound(X)  To UBound(X) - 1
' place the above For I loop here
Next J
```

Computing the Number of Comparisons for Each Round. We still need to compute H before the For I loop is reached. As stated previously, the first time H should have a value of one less than the upper bound of the array and should decrease by 1 in each subsequent round. This can be done by setting its initial value before the For J loop and decreasing it by 1 inside the J loop:

```
H = UBound(X)
For J = LBound(X) To UBound(X) -1
     H = H - 1
     ', place the above For I loop here
Next J
```

The Bubble Sort Sub Procedure. A sort routine is best written as a separate Sub procedure, which can then be called by any other procedure that needs a sort operation. Following this consideration, the complete Bubble Sort routine can be presented as follows:

```
Sub BubbleSort(X() as Long)
Dim I as Long
Dim J as Long
Dim H as Long
Dim Temp as Long
     H = UBound(X)
     For J = LBound(X)  To UBound(X) -1
          H = H - 1
          For I = LBound(X) To H
               If X(I) > X(I + 1) Then
               ' out of order; swap
                    Temp = X(I)
                    X(I) = X(I + 1)
                    X(I+1) = Temp
               End If
          Next I
     Next J
End Sub
```

Testing the Procedure. To test the procedure, you can design a visual interface similar to the one shown in Figure 9.1. As you may infer, the visual interface includes the following:

1. A frame, which contains a text box and a command button. The text box is named txtNumber and will be used to specify the upper bound for the array to be sorted. The command button is named cmdGenerate and has the caption "Generate." This button will be used to generate the random numbers specified in the text box txtNumber.
2. Another command button with the caption "Bubble Sort." This button is named cmdBubbleSort and will be used to initiate the sorting.
3. A list box, which is named lstResults. This will be used to show the sorting results.

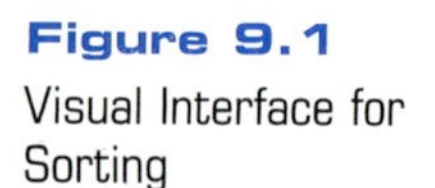

Figure 9.1
Visual Interface for Sorting

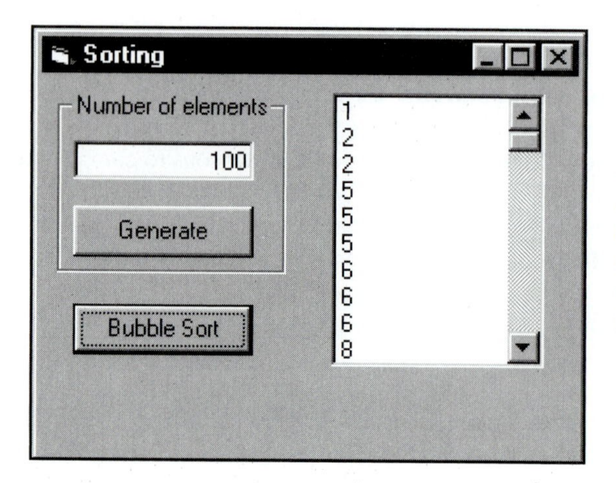

With the controls in this form properly named and the code in this subsection properly entered, you should be able to test the Bubble Sort procedure by entering a number, clicking the Generate button, and then clicking the Bubble Sort button. The list box should show the results.

How the Testing Project Should Work. When the program starts, the user is expected to enter a number in the text box. When he or she clicks the Generate button, your program will set the upper bound of the array X() to the number in the text box and generate random numbers to populate the entire array. The values of the random numbers will be in the range of 0 to this number. When the user clicks the Bubble Sort button, your program will call the Bubble Sort Sub procedure and populate the list box with the sorting results.

Declaring the Array. Because the array X() to hold the random numbers will be used in several procedures, it should be declared at the form level. In addition, its upper bound will change, depending on the number the user enters in the text box. Thus, it should be declared as a dynamic array. Its declaration in the form module should appear as follows:

```
Option Explicit
Dim X() As Long
```

Generating the Random Numbers. The random numbers will be generated when the user clicks the Generate button. The button's Click event procedure can appear as follows:

```
Private Sub cmdGenerate_Click()
Dim Number As Long
Dim I As Long
    Randomize
    Number = Val(txtNumber.Text) 'Take the number from the user
    ReDim X(Number) 'Set X()'s upper bound to Number
    For I = 0 To Number
        X(I) = Rnd * Number  'Populate X() with random numbers
    Next I
End Sub
```

In this procedure, the number entered in the text box is assigned to the variable Number. Then, X() is dynamically dimensioned with its upper bound set to Number. In the For loop, each element of X() is assigned a random number. Because the Rnd function generates a random number in the range of 0 and 1, multiplying this number by Number should result in a value in the range of 0 to Number. Notice that to avoid having the same random number sequence each time the project starts, the Randomize statement is used to randomize the sequence.

Calling the Sorting Sub and Displaying the Results. When the user clicks the Bubble Sort button, your program should call the Bubble Sort Sub procedure and display the results. This event procedure appears as follows:

```
Private Sub cmdBubble_Click()
Dim I As Long
Dim TheTime As Single
    TheTime = Timer
    BubbleSort X() 'Call BubbleSort to sort the array
    Debug.Print Timer - TheTime
    lstResults.Clear 'Clear all previous data
    For I = 0 To UBound(X)
        ' Populate the list box with sorted data
        lstResults.AddItem X(I)
    Next I
End Sub
```

You can test your Bubble Sort procedure with the visual interface in Figure 9.1 and the preceding event procedures. Run the project. Enter a number in the text box. Click the Generate button and then the Bubble Sort button. You can then inspect the numbers in the list box to ensure that they are in order. (*Note:* Be sure that the list box's Sorted property is set to False, the default.)

Computing Time Used. Notice that to see how much time the sort routine takes, two additional statements have been added. First, before calling the Bubble Sort procedure, TheTime (declared as Single) is assigned a value returned by the ***Timer function***, which returns a value (of the Single type) in seconds that represents the current time. After the Sub is called, TheTime is subtracted from Timer to obtain the time it takes to perform the sorting. The result is printed in the debug window. Although this is a fairly crude way of determining the time consumed, it should give you a good idea about sorting efficiency of a particular algorithm.

Notice also that the list box is first cleared with its ***Clear method*** before it is populated with the sorted data. This is necessary because the user may click the Bubble Sort button several times in the duration of the program. Without that statement, the new sorted results will be mixed with the previous ones, making it difficult to examine the results.

A Remark on Sorting Efficiency. The speed of a sorting algorithm depends mainly on two factors:

1. The number of comparisons
2. The amount of data movements

Recall that the number of comparisons involved in bubble sort varies from round to round, ranging from n –1 in the first round to 1 in the last round. Thus, the total is 1 + 2 + ... + (n –1) = n (n-1)/2. This number is in the order of n^2 and can become huge when n is large. In addition, the number of data movements can be equally huge. If you inspect the process closely, you should find that a big element located on the left side will take many swaps before reaching its final position on the right side of the array. *Bubble sort is considered the least efficient sorting algorithm.*

Simple Selection Sort. One way to alleviate the data movement problem in the bubble sort algorithm described is to select the proper element for one position at a time; that is, instead of comparing neighboring elements in each round, the program can compare one fixed element with other elements. For example, we can start with finding the largest element in the array by comparing the last element with all other elements. If the other element is greater than this last element, the two elements are swapped. The new element in the last position is then considered the new champion until another element in the array is found to be greater. At that time, another swap will take place. This modification should reduce the number of swaps and is left to you as an exercise.

Straight Insertion Sort

Imagine that in the sorting process, an additional array is used for output purposes. Each element from the original (input) array is placed into the output array in sorted order. When all elements from the original array are moved to the output area, the sorting is complete. To ensure that a new element from the input array is placed in the output array "in sorted order," it is compared with the elements already in the output array to determine its proper position. Once this position is identified, this new element is inserted in that position. This algorithm can be illustrated as follows.

The first element is moved into the output area.

Position	1	2	3	4	5
Input (Original)	38	51	23	56	34
Output	38				

Then the second element, 51, will be moved to the output area. It is first compared with the existing element in output, 38. Because 51 is greater, it is placed at the end of the output area, resulting in the following:

Position	1	2	3	4	5
Input (Original)	38	51	23	56	34
Output	38	51			

Now, the third element will be moved. When it is compared with the elements in the output area, we find that it should be inserted at position 1. Thus, the result will appear as follows:

Position	1	2	3	4	5
Input (Original)	38	51	23	56	34
Output	23	38	51		

23 is inserted at position 1.

This process continues until all elements in the original array are moved into the output area. In actual implementation, there is no need to set aside another array for output purposes. Recall that the number of output elements is equal to the number of elements already moved from the input array. Because all the elements in the output area are also the same as those already moved from the input array, the area in the input array can be used to hold the output.

The algorithm involves two major activities when an element is "moved" from the input area to output:

1. Determining the proper position of the new element
2. Inserting the new element in its proper position

We can write a function (e.g., FindPos) to find the proper position for the new element and a Sub procedure to perform the insertion.

The ***FindPos function*** will search the output area sequentially until the new element is less than the element in the output or the output area is exhausted. Either of these conditions identifies the new element's proper position. For example, if the output area has 38 and 51 and the new element is 23, the function should return the first position (e.g., 1) as shown here.

Position	1	2	3
Output	38	51	

23 should be inserted here; thus, 1 (the position) should be returned.

The code appears as follows:

```
Function FindPos(X() as Long, V as Long, L as Long) as Long
' This function searches and returns the proper position
' for a value V in an array whose elements in the range of its
' lower bound and (L - 1)th position are sorted (L is imagined
' to be the extra position to accommodate an additional element
' to be inserted)
Dim I as Long
    For I = LBound(X) to L - 1
        If V < X(I) Then
            FindPos = I
            Exit Function
        End If
    Next I
    FindPos = L
End Function
```

The Insert Sub Procedure. Assume P is the position in the array X() at which to insert the Lth element. Then all elements starting at P through L – 1 will need to be shifted to the right by one position first. The Lth element can be placed at the Pth position to complete the insertion. The steps can be depicted as follows.

Step 1: Move elements to the right.

Position	1	2	3
Output	38	51	

Step 2: Insert the new element.

Position	1	2	3
Output	23	38	51

A Sub procedure to insert X(L) into the sorted output area can be written as follows:

```
Sub Insert(X() as Long, P as Long, L as Long)
' This procedure performs an insertion of X(L) at position P of
' Array X(); L is also the upper boundary of the sorted area
Dim I as Long
Dim Temp as Long
    Temp = X(L)   ' keep the element to be inserted
    ' Move every element in the range of p to L - 1
    ' by one position to the right
    For I = L - 1 to P Step -1
        X(I + 1) = X(I)
    Next I
    ' Insert the new element at position P
    X(P) = Temp
End Sub
```

Note that in this routine L serves two purposes. The element in this position is the one to be inserted. In addition, L identifies the upper boundary of the area where an insertion is to take place. Notice also that the elements are moved to the right, last elements first to avoid overwriting existing data.

The Insertion Sort Procedure. The Insertion Sort Sub procedure can be implemented by calling these two procedures iteratively:

```
Sub InsertionSort(X() as Integer)
Dim I as Long
Dim P as Long
    For I = LBound(X) + 1 to UBound(X)
        P = FindPos(X(), X(I), I)   'Find position for X(I)
        ' Insert X(I) to position P of the sorted area
        Insert X(), P, I
    Next I
End Sub
```

Notice that the For loop starts with LBound(X) + 1, the second position of the array. The first element does not need to be sorted. Within the loop, the FindPos function is used to identify the proper position of X(I). The area to search for this position is between LBound(X) and I. (The area between the lower bound and I – 1 contains the sorted elements. X(I) should be placed at position I if it is greater than all elements in this area.) Once this proper position, P, is identified, the Insert Sub procedure inserts X(I) into the output area with an upper boundary set at I.

Insertion Sort Versus Bubble Sort. When data in the array are placed randomly, this algorithm requires fewer comparisons than bubble sort. As a new element is compared with the elements in the sorted output area, the expected number of comparisons is half of the elements in the sorted area, whereas the previous two algorithms require comparisons of all possible pairs of elements. Because data movements in insertion sort involves shifting positions (to the right) rather than swapping, fewer data movements are needed than in the preceding algorithm. Thus, straight insertion sort is faster than bubble sort.

Testing Insertion Sort. The simplest way to test this algorithm is to use the same interface and event procedures as for the bubble sort:

1. Add the three procedures presented in this subsection (the FindPos function, the Insert sub, and the InsertionSort sub) to the same form module (code window).

2. Add another command button to the form. Name it cmdInsertionSort and set its Caption property to "Insertion Sort."
3. Add the following event procedure:

```
Private Sub cmdInsertionSort_Click()
Dim I As Long
Dim TheTime As Single
    TheTime = Timer
    Debug.Print T
    InsertionSort X() 'Call InsertionSort to sort the array
    Debug.Print Timer - TheTime
    lstResults.Clear 'Clear all previous data
    For I = 0 To UBound(X)
        lstResults.AddItem X(I) 'Add sorted element to the list box
    Next I
End Sub
```

Notice that the only difference between this procedure and the cmdBubbleSort Click procedure is the statement that calls the sort routine. Here, the Sub procedure, InsertionSort (instead of BubbleSort), is called.

To test the InsertionSort Sub, you can do the following:

1. Enter a number in the text box.
2. Click the Generate button.
3. Click the Insertion Sort button. (Be sure to skip the Bubble Sort button to obtain "fair" results.)

To obtain a "truly fair" comparison between the two sorting algorithms, you should populate the same random numbers in two different arrays. Each array can then be sorted by each sorting routine to obtain the sorting time. Such a modification is left to you as an exercise.

Binary Insertion Sort. The number of comparisons in the preceding algorithm can be further reduced if the binary search algorithm is used to search for the position for a new element. The binary search algorithm is explained in the subsection "Sequential Search and Binary Search" in this section. Implementing this sorting algorithm is left to you as an exercise.

Shell Sort

You may have noticed that in bubble sort, each element is moved toward its proper position one swap at a time. Many swaps are usually involved before each element reaches its final position. One approach to improve this slow movement is to initially perform the comparisons of an element with another approximately half the array away. A swap of these two elements will thus accomplish a "big move." The comparisons continue until no further swap is called for. This interval of comparisons can then be cut by half. The same process is repeated. Eventually, the interval will be equal to one. When it finally finishes the comparisons with this interval, we can be sure that all elements are sorted in order. (At this stage, the sort is similar to the bubble sort but requires much fewer swaps and rounds of comparison.)

The following example illustrates how Shell sort is performed:

Position	1	2	3	4	5
Value	38	51	23	56	34

The initial interval is computed to be slightly smaller than half of the array; that is, 2 in this case. The first element, 38, is then compared with the third element, 23. Because the two elements are out of order, they are swapped:

Position	1	2	3	4	5
Value	23	51	38	56	38

Then the second element, 51, is compared with the fourth element, 56, and 38 with 34, resulting in another swap:

Position	1	2	3	4	5
Value	23	51	34	56	38

The comparisons have reached the end. Because the current round resulted in swaps, another round of comparisons with the same interval should be performed; that is, 23 with 34, 51 with 56, and 34 with 38. No swap occurs. So, the interval is reduced by half to 1 and another round of comparisons is performed until no swap occurs.

Assume X() is the array to be sorted. We can first compute the interval as follows:

```
Interval = (UBound(X) - LBound(X)) / 2
```

(Note that the resulting quotient will be rounded. Thus, for an array of an even number of elements, the initial interval will be half of its size.)

A For loop as shown here should complete a round of comparisons:

```
For I = LBound(X) to UBound(X) - Interval
     If X(I) > X(I + Interval) Then
     ' Out of order, swap
         Temp = X(I)
         X(I) = X(I + Interval)
         X(I + Interval) = Temp
     End If
Next I
```

The For statement sets the position of the element on the left to be compared and starts at the lower bound of the array. It should end when I + Interval is greater than the upper bound of X; that is, I should go as high as I + Interval = UBound(X). Thus, the ending value for I is Ubound(X) – Interval.

This loop is to be repeated until no swap occurs. To keep track of swaps, we can use a Boolean variable, Swapped. The variable can be set to False before executing the For loop. If a swap occurs, it is set to True. Before the outer loop is repeated, this variable can be tested and another round of comparisons is performed only if Swapped is True:

```
Do
     Swapped = False
     For I = LBound(X) to UBound(X) - Interval
          If X(I) > X(I + Interval) Then
          ' Out of order, swap
              Temp = X(I)
              X(I) = X(I + Interval)
              X(I + Interval) = Temp
              Swapped = True
          End If
     Next I
Loop While Swapped
```

When the outer loop is finished, it is time to reduce the interval size by half and repeat another round of comparisons until the interval size is zero. The entire sort procedure using the Shell sort algorithm should appear as follows:

```
Sub ShellSort(X() As Long)
Dim Interval As Long
Dim I As Long
Dim Swapped As Boolean
Dim Temp As Long
     Interval = (UBound(X) - LBound(X)) / 2
     Do Until Interval = 0
          Do
               Swapped = False  ' assume no swap
                For I = LBound(X) to UBound(X) - Interval
                    If X(I) > X(I + Interval) Then
```

```
                        ' Out of order, swap
                           Temp = X(I)
                           X(I) = X(I + Interval)
                           X(I + Interval) = Temp
                           ' Swap occurs, so set swapped to true
                           Swapped = True
                        End If
                   Next I
              Loop While Swapped
              ' Reduce the interval by half
              Interval = Int(Interval / 2)
         Loop
    End Sub
```

You can implement a test procedure by following the same steps as outlined in the preceding subsection. Test the program. You should find that this algorithm is much faster than those previously discussed.

Quick Sort

You may recall that in bubble sort, in each round of comparisons, the algorithm attempts to identify which element in the array should be moved to a destination position. In other words, a destination is waiting for an element that "qualifies." In quick sort, the goal is inverted. The algorithm looks for the proper position for the given data element at hand. Specifically, when the sorting operation starts, the first element in the array is considered the pivotal element. The algorithm looks for the proper final position in the array to place this pivotal element. This is done by first comparing the pivotal element with the array elements backward (right to left) until the pivotal element is greater than the element in the array. The pivotal element is swapped with this element. Then, the pivotal element (in its new position) is compared with elements in the array forward (left to right) until it is found to be smaller than another element in the array. A swap takes place. Then the comparisons go backward again.

The backward-forward sequence of comparisons/swaps continues until all elements in the array have been compared with the pivotal element. At this point, no element on the left side of the pivotal element is greater than and no element on its right is less than the pivotal element. The pivotal element has found its proper position. This process also ensures that all elements on the left side are smaller than all elements on the right side of the pivotal element; no further sorting between the two sides is necessary. The elements on each side can then be sorted separately using the same algorithm.

The following example illustrates how the pivotal element is placed in its proper position.

Position	1	2	3	4	5
Value	38	51	23	56	34

The first element, 38, is the pivotal element. At first, the comparisons start from right to left until the pivotal element is greater than the element in the array. This occurs immediately when 38 is compared with the fifth element, 34. A swap takes place:

Position	1	2	3	4	5
Value	34	51	23	56	38

Now, comparisons turn forward. (Notice that 38 is the pivotal element.) The second element, 51, is compared with 38. They are out of order. Another swap takes place:

Position	1	2	3	4	5
Value	34	38	23	56	51

Then, comparisons go backward again. 38 is compared with 56, then with 23, where another swap takes place:

Position	1	2	3	4	5
Value	34	23	38	56	51

At this point, all elements have been compared with 38. The pivotal element has found its proper position. Note that all elements on its left side are smaller than 38 and all elements on its right side are greater. The subarrays on both sides (as depicted in the following table) can be sorted by the same algorithm:

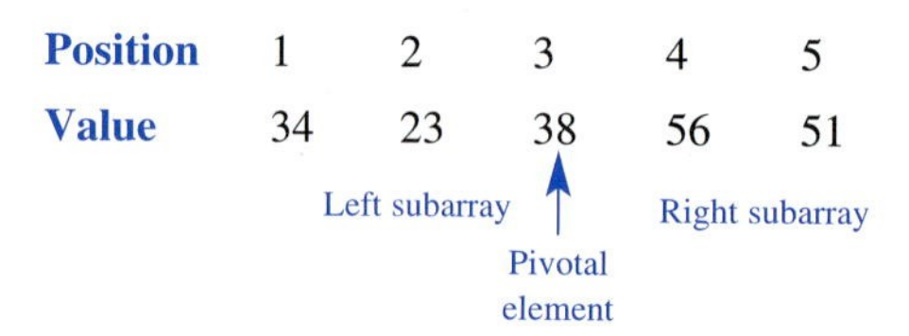

Position	1	2	3	4	5
Value	34	23	38	56	51

Header for Quick Sort. Before we start coding for this algorithm, we should note that we will use the same procedure to sort subarrays. This means that this sort Sub procedure will have to call itself; that is, it will be a recursive procedure. Each subarray has a different range of elements to sort. The range can be defined by the beginning and ending positions of the subarray. Thus, the header of this Sub procedure should look a bit different from the previous sort procedures:

```
Sub QuickSort(X() as Long, BegPos as Long, EndPos as Long)
```

where *X()* is the array to be sorted and *BegPos* and *EndPos* define the range of the subarray to sort. Of course, when the routine is initially called, these variables will cover the entire range—LBound(X) and UBound(X)—of the array.

We will use two variables, I and J, to keep track of the positions for forward and backward comparisons, respectively. Initially, I starts at the beginning of the range and J starts at the end:

```
I = BegPos
J = EndPos
```

The first element is the pivotal element:

```
Pivot = X(I)
```

Comparing Backward. The comparisons will first go backward. For any element J in the array, if it is found to be greater than or equal to Pivot, we will go one position to the left; otherwise, a swap takes place and the backward comparison ends:

```
If Pivot =< X(J) Then
' In order, go one position left
    J = J - 1
Else
' out of order; swap and terminate the loop
    X(I) = X (J)
    X(J)= Pivot
    Exit Do
End If
```

Note that before the swap, X(I) and Pivot are the same. There is no need to assign X(I) to Pivot in the swap process. This comparison routine should be enclosed in a Do loop. If the comparisons exhaust all the items (i.e., I = J), the loop should also end. Thus, the complete code for backward comparisons should appear as follows:

```
Do Until I >= J
    If Pivot <= X(J) Then
    ' In order, go one position to the left
        J = J - 1
```

```
        Else
        ' out of order; swap and terminate the loop
            X(I) = X (J)
            X(J)= Pivot
            Exit Do
        End If
    Loop
```

Comparing Forward. Once this loop ends, the process should proceed to the next phase to compare forward. The code can be written in a similar fashion as follows:

```
    Do Until I >= J
        If Pivot >= X(I) Then
        ' In order, go one position to the right
            I = I + 1
        Else
        ' out of order; swap and terminate the loop
            X(J) = X (I)
            X(I)= Pivot
            Exit Do
        End If
    Loop
```

Again notice that at this point before the swap, Pivot and X(J) are the same (see the swap in the preceding loop). There is no need to assign X(J) to Pivot at the beginning of the swap.

The Outer Loop. The preceding two loops should be repeated as long as some elements still have not been compared with Pivot; that is, another (outer) loop as shown next should enclose the two preceding loops :

```
    Do Until I >= J
    ' Place both of the above loops here
    Loop
```

Sorting the Subarrays. The preceding code completes the process of placing the pivotal element in its proper position. As stated at the beginning of this subsection, once this is done, the subarrays on both sides of the pivotal element can be sorted using the same algorithm. Thus, the following two lines of code should be placed immediately after the preceding loops:

```
    QuickSort X(), BegPos, J - 1  'Sort the subarray on left side
    QuickSort X(), J + 1, EndPos ' sort the subarray on right side
```

Terminating the Procedure. The procedure so written will continue to call itself unless we provide additional code to end the recursive process. The procedure should discontinue further sorting under the following circumstances:

1. There is only one element in a subarray; therefore, there will be no need to sort.
2. There are only two elements in a subarray, so we can perform a simple comparison to see whether they are out of order. If so, a swap can be performed. Otherwise, nothing further needs to be done. In either case, there is no need to perform additional sorting.

This analysis suggests the following code:

```
    If EndPos - BegPos < = 0 Then Exit Sub 'One or fewer elements,
                                           ' no need to sort
    If EndPos - BegPos = 1 Then
    ' This subarray has two elements, check to see if they are
    ' out of order
        If X(BegPos) > X(EndPos) Then
        ' Out of order, swap
            Temp = X(BegPos)
            X(BegPos) = X(EndPos)
            X(EndPos) = Temp
        End If
        Exit Sub
    End If
```

These lines should be placed at the very beginning of the procedure.

The Better, the Worse. The code just presented basically completes the quick sort algorithm in its original form. When used to sort an array with random elements, it is very fast because this method preserves the results of comparisons and involves few unnecessary data movements. Recall that all elements found to be smaller than the pivotal element are placed on its left and all elements greater are on its right. Thus, none of the elements on the left need to be compared with those on the right, eliminating many unnecessary comparisons that occur in bubble sort. The process of searching for the proper position of the pivotal element also moves each element near its proper position. However, when used to sort an array that is already in order, the number of comparisons degenerates to bubble sort because at the end of each round, the pivotal element is placed at the beginning of the array, resulting in only one side to be sorted. The next pivotal element will again be compared with the remainder of the entire array.

Solving the Paradox. One proposal to alleviate this problem is to select a random element (instead of the first element) as the pivotal element. Another proposal is to use the midpoint of the array as the pivotal element. If we use this second approach, we will first swap the midpoint element with the first element and then proceed with the sorting as previously presented. That is, we will add the following lines:

```
M = Int((BegPos + EndPos) / 2 ) 'Find mid point
' Use mid point element as the pivotal element
' Also swap the mid point element with the first element
Pivot = X(M)
X(M) = X(BegPos)
X(BegPos)= Pivot
```

These four lines will replace the line Pivot = X(I) presented previously.

The Stack Space Issue. Another issue concerning quick sort is the amount of stack space needed. The Sub procedure calls itself when sorting the subarrays on both sides of the pivotal element. The parameters passed to the procedure itself are kept in the memory "stack." If not carefully managed, the routine can run out of stack space before the sort routine is complete. The solution is to ensure that the shorter subarray is sorted first. Sorting of shorter arrays can be resolved sooner because their subarrays will reach two or few elements much more quickly. To implement this solution, the calls to sort the subarrays can be rewritten as follows:

```
If J - BegPos <= EndPos - J Then
    ' Left side is shorter, sort it first
    QuickSort X(), BegPos, J - 1  'Sort the left subarray
    QuickSort X(), J + 1, EndPos ' sort the right subarray
Else
    ' Right side is shorter, sort it first
    QuickSort X(), J + 1, EndPos ' sort the right subarray
    QuickSort X(), BegPos, J - 1  'Sort the left subarray
End If
```

The complete Quick Sort routine as modified appears as follows:

```
Sub QuickSort(X() as Long, BegPos as Long, EndPos as Long)
Dim Temp as Long
Dim Pivot as Long
Dim M as Long
Dim I as Long
Dim J as Long
    If EndPos - BegPos < = 0 Then Exit Sub 'One or fewer elements,
                                             ' no need to sort
    If EndPos - BegPos = 1 Then
    ' This subarray has two elements.
    ' Check whether they are out of order
        If X(BegPos) > X(EndPos) Then
        ' Out of order, swap
```

```
                Temp = X(BegPos)
                X(BegPos) = X(EndPos)
                X(EndPos) = Temp
            End If
            Exit Sub 'No need to do anything more
        End If
        ' Here is the typical quick sort
        I = BegPos   ' set initial left position for forward comparisons
        J = EndPos   ' set initial right position for backward comparisons
        M = Int((BegPos + EndPos) / 2 ) 'Midpoint of array
        Pivot = X(M)      ' Use midpoint of array as pivotal element
        X(M) = X(BegPos)  ' Swap midpoint with first element
        X(BegPos) = Pivot
        ' Find the proper position for Pivot
        Do Until I >= J
            ' Check backward
            Do Until I >= J
                If Pivot <= X(J) Then
                ' In order, go one position to the left
                    J = J - 1
                Else
                ' out of order; swap and terminate the loop
                    X(I) = X (J)
                    X(J)= Pivot
                    Exit Do
                End If
            Loop
            ' Check forward
            Do Until I >= J
                If Pivot >= X(I) Then
                ' In order, go one position to the right
                    I = I + 1
                Else
                ' out of order; swap and terminate the loop
                    X(J) = X (I)
                    X(I)= Pivot
                    Exit Do
                End If
            Loop
        Loop
        ' Sort subarrays
        If J - BegPos <= EndPos - J Then
            ' Left side is shorter, sort it first
            QuickSort X(), BegPos, J - 1  'Sort the left subarray
            QuickSort X(), J + 1, EndPos ' sort the right subarray
        Else
            ' Right side is shorter, sort it first
          QuickSort X(), J + 1, EndPos ' sort the right subarray
          QuickSort X(), BegPos, J - 1  'Sort the left subarray
        End If
    End Sub
```

This completes the discussion of the quick sort algorithm. The next subsection presents sample empirical performance results of various sorting algorithms. You should find the quick sort algorithm gets its name for a good reason.

Comparison of Performance

As you can see, some of the algorithms are pretty simple, whereas others are more involved. In general, if two algorithms give the same performance, we would rather use the simpler one. The additional complexity can be justified only with better performance. So, how do they compare in terms of speed? The table on p. 356 shows the time used to sort varying number of elements by these algorithms (including the two mentioned but not discussed in detail) using a Pentium II 233 MHz machine.

Number of Elements	Bubble Sort	Selection Sort	Insertion Sort	Binary Insertion Sort	Shell Sort	Quick Sort
1,000	1.27001	0.59999	0.39001	0.22001	0.10998	0.009882
2,000	5.16002	2.41999	1.54001	0.99003	0.21998	0.005000
4,000	20.9200	9.56002	6.32002	3.73002	0.60998	0.15999
8,000	83.6500	38.11996	25.4300	14.6700	1.47999	0.28001
16,000	334.5500	152.64000	101.56	58.3301	3.83998	0.50001

The left most column shows the number of long integer numbers (generated by the formula Rnd * N) being sorted. The numbers in the table are time in seconds. Because the numbers are randomly generated, the results can be different if you attempt to replicate the experiments. However, you should be able to make several general observations:

- Quick sort and Shell sort far outperform the other algorithms.
- As the number of elements to sort doubles, the first four algorithms approximately quadruple the time used, whereas the latter two algorithms slightly exceed twice the time.

The nearly linear relationship between the number of elements to sort and time required suggests that the last two algorithms are not only more efficient but also "steadier" performers.

Sequential Search and Binary Search

Once data in an array are sorted in order, they can be searched with more efficient algorithms. Data presented randomly can be searched only sequentially. The table lookup example given previously (e.g., looking for the phone number given an employee's name) shows how a sequential search can be coded. The average number of comparisons required to find an item will be half of the number of elements in the array.

Improved Sequential Search with Sorted Data. The number of comparisons can be reduced if the data are arranged in order, even with the same sequential search method. How? Because the data are in order, if the data in the array is found to be greater than the search key, there is no need to search further. All data beyond this point will be greater than the search key. Thus, the search can be terminated with the conclusion: data not found. This idea can be implemented with the following code for the same lookup problem (assuming employee names are sorted in ascending order):

```
Private Sub cmdSearch_Click()
Dim Name As String
Dim I As Integer
     Name = txtName.Text
     For I = 0 To EmployeeCount -1
          If Name = Employees(I) then
               MsgBox "The phone number for " & Name _
                 & " is " & Format$(Phones(I), "(000)-000-0000")
               Exit Sub
          ElseIf Name < Employees(I) Then
          ' The name in array is greater than the search key;
          ' There's no such an employee
               Exit For
          End If
     Next I
     MsgBox "Employee name " & Name & " not found."
End Sub
```

The Binary Search. Actually, the preceding search can be even more efficient if the binary search algorithm is used. This algorithm begins by setting the lower and upper boundary of the search to the entire range of the array. It then starts the search at the midpoint of the array. If the search key is greater than the data at the midpoint, the item being searched (if it exists) must be in the upper half of the array; the lower boundary can be adjusted to this midpoint. On the other hand, if the search key is less than the element in the array, the item being search must be in the lower half. Thus, the upper bound is adjusted. The midpoint of this new search boundary is then computed. The search continues, each time narrowing the search boundary by half until the item is found or there is only one item in the range (lower and upper bounds are the same; this means data for the search key does not exist). This algorithm is similar to the half interval method introduced in Chapter 7, "Repetition," to find a numerical solution for a mathematical function. (See Figure 7.3 for a sketch of the algorithm.) Using this algorithm, the preceding lookup problem can be coded as follows:

```
Private Sub cmdSearch_Click()
Dim Name As String
Dim I As Integer
Dim Lower As Integer
Dim Upper As Integer
    Name = txtName.Text
    Lower = 0
    Upper = EmployeeCount -1
    Do
        I = Int((Lower + Upper) / 2) 'Compute the mid point
        If Name = Employees(I) then
            MsgBox "The phone number for " & Name _
              & " is " & Format$(Phones(I), "(000)-000-0000")
            Exit Sub
        ElseIf Name > Employees(I) Then
        ' the name in array is less than the search key;
        ' Adjust the lower bound
            Lower = I + 1
        Else
        ' The name in array is greater than the search key;
        ' Adjust the upper bound
            Upper = I - 1
        End If
    Loop Until Lower = Upper
    If Name = Employees(Upper) Then
    Msg Box "The phone number for " & Name _
        & " is " & Format$(Phones(I), "(000)-000-0000")
    Else
    MsgBox "Employee name " & Name & " not found."
    End If
End Sub
```

Notice that after the Do loop, Name is compared with Employees(Upper) to determine for the last time that the name is actually not in the array. This is necessary because when Lower and Upper reach the same value, a new I value has not been computed. Before leaving this example, we should note that the binary search method is commonly used. Thus, in developing your projects, you should consider writing the search as a function that will take a sorted array and the search key as its parameters and will return the position of the search key in the array. This should be done particularly when you anticipate that more than one routine will need to use the search. The function can also easily be copied into another project that needs the same functionality. Other ideas of reusing the code are presented in Chapter 11, "Menus and Multiple Form Applications"; Chapter 12, "Object-Oriented Programming"; and Chapter 14, "Beyond the Core." Converting the preceding search routine into a Function procedure is left to you as an exercise.

9.4 Control Arrays

Like variables, controls can also be set up as arrays. We first discuss how you can set up control arrays. Then, we explore some sample uses of control arrays.

Creating a Control Array at Design Time

You can create a control array at design time either by changing the name of the controls or by performing the copy and paste method.

The Changing Control Name Method. Here is a walk-through to create a control array with five text boxes named txtCashFlow by changing the name of controls. Follow these steps:

1. Draw five text boxes in a form. Align them top-down neatly.
2. Change the name of Text1 to txtCashFlow.
3. Set the Index property of txtCashFlow to 0.
4. Change the name of Text2 to txtCashFlow. (Press the Enter key when you finish.) Inspect its Index property. It should automatically show a value 1.
5. Change the name of all remaining text boxes the same way as in number 4. When you complete changing the names of these text boxes to txtCashFlow, you have created a text box array named txtCashFlow.

In summary, to create a control array by changing the name of the controls, you first set the Name property of the first control and set its Index property to 0 or any positive number (which will be used as the lower bound of the array index). Then change the name of the remaining controls to the same as the first control.

The Copy and Paste Method. You can also create a control array by using the copy and paste method. To create the same control array as just described using this method, follow these steps:

1. Draw one text box on the form.
2. Name the text box txtCashFlow.
3. Highlight the text box. Then either click the Copy option in the Edit drop-down menu or right-click on the text box to obtain the pop-up context menu. Then select the Copy option.
4. Right-click on the form and select the Paste option. (Or, select the Paste option from the Edit drop-down menu.)
5. You will be asked to confirm that you do want to create a control array. Click the Yes button.
6. You will see a new text box shown in the upper-left corner of the form. Move it to the position you want it to be.
7. Repeat numbers 4 through 6 until you create five text boxes. (The computer will only ask you once whether you want to create a control array.)

This second method is the "standard" way of creating a control array. Because all the properties of the additional elements are copied from the original control, this method has the advantage of creating an array of uniform characteristics (property settings) easily.

When you use the copy and paste method to create a control array, be sure that you set all the properties to your specs before starting the copy and paste process. Because all the properties are automatically copied from their original for the subsequent elements, setting the properties for the original beforehand can save you a lot of time and effort as well as prevent the necessity to hunt for "mysterious errors."

Referencing Elements of a Control Array. Once the control array is created, you can refer to each individual control in the same manner as in the variable array. For example, txtCashFlow(3) refers to the fourth text box in the array. txtCashFlow(N) (N being a variable) will refer to the N+1th element in the control array and can refer to a different element when the value of N changes.

Creating a Control Array at Runtime

You can also create control arrays dynamically at runtime. To do so, follow these steps:

1. Draw a control of interest (e.g., a text box) on the form.
2. Set its Index property to the desired lower bound of the array (usually the Index is set to 0, but you can set it to any positive number).
3. Use the load command in the code to load the additional controls for the array.
4. Move the loaded controls to the desired position in the form using the Move method.
5. Set the loaded control's visible property to True.

Assume that you have (1) drawn a text box on the form, (2) set its Name property to txtCashFlow, and (3) set its Index property to 0. The following code will create four additional elements for txtCashFlow array and align them vertically.

```
Private Sub Form_Click()
Dim I As Integer
Dim X As Integer
Dim Y As Integer
Dim H As Integer
     X = txtCashFlow(0).Left
     Y = txtCashFlow(0).Top
     H = txtCashFlow(0).Height + 10
     For I = 1 To 4
          Load txtCashFlow(I)   'Create a new text box
          ' Compute the vertical position for the new control
          Y = Y + H
          ' Place the new text box in proper position
          ' (vertically below the preceding one)
          txtCashFlow(I).Move X, Y
          ' Make the new control visible
          txtCashFlow(I).Visible = True
     Next I
End Sub
```

The variables X and Y are used to locate the newly loaded controls and are initially assigned with the original control's left and top properties, respectively. In the loop, the (I+1)th element of the control array is loaded by the Load statement. The vertical position for the new control, Y, is computed by adding the height of the control plus 10 twips so that there is some vertical space between controls (see Figure 9.2 for a sketch). (*Note: Twips* are the default measuring unit for the VB visual interface. One inch equals 1,440 twips.) Then the newly loaded control's upper-left corner is set at the coordinate (X, Y) using the Move method. This should vertically align the controls because all of them will have the same horizontal position (the same Left property with a value X). The control's Visible property is then set to True so that the control will appear.

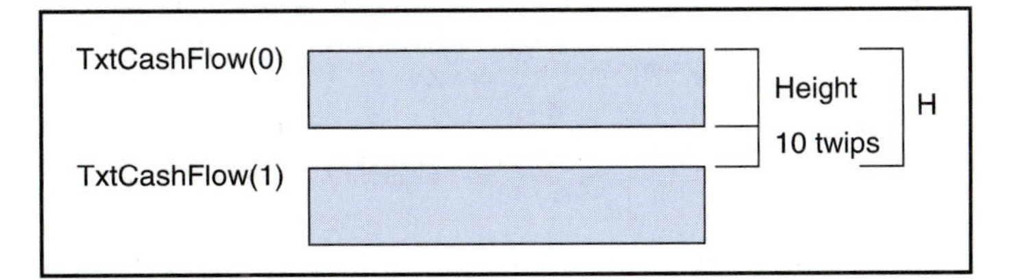

Figure 9.2
Layout of the Text Boxes

In a way, the creation of a control array at runtime appears to run against the "spirit" of VB. The key feature of VB is that the developer has tools to create/design the visual element of a project at design time. However, there are situations in which you may have to resort to creating a control array at runtime. For example, the number of controls to be placed on a form may not be known until runtime; that is, the size of the array may have to depend on the user or other input.

Sample Uses of Control Arrays

Why use control arrays? In many cases, their use helps simplify the code. The following three examples represent a sample of their uses.

Simplified Code for Data Movement. Consider the text box array txtCashFlow that was created in the previous illustration. Cash flow data entered by the user can be used for the computation of the net present value or other values for capital project evaluation. Data in the controls, however, are not (should not be) used directly for computations. They are first assigned to variables, (in this case, an array variable), which are then used in the computations. Assume the array CashFlow has been declared properly. The following lines of code will move the data from the control array to the array variable:

```
For I = 0 To 4
    CashFlow(I) = Val(txtCashFlow.Text(I))
Next I
```

Coding this way also provides greater flexibility. When the upper and lower bounds of the arrays (the variable and the control) change, the counter of the loop can be changed easily, especially if the starting and ending values are set by variables. In contrast, if either the controls or the variables are not set up as arrays, the change in the upper and lower bounds (number of data elements) will call for a change in the program by adding or deleting some statements.

Code Minimization. When controls are set up as arrays, the header of their event procedures also change, with an additional Index parameter passed to the procedures. For example, the KeyPress event procedure for a single control (e.g., txtNumber) appears as follows:

```
Private Sub txtNumber_KeyPress(KeyAscii As Integer)
```

The same procedure for the control array txtCashFlow will appear as follows:

```
Private Sub txtCashFlow_KeyPress(Index As Integer, _
    KeyAscii As Integer)
```

The Index parameter here refers to the Index of the control for which this event is raised; for example, when txtCashFlow(0) has a KeyPress event, the Index parameter will have a value of 0.

If your code will apply to all controls in the array, you can safely ignore the value of Index. Thus, the following code to ensure that all keys entered are numeric will apply to all controls in the array:

```
Private Sub txtCashFlow_KeyPress(Index As Integer, _
    KeyAscii As Integer)
    Select Case KeyAscii
    Case Is < vbKeySpace
    ' Control keys, no problem
    Case vbKey0 To vbKey9
    ' Numeric keys, no problem
    Case Else
    ' Non-numeric keys, display error message
        MsgBox "Numeric keys only, please."
    ' and suppress the key
        KeyAscii = 0
    End Select
End Sub
```

This code is sufficient to handle the potential key problems for *all* text boxes in the array without the need to provide the code for each individual control.

Identifying the Last Element Having an Event: Which Option Button Is On? Occasionally, you may need to identify the control that has an event raised most recently. For example, you may need to know which option button in a group was last clicked. Assume that you use four option buttons for the user to specify the depreciation method for fixed assets. These four methods are the straight-line, double declining balance, ACRS, and the modified ACRS methods. When the user clicks the "Compute" command button, your program will need to identify the depreciation method specified before the computation of depreciation can proceed. Without the use of a control array for the depreciation methods, you will need to give the code to test the Value property of each control to identify the option button clicked.

On the other hand, with the use of a control array for these option buttons, you have other ways. For example, you can use a loop to identify which option button's Value property is True. Still another way is to use a form-level variable and assign it the Index value of the control array in the array's Click event. The following code illustrates how this is done (assuming the control array is named optDepreMethod).

```
' Module level declaration
Option Explicit
Dim DepreMethod As Integer

Private Sub optDepreMethod_Click(Index As Integer)
' Keep the index of the current button clicked
    DepreMethod = Index
End Sub
```

The assignment statement inside the event procedure identifies the depreciation method (its index) that is last clicked. The variable DepreMethod can then be used in the command button Click event to guide the computation of depreciation as shown in the following code:

```
Private Sub cmdCompute_Click()
' DepreMethod has the index of the option button that was last clicked
    Select Case DepreMethod
    Case 0
    ' Place code for straight line depreciation here
    Case 1
    ' Place code for double declining balance here
    Case 2
    ' Place code for ACRS here
    Case 3
    ' Place code for modified ACRS here
    End Select
End Sub
```

This approach can reduce the lines of code in identifying the control in question. However, the drawback is that the code may no longer be as clear. One way to improve its readability is to replace the literal constant with named constant. For example, you can declare the constant name dmACRS with a value of 2 to represent the ACRS method. Also, as always give plenty of comments to clarify the purpose of your code.

9.5 Two-Dimensional Arrays

As stated at the beginning of this chapter, array variables can have more than one dimension. Let's consider the case of two-dimensional variables. The syntax to declare a two-dimensional variable is as follows:

```
Dim Name([LB1 To] UB1, [LB2 To] UB2) [As Type]
```

where *Name* = any legitimate variable name

LB_n = lower bound for the nth subscript

UB_n = upper bound for the nth subscript

Type = any valid data type

As you can see, the only difference between a two-dimensional array and one-dimensional array is the number of subscript(s). When a variable has more than one subscript, the subscripts are separated by commas. The following are examples of valid declarations of two-dimensional arrays:

```
Dim A(9, 9) As Integer
Dim Weights(62 To 76, 2) As String
Dim Tuition(1 To 18, 1 To 3) As Single
```

The first line declares a 10 × 10 Integer array, A, depicted as follows:

A(0, 0)	A(0, 1)	A(0, 2)	...	A(0, 9)
A(1, 0)	.	.	.	A(1, 9)
.	.	.	.	.
A(9, 0)				A(9, 9)

Note that when the lower bound of a subscript is not declared, it defaults to 0.

The second line declares a 15 × 3 Weights String table depicted as follows:

Weights(62, 0)	Weights(62, 1)	Weights(62, 2)
Weights(63, 0)	.	.
.	.	.
Weights(76, 0)		Weights(76, 2)

The third line declares a 18 × 3 Tuition table depicted as follows:

Tuition(1, 1)	Tuition(1, 2)	Tuition(1, 3)
Tuition(2, 1)	.	.
.	.	.
Tuition(18, 1)		Tuition(18, 3)

How are two-dimensional arrays used? They can be used to represent various kinds of two-dimensional data. The following discussion explains how they can be used to represent tables, matrices, and even game boards.

Tables

Let's revisit the weight watcher example from the first section. The weight table shown there was only for males with a medium frame. What happens to the small- and large-frame males? Actually, the complete weight table appears as follows:

Height (in Shoes)	Small Frame	Medium Frame	Large Frame
5'2"	112–120	118–129	126–141
5'3"	115–123	121–133	129–144
5'4"	118–126	124–136	132–148
5'5"	121–129	127–139	135–152
5'6"	124–133	130–143	138–156
5'7"	128–137	134–147	138–156
5'8"	132–141	138–152	147–166
5'9"	136–145	142–156	151–170
5'10"	140–150	146–160	155–174
5'11"	144–154	150–165	159–179
6'	148–158	154–170	164–184
6'1"	152–162	158–175	168–189
6'2"	156–167	162–180	173–194
6'3"	160–171	167–185	178–199
6'4"	164–175	172–190	182–204

Refining the Weight Watcher Project. We can design a project similar to the previous one with this "more complete" set of data to respond to any normal-weight queries. The weights shown in the preceding table can be read into a two-dimensional array. The user can specify the height and the frame size and then click a "Show Normal Weight" command button.

The program can then retrieve a "cell" (an element) from the table and display it in a label. The visual interface appears as in Figure 9.3.

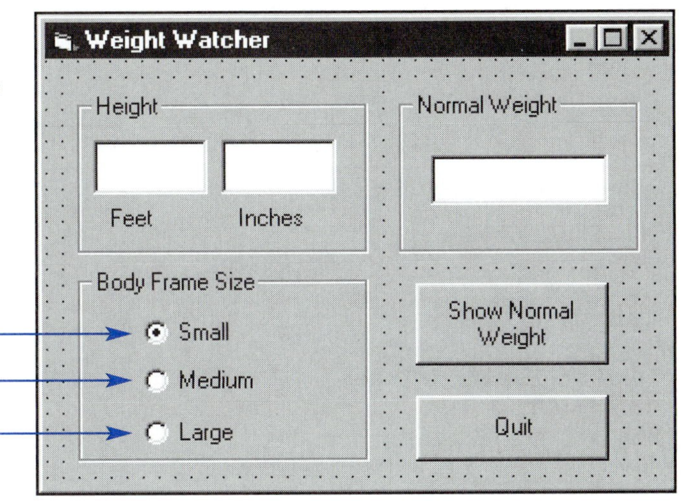

Figure 9.3
Visual Interface for the Weight Watcher Project

These option buttons are named optBodyFrame(0), optBodyFrame(1), and optBodyFrame(2). The advantage is that you can identify which one is clicked with one line of code, as explained in the text.

The following table lists the controls and properties used in the code.

Control	Property	Setting	Remarks
Text box	Name	txtFeet	To specify height
Text box	Name	txtInches	
Label	Name	lblNormalWeight	To display normal weight for the given height
Option buttons (array indexed from 0 to 2)	Name	optBodyFrame	To specify body frame
	Caption	Small, Medium, and Large for array element 0, 1, and 2, respectively	
Command button	Name	cmdShow	To initiate the computation and display of normal weight
	Caption	Show normal weight	
Command button	Name	cmdQuit	To terminate the program
	Caption	Quit	

Code Requirements. What are the required actions for the project?

1. As soon as the program starts, the weight table needs to be read in from a file; that is, the weight array Weights() needs to be populated with data.
2. When the user clicks the "Show Normal Weight" command button, the program needs to do the following:
   2.1 Convert the height into inches.
   2.2 Identify the option button clicked for the frame size.
3. Use the numbers obtained in number 2 to retrieve and display the weight data in the label.

Coding the Project. Let's now consider the code for the project. The first step is to populate the Weights() table as the project starts. Assume the data file has been created in a manner suitable for the Input statement. Further assume that the heights in the file are in inches. That is, the file appears as follows:

62, "112-120", "118-129", "126-141"

63 ...

.

.

76 ... "182-204"

The table can then be populated as follows:

```
Option Explicit
Dim Weights(62 To 76, 2) As String
Private Sub Form_Load()
Dim I As Integer
Dim Height As Integer
Dim WeightFile As Integer
' Open weight file
WeightFile = FreeFile
Open "MaleWeights.txt" For Input As #WeightFile
' Populate the weight table
    For I = 62 to 76
        Input #WeightFile, Height, _
          Weights(I,0), Weights(I, 1), Weights(I, 2)
    Next I
End Sub
```

Note that the second subscript of weight has a range from 0 to 2. We use the columns 0, 1, and 2 to store the weights for small, medium, and large frames, respectively. Thus, Weights(76,2) refers to the normal weight for a male with a height of 6'4" and a large frame; that is, 182–204. Also note that because the heights are implicitly represented by the first subscript of Weights(), there is no need to store the height data with another array. Thus, the height data in the file are read without being stored as an array. At the end of the loop, the variable Height will have only one value (the last value read), 76.

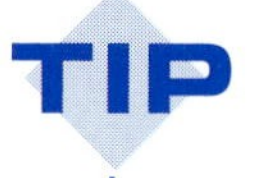

In this example, there is another (and better) way to read the weights into the Weights() array as shown here:

```
Do Until EOF(WeightFile)
    Input #WeightFile, Height
    Input#WeightFile, Weight(Height,0),Weight(Height,1), _
      Weight(Height,2)
Loop
```

The first Input statement reads the height. Then the second Input statement uses the value of Height as the first subscript of the Weight array. Thus, when the Height (the first element in the line) is 63, the second Input statement will place the weight data in Weight(63,0), Weight(63,1), and Weight(63,2). The weight data will always be stored in the correct positions in the array, even if the content of the file has been changed. Also, if the array has been declared to accommodate a wider range of heights, you will never have to worry about revising the program when weights for other heights are added to the file.

When the Show button is clicked, the program needs to convert the height to inches and identify which of the frame option buttons is clicked. Converting the height is easy, as shown in the previous example:

```
Inches = Val(txtFeet.Text) * 12 + Val(txtInches.Text)
```

But how do we identify which option button was last clicked? We will use the approach shown in the subsection "Which Option Button Is On?" That is, the option buttons in the preceding interface are set up as a control array, named optBodyFrame, with the Index 0, 1, and 2 representing small, medium, and large, respectively. We will use the variable BodyFrame to identify the button clicked. We can then code the option buttons' Click event procedure as follows:

```
Private Sub optBodyFrame_Click(Index As Integer)
    BodyFrame = Index 'Keep the index of the button clicked
End Sub
```

Finally, how do we identify which weight to show? The element (cell), Weights(Inches,BodyFrame) should give the weight that corresponds to the height and body frame "computed" previously. The complete code of the project should appear as follows:

```
Option Explicit
Dim Weights(62 To 76, 2) As String
Dim BodyFrame As Integer

Private Sub Form_Load()
Dim I As Integer
Dim Height As Integer
Dim WeightFile As Integer
' Open weight file
    WeightFile = FreeFile
    Open "MaleWeights.txt" For Input As #WeightFile
' Populate the weight table
    For I = 62 to 76
        Input #WeightFile, Height, _
          Weights(I,0), Weights(I, 1), Weights(I, 2)
    Next I
End Sub

Private Sub optBodyFrame_Click(Index As Integer)
    BodyFrame = Index 'Keep the index of the option button '
                      clicked
End Sub

Private Sub cmdShow_Click()
Dim Inches As Integer
    ' Convert height to inches
    Inches = Val(txtFeet.Text) * 12 + Val(txtInches.Text)
    ' Display result in label
    lblNormalWeight.Caption = Weights(Inches, BodyFrame)
End Sub
```

Can you see the benefits of using a table (array) for selection? Without the Weights table as an array, the alternative will be to code the project using the Select Case structure. Compare this solution with the solution to the tuition problem illustrated in Chapter 5, "Decision." Using that approach, you will also need to nest the Select Case structure because the selection involves two factors, the height and the body frame size. The code will be much longer and not as neat or elegant.

Matrices

A matrix consists of a rectangular array of numeric elements in rows and columns. It is mainly used in matrix algebra to handle various linear algebraic problems. The two-dimensional array fits exactly the definition of a matrix and can be used to represent the matrix to perform any matrix operations. For example, by definition, adding two matrices calls for the addition of the corresponding elements in the two matrix operands. Suppose the two matrices as represented by 2 two-dimensional arrays are A and B. The matrix operation A + B will mean performing A(I, J) + B(I, J) for the entire range of both subscripts. A and B should be required to be declared with the same dimensions. The following Sub procedure adds the two matrices and gives the results to C, another matrix that is expected to have the same dimensions as A and B.

```
Sub MatrixAdd(A() As Double, B() As Double, C() As Double)
Dim I As Integer
Dim J As Integer
```

```
        For I = LBound(A, 1) To UBound(A, 1)
            For J = LBound(A, 2) To UBound(A, 2)
                C(I, J) = A(I, J) + B(I, J)
            Next J
        Next I
    End Sub
```

In this procedure, the loop counters I and J are set to start from the lower bound to the upper bound of their respective subscripts.

Notice the arguments used in the LBound and UBound functions. When the array has more than one subscript, you can specify the subscript number for which you want the boundary. LBound(A, 1) tells the function to return the lower bound of the first subscript; and UBound(A, 2) tells the function to return the upper bound of the second subscript. When the optional second parameter (the subscript number) is omitted, the first subscript is the default.

Game Boards

Two-dimensional arrays can also be used to represent boards used in games that call for the placement of different markers or stones on the board. For example, in a tic-tac-toe game, two players will mark alternately on a 3 × 3 board with X's and O's. The first player who can place three of the same marks in a straight line (vertically, horizontally, or diagonally) wins the game. You can use a two-dimensional variable (e.g., Status) to keep track of the marks that the players place on the board while your program "draws" the marks on the screen. For example, when the first player places an X mark on position (1,1), you can code the following:

```
    Status(1, 1) = 1
```

You can use any nonzero value to represent one side and another value (e.g., -1) to represent the other side. A zero value in a position will indicate that the position is not yet marked (occupied) and is available; otherwise, an attempt to mark the position will be considered illegitimate. Each time a player marks a position, your program will need to determine whether your program can declare him or her the winner.

In addition to keeping track of the status internally, you will also need to consider how the game should be represented "externally"; that is, what will be used to represent the board and the marks on the screen. One way is to actually draw the X and O marks on a picture box, which can be used to represent the board. You should be able to do this after you study Appendix B, "Graphics, Animation, Drag and Drop." An easier way (which uses more computer resources) is to use an array of nine labels to represent the nine positions on the board. (Again, you can use a picture box as the board.)

To illustrate how this can be done, let's actually develop a project for the game.

The Visual Interface. When your program starts, the visual interface can appear as in Figure 9.4. The interface requires the following controls:

1. A picture box. This control will serve as the game board.
2. A label array. At design time, you need to draw only one label in the picture box. Be sure to draw this control in the picture box so that the latter is the container of the label. (Do not just create a label and drag it into the picture box.)

The following table lists selected property settings for these controls.

Control	Property	Setting	Remarks
Picture box	Name	PicBoard	To serve as the game board
Label	Name	lblMark	To show the mark
	Caption	(Cleared)	
	Font	Courier New 24	
	Alignment	2 - Centered	To center the mark
	BorderStyle	1 - Fixed Single	To show the label as a square
	Index	1	First element of the array

Notice that the lowest index for the label is set to 1, not 0. This has some implication to the computation formula for each label's position.

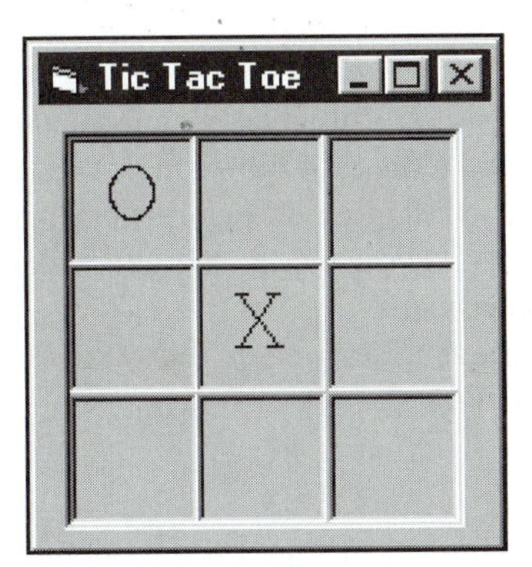
Tic Tac Toe
O
X

Figure 9.4
The Tic-Tac-Toe Game in Action

As the players take turns in marking the board (by clicking the square), your program displays the proper marks and declares the winner when one player is able to place three of the same marks in a straight line.

Setting up the Tic-Tac-Toe Board. When your program starts, the board (picture box) should appear with 3 × 3 blank squares. These squares are labels in an array. When your program starts, it needs to do the following:

1. Make sure that the board is square. You can use code to assign the picture box's width setting to its Height property to accomplish this.
2. Compute the dimension of each "square" (label) so that the nine squares will fit in the board. Each label should be one-third of the board in width and height.
3. Position the squares (labels) in the board. The label's Move method can be used. The challenge is computing the position of these squares. The following discussion focuses on this aspect first.

Determining the Positions of the Squares. While the labels are indexed as one to nine, they are placed squarely in a 3 × 3 area as shown in Figure 9.5. The first "view" takes a sequence of numbers, whereas the second view requires a coordinate.

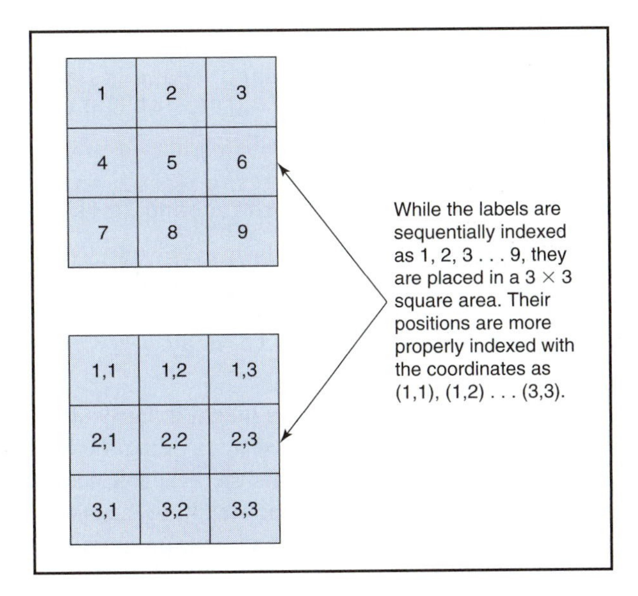
1
2
3
4
5
6
7
8
9
1,1
1,2
1,3
2,1
2,2
2,3
3,1
3,2
3,3
While the labels are sequentially indexed as 1, 2, 3 . . . 9, they are placed in a 3 × 3 square area. Their positions are more properly indexed with the coordinates as (1,1), (1,2) . . . (3,3).

Figure 9.5
Different "Views" of the Squares

To convert from one view to the other, we can write two general procedures: one to convert from the sequence number to the coordinate (call it ItoXY) and another to convert from the coordinate to the sequence number (call it XYtoI).

The ItoXY procedure can be written as a Sub as follows:

```
Sub ItoXY(I As Integer, X As Integer, Y As Integer)
    X = (I - 1) Mod 3 + 1
    Y = Int((I - 1) / 3) + 1
End Sub
```

Note that X gives the horizontal position of the two-dimensional coordinate. You can verify that the formula will produce 1, 2, 3, and repeat for the sequence 1, 2, 3 ... 9. These are the numbers for the second subscript in the second diagram in Figure 9.5. The formula for Y should yield 1 for the sequence numbers 1, 2, and 3; and 2 for 4, 5, and 6; and so on. Thus, Y gives the vertical coordinate of the two-dimensional board.

The XYtoI procedure can be written as a function as follows:

```
Function XYtoI(X As Integer, Y As Integer) As Integer
    XYtoI = (Y - 1) * 3 + X
End Function
```

You can verify that for each coordinate (X, Y) the formula in the function produces the correct sequence number for the corresponding diagram in the first diagram in Figure 9.5.

In general, when a procedure returns a value, it is more convenient to code it as a function. However, when it affects more than one value, a Sub procedure is more convenient. Once these procedures are available you can use them to compute the positions of the squares (labels).

Positioning the Squares. As soon as the project starts, the squares should be placed in the game board in their proper positions. The code to perform this should be placed in the Form Load event procedure as follows:

```
Option Explicit
Dim Player As Integer
Dim Status(1 To 3, 1 To 3) As Integer
Private Sub Form_Load()
Dim X As Integer
Dim Y As Integer
Dim W As Single
Dim H As Single
Dim I As Integer
    picBoard.Height = picBoard.Width 'Make the board square
    W = picBoard.ScaleWidth / 3 'Width for the square
    H = W 'Height for the square (same as width)
    'Position and set the size for 1st label
    lblMark(1).Move 0, 0, W, H
    For I = 2 To 9
        Load lblMark(I) 'Load the label into memory
        ItoXY I, X, Y 'Find the coordinate for this label
        'Position the label
        lblMark(I).Move (X - 1) * W, (Y - 1) * H
        lblMark(I).Visible = True 'Make the square visible
    Next I
    Player = 1 'First player to play
End Sub
```

The computation of each label's width and height is fairly straightforward. W, the variable used to keep the width of the label, is obtained by dividing the ScaleWidth of the picture box. Recall that the ScaleWidth property represents the available interior width. The result is also assigned to H, the variable used to represent the Height of the label. (Using this variable is actually redundant but might add to the readability of your program.) The statement:

```
lblMark(1).Move 0, 0, W, H
```

moves the first label to the upper-left corner of its container (the picture box) and sets the label's width and height to W and H, the value computed previously.

In the For loop, I starts from 2 and ends with 9. These values are used to load the second through the ninth labels in the array. The sequence number I is then converted to X and Y using the ItoXY Sub procedure discussed previously. The statement:

```
lblMark(I).Move (X - 1) * W, (Y - 1) * H
```

moves the current label to the coordinate represented by (X, Y). Note that in computing the actual position, both X and Y are subtracted by 1 because the first position has a coordinate of (1, 1). Subtracting 1 gives the number of positions from the first position. Because each label has a width and height of W and H, the positional values are multiplied by these values to obtain actual coordinates in twips.

Note that we have also declared two form-level (module-level) variables. Player will be used to keep track of the side to play, and the array Status will be used to record the status of the positions on the board as explained previously. These two variables are used in several procedures.

Playing the Game. As the players take turns to click a position (square) on the board, the computer should determine whether the selection is legitimate. If the square has already been marked, the computer should signal an error. In the following procedure, this is accomplished by sending a "Beep" sound with the ***Beep statement***. The procedure should terminate.

On the other hand, if the selection is legitimate, the computer should display the mark for the player. When the first player clicks a square, an X mark will be displayed; when the second player clicks a square, an O mark will be displayed. In addition, the variable Status should record this mark. The label array's Click event procedure appears as follows:

```
Private Sub lblMark_Click(Index As Integer)
Dim X As Integer
Dim Y As Integer
     ItoXY Index, X, Y 'Find the position clicked
     If Status(Y, X) Then
     ' Position already marked, beep and do nothing
         Beep
         Exit Sub
     End If
     Status(Y, X) = Player 'Record the mark
     ' Mark the position
     Select Case Player
     Case 1
     ' If current player is the first player, place an "X"
         lblMark(Index).Caption = "X"
     Case -1
     ' If current player is the second player, place an "O"
         lblMark(Index).Caption = "O"
     End Select
     FindWinner 'Determine if a player wins
     Player = -Player 'Change hand
End Sub
```

Notice the statement at the end of the procedure:

```
Player = -Player 'Change hand
```

This statement changes the sign of the value for Player. Thus, in effect, we are using 1 to represent the first player and –1 to represent the second player. These values are used in the Select Case block to determine which mark to display in the label clicked.

After each mark (click), the computer should also determine whether the current player should be declared the winner. This is done by calling a Sub procedure named FindWinner.

Determining the Winner. There are several ways to determine whether the current player wins the game. The most straightforward way is to check to see whether any of the straight lines has three marks of the same kind. You can check the Status array for this purpose. Note that zeros should not be considered marks.

To determine whether the diagonal down right positions have three of the same marks, you can code the following:

```
Dim ThePlayer As Integer
    ' Diagonal down right
    If Status(1, 1) Then
        ThePlayer = Status(1, 1)
        If Status(2, 2) = ThePlayer And _
        Status(3, 3) = ThePlayer Then
        MsgBox lblMark(XYtoI(1, 1)).Caption & _
        " is the winner"
        Exit Sub
    End If
    End If
```

The preceding code gets the value of the upper-left position, Status(1,1), and checks whether it is nonzero. If so, it checks to see whether both of the other squares on the diagonal are of the same value. If so, the program declares the winner with the mark displayed at position (1, 1). The left down diagonal can be checked in a similar manner.

You can use the same approach to check whether a row has three of the same marks. Because the three rows can be checked in the same manner, you can use a For loop to perform the task. The code appears as follows:

```
' Row wise
    For I = 1 To 3
        If Status(I, 1) Then
            ThePlayer = Status(I, 1)
            If Status(I, 2) = ThePlayer And _
              Status(I, 3) = ThePlayer Then
                MsgBox lblMark(XYtoI(I, 1)).Caption & _
                " is the winner"
                Exit Sub
            End If
        End If
    Next I
```

Declaring the Winner: The Complete Procedure. Overall, the procedure should check four possible different types of "three of the same marks." These include diagonal down right, diagonal down left, row wise, and column wise. Note that the latter two include all rows and all columns. The complete procedure should appear as follows:

```
Sub FindWinner()
Dim I As Integer
Dim ThePlayer As Integer
    ' Diagonal down right
    If Status(1, 1) Then
        ThePlayer = Status(1, 1)
        If Status(2, 2) = ThePlayer And _
          Status(3, 3) = ThePlayer Then
            MsgBox lblMark(XYtoI(1, 1)).Caption & _
            " is the winner"
            Exit Sub
        End If
    End If
    ' Diagonal down left
    If Status(1, 3) Then
        ThePlayer = Status(1, 3)
        If Status(2, 2) = ThePlayer And _
          Status(3, 1) = ThePlayer Then
            MsgBox lblMark(XYtoI(1, 3)).Caption & _
            " is the winner"
            Exit Sub
        End If
    End If
```

```
        ' Row wise
        For I = 1 To 3
            If Status(I, 1) Then
                ThePlayer = Status(I, 1)
                If Status(I, 2) = ThePlayer And _
                  Status(I, 3) = ThePlayer Then
                    MsgBox lblMark(XYtoI(I, 1)).Caption & _
                    " is the winner"
                    Exit Sub
                End If
            End If
        Next I
        ' Column wise
        For I = 1 To 3
            If Status(1, I) Then
                ThePlayer = Status(1, I)
                If Status(2, I) = ThePlayer And _
                  Status(3, I) = ThePlayer Then
                    MsgBox lblMark(XYtoI(1, I)).Caption & _
                    " is the winner"
                    Exit Sub
                End If
            End If
        Next I
    End Sub
```

Additional Remarks. Of course, the preceding program can be improved in several ways:

- After the program declares a winner, the board and the status array can be cleared for another game. In addition, a command button can be provided for the user to click to start a new game. (The game can end without a winner.)
- The "squares" can be made to look nicer with more attractive colors.
- Additional routines can be added so that the computer can play the game against a single user.

These desirable enhancements are left to you as an exercise. Note that the tic-tac-toe game is fairly simple compared with many other games. There are various challenges to the programmer to program a board game. Suffice it to say that the two-dimensional array can be handily used to represent the state of the board.

9.6 Additional Notes on Arrays

The preceding discussion focuses on the practical uses of arrays. This section presents several additional matters/issues concerning arrays that deserve your attention.

Default Lower Bound and Option Base 1

We have stated that if a variable is declared without explicitly indicating its lower bound, the default lower bound will be 0. Thus, the statement:

```
Dim A(9) As Integer
```

will in effect declare the array A to have a subscript range of 0 to 9. The default lower bound of all arrays in a form can be changed to 1 if you place an ***Option Base 1*** statement in the general declaration section. (Note that you must place this statement before any Dim statement that declares an array.) For example, the following statements will declare the array variable Scores to have a subscript range of 1 to 50:

```
Option Explicit
Option Base 1
Dim Scores(50) As Integer
```

That is, in this case, the statement:

```
Print LBound(A)
```

will display a value of 1 instead 0. (Place this line in the Form Click event and test the result.)

Preserving Data in ReDim

Each time you use the ReDim statement to change the size of an array, the previous content of all elements will be reinitialized (to 0 for numeric variables and to zero-length string for string variables) and lost. However, you can preserve their previous contents by using the keyword "Preserve" in the ReDim statement. For example, assume a form-level array variable Students() has been previously populated with text strings and you would like to expand its size by doubling its upper bound without losing its previous contents. You should be able to accomplish this by the following statement:

```
ReDim Preserve Students(2 * UBound(Students))
```

Clearing the Content of an Array: The Erase Statement

You can clear (reinitialize) the contents of an array (declared with the Dim statement) by using the Erase statement. For example, suppose the array variable Employees has been populated with a department's employee names and you would like to clear its contents so that you can populate it with the employee names of another department. You should be able to clear the array variable's previous contents by coding the following:

```
Erase Employees()
```

Note that the pair of parentheses following the name of the array variable are optional.

If an array is created with the ReDim statement (i.e., it is created dynamically), the Erase statement will not only clear the array's previous contents but also reduce the array to zero elements. That is, Erase in effect releases the memory previously occupied by the array variable.

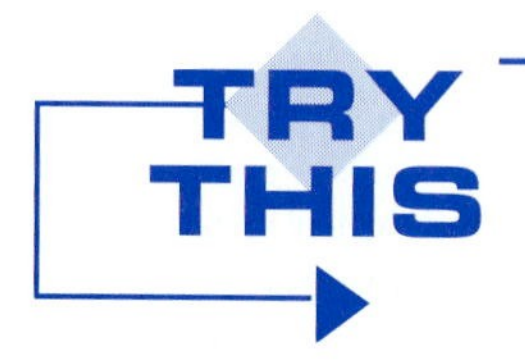

Enter the following code in a new form:

```
Option Explicit
Private Sub Form_Click()
Dim A(100) As Long
    ReDim B(100) As Long
    Debug.Print "UBound(A)="; UBound(A)
    Debug.Print "UBound(B)="; UBound(B)
    Erase A, B
    Debug.Print "UBound(A)="; UBound(A)
    Debug.Print "UBound(B)="; UBound(B)
End Sub
```

Run the project and click the form. You will encounter a "Subscript Out of Range" error with the last Debug.Print statement highlighted. The immediate window should show 100 as the upper bound for A before and after the Erase statement. However, after the Erase statement, the dynamic array B no longer has any element in it. Thus, you get the error message.

Appropriate Use of Arrays

As you can see from all the preceding examples, arrays can be very useful and powerful. Often, they are used in conjunction with loops. For this reason, arrays tend to be overused by the beginner when the program calls for the use of loops. As an illustration, suppose we would like to read a file and list its content. Simple? Assume the file (named DataFile) has been opened. After learning about arrays, a beginner would tend to code as follows:

```
Dim DataRec(1 To 5000) As String
Dim Counter As Integer
Dim I as Integer
```

```
Do Until EOF(DataFile)
     Counter = Counter + 1
     Line Input #DataFile, DataRec(Counter)
Loop
For I = 1 To Counter
     lstRecords.AddItem DataRec(I)
Next I
```

That is, the entire file is read in and kept in the memory before each record is added to the list box lstRecords for display. If the data in a file can be handled in one single pass (reading from the beginning through the end), there is actually no need to use an array.

The same goal can indeed be accomplished with the following code:

```
Dim DataRec As string
Do Until EOF(DataFile)
     Line Input #DataFile, DataRec
     lstRecords.AddItem DataRec
Loop
```

Arrays use much more memory than scalar variables. When there is no need to use arrays, they should be avoided. In general, you will need an array if the group of data will need to be worked on back and forth (usually more than one time) or randomly such that the order cannot be predicted. Hopefully, the examples in this chapter have shown you the proper context where arrays are called for.

9.7 An Application Example

Accumulating Total Sales by Product

We conclude this chapter with an application example, which requires the accumulation of total sales by product.

The Project. Your company sells 25 different products. The sales transactions are kept in a sequential file. Each record contains a field representing the product (product code) and another field for the sales amount. These records are kept in ascending order by the transaction date (thus, not by the product code). You are interested in obtaining the total sales by product. The results should be displayed in a list box.

Algorithm

How can the sales be accumulated by product when the file is not sorted in the order of product code? There are several ways, each with variations in details. We will follow an approach that uses two arrays, one to keep track of the product codes already encountered and the other to accumulate total sales for the corresponding products. This can be depicted as follows:

Product Codes

D	A	C	...	K

Sales by Product

Sales for D	Sales for A	Sales for C	...	Sales for K

How do we keep track of product codes? As each record is read, its product code is compared with the ones already in the product code array. The number of codes already in the array can be tracked by a counter variable (e.g., ProductCount). If the current product code is not found, ProductCount should be increased by 1 and the current (new) product code placed in this position. This approach is similar to the first method of generating a random lottery number discussed previously.

How do we accumulate the sales for the corresponding product? The preceding search for the product code should give the position of the product code in the array. Let's call the position ProductPos. This value can then be used as the subscript for the array SalesByProduct to add the current sales. That is, the total sales by product can be accumulated with the following statement:

```
SalesByProduct(ProductPos) = SalesByProduct(ProductPos) + Sales
```

Coding the Project

Suppose the routine to perform the computation is invoked when the user clicks the button named cmdCompute. This routine should do the following:

1. Read the sales records.
2. Build the product code array and accumulate the total sales by product.
3. Display the results in a list box.

Because the accumulation of sales hinges on the successful creation of the product code array, let's consider this aspect in more detail. To show how this array can be built, we will assume the first few records in the file as follows. For simplicity, we will pay attention only to product code.

Record No.	Product Code	Sales Amount (Not Shown)
1	D	
2	A	
3	D	
4	C	

When the first record is read, the product code array is empty and the product count is zero. The current product code in record one (i.e., D) will be compared with all elements in the product code array, which is still empty. Thus, D is not found. We will then increase the product count by 1 and place D in this position of the product code array. The state in the memory can be represented as follows:

Record No.	Product Code	Product Count	Content of Product Codes (Array)
1 (before processing)	D	0	(Empty)
1 (after processing)	D	1	D

After the second record is read and before it is processed, the memory state will be the same as after processing the first record, except for the current product code from the record, which is now A. The same steps just outlined will be repeated. Again, A is not found in the array. Thus, the product count will be increased by 1. The product code A is added to the array. The states of memory should be as follows:

Record No.	Product Code	Product Count	Content of Product Codes (Array)
1 (before processing)	D	0	(Empty)
1 (after processing)	D	1	D
2 (after processing)	A	2	D, A

When the third record is read, the current product code will be D, which is already in the array. Thus, there will be no change to the product codes array. The product code position will be identified and used to accumulate the sales amount.

Because the product codes can appear in any order, they will be searched sequentially. The search routine appears as follows:

```
For I = 1 To ProductCount
      If ProductCode = ProductCodes(I) Then
    ' A match is found, set the product position and
      ' terminate the loop
        ProductPos = I
        Exit For
    End If
Next I
```

If the product code is not found, we will need to add it to the array. As shown in the lottery number example, to determine whether the product code is in the array, we will need an indicator. Here, we will use the value of ProductPos for this purpose.

How? As shown in the preceding code, if the product code is found, ProductPos will be set to its position in the array. The position has to be in the range of 1 to ProductCount. If we set ProductPos to ProductCount + 1 before the loop, we can check whether this value has changed. If it has not changed, the product code is not found and we can add the current product code to the array. Thus, the code can appear as follows:

```
ProductPos = ProductCount + 1
For I = 1 To ProductCount
    If ProductCode = ProductCodes(I) Then
    ' Product code is found, get this position and exit the loop
        ProductPos = I
        Exit For
    End If
Next I
If ProductPos = ProductCount + 1 Then
' No change in product pos as initially set.
' This means the product code is not found
' Update count and add the code to array
    ProductCount = ProductPos 'Increase count by 1
    ' and keep the current code in the array
    ProductCodes(ProductPos) = ProductCode
End If
```

The preceding code deals with a product code read from a record. Of course, we will need to open and read the file. Reading the entire file will take another loop, which should be the outer loop of the preceding routine. For simplicity, we assume that each transaction in the file has only two fields: product code and sales. We further assume that the file is created in a manner suitable for the Input statement. The following code should carry out the project's requirements:

```
Private Sub cmdCompute_Click()
Dim I As Integer
Dim SalesFile As Integer
Dim ProductPos As Integer
Dim ProductCount As Integer
Dim ProductCode As String
Dim Sales As Double
Dim ProductCodes(1 To 25) As String
Dim SalesByProduct(1 To 25) As Double
' Step 1: Open sales file
    SalesFile = FreeFile
    Open "C:\Sales\Sales.txt" For Input As SalesFile
' Step 2: read and accumulate sales by product
    Do Until EOF(SalesFile)
        Input #SalesFile, ProductCode, Sales
        ' Search for the product code in Product codes array
        ' Assume this product code is not in array;
        ' in that case the product position will be one more
        ' than the current count
        ProductPos = ProductCount + 1
```

```
                For I = 1 To ProductCount
                    If ProductCode = ProductCodes(I) Then
                    ' Product code is found, get this position
                    ' and exit the loop
                        ProductPos = I
                        Exit For
                    End If
                Next I
                If ProductPos = ProductCount + 1 Then
                ' No change in product pos as initially set;
                    ' this means the product code is not found
                    ' Update count and add the code to array
                    ProductCount = ProductPos 'Increase count by 1
                    ' and keep the current code in the array
                    ProductCodes(ProductPos) = ProductCode
                End If
            ' Add current sales to corresponding total
                SalesByProduct(ProductPos) = _
                    SalesByProduct(ProductPos) + Sales
        Loop
    ' Step 3: Show results in the list box
        For I = 1 To ProductCount
            lstSales.AddItem ProductCodes(I) & vbTab & _
              SalesByProduct(I)
        Next I
    End Sub
```

The procedure begins with opening the sales file for input. Then in the outer loop, the product code and sales in each record are read. Next comes the routine to search for the product code and set the value for the product position, including handling the addition of a new product code. Then, the statement:

```
SalesByProduct(ProductPos) = SalesByProduct(ProductPos) + Sales
```

adds the current sales to the total sales at the position ProductPos. If the current product code is D (refer to the diagram at the beginning of the example), ProductPos should have a value of 1. Thus, the statement will in effect appear as follows:

```
SalesByProduct(1) = SalesByProduct(1) + Sales
```

Consequently, the current sales will be added to the first element (which corresponds to the position of Product D) of the array SalesByProduct. In sum, this statement tells the computer to add current sales to the total sales of the current product code.

Finally, step 3 uses a For loop to populate the list box with the accumulated sales by product using the AddItem method. If the Sorted property of the list box is set to True, the list box will show the sales in ascending order by the product code.

As stated at the beginning of this example, other algorithms can be used to solve the same problem. For example, you can sort the file by product code first. Then, the accumulation of sales by product basically involves going through the sorted data arrays in sequential order and adding the sales with the same product code together. The implementation of this algorithm is left to you as an exercise.

Summary

This chapter presents arrays and their uses. You have learned how arrays can be declared and have been introduced to various uses of one-dimensional arrays. You have also learned several sorting algorithms. Sorting is an interesting and important use of arrays. Sorted data can be searched much more efficiently by the use of the binary search algorithm.

You have also learned how control arrays can be created at design time and runtime, as well as how they can be used to minimize code and improve program elegance. The uses of two-dimensional arrays are also mentioned with brief illustrations.

This chapter also shows an application example to illustrate how arrays can be used to accumulate sales by product. The same method can be applied to various similar problems; for example, accumulating expenses by department, total assets by account, and product purchase costs by vendor, and so on.

Recall that the structure of the array is very simple. It is just a collection of individual elements indexed with one or more subscripts. Yet, the applications of arrays to programming problems can be so powerful, complex, and fascinating. It is hoped that the examples given in this chapter provide you with a good foundation in further developing your programming skills.

Visual Basic Explorer

9-1. Range of Subscript Declaration. In the general declaration section, try the following statements in a new form and run the project ('comment out the ones that the computer refuses to accept):

```
1. Dim A(-100) as Integer
2. Dim B(0 to -100) as integer
3. Dim C(-100 to 0) as Integer
4. Dim D(-100 to - 50) as integer
```

Which one(s) does the computer accept? What do you infer as the general rule concerning the declaration of subscripts for an array variable?

9-2. Relative Position of a Named Constant for Use. Try separately each of the following pairs of statements in the general declaration section in a new form and run the project:

```
1. Const HUNDRED As Integer = 100
   Dim A(HUNDRED) As Integer
2. Dim A(HUNDRED) As Integer
   ConstHUNDRED As Integer = 100
```

Does the computer accept both? What do you infer as the rule concerning the use of a named constant in the declaration of an array?

9-3. Use of a Variable for Array Declaration. Place the following code in the general declaration section of a new project:

```
Dim N as Integer
```

Then type in the following code for the Form Click event procedure:

```
Private Sub Form_Click()
    N = 10
    Dim A(N) As Integer
    Debug.Print LBound(A); UBound(A)
End Sub
```

Run the project and click the form. What does the computer say?

9-4. Static Arrays. Can you declare a static array in a procedure? If so, how is it different? You can try the following code and find out.

```
Private Sub Form_Click()
Dim I As Integer
Dim A(5) As Integer
Static B(5) As Integer
    For I = 0 To 5
        A(I) = A(I) + 1
        B(I) = B(I) + 1
    Next I
    Print "A:";
    For I = 0 To 5
        Print A(I);
    Next I
    Print
```

```
        Print "B:";
        For I = 0 To 5
            Print B(I);
        Next I
        Print
    End Sub
```

Run the project and click the form several times. Do you see any differences between the values of elements in arrays A and in B?

9-5. The Option Base Statement. Try the following code:

```
Option Base 1
Private Sub Form_Click()
Dim A(10)
    Debug.Print LBound(A)
End Sub
```

What does the LBound function return? Is it 0 or 1? What does the statement, "Option Base 1" mean? Try some other constant in place of 1 in this statement and see what the computer says. (It expects only either 0 or 1.)

9-6. Use of ReDim. Change the Dim statement in the event procedure in 9-3 to the following:

```
ReDim A(N) as Integer
```

Run the project and click the form. Any error message? Check the immediate window. What numbers do you see?

9-7. Use of ReDim. (continued from 9-6). Revise the procedure in 9-6 as follows:

```
Option Base 1
Private Sub Form_Click()
    N = 10
    ReDim A(N) As Integer
    Debug.Print LBound(A); UBound(A)
End Sub
```

Run the project and click the form. What numbers do you see in the immediate windows?

9-8. Using Functions to Declare Subscript Range. Place the following code in the general declaration area of a new project:

```
Dim A(1 to 100) as Integer
```

Then type in the following code for the Form Click event procedure:

```
Private Sub Form_Click()
    ReDim B(LBound(A) To UBound(A)) As Double
    Debug.Print LBound(B); UBound(B)
End Sub
```

Run the project and click the form. What do you see in the immediate window? What do you learn from this exercise? The range of an array subscript in a ReDim statement can be any expression as long as the results are legitimate.

9-9. Changing the Data Type of an Array. Place the following code in the general declaration section of a new project:

```
Dim A() as integer
```

Then enter the following code in the Form Click event procedure:

```
Private Sub Form_Click()
    ReDim A(10) as Double
End Sub
```

Will VB allow you to change data type in a ReDim statement? Run the project and click the form to find out.

9-10. Content of an Array After ReDim. Draw a command button on a new form. Name it cmdReDim and set its Caption property to "Re Dim." Then enter the following code:

```
Option Explicit
Dim A() As Integer

Private Sub Form_Click()
Dim I As Integer
    ReDim A(10)
    For I = 0 To 10
        A(I) = Int(Rnd * 100)
    Next I
    ShowMe A()
End Sub

Private Sub cmdReDim_Click()
    ReDim A(12)
    ShowMe A()
End Sub

Sub ShowMe(X() As Integer)
Dim I As Integer
    For I = LBound(X) To UBound(X)
        Debug.Print X(I);
    Next I
    Debug.Print
End Sub
```

Run the project and click the form. What numbers do you see in the immediate window? Now click the ReDim button. What numbers do you see in the immediate window?

9-11. Preserving Content of an Array After ReDim. Change the cmdReDim Click event procedure in the preceding exercise (9-10) as shown next (add the Preserve key word to the ReDim statement). Run the project again. Click the form. What numbers do you see? Click the Re Dim button. What numbers do you see? What difference does the keyword "Preserve" make?

```
Private Sub cmdReDim_Click()
    ReDim Preserve A(12)
    ShowMe A()
End Sub
```

9-12. Changing the Number of Subscripts and the Preserve Keyword. Change the event procedure in 9-11 to the following:

```
Private Sub cmdReDim_Click()
    ReDim Preserve A(4, 4)
End Sub
```

Run the project and click the Re Dim button. Any error message? End the execution. Then start it again. This time click the form first and then click the Re Dim button. Any error message? You cannot use the Preserve keyword when you change the number of subscripts in the ReDim statement.

9-13. ReDim and Preserve with a Multidimensional Array. Bring a command button onto a new form. Name it cmdReDim and set its Caption property to "Re Dim." Then enter the following code:

```
Option Explicit
Dim A() As Integer

Private Sub Form_Click()
    ReDim A(10, 10)
End Sub
```

```
Private Sub cmdReDim_Click()
    ReDim Preserve A(10, 4)
End Sub
```

Run the project. Click the form and then click the Re Dim button. Any error message? Now change the ReDim statement in the cmdReDim Click event procedure to the following:

```
ReDim Preserve A(4, 10)
```

Run the project. Click the form and then click the Re Dim button. Any error message? You can change the second (last) subscript but not the first (others) in a ReDim statement with the Preserve keyword.

9-14. Returning an Array from a Function. Can a function return an array? Yes, with VB6. The following function will return a sequence of 1, 2, 3, ... I in an array.

```
Option Explicit
Function Sequence(N As Integer) As Integer()
Dim I As Integer
ReDim A(1 To N) As Integer
    For I = 1 To N
        A(I) = I
    Next I
    Sequence = A()
End Function
```

Note how the function is declared. Note also the last line within the procedure. The entire array of A is assigned to the function.

To test the function, enter the preceding code in the code window. Also enter the following Form Click event procedure.

```
Private Sub Form_Click()
Dim B() As Integer
Dim I As Integer
    B = Sequence(5) 'Generate a sequence of 1, 2, ...5
    For I = LBound(B) To UBound(B)
        Print B(I)
    Next I
End Sub
```

Note how B is declared and assigned. Run the project and click the form. What do you see?

9-15. Passing an Array By Val. Enter the following line in the code window:

```
Sub PrintArray(ByVal A() As Variant)
```

What response do you get from the compiler? Can you pass an array by value then?

9-16. Type Checking and the Variant Type. Try the following code:

```
Sub PrintArray(A() As Variant)
Dim I As Integer
    For I = LBound(A) To UBound(A)
        Print A(I);
    Next I
    Print
End Sub

Private Sub Form_Click()
Dim MyIntArray(2) As Double
Dim MyStrArray(2) As String
Dim I As Integer
    For I = 0 To 2
        MyIntArray(I) = I
        MyStrArray(I) = Chr$(65 + I)
```

```
        Next I
        PrintArray MyIntArray
        PrintArray MyStrArray
    End Sub
```

Are the calls at end of the Form Click event successful? VB imposes strict data type matching to ensure an error-free execution and does not automatically convert the argument into the data type expected of the parameter(s) in a general procedure. Now, change the header for PrintArray to the following:

```
    Sub PrintArray(A As Variant)
```

Note that the pair of parentheses following the parameter A were removed. Run the project again. Does it execute this time? Are the results correct? The entire array passed to the procedure is taken as a single Variant variable, which by itself can be an array! See the power of the Variant data type and the potential danger of misusing it? (Contributed by Ben Wu, Indiana University.)

Exercises

9-17. Random Roll Calls with Repetition. Create a text file with a class roll of 15 names, one line each (use Notepad and save the result). Draw a command button on a new form. Name the button cmdCall and set its Caption property to "Call." Develop the code to perform the following:

1. As soon as the program starts, populate an array named Students with the names in the file; that is, you need to open the file and then read all the names into the Students array.
2. When the user clicks the Call button, a student's name drawn randomly from the array will be displayed with the MsgBox. The name of each student can be repeated.

9-18. Random Roll Calls Without Repetition. Modify the program in 9-17 so that the following is true:

1. The number of students in the file may change and the array Students will accommodate a "huge" class (400 students).
2. When the user clicks the Call button, a student's name drawn randomly from the array will be displayed with the MsgBox. The name of each student cannot be repeated.

(*Hint:* This is a "sampling without replacement" problem.)

9-19. Computing the Value of a Polynomial Function. Write a Function procedure to compute the value of a polynomial function of any degree. The header should appear as follows:

```
    Function Polynomial(A() As Double, X As Double) as Double
```

where *A()* is an array containing the coefficients of the polynomial function and *X* is the value of the variable in the polynomial function.

For example, given the following function:

$f(x) = 3x^4 + 10x^3 - 12x^2 + 5x - 20$

the array parameter A should contain 3, 10, -12, 5, and -20.

The function should return the value given any value of x. Test the result using 1 and 2 individually as the value of x.

9-20. Computing Average, Max, and Min. Draw two command buttons on a new form. Name them cmdPopulate and cmdCompute. Give each its proper caption. Provide the code to ensure that the following occurs:

1. When the Populate button is clicked, the array Scores is populated with random integers ranging from 65 to 100. The array should have 60 elements.

2. When the Compute button is clicked, the average, high, and low of the scores are computed and displayed in a message box.

9-21. Finding the Two Largest Numbers. Modify the preceding exercise (9-20) so that when the Compute button is clicked, the two highest scores are displayed in a message box.

9-22. Finding the n (n <=5) Largest Numbers. Modify the program in 9-21 so that when the Compute button is clicked, the n highest scores are displayed in a message box. The number n is specified by the user in a text box named txtNumber (add this control to the form). (*Hint:* Use another array [call it Highest] to keep track of the n highest scores. Refer to the insertion sort algorithm for hints to populate this array, treating this array as the "sorted output." (Note, however, that the highest value should be placed at the first position.)

9-23. Which Checks Are Still Outstanding? Suppose you have written 100 checks, numbered 1001 through 1100, in a month. When you receive the monthly statement from the bank, you add the check numbers that have been returned to a file. Design a project that will show you the checks that are still outstanding when your program reads through the "checks returned" file.

9-24. Who Has Not Yet Checked in? In an exclusive club meeting, all 200 members are all expected to attend. As each member checks in, he or she reports his or her membership number (501 to 700). Assume the check-in procedure is computerized. The user is to enter a membership number and then click the Check In button. At any time, you can request the list of members (membership numbers) who are still "outstanding." The "outstanding" list should be populated in a list box. Note that a member is not allowed to check in twice. (Your program should detect this error.)

9-25. Counting Frequency of Random Numbers Ranging from 0 to 99. Modify the frequency-counting example in this chapter so that the random numbers involved are 0 through 99, instead of 0 through 9. Display the results in a list box.

9-26. How Many Times Did Each Patient Visit the Clinic Last Year? A clinic maintains a file recording all patient visits. The file is arranged in ascending order by date (first field of each record). Other fields in each record include the patient number (second field) and the diagnosis code. The physician would like to know how many times each patient visited the clinic last year. The patient number ranges from 20,001 to 25,000.

Develop a project that can provide this information. Display the results in a list box. Each line in the list box will give the patient number and the number of times the patient visited the clinic. (*Note:* For simplicity, use random numbers in the range of 20,001 and 25,000 to represent the patient numbers.)

9-27. Searching for a Number in an Array and Returning the Position. Draw a text box and command button on a new form. Name the text box txtNumber and the command button cmdSearch. Clear the Text property of the text box. Set the command button's Caption property to "Search." Then provide the code to accomplish the following:

1. When the project starts, populate an array (named EmployeeNos) of 10,000 elements with random numbers ranging from 10,000 to 50,000. Each number in the array should be unique.
2. Write a function to search for a number in an array. It should return the position of the array in which the number is found. Otherwise, it should return a value of –1. The header of the function should appear as follows:

```
Function FindPos(Numbers() As Long, SearchKey As Long) _
    As Long
```

3. When the user clicks the command button, the computer searches for the number entered in the text box in the array (by using the function developed in number 2) and displays a message similar to the following if the number is found:

   `Employee no. 10538 is found in position 92 of the array.`

   If the number is not found, the message should appear as follows:

   `Employee no. 30348 is not found in the array.`

9-28. Lookup: Your Grade Given a Score. Suppose a teacher has the following grading system:

Score Range	Grade
88 and over	A
75–87	B
60–74	C
Below 60	D

Instead of using the Select Case structure, you would rather use two arrays to handle this problem. Develop a project that will display the grade in a message box when the user enters a score in a text box named txtScore and clicks a button named cmdGrade. (*Hint:* You need to keep only the lower score of each grade to decide the grade.)

9-29. Lookup: City/Township Given a Zip Code. This exercise represents an alternative programming solution to Exercise 7-30. You can download a complete US zip code list from the following Internet URL:

http://www.qrz.com/files/misc/zipcodes.txt

Save the file in your favorite folder. Each line in the file contains a zip code followed by a comma, a blank space, and the township, county, and state code, as the following lines show:

10081, New York, New York, NY

10087, New York, New York, NY

The file is arranged in ascending order by zip code.

You are to develop a project that will display the name of the city/township in a label when the user enters a zip code in a text box and clicks a command button captioned "Search."

You can read the complete file and populate the zip code information in two arrays as soon as the program starts. One array will hold the zip codes, while the other holds the corresponding names of city/townships (including state codes). Because the zip codes are arranged in ascending order, your search should use the binary search algorithm. Also, it will be a good idea to write the search routine as a function that will return the position of the zip code (search key) in the zip code array. This position value can then be used to obtain the name of the corresponding city name. Also, if the zip code is not found, the function should return a value of –1. (*Note:* If multiple townships share the same zip code, the function should return the first position.)

9-30. Probability of at Least Two Persons with the Same Birthday in a Gathering with 34 People. What is the probability that in a party of 34 people, at least two people will have the same birthday? Develop a project to simulate (approximate) this probability. You can set up an array with 365 elements, each representing a day in the year. Generate 34 random days in the year (with a value range from 1 to 365) and use the array to keep track of how many birthdays fall in each day. If any day (element in the array) has more than 1 count, you have found at least one incident of "the same birthday" in this experiment.

Now, if you do this experiment 1,000 times and count the number of times you find the occurrence of "the same birthday," you can approximate the probability by dividing the count by 1,000.

9-31. Probability of at Least n Persons with the Same Birthday in a Gathering of p People. Modify the program in 9-30 so that the number of people having the same birthday and the number of people in a party can be any number specified by the user.

9-32. Probability of Exactly n (n = 2 to p) Persons with the Same Birthday in a Gathering of p People. Consider the experiments in 9-31. How many times do 2, 3, 4, ... p people have the same birthdays? (*Hint:* Use another array to count the frequency of the counts that are greater than 1.)

9-33. Chances of Winning. Assuming that as a blackjack player, you have 49% probability of winning a hand, develop a project to allow yourself to approximate the probability of winning exactly 30, 31, 32, ... or more hands out of 50. Use the Monte Carlo simulation method illustrated in the chapter.

9-34. Good Product Units from a Sequential Process. Suppose a product takes two processes to complete. A batch of raw materials is placed at the beginning of the first process. At the end, units are inspected for quality. Good units are then placed into the second process. At the end, another inspection is performed. Assuming the probabilities of obtaining good units are 97% and 98% for processes 1 and 2, respectively, develop a project to compute the probability of obtaining at least g (e.g., 1,000) good units when r (e.g., 1,100) units of raw materials are placed in production at the beginning of process 1. (Show separate probability for each good unit count; e.g., 1000, 1001, ... and so on.)

9-35. Parse a Text String into Words. Assume that a text string contains several/many words, all separated by blank spaces (can be one or more between two words). Write a Function procedure that will parse the string and extract all words in the string and return them in an array. The text string will be passed to this function as a parameter. (*Hint:* See 9-14 for a function returning an array. *Note:* In VB6, there is a new function, Split, that can perform this requirement. Do not use that function. Create one "from scratch" for yourself.)

9-36. List All Prime Numbers up to 60,000. Write a Sub procedure that will list all the prime numbers from 1 to 60,000. A prime number is one that can be evenly divided only by 1 or itself. The first smallest prime numbers are 1, 2, 3, 5, and 7. (*Hint:* Identify these numbers from the smallest. Use an array to store all the identified prime numbers. Test whether a number is a prime number by checking the remainder of this number divided by all the identified prime numbers. If a number cannot be evenly divided by any prime numbers that are less than the square root of this number, this number is a prime number.)

Test your program as follows:

1. Draw a command button and a list box on a new form.
2. When the user clicks the button, the event procedure should call your prime number procedure to obtain the results. Populate the results in the list box mentioned in number 1.

9-37. Revisiting the "Rotating Banner" Project. Refer to 2-22. Change your design so that it uses one label control array instead of two labels for the banner. (*Hint:* At design time, set up only one label control as the banner and set its Index property to 0 so that the label becomes the first element in a control array. Then load the second label by code.)

9-38. Load Text Boxes, Obtain Cash Flow, and Compute the Net Present Value of an Investment Project. Develop a project to calculate the net present value of an investment project. When your program starts, the form has two text boxes (with proper labels) and one command button. The text boxes expect the user to enter the required rate of return for the project and the expected life of the project. As soon as the user finishes entering the expected life (by pressing the Enter key), your program should show additional text boxes (with proper labels) for the user to enter the cash inflow for each period of the expected life. Note the total number of text boxes should be one more than the number of periods so that the user can also enter the amount of initial investment. When the user clicks the Compute button, your program computes and displays the net present value in a label, which should appear like a text box.

9-39. Computing the Internal Rate of Return for a Project. For a typical simple project that has a negative initial cash flow (investment) followed by a series of positive cash flows, there is a rate that makes the net present value of the project equal to zero. This rate is referred to as the internal rate of return. You are to design a project that will compute the internal rate of return for a project based on the same setting as given in 9-38. (Change the label "Required rate of return" to "Initial guess." Or, delete this label and the related text box.)

9-40. Revisiting the Tuition Computation Problem. Consider the tuition computation problem presented in Chapter 5 again. Design a project to carry out the "computation" using an array to hold the tuition data. The interface should appear the same as in the second approach.

9-41. Weight Watcher Program Continued. Here is the normal weight table for women. Modify the weight watcher program presented in the text so that you can also inquire about women's normal weight, given the height. You will need to add two option buttons for the user to indicate the gender of the person of interest. (*Hint:* This can be handled several ways. One way is to use two tables to store the weights: one for men and another for women. The table to look up the weight will then depend on which of the option buttons for gender is clicked.)

Height	Small Frame	Medium Frame	Large Frame
4'10"	92–98	96–101	104–119
4'11"	94–101	98–110	106–122
5'	96–104	101–113	109–125
5'1"	99–107	104–116	112–128
5'2"	102–110	107–119	115–131
5'3"	105–113	110–122	118–134
5'4"	108–116	113–126	121–138
5'5"	111–119	116–130	125–142
5'6"	114–123	120–135	129–146
5'7"	118–127	124–139	133–150
5'8"	122–131	128–143	137–154
5'9"	126–135	132–147	141–158
5'10"	130–140	136–151	145–163
5'11"	134–144	140–155	149–168
6"	138–148	144–159	153–173

9-42. Binary Search for a Match. It is well know that when searching a sorted array, the binary search algorithm is much more efficient than the sequential search. Write a binary search function with the following header:

```
Function BinarySearch(X() As Long, SK As Long) as Long
```

where *X()* is a sorted array and *SK* is the value (search key) to search for.

The function will return the position of the array at which SK is found. If SK is not found in the array, the function will return a value of –1.

9-43. A Possible Improvement on the Bubble Sort. A suggested method to improve the performance of the bubble sort is to add a counter in the inner loop. The counter will count the number of swaps. If there is no swap after the loop is complete, the counter will be zero. This will be an indication that all the elements in the array are already in order. Thus, the process can be terminated immediately. The counter adds overhead to the sorting process but allows the algorithm to perform faster when the array to be sorted is already pretty much in order. Modify the code in the text to implement this improvement.

9-44. Simple Selection Sort. Write a Sub procedure to perform the simple section sort as described in the chapter.

9-45. Reverse Simple Selection Sort. The simple selection sort as described previously has an alternative. Instead of selecting the largest element first, we can start with selecting the smallest element first (and placing it in the first position of the array). You can then proceed to find the second, third,... and n^{th} smallest elements in the same manner. Modify the program presented in 9-44 to implement this alternative sorting algorithm for simple selection.

9-46. Binary Insertion Sort. Write a Sub procedure to perform the binary insertion sort as described in the chapter.

9-47. Improved Shell Sort. Empirical studies have found that Shell sort is most efficient when the intervals of sort are computed as follows:

$\text{Interval}_1 = 1$

$\text{Interval}_{k+1} = 3 \times \text{Interval}_k + 1$

And stops when $\text{Interval}_{k+2} >$ Number of elements to be sorted

That is, the intervals can be computed as follows:

K Value	Interval
1	1
2	3 × 1 + 1 = 4
3	3 × 4 + 1 =13
4	3 × 13 + 1 = 40
5	3 × 40 + 1 =121
6	3 × 121 + 1 = 364

An array with 300 elements should be sorted with the sort intervals set to 40, 13, 4, and 1 according to this table (because two steps below it, the interval [364] is greater than the number of elements [300]). Modify the Shell Sort routine as presented in the text to implement this improvement.

9-48. Reverse Quick Sort. You may have noticed that in the quick sort algorithm, if you use the last element in the array (instead of the first element) as the pivotal element, the comparisons should start forward first until a swap is called for; followed by backward comparisons. Thus, the backward/forward comparison sequence in search for the proper position for the pivotal element as presented in the text is changed to a forward/backward sequence. Just for the fun of it, revise the quick sort procedure to implement this modification.

Projects

9-49. Demand During Lead Time with Random Lead Time Days and Random Daily Demand. The demand for a product during a lead time period (between the day you place a purchase order and the day you actually receive the goods you have ordered) is affected by two factors: the lead time in days and the demand in each of these days. The lead time period (in days) is subject to a random distribution, as is the demand each day during this period. Suppose the lead time period has a probability distribution as follows:

Lead Time (No. of Days)	Probability	Cumulative Probability
13	.3	.3
14	.5	.8
15	.2	1.0

Also assume the daily demand for the product is subject to the following probability distribution:

Daily Demand in Units	Probability	Cumulative Probability
30	.2	.2
31	.6	.8
32	.2	1.0

If you inspect the two tables, you should see that the total demand during each lead time period can vary from 390 (13 × 30) to 480 (15 × 32), subject to a joint probability distribution. You are to develop a project to simulate (approximate) the probability of demand during lead time for this company. Your output should appear as follows:

Demand During a Lead Time Period	Probability
390	0
391	.01
392	.
.	.
.	.
480	0

(*Hint:* Consider the simulation for the actual demand for a day. If you draw a random number and it turns out to be .5, you can "assert" that the demand for that day is 31. You draw this conclusion because the number falls in the cumulative probability that includes 31. Similarly, if the random number is .9, you can claim the demand for that day is 32. Thus, to simulate daily demand, you can use two arrays: one holding the cumulative probability and another holding the daily demand. Once you obtain a random number, you can search the cumulative probability array and identify the position, which is used to obtain the actual daily demand from the daily demand array. If you repeat this simulation for a lead time period and add all the daily demand, you will come up with the demand for a lead time period. But how do you know the days of a lead time period? You use the same simulation method but a different pair of arrays (refer to the first table for needed data). If you repeat the simulation for 1,000 lead time periods, you will be able to count the number of times each demand quantity occurs.)

9-50. Finding Connected Groups in a Go Game Board. A Go game board has a dimension of 19 × 19 lines. Two players take turns in placing their stones (black versus white) on the intersections. The objective is to occupy as big a territory as possible. A group of isolated stones of one player is captured if it is completely surrounded by the opponent's stones without empty intersections inside the group.

One aspect of programming the game is to identify the groups of stones that are "connected." Two stones of the same side (color) are connected if both are on the same line (vertical or horizontal; i.e., on the row or column) and next to each other on the other dimension. For example, the two stones at (9,10) and (9,11) are connected because they are on the same row and next to each other by column. Many stones placed on the board can be connected to one another vertically and horizontally to form a group.

The Challenge: When your program starts, the user will enter the number of stones to be placed on the board (use a text box for this purpose). Your program will proceed to simulate where these stones are placed on the board. The next step is the key challenge: to identify the number of connected groups (as described) and the stones belonging to each group. To simplify the problem, assume all stones on the board are of the same color (played by the same player).

Internal Representation: Various schemes can be used to represent the status of the game board internally. For example, an intersection, Board(x, y) has a value zero if it is not occupied by either side and has a value of –1 if occupied by the Black side and a value of 1 if occupied by the White side. Because you are assuming only one side is playing, you can use either –1 or 1 to indicate that a stone has been placed at the intersection.

Simulating the Intersection Points Occupied (Played): You can use a pair of random numbers to simulate the intersection point at which the player places the stones. More specifically, if you declared the Board as Board(1 to 19, 1 to 19), you will need to generate a pair of random number Row and Col, each within the range of 1 to 19. Notice that an intersection may have been occupied already. In that case, another pair of Row and Col must be generated until an empty intersection is found. Refer to the "Sampling Without Replacement" subsection in Section 9.2 for hints to identify whether a number has already been selected.

A Hint: Note that a stone may be connected to as many as four other stones, which can in turn be connected to other stones. It would be much easier to use a recursive procedure to identify the group. However, you will need to avoid "double counting," which involves including an intersection that has already been included/connected. (This will result in an endless connection loop.) Use another array (with the same dimension as the board) to identify the group to which a particular intersection belongs.

Displaying Results: Use a list box to show the result. One way to show the results is as follows:

Group 1:
1, 1
1, 2
1, 3
2, 1
3, 1

Group 2:
10, 12
11, 12
12, 12

where each pair of numbers represents the coordinate of the intersection. Enjoy your challenge!

9-51. Sorting Records, Not Just the Sort Keys. The presentation in the text focused only on sorting an array (consisting of the sort keys). In most of the real-world applications, sorting is done for an array of records, not just the sort keys of the records. Imagine a student file represented by three (and of course, can be more) arrays: Names(), SSN(), and Scores(). We would like to sort the file by Scores(). We certainly are not interested in writing a special sorting routine to actually sort all these arrays by Scores(). Otherwise, we would have to write a special sorting routine for each sorting problem we encounter. We would rather have a routine general enough to handle all different situations. How can this be accomplished? Usually, it is done by associating the sort keys with their original positions in the array. Consider this example:

Sort Keys (Score) Before Sorting	Original Position in Array
91	1
85	2
98	3
76	4
89	5

After sorting, if the original positions continue to be associated with the sort keys, the table will appear as follows:

Sort Keys (Score) After Sort	Original Position in Array
76	4
85	2
89	5
91	1
98	3

The original positions can then be used to retrieve data in other arrays that are not physically moved in the sort process but can now be presented in the order of the sort keys. (See the illustration near the end of this problem.)

To accomplish this, the sort routine should be modified to accept another array used to hold the original positions and arrange these positions at the same time the sort keys are being sorted.

For example, we can modify the Bubble Sort procedure presented in the text as follows:

```
Sub BubbleSort(X() as Long, RecPos() as Long)
' RecPos() is an array holding the record positions associated with
the sort keys
Dim I as Long
Dim J as Long
Dim H as Long
Dim Temp as Long
    H = UBound(X)
    For J = LBound(X)  To UBound(X) -1
        H = H - 1
        For I = LBound(X) To H
            If X(I) > X(I+1) Then
            ' out of order; swap the sort keys
                Temp = X(I)
                X(I) = X(I+1)
                X(I+1) = Temp
                ' Note: the following lines are newly added
                ' swap the position pointers
                Temp = RecPos(I)
                RecPos(I) = RecPos(I+1)
                RecPos(I+1) = Temp
            End If
        Next I
    Next J
End Sub
```

Assume the arrays Names(), SSN(), and Scores() have been properly populated (filled with data). An event procedure (e.g., cmdSort_Click), which uses the Bubble Sort routine, can be coded as follows:

```
Private Sub cmdSort_Click()
ReDim RecPos(LBound(Scores) to UBound(Scores))
Dim I as Long
Dim P as Long
    ' set up the record position array
    For I = LBound(Scores) To UBound(Scores)
        RecPos(I) = I
    Next I
    ' call the sort routine
    BubbleSort Scores(),RecPos()
```

```
        ' show data in sorted order on the form
        For I = LBound(Scores) To UBound(Scores)
            P = RecPos(I)   'P holds the record position
                            ' corresponding to the sorted key
            Print Names(P); SSN(P); Scores(I)
        Next I
    End Sub
```

Note that the arrays Names() and SSN() are retrieved by P, whereas Scores() is retrieved by I. The latter has been sorted in proper order, but the former two have not been sorted. However, their record positions (P) have been arranged in the same order as Scores.

Required. Modify the Quick Sort procedure presented in the text to have this record sorting capability. Test your modified procedure to sort the zip code file discussed in 9-29 by township. Show the first 10,000 sorted records in a list box.

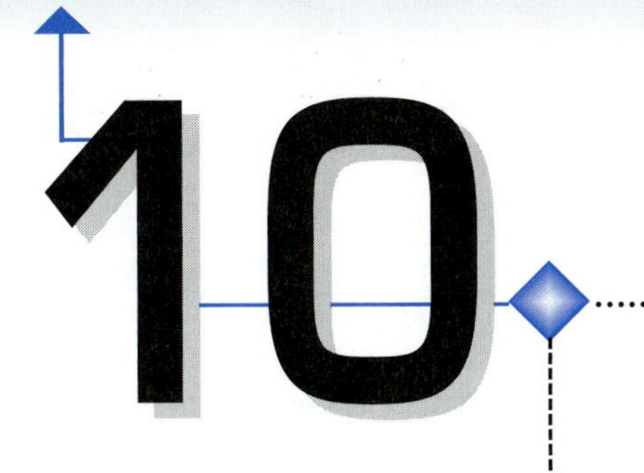

10 Special Topics in Data Entry

This chapter considers various issues related to the user interface/data-entry screens. We focus on designing data-entry screens that can facilitate user efficiency and "satisfaction" with data entry/interaction. As pointed out in Chapter 1, "Introduction," VB programs operate in the graphical user interface (GUI) environment. Design under this environment is different from the traditional DOS character/keyboard based environment. We first present important principles that guide the design of the GUI. Several of these principles have been presented and observed in our programming practices in previous chapters. In this chapter, we further illustrate how some of these principles can be implemented in your programs.

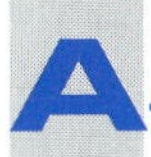

After completing this chapter, you should be able to:

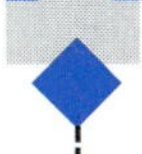

- Enumerate important principles of a sound GUI design.
- Provide code to enable the user to use the navigation keys (e.g., Enter key, up-arrow and down-arrow keys) in a more "traditional" way by using the SendKeys statement.
- Set up access keys for various VB controls to enable the user to move around the data-entry screen more freely and efficiently.
- Implement data entry error-checking routines at three different levels: individual key, field, and screen (form) levels.
- Implement error trapping and handling for your program to be more robust and user-friendly.
- Design and implement visual feedback in a program that involves lengthy processes.

10.1 Principles of GUI Design

Designing a GUI is more an art than a science. However, there are principles that can be used to guide a sound design. An interface design that follows these principles strictly will result in a much more efficient, effective, and accurate data-entry screen. These principles include simplicity and clarity, flexibility, consistency, immediate feedback, forgiveness, and pleasant appearance. Let's consider each of these principles in more detail.

Simplicity and Clarity

All user interfaces (data-entry screens) should have *a simple and clear layout*. For example, each data field should be accompanied by a caption that clearly indicates what is to be entered. To enhance neatness of the layout, logically related data should be grouped together within a container such as the frame or picture box. When many data fields are required, further grouping can be accomplished by using the tab control.

Minimal Keystrokes. From the user's viewpoint, simplicity implies that the screen is easy to use. One aspect of this is to require the minimal number of keystrokes by the user to complete the task. You should consider alternatives to text boxes to obtain data from the user. For example, check boxes instead of text boxes can be used where the user is expected to answer yes or no. Option buttons or combo boxes can be used for mutually exclusive choices in place of text boxes for the user response. In any case, default values or settings can also be provided.

Recognition Versus Recall. In addition, you should bear in mind that it is much easier for the user to recognize than to recall an item. Thus, when the user is expected to "enter" an item that is already available to your program (e.g., an item that already exists in a database), it will be helpful if a list box or combo box is used to present data items for the user to choose from. If the list of existing items is too long (e.g., customer numbers of an accounts receivable file with thousands of records), a custom dialog box can be provided to facilitate the search for the correct item.

Clear Labeling and Messages. Clarity also means various buttons for important actions should be captioned explicitly. For example, a command button to save data should be labeled "Save," not "OK." The latter should be used only when the user is requested to acknowledge a message.

We have considered all these points throughout the book and stressed their uses in Chapter 3, "Some Visual Basic Controls and Events," when introducing various VB controls for user interface design. In addition, we have attempted to observe this principle in all our examples. The previous discussion serves as a reminder of this principle.

Flexibility

Your program should provide the user with flexibility in *mobility* and in *customizing* the screen. The user should be given the freedom to move around the screen without undue restrictions. When the user uses the mouse, he or she can click on any object on the screen. Thus, the mobility is not an issue. What if the user prefers to use the keyboard? We should also provide a means for the user to move around easily using this method. This can be accomplished by setting up "access keys." The implementation of access keys is presented in this chapter.

Providing flexibility should be balanced against data accuracy and "safety." For example, as soon as the user enters a wrong type of key (e.g., a letter in a numeric field), a message should be clearly displayed. Indeed, you should regard helping the user catch an entry error at the earliest possible point as a user-friendly design. This will guide the user to enter correct data and avoid unnecessary keying attempts. In Section 10.4, we present error-checking techniques.

Customization and Safety. Under certain circumstances, it is also desirable to provide the user with the ability to customize. For example, the size of a column in a report onscreen can be made adjustable. The tone and loudness of audio feedback (some users may even prefer none) can also be made adjustable. For "safety" reasons, allowing the user to customize screen or VB control colors may not be desirable. At least, you should provide code to guard against choosing the same color for both foreground and background, which renders all entered data invisible.

Consistency

All data-entry screens should have *consistent appearance*. This includes the location of menus, command buttons, and icons. Consistent screens make it much easier for the user to anticipate, identify, locate, and respond to relevant items. Wording and terminology displayed in labels and messages should also be consistent. Questions and prompts should be consistent in soliciting responses from users. For example, if a question is worded such that a "no" answer from the user means that the program should not quit, all questions in a similar context should be worded in the same manner.

Consistent Behavior. Consistency also means that all function keys and navigation keys should behave the same way throughout all screens. For example, if the up-arrow and down-arrow keys are programmed to move up and down the data fields in one screen, they should behave the same way in all other screens. This eliminates the uncertainty in the user's mind in anticipating the responses from the computer.

Immediate Feedback

By nature, human beings need feedback. Imagine that you are on the phone talking for several minutes without hearing any voice from the other end. Won't you pause and ask, "Hello! Are you still there?" Similarly, the user may start to click various buttons or press different keys when he or she sees no response from the computer after clicking a button. Many unexpected consequences might ensue if your program has already started the action after the first click. The importance of immediate proper feedback cannot be overemphasized.

Visual Feedback for Long Processes. When the user clicks a button to initiate a process that may take 1 or 2 seconds to complete, the program should change the mouse pointer to hourglass to indicate that an activity is being carried out. A slightly longer process should display a status message. A process requiring more than just a few seconds to complete should display a progress bar to show the progress. All these provide a visual feedback to the user and create a perception of "faster" process/response by the computer. Section 10.6 demonstrates how these can be implemented in VB.

Immediate Message for Entry Errors. When entering data, if the user presses a key not expected by the program (e.g., wrong data type), a message should be displayed so that the user is informed and can avoid attempting the same thing unsuccessfully. Indeed, any type of data-entry errors should be identified as soon as practicable.

Minimizing Unnecessary Effort. If the user is not expected to enter any data on a particular screen, either the screen should not be made available to him or her or it should be shown on a read-only basis. In no case should the user be allowed to enter the data, only to be informed of his or her ineligibility when he or she is ready to save.

Forgiveness

As human beings, we all make unintentional mistakes. It is unavoidable that the user will press the wrong key or click the wrong button. When a serious consequence can ensue, your program should protect the user from these types of errors.

Protecting Against Potential Loss of Data. For example, when the user takes an action that can mean loss of data, a warning message with a request to confirm the action should be displayed. Thus, if the user clicks a button to delete a file, a message should appear to confirm the action before the file is actually deleted. Also, when a large quantity of data onscreen is deleted, a way to "undo" should also be provided. In addition, if the user decides to leave a screen with unsaved data, a message should be displayed to warn the user of the potential loss of data and an option should be provided for the user to go back to the screen.

Guard Against Abrupt Program Termination. Sometimes, a "wrong answer" from the user can cause operational problems (e.g., division by zero) to the computer. Your program can be terminated abruptly. A program that behaves this way cannot be considered user-friendly. Thus, you should provide code to take care of potential problems of this nature. This chapter explains how to handle user errors that can cause your program to end abruptly.

Pleasant Appearance

The screen should appear harmonious in color and use of space, drawing the user's attention to the most important element of data on the screen. Colors and graphics that distract attention should be avoided. Although this principle appears to be easy to appreciate, people do vary in their taste. I have seen many "interesting" designs meant to be an enhancement for the presentation by the students. It would seem advisable to seek opinions from experienced graphic designers when one has some "unconventional" design in color and graphics.

The following table summarizes this discussion and indicates how each principle is treated in this chapter.

Principle	Applicable Objectives and Suggestions	Remark/Disposition
Simplicity and clarity	Has simple design and clear screen layout	Chapter 3 provides general guidelines. This principle is observed throughout the text.
	Requires minimal keystrokes for data-entry screens	
	Provides clues for easy recognition of required items	
	Provides clear labeling and instruction	
Flexibility	Allows users maximal latitude in moving around the screen	Section 10.2 discusses design of a user-friendly keyboard.
	Provides ways to customize	A few examples in the text touch the surface of customization.
Consistency	Has consistent appearance	The principle is considered only in general. No technical issue is explicitly treated in this text.
	Implements consistent behavior	
Immediate feedback	Provides visual cues and messages in long processes	Section 10.6 discusses different means of visual feedback.
	Provides immediate messages for errors in data entry	Section 10.4 discusses handling three levels of error checking.
Forgiveness	Warns users of potential loss of data Guards against potential computer problems and loss of data	Section 10.3 illustrates the detection and caution of potential loss of data. Section 10.5 illustrates handling user errors that can cause problems for the program.
Pleasant appearance	Has harmonious screen layout and color	Not treated in this text.

As you can see from the table summary, most of these principles are generally observed wherever they are applicable throughout this book. As indicated, the following sections consider the implementation of some of these principles.

10.2 Designing a User-Friendly Keyboard

One principle stated in the preceding section is that the user should be provided with maximal allowable freedom in mobility around the screen. In data-entry applications, the user usually relies on the keyboard, rather than on the mouse, to perform various activities. One important consideration of this aspect is that the user may expect a particular key to behave in a certain way, which may not be considered "standard" in the Windows environment. For example, the user may expect the cursor (focus) to move to the next data field (control) when he or she presses the Enter key, a habit that he or she has had since the DOS era. Under the Windows environment, the Tab key is used for the same purpose, whereas the Enter key is usually associated with a command button (e.g., "Save"). Should we then tell the user to change the habit and consider the matter "closed"? This will appear to ignore the user's need and should not be considered as a user-friendly attitude. This section considers a few of these issues with code solutions.

Handling the Enter Key

We begin with the issue cited in the introductory paragraph of this section. How do we make the Enter key move the focus to the next control?

There are ways to change the behavior of the Enter key. For example, for each control, you can test whether the key pressed is the Enter key. If so, you can use the SetFocus method to set the focus to the next control. However, such an approach is tedious to implement. To set the focus, you will need to identify the control involved. In addition, a group of similar code will need to be repeated for each of the controls involved.

The SendKeys Statement. There is a simpler way. It involves the use of the SendKeys statement, which allows the program to emulate sending keystrokes to the active window (control) as if the keys were pressed by the user. The SendKeys statement has the following syntax:

```
SendKeys KeysToSend[,Wait]
```

The Wait parameter is a Boolean value that specifies whether the execution should wait until the keys are processed. A value of True indicates that the keys must be processed before execution will continue to the next statement. The default is False. The following statement will send the text string "abcd" to txtName when it has the focus:

```
Private Sub txtName_GotFocus()
    SendKeys "abcd"
End Sub
```

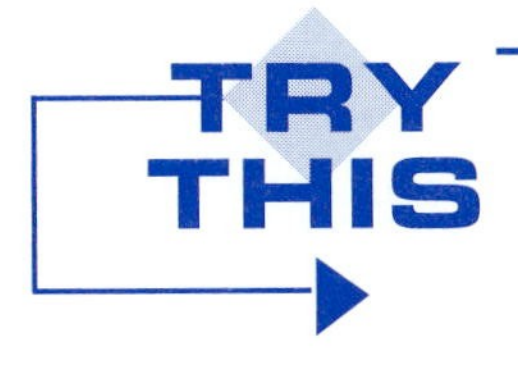

Draw three text boxes on a form. Name the second one txtName. Then enter the following code:

```
Private Sub txtName_GotFocus()
    SendKeys "abcd"
End Sub
```

Run the project. Keep pressing the Tab key to move the focus around. The text string should be added to txtName each time the control receives the focus.

Keys that are not displayed (e.g., Tab, Home, and Delete) should be coded with a special code enclosed in a pair of braces. For example, the following code will send a Tab key to the active window (control):

```
SendKeys "{tab}"
```

The Windows will then process the key accordingly. Because a normal Tab key moves the focus to the next control, that statement will bring the same effect. Recall that the named system constant vbTab represents the Tab key, Chr$(9). Thus, the following statement will accomplish the same:

```
SendKeys vbTab
```

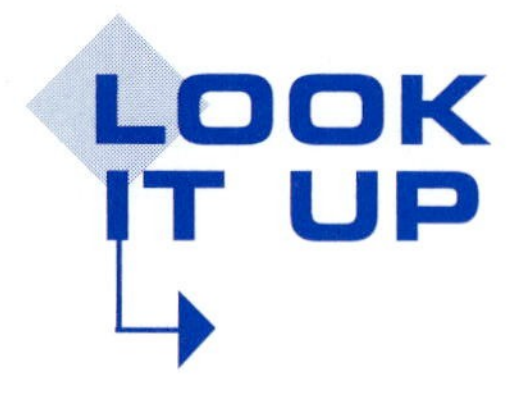

You can find the complete set of special keys and their corresponding codes for the SendKeys statement in the Index tab of the online Help file by looking for the keyword "SendKeys." Also note that keys such as %, ^, and + have special meanings to SendKeys. To send them as their original keystrokes, you should enclose them in a pair of braces, too. For example, to send a "+" key, you code the following:

```
SendKeys "{+}"
```

"Converting" the Enter Key. The Enter key can be trapped in the KeyPress event. If we use the SendKeys statement to send a Tab key in its place, we in effect convert the Enter key to the Tab key. This will move the focus to the next control. For example, if a form has a text box named txtID, we can code the procedure as follows:

```
Private Sub txtID_KeyPress(KeyAscii as Integer)
' check for the Enter key
    If KeyAscii = vbKeyReturn then
        SendKeys vbTab   ' send a tab key to emulate tabbing
        KeyAscii = 0  'Nullify the key to kill further processing
    End If
End Sub
```

In the procedure, if the Ascii value of the pressed key is equal to vbKeyReturn, a Tab key is sent from the program to emulate the pressing of that key by the user. This should cause the Windows operating system to process the key and "tab" to the next control. Notice that the parameter KeyAscii is assigned a value of zero afterward. This suppresses the key actually pressed by the user. There will be no further processing of the Enter key. Without such a statement, the system will continue to process the key and you will hear a beep.

Although the preceding code will work, you will soon find a lot of repetitive code to handle the key if the form contains many controls. One elegant way to avoid such a situation is to place the same code in the ***Form_KeyPress event*** procedure. A form cannot receive focus when there are controls on it. However, it can intercept the keys from most controls and handle these keys before passing them to the controls when its ***KeyPreview property*** is set to True. Thus, a generic Enter key handler can be created by do the following:

- Setting the form's KeyPreview property to True
- Providing the following code:

```
Private Sub Form_KeyPress(KeyAscii as Integer)
    ' check for the Enter key
    If KeyAscii = vbKeyReturn then
        SendKeys vbTab   ' send a tab to emulate tabbing
        KeyAscii = 0  'Nullify the key to kill further processing
    End If
End Sub
```

Many VB projects with the preceding code fail to work properly because the programmer forgets to set the form's KeyPreview property to True. Wherever the Form_KeyPress event procedure is used, make sure this property is set to True.

Auto Tabbing

Many programs move focus to the next field when the current field is filled. This saves the user the need to press the Enter key. The masked edit box will behave this way when its ***AutoTab property*** is set to True.

The text box can be programmed to work the same way if its ***Max Length property*** is set to its proper value. Because the focus is expected to move to the next control after the key is entered, an event procedure to consider to place the code is the ***Change event***. For example, using the same SendKeys "trick," we can implement auto tabbing for the text box named txtID as follows:

```
Private Sub txtID_Change()
    If txtID.SelStart>=txtID.MaxLength then
        SendKeys vbTab 'Tab to the next control
    End If
End Sub
```

The SelStart property gives the cursor position of the control. The If statement checks if this position is equal to or greater than the text's MaxLength. If so, a Tab key is sent, resulting in a move of the cursor to the next control.

To make a masked edit box automatically tab to the next control after it is filled with data, set its AutoTab property to True.

Although this code should work, we need to consider two issues: First, experienced programmers are reluctant to suggest placing code in the Change event because of the potential of encountering unexpected results. This is because when there is a change in txtID.Text (e.g., some value is assigned to it, not necessarily by a key pressed by the user), this event is triggered. Thus, there is always that potential that a Tab key is sent unexpectedly by this procedure.

Second, if a form has many text boxes, there will be a lot of repetitive code. You could minimize the code repetition if there were a way to handle the Change event for all controls at the form level. However, there's no Change event for all controls at the form level.

You could indeed move the code to the form's ***KeyUp event*** to handle this, with an understanding that it will look a bit "unnatural":

```
Private Sub Form_KeyUp(KeyCode As Integer, Shift As Integer)
    If TypeName(ActiveControl) = "TextBox" Then
        If ActiveControl.SelStart  >= ActiveControl.MaxLength Then
            SendKeys vbTab
        End If
    End If
End Sub
```

The KeyUp event occurs when the user releases the key pressed. It occurs after the Change event. The event procedure has two parameters: KeyCode and Shift. The KeyCode is an integer value that represents the key position in the keyboard. The Shift parameter is a Flags value that indicates the state of the three "shift" keys: Shift, Ctrl, and Alt keys. The following table shows how this parameter is used.

Bit Position	Key Masked	Value When the Key Is Pressed
0 (lowest bit)	Shift	1
1	Ctrl	2
2	Alt	4

The preceding routine, however, does not involve checking for either the KeyCode or Shift value because all we are interested is the cursor position. *When the form's KeyPreview property is set to True, this code should work for all text boxes in the form.*

Notice that there is an If statement that checks to ensure that the active control is a text box. Many controls can have the KeyUp event, but not all of them have the MaxLength property. Testing this property for those controls that do not have it will result in an error.

The preceding routine may not work properly under certain special situations. A better solution is provided in Chapter 14, "Beyond the Core," in which the use of API (application program interface) is introduced.

Arrow Keys Up and Down

In a similar fashion, in a form that has controls vertically aligned, the user may expect to use the up-arrow and down-arrow keys to navigate up and down among the fields. The SendKeys statement discussed can again be used to do the trick. However, the arrow keys are not trappable in the KeyPress event. Instead, they can be trapped in the ***KeyDown event***, which occurs before the KeyPress event. Again, a form-level KeyDown event is available and can be used to intercept all keys meant for the various controls for input purposes (e.g., text boxes, masked edit boxes) The Form KeyDown event has the same header as the KeyUp event:

```
Private Sub Form_KeyDown(KeyCode As Integer, Shift As Integer)
```

Where the *KeyCode* and *Shift* parameters have the same meaning and values as those in the KeyUp event.

The left-, up-, right-, and down-arrow keys have the key code values 37, 38, 39, and 40, respectively. Their corresponding named constants are vbKeyLeft, vbKeyUp, vbKeyRight, and vbKeyDown. We can check for the up- and down-arrow keys and handle them with the SendKeys statement in a manner very similar to the way we handle the Enter key:

```
Private Sub Form_KeyDown(KeyCode As Integer, Shift As Integer)
    Select Case KeyCode
    Case vbKeyUp
    ' Arrow key up; replace it with the Shift+Tab key
        SendKeys "+{tab}"  'Send Shift+Tab key
        KeyCode = 0  'Suppress the up-arrow key
    Case vbKeyDown
    ' Arrow key down; replace it with the tab key
        SendKeys vbTab 'Send tab key
        KeyCode = 0 'Suppress the down-arrow key
    End Select
End Sub
```

Notice that the down-arrow key is handled in exactly the same way as the Enter key. Note also that some of the keys used in the SendKeys statement have special meanings. For example, the "+" sign represents the Shift key, and the "%" symbol represents the Alt key. As explained previously (in a Look It Up box), if you mean to send a "+" as a "+" sign (instead of the Shift key), you need to enclose the key in a pair of braces, as "{+}." The up-arrow key has a named constant vbKeyUp. When this key is pressed, the code will send Shift+Tab to inform the system to move the cursor up (to the preceding control.)

In this and the preceding subsection, we ignore the possibility that the Shift key is pressed. In some cases, when that key is pressed, some "unexpected" result can occur. A better alternative than using the SendKeys statement is presented Chapter 14.

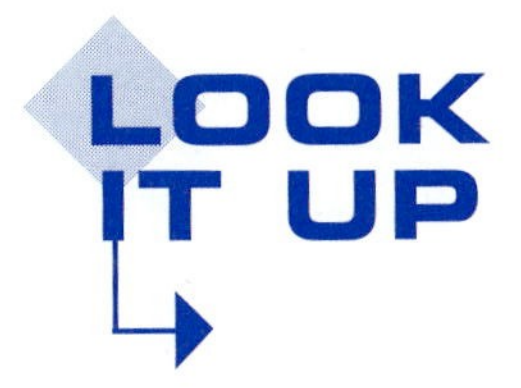

A complete list of the named constant and actual key code value for all keys can be found by searching the keyword "key code constant" in the Index tab of the online Help file.

Providing Access Keys

As discussed at the beginning of this chapter, providing the user with maximal mobility should mean that the user can move from one data-entry box to another wherever it may be in the form with the keyboard, not just with the mouse. You can accomplish this by providing the user with the access keys. This implementation does not even require any code. It involves creating the "access keys" and setting up the proper tab orders for the controls.

Accessing a Control with the Caption Property by Key. A control that has the Caption property can have an access key if you place an "&" before the letter in the caption that you want it to be the access key. For example, suppose you have three controls on the forms: chkStudent (a check box), optMale (an option button), and optFemale (another option button) with the following captions: Student, Male, and Female, respectively. If you set these three captions to &Student, &Male, and &Female, respectively, you should see that S, M, and F in each respective control is underlined (Figure 10.1). Now, when you run the project, pressing Alt+S, Alt+M, Alt+F (in any order) will allow the focus to move to chkStudent, optMale, and optFemale, just like the way you use the mouse to click on it.

Figure 10.1
A Visual Interface with Access Keys

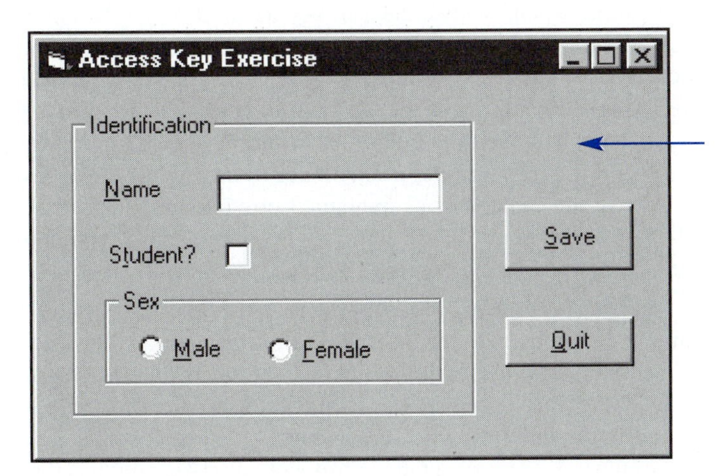

Here is a form with proper access keys. Notice the letter in each caption is underlined. Pressing Alt+<underlined letter> will move focus to that control. To underline the letter, place the "&" sign before the letter when you set the Caption property. The TabIndexes for lblName and txtName are set to 0 and 1, respectively. (They must be consecutive to work properly.)

Accessing a Control Without the Caption Property by Key. What if the control you want to move to does not have a Caption property (e.g., the text box, combo box, or list box)? In general each of these controls is accompanied by a label control that indicates its content or purpose. For example, a text box named txtName most likely will be accompanied by a label with the caption "Name." To provide the access key functionality for the text box, you can do the following:

1. Set the access key to the label (e.g., set the caption to &Name).
2. Set the TabIndex for the label and the text box in sequence (e.g., set the TabIndex properties for the label and the text box to 0 and 1, respectively).

At runtime, the label does not receive focus. Any focus set to it will be given to the next control that can receive focus. Thus, setting the TabIndex property for the label and the text box right next to each other will allow the text box to receive the focus when the user presses the access key in the label.

Figure 10.1 shows a simplified data-entry form with access keys properly set up. Draw the same as a practice. Notice the following points in particular:

- Place the "&" before the letter that is underlined in the caption of each control.
- Ensure that the label with the caption "Name" has its TabIndex property set to 0 and that the Name text box has its TabIndex property set to 1. The TabIndex sequence is very important for a control that relies on another control with the Caption property to receive the focus.
- Run the project after completing the visual interface. Test to ensure that the access keys work properly.

Note also that the "Student" check box has its caption placed before the check box. Set its Alignment property to 1 (Right Justify) to show this effect. (There is no need to add a label.)

Using the SSTab Control

In Chapter 3, we presented the SSTab control as a container that can be used for a data-entry screen that has to handle a large number of data-entry fields. You should be aware of the following issues when using the SSTab in your project:

- All controls that you place on the tab control must have their positions fixed at the design time. That is, you are not allowed to move the controls' position by code. Otherwise, the results can be unpredictable.
- Whichever tab you leave on top at the design time is the tab that appears on top at runtime. This may not necessarily be the first tab of the control. Thus, you must take care to ensure that the tab you leave on top before running the project is truly the one you mean to show when the tab appears.
- At runtime, when you use the Tab key to tab through the controls inside a tab control, the current tab (caption) will receive the focus after the last control on the tab is tabbed (not the next tab of the control). Using the keyboard, to move to the next tab, you can press Ctrl+Tab only while the tab has the focus. This can prove to be very inconvenient.

  One way to solve this problem is to set the access key to each tab. This can be done by placing an "&" sign before the letter to be used as the access key in the tab caption in exactly the same way as explained previously. Recall that the tab captions of the tab control can be set in the control's Properties page, which is accessible by clicking the Custom box in the control's Properties window.
- In general, the user is not really interested in the tab caption when engaging in data-entry operations. He or she would rather get to the first control in each tab immediately after accessing (clicking) the tab of interest. One way to do this is to use to ***SetFocus method*** to set the focus on the first control in each tab. The code can be placed in the tab control's Click event.

  To illustrate, assume a tab control named sstAccount has three tabs. The first control in each tab respectively is: txtAccountNo, txtInsuranceID, and txtEmployerID. The code will appear as follows:

```
Private Sub sstAccount_Click(PreviousTab As Integer)
    Select Case sstAccount.Tab
    Case 0
```

```
' Set focus on the first control in the first tab
        txtAccountNo.SetFocus
    Case 1
' Set focus on the first control in the second tab
        txtInsuranceID.SetFocus
    Case 2
' Set focus on the first control in the third tab
        txtEmployerID.SetFocus
    End Select
End Sub
```

Note that the tab count starts with zero. Note also that if each tab caption has an access key, then pressing the access key will raise the Click event, causing the preceding procedure to execute. This will make the keyboard operation quite efficient.

In addition, the Click event has a parameter PreviousTab. You may have a situation in which certain conditions in a tab must be met before you will let the user leave that tab. You can use this parameter to perform the necessary check and even to return to the previous tab. For example, suppose in the preceding case that it is mandatory that an account number be entered before other tabs can be accessed. You can insert the following code before the Select Case statement:

```
If PreviousTab = 0 Then
    If Val(txtAccountNo.Text) = 0 Then
        ' Account number not yet entered
        sstAccount.Tab = PreviousTab 'Return to previous tab
    End If
End If
```

10.3 Additional Considerations

This section considers the potential loss of data on the screen when the program quits. The user may have clicked a "wrong" (Quit) button unintentionally after a screenful of data has been entered but not yet saved. To guard against such a possibility, you should detect and warn the user of unsaved data, and allow the user to back out of the Quit command.

Detecting Unsaved Data

When the user pushes the Quit button, a user-friendly program should warn the user of the possibility of losing data if such a situation exists. Thus, your code should first check to see whether the current screen contains any entered data. If you are sure that the user will rely on the keyboard exclusively to enter data, one possible approach to detect unsaved data is to set up a Boolean variable at the form level (module level) and use it to keep track whether any key has been pressed. The following code fragments illustrate this approach.

In the general declaration section:

```
Option Explicit
Dim KeyPressed as Boolean 'Declare a module level variable
```

In the routine that saves the data:

```
KeyPressed = False 'data have been saved; all keys are "cleared"
```

In the Form_KeyPress event procedure (*note:* remember to set the form's KeyPreview property to True):

```
KeyPressed = True
```

This approach should detect all data entered through the keyboard. However, it will not detect data obtained by copy (or cut) and paste. Because all changes to text boxes and masked edit boxes will trigger the Change event, an alternative is to place the preceding statement in the Change event of each control. This approach should work elegantly if the number of text boxes and masked edit boxes on the form is fairly small.

If the form contains many text boxes and masked edit boxes and if they are cleared when saved, an alternative is to check whether any control contains any data. The following code fragment should set the variable NotYetSaved to True if any nonblank edit box is found.

```
Dim Ctrl As Control
Dim NotYetSaved As Boolean
    For Each Ctrl In Controls
        Select Case TypeName(Ctrl)
        Case "TextBox"
            NotYetSaved = Len(Trim$((Ctrl.Text)) > 0
        Case "MaskEdBox"
            NotYetSaved = Len(Trim$((Ctrl.ClipText)) > 0
        End Select
        If NotYetSaved Then Exit For
    Next Ctrl
```

This routine uses the For Each loop to enumerate through all controls in the form and test whether each text box or masked edit box contains any nonblank data. If one is found, the variable NotYetSaved is set to True and the loop is terminated. This routine can be placed in either the QueryUnload or Unload event (explained in the next subsection) to detect unsaved data.

Handling Unsaved Data When the Program Is Quitting

When the user clicks the close (x) button on the form's control box or when your code executes the Unload statement, two events will be triggered: the form's ***QueryUnload*** and the ***Unload events***. The QueryUnload event occurs before the Unload event. Both events provide a Cancel parameter that can be used to cancel the unloading operation. The former provides an additional parameter that indicates the source of the unloading operation, but the latter does not. This parameter can be useful in some cases. Thus, it is desirable to become acquainted with this event procedure, which has the following header:

```
Private Sub Form_QueryUnload(Cancel As Integer, UnloadMode As _
    Integer)
```

where *Cancel* = an integer parameter your code can assign a value; if it is assigned with a nonzero value, the form's unload operation will be canceled

UnloadMode = an integer value indicating the source that triggers the unloading operation

The most common causes of unloading are the following:

- vbFormControlMenu (0): The user clicks the Close button in the form's Control box.
- vbFormCode (1): The code executes an Unload statement.

When you want your code to detect whether there are unsaved data on the form, it is not necessary to check the unload mode. Thus, either of the two events can be used. For familiarity, suppose you use the QueryUnload event and assume you use the first approach in the preceding section. You can code the following:

```
Private Sub Form_QueryUnload(Cancel As Integer, UnloadMode As _
Integer)
Dim Ans as Integer
    If KeyPressed then
        Ans = MsgBox("Data not yet saved.  Ok to quit?", _
          vbYesNo + vbQuestion)
        If Ans = vbYes Then
        Else
            Cancel = True 'Cancel unload
        End If
    End If
End Sub
```

The statement in the form's KeyPress event procedure in the preceding section will ensure that the Boolean variable KeyPressed will reflect keys entered after data are saved. In the QueryUnload procedure, this variable is tested. If it is True, there are unsaved data. The MsgBox function is then used to warn the user and obtain the user's direction. If he or she decides it is okay to quit, Ans will have a value vbYes (6). If not, the Cancel parameter is assigned a nonzero value so that the unload operation will be canceled.

If you use the last approach presented in the preceding section, you can insert that fragment of code in this QueryUnload event procedure. In addition, the variable Keypressed in this procedure should be replaced with NotYetSaved. The following layout shows how the code should be arranged:

```
Private Sub Form_QueryUnload(Cancel As Integer, UnloadMode As _
  Integer)
Dim Ans as Integer
'Place the code in the preceeding section to set NotYetSaved here
    If NotYetSaved Then
        'Place the code inside the "If KeyPressed" block here.
    End If
End Sub
```

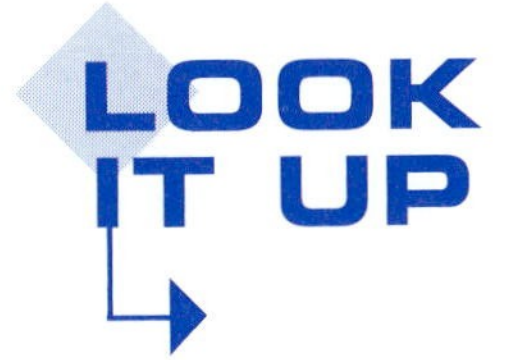

Use the keyword "QueryUnload Event" to search the Index tab of the online Help file. Its "Visual Basic Reference" page lists additional causes of unloading the form.

10.4 Checking for Data-Entry Errors

From the user's viewpoint, he or she wants to be informed of an error at the point of its occurrence. This enables the user to make the correction immediately without having to look back for the source data. Thus, the timing in checking for the error is exactly at the point of the error. An error can occur at one of the following three points:

1. When the user presses a key
2. When the user leaves a data field
3. When the user signals that the screen entry is complete, which usually occurs when the user clicks a command button such as "Save" or "OK"

This section considers checking for errors at each of these three points.

The concepts and techniques involved in this section can be complicated. The most effective way to learn the materials is to work along as you read. Your understanding of the materials will be much deeper if you do so.

To illustrate how error checking can be implemented at each of the three levels, we will use a simplified W-4 data-entry form as an example. Its visual interface appears in Figure 10.2.

Figure 10.2
Simplified W-4 Data-Entry Form

The Mask property is set to expect the Month being entered as a three-letter string, just to illustrate a generalized error checking for the masked edit box.

The following table gives the controls used for the data fields and the settings of certain selected properties.

Field	Control	Property	Setting	Remark
Employee Number	Text box	Name	txtEmpNo	4 digits, numeric
Employee Name	Text box	Name	txtEmployeeName	Last, First Init.
Date of Employment	Masked edit box	Name Mask	mskDateOfEmp ##-???-####	To illustrate mask checking
Zip Code	Combo box	Name	cboZipCode	User can select or enter a new zip code
Number of Dependents	Text box	Name	txtDependents	3 digits, numeric

The TabIndex properties of these controls are properly set by "row" and top-down; that is, the label with the caption "Employee Number" has a TabIndex of zero; txtEmpNo, 1; and so forth.

Notice in particular that the masked edit box mskDateOfEmp has a mask "##-???-####," which expects two digits for the day of the month, three characters for the month, and four digits for the year. Some programmers maintain that such a field design ensures no confusion between month and day. However, it can also cause inconvenience to the user. It requires the user's familiarity. In addition, correcting an entry error can take additional effort. We use the design here simply for the purpose of illustrating how to handle a mask with mixed key types.

Notice also that we assume when the program starts, the combo box cboZipcode will be populated with zip codes stored in the employee database. However, the user can either select a zip code from its list box or enter one directly.

When the User Presses a Key

What kind of data-entry errors can your program detect at this level? Because all your program knows is the key the user presses, your program will not be able to tell whether the entire data field is valid. However, your program should be able to identify whether the key is numeric or alphabetic. Thus, when the user presses an alphabetic key and the data field is numeric, your program should be able to identify this type of error and inform the user accordingly.

Several types of VB controls accept key input: text boxes, mask edit boxes, and combo boxes. Checking for errors for each of these controls involves slightly different considerations. Let's consider the text box first.

Working with Text Boxes. Not all the keys pressed by the user are data input. For example, the user may press a control key, a navigation key, or a function key. Only the alphanumeric keys are meant for input. These keys can be checked for validity in the familiar KeyPress event, which has the following header:

```
Private Sub Object_KeyPress (KeyAscii as Integer)
```

where *object* refers to a textbox.

The Ascii value of the key the user presses is passed to this procedure, where you can write code to check for specific types of key errors. For example, if a textbox is intended for numeric data only but the user presses an alphabetic key, the program should catch the error and display a message. The code to check for numeric keys has been illustrated in Chapter 5, "Decision." The code to check for the text box txtNumber is reproduced as follows:

```
Private Sub txtNumber_KeyPress(KeyAscii as Integer)
     Select Case KeyAscii
     Case Is < vbKeySpace
     ' These are control keys; ignore
     Case vbKey0 To vbKey9
     ' These are numeric keys; ignore
```

```
        Case Else
        ' These are neither control keys nor numeric keys;
        ' display an error message and suppress the key
            MsgBox "Numeric key only, please."
            KeyAscii = 0
        End Select
    End Sub
```

For our example, the preceding routine can easily be modified to suit our needs. For example, the same code can be changed to check for numeric keys for txtEmpNo and txtDependents. You can copy the same code but change the procedure headers as follows:

```
Private Sub txtEmpNo_KeyPress(KeyAscii as Integer)
     ' Copy and Paste the same code from above
End Sub
Private Sub txtDependents_KeyPress(KeyAscii as Integer)
     ' Copy and Paste the same code from above
End Sub
```

In a similar fashion, an event procedure can be written to check for alphabetic keys for the text box named txtEmpName. The code is given as follows:

```
Private Sub txtEmpName_KeyPress(KeyAscii as Integer)
     Select Case KeyAscii
     Case Is < vbKeySpace
     ' Control key.  Ignore it.
     Case vbKeyA to vbKeyZ, 97 to 122
     ' Uppercase and lowercase alphabets.  Need to do nothing
     Case Else
     ' Not an alphabetic key. Display an error message and nullify it.
          MsgBox "Alphabet keys only, please."
          KeyAscii = 0
     End Select
End Sub
```

Note that there are no predefined constant names for the lowercase alphabetic keys. For simplicity, we use their Ascii key code values in the code. For clarity, you should provide your own symbolic names for these keys.

Handling Some Special Characters. Note also that the code allows for alphabets only. However, the text box for employee names should also allow spaces, commas, and periods. Thus, we can add the following "Case" statement:

```
Case vbKeySpace, 44, 46
' Space, comma, and period. Ignore.
```

You may have noticed that we use the literal constants for comma and period. There are no predefined constant names for comma or period, although space is defined as vbKeySpace. An alternative is to use code Asc(",") and Asc(".") in place of the literal constants. This in effect uses the Asc function to generate the Ascii values. The code appears clear. However, it will execute a bit slower because function calls are involved. Yet, another alternative is to declare the key codes for the two characters in the program with names such as keyComma and keyPeriod. Then they can be used along with vbKeySpace in the preceding line. For simplicity and clarity, we will use the following code for all later discussion:

```
Case vbKeySpace, Asc(","), Asc(".")
' Space, comma, and period. Ignore.
```

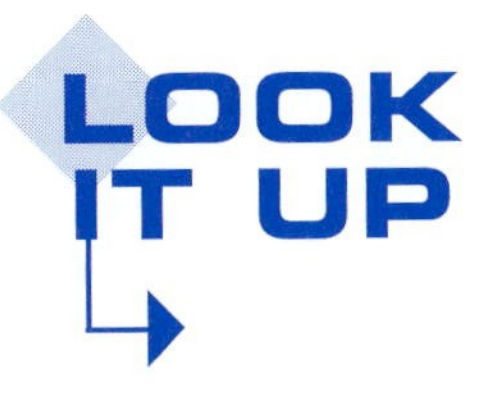

Search the Index tab of the online Help file using the keyword "Keycode constant." You should be able to see all key code constants that are predefined with names. You should take advantage of them whenever you need to reference them in your code. The use of named constants in code enhances the code's readability and clarity as we have repetitively pointed out.

The Ever-Present Repetitive Code. The preceding coding strategy, which includes error-checking code in each control's KeyPress event procedure, will work fine as long as the number of text boxes on a form is limited. However, when the number grows large, you will soon find the code for the project becomes pretty fat. There will be a lot of duplicate code because each text box checking for the same type of errors will have to repeat exactly the same code in its own KeyPress event procedure. (You may have already noticed the problem for txtEmpNo and txtDependents.)

Minimizing Code for Key Verification. Two strategies can be used to minimize the code. One approach is to move the preceding code into independent Sub procedures (call them CheckNumeric and CheckAlphabet) and replace the code in the event procedure with a Sub call. The code structure under this strategy will appear as follows:

```
'(In the General Section:)
Private Sub CheckNumeric(KeyAscii as Integer)
' move the code under txtNumeric here
    Select Case KeyAscii
    Case Is < vbKeySpace
    ' This is a control key.  Ignore it.
    Case vbKey0 to vbKey9
    ' The key is between "0" and "9".  No need to do anything.
    Case Else
    ' This key is not numeric, display an error message
        MsgBox "Numeric data only, please."
        KeyAscii = 0
    End Select
End Sub

Private Sub CheckAlphabet(KeyAscii as Integer)
' move the code under txtEmpName_KeyPress here
    Select Case KeyAscii
    Case Is < vbKeySpace
    ' Control key.  Ignore it.
    Case vbKeyA to vbKeyZ, 97 to 122
    ' Uppercase and lowercase alphabets.  Need to do nothing
    Case vbKeySpace, Asc(","), Asc(".")
    ' Space, comma, and period. Ignore.
    Case Else
    ' Not alphabetic key. Display an error message.
        MsgBox "Alphabet only, please."
    'Nullify the key pressed.
        KeyAscii = 0
    End Select
End Sub

'(The event procedures:)
Private Sub txtEmpNo_KeyPress(KeyAscii as Integer)
    CheckNumeric KeyAscii
End Sub

Private Sub txtDependents_KeyPress(KeyAscii as Integer)
    CheckNumeric KeyAscii
End Sub

Private Sub txtEmpName_KeyPress(KeyAscii as Integer)
    CheckAlphabet KeyAscii
End Sub
```

This strategy works well when the number of text boxes is moderate. The code looks pretty neat already, although you will have to insert the code to call the proper error-checking routines in each KeyPress event procedure. Try the preceding code before continuing.

Key Verification with Form KeyPreview. The other strategy for code minimization with key verification requires no code in the event procedures but the setting of the Tag property of each control. This strategy takes advantage of the form's KeyPreview capability.

As explained in Section 10.2, when the form's KeyPreview property is set to True, all keys that are meant for the text boxes are first "previewed" by the form in the Form KeyPress event. Thus, if we can identify what type of data the current control (text box) expects, we can call the proper error-checking routine (as written previously) accordingly.

The code will be too cumbersome if the name of each control has to be identified individually in this event procedure. Fortunately, all we need to know is the data type (numeric or alphabet) the data field (control) allows. This can be accomplished by setting the control's Tag property to a predetermined value that identifies the particular type. For example, we can use "N" tag for numeric data and "A" tag for alphabetic data. The ***Tag property*** is an "extra" property provided for the programmer's use and is not used by the control itself; that is, setting the property to any value does not in any way affect the control's behavior or appearance. Thus, you can use it for any purpose you see fit.

To illustrate how to implement this strategy, at design time, we can first set the Tag property of txtEmpNo and txtDependents to "N" and that of txtEmpName to "A." Then, instead of inserting any code in each control's KeyPress event procedure, we provide the following code:

```
Private Sub Form_KeyPress(Key Ascii as Integer)
    Select Case ActiveControl.Tag
    Case "A"
        CheckAlphabet KeyAscii
    Case "N"
        CheckNumeric KeyAscii
    End Select
End Sub
```

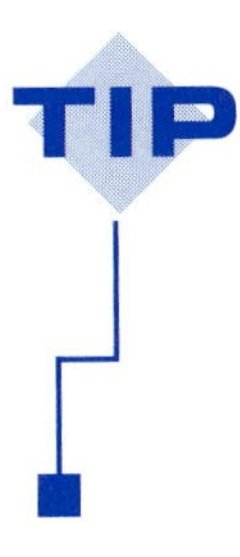

When you place the key verification code in the Form KeyPress event, you no longer need the code in the KeyPress event of each control. Remove these event procedures from your code window, but remember to do the following:

- Set the form's KeyPreview property to True.
- Set the Tag property of txtEmpNo and txtDependents to "N" (without quotes).
- Set the Tag property of txtEmpName to "A" (without quotes).

The ActiveControl. In the preceding event procedure, ActiveControl in the Select statement refers to the VB control that is currently active when the key is pressed. VB's ability to recognize "***ActiveControl***" makes the code much more concise. ActiveControl.Tag refers to the Tag property of the active control. This property should be set at design time as explained previously.

Providing Additional "Type" Checking. The code for CheckAlphabet and CheckNumeric Subs should remain the same. All additional text boxes that require data type checking will only need to have their Tag properties set to either N or A according to their expected data type. When more data types are used, additional tag values and error-checking Subs can be added under this strategy. For example, the preceding CheckNumeric Sub allows only integers. If another text box allows the decimal point, it will be proper to add another Sub (e.g., CheckDecimal). Then another Tag value like "D" can be used for this purpose. The implementation of this additional capability is left to you as an exercise.

Note that if you use this last strategy but set no Tag value for a control, no error checking will be performed on the key pressed in this control.

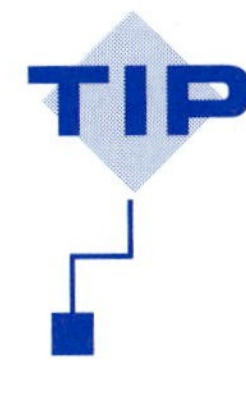

Always make sure that the form's KeyPreview property is set to True when you have code in the form's KeyPress event procedure. Many times, the code in the form's KeyPress fails to execute, not because of any error in the code but because the developer neglected to set this property to True. Also, if you mean to have a textbox checked for data type error when you use the KeyPress event procedure, be sure to have its Tag property set properly.

In summary, if a data-entry form has only a few text boxes, error checking can be coded in the control's KeyPress event procedure. However, if the form contains many text boxes, a strategy that works well is to set each control's Tag property to a predetermined value and then invoke the error-checking routine in the Form KeyPress event procedure by matching the Tag value. In this case, the form's KeyPreview property must be set to True.

Working with Masked Edit Boxes. As you already know, masked edit boxes are useful in filtering out data-entry errors when a data field has a specific pattern such as dates or Social Security numbers. At design time, you can set the Mask property to the desired pattern, such as "###-##-####" for Social Security numbers. This masked edit box will deny the entry of any nonnumeric key. To keep the user informed, you should display a message when a wrong key is pressed.

One possible solution is to place code in the ***ValidationError event***, which is raised when the user presses a key not allowed for the mask. For example, assume you have a masked edit box named mskSSN with its Mask property set to "###-##-####." The event procedure can be coded as follows:

```
Private Sub mskSSN_ValidationError(InvalidText As String, _
    StartPosition As Integer)
        MsgBox "Number only, please."
End Sub
```

Similar code can be provided for a masked edit box that allows only alphabetic data. Notice, however, that the preceding code works fine with VB5 but will trap the user in an endless loop of error messages with VB6, rendering this event useless.

An alternative is to place the code in the control's KeyPress event. This approach will make handling the mask edit box exactly the same as handling the text box, assuming the control expects only one type of data (e.g., numeric or alphabet). For example, using the second approach illustrated previously, you can use the following code to verify keys for mskSSN.

```
Private Sub mskSSN_KeyPress(KeyAscii As Integer)
    CheckNumeric KeyAscii
End Sub
```

A Mask with Mixed Keys. A different coding scheme will be needed when a mask requires more than one type of data. In our example, mskDateOfEmp has a mask "##-???-####," suggesting that the first two positions and the eighth through the eleventh positions require numeric keys, whereas the fourth through the sixth positions call for alphabetic keys.

In this case, to be able to inform the user of the type of the expected key, the mask character must be identified. The error message will depend on the mask character. The code in the KeyPress event procedure can appear as follows:

```
Private Sub mskDateOfEmp_KeyPress(KeyAscii As Integer)
Dim KeyPos As Integer
Dim MaskChar As String
    KeyPos = mskDateOfEmp.SelStart + 1 'Cursor Position
    MaskChar = Mid$(mskDateOfEmp.Mask, KeyPos, 1)
    Select Case MaskChar
    Case "#"
        CheckNumeric KeyAscii
    Case "?"
        CheckAlphabet KeyAscii
    End Select
End Sub
```

The procedure begins with obtaining the position in which the current key is being entered. Recall that the SelStart property gives the cursor position. However, SelStart starts with a value of 0 for the first position. To extract the corresponding mask character, you will need to use the Mid$ function, which considers the first position of a string position 1 rather than 0. Thus, 1 should be added. The Select Case block uses the extracted MaskChar to determine which Sub procedure to call. It will call CheckNumeric if the mask character is "#"; if the mask character is "?" it will call CheckAlphabet.

You will soon discover that when the number of masked edit boxes in the form is large, using this approach to check for key errors can easily make the code fat. In addition, the tedious task of "getting the code done right" can become challenging. An alternative is to write a generalized Sub procedure. The code can appear as follows:

```
Sub CheckMask(KeyAscii As Integer, mskControl As MaskEdBox)
Dim KeyPos As Integer
Dim MaskChar As String
    KeyPos = mskControl.SelStart + 1
    MaskChar = Mid$(mskControl.Mask, KeyPos, 1)
    Select Case MaskChar
    Case "#"
        CheckNumeric KeyAscii
    Case "?"
        CheckAlphabet KeyAscii
    End Select
End Sub
```

This Sub procedure requires the calling procedure to pass both the key just pressed and the mask edit control involved. It should be called from the control's KeyPress event. To use it to check the keys for the date of employment, you will code the following:

```
Private Sub mskDateOfEmp_KeyPress(KeyAscii As Integer)
    CheckMask KeyAscii, mskDateOfEmp
End Sub
```

Key Validation Using the Form KeyPress Event. Actually, the CheckMask Sub procedure can also be invoked from the Form KeyPress event. Assume an "M" (hinting "masked") is set as the Tag property for each masked edit box. You can modify the previous Form KeyPress event procedure as follows:

```
Private Sub Form_KeyPress(KeyAscii As Integer)
    Select Case UCase$(ActiveControl.Tag)
    Case "A"
        CheckAlphabet KeyAscii
    Case "N"
        CheckNumeric KeyAscii
    Case "M"
        CheckMask KeyAscii, ActiveControl
    End Select
End Sub
```

In the Select Case statement, the UCase$ function is used so that the procedure is not case sensitive. Setting the Tag property with an uppercase or lowercase will not cause any problem.

Notice that ActiveControl is the second argument passed to the CheckMask procedure. Recall that CheckMask expects a masked edit box as the second parameter. We assume that a control whose Tag property is set to "M" is a masked edit control.

Working with Combo Boxes. When a combo box's Style property is set to Dropdown Combo (the default setting with a value 0) or Simple Combo (1), the box's text can either take on a selection from the list in the combo box or be entered by the user. If the text is entered, the combo box is equivalent to a text box. Thus, the same error-handling techniques discussed in the text box section can be applied in exactly the same manner. For example, if you use the strategy of setting the Tag property and the combo box allows only alphabetic keys, you can simply set the Tag property of this combo box to "A" without any additional code. In our example, the Tag property of cboZipCode should be set to "N" so that the control can be checked for numeric keys.

Checking for Errors at the KeyPress Level: A Recapitulation. If a form has only a few controls, you can use the strategy of checking for valid keys for each control individually. However, when the form has many controls, one strategy that minimizes the code is to take advantage of the form's KeyPreview feature. To perform the error-checking routine at the KeyPress level using this strategy, you should do the following:

- Set the form's KeyPreview property to True.
- Provide the error-checking procedures, each accepting only specific groups of keys. For our example, you should have three Sub procedures: CheckNumeric, CheckAlphabet, and CheckMask.
- Set the Tag property of each control according to the type of keys allowed. For our example, the Tag property should be set as follows:

Control	Tag Property Setting
txtEmpNo	N
txtEmpName	A
mskDateOfEmp	M
cboZipCode	N
txtDependents	N

- In the form's KeyPreview event procedure, call the error-checking procedures according to the Tag property of the active control to be checked.

This strategy requires a minimal amount of code and maintenance. When you add more VB controls to the form, chances are you need to do nothing about the code but just set their Tag properties. Remember to set the form's KeyPreview property to True to ensure that the form's KeyPress event procedure is activated properly.

When the User Is Done with the Field

Even if each individual key entered has been checked as illustrated, the resulting data field may not necessarily be valid. The user can leave the data field prematurely, resulting in incomplete data, or the entered field may correspond to no reality; for example, 02-DDD-1982 might have been entered as a date. Thus, checking errors at the KeyPress level does not eliminate the need to check for errors at the field level.

The LostFocus Event and the Endless Error Trap. When the user finishes entering the data in data field, he or she will proceed to the next task by leaving the VB control (that field). A ***LostFocus event*** for that control is then raised. Before VB6, this is the event in which the field-level data validation code is placed. In general, it is desirable to reset the focus to the control that lost the focus when some error is found in the field. However, the LostFocus event by definition is not raised until another control receives the focus (which then becomes the currently active control). Thus, resetting the focus back to the original control will also cause the currently active control to lose focus. Now, if this control also has a field-level error-checking routine in its LostFocus event and if this field has an error, the procedure will also reset the focus, causing the original control to lose focus again. The user is then trapped in an endless loop of error messages. You can experience this problem in one of the Visual Basic Explorer exercises (10-8) at the end of this chapter. There, we also offer some possible solutions.

VB6 introduces a pair of features that help eliminate this problem: the ***Validate event*** and the ***CausesValidation property***. The Validate event occurs before another (the target) control receives the focus (thus also before the current control loses focus). The CausesValidation property of the target control, when set to True, will cause the original control's Validate event to be raised. The following paragraphs explain how this pair of features can be used to perform field-level data validation.

Checking for Missing Data. Occasionally, the user may even leave a field without keying anything, even though data is required for the field. To check for this error, an independent function can be written. The function can then be called from the Validate event of any control whose data entry is required, not optional. In our example, txtEmpNo should not be allowed to be blank. The code to check for missing data can appear as follows:

```
Private Sub txtEmpNo_Validate(Cancel As Boolean)
    If Missing(txtEmpNo.Text) Then
        MsgBox "Must have employee number to proceed."
        Cancel = True
    End If
End Sub

Private Function Missing(Text as String) as Boolean
    Missing = Len(Trim$(Text)) = 0
End function
```

In the text box's Validate procedure, the Missing function is called to check for missing data. If the function returns a value of True, an error message is displayed. In addition, the event's Cancel parameter is set to True. When this Boolean parameter of the Validate event procedure is set to True, the control will retain the focus, without causing any other events (e.g., another control's LostFocus event) to fire.

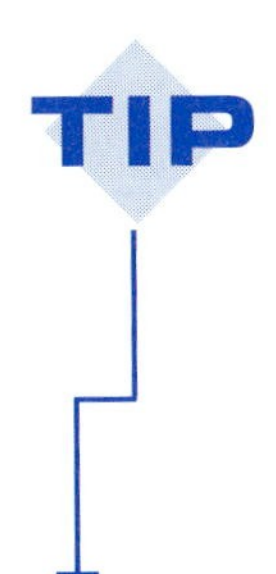

If you check the keyword "Validate event" in the Index tab of the online Help file, you will find that it has a different header as follows:

```
Private Sub object_Validate(KeepFocus As Boolean)
```

That is, the parameter is named KeepFocus, not Cancel. However, the template provided by the VB IDE has indeed Cancel as the parameter. Admittedly, KeepFocus reads much clearer and should be used. You can change the parameter name without affecting the actual result. We choose to use Cancel so that you won't be confused when you obtain the event template in the VB IDE.

Will this Validate event be fired all the time when the user attempts to leave the text box? It depends on the setting of the CausesValidation property of the target control that the user is attempting to move to. For example, if the user is moving the focus to the text box named txtEmpName, which has its CausesValidation property set to True (default), the preceding Validate event will be fired. On the other hand, if the user clicks on the command button named cmdDelete, whose CausesValidation Property is set to False, the preceding Validate event procedure will not be triggered.

Setting for the CausesValidation Property. For each control that requires checking errors at the field level, we will place the error-checking code in its Validate event procedure. However, should we set the CausesValidation property of all controls in a form to True? In general, before the user moves the focus from one data-entry box to another, you want to be sure that the current control has valid data. Thus, we can set this property to True for all VB controls used for data input. This is not the case for some command buttons. For example, consider the case of a "Quit" button. If its CausesValidation property is set to True, when the user decides to quit in the middle of a data field, this field's validation procedure will be triggered, insisting that the user enters valid data before quitting. Annoying, isn't it? In general, this property of the command buttons should be set to False, except for the Save button. All data to be saved should be validated. Setting the button's CausesValidation property to True ensures that the current data field's Validate event will be triggered.

Set the CausesValidation property of all controls to True (default) except for the command buttons for delete, quit, or browse operations.

The "Missing" function compares the length of the trimmed text with 0 and returns a "True" or "False" value depending on whether the comparison result is true or false. Note that the first "=" sign in the formula denotes "assignment," whereas the second "=" sign calls for the comparison of the length with 0. The Trim$ function will return a zero-length string when the argument text is a string containing only spaces. The Len function will then return a zero. The comparison will result in a value "True," which is then assigned to "Missing," which is in turn returned to the calling procedure.

Because it is easy to check for missing data directly in a Validate event procedure, one might want to place the code directly in the event procedure, instead of using the Missing function. He or she might question the desirability of a coding structure as shown previously. One reason for showing such a code structure is to illustrate how error conditions common to many controls can be put together. In addition, the previous approach has an advantage of code consistency; all error conditions common to several controls can be coded in a similar manner. Only errors unique to a particular control will be written as additional error-checking code in the Validate event procedure.

For our example, all data-entry boxes should require data. Therefore, you should provide code in the Validate event of each control. The code for mskDateOfEmp should appear as follows:

```
Private Sub mskDateOfEmp_Validate(Cancel As Boolean)
    If Missing(mskDateOfEmp.ClipText) Then
        MsgBox "Please enter date of employment.", vbInformation
        Cancel = True
        Exit Sub
    End If
End Sub
```

Notice the ClipText property, not the Text property, is used to check for missing data. As you may recall, the ClipText property gives only the data (keys) that the user has entered and excludes the literal constants that the mask automatically provides, whereas the Text property includes all these characters.

All other controls can be checked for missing data in the same manner as the Validate event procedure for txtEmpNo. The code is left to you as an exercise.

Other Types of Errors. In general, each data field has its unique requirement in addition to some common error conditions such as missing data. At this error-checking level, there is no elegant way similar to using the Form KeyPress event procedure illustrated previously to factor out the code for even the common error conditions. The following is all you can do to minimize code:

1. Write independent function procedures to return a value signaling an error condition.
2. Call the pertinent functions from the Validate event procedures. These event procedures can test the returned values and perform proper actions accordingly.

Two built-in functions that can be potentially useful to checking data field errors are ***IsDate*** and ***IsNumeric***. The former can be used to test whether a data field (especially a masked edit control) is a valid date. For example, the following code can be placed in the Validate event procedure for a masked edit box named mskDate. It will display an error message when the control contains an invalid date.

```
If IsDate(mskDate.Text) Then
' The field appears acceptable, check the month.
    If Val(Left$(mskDate.Text, 2)) <= 12 Then
    ' This is a valid date.  Do nothing.
    Else
    ' The date is not really valid.  Display an error message.
        MsgBox "Please enter a valid date."
        Cancel = True
    End If
Else
    MsgBox "Please enter a valid date."
    Cancel = True
End If
```

In the preceding code, we assume that the masked edit box expects a date in the format mm/dd/yyyy. The IsDate function accepts a date in either the mm/dd/yyyy format or the dd/mm/yyyy format. Thus, both "02/28/1998" and "28/02/1998" will be considered valid. To be sure that the entered date conforms to the first format, the code checks the first two digits (for month) in the field to ensure that it is not greater than 12. Note that the code will not be suitable for our W-4 form example because of the different mask setting.

The IsNumeric function checks whether a data field is a valid numeric field. For example, IsNumeric("1X3") will return a value False, whereas IsNumeric("23.5") will return a value True. This function can be used in a manner similar to the code for IsDate.

You may wonder how a field can still go wrong if each key has been checked for numeric data type. It probably won't if it allows only numeric keys. However, if the field allows a decimal point, the code to check for numeric keys will need to be modified to accept the decimal point. If no additional care is taken to check for more than one decimal point in the field, the user might just happen to leave two or more decimal points. In this case, the IsNumeric function will come in handy as a final check for the field.

When You Are Not So Sure. Sometimes, as the user leaves a control, you may find it desirable to warn him or her about certain conditions but not necessarily insist that the user enter a "correct" value. For example, the user may enter 12 in the text box for the number of dependents, named txtDependents. We cannot be sure that the user means 12. Perhaps, he or she meant to enter either 1 or 2 and by mistake left both in. Or, perhaps, he or she does have 12 dependents. In such situations, rather than assuming the user is in error or accepting the data outright, you can call to the attention of the user and ask if the data should be accepted. Using the MsgBox function can conveniently implement this design concept. The code can appear as follows:

```
Private Sub txtDependents_Validate(Cancel As Boolean)
Dim N as Long
Dim Ans as Long
    N = Val(txtDependents.Text)
    If N > 5 Then
        Ans = MsgBox("Number of dependents = " & N & _
          ".  Ok to accept?", vbYesNo + vbQuestion)
        If Ans = vbYes Then
        ' Ok. Do nothing.
        Else
        ' Not Ok to accept the number
            Cancel = True 'Retain focus
        End If
    End If
End Sub
```

Use the MsgBox function to prompt for a proper response from the user when the number of possible choices is no more than three.

The first argument of the MsgBox function displays the number of dependents and asks whether it is OK to accept this value. The next argument makes MsgBox display both the "Yes" and "No" button as well as the "?" icon in the message box. If the user clicks the "Yes" button, the MsgBox returns the value vbYes (6); otherwise, it returns the value vbNo (7). The returned answer value is assigned to the variable Ans. The computer then checks whether the Ans is vbYes. If not (suggesting not to accept the entry), it resets the focus to this control. Otherwise, nothing is done, suggesting that the user's action is accepted. Figure 10.3 shows how the program reacts to a sample entry with a questionable value entered for the number of dependents field.

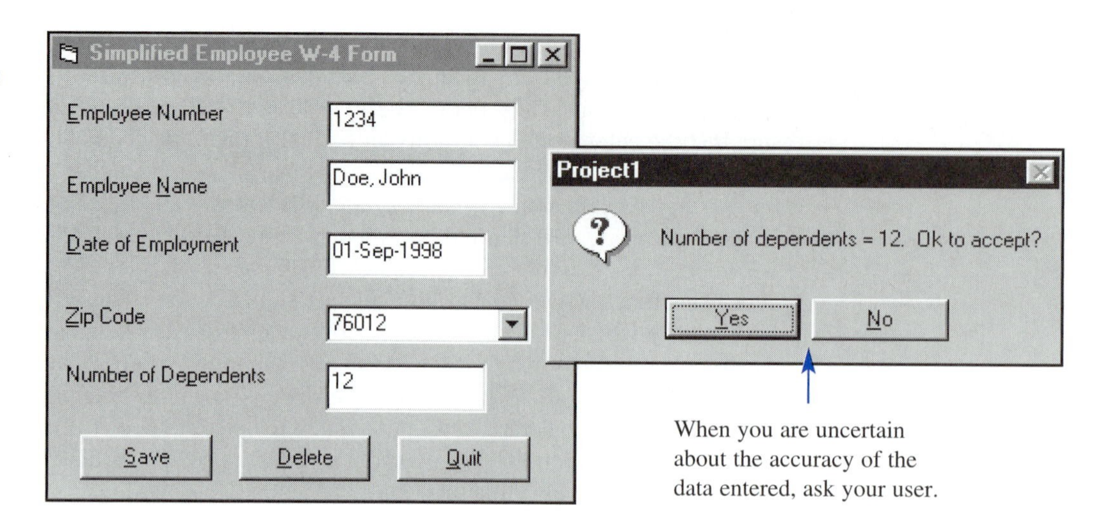

Figure 10.3
Confirming a Value in a Data-Entry Field

When the User Is Ready to Proceed

It would seem that if all data fields have routines to check for keys pressed and Validate event procedures to check for field-level errors, the resulting data screen should be fine when the user is ready to proceed (save, for instance). Not so! For example, the user may complete the first data field correctly and proceed to save the screen, leaving all other fields in the form blank. None of the KeyPress and Validate event procedures written for all subsequent controls would have been triggered.

One possible strategy to ensure that all data fields are entered is to allow the user to proceed only to the next control in the form. Although it is not hard to implement such a strategy, it is too restrictive and is not considered user-friendly. This is particularly true when the user is updating a record with only a minor correction. Imagine the trouble of tabbing through a score of data fields to correct an error and then having to tab through another bundle of fields before you reach the "Save" button!

Calling the Validate Event Procedures from the Save Click Event. Another strategy is to call all the Validate procedures one by one in the "Save" button Click event procedure. This would appear to work. However, if you simply list all the Validate event procedures in the command Save Click event procedure, you may soon find the project behaves strangely.

To illustrate, assume you have had all the Validate event procedures written for the controls in our example (txtEmpNo, txtEmpName, mskDateOfEmp, cboZipCode, and txtDependents). You can gain this experience, now. First, add the following code (which calls the Validate event procedure of all controls):

```
Private Sub cmdSave_Click()
Dim Cancel As Boolean
    txtEmpNo_Validate Cancel
    txtEmpName_Validate Cancel
    mskDateOfEmp_Validate Cancel
    cboZipCode_Validate Cancel
    txtDependents_Validate Cancel
    MsgBox "Data saved."   ' Just pretending
End Sub
```

Run the project. Enter a number in the Employee Number field. Then click the "Save" command button. You should see a sequence of error messages followed by "Data saved." before you are given a chance to enter any data.

Recall that before this "experiment," everything appears to work fine; that is, when a text box was blank, an error message was displayed and the focus was reset if you tried to proceed to the next data field. Why then does calling each Validate event procedure in sequence not seem to work properly? The mystery lies in the fact that these Validate procedures are now called and executed one right after another, whereas in the previous case, each of them is triggered by the control's Validate event itself. Previously, as soon as the Validate event procedure finishes, execution control is returned to the system, which waits for another event to be raised. Calling these Validate procedures one after another does not allow execution control to return to the system even when some error is detected.

There is another problem. Because these procedures are called from the command button's Click event, not by the system when the events are fired, the Cancel parameter passed to the procedures are not used by the system to reset the focus but simply returned to the Save button's Click event procedure.

Tricking the System to Trigger the Validate Event. The only way to ensure that Validate event procedures behave properly is for the system to trigger each of them. Is there a way to trick the system into action by code to fire those Validate event procedures? Recall that to trigger these procedures manually (initiated by the user), the focus should first be set on the first entry box (in our case, txtName). Then the user will press the Tab key repetitively until the Save button is reached. By code, we can set the focus on the first entry box by the SetFocus method. To tab through the controls, we can use the SendKeys statement to send the Tab key as we did in previous sections. To repeat tabbing, we can use a loop. Thus, our "first approximation" using this approach should appear as follows:

```
Private Sub cmdSave_Click()
    TxtEmpNo.SetFocus 'Set focus on the first control
    Do Until ActiveControl.TabIndex >= cmdSave.TabIndex
        SendKeys vbTab  'Send the tab key to move focus
    Loop
    MsgBox "Data saved."   ' Pretending
End Sub
```

In the procedure, we first set the focus on the first text box, txtEmpNo (which then becomes the active control). Inside the loop, the SendKeys statement sends a Tab key. If everything works as anticipated, the focus will move to the next control. As the focus moves, ActiveControl will refer to the control currently receiving focus. The "Until" clause in the Do statement tests to ensure that all controls (for input) have been tabbed through by comparing the TabIndex of the active control with that of the command button (cmdSave). If it is greater or equal, all the controls for input must have been tabbed through. The focus is back on the Save command button. (*Note:* Before testing the procedure, make sure that the TabIndex properties of all the controls are set properly.)

Run the program and click the Save button. You will notice that the computer locks up. Press Ctrl+Break to break the process. End the program.

What happened? Why doesn't the SendKeys statement work? Recall that the statement emulates a key being sent to the Windows operating system. As your program is busily executing the loop, the operating system is not given the time to process the Tab key(s) sent by your program. To ensure that the operating system is given time to handle the environment (e.g., processing keys entered and mouse clicks by the user or updating the screen appearance), you need to release the execution control to the operating system.

The DoEvents Statement. The statement to fulfill this is the ***DoEvents statement***. When execution reaches this statement, VB will release the control to the operating system. As soon as the system finishes its work, execution control will return to the statement immediately following the DoEvents statement. Thus, the preceding loop should be modified as follows:

```
Do Until ActiveControl.TabIndex >= cmdSave.TabIndex
    SendKeys vbTab  'Send the tab key to move focus
    DoEvents 'Release control to the Windows operating system
Loop
```

If you test run the program again and click the Save button without entering any data, it still does not work properly. This time, it continues to display the message "Must have employee number to proceed." In addition, the focus remains set on the text box for employee number. (Press Ctrl+Break and end the program again.)

What went wrong this time? Let's examine the loop again. The SendKeys statement sends the Tab key. With the DoEvents statement, the operating system is able to attempt to move the focus to the second control. However, an error (missing data) is then detected in the txtName's Validate event, causing the error message to be displayed and the control to retain the focus. The loop is then executed another time with the same sequence of events. Thus goes the endless loop. What we need now is to exit the loop (indeed, the procedure) when an error is detected.

"Signaling" Error from the Validate Procedures. We need to find a way for the Validate procedures to inform the loop when an error is detected. This can be done by setting up a form-level Boolean variable (e.g., BadField). When each of the Validate procedures is triggered, if an error is found, the procedure can set the variable to True. The variable can be set to False at the beginning of the loop. Inside the loop, an If statement can be used to test whether the variable is True. If so, the execution control should be returned to the system level (Exit Sub) so that the user can correct the error. Thus, the command's Click event procedure should appear as follows:

```
Private Sub cmdSave_Click()
    TxtEmpNo.SetFocus
    BadField = False
    Do Until ActiveControl.TabIndex >= cmdSave.TabIndex
        SendKeys vbTab  'Send the tab key to move focus
        DoEvents 'Release control to the Windows operating system
        If BadField Then Exit Sub 'If field is bad, then terminate.
    Loop
    MsgBox "Data saved."  ' Pretending
End Sub
```

The txtEmpNo Validate procedure should look like the following:

```
Private Sub txtEmpNo_Validate(Cancel As Boolean)
    If Missing(txtEmpNo.Text) Then
        MsgBox "Must have employee number to proceed."
        Cancel = True  ' Retain focus
        BadField = True 'Signal an error has been encountered
    End If
End Sub
```

Of course, *all other Validate procedures should include the statement to assign True to BadField where an error is detected.* (Place the statement immediately below Cancel = True.) In addition, in the general declaration section, the variable BadField should be declared as follows:

```
Dim BadField as Boolean
```

This statement makes the variable BadField a form-level (module-level) variable; that is, it is recognized by all procedures in the form. Once you complete this revision, test your program again. It should work properly.

To summarize, at the screen level, there is an elegant way to trigger all the Validate procedures to ensure that all data-entry boxes contain valid data. This is accomplished by doing the following:

1. Setting the focus on the first data-entry box using the SetFocus method
2. Assigning False to a form-level error flag (we called it BadField) before the loop
3. Repetitively sending the Tab key followed by a DoEvents statement to tab through all data-entry boxes so that the Validate procedures are triggered
4. Testing in the loop whether the error flag (BadField) is True; and if so, exiting the procedure (note that steps 1 through 4 should be done in the cmdSave procedure)
5. Setting the error flag (BadField) to True in the Validate procedures where errors are found

10.5 Handling Errors

Consider the following program:

```
Option Explicit
Private Sub cmdSave_Click()
Dim TextFile As Integer
    MsgBox "Please insert a blank diskette in drive A. " _
      & "Click the OK button when ready."
    TextFile = FreeFile
    Open "a:\TextFile.txt" For Output As #TextFile
    Print #TextFile, txtContent.Text
    Close #TextFile
End Sub
```

A User's Nightmare

As you can see, the preceding program saves whatever the user types in a text box named txtContent onto a file named TextFile.txt in Drive A. Before the Save operation starts, you are careful enough to inform/remind the user to insert a blank disk in Drive A and click the OK button when everything is set. The program has no syntax error or logic error; thus, it appears to be bug free. Does this mean that it will work without any problem? Yes, until a careless user forgets to insert a disk before he or she clicks the OK button in the message box. Then the system displays a message box showing error #71, "disk not ready." The program is then terminated, giving the user no "recourse." If this program has been compiled and is being run from Windows, it will completely disappear from the screen.

Although it is not the program's (or programmer's) fault in handling the disk, a program that behaves this way is not considered user-friendly. As explained in Section 10.1, a sound GUI program should be forgiving; that is, it should not "punish" the user for his or her mistake. Imagine that the user has spent 3 hours working on the text that represents an important document. Clicking the Save button was the last step to complete the job!

The On Error Statement

So, what code can you provide to prevent something like this from happening? The statement to use is the On Error statement, which was briefly introduced in Chapter 5. The technique is referred to as error trapping/handling. The On Error statement can take one of the following syntax forms:

```
On Error GoTo Line
On Error Resume Next
On Error GoTo 0
```

where *Line* represents a line label representing the code location to handle the error.

The second line, "On Error Resume Next," tells the computer to ignore the current error and proceed to the statement next to the one where the error occurs. The third line, "On Error GoTo 0," disables the error handler; that is, from this line on, all the errors will be treated as if none of the On Error statements had been coded in the procedure.

To see how the On Error statement works, let's modify the preceding program as follows:

```
Option Explicit
Private Sub cmdSave_Click()
Dim TextFile As Integer
    On Error GoTo HandleError
    MsgBox "Please insert a diskette in drive A. " _
      & "Click the OK button when ready."
    TextFile = FreeFile
    Open "a:\TextFile.txt" For Output As #TextFile
    Print #TextFile, txtContent.Text
    Close TextFile
    Exit Sub 'So that execution will not drop below this line.
```

```
HandleError:
    If Err.Number = 71 Then
        ' disk not ready error
        MsgBox "Please be sure a diskette has been inserted. " _
        & "Click the OK button when ready. ", vbExclamation
        Resume
    Else
        MsgBox "Error no. " & Err.Number & " " _
          & Err.Description & ".  Text has not been saved." _
            , vbInformation
    End If
End Sub
```

The On Error statement is placed at the beginning of the procedure. From that point on, the error handler is enabled. That is, at runtime, an error in any statement following the execution of the On Error statement will cause the execution control to branch to the line with a label referenced in the On Error statement (in this case, HandleError). For example, in this procedure, an error in the Open statement caused by the user's failure to insert a disk will cause the execution to jump to the line label HandleError.

The Line Label Statement

Notice how the line label HandleError is constructed. The line label name must be placed at the beginning of a line and must immediately be followed by a colon (:). Then, any GoTo statement referring to this label will cause the execution to branch to this line. Notice also that in the line that references this line label, there is no need to place a colon after it. That is, you code:

```
On Error GoTo HandleError
```

instead of:

```
On Error GoTo HandleError:
```

Finally, also notice that there is an Exit Sub statement before the HandleError line. The statement is added so that in the normal course of operation (without an error), the execution will not drop through the routine to handle errors.

The Err Object

Before explaining how the error-handling routine in the procedure works, let's take a look at the Err object first. This object deals with runtime errors. It can be used to raise or clear an error. When an error occurs, it contains information such as the error number (Err.Number) and description (Err.Description) that explains the nature of the error. In deciding what the proper action is to take, the code must first check to ascertain the error number. If there is a need to inform the user of the problem, the Description property of the Err object can be most suitable. Thus, the Err object can be useful in error handling.

How the Error Handler Works

How does the error-handling routine in the preceding procedure work? It first checks whether the error number is 71, which is the "disk not ready" error. If this is the case, a message instructing the user to insert the disk is displayed. The Resume statement following the message will branch the execution back to the line where the error occurs (i.e., the Open statement), allowing another attempt to open the file. If the error number is not 71, the code will simply display the error number and description. It also informs the user that the data is not saved. Because the next statement after the message is the End Sub statement, the execution control returns to the caller (in this case the system). Once exiting the procedure (cmdSave_Click), the error handler is disabled; that is, the On Error statement no longer has its effect.

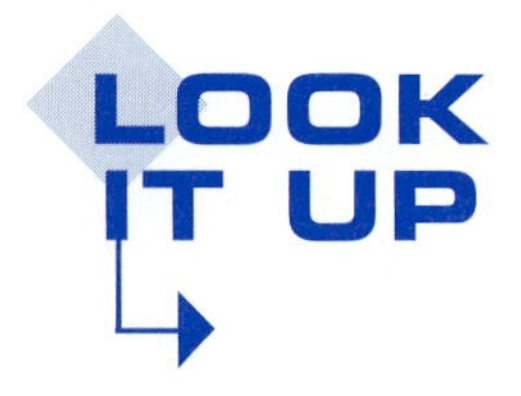

To find the error number of particular interest to you, select the Contents option in the online Help menu. Then double-click the following items in sequence when each appears on the left side of the Help screen:

MSDN Library Visual Studio 6.0
Visual Basic Documentation

Reference
Trappable Errors
Core Visual Basic Language Errors

You should see a long list of errors along with their respective descriptions. Error numbers 52 through number 76 are pertinent to file I/O operations and can be of particular interest to you.

Admittedly, the error handler presented here is very crude. For example, the error number can be replaced with a more descriptive named constant. In addition, we can check for more possible errors commonly associated with disk I/O operations, such as disk full (error number 61) or permission denied (error number 70; disk is write-protected). Furthermore, you may want to handle the disk not ready in a different manner. For example, you can do the following:

1. Inform the user as to the nature of the problem.
2. Provide the user alternative actions that he or she can choose; for example, retry, ignore, or abort.
3. Branch based on the user's response. Resume, Resume Next, and Exit Sub should correspond to retry, ignore, and abort, respectively.

Our presentation is only for the purpose of illustrating the code structure for error handling. The desired refinement is left to you as an exercise.

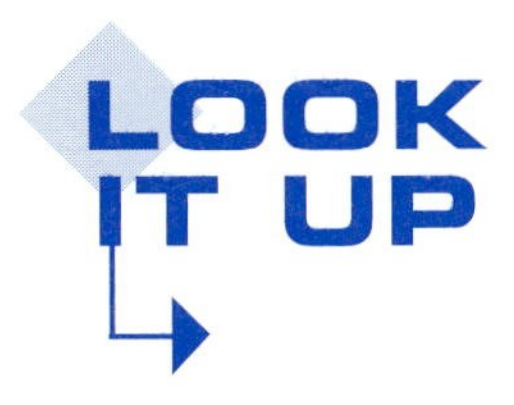

The online Programmer's Guide in the Help file has a thorough discussion on error handling. It even presents a framework for "generalized" error handling. To study the guide, click any of the first three options in the Help menu. Then at the center of the Help screen, click the following highlighted items (links) in sequence when each appears:

Visual Basic
Programmer's Guide
What Can You Do with Visual Basic
Debugging Your Code and Handling Errors

You should see a long list of topics. The first seven topics are particularly pertinent and helpful in this respect.

10.6 Providing Visual Clues

Imagine that you are using a program written by someone else. The program will process a large database in a complex manner and will take a few hours. When you click the "Start Process" button, you see nothing taking place. What will be your reaction? We will tend to think that maybe we did not click the button properly or, for whatever reason, that the computer did not register the click. Thus, we will most likely click the button one more time. If nothing happens again, we will click it again and again . . . What if it turns out that the program actually has started the process on the first and all subsequent clicks? It may take several days before all the repeated processes are completed. For fear that the program may have been so (carelessly) designed that it can ruin your database if you attempt to stop the process, you may have no choice but wait.

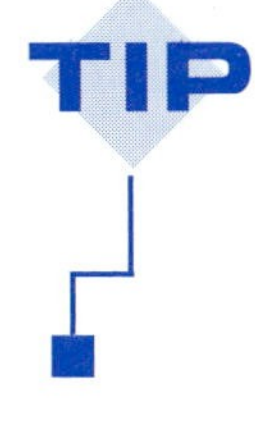

When a process should be carried out only once in the duration of the project, be sure to disable the command button that initiates the process once it is started. For example, assume that the command button to initiate a process is named cmdProcess. Then you should insert a statement to disable the button in its Click event as follows:

```
Private Sub cmdProcess_Click()
    CmdProcess.Enabled = False
```

continues

```
        ' Other statements to start to process
    End Sub
```

A long process can be handled similarly even if it can be initiated more than once. In the latter case, insert a statement to enable the button at the end of the Click event procedure.

What do you wish that this program had provided? Immediate visual feedback! When we clicked the button, if it had somehow "acknowledged" the click (e.g., by disabling that button), we would not have clicked the button another time. (Furthermore, the program should not start the process the second time.) Because it is a long process, we would rather the computer tell us where the process is as it progresses. Finally, in each processing step, the computer should inform us of the percentage of completion. All of these steps assure us (as the user) that everything is progressing without any problems, alleviating our anxiety in deciding what to do next (if anything).

Listing Prime Numbers: An Illustrative Example

Now, put yourself in the position of the programmer; how would you implement the preceding "wish list"? To answer this, let's consider a simpler example. You have a program to compute and list all the prime numbers up to the number the user specifies in a text box named txtUpperLimit. The results will be displayed in a list box named lstPrimes. The program will start the computation/listing process when the user clicks the "Compute" button (named cmdCompute). The original program appears as follows:

```
Option Explicit
Dim Primes() As Long
Private Sub cmdCompute_Click()
    ComputePrimes Val(txtUpperLimit.Text)
End Sub
Sub ComputePrimes(N As Long)
Dim I As Long
Dim J As Long
Dim Ib As Long
Dim SquareRoot As Long
Dim PrimeCount As Long
Dim IsPrime As Boolean
Dim NumbersToDisPlay As Long
' Step 1: Compute prime numbers up to upper limit
    ReDim Primes(1 To N / 2)
    lblStatus.Caption = "Computing prime numbers"
    Primes(1) = 1 'We know 1 and 2 are prime numbers.
    Primes(2) = 2
    PrimeCount = 2
    For I = 3 To N Step 2
        SquareRoot = Sqr(I)
    ' The following loop test if I is a prime number
        IsPrime = True 'Assume I is a prime
        For J = 3 To PrimeCount
            If (I Mod Primes(J)) = 0 Then
           ' I can be evenly divided by a prime. It's not a prime
                IsPrime = False
                Exit For
            ElseIf SquareRoot < Primes(J) Then
            ' I cannot be evenly divided beyond this number
            ' I is a prime number
                Exit For
            End If
        Next J
        If IsPrime Then
        ' I is a prime number; add to the list
            PrimeCount = PrimeCount + 1
            Primes(PrimeCount) = I
        End If
    Next I
```

```
' Step 2: Show results in the list box
    lstPrimes.Clear  'start the list box afresh
    lstPrimes.Visible = False 'To speed up the operation
    ' The next 3 lines ensure that only the largest 32000 primes
    ' are displayed in the list box
    Ib = PrimeCount – 32000
    If Ib < 1 Then Ib = 1
    NumbersToDisplay = (PrimeCount - Ib) + 1
        For I = Ib To PrimeCount
            lstPrimes.AddItem Primes(I)
    Next I
    lstPrimes.Visible = True 'Show the list box
End Sub
```

The event procedure is triggered when the user clicks the "Compute" button. The procedure simply calls the ComputePrimes procedure to perform the computation using the number in the text box (txtUpperLimit) as the argument. This Sub procedure also populates the list box with the prime numbers found in the procedure. Additional details are discussed in the following subsection.

As a technical side note, notice the routine to populate the list box. Each time an item is added to the list box, the control updates its appearance. This can take up a lot of time. You can speed up the process by setting the control's Visible property to False before the loop and then setting the same property back to True after everything is populated. The control will not attempt to update its appearance when it is not visible.

The Prime Number Computing Algorithm

The prime number computation Sub consists of two major steps: computing the primes and showing the primes in the list box. As you know, a prime number is one that can be evenly divided only by the number 1 and itself. The first two prime numbers are 1 and 2. A loop (For I = 3 to N) is set up to examine every odd number starting from 3 through the specified upper limit. Inside the loop, the number is examined by testing whether it can be evenly divided by any previously found prime numbers, using yet another loop (For J = 3 To PrimeCount). As soon as the number is found to be evenly divisible by a prime number, the IsPrime flag is set to False and the inner loop is terminated (Exit For). If the number cannot be evenly divided by any prime number up to the number's square root, it must be a prime number. As each prime number is found, it is added to the prime number list.

In the step to show the list of the prime numbers, note that the list box has an upper limit of holding approximately 32K items. To avoid exceeding its capacity, we elect to show only the last 32,000 prime numbers found in the computation. Also, to simplify the program focus, the code assumes that the user always enters a valid upper limit before clicking the button.

This program can take a long time if the user enters a large number as the upper limit. Let's consider how the visual feedback can be implemented.

The Mouse Pointer

When you test the program, if you enter a number that exceeds 100,000 in the text box, you will start to sense that it takes "a while" for the computer to complete the task. (Depending on the speed of your computer, the specific threshold value may vary.) To provide some visual clue to the user that the process has started, the mouse pointer's appearance can be changed. Typically, when the computer is waiting for the user to take actions, the mouse pointer is the default (normal) one. Once a process has started, you would signal to the user to wait. The typical mouse pointer used for this purpose is the hourglass. ***MousePointer*** is a property that can be referenced with the following syntax:

```
Object.MousePointer
```

where *Object* can be Screen, Form, or any control. If omitted, the form (Me) is the default. The MousePointer property has an integer value that represents the shape of the mouse pointer. For example, the named constant vbDefault (0) is the value for the default mouse pointer; vbHourglass (11) is the named constant for the hourglass.

To signal to the user to wait, when the computation for the prime numbers starts, we can modify the command's Click event procedure as follows:

```
Private Sub cmdCompute_Click()
Dim MousePointerUsed As Integer
    MousePointerUsed = MousePointer 'Save current mouse pointer
    MousePointer = vbHourglass 'set mouse pointer to "Wait"
    ComputePrimes Val(txtUpperLimit.Text)
    MousePointer = MousePointerUsed 'Restore mouse pointer
End Sub
```

In this modified procedure, the current mouse pointer is preserved with a variable named MousePointerUsed. Then the MousePointer property is assigned the value vbHourglass. At this point, the mouse pointer is turned into the hourglass shape. The prime number computation/listing procedure is then called. Once the process is complete, the mouse pointer is restored to its original value. We restore the mouse pointer to its original shape, instead of assigning the default value (vbDefault), to preserve the user's preference. Some users may have assigned a different mouse pointer to his or her computer as a matter of personal taste.

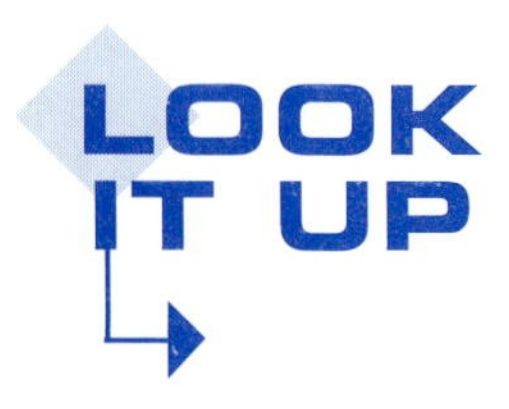

Use the keyword "MousePointer Property" to search the Index tab of the online Help file. The page lists all available settings (0 through 15 and 99) and the descriptions for the mouse pointer. These settings can be helpful in providing visual cues to the user when your application involves graphic operations.

Messages for Progress Status

It is also a good practice to display a message indicating the status (what is taking place) before a long process is undertaken. If a process involves multiple steps, displaying a message at the beginning of each step will make the user feel that the process is going even faster. This can easily be implemented. For example, in the preceding example, you can draw a label on the form. Assume you have named it lblStatus. Then before calling the Sub function, you can add a line to the code as follows:

```
lblStatus.Caption = "Computing prime numbers.  Please wait."
```

It goes without saying that if the event procedure involves more than just calling the prime number computation routine, you should add a line to change the labels' captions before calling each of these additional procedures. Indeed, in the prime computation function, there are two major steps: performing the computation and listing the results. We can add the following statements at the beginning of these steps:

```
(At the start of prime computations:)
lblStatus.Caption = "Computing prime numbers."

(At the start of adding prime numbers to the list box:)
lblStatus.Caption = "Populating the list box with prime numbers."
```

The Progress Bar

If a process takes a long time to complete, simply displaying the steps being performed is not enough. The user may still be uncertain as to how far the process has progressed. Even a 2-second wait may appear "very long" to the user. To assure the user that the process has been going fine, you can add a ***progress bar*** to your project and use it to display the percentage of completion. The progress bar has a rectangular shape and is used to display the progress in a lengthy process. You can make the progress bar gradually fill its rectangle with the system highlight color by changing its Value property as the process progresses. Figure 10.4 shows the progress bar icon and the control in action when used in the prime number computation project.

Adding the Progress Bar to Your Project. The progress bar is not an intrinsic control and must be added to your project. It belongs to the group of Microsoft Windows common controls 6.0. To add the progress bar to the prime number computation project:

1. Add Microsoft Windows Common Control 6.0 to the project.
   1.1 Click the Project menu and select the Components option.
   1.2 Check the "Microsoft Windows common controls 6.0" item.
   1.3 Click the OK button. The entire group of controls will appear in your toolbox.
2. Draw a progress bar on the form.
3. Change the control's name to prgStatus, using the control's Properties window.

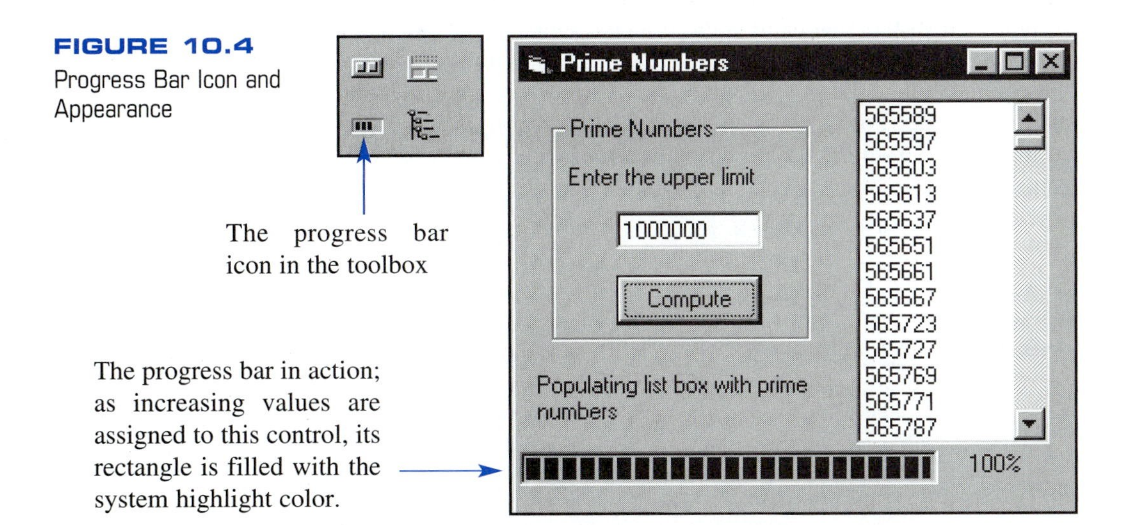

FIGURE 10.4
Progress Bar Icon and Appearance

The control has ***Max*** and ***Min properties*** with default values of 0 and 100, respectively. Because these can conveniently be used to represent percentages, they can be left unchanged. It has a Value property that is accessible only at runtime. As mentioned, setting this property will make the progress bar fill its rectangle with the system highlight color. Thus, to show the progress, you can compute the percentage of the progress and set the Value property of the progress bar accordingly.

Use "prg" as the three letter prefix to name the progress bar.

Using the Progress Bar. Because the actual computations are carried out in the function, you should modify the code in the ComputePrimes function to use the progress bar. In addition to filling the progress bar, the code should also display the percentage value, using a label named lblPercent. To compute the percentage, we will need to declare a variable, Percent. Also, to avoid continuously assigning the same percentage to the progress bar and the label (operations involving control properties take up much more time than involving variables), we will use another variable, PrevPercent, to test for the change. What percentage do we compute? We will take a crude approach by using the number of numbers examined (N); that is:

```
Percent = (I / N) * 100
```

This value will not be assigned to the progress bar or the label until it changes by a percentile. You can determine whether it has changed by comparing its value with PrevPercent. Thus, you can code the following:

```
If Percent > PrevPercent Then
'Percentage has changed,
    prgStatus.Value = Percent 'Fill progress bar with new value
    lblPercent.Caption = Percent & "%" 'Show the value in label
    PrevPercent = Percent  'Update the value of PrevPercent
    DoEvents 'Allow the OS time to update screen
End If
```

Inside the If block, the computed value of Percent is assigned to the progress bar's Value property as well the label's Caption property. Also, it is assigned to PrevPercent so that PrevPercent can be used again to detect changes in the value of Percent. Notice that we also include a DoEvents statement in the If block. This is to ensure that the Windows operating system is given time to update the screen (e.g., label captions) while the program is looping through the computations. The percentage computation along with the If block can be placed immediately below the "For I" statement (inside the outer loop).

In a similar fashion, the progress in populating the list box with the prime numbers can be coded. The revised Sub procedure is as follows:

```
Sub ComputePrimes(N As Long)
Dim I As Long
Dim J As Long
Dim Ib As Long
Dim NumbersToDisplay As Long
Dim NumberCount As Long
Dim SquareRoot As Long
Dim PrimeCount As Long
Dim IsPrime As Boolean
Dim Percent As Integer
Dim PrevPercent As Integer
    ' Step 1: Compute prime numbers up to upper limit
    ReDim Primes(1 To N / 2)
    lblStatus.Caption = "Computing prime numbers"
    Primes(1) = 1 '1 and 2 are known prime numbers
    Primes(2) = 2
    PrimeCount = 2
    prgStatus.Visible = True ' Show the progress bar
    For I = 3 To N Step 2
        Percent = (I / N) * 100 'compute percent
        If Percent > PrevPercent Then
        ' Percentage has changed
            prgStatus.Value = Percent 'Fill progress bar
            lblPercent.Caption = Percent & "%" 'Update the label
            PrevPercent = Percent 'Update PrevPercent
            DoEvents 'Allow OS time to update screen
        End If
        SquareRoot = Sqr(I)
    ' The following loop test if I is a prime number
        IsPrime = True
        For J = 3 To PrimeCount
            If (I Mod Primes(J)) = 0 Then
            ' not a prime
                IsPrime = False
                Exit For
            ElseIf SquareRoot < Primes(J) Then
            ' I will have no chance to be evenly divided
            ' beyond this prime number
            ' This is a prime number
            Exit For
            End If
        Next J
```

```
            If IsPrime Then
            ' I is a prime number; add to the list
                PrimeCount = PrimeCount + 1
                Primes(PrimeCount) = I
            End If
        Next I
        ' Step 2:  Show results in the list box
        lstPrimes.Clear  'start the list box afresh
        lstPrimes.Visible = False 'To speed up the operation
        Ib = PrimeCount - 32000
        If Ib < 1 Then Ib = 1
        NumbersToDisplay = (PrimeCount - Ib) + 1
        lblStatus.Caption = "Populating list box with prime numbers"
        DoEvents
        PrevPercent = 0
        For I = Ib To PrimeCount
            NumberCount = NumberCount + 1
            Percent = (NumberCount / NumbersToDisplay) * 100
            If Percent > PrevPercent Then
                prgStatus.Value = Percent
                lblPercent.Caption = Percent & "%"
                PrevPercent = Percent
                DoEvents
            End If
            lstPrimes.AddItem Primes(I)
        Next I
        lstPrimes.Visible = True
    End Sub
```

Summary

You have been introduced to several selected topics in data entry/user interface. This chapter began with a brief explanation of the principles of a sound GUI design, which include simplicity and clarity, flexibility, consistency, immediate feedback, forgiveness, and pleasant appearance. You have now become aware of several issues related to the use of keyboard in the context flexibility and mobility. These include handling the Enter key, up- and down-arrow keys, auto tabbing, and the use of access keys. You have learned the technique to convert by code one key (pressed by the user) to another to enhance flexibility for the user, using the SendKeys statement. You have also learned the issues related to and possible solutions to the use of the SSTab control.

In the context of forgiveness, you have been introduced to a way to detect unsaved data and to prompt the user for proper actions before a form unloads. You have also learned an error-trapping technique to ensure that the program is robust and to minimize the chance that it terminates unexpectedly and abruptly when an error is encountered. The technique involves the use of the On Error statement.

You have studied checking for user data-entry errors at different levels. These include (1) when the user presses a key (the key press level), (2) when the user leaves a data field (the field level), and (3) when the user claims that the entry onscreen is complete (the screen level). At the key press level, an elegant way to check for errors is to enable form KeyPreview (by setting the property to True). You can then use the form's KeyPress event to call the appropriate error checking procedure. This technique involves setting each control's Tag property according to its expected data type. The Tag settings are the criteria in the event procedure to call the proper error-checking procedure.

When the user leaves a field, the control's Validate event is fired if the oncoming control's CausesValidation property is turned on. Thus, the Validate event is the procedure to place code for checking for errors at the field level. In general, the CausesValidation property of the data-entry boxes should be set to True, whereas that of most command buttons should be set to False.

To ensure that all data have been entered and are valid, each Validate event procedure must be invoked again when the user proceeds to the next step (e.g., to save). One trick to accomplish this is to set the focus on the first data-entry box and then use the SendKeys statement to emulate pressing the Tab key by the user. You should be aware that the operating system must be given time to process the Tab key. To release the execution control to the operating system, be sure to include the DoEvents statement. In addition, once an error is detected in a Validate event procedure, the procedure that performs the SendKeys statement should immediately be terminated (Exit Sub) to allow the user to make corrections.

Finally, you have understood the user's need for feedback when the process involved in the program is lengthy. The visual feedback includes changing the mouse pointer's appearance, displaying a status message at the beginning of each major step, and using the progress bar to show the progress. The prime number computation example has illustrated how each of these feedback techniques could be implemented.

Visual Basic Explorer

10-1. Ampersand in the Caption Property of the Label. Draw a label on a form. Set its Caption property to "John & Jane's Income." What do you see? Why is there an underline (_) in the label? (Because "&" is used to set the access key for the label.) Now try "John && Jane's Income." What do you see this time?

10-2. Ampersand in the Caption Property of the Command Button. Draw a command button on a form. Set its Caption property to "Pick & Save." What do you see? You should see an underline (_) just as in the case of the label. So, how do you get the "&" symbol to show on a caption? Look to the preceding exercise for the answer. Indeed, all the Caption properties (if they exist) for all controls behave the same way in this respect. Try the check box and the option button to prove or disprove this assertion.

10-3. Access Key of the Command Button. How does the access key of the command button work? When the user presses its access key, is its Click event fired or does it just get focus? To answer, draw a command button and a text box on a form. Name the command button cmdSave and set its Caption property to "&Save." Enter the following code:

```
Option Explicit
Private Sub cmdSave_Click()
    Debug.Print "Click"
End Sub
Private Sub cmdSave_GotFocus()
    Debug.Print "Got focus"
End Sub
```

Run the project. Make sure the focus is set on the text box. Then press Alt+S. Check the immediate window. You should see both events fired. Also, which event is fired first? (*Note:* You might be tempted to replace Debug.Print with MsgBox in the preceding code. Why not? Try it. You should see some difference in the results. MsgBox sometimes takes away some events that are actually fired. Beware!)

10-4. Key Code Values of Various Keys. Want to know the key code values of various keys? Draw a text box on a form. Name it txtTest. Enter the following code:

```
Private Sub txtTest_KeyDown(KeyCode As Integer, Shift As  Integer)
    Debug.Print "Key code = " & KeyCode & ". Shift = " &  Shift
End Sub
```

Run the project and try the following keys:

Arrow keys (of all directions) with and without the Shift key

1 (one) on the regular keypad with and without the Shift key

1 (one) on the numeric keypad with and without the Shift key

Esc

F3 and F4 (be aware that some function keys can get activated in the IDE)

Page Up and Page Down

"A" with and without the Shift key

Enter on both the keyboard and the numeric keypad

Which key code values surprise you? (How about the 1's on different keypads and "A" with and without the Shift key?)

10-5. Sequence of Keyboard Events. When a key is pressed on a command button, what keyboard events are fired and in what sequence? To obtain the answer, draw a command button on a form. Name it cmdTest and set its caption to "Test." Enter the following code (the count is added to give you a clearer messages):

```
Private Sub cmdTest_Click()
Static Count As Integer
    Count = Count + 1
    Debug.Print "Command Click " & Count
End Sub
Private Sub cmdTest_KeyDown(KeyCode As Integer, Shift As _ Integer)
Static Count As Integer
    Count = Count + 1
    Debug.Print "Command Key Down " & Count
End Sub
Private Sub cmdTest_KeyPress(KeyAscii As Integer)
Static Count As Integer
    Count = Count + 1
    Debug.Print "Command Key Press " & Count
End Sub
Private Sub cmdTest_KeyUp(KeyCode As Integer, Shift As _ Integer)
Static Count As Integer
    Count = Count + 1
    Debug.Print "Command Key Up " & Count
End Sub
```

Run the project. Set the focus on this command button. Press several alphabetic keys. What events are fired? In what sequence? Press the spacebar. Compare the results with the previous keys. Any difference? Pressing the spacebar also triggers the Click event.

10-6. Access Key and Keyboard Events. Modify the Caption property of the command button in the preceding exercise to "&Test." Test the project again. Do you observe any differences between the results you obtain here and previously? (Not really.) This time also try to press Alt+T while the command button has the focus. Try another time while the command button does not have the focus. Compare the results between with focus and without focus. (Is there a Click event? a KeyPress event?) Also compare the results of each with the previous ones.

10-7. Keyboard Events and Key Preview. Modify the preceding project in the following manner:

1. Set the form's KeyPreview property to True.
2. Add the Keyboard event procedures for the form, each paraphrasing the counterpart of the command button as follows:

```
Private Sub Form_Click()
Static Count As Integer
    Count = Count + 1
    Debug.Print "Form Click " & Count
End Sub
Private Sub Form_KeyDown(KeyCode As Integer, Shift As _ Integer)
Static Count As Integer
    Count = Count + 1
    Debug.Print "Form Key Down " & Count
End Sub
```

```
Private Sub Form_KeyPress(KeyAscii As Integer)
Static Count As Integer
    Count = Count + 1
    Debug.Print "Form Key Press " & Count
End Sub

Private Sub Form_KeyUp(KeyCode As Integer, Shift As _ Integer)
Static Count As Integer
    Count = Count + 1
    Debug.Print "Form Key Up " & Count
End Sub
```

Run the project. Press an alphabetic key. What events are triggered? In what order? Each command event is preceded by a form event of the same kind; for example, the command's KeyDown event is preceded by the form's KeyDown event. Were you expecting that all form Keyboard events would precede all the command Keyboard events?

Turn off the form's KeyPreview property and try the same steps again. Do you see any form Keyboard events? (You should not.)

10-8. The Endless Error Message Trap. Draw two text boxes on a new form. Clear the text in each box. Place the following code in the code window:

```
Option Explicit

Function Missing(Text As String) As Boolean
    Missing = Len(Trim$(Text)) = 0
End Function

Private Sub Text1_LostFocus()
    If Missing(Text1.Text) Then
        MsgBox "Must have data to proceed."
        Text1.SetFocus
    End If
End Sub

Private Sub Text2_LostFocus()
    If Missing(Text2.Text) Then
        MsgBox "Must have data to proceed."
        Text2.SetFocus
    End If
End Sub
```

The code is meant to be used to check for missing data and reset the focus for each text box. As explained in the text, the LostFocus event is where to check for field-level errors before VB6's arrival. Run the project. Without entering any data, tab to the next control. You will be trapped in an endless error message loop. The reason is given in the text.

How can you solve this problem? One way to avoid the trap is to allow the user to move back to any previous control without checking for errors. If you insert the following line in Text2's LostFocus event before the If statement, the trap will not occur:

```
If ActiveControl.TabIndex < Text2.TabIndex Then Exit Sub
```

10-9. Where Is the Error? Draw a command button on a new form. Name the command button cmdCompute. Set its Caption property to "Compute." Then enter the following code:

```
Option Explicit
Private Sub cmdCompute_Click()
Dim Area As Double
Dim Width As Double, Height As Double
    On Error GoTo InformProblem
    Area = 10
    Height = ComputeHeight(Area, Width)
    MsgBox "The height is " & Height
    Exit Sub
```

```
InformProblem:
    MsgBox Err.Number & " " & Err.Description _
      & ". Problem ignored.", vbInformation
    Resume Next
End Sub
Function ComputeHeight(Area As Double, Width As Double) _
    As Double
    ComputeHeight = Area / Width
End Function
```

Run the project. What messages do you see? Why is the Height zero (according to the message)? Now, comment out the On Error statement in the Click event procedure. Run it again. Where do you see the problem (error message)? The ComputeHeight function has a division by zero error because the parameter Width has a zero, which is passed by the Click event procedure.

In the original code, the error handler in the Click event procedure is enabled before the ComputeHeight function is called. The error occurs in the function. However, there is no error handler in that procedure. Thus, the error is returned to the caller (Click event), which then jumps to its error handler. Because the error handler uses the "Resume Next" statement after displaying the error message, the next statement executed is the MsgBox statement, which displays the value of Height. Height has not yet been assigned any value because of the error in the function. Thus, the message displays a zero for the height.

Exercises

10-10. A Visual Interface with Access Keys. Your company's fixed asset application program requires the following data fields:

Field Name	Description	Control
Asset ID	Has a mask: AAA9999 Where *A* = Any letter *9* = Any digit	Masked edit box
Description	Alphanumeric field for asset description (maximum 32 characters)	Text box
Location	City name such as New York, Dallas, and Los Angeles (maximum 16 characters)	Combo box
Depreciable?	Yes/No to indicate whether asset is depreciable	Check box
Depreciation Method	0-No depreciation 1-Straight-line depreciation 2-ACRS depreciation	Option buttons
Cost	Numeric field (allow up to 99,999,999.99)	Text box
Life	Economic useful life in years (four digits maximum)	Text box

Design a data-entry screen for this application. The form should also include two command buttons: one to save data and another to Quit. All controls must be assigned a proper access key for the user to access the field using the keyboard. Provide code to handle only the Quit button.

10-11. A User Interface That Moves Focus with the Up-Arrow, Down-Arrow, and Enter Keys. (continued from 10-10). Add code to the preceding project so that when the user presses the Enter key or down-arrow key, the focus will move to the next field, and when the user presses the up-arrow key, the focus will move to the preceding field. Also, when the field is "filled" (reaches maximum length), the focus should automatically move to the next field (control).

10-12. Programming a User Interface Involving the SSTab. (modified from 10-10 and 10-11). Redesign the visual interface for 10-10. Use an MS SSTab as a container for the data fields. Make the SSTab show two tabs: one with the caption "Asset ID" and the other with the caption "Depreciation." The first tab will contain the first three fields, and the second will contain the last four fields. The command buttons should be placed on the form, not on either tab.

Again, all controls should have access keys. In addition, the SSTab should behave as follows:

- When the user clicks a tab (or reaches the tab using its access key), the focus should be set on the first control on that tab.
- When the user "completes" the last fields on the tab (by pressing the Enter or down-arrow key), the focus should move to the next "logical" VB control. That is, the focus should move to the Depreciable field when the user presses the Enter key in the location field and to the Save button when in the Cost field.
- The Asset ID field must contain something before the user is allowed to move to the next tab.

10-13. Check for Numeric Keys. Develop a Sub procedure that will ensure that the key entered is a numeric key. A nonnumeric key will trigger the MsgBox to display an error message. The "bad" key should be suppressed. Test this Sub by a call from the form's KeyPress event. Set the Tag property to "N" (numeric) of the VB control to be used to test for this purpose.

10-14. Check for Numeric Keys with Decimal Point. Add another Sub to the preceding project. This Sub should accept the numeric keys and one (and only one) decimal point in a VB control. An unacceptable key should trigger the MsgBox to display an error message. The "bad" key should be suppressed. Test this Sub by a call from the form's KeyPress event. Set the Tag property to "D" (decimal) of the VB control to be used to test for this purpose.

10-15. Check for Currency Data. Add another Sub to the preceding project. This Sub should accept the numeric keys, dollar sign ($) if it is the first character in the field, commas, and one decimal point. An unacceptable key should trigger the MsgBox to display an error message. The "bad" key should be suppressed. Test this Sub by a call from the form's KeyPress event. Set the Tag property to "C" (currency) of the VB control to be used to test for this purpose.

10-16. Check for Alphabetic Keys. Add another Sub to the preceding project. This Sub should accept only space and alphabetic keys. An unacceptable key should trigger the MsgBox to display an error message. The "bad" key should be suppressed. Test this Sub by a call from the form's KeyPress event. Set the Tag property to "L" (letter) of the VB control to be used to test for this purpose.

10-17. Enforcing Uppercase Alphabetic Keys. Add another Sub to the preceding project. This Sub should accept only space and alphabetic keys. All lowercase letters will automatically be converted to uppercase letters. An unacceptable key should trigger the MsgBox to display an error message. The "bad" key should be suppressed. Test this Sub by a call from the form's KeyPress event. Set the Tag property to "U" (uppercase) of the VB control to be used to test for this purpose.

10-18. Alphabetic and Numeric Keys Only. Add another Sub to the preceding project. This Sub should accept space, alphabetic, and numeric keys (but not any special characters). All lowercase letters will automatically be converted to uppercase letters. An unacceptable key should trigger the MsgBox to display an error message. The "bad" key should be suppressed. Test this Sub by a call from the form's KeyPress event. Set the Tag property to "X" (cross) of the VB control to be used to test for this purpose.

10-19. The Name Enforcer, Again. Add another Sub to the preceding project. This Sub should act as the name enforcer. That is, it will accept spaces, letters, a comma, a period, and hyphens and will automatically convert the first letter of each word to the uppercase letter. An unacceptable key should trigger the MsgBox to display an error message. The "bad" key should be suppressed. Test this Sub by a call from the form's KeyPress event. Set the Tag property to "E" (enforcer) of the VB control to be used to test for this purpose.

10-20. The Mask Handler. Add another Sub to the preceding project. This Sub handles keys based on the Mask property of the masked edit box. An unacceptable key should trigger the MsgBox to display an error message. The "bad" key should be suppressed. Test this Sub by a call from the form's KeyPress event. Set the Tag property to "M" (masked) of the VB control to be used to test for this purpose.

10-21. The Check Date Function. Write a function that will ensure that a text string parameter is a valid date field. (Only a string with the mm-dd-yyyy format should be considered valid.) If so, the function returns a value of False. Otherwise, an error message is displayed and the function returns a value of True. Name the function CheckDate. Test this function by creating a masked edit box for date entry. When the user leaves the control, your code should check if the date entered is valid. If not, the focus should be reset to this control.

10-22. The Check Numeric Function. Write a function that will ensure that a text string parameter is a valid numeric field. If so, the function returns a value of False. Otherwise, an error message is displayed and the function returns a value of True. Name the function CheckNumeric. Test this function by creating a text box for date entry. When the user leaves the control, your code should check whether the text box contains a valid number. If not, the focus should be reset to this control.

10-23. The Range Checker. Write a function that will ensure that a number is within a specified range. Name this function CheckRange. The function takes three parameters: the number, the lower bound, and the upper bound of the number. If the number is within the range of lower and upper bound, the function returns a value of False. Otherwise, it returns a value of True. Test this function with a text box. Assume the valid range of this number is 20,000 to 30,000, inclusive. When the user leaves this control, your code should check to ensure the value is within the range. If it is not, your routine will display an error message and reset the focus to this control. Note that the keys entered in this text box should be checked for valid numeric keys first.

10-24. Check Digit. Many programs use the check digit to check the validity of an ID number, such as the bank account number or credit card number. The check digit is usually generated by multiplying each individual digit in the ID number by a sequence of "multipliers," which are prime numbers 1, 3, 5, and so on, starting with 1 at the lowest digit. The products (multiplication results) are then summed. The total is then divided by yet another (higher) prime number. The resulting remainder (or its complement) is then used as the check digit. This method of computing the check digit can be shown as follows:

Account number						
	7	5	3	6	9	8
Multiplier						
	11	7	5	3	2	1
Results						
	77	35	15	18	18	8

Total of results = 77 + 35 + 15 + 18 +18 + 8 = 171
Remainder of 171/13 = 2

This digit is then attached as a part of the account number and given to the account holder. Thus, the preceding account number will be 7536982.

When entering a transaction for this account, this number is entered. The same check digit computation routine is used to ensure that the account number is entered correctly.

Write a function to generate the check digit using the method described. Call the function GenerateDigit. Then write another function to verify the accuracy of an ID number. Call it CheckDigit. It should return a value of True when the check digit is invalid.

To test the functions, draw two command buttons and a text box on a form. Name the command buttons cmdGenerate and cmdCheck and set their captions to "Generate" and "Check," respectively. Name the textbox txtIDNumber. Then provide the code to perform the following:

- When the user clicks the Generate button, your code will generate the check digit for the ID number entered in the text box. (Note that the ID number must be six digits long.) If the resulting check digit is a two-digit number, your program should advise the user that the ID number should not be used. Otherwise, the check digit should be displayed.
- When the user clicks the Check button, your code should use the CheckDigit function to verify the number given in the text box. (The user is expected to include the check digit as the last digit of the ID number.) If the check digit is correct, your program will display the message "Accept the ID number." Otherwise, it should display the message "The ID number is not valid."

10-25. Consistency Test and More. In the W-4 form of a payroll system, the screen has the following fields:

Field Name	Control	Control Name
S-S-N	Masked edit	mskSSN
Employee Name	Text box	txtName (Last, First Init.)
Date of Birth	Masked edit	mskDOB (mm-dd-yyyy)
Date of Employment	Masked edit	mskDOE (mm-dd-yyyy)
No. of Dependents	Text box	txtNoOfDependents

Design a project for this data-entry screen and provide code to ensure that all data entered are valid before the record is saved. The error-checking routine should include at least the following:

- All keys entered should be checked immediately to ensure they are of the proper type. For the employee name, the first letter of each word should be uppercased. Invoke all key error-checking routines from the form's KeyPress event.
- When the user leaves a field, your code should ensure that the field is properly entered. This means:
  - None of the fields should be left blank.
  - S-S-N should have nine digits entered by the user.
  - Employee name should have a comma separating the last name and first name.
  - Dates entered must be valid.
  - If the number of dependents is "excessive," your code should verify with the user before accepting the number.
- The company has a policy not to hire anybody younger than 18 years old. The dates entered should be cross-checked to "enforce" this policy.
- When the user "finishes" the screen by clicking the "Save" button, all fields should be checked for validity again. If everything is checked to be valid, your program

should display "Data Saved" without actually saving the data. Then, the screen should be cleared.

10-26. Protecting Against Disk-Handling Errors. Modify the error-handling routine in Section 10.5 so that all potential disk errors are properly handled. For example, disk full or bad sectors should be detected. Your program not only should inform the user of the problem and suggest remedial action(s) (e.g., inform the user to insert another diskette) but also should provide a choice to quit when the user opts to do so.

10-27. Visual Feedback. Refer to Exercise 9-34. The project computes the probability of good output units in a two-process production setting, using the Monte Carlo simulation technique. Set the number of experiments to 100,000. This will take a "long time" to complete the simulation. Implement the following visual feedback for the project:

1. Change the mouse pointer's appearance at the beginning of the simulation.
2. Use a label to indicate that the simulation is in progress.
3. Use a progress bar and a label to indicate the percentage of computations completed as the simulation progresses.

Projects

10-28. Refer to Project 3-30 in Chapter 3. Complete the following additional requirements for the project:

1. Allow the user to use the Enter key to move to the next control.
2. Allow the user to use the up- and down-arrow keys to move up and down through the controls on the form.
3. Allow the masked edit boxes and text boxes to auto tab to the next control when all required keys in the field have been entered. (Note that masked edit boxes have the AutoTab property. Setting this property to True will enable the auto tabbing without any code.)
4. Set up the access keys so that the user can "jump" among different controls in the form using the keyboard.
5. Provide code to check for all controls in the form such that when a wrong key is pressed in a control, a message is displayed and the key is suppressed.
6. Provide code to perform the field level checks for the following fields:

Field	Type of Errors to Check
Place of Birth	No blank space
Date of Birth	Valid date; respondent at least 18 years old
Number of Children	Valid range is between 0 and 9; prompt for Confirmation if greater than 9

7. When the user clicks the Save button, all three fields presented in item 6 should be checked to ensure validity. (*Hint:* This is the screen-level data validation.)

10-29. Refer to Project 3-31 in Chapter 3. Complete the following additional requirements for the project:

1-5. Replicate requirements 1 through 5 as listed in 10-28.

6. Provide code to perform the field level checks for the following fields:

Field	Type of Errors to Check
Name	No black space
Date of Birth	If entered, valid date and older than 18

Field	Type of Errors to Check
Address	No blank space
Date Dues Paid	Valid date; no older than 5 years; not a future date

7. When the user clicks the Save button, all the four fields presented in item 6 should be checked to ensure validity.

10-30. Refer to Project 3-32 in Chapter 3. Complete the following additional requirements for the project:

1-5. Replicate requirements 1 through 5 as listed in 10-28.

6. Provide code to handle the SSTab such that when a tab is clicked, the first control in the tab receives the focus.
7. Provide code to perform the field level checks for the following fields:

Field	Type of Errors to Check
Name	No black space
Insured's Address	No blank space
City	No blank
State	No blank
Zip Code	No blank
Date of Birth	Valid date and older than 18
Sex	Must select one

8. When the user clicks the Save button, all the fields in item 7 should be checked to ensure validity.

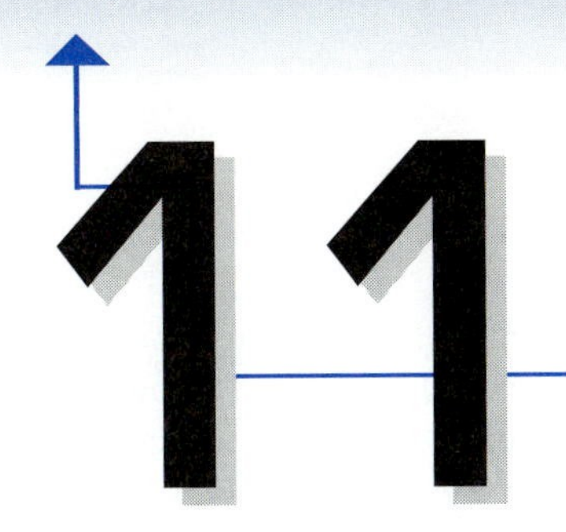

11 Menus and Multiple-Form Applications

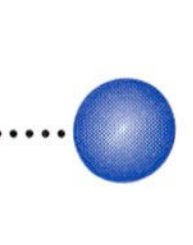

The previous chapters focused on projects involving only one form. This chapter deals with topics related to large projects. In large projects:

- Many forms are used.
- Because many program functions (capabilities) must be provided, menus are used in place of command buttons.
- Many similar activities/functions will be called for in different forms. Thus, there are plenty of opportunities to reduce redundant code. This requires careful analysis and design of the project.

The purpose of this chapter is to present techniques to handle all these aspects.

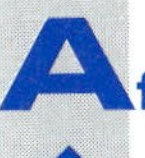

After completing this chapter, you should be able to:

- Create menus.
- Follow proper guidelines in creating menus.
- Add forms to a project.
- Designate a startup object for the project.
- Start, hide, or unload a form.
- Ensure that all forms in the project are unloaded when the project ends.
- Design and implement ways to share data among forms.
- Create and code MDI applications.
- Appreciate and observe design principles for large projects.

11.1 The Menu Control

When your application needs to provide many capabilities from which the user can choose to perform, it will not be practical to use command buttons to trigger these functions. The buttons can clutter the form quickly, making the form(s) look messy, thus making it difficult for the user to locate the needed function/button. In such cases, the menu will be a good alternative.

Creating a Menu

You have seen menus in action in various Windows applications. The VB IDE that you have been working with has a menu bar on which many menus are presented. You can create a similar menu bar and menus in your applications by using the menu editor in the IDE.

Design Considerations. Before you start to create menus for your application, you should carefully analyze your application to identify all capabilities it needs to provide. Each capability/function that the user can select to perform will typically become an option in one of the menus. You will then decide how these capabilities should be grouped. There can be various ways to group them. The most important consideration should be how *logical* (natural) the menus appear to the user. Another consideration is *consistency* with all other Windows applications.

To illustrate, consider a receivable application system for a family clinic. The application is used to keep track of patients' visits and the resulting fees. In most cases, the patients are insured. An insurance company pays the major portion of the fees, and the patient is responsible for a fixed co-pay amount. To obtain payments from the insurance company, the clinic needs to file an insurance claim form for each patient visit, which requires various types of information concerning the patient, the insured, the diagnosis, and the treatment. In many cases, the person who is actually responsible for the "account" (payment) is not the patient but somebody else (e.g., the patient's parent, who is the insured). Thus, the application system must maintain records concerning not only the visits but also all data pertinent to the patients, accounts, insurance companies, as well as the relationships among these "entities." In addition, to support the recording of patient visits, the application system needs to maintain code tables for diagnoses as well as treatments (services provided).

The maintenance of records for all the aforementioned activities and entities requires the following:

- Screens (forms) for data-entry operations
- Reports of various activities (patient visits and payments as well as insurance remittance) for review and verification
- Screens to view activities and entities in files
- Claim forms for fee reimbursement
- Other utility functions for file maintenance operations and system customizations

How should all these functions be grouped for menus? Programmers tend to group functions by their program types; for example, report-generating procedures are grouped together under the menu Reports. However, this approach of grouping may not be most intuitive to the user, who tends to think along the line of business activities. For example, the user most likely would rather see all the software capabilities related to insurance grouped under the menu Insurance. This menu can include procedures and forms that perform maintenance of insurance company information, list insurance companies, print claim forms, as well as generate reports for all outstanding claims.

When designing menus for an application, keep in mind that you develop the application for the user to use. Only those applications that fit the user's needs and meet his or her application requirements are used and considered successful.

Along the line of designing a menu system that appears "natural" (intuitive) to the user, you should also consider its consistency with other applications. For example, most users are likely to be well acquainted with the word processing software as well as other Windows applications.

These applications have the familiar File, Edit, and Help menus. Thus, as long as your application needs to provide similar functions, they should be incorporated in a similar manner. This will alleviate the user's needs to learn to navigate around your software system.

When designing a menu structure, group menu items by their intuitive appeal to the user first. This usually means a menu structure should resemble the grouping of business activities, instead of program functionality. The user will find such structure much easier to work with.

Using the Menu Editor. Once you have designed the menus for your application, you can use the VB's menu editor to create the menus. To start the menu editor:

1. Make sure that the form or a control on it, not another window (e.g., the code window), has the focus of the IDE.
2. Do one of the following:
   - Click the Menu Editor Icon in the toolbar (Figure 11.1).
   - Click the Tools menu; then select the Menu Editor option.
   - Press Ctrl+E.

Figure 11.1
The Menu Editor Icon

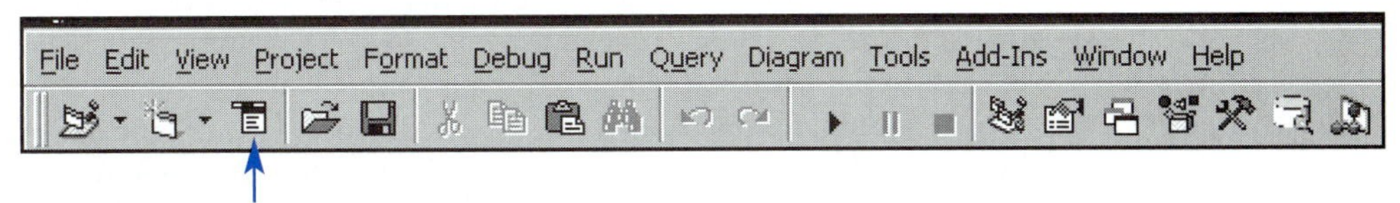

Click the Menu Editor Icon to start the menu editor.

The Menu Editor dialog box will appear as in Figure 11.2.

Figure 11.2
The Menu Editor Dialog Box

Menu Editor

Caption: | OK
Name: | Cancel
Index: | Shortcut: (None)
HelpContextID: 0 | NegotiatePosition: 0 - None
Checked | Enabled | Visible | WindowList
Next | Insert | Delete

The boxes in the upper portion of the dialog box allow you to set various properties for the menu. Let's now take a closer look at each of these boxes.

The ***Caption box*** is used to set the caption of the menu that will appear on the menu bar or as an option in the menu. For example, if you set the caption to "File," then "File" will appear on the menu bar. You can place an ampersand sign ("&") before a letter to make the letter underlined, a recommended design choice. At runtime, the user can access this menu by pressing Alt+<the underlined letter>, which is recognized as the access key of the menu item.

If you have an item that requires the user to provide additional information to complete the operation, observe the guideline that an ellipsis (. . .) follow the text. For example, the typical Open option under the File menu will call for the user to specify the filename. Thus, the caption in the box should be "&Open . . ."

The ***Name box*** is where you specify the name of the menu. This name is like the Name property for any control. In your code, you refer to the menu by this name. If you decide to use a ***menu array*** (which behaves exactly like a control array), you can set the index value in the ***Index box***. *All menu elements in an array must have the same menu name, and their index values must be consecutive, beginning with zero.* Menu arrays, like other control arrays, can diminish your code clarity and add problems to code maintainability. You should use menu arrays only when your code needs the flexibility of an array or when the menu contains items of the same nature. A good example of using the menu array is to show the most recently saved files.

You can select a shortcut key from the ***Shortcut combo box***. If you select one, the user can access this menu item directly by pressing this key (a key with a combination of Ctrl+<the letter selected>) without having to click through various levels of menus.

If you check the ***"Checked" check box*** for a menu item, this item will have a check mark placed in front of its caption during runtime. This Checked property is available at both design time and runtime. Thus, you can use code to show or remove the check mark by assigning True or False to this property.

Note that this property can be set only for options at the lowest level of the menu structure (hierarchy). For example, suppose the Player menu of a game program consists of two options: (1) human to play first and (2) computer to play first. You will be able to check either of these two options. However, you cannot check the Player menu itself because this item is not the lowest level in the menu hierarchy.

The Enabled and Visible properties are the familiar properties that you have worked with many times. Setting the Enabled property to False will disable the menu. You disable a menu item when it is incompatible with the current operating environment. Setting the Visible property to False will make the menu item disappear from the menu (or menu bar). This is typically done for a pop-up menu to be discussed later.

The left- and right-arrow buttons in the midleft section of the menu editor allow you to control the level of menus. When you start to construct a menu (e.g., File), it begins with the top level. Those menu options under this menu (e.g., New, Open) will be the second level. To add items at this level while you are at the top level, click the right-arrow button. When you are ready to go back to the previous level, click the left-arrow button.

The up- and down-arrow buttons move a menu item in the menu list up or down by one position; that is, the button makes the current menu item exchange the position with the one above or one below. The Next button moves the focus to (highlights) the next menu item. The Insert button inserts a new menu item in the menu list, and the Delete button deletes the current item from the menu list. Finally, the list box at the bottom lists all existing menu items that you have created. You can actually see the list building up while you are adding more items to the menu list.

Creating a File Menu Step by Step. To illustrate how the menu editor works, suppose you need to create a File menu that consists of four options: New, Open, Close, and Exit. You will do the following:

1. Start the menu editor. Press Ctrl+E. Again, recall that the menu editor can be activated only when the form or a control on it has the focus of the IDE.

2. Enter "&File" in the Caption box. This will make File" appear as the menu in the menu bar. (Notice that the first letter in File, F, is underlined.)
3. Enter mnuFile in the Name box. The MS menu naming guide suggests that menu names start with the prefix "mnu" as a part of the object-naming convention. Once you enter the name, you have created the File menu item. All other properties for the menu item can take their default settings.
4. Click the Next button to go to the next menu item.
5. Click the right-arrow button to move to the lower level of menus. This will allow us to create New, Open, etc., at the next level of menu items (as menu options).
6. Enter "&New" in the Caption box and mnuFileNew in the Name box to create the New option. The MS menu naming guide suggests that a lower-level item include the name of its upper level as a part of its name. Thus, you name the New item in the File menu mnuFileNew.
7. Click the Next button.
8. In a similar fashion, you can create menu items for Open, Close, and Exit. Make sure that the caption for Open is entered as "&Open..." to indicate that this item requires the user input. (Note the ellipsis at the end.)
9. Click the OK button to exit the menu editor when all items are entered properly.

Adding a Separator Line. You should be able to see File appear in the menu bar of your form. If you click the menu, you should be able to see all the menu options (New, Open, and so on) in the drop-down menu list. Examine the menu list carefully. You may wish to add a line (separator) between Exit and all other items above it because this item and others appear to logically belong to different categories. You can create a separator in the menu list by entering a dash (-) in the Caption box in place of any regular text and giving a name as if it were a menu item. To insert a separator line, you can do the following:

1. Start the menu editor again.
2. Click E&xit in the list box at the bottom (assuming E&xit is what you have entered).
3. Click the Insert button. This will insert a menu item before Exit.
4. Enter a dash (-) in the Caption box and mnuFileLine1 in the Name box.
5. Click the OK button to exit.

Figure 11.3 gives the resulting menu after adding the separator line.

Figure 11.3
Menu Items in the Menu Editor List Box and in the Form

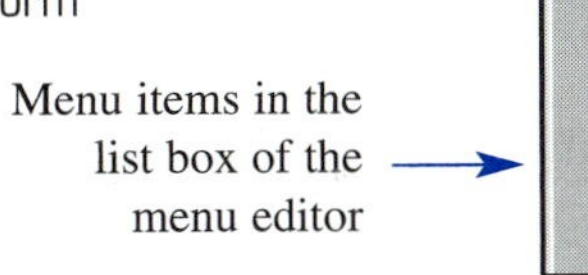

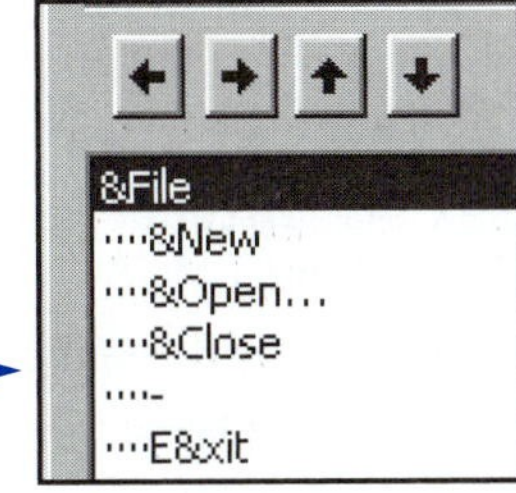

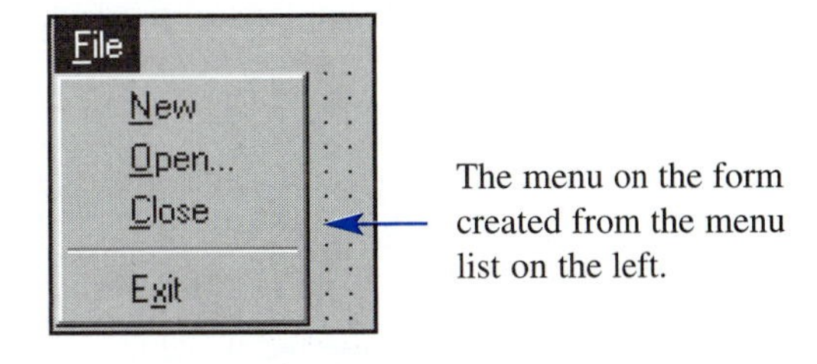

Adding New Menu Items in the Menu Bar. When you are ready to add another menu to the menu bar (i.e., create another top-level menu), you will need to use the menu editor again. You will then do the following:

1. Click the last item in the list box (in this case, E&xit again).
2. Click the Next button to move to the next item.
3. Click the left-arrow button so that the menu level is moved up by one level.

Once you are there, you will enter the new menu in exactly the same manner as you did to create the File menu.

Pop-Up Menus

In some cases, you may find that some menus do not belong to the menu bar. They should be available only in certain situations. Because these menus appear only under certain contexts, they are recognized as context menus. They should be constructed as pop-up menus.

You can create pop-up menus in the same way as you create a regular menu; that is, you create the top-level menus with their lower-level menu options by following exactly the same steps. (Note that *a pop-up menu must have at least two levels of menus.*) Pop-up menus are included in the same menu list as the regular menus. (There is no separate menu list in the form for pop-up menus.) Because these pop-up menus usually do not belong to the menu bar, you should check off its Visible property so that they will not appear in the menu bar. Then at runtime, you use the ***PopupMenu method*** to activate the menu of interest. The PopupMenu method has the following syntax:

```
[Object.]PopupMenu menuname [, flags][, x] [, y] _
    [, boldcommand]
```

where *Object* = the name of the form in which the menu is to appear; if omitted (usually is), the current form is the default

Menu name = the name of the menu to pop up

Flags = a number that specifies how the menu should be aligned with a specific point in the form and how the menu should respond to clicks (The named constants for alignment are vbPopupMenuLeftAlign, vbPopupMenuCenterAlign, and vbPopupMenuRightAlign. The named constants for click response are vbPopupMenuLeftButton [menu item will respond to a left button click] and vbPopupMenuRightButton [menu will respond to both left and right button clicks].)

x, y = the position at which the menu is to appear; if omitted, the menu will appear at the position at which the mouse click occurs; the alignment with this position depends on the constant you specify for alignment as previously indicated

Boldcommand = the menu item to appear in boldface font

Usually, pop-up menus appear only when the user clicks the right mouse button on a particular object. The most appropriate event to test for the mouse button to pop up a menu is the ***MouseUp event***. Several events are associated with the mouse actions: MouseDown, Click, Double-click, MouseMove, and MouseUp. The Click and Double-click events do not provide a parameter to test the button. The MouseMove event occurs anytime the mouse moves, even when none of the mouse buttons is pressed. The MouseUp event occurs when the mouse button is released. It represents where the mouse finishes its action and therefore is where the user expects the "action" to take place (a menu to pop up). The MouseUp event has the following header:

```
Private Sub object_MouseUp([Index As Integer,] _
    Button As Integer, Shift As Integer, X As Single, Y As Single)
```

where *object* = form or some applicable controls such as the text box or command button

Index = the Index value of the object in an object array; omitted when the object does not belong to an array

Button = a value indicating the mouse button pressed; the named constants for the buttons are vbLeftButton (1), vbRightButton (2), and vbMiddleButton (4); you can use these constants to test which mouse buttons are pressed

Shift = a value that represents the state of the Shift, Ctrl, and Alt keys; the named constants for these key masks are vbShiftMask (1), vbCtrlMask (2), and vbAltMask (4); you can use these constants to test which shift keys are pressed (Note that these values are different from these keys' key code values.)

x, y = the horizontal and vertical coordinate of the mouse position

Just as an illustration, assume you have created the File menu previously discussed. To see how the PopupMenu method works, you can test the following code:

```
Private Sub Form_MouseUp(Button As Integer, Shift As Integer, _
  X As Single, Y As Single)
    If Button = vbRightButton Then
      PopupMenu mnuFile, vbPopupMenuLeftAlign, , , mnuFileOpen
    End If
End Sub
```

You should be able to observe the following:

- The menu will pop up when you right-click on the form because the code is placed in the form's (not a control's) MouseUp event.
- The menu will not pop up if you start the right-click in an object other than the form (i.e., a control), even if you drag the mouse to the form to release the button.
- The menu will pop up if you start the right-click in the form even if you drag the mouse to a control.
- The menu's left edge will align with the position where you release the mouse button. That position is the default when the (x, y) coordinate is not specified. The alignment is on the left (the default) as specified by the constant vbPopupMenuLeftAlign.
- Using the left mouse button will not cause the menu to pop up because the code tests to ensure that the right button is pressed before displaying the menu.
- The Open menu option will appear in boldface font because it is the one specified in the "bold command" parameter (see Figure 11.4).

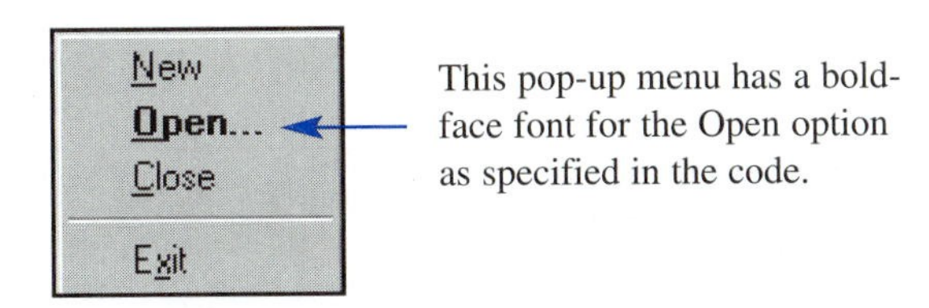
New
Open...
Close
Exit
This pop-up menu has a bold-face font for the Open option as specified in the code.

Figure 11.4
A Sample Pop-Up Menu

Invoking an Action

The menu control has only one event, the Click event, which occurs when one of the following three situations occurs:

- The menu item is clicked.
- The menu's access key (Alt+<the underlined letter in the caption>) is pressed.
- The menu's shortcut key (Ctrl+<letter as specified in its shortcut key property>) is pressed.

Coding the event is the same as coding for the Click event of a command button. For example, the code for the menu mnuFileExit with the caption "Exit" will be as follows:

```
Private Sub mnuFileExit_Click()
    Unload Me
End Sub
```

Levels of Menus

VB allows you to create menus up to four levels. However, keep in mind that as the levels of menu increase, they could become very confusing to the user. When you are designing the menu structure, avoid a design that goes beyond three levels.

Occasionally, a submenu is used for the choice of settings of the operating environment such as the background color or font for an object. In such cases, a custom dialog box (a form created to ascertain specifications from the user) with option buttons and check boxes can be used as a substitute and usually is a better alternative.

11.2 Multiple-Form Applications

In the previous chapters, the projects we worked on were all single-form projects. We ignored the possibility that a project may require more than one form. In most practical applications, however, a project can involve many forms, each performing a special task, such as displaying a report or working as a data-entry screen. This section considers issues related to multiple-form applications.

Adding a Form to a Project

When you start a new standard EXE project, a new form is automatically provided. To add an additional new form to the project:

1. Click the Add Form icon in the toolbar or select the Add Form option in the Project menu. An Add Form dialog box will appear.
2. In the New tab, select Form.
3. Click the Open button or just double-click the Form icon in the tab.

Switching Among Forms and Code Windows. The form that you add to the project most recently is the one that will appear on top in the center of the IDE. The code window (module) will also be associated with this form.

To switch to another form, double-click the form name in the Project Explorer window or click the form name and then click the form icon. To switch to another code window directly, click its form name and then click the View Code icon in the Project Explorer window. You can also use the Window menu to select the desired object (form or code module) from the open object list (see Figure 11.5).

Figure 11.5
Different Ways to Switch Forms or Code Windows

Select the objects in this window and click the icon on the top to make it appear in the IDE window.

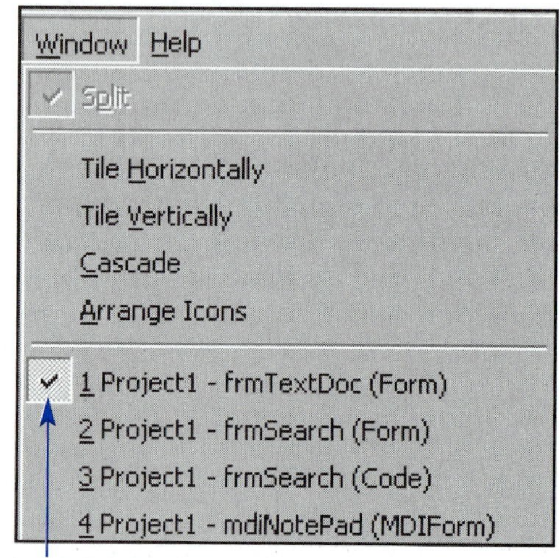

Or, click the object in this list to make it show in the IDE window.

Starting Up and Calling a Form

When your project starts, only one form will automatically start. The default startup form is the first form that you create in the project. To start up with another form in the project, you will need to specify it in the Project Properties dialog box. To start the dialog box:

1. Click the Project menu.
2. Click the Project 1 Properties option (last one in the menu).

The dialog box appears as in Figure 11.6.

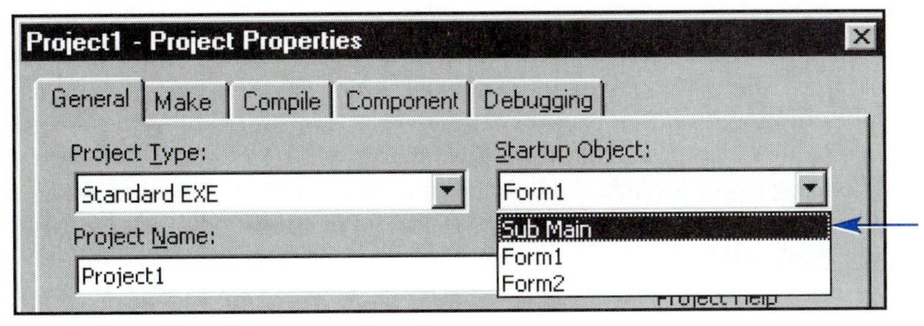

Figure 11.6
Project Properties Dialog Box

You can select the object from this list as the startup object. This list should include all forms in the project plus Sub Main.

You can then click the drop-down arrow on the Startup Object box and select the form. Notice that in the drop-down list, in addition to all the forms you have created, there is also an item called "Sub Main." The use of this procedure is discussed in the subsection "The Standard Module".

The Show Method. If only one form will start up, how do you make the other forms appear? You use the form's ***Show method***. The show method has the following syntax:

```
Object.Show [style] [, ownerform]
```

where *Object* = the form to show

Style = a value indicating whether the form is to be modal or modeless; if omitted, modeless is the default

Owner form = the name of the form that "owns" the form to show (Because the form that "owns" the form to show should be the current form, Me is the name to appear here. This parameter is normally omitted.)

To illustrate, assume that you have created several forms for the Clinic project discussed the preceding section. The first form is named frmClinicMenu, which is the startup form. Another form is named frmAccount to be used for account data entry/edit. In frmClinicMenu, there is a menu item named mnuAccountEdit with the caption "Account entry/edit." Obviously, when the user clicks the Account menu option, he or she expects to see an account form to enter/edit account data. Thus, the code for the Click event of the menu item should appear as follows:

```
Private Sub mnuAccountEdit_Click()
    frmAccount.Show  'display the account form
End Sub
```

The execution of this code will make frmAccount appear. Note that a form needs to be loaded into memory before it can be shown. However, there is no need to explicitly load the form. If a form is not loaded before the Show method is invoked, it will be automatically loaded first.

Modal and Modeless Forms

The preceding code will show the form in ***modeless style***, the default. A form can be displayed in either ***modal*** or ***modeless style***. When displayed as a modeless form, it acts independently of the form that invokes it. All remaining code in the procedure that invokes the form will continue to execute. In addition, the user can change focus among all forms that appear by clicking on the form of interest.

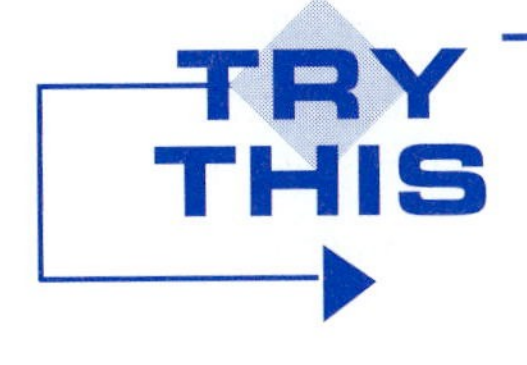

Create two forms in a project. In the first form, draw a command button. Name it cmdShow and set its Caption property to "Show Form 2." Place the following code in the first form:

```
Private Sub cmdShow_Click()
    Form2.Show
    Debug.Print "Form2 has been called."
End Sub
```

continues

Run the project and click the button. You should see that the message appears in the immediate window while the second form appears on top. (The message does not wait until the second form is "finished.")

Click on the first form. It should appear on top again. Click the forms alternatively. Whichever is clicked will appear on top. Click the close (x) button of the first form. The second form does not quit although the first form does. Modeless forms are independent of each other.

Modal Form and Custom Dialog Box. On the other hand, a modal form will stay on top of the current application. No other forms in the same project can get focus until this form is either unloaded or hidden. In addition, the remaining code in the procedure that invokes the modal form will not be executed until the modal form is either unloaded or hidden.

Modal forms are usually used as custom dialog boxes. A ***custom dialog box*** is a form that is designed to solicit special input from the user. For example, in an account data-entry form, the user may have difficulty recalling the account number of an account although the account name is known. In such a case, you may provide a special "lookup" button that the user can click to look for the account number given an account name. When the button is clicked, another form is displayed to help the user search for the account number. The form designed for such purposes is recognized as a custom dialog box (as opposed to the common dialog box, which is provided by VB to help your code obtain certain information commonly required for input/output operations).

Unloading and Hiding Forms

Recall that to unload a form, you use the Unload statement, which has the following syntax:

```
Unload FormName
```

Recall also that if the code to unload the form is in the code module of the same form, the code will appear as follows:

```
Unload Me
```

A form can be unloaded not only by code as just shown but also by the user's clicking the close button on the form's title bar.

Hiding a Form. To hide a form, use the Hide method, which has the following syntax:

```
Object.Hide
```

where *Object* represents the form to hide. Again, if the code is in the code module of the same form, to hide the form, you will code the following:

```
Me.Hide
```

Differences Between Unloading and Hiding a Form. Both unloading and hiding a form will make the form disappear. However, there are several differences between the two actions:

- The visual element of an unloaded form is destroyed. Property settings of the controls in the form are no longer available.
- A hidden form remains in memory. Controls in the form can still be accessed.
- The unloaded form will no longer be in memory, whereas the hidden form will continue to occupy memory.
- It takes longer to show an unloaded form than a hidden form because the unloaded form will have to be loaded into memory first.

The Visual and Code Elements of the Form. At this point, it is important to differentiate the visual element of the form and its code module (window). We have been viewing the visual element and the code of the form as one unit. However, their life cycles are not exactly the same. The following events are associated with the life cycle of the form:

- *Initialize:* This is the earliest event of the form. Only its code module is in the memory. All forms must go through this stage before coming into existence.
- *Load:* This event occurs when the visual element of the form is brought into the memory. A form can be loaded either explicitly by using a Load statement or implicitly by using a reference to the form or a control on the form. Code in the Form Load event will be triggered when the form loads.
- *Unload:* The visual element of the form can be unloaded by using an Unload statement or by clicking the close (x) button in the control box of the form. The visual element is destroyed. All property settings of the controls in the form will no longer be available. However, its code module remains intact; that is, data in public or form-level variables are still available. To destroy the code module (thus, release the resources it uses), you must set the form to Nothing. For example, the following statements will not only unload but also destroy the code module of the form named frmTest (i.e., it will destroy both the visual and code elements):

```
Unload frmTest 'Destroy the visual element
Set frmTest = Nothing 'Destroy the code module
```

- *Terminate:* At this stage, both the visual element and code module of the form are completely destroyed. The system resources previously used by the form are released.

Visual Basic Explorer 11-10 provides a hands-on exercise for you to explore and understand the sequence of form events and the availability of data in the form. A clear understanding of the form's life cycle enables you to know what data are available at different stages so that you can design code that performs accurately.

The Form Activate Event. Because it takes time to reload a form, to improve performance, you may find it desirable to hide (instead of unload) a form when it should no longer appear. You can then use the form's Show method to display the form when it is called again. Often, you will find it desirable to reset the state of the form. For example, you may want to set the focus on the first control in the form. Such a state is "automatic" when the form is first loaded. However, when the form is hidden, all the states of the form are kept "as is." Therefore, when it is shown again, the focus may not necessarily be on the first control. To ensure this state, you may want to place code in the Form Activate event. For example, if the form's first control is mskDate, you will code the following:

```
Private Sub Form_Activate()
    mskDate.SetFocus
End Sub
```

The ***Form Activate event*** occurs when the form becomes the active window. Thus, when you use the Show method to display the form, the Form Activate event will ensue. However, each time the form is activated, this event occurs; that is, it can occur many times in the duration of the form's life. (In contrast, the Form Load event occurs only when the form is being loaded; i.e., it occurs only once in the form's life cycle.)

You should also be aware that the Activate event can also occur in various contexts. For example, unloading/hiding another form currently on top of it or user actions such as clicking on it will activate the form, thus causing the event to be raised.

To illustrate the effect, consider a multiple-form application in which a data-entry form contains several fields for a payroll data-entry application. The first field is the date field (named mskDate); the second field is the employee ID field (named txtEmployeeNo). On the side of this second field is a "Search" command button (named cmdSearch) that the user can click to invoke another form (a custom dialog box named frmFindID) to find the employee ID given to an employee name. For simplicity, assume that this dialog box will always be hidden when the user clicks the Done button after the employee ID is found. The control to hold the result is named txtEmployeeNo (see Figure 11.7). The code in the data-entry form may appear as follows:

```
Private Sub Form_Activate()
' This form will be hidden later.
' To ensure the focus is set to the first control in the form
' when the form reactivates, I code:
    mskDate.SetFocus
End Sub

Private Sub cmdSearch_Click()
' If the user wants to use the dialog box to find the employee
' ID, he or she will click the command button, cmdSearch.
' Display the dialog box as modal so that the next two statements
' will be executed only after the dialog box disappear
    frmFindID.Show vbModal
' Assuming the dialog box is hidden, I can still get the content
' of the control in it
    txtEmployeeNo.Text = frmFindID.txtEmployeeNo.Text
    txtEmployeeNo.SetFocus  'Set the focus on the ID field
End Sub
```

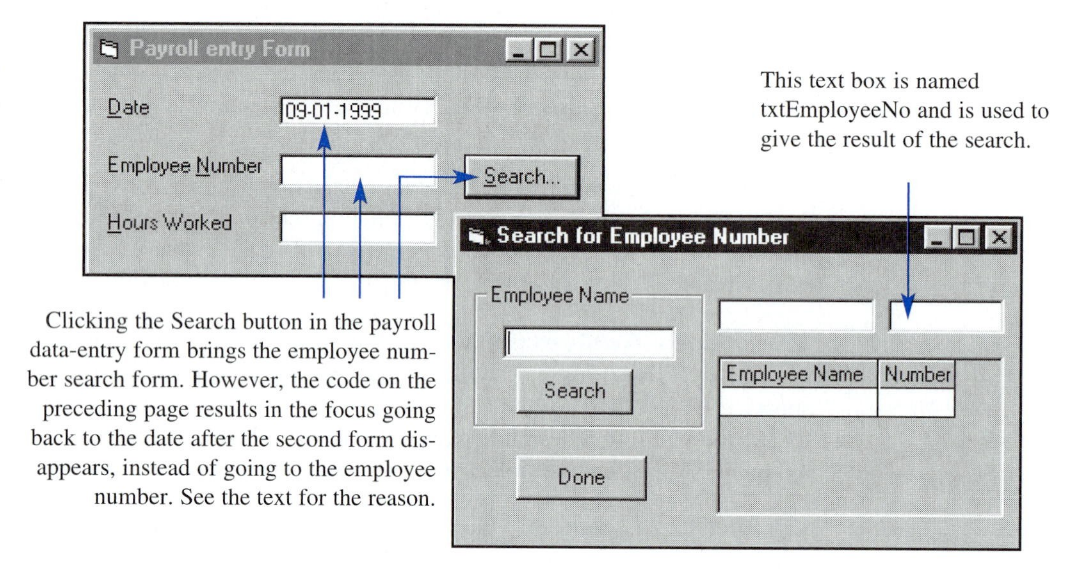
Payroll entry Form
Date
09-01-1999
Employee Number
Hours Worked
Search...
This text box is named txtEmployeeNo and is used to give the result of the search.
Search for Employee Number
Employee Name
Search
Done
Employee Name
Number
Clicking the Search button in the payroll data-entry form brings the employee number search form. However, the code on the preceding page results in the focus going back to the date after the second form disappears, instead of going to the employee number. See the text for the reason.

Figure 11.7 User Interface for a Payroll Application

After the user clicks the Search command button, finds the employee ID with the dialog box, and quits from it, which control in the data-entry form will get the focus? By inspecting the code in the command's Click event procedure, we will expect txtEmployeeNo will get the focus. Not exactly! The masked edit gets the focus. How does this happen? Here is the sequence of events after the user clicks the Search command button:

1. frmFindID is called. The focus is shifted to the custom dialog box (frmFindID).
2. After finding the employee ID, the user clicks the Done button in the dialog box, causing it to hide.
3. The next two statements in the Click event procedure are executed.
4. The data-entry form is reactivated because it lost the focus to the dialog box and it regains the focus when the dialog box is hidden. Thus, the Form Activate event is raised.
5. The data-entry Form Activate event procedure is executed, causing the focus to be set on mskDate.

To test the effect of the preceding code, follow these steps to design the visual interface:

1. Start a new project. There should be only one form in the project.
2. Name the form frmPayrollEntry. Set its Caption property to "Payroll Entry Form."

3. Draw three labels, one masked edit box, two text boxes, and a command button on the form. Take care of their sizes and locations as shown in the Payroll Entry Form in Figure 11.7.
4. Set the captions for the labels and the command button as shown in the visual interface. Notice that each caption has an underlined letter. Place an "&" before that letter as a practice to set up the access keys.
5. Name the masked edit box mskDate; the first text box, txtEmployeeNo; the second text box, txtHoursWorked; and the command button, cmdSearch.
6. Add the preceding two event procedures to the form: Form Active and cmdSearch Click.
7. Add a new form to the project. Click the Add Form icon in the toolbar. Then click the Open button in the Add Form dialog box.
8. Name the new form frmFindId. Set its Caption property to "Search for Employee Number."
9. Draw a text box on the form. Name it txtEmployeeNo. (See Figure 11.7 for its location.)
10. Draw a command button on the form. Set its Caption property to "Done" and name it cmdDone. Add the following event procedure:

```
Private Sub cmdDone_Click()
     Me.Hide
End Sub
```

11. You can add all other controls on the form. However, they are not needed to test the preceding code.

Run the project. To see the effect:

1. Click the Search button. The second form (frmFindID) should appear on top.
2. Enter a number in txtEmployeeNo to imitate the search result.
3. Click the Done button.
4. Inspect the result on the first form. You should see the "found" employee number in the employee number text box. However, the blinking cursor appears in the masked edit box, not in the employ number box as explained previously.

Avoiding Unexpected Execution of the Activate Event. The preceding result is unexpected. If you have to use the Form Activate event to handle specific situations, you will need to design code to avoid this unexpected consequence. One way is to use a form-level variable to indicate the state of the form and to allow the code in the Form Activate event to execute only when the state is "right." In the preceding example, you want the Activate event procedure in frmPayrollEntry to execute only when the form gets reactivated from the "hidden" state. Assume the code to hide the form is placed in the Quit button (cmdQuit). Your code scheme in the "Payroll Entry Form" to avoid the unexpected result can be as follows:

```
Option Explicit
' Declare a form level variable to indicate hiding state
Dim Hiding As Boolean
Private Sub cmdQuit_Click()
    Hiding = True ' I'm hiding now
    Me.Hide
End Sub
Private Sub Form_Activate()
    If Hiding Then
    ' I'm getting activated from a hiding state
        mskDate.SetFocus 'Set focus to the first control
        Hiding = False 'Now I'm activated.
        'Turn the indicator off.
    End If
End Sub
```

Notice that the preceding code assumes that frmPayrollEntry is invoked by yet another form. To test it, do the following:

1. Modify the code in the Form Activate event procedure in frmPayrollEntry as indicated.
2. Add a command button to the form. Set the button's Caption property to "Quit" and name it cmdQuit. Add the cmdQuit Click procedure as shown previously.
3. Add a new form to the project. Name the form frmPayrollMenu.
4. Create a menu with the caption "Activities" and name it mnuActivities.
5. Create an option under the Activities menu. Name the option mnuActivitiesEntry and set its Caption property to "Payroll Entry."
6. Enter the following code:

```
Private Sub mnuActvitiesEntry_Click()
    frmPayrollEntry.Show
End Sub
```

7. Make frmPyarollMenu the startup object. The steps have been outlined in the subsection "Starting Up and Calling a Form."

You may still want to wait until you read "Ending a Project" (which follows) and add another event procedure in frmPayrollMenu before testing the project.

Ending a Project. In Chapter 2, "Introduction to Visual Basic Programming," there was a brief discussion about how to end a project. It was suggested that the Unload statement be used instead of using the End statement. The End statement unloads all forms for the project. No events such as Unload or QueryUnload will be raised when the End statement is executed. The project terminates immediately. This can cause problems. For example, there may be still open forms with unsaved data. Because the Unload and QueryUnload events will not be raised, there will be no way to warn the user or to save the data. On the other hand, the Unload statement will not cause this problem.

However, unloading the startup form does not automatically unload other forms, whether they are shown or hidden. These forms continue to use computer resources and can cause memory leaks (a term used to describe a situation in which memory is being occupied by some objects that are doing nothing meaningful, while the occupied memory cannot be used for any other useful purposes). To ensure that all forms in the project are unloaded when the main (startup) form unloads, there should be a routine in the QueryUnload or Unload event procedure to enumerate and unload these forms. The procedure can appear as follows:

```
' Place this procedure in the startup form
Private Sub Form_QueryUnload(Cancel As Integer, _
    UnloadMode As Integer)
Dim Frm As Form
    For Each Frm In Forms
        Unload Frm
        Set Frm = Nothing
    Next Frm
End Sub
```

The code uses the For Each loop to enumerate through all forms in the Forms collection that are still being loaded (either shown or hidden). It then unloads the form identified. In addition, it uses the Set statement to destroy the code in the form. This will completely clear the form and its code module from the memory. One of the Visual Basic Explorer exercises at the end of this chapter provides a hands-on illustration of the differences of the End statement and the Unload statement in their behavior.

The QueryUnload and Unload Events. While a form is being unloaded, its QueryUnload and then Unload events will be raised. In the startup form, either of these events can be used to unload all forms that are still loaded. Either of these events can also be used by all forms to check for unsaved data or other conditions that need to be taken care of before the form unloads. The differences between QueryUnload and Unload events include the following:

- The QueryUnload event is raised before the Unload event.
- Both provide a Cancel parameter, which can be used to cancel the unloading operation by setting it to a nonzero value. However, as discussed in Chapter 10, "Special Topics in Data Entry," the QueryUnload event procedure provides an additional parameter, UnloadMode, which allows your code to identify the cause of the unloading.

If you still want to use the End statement to terminate a project, be sure that the statement is placed only in the startup form. Using this statement in a form other than the startup form can cause your program to crash.

Sharing Data Between Forms

In multiple-form applications, frequently data need to be passed (shared) among forms. Data can be stored in variables or in the properties of VB controls. A control property in one form can be referenced in another form by the syntax:

```
FormName.ControlName.Property
```

Thus, to display the Text property of the text box txtName on the form frmAccount, you can code in another form (e.g., a form to prepare a report) as follows:

```
MsgBox "The account name is " & frmAccount.txtName.Text
```

Declaring Global Variables. Variables in a form declared with a Dim statement cannot be accessed by another form. To make a variable accessible by other forms, you need to declare it with the keyword ***Public*** instead of Dim. For example, to make the variable AccountName in frmAccount available to other forms, you can code in the general declaration section as follows:

```
Option Explicit
Public AccountName As String
```

In other forms, you can refer to this variable by the following syntax:

```
FormName.VariableName
```

Thus, to display the AccountName in frmAccount in another form, you will code the following:

```
MsgBox "The account name in form account is " _
    & frmAccount.AccountName
```

Potential Problems with Accessing Data in a Form Directly. When you refer to data in another form directly as just shown, you should be aware of the following:

- To obtain the correct result at the time the statement is executed (1) the form being referenced must be still in memory (not yet unloaded) if you are referencing the value (setting) of a control property and (2) the code module of the form must be still in memory if you are referencing the value of a public variable. That is, a statement to set the form to Nothing has not yet been executed.
- If the form has already been unloaded, the form will be reloaded when its name is referenced. (There will be no error messages.) The property settings of all controls will be reinitialized; thus, the result may not be as expected. If the form has been

destroyed, the public variables will also have been reinitialized. In both cases, the form may not show, but it will remain in the memory.

Keeping a Form from Unloading. Ensuring that a form remains in memory can become fairly complicated. For example, although you may use the form's Hide method in code to ensure that the form you will make reference to later remains in memory, this may not be enough. The user may use the Close (x) button to unload the form. You can solve this problem by one of the following approaches:

- Set the form's BorderStyle to None. In this case, the form will show no title bar (therefore no control box). The form's appearance may not be exactly what you want. In addition, this does not apply to a form that has a menu bar.
- Set the form's ControlBox property to False. Doing this eliminates the user's flexibility to maximize or minimize the form.
- Place code in the form's QueryUnload event to check whether the user initiates the unloading and, if so, to cancel the operation. This can be done as explained next. However, it takes extra code and effort.

Recall that the QueryUnload event procedure has the following header:

```
Private Sub Form_QueryUnload(Cancel As Integer, _
     UnloadMode As Integer)
```

The first parameter can be used in the code to cancel the unloading operation by assigning a nonzero value to the parameter. The second parameter pertains to the unload mode, which gives the cause of the unload action. This value will be zero (vbFormControlMenu) if the unload is caused by the user's clicking the Close button. Thus, you can check whether this is the case. If so, you can cancel the unload operation but hide the form. The code will appear as follows:

```
Private Sub Form_QueryUnload(Cancel As Integer, _
     UnloadMode As Integer)
     If UnloadMode = vbFormControlMenu Then
     ' The user clicked the close button
          Me.Hide  'hide the form
          Cancel = True  'and cancel the unload operation
     End If
End Sub
```

As you can see, the code is fairly simple. However, you will need to take care of this for every form whose control properties will be accessed by other forms.

There is another way by which data can be shared by all forms. This involves the use of the standard module, which is discussed in the next section.

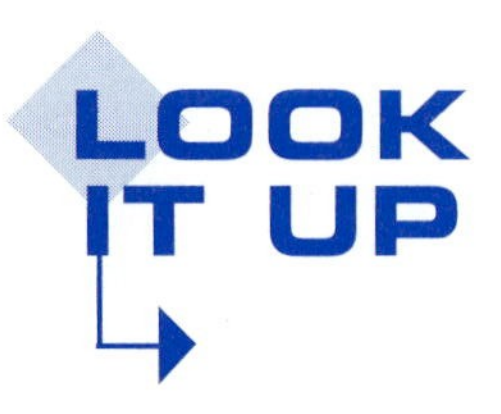

The keyword "QueryUnload event" for visual basic reference in the Index tab of the online Help file provides explanation of the QueryUnload event. Various values for the cause of the UnloadMode are listed and explained.

The Standard Module

The code you place in a form's code window is kept in a ***code module*** recognized as the form module. Form modules are saved with a ".frm" file extension. Other kinds of code modules also exist. The ***class module*** is used to store code for a "class," which is the foundation of objects. The class module is saved with a ".cls" file extension. The use of the class module is discussed in Chapter 12, "Object-Oriented Programming." Finally, the ***standard module*** is used to contain code and data common to other code modules, especially forms. The standard module is saved with a ".bas" file extension.

The standard module contains only code and variables. It has no form or any container in which you may place any control or visible object. However, you can use it to keep procedures and data that are global in nature. These elements can then be accessed by all modules (form, standard, and class modules) in the project. Indeed, if none of the global procedures placed in a standard module make reference to any specific objects in a project, the module can be reused in other projects as well. All you have to do is to add such a module to the project that needs the procedures in it.

Adding Standard Modules to a Project. To add a new standard module to a project:

1. Click the Project menu. Select the Add Module option and the Add Module dialog box will appear.
2. Select the New icon in the New tab. Then click the Open button. (To add an existing module, select the Existing tab. Then browse through the file system to find the module to add.)

The default name for the first new standard module is Module1. You can change its name to a more meaningful one in the same manner as changing a form name; that is, click the module name in the Project Explorer window and then change the Name property in the Properties window.

A project can have as many standard modules as you need. In a very large project, you may find it desirable to include more than one module, each specialized in a particular aspect. Procedures that are useful to all projects should be placed in a module (or modules) separated from procedures that are to be used only by forms in a particular project. Modules arranged in this manner can enhance their reusability.

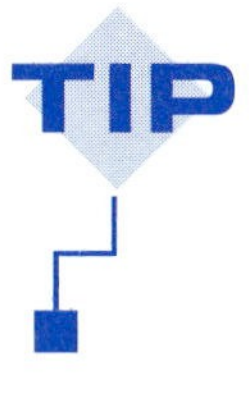

Assign each standard module a unique and meaningful name as you would for a form. Use "mod" as the three-letter prefix for the name of the standard module. This makes it easier to identify the use of the module. When you need to add such a module to another project, you will encounter fewer problems. Standard modules of the same name cannot be included in the same project.

Declaring Variables and Procedures in a Standard Module. You can declare variables and procedures in a standard module in the same way as in a form module. Similar rules for scope and duration apply:

- Variables declared within a procedure are recognized only within the procedure. Variables declared with a Dim statement in the procedure are reinitialized each time the procedure is called. Variables declared with a Static statement retain their values until the project ends.
- Variables declared at the module level with a Dim statement are recognized by all procedures in the module but are not accessible to other forms or modules. These variables retain their values until the project ends.
- Variables declared with a Public statement are recognized by all procedures in the module and are also accessible to other forms or modules. Thus, *Public variables have a global scope*. These variables retain their values until the project ends.
- Public variables can be declared only in the general declaration area. Static variables can be declared only inside a procedure.

Most of these rules are similar to those explained in Chapter 4, "Data, Operations, and Built-In Functions."

Duration of the Standard Module and Form Module. One difference between the standard module and the form is their time duration. The standard module exists throughout the entire life of the project, whereas the form can be unloaded and destroyed before the project ends (or loaded after the project starts). Thus, global and module-level variables in the standard module exist for the entire life of the project, whereas in the form, they exist for the entire life of the form, which can be shorter than the life of the project.

Private Variables. In contrast to the keyword Public, there is also the keyword Private, which can be used to declare module-level (including form-level) variables. Variables declared this way are equivalent to being declared with the Dim statement at the module level.

Public and Private Procedures. The keywords Public and Private are also used to define the scope of Sub and Function procedures. A procedure that begins with the keyword Public is recognizable and accessible to all other modules, whereas a Private procedure is accessible only in the module that contains the procedure. For example, consider the following two procedures:

```
Public Sub FirstProc()
    'Statements
End Sub
Private Sub SecondProc()
    'Statements
End Sub
```

FirstProc can be called from any other modules, but SecondProc can be used only within the module.

Also, a procedure that is not preceded by the Public or Private keyword is a Public procedure by default. These rules of declaration for procedures apply to procedures in forms as well.

Calling Procedures in Another Module. To call a Public procedure in a standard module, the syntax is exactly the same as if the procedure were in the same form (or standard module). Thus, to call FirstProc from a form, you will code the following:

```
FirstProc
```

To call a Public procedure in a form, you must qualify the procedure with the form name. For example, assume in a form named frmAccount, there is a public function ComputeBalance, which requires an account number as its parameter and returns a value as the account balance. To use the function from another module (form or standard module), you can code the following:

```
AccountBalance = frmAccount.ComputeBalance(AccountNumber)
```

Of course, here we assume that AccountBalance and AccountNumber have been properly declared and that AccountNumber has been assigned a proper value.

Another Way to Share Variables Among Modules. We have mentioned potential problems with accessing data in a form directly because of the possibility that the form is destroyed or unloaded prematurely. One possible solution is to use a standard module in which you can place all variables to be shared by various forms. The form that provides the value can then assign it to the variable in the standard module. Once this is done, whether this form is unloaded or destroyed is no longer a concern. All other forms or modules can access the value simply by referencing the variable in the standard module.

In our previous example, various forms need to access the Text property of txtName in the form frmAccount. To use the standard module as the bridge to keep the data, you can first add a declaration in the module as follows:

```
Public AccountName As String
```

Then in frmAccount, you can assign the value as follows:

```
AccountName = txtName.Text
```

From then on, in all other forms or modules, you can use the value regardless of the state of frmAccount. Your code in these modules can appear as follows:

```
MsgBox "Account name is " & AccountName
```

Notice that the (standard) module name does not need to be referenced. The variable name alone is sufficient in most cases.

Variables and Procedures in Multiple Modules. As noted, you can have more than one standard module in a project. Can you then declare the same Public variable (and procedure) names in these modules? Yes. If you declare the same Public variable (procedure) name in two standard modules, this name actually represents two different variables (or procedures) in the two modules. To refer to each variable or procedure, you will need to qualify the variable name with the module name. For example, suppose the variable name AccountName is declared as Public in two modules: modAccounts and modInsurance. To refer to that variable in modAccounts from another module, you will need to code the following:

```
modAccounts.AccountName
```

Thus, the syntax in referring to these variables/procedures is the same as that for those Public variable/procedure names declared in a form. If you fail to qualify the variable name with the module name when the former appears in more than one module, you will encounter an "ambiguous name detected" error message, as shown in Figure 11.8.

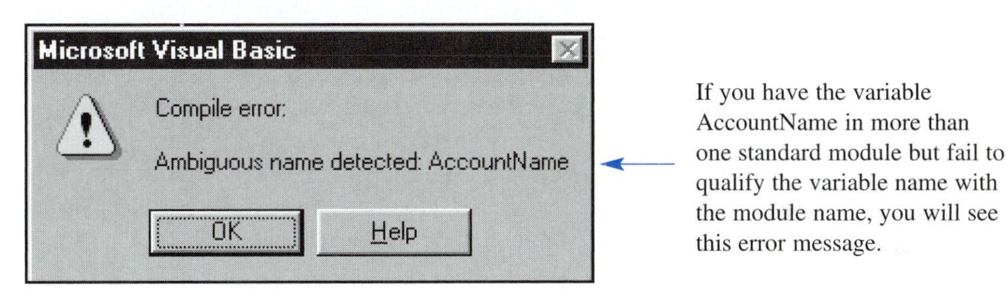
Microsoft Visual Basic
Compile error:
Ambiguous name detected: AccountName
OK
Help
If you have the variable AccountName in more than one standard module but fail to qualify the variable name with the module name, you will see this error message.

Figure 11.8
"Ambiguous Name Detected" Error Message

Using Sub Main as the Startup Object. The standard module can also contain a special procedure, ***Sub Main***. This procedure can then be designated as the startup object in place of a form. Usually, this is done when the main form will take a long time to load. To alleviate the user's anxiety while waiting for the program to start, the Sub Main procedure is started first. This procedure then displays another form while loading the main form. The first form, recognized as the "splash form," usually displays a logo of the software product for a few seconds and then disappears. By this time, the main form is loaded into memory and is then shown. You have seen such an arrangement in action: VB6 starts with a splash form before its IDE appears on the screen to work with you.

The code in Sub Main can appear as follows:

```
Public Sub Main
Dim TimeToEnd As Date
' Invoke the splash form
    frmLogo.Show
' Set Ending time (4 seconds from now)
    TimeToEnd = DateAdd("s", 4, Now)
' Load the main form. (Assume the name is: frmAppMainMenu)
    Load frmAppMainMenu
' Wait until time is up
    Do Until Now >= TimeToEnd
        DoEvents 'Release time to the system
    Loop
```

```
    ' Unload the splash form
        Unload frmLogo
        Set frmLogo = Nothing
    ' Display the main form
        FrmAppMainMenu.Show
End Sub
```

Notice the loop where the wait is. The loop will ensure that at least 4 seconds has elapsed before dropping the execution control down to the next statement. A DoEvents statement is placed inside the loop to release the time to the Windows operating system to handle various activities while your program is waiting. This is not only desirable but also necessary and important in this case. If the execution control is not released, your program will be busy doing nothing but looping, while nothing else in the system, including loading the main form, is taking place. This would have defeated the main purpose of using the splash form.

Again, the Sub Main procedure should be placed in a standard module. There can be only one Sub Main procedure in a project. You will still need to designate it as the startup object for it to perform as expected.

A Multiple-Form Example

To illustrate how to code an application with multiple forms, let's consider an example. This project involves a number guessing game. When the project starts, the program displays an instruction explaining how to play the game and instructs the game player (user) to enter his or her name and click the Ready button to proceed (to go on to the next form).

The second form has two command buttons: "Play a Game" and "Quit." When the first button is clicked, a label and a text box are enabled. In addition, a number in the range of 1 to 1,000 is selected at random, which will be the number for the player to guess. The label instructs the player to enter a number in the text box and press the Enter key when complete. The program then checks whether the entered number is equal to the selected random number. If so, it displays the message "That's right!" with the player's name and informs the player of the number of times he or she tried and for how long before the correct number was obtained. If the guessed number is not equal to the random number selected, a label below the text box gives a hint indicating whether the actual number is higher or lower.

Designing the Interface. The two forms of this project appear as in Figure 11.9. The following table explains the names and purposes of the forms and controls.

Object	In Form	Name	Purpose
Form		frmGuess	The startup form; contains the game instructions
Text box	frmGuess	txtPlayer	To obtain the player's name
Command button		cmdReady	To invoke the game form frmGame
Command button		cmdQuit	To end the project
Form		frmGame	The actual game form
Command button	frmGame	cmdGame	To start a new game
Text box		txtNumber	For the player to enter a guessed number (*Note:* Also set its Enabled property to False.)
Label		lblGuess	The label for txtNumber (*Note:* Also set its Enabled property False.)
Label		lblHint	To display a hint telling whether the actual number is higher or lower than the guessed one
Command button		cmdBye	To make the frmGame disappear (Focus goes back to the main form)

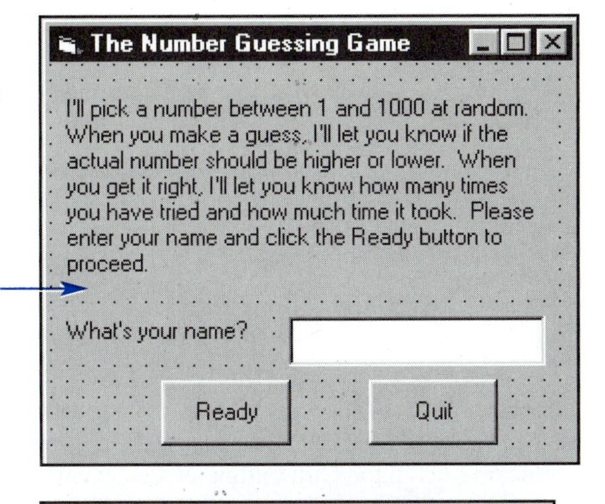

Figure 11.9
Visual Interface of The Number Guessing Game

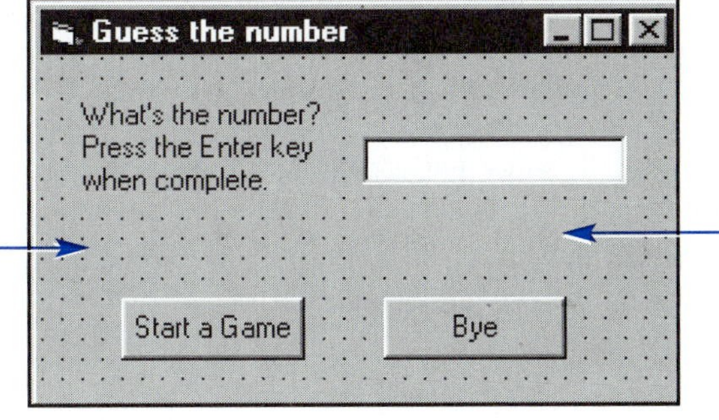

Coding the Project. Let's look at what *should* happen in the startup form. As you would expect, when the project starts, the startup form should appear and wait for the player to enter his or her name and click the Ready button. The Click event procedure should do the following:

1. Check to ensure the name is entered.
2. Show the second form (frmGame) if the name is present.

Thus, the procedure should appear as follows:

```
Private Sub cmdReady_Click()
    If Len(Trim$(txtPlayer.Text)) = 0 Then
    ' No name is entered, display a message.
        MsgBox "Please enter your name to proceed."
    ' Set focus on the text box
        txtPlayer.SetFocus
        Exit Sub
    End If
' Display the number guessing form
    frmGame.Show
End Sub
```

Notice that the game form frmGame is invoked from the main form's cmdReady Click event procedure with the following statement:

```
frmGame.Show
```

At the end of the game, when the user clicks the Quit button in the main form, the program should unload. Thus, the following familiar code should appear as follows:

```
Private Sub cmdQuit_Click()
    Unload Me
End Sub
```

Ensuring All Forms Are Unloaded. In addition to the preceding code, in a multiple-form application, you should take care to *ensure that all remaining forms are unloaded when the main (startup) form unloads*. Therefore, the following code should also appear:

```
Private Sub Form_QueryUnload(Cancel As Integer, _
  UnloadMode As Integer)
Dim Frm As Form
    For Each Frm In Forms
        Unload Frm
        Set Frm = Nothing  'Destroy the code module, too.
    Next Frm
End Sub
```

Notice that the routine to unload all forms is placed in the QueryUnload (or Unload) event, not in the Quit button's Click event. The code in the QueryUnload event is executed either when the code initiates the unloading (as in the Quit button's Click event) or when the user clicks the Close button in the control box. In contrast, the code in the Quit button's Click event is executed only when the user clicks that button.

Because there is only one other form in the project, why use a loop? Can't we just unload the other (game) form? Yes, you can. However, when you decide to have more forms in the project in the future, you will need to revise the code, requiring additional maintenance care and effort. On the other hand, the code using the loop is highly reusable and so general that there will be no maintenance problem in the future. Again, all three preceding event procedures should be placed in the first form's (frmGuess') code module.

Starting the Game. Now, let's look at the procedures in the second form, frmGame. The text box (txtNumber) to enter the guessed number and its label (lblGuess) should be disabled at design time so that the player cannot enter the number before the program is ready for a game (i.e., the number to be guessed needs to be set first.) So, when the "Start a Game" button is clicked, the preceding two controls are enabled with the following statements:

```
txtNumber.Enabled = True
lblGuess.Enabled = True
```

A random number in the range of 1 to 1,000 should be picked and kept in the variable TheNumber. The statement should appear as follows:

```
' Pick a random number between 1 and 1000
TheNumber = Int(Rnd * 1000) + 1
```

Also, the text box is cleared and the focus is set on it, ready for the user to guess the number:

```
txtNumber.Text = ""
txtNumber.SetFocus
```

Finally, the start time should be "recorded" using the timer function for later computation of time used:

```
StartTime = Timer 'Start counting elapse time
```

Because both the start time and the random number are to be shared by other procedures, they should be declared at the form level. The complete procedure appears as follows:

```
Option Explicit
Dim TheNumber As Integer
Dim StartTime As Single

Private Sub cmdGame_Click()
    Randomize  ' Use a new seed for the random number series
    ' Enable the text box for guessing
    txtNumber.Enabled = True
    lblGuess.Enabled = True
    ' Pick a random number between 1 and 1000
    TheNumber = Int(Rnd * 1000) + 1
    txtNumber.Text = ""
```

```
    txtNumber.SetFocus
    StartTime = Timer 'Start counting elapse time
End Sub
```

Responding to an Entered Number. The player is instructed to press the Enter key after entering a number in the text box (see the interface design). Therefore, the code to check whether the number entered is correct is placed in the text box's KeyPress event. The procedure will be executed only when the Enter key is pressed.

The entered number should be compared with the number to be guessed (TheNumber). If the two match, a "That's right!" message (along with the player's name) is displayed. The count for the number of trials is reset, and another game can be played. Otherwise, the program shows a hint (either "Higher" or "Lower") depending on the comparison. The code appears as follows:

```
Private Sub txtNumber_KeyPress(KeyAscii As Integer)
Static Count As Integer
Dim TheAnswer As Integer
' This procedure compares the answer entered with TheNumber
' Perform this routine only when the Enter key is pressed
    If KeyAscii <> vbKeyReturn Then Exit Sub
    KeyAscii = 0 'Suppress the Enter key
    Count = Count + 1
    TheAnswer = Val(txtNumber.Text)
    If TheNumber = TheAnswer Then
        lblHint.Caption = ""   ' The answer is right.
                               ' Clear the hint.
        MsgBox "That's right! " & frmGuess.txtPlayer.Text & _
          vbCrLf & "It takes you " & Count & " trials " & _
          vbCrLf & " for " & Timer - StartTime & "seconds " & _
          vbCrLf & " to get the correct number."
        Count = 0  'Clear the counter
        cmdGame_Click ' Start another game
    ElseIf TheNumber < TheAnswer Then
        lblHint.Caption = "Lower"
    Else
        lblHint.Caption = "Higher"
    End If
' Highlight the previously entered number
    txtNumber.SelStart = 0
    txtNumber.SelLength = Len(txtNumber.Text)
End Sub
```

The meaning of the code should be apparent. Pay particular attention to the way the player's name in the previous form is referenced in the first line of the MsgBox statement. The control's name is qualified by the form name (with a dot). Thus, the text property of that text box is coded as follows:

```
frmGuess.txtPlayer.Text
```

Quitting the frmGame Form. When the player clicks the Bye button, the form should unload. Thus, the familiar code appears again:

```
Private Sub cmdBye_Click()
    Unload Me
End Sub
```

Again, Why Was the QueryUnload Event Procedure Used? Recall that in the first (startup) form, there is code in the QueryUnload event that ensures that all forms in the project are unloaded. However, if this second form is unloaded by code already and the player's clicking the Close button in the control box will also unload it, why is there a need for the code in that QueryUnload event?

Recall that forms that are not invoked as modal work independently of each other. The user can switch between the two forms at will by clicking on the desired form. Thus, the player can set focus on the startup form (and then click the Quit or Close button) while the game form continues to appear. This can cause some problems. Recall also that when a form's name is referenced in some other module, the form will automatically be loaded, although not shown. The form's existence in the system will never be observable and can cause memory leak. This can happen in our example if the first form is allowed to unload without unloading the second form (the first form's txtPlayer is referenced in the second form).

In a more complex project, the possibility of loading a form "unintentionally" can be very high. The code in the QueryUnload event of the startup form ensures that all forms are unloaded and that their code modules are destroyed, whether the forms appear or not.

Should the code in the cmdBye Click event also include the following statement?

```
frmGuess.Show
```

There is no need. The existing code structure ensures that the startup form must exist if the game form exists. The startup form will automatically get the focus when the user quits the game form.

11.3 MDI Applications

In the preceding section, the forms used in a project have no parent-child relationship with each other. Each form presents itself as a "single document"; that is, only one document of a similar nature appears in the project at one time. Applications involving forms of this kind are referred to as ***single document interface (SDI) applications***. Most of the real-world applications are of this type. Some applications involve forms of ***multiple document interface (MDI)***. Several documents of similar nature are loaded in different windows of the same project at the same time. The familiar applications of this kind are word processing and spreadsheet applications. Additional examples of this style of applications include the following:

- Real estate property listing in which several real properties can be shown for review and comparison
- Graphic design in which multiple pictures can be shown for cropping, cutting, pasting, and other drawing/painting operations
- Music composition in which multiple pieces of music can be displayed for the composer to analyze or to cut and paste like in word processing operations

In these applications, multiple "documents" can be loaded. Each document appears on a window (form) and handles different data (document) but behaves in the same manner and shares the same menu bar. All these documents are child forms of the MDI (parent) form. There is a parent-child relationship between these documents and the MDI form.

Differences Between MDI and SDI in Behavior

You can tell whether an application is SDI or MDI by the manner the forms (documents) interact with each other. Here is a selected list of the differences in their behavior and restrictions:

- MDI child forms stay within the boundary of their parent form, whereas SDI forms can appear on any part of the screen, independent of each other's location.
- When the MDI parent form is minimized, all child forms are also minimized, whereas minimizing an SDI form does not affect any other forms.
- When an MDI child form is minimized, its icon stays within the boundary of the MDI (parent) form. When an SDI form is minimized, its icon appears on the taskbar of the Windows system.
- There can be only one MDI parent form in a project. However, you can have as many SDI forms as you want in a project.

Creating an MDI Application

To create an MDI application:

1. Add an MDI (parent) form to your project.
2. Indicate the form(s) that will be used as MDI child form.

Here are the steps:

1. To add a new MDI form:
    1.1 Select the Add MDI Form option in the Project menu. The Add MDI dialog box will appear.
    1.2 Select the New tab in the dialog box and click the Open button.

A project can have only one MDI (parent) form. (You will see the Add MDI Form menu option disabled after adding one.)

2. To include a form as an MDI child form, set its MDIChild property to True. If all documents in your application are of the same type (e.g., a word processor works only on the same type of "documents"), you will need only one MDI child form. Multiple copies of the same form can be loaded to handle different documents. The technique to load several copies of the same form is discussed in the next section. However, you can have more than one child form in an MDI project. In this case, each child form should have a different user interface.

Note that the MDI (parent) form can contain only menus, controls with the Align property, and controls that do not appear at runtime (e.g., the timer). Thus, none of the controls typically used for data entry (e.g., the text box, option button, check box) can be placed on such a form. At runtime, the MDI serves as the container of all its child forms.

On the other hand, because an MDI child form is just a form with its MDIChild property set to True, you can treat it exactly like a regular form. However, an MDI child form cannot be shown as a modal form.

11.4 Coding an MDI Project: An Example

To illustrate the special issues involved in an MDI project and how it is put together, let's consider a simplified example. We will create a program that behaves pretty much like the Notepad except that the program will be able to handle multiple documents. Thus, you are creating an MDI project. This will involve the following the major steps:

1. Designing the features of the program
2. Creating the MDI interface
3. Implementing the features

Features of the Project

Here are the list of features/capabilities the project is expect to provide:

- As a Notepad application, the program will mainly work with a text file with a ".txt" extension. It will allow the user to use other file extensions as long as the file itself contains only text.
- When the project starts, no document will be displayed until the user chooses either to create a new document (New) or open an existing document (Open) from a File menu. Thus, there will be only one menu (the File menu) on the menu bar when the program starts or when there is no open document.

- When there is (are) open document(s), two additional menus, Find and Window, will appear. The Find menu enables the user to search for a text with a custom Search dialog box. The Window menu provides options to arrange the documents, such as cascade or tile. In addition, it also provides a list of open documents, of which the user can select one to work on. In addition, the File menu will be expanded to include the Save and Close options.
- When a document is being closed (child form being unloaded), the program will prompt the user whether to save the document if there is any change to the text. When the application (project) is being closed, all open documents will be handled similarly.

Creating the Interface

Let's now consider the details in the user interface.

Forms and Modules. Because the project is an MDI application, we will need to add an MDI form to the project. We will need an MDI child form to handle the text document(s). Also, we will need another form to serve as the Search dialog box. In addition, a standard module will be used to hold various procedures (Subs and Functions) and variables to be shared by the forms in the project. Here are the steps:

1. Add an MDI form to the new project.
   1.1 Select the Add MDI Form option from the Project menu. Then select the New icon in the New tab from the Add MDI Form dialog box. Click the Open button.
   1.2 Name this form mdiNotePad.
   1.3 Set this form as the startup object for this project. Select the Project1 Properties option in the Project menu and change the startup object in the Project Properties dialog box.
2. Add a common dialog box to the MDI form. It will be used to prompt the user for a filename to save or open.
   2.1 Add the common dialog box icon to the project. Click the project menu and select the Components option. Check the item "Microsoft Common Dialog Control 6.0" in the Components dialog box and click the OK button.
   2.2 Double-click the common dialog icon to make it appear on the MDI (parent) form. Change the common dialog box's name to cdlFile.
3. Set the MDIChild property of the first (regular) form to True. You can find and set this property in the form's Properties window, like most of the form's properties. This form will then be used as the document form. Name this form frmTextDoc.
4. Add one additional form. This form will be used as the custom dialog box to perform a text search.
   4.1 Select the Add Form option from the Property menu. Then in the Add Form dialog box, select the Form Icon in the New tab, and click the Open button.
   4.2 Name this form frmSearch. Dialog boxes should stay on top of the application when invoked. Thus, the form will be shown as a modal form. (Do *not* set this form's MDIChild property to True.)
5. Add a standard module.
   5.1 Click the Project menu and select the Add Module option.
   5.2 Select the New tab in the Add Module dialog box and click the Open button.
   5.3 Name the module modMDIProcs.

This module will be used to hold variables and procedures shared by the forms in the project. Several procedures in both the MDI parent and child forms call for the same code. A few variables used in the custom dialog box will also be preserved here so that unloading that form will not cause problems.

Designing the Menu Bar(s). The preceding description of the menu bar sounds more complex than it actually is. In an MDI application, when there is no active child form or when the child form does not have a menu, the menu bar in the MDI form appears. Once the child form is activated, its menu bar will replace the MDI form's; that is, the child form's menu bar does not appear on the form itself but replaces the one on the MDI form. Thus, the previous description simply implies that there should be two menu bars: one on the MDI form and one on the child (document) form; each is described as follows:

- The MDI has one menu, File (named mnuFile), with three options: New, Open, and Exit and are named mnuFileNew, mnuFileOpen, and mnuFileExit. There should be a line (separator) between Open and Exit, as shown in Figure 11.10. (Follow the steps outlined in Section 11.1 to create this menu.)

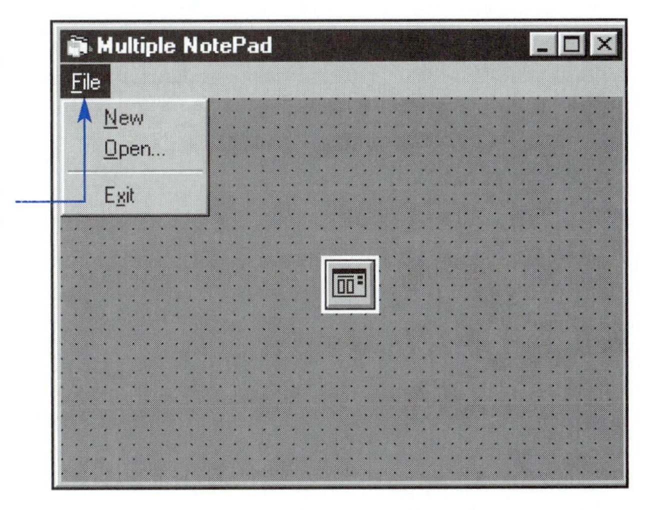

Figure 11.10
Visual Interface for the MDI Form

Here's the MDI (parent) form with a File menu and a common dialog box.

- The child form has three menus: File, Find, and Window. (See Figure 11.11 for the sample interface. Follow the steps outlined in Section 11.1 to create these menus.)
  - The File menu has five options: New, Open, Save, Close, and Exit. Again, there should be a separator between Close and Exit. Name the Save and Close menus mnuFileSave and mnuFileClose, respectively. Give all other items in the File menu the same names as those in the MDI form.
  - The Search menu will have no option. Clicking it will invoke the Text Search dialog box.
  - The Window menu will have two options plus the list of open documents. The two options deal with how the open documents should appear in the MDI parent window. These are Cascade and Tile and should be named mnuWindowCascade and mnuWindowTile, respectively.

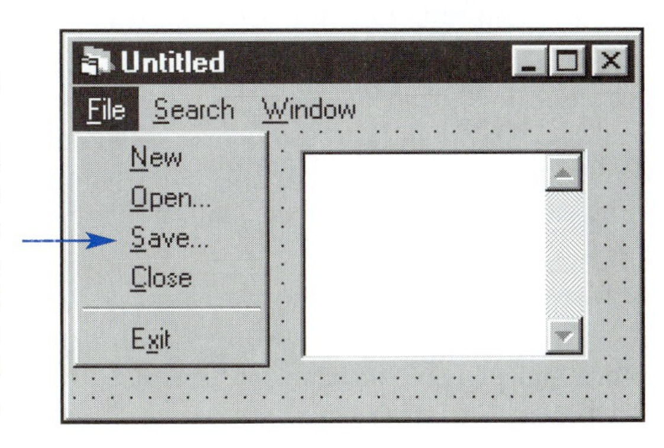

Figure 11.11
Visual Interface for the MDI Child Form

Here is the MDI child form with three menus and a text box. The Window menu has two options (Cascade and Tile) with the Window List check box checked (see Figure 11.12).

Recall that there is a check box in the menu editor Windowlist (see Figure 11.12). This box can be checked only in MDI applications. When it is checked for a menu, the captions of all open documents (windows) will automatically appear as a list in the last part of this menu. The document selected from the list will appear on top in the MDI workspace and become the active window. For our example, check the Windowlist check box for the Window menu.

Figure 11.12
The Window Menu with the WindowList Check Box Checked

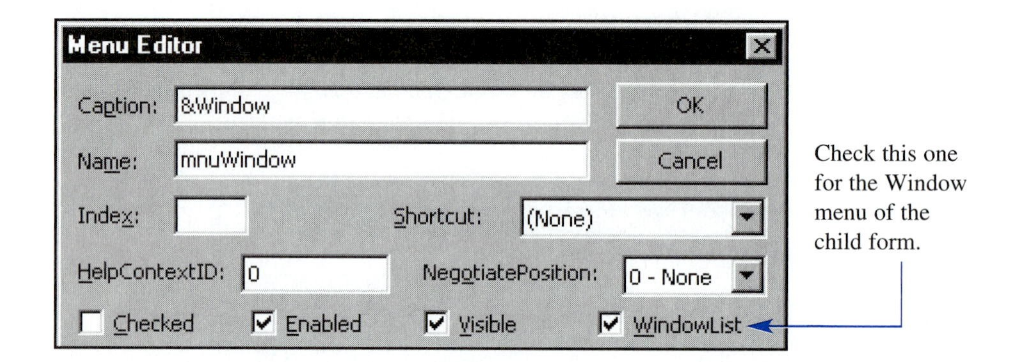

The Document on the Child Form. Because the child form will be used to handle the text document, the control to display the document should be placed in this form. The controls that are suitable for this purpose include the text box and the ***rich text box control***. For our purpose, the familiar text box will be used to display the document.

So, add a text box on the child form. Name the text box txtDocument. Also, set its MultiLine property to True and the ScrollBars property to Vertical. This will enable the text box to display and handle the document properly.

Note that you cannot place the text box on the MDI (parent) form because the former does not have an Align property. Actually, the MDI form can serve only as the container of its child form(s). Multiple copies of the child form can be loaded and displayed within the MDI form to handle different documents. Thus, placing a text box on the MDI form will not make much sense anyway.

The Custom Search Dialog Box. We discuss details of this form in the subsection "Building the Find Dialog Box."

Coding the Project

Now, we have three forms and a standard module to write code. By the sheer number, the project appears pretty complex already. As we start to discuss the code to write, be aware of the specific module in which the code is to be placed.

Handling Events in the MDI Form

Let's consider the code in the MDI form first. This form has three options in the File menu: New, Open, and Exit.

It is fairly straightforward to code the event procedure for Exit. Like the SDI application, the Unload statement should be used. In MDI applications, this statement is even more powerful. When the MDI form unloads, all its child forms will also unload without any additional code. Those Unload and QueryUnload events for the MDI form as well as the child forms will all be raised. Thus, the mnuFileExit Click event procedure will contain the familiar unload statement as follows:

```
Private mnuFileExit_Click()
    Unload Me
End Sub
```

Should there be any code in the QueryUnload event? The major concern when unloading the main (startup) form of the project is to ensure that all other forms will also unload. Because the child forms will automatically be unloaded, there is no need to worry about them. However, there is also a custom dialog box (frmSearch), which is not an MDI child form. Is there a possibility that this form remains loaded in memory? This is discussed in the subsection "Building the Find Dialog Box."

The New and Open Menu Options. Both the New and Open menu options also appear in the child form. The code for each respective menu option will be the same. Thus, rather than providing the specific code for these menu options in the MDI form, we should place the code as Subs in the standard module. The menu's Click event procedure will simply call the proper Sub in the standard module. Therefore, the code appears as follows:

```
Private Sub mnuFileNew_Click()
    OpenNewDoc
End Sub
Private Sub mnuFileOpen_Click()
    OpenExistingDoc
End Sub
```

Coding the Procedures in the Standard Module

Let's consider the procedures in the standard module called from the MDI form. The OpenNewDoc Sub should do the following:

- Load a new child form and display it as a new window in the MDI form.
- Make the child form's title bar display "Untitled1," "Untitled2," and so on.

Loading a New Child Form. To load and display a new form:

1. Declare a form object variable.
2. Associate this variable with a new form using the Set statement.
3. Use this variable to reference the new form to perform required actions.

To declare a form object, code the following:

```
Dim frmDocument as Form
```

The variable frmDocument is declared to be of the (generic) form type. A variable so declared can be associated with any types of forms. Recall that when declaring variables, you can make the code more efficient by declaring the variable type as specific as possible. This form variable will be associated with the form template frmTextDoc (the name for the child form) that you have created at design time. Thus, to make your code more efficient, you can code the following:

```
Dim frmDocument as frmTextDoc
```

In the declaration, frmDocument is a variable, whereas frmTextDoc refers to the form template that you have created at design time.

Once you have the form variable defined, you can create a new form by coding the following:

```
Set frmDocument = New frmTextDoc
```

The Set statement associates the form variable frmDocument with the form object frmTextDoc. Notice the New keyword in the statement. This keyword creates a new object, in this case, a new child form.

To set the form's title bar (caption), code the following:

```
frmDocument.Caption = "Untitled" & Forms.Count
```

Note that there is a ***form collection***, Forms, in the project. Its Count property gives the number of forms loaded in the project. As new forms are created, the count increases. This number is concatenated with the constant literal "Untitled" to form the title in the form's title bar. The complete code to show a new form (document window) appears as follows:

```
Public Sub OpenNewDoc()
Dim frmDocument As frmTextDoc
```

```
        Set frmDocument = New frmTextDoc
        frmDocument.Caption = "Untitled" & Forms.Count
        ' Fill the area in the MDI form with this new form
        frmDocument.WindowState = vbMaximized
        frmDocument.Show  'Display the form
    End Sub
```

As stated, this procedure should be placed in the standard module.

Referencing the Active Form. Each time this procedure is executed, a new form is created. Note that the variable frmDocument is declared within a procedure and thus is recognized only in this procedure. So, how do you refer to the form in other procedures? Recall that there can be several copies of the same form. The child form that is on top is the active form of the MDI (parent) form. Thus, in the standard module, this child form can be referred to as follows:

```
mdiNotePad.ActiveForm
```

In the MDI (parent) form, you can simply refer to it as follows:

```
ActiveForm
```

Loading an Existing Document. Now let's consider the OpenExistingDoc procedure. This procedure is expected to open an existing document. The specific steps should include the following:

1. Open the file for input.
2. Create a new child form.
3. Read the entire file into the text box in the child form.
4. Assign the child form's caption with the filename.
5. Maximize and display the form.
6. Close the file.

The first three steps actually open and display the existing document. The fourth step displays the document name (filename) in the child form's title bar. Steps 5 and 6 take care of additional program details.

To open a file, your program must know the filename, which should be provided by the user. This is commonly done using the common dialog box. Assume a function, GetOpenFileName, for such a purpose is available. Then, the OpenExistingFile procedure can appear as follows:

```
Public Sub OpenExistingDoc()
Dim FileNo As Integer
Dim FileName As String
Dim frmDocument As frmTextDoc
    FileName = GetOpenFileName  'Get the filename to load
    If Len(FileName) > 0 Then
        ' Create a new child form to hold the existing document
        Set frmDocument = New frmTextDoc
        ' Open the text file
        FileNo = FreeFile
        Open FileName For Input As #FileNo
        ' Read the entire file into the text box.
        frmDocument.txtDocument.Text = Input(LOF(FileNo), FileNo)
        ' Assign the filename to the form's caption
        frmDocument.Caption = FileName
        frmDocument.WindowState = vbMaximized   ' Use the entire
                                                ' MDI area
        frmDocument.Show    'Display the document
        Close FileNo 'Close the source document file
    End If
End Sub
```

This procedure calls the function GetOpenFileName to obtain an existing file. The function will return the filename if the user selects one; otherwise, a zero-length string is returned. In the

OpenExistingDoc Sub, the code checks to ensure that a valid filename is returned. If so, it proceeds to perform the remaining tasks as outline.

Obtaining the Filename. Coding for the function GetOpenFileName should be similar to the code example in Chapter 6, "Input, Output, and Procedures" (using the common dialog box), and appears as follows:

```
Public Function GetOpenFileName()
' Ask for a file to open using the common dialog in mdiForm
' Make sure that the cancel error property is set to True.
' Error will be raised if user cancels the dialog.
   Const FileFilter As String = "Text File (*.txt)¦*.txt¦" _
      & "All Files (*.*)¦*.*"
    On Error GoTo DoNothing
    mdiNotePad.cdlFile.Filter = FileFilter
    ' File must exist to be opened.
    mdiNotePad.cdlFile.Flags = cdlOFNFileMustExist
    mdiNotePad.cdlFile.ShowOpen
    GetOpenFileName = mdiNotePad.cdlFile.FileName
DoNothing:
End Function
```

Note how the common dialog box in the MDI (parent) form is referenced in the procedure. A control in an MDI form is referenced in exactly the same way as in any ordinary form. The syntax for referencing a control in a form is explained in the preceding section. The code dealing with the use of the common dialog has been explained in the I/O section of Chapter 6. Note again that both of the preceding procedures should be placed in the standard module.

Handling the Events in the Child Form

Events in the child form can be classified into three major categories:

1. When the form size changes by code or by user actions
2. When the form is unloaded
3. When one of the menu options in the form is clicked

Taking Care of Form Resizing. Let's consider the event of form size change first. Why is this of concern? Recall that a text box is used in the form to display the document. Basically, you would like the text box to occupy the entire available area of the form, regardless of the size (or state) of the form. The user may set the child form to normal, maximized, or minimized. The size of the text box should be adjusted accordingly. We can use the text box's Move method to change its size to the available space of the form. When the form's size changes, its ***Resize event*** is raised. Thus, the code to adjust the size of the text box will appear as follows:

```
Private Sub Form_Resize()
    txtDocument.Move 0, 0, Me.ScaleWidth, Me.ScaleHeight
End Sub
```

Of course, this event procedure should be placed in the child form's (frmTextDoc's) code module.

Unloading the Child Form. The active child form (the one currently on top) will unload when the user clicks the Close button on the child form's control box. It should also be unloaded when the user clicks the Close option in the File menu. To unload the child form in the Close menu Click event, you can use the familiar unload statement as follows:

```
Private Sub mnuFileClose_Click()
    Unload Me
End Sub
```

Safeguarding Unsaved Data. When the child form unloads, your code should prompt the user whether to save changes made to the document, if they occur. The prompt should be coded in the QueryUnload (or Unload) event. But how can you tell if there is any changes made to the document? The document is changed when the content of the text box is changed. When this happens, the text box's Change event is raised. You can create a form-level Boolean variable (e.g., TextChanged) to keep track of the change. If there is a change in the text box, the variable will be set to True. When the document is saved, the variable should be set to False. The code to declare the variable and set it to True can appear as follows:

```
' In the general declaration area
Dim TextChanged As Boolean

Private Sub txtDocument_Change()
    TextChanged = True
End Sub
```

Then in the QueryUnload event, you can code the following:

```
Private Sub Form_QueryUnload(Cancel As Integer, _
    UnloadMode As Integer)
Dim Ans As Integer
    If TextChanged Then
        Ans = MsgBox("Save changes in " & Me.Caption & "?", _
          vbQuestion + vbYesNo)
        If Ans = vbYes Then
            SaveDoc
        End If
    End If
End Sub
```

The code to set the variable to True is placed in the text box's Change event. Admittedly, the Change event will also be raised when an existing document is read into the text box. In this case, the text has not really changed. Therefore, the Boolean variable should not be set to True. The technique to take care of this fine point is left to you as an exercise (see Exercise 11-17).

You may then be wondering why place the code in the Change event instead of KeyPress or KeyDown event. Recall that our goal is to detect any changes in the text box. A key (e.g., Esc key) that triggers the KeyPress and/or the KeyDown event does not necessarily cause a change in the text box. In addition, not all the changes in a text box are done through the keyboard. For example, the user can use the mouse to perform cut, copy, and paste operations. None of these will trigger any keyboard events, whereas the Change event will capture the change.

Note that the variable TextChanged is a form-level (module-level) variable and is associated with the active form. When multiple copies of the child form are loaded, each form will have its own "TextChanged" variable. Each will maintain its own state, independent of each other. All the event procedures starting from the subsection titled "Handling the Events in the Child Form" should be placed in the child form's code module.

Handling the Menu Click Events in the Child Form. The child form has three menus: File, Find, and Window. Events in each menu are discussed next.

Events in the File Menu. The File menu has New, Open, Save, Close, and Exit options. The Click events for the New, Open, and Exit options should be exactly the same as those for the MDI form. All code for these menus must be repeated in this child form. Add the code now if you are following the example. Also, the code for the Close menu has been discussed in the preceding subsection.

How should the Click event for the Save menu option be coded? To be consistent with those events for New and Open options, this event procedure should call a Sub in the standard module to handle the saving of a file. The event procedure can appear as follows:

```
Private Sub mnuFileSave_Click()
    SaveDoc
End Sub
```

The actual code for SaveDoc to be placed in the standard module should resemble its counterpart, OpenExistingDoc, and thus is left to you as an exercise.

The Find menu's Click event should bring up the Search dialog box (form) for the search of a specified text. The form is named frmSearch. Recall that dialog boxes should be displayed as a modal form because it is expected to provide the calling form with data and should remain on top until it disappears (is unloaded or hidden). The code to handle the Click event for the Find menu appears as follows:

```
Private mnuFind_Click()
    frmSearch.Show vbModal ' Call the Find dialog box
End Sub
```

The Window menu has two options: Cascade and Tile, which refer to how the child forms should be arranged in the MDI workspace. Recall that the code in the OpenExistingDoc Sub to create a new child form includes a statement to maximize the child form. This in effect makes the newly created child form occupy the entire workspace of the MDI form. When several documents are open, this Window menu allows the user to choose a different layout of the documents: either cascade or tile. The *MDI form has the **Arrange method***, which can be used to display child forms in several different ways. The Arrange method has the following syntax:

```
Object.Arrange layout
```

where *Object* is a name that represents an MDI form and *Layout* is the arrangement for the child forms in the MDI workspace, such as cascade, title horizontally or vertically, and so on.

The named constant for the cascade arrangement is vbCascade. The documents can be tiled in two ways: horizontally or vertically. Assume the preferred way for arranging the documents is horizontally. The named constant is vbTileHorizontal. Thus, the code to handle the cascade and tile Menu Click event will appear as follows:

```
Private mnuWindowCascade_Click()
    mdiNotePad.Arrange vbCascade
End Sub
Private Sub mnuWindowTile_Click()
    mdiNotePad.Arrange vbTileHorizontal
End Sub
```

All the preceding event procedures should be placed in the child form frmTextDoc.

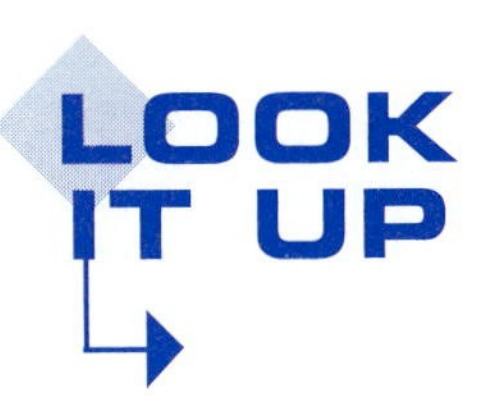

For information about the exact values and their uses of the parameter of the Arrange method for the MDI form, look up the keyword "Arrange method" in the Index tab of the online Help file.

Building the Find Dialog Box

Now let's turn our attention to the form (frmSearch) to be used to find the specified text in the document. Figure 11.13 shows the visual interface of this custom dialog box, which should behave in the following manner:

- When the user enters the search text in the text box and clicks the "Find Next" button, it should find and highlight the text in the document that matches the search text.
- When the user clicks the "Find Next" button another time, it should highlight the next match. When there is no (or no more) text in the document that matches the search text, a message "Text not found" is displayed.
- When the user clicks the Cancel button (or the Close button on the title bar), the form should disappear.
- When the user clicks the Find menu in the MDI child form again, this dialog box (form) will show the previous search text in the text box. This form should also "remember" the position of the text in the document that was previously highlighted so that any repeated search will start from there.

Thus, this form should have the following controls:

- A text box (accompanied by a properly captioned label), which will be used by the user to enter the text to find. Name it txtSearch.
- A command button with the caption "Find Next." The user will click this button when he or she finishes entering the search text and is ready to search. Name this command button cmdFind.
- Another command button with the caption "Cancel." The user will click this button when he or she is done with the search. Name this button cmdCancel.

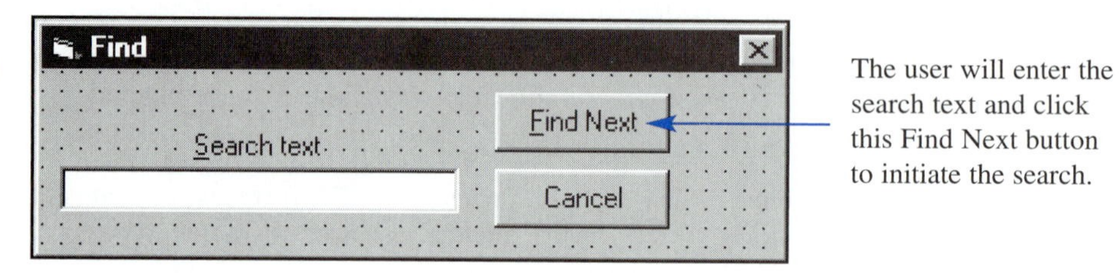

Figure 11.13
The "Find" Custom Dialog Box

The user will enter the search text and click this Find Next button to initiate the search.

Unload or Hide. An important consideration in coding this form is whether it will be unloaded or just hidden when the user clicks the Cancel button. If the form will be hidden, to be consistent (for simplicity of handling the code), we need to ensure that when the user clicks the Close (x) button, the unload operation is canceled and the form is hidden. The code to handle this is illustrated in the preceding section. Then when the project ends (the MDI form is unloaded), the MDI form will need to ensure that this form is also unloaded.

On the other hand, if frmSearch is unloaded when the Cancel button is clicked, there will be no special need to handle its Close button. In addition, because this dialog box is invoked as a modal form, it will remain on top until it is unloaded. Thus, the MDI form will have no need to ensure that this form is unloaded. However, we need to find a way to keep the values of some variables when the form unloads. In particular, two values need to be preserved: the search text and the position at which the search text is last found (highlighted).

Because this form is fairly "light" (with very few controls and little code), there will be no noticeable performance difference between unloading or hiding the form. We will use the unload approach. We can then use this case to illustrate the technique to use the standard module to preserve data. The code for the Cancel command button should appear as follows:

```
Private Sub cmdCancel_Click()
    Unload Me
End Sub
```

Coding for the Find Operation. The "Find Next" event procedure should take care of the following steps/situations:

- It should check to ensure that there is search text in the text box. If there is no search text, the procedure should display the message "Please enter search text" and exit.
- It should also check to see whether the current search is a continuation of a previous search. This can be determined by comparing the current search text with the previous one. If they are the same, it is a continuation and the search should start from the previously highlighted position plus the length of the search text. Otherwise, it is a new search and should start from position one.
- The actual search should use the start position just determined. If no text in the document is found to match the search text, the message "Text not found" should be displayed. Otherwise, the text found in the document should be highlighted. As explained in Chapter 3, "Some Visual Basic Controls and Events," highlighting can be accomplished by setting the text box's SelStart and SelLength properties.
- The preceding search text and the highlighted position should be preserved for the next round. These variables will be preserved in the standard module in which two Public

variables are declared for this purpose: FindCurrText (as string) and FindBegPos (as integer). These two variables can actually be used in the preceding search/find operation without other additional variables as shown in the following code.

So, we will begin by coding the following two lines in the general declaration area of the *standard module*:

```
Public FindCurrText As String
Public FindBegPos As Long
```

The "Find Next" (cmdFind) event procedure (*in frmSearch*) can be coded as follows:

```
Private Sub cmdFind_Click()
Dim SearchText As String
     ' Search text will be held in a variable for ease
     ' and efficiency of code
     SearchText = txtSearch.Text
     If Len(SearchText) = 0 Then
     ' no text to search for
        MsgBox "Please enter search text.", vbInformation
        Exit Sub
     End If
     If UCase$(SearchText) <> UCase$(FindCurrText) Then
     ' Search text has changed.  Start over.
        FindBegPos = 1
        FindCurrText = SearchText
     Else
     ' Continued search. Start from the position after
     ' the current "word"
        FindBegPos = FindBegPos + Len(SearchText)
     End If
     ' Find the next position by using the Instr function
     FindBegPos = InStr(FindBegPos, _
       mdiNotePad.ActiveForm.txtDocument, FindCurrText, _
         vbTextCompare)
' Is the search text found?
     If FindBegPos = 0 Then
        MsgBox "Text not found.", vbInformation
     Else
     ' Highlight the text found.
        mdiNotePad.ActiveForm.txtDocument.SelStart = _
           FindBegPos - 1
        mdiNotePad.ActiveForm.txtDocument.SelLength = _
           Len(FindCurrText)
     End If
End Sub
```

Pay particular attention to the way the text box in the child form is referenced (starting at the second half of the code). In the search/find form, all it knows is that it is dealing with the active child form of the MDI form. There is no particular form (object) variable for the child form for reference. Thus, the child form is referenced as follows:

```
mdiNotePad.ActiveForm
```

The following is how to reference the text box:

```
mdiNotePad.ActiveForm.txtDocument
```

Displaying Previous Search Text. When the search form is unloaded and invoked later, the controls in the form lose their previous contents. The search text box will no longer have the text previously entered by the user. The two variables in the standard module, FindCurrText and FindBegPos, help preserve the values. As soon as the form reloads, the previous search text can be assigned back to the search text box. Thus, in the dialog box form (frmSearch), you can code the following:

```
Private Sub Form_Load()
     txtSearch.Text = FindCurrText
End Sub
```

Highlighting Text in a Text Box Without Focus. If you test the code now, you may find that the text found in the document (child form) is not highlighted. This occurs because the default setting for the HideSelection property of the text box is True, allowing it to highlight only when it has the focus. However, the search form is the object that remains on top and has the focus. To have the text box of the child form highlighted without the focus, set the control's HideSelection property to False.

Notice that the search is not case sensitive. This is accomplished by using the UCase$ function of both the current search text and previous text in their comparison. Also, the last parameter of the Instr function for the search is specified as vbTextCompare, meaning the search will ignore the case.

A Few Design Notes. Usually, a dialog box is used to provide a service/data, as is the case here. As such, it should stop at the point where the data is generated and leave the remaining task of using the data to the calling procedure/form to handle. Such a design will make the code much neater and reusable by other procedures, forms, or even projects. However, the problem at hand, for the dialog box to highlight the text found in the calling form while continuing to stay on top (invoked as a modal form), makes such a design tricky. The code (based on the current design) is also used to illustrate how the child form is referenced in other modules. As such, the code in the dialog box loses its general applicability. It should be considered as a "specialized" dialog box, providing a specific service only to the current project. A possible solution to make this dialog box general is given as an exercise at the end of this chapter.

You may also recall that the function GetOpenFileName in the standard module refers directly to the common dialog box in the MDI form. Again, the purpose of such a design is to show how a control in the form can be referenced. For the function to be reusable, a better design will be to require a common dialog control as a parameter of the function. The refinement is left to you as an exercise.

Summary of Procedures. This example includes three forms and one standard module. The code involves many procedures and a lot of details. The following table provides a summary of the procedures in different modules.

Form/Module	Procedure	Procedure Type	Remark
MDI parent	`mnuFileNew_Click`	Event	Calls OpenNewDoc in the standard module
	`mnuFileOpen_Click`	Event	Calls OpenExistingDoc in the standard module
	`mnuFileExit_Click`	Event	Quits
Standard module	`OpenNewDoc`	General Sub	Creates a new document window (child form) in the MDI form
	`OpenExistingDoc`	General Sub	Reads an existing document into a document window (child form) in the MDI form
	`GetOpenFileName`	General Sub	Uses the common dialog box in the MDI form to prompt the user for a file path
	`SaveDoc`	General Sub	Not shown; for you to add
Child form (frmTxtDoc)	`mnuFileNew_Click`	Event	Calls OpenNewDoc in the standard module
	`mnuFileOpen_Click`	Event	Calls OpenExistingDoc in the standard module
	`mnuFileExit_Click`	Event	Closes a document (child form)

Form/Module	Procedure	Procedure Type	Remark
	mnuFileSave	Event	Calls SaveDoc in the standard module
	mnuFileCose_Click	Event	Unloads the child form
	mnuFind_Click	Event	Calls frmSearch
	mnuWindowCascade_Click	Event	Cascades child forms
	mnuWindowTile_Click	Event	To tile child forms horizontally
	Form_Resize	Event	Adjusts the text box size
	Form_QueryUnload	Event	Prompts to save unsaved data
	txtDocument_Change	Event	Keeps track of text changes
Custom dialog	cmdCancel_Click	Event	Unloads the search form
box (frmSearch)	cmdFind_Click	Event	Searches and highlights text
	Form_Load	Event	Places previous search text in the search text box

Creating MDI Applications: A Recap

The MDI Notepad application involves many programming aspects. The following table summarizes the essentials to the creation of an MDI application.

Objective	What to Do	Remarks
To create an MDI application	Add the MDI form to the project.	You may want to set the startup object to the MDI form. Click the Project menu and select the (Project1) Property option to access the Project Properties dialog box.
To make a form a child window of the MDI application	Set the form's MDIChild property to True.	
To change the menu bar with the presence of a child form	Create menus in both the MDI and child forms.	When the child form is active, its menu replaces the MDI's.
To make a menu show the titles of child forms	Check the WindowList property of the menu in the child form.	

To create a new document (child window)	1. Declare a form variable.
	2. Set the variable to a New child form.
		For example:
		`Dim MyForm as frmTextDoc`
		`Set MyForm = New frmTextDoc`

To open an existing document	1. Perform the two steps to create a new document.
	2. Open the existing file.
	3. Read the file content into the text box in the child form.
		For example, add the following code:
		`Dim ExistingDoc As Integer`
		`ExistingDoc = FreeFile`
		`Open "C:\Temp\Demo.Txt" For _`
		`Input As #ExistingDoc`
		`txtDoc.Text = _`
		`   Input(LOF(ExistingDoc), _`
		`   ExistingDoc)`

To share variables and procedures among forms	Use Public variables and procedures in a standard module.	These elements alleviate the need to consider whether the form is loaded.
To reference a control in the MDI form	Use the following familiar syntax: `MDIForm.Control`	For example: `mdiNotepad.cdlFile.ShowOpen`

Objective	What to Do	Remarks
To reference a control in the active child form	Use the following syntax: `[MDIForm.]ActiveForm.Control`	For example: `Print mdiNotepad. _ ActiveForm.txtDoc.Text` *Note:* In the MDI form, reference to the MDI form name can be omitted.
To cascade or tile child windows	Use the MDI form's Arrange method.	For example: `mdiNotePad.Arrange vbCascade`

Additional Remarks

As you start to review this "notepad" application, you may have realized that MDI is an interface style choice. If the user needs to refer to more than one document in an application that handles only a single document (e.g., the MS Notepad), he or she can load another copy of the application. However, if your application often involves multiple documents, it will be much easier for the user to work with an MDI interface. Your interface style choice should be based on this consideration.

In the preceding section, we noted that a standard module could be used to provide specific services to other forms (e.g., holding Public variables or procedures usable to various forms). In other cases, the procedures in the module can be made reusable if the code makes no specific reference to other modules. Apparently, the standard module in the example project is used for the former purpose and therefore will not be reusable for other projects.

Admittedly, the project is highly simplified. The main purpose is to illustrate the key issues particularly pertaining to an MDI project. Hopefully, by working with the example, you have a good understanding of the use and design of MDI applications.

You can, of course, add several enhancements to the program. For example, you can do the following:

- Add the code to save a document.
- Add the "find and replace" capability to the custom dialog box.
- Include an Edit menu. (Note though that the Edit Context [pop-up] menu is automatically supported by VB for the text box.)
- Show the saved document names (filenames) at the bottom of the File menu.
- Remedy the limitation of the text box, which cannot handle more than 64K bytes of data. Thus, you can either add a routine to reject an "oversized" file or replace the text box with the rich text box (which does not have such a size restriction).

All of these are left to you as an exercise.

VB6 comes with sample code for various applications. One of these pertains to the use of the MDI form for the Notepad application, which is much more complete than our illustration. You may want to study the code there, too. A careful comparison of the code between the two "versions" can yield additional insight.

11.5 Designing a Large Project

As the size of a project grows, various problems and issues that do not seem obvious in a small project will start to surface. In some cases, efforts to "patch" the code can induce even more problems. Most of these problems relate to repetitive code, entangled code, and the "hidden bugs" that appear to be too many to ignore but too undetectable to catch. Thus, in developing a large project, it pays to put in a lot of effort up front by carefully analyzing the requirements and designing the framework before any single line of code is started. The following are a few pointers worth careful consideration.

Modular Design

With the huge size of code, it is easy to get into a situation in which code in different procedures are "entangled"; that is, code in two or more procedures (or modules) may make reference to each other directly. The logic for such code structure becomes difficult to trace. Such code structure can cause great difficulty for maintenance. A minor change in the program requirements can call for a huge amount of maintenance effort.

For example, imagine a form (named frmEmployee) with a text box to enter the employee number. A command button is provided to invoke a custom dialog box (named frmSearchEmpNum), which allows the user to search for the employee number given a name. The dialog box is invoked in a typical manner:

```
Private Sub cmdEmpSearch_Click()
    frmSearchEmpNum.Show vbModal
End Sub
```

However, the Form Unload event procedure in frmSearchEmpNum appears as follows:

```
Private Sub Form_Unload()
    frmEmployee.txtEmpNum.Text = txtEmpNum.Text
End Sub
```

Notice that this event procedure places the employee number in the target text box before the custom dialog box unloads. Such a design can cause several problems. First, if the target text box, for whatever reason, has to change its name or to be moved to another form, the code in the dialog box will have to be changed. Second, the dialog box is extremely "specialized." It can provide service to only one control. If another text box in the same project needs the same service, either another dialog box with nearly the same code will have to be developed or the code in the dialog box must be modified to identify the new target text box, making the code unnecessarily complex. Its maintainability and general applicability become an issue.

When developing code for large projects, be particularly careful in design to ensure that code in each procedure remains independent of each other. As implied in the previous discussion, to accomplish this, you should observe these rules:

- Avoid referencing objects in other forms or modules directly.
- Avoid declaring and sharing variables of a broader scope than necessary. In other words, declare and use variables with a scope as narrow as possible.

Procedures designed this way can then become the building block of a large project. Such a design is recognized as modular design.

Following this design approach, several alternatives to the preceding "problem" example can be considered:

- The dialog box places the result (employee number) in a Public variable either in the form module or in a standard module. The calling procedure can then obtain the result from the Public variable.
- The dialog box hides (instead of unloading) itself after completing the task. The calling procedure can then obtain the result directly from the control in the dialog box that holds the result.
- The dialog box provides a Public procedure (e.g., EmployeeSearch) that takes the target text box in the calling form as the parameter. The result can then be placed in this control. The calling procedure calls EmployeeSearch in the custom dialog box instead of invoking the dialog box itself. Note that because the target control is passed as a parameter, any similar controls can be passed to the procedure in the dialog box. A project at the end of this chapter explores this design alternative.

In any of these design alternatives, any change (to the name of the control that needs the service) in the calling procedure will require no change in the code in the dialog box. In addition, any other text box requiring the same service can conveniently call the same dialog box.

"Factoring" to Minimize Code

Another problem in large projects is the potential of repeated code. Several forms can require the same computations and perform similar activities. Indeed, even in the same form, several procedures can require similar code to perform certain activities. Copying similar code to handle the repetitive needs not only can be boring and time-consuming but also can be error prone. In addition, the sheer number of lines of code can create problems for maintenance. Each time a revision of the repeated code is called for, the same "correction" will have to be done many times, increasing yet another possibility of introducing more errors.

As illustrated in the MDI application example, one way to alleviate this problem is to analyze the program requirements carefully and code the required activities as Public general procedures in a standard module. Any event that needs to handle the activities can then simply call that procedure. The code to open a new document and an existing file serves as a good example.

An important advantage of this "factoring" approach is that if there is any error or required revision of the code, you need to look at only one place for the correction. All procedures that use the function will automatically be corrected. The effort required for the revision is minimized, with much less chance to introduce additional errors.

"Layered" Standard Modules

The concept of modular design and code reusability can be carried out further by using multiple standard modules in a project. Some standard modules can be used to contain code and data that are particularly related to the current project, whereas others can be used to contain procedures that are useful to many projects. Procedures in each type of standard modules can be further classified by their commonality. For example, procedures that deal with files can be placed in one module. Modules of this nature can be added to any project that needs their capabilities.

Object-Oriented Programming

An additional approach to handling a large project is the use of the object-oriented programming technology. An object is a unit of code with data. It presents itself as a single unit (object or entity). A programmer using the object does not need to know anything about its inner working other than its interfaces: properties, methods, and events. A big project that involves a team can be divided into several subprojects (units). These units can then be coded as objects. The project can then be assembled by putting the objects together, allowing all to interact with each other through their defined interfaces. Object-oriented programming is discussed in detail in Chapter 12.

ActiveX Components

Many of the objects created in the development of a project can also be used in many different projects. Conversely, a new project can be developed more easily if it can use many of the existing objects. Thus, in the development of large projects, the reusability of code is an important consideration. When these objects are created and compiled in accordance with the ActiveX specification, these objects are reusable and can be incorporated into a new project easily. The use and creation of ActiveX components are explored in Chapter 14, "Beyond the Core."

Summary

This chapter deals with topics related to large projects, which typically involve the use of menus and many forms. We have considered how to design and create menus as well as how to work with projects with multiple forms (SDI or MDI). We have discussed most of the issues pertaining to MDI projects by working through an MDI Notepad example. Hopefully, such a treatment enables you to see the context of the problems/issues at hand more clearly. It is important that you actually work (not just read) through the examples to gain a good insight. The chapter concludes with some suggestions for handling large projects. Although you may not be working on any large project currently, you should treat all your programming endeavors as "large" and follow these suggestions faithfully. A good habit developed now will pay you big dividends in the future.

Visual Basic Explorer

11-1. Sequence of Mouse Events. Four events can be associated with a mouse click: Click, MouseDown, MouseUp, and MouseMove. However, which event precedes which? Use a debug statement in each of these events for a form to find out; for example, code the Form Click event as follows:

```
Private Sub Form_Click()
    Debug.Print "Form click event is raised."
End Sub
```

(Code similarly for the other event procedures.)

Run the project and move the mouse around while clicking the form. List the events in sequence of their occurrence.

11-2. Who Gets the Mouse Events? In the preceding project, add a text box on a form. Add the four mouse event procedures for the text box and paraphrase the Debug.Print statement; for example, "Text box Click event is raised." Then try the following actions and observe the messages in the immediate window:

1. Press and release the mouse button in the form.
2. Press and release the mouse button in the text box.
3. Press the mouse button in the form and release it in the text box.
4. Press the mouse button in the text box and release it in the form.

11-3. Are Menus Controls? In a new form, set up a File menu with Open, Close, and Exit as its options by following the example in this chapter. Draw a command button. Name it cmdShowControls and set its Caption property to "Show Control Names." Enter the following code:

```
Private Sub cmdShowControls_Click()
Dim Ctrl as Control
    For Each Ctrl In Controls
        Debug.Print Ctrl.Name
    Next Ctrl
End Sub
```

Run the project and click the button. Do the menu names appear in the immediate window? What else do you see?

11-4. Resizable and Nonresizable Forms. The form has a BorderStyle property that may interest you. Run a project with a new form. Can you resize the form by dragging an edge from one of its sides? End the program.

Set the form's BorderStyle property to vbFixedSingle (1). Run the project again. This time, can you resize the form?

The form's BorderStyle can have several other settings. Some of these deal with how the form will (not) appear on the Windows' taskbar. Refer to BorderStyle property in the Index tab of the online Help file for details.

11-5. Is the Minimized Form Idle or Active? Does a minimized form continue to work? To test, draw a text box in a new form. Name the text box txtElapse. Clear its Text property. Enter the following code:

```
Option Explicit
Private Sub Form_Resize()
Dim ComeBackTime As Date
```

```
        If Me.WindowState = vbMinimized Then
            ComeBackTime = _
              DateAdd("s", Val(txtElapse.Text), Now)
            Do Until Now > ComeBackTime
                DoEvents
            Loop
            Me.WindowState = vbNormal
        End If
    End Sub
```

Run the project. Enter a number in the text box. Click the Minimize button on the form's title bar. The form should "come back" in the number of seconds specified in the text box. A minimized form is not really idle, is it?

11-6. Unloading or Ending Multiple Forms. How does Unload differ from End in terminating a project with multiple forms? To test, draw three command buttons on the form. Name them cmdLoad, cmdUnload, and cmdEnd. Set their Caption properties to "Load," "Unload," and "End," respectively. Enter the following code:

```
Option Explicit
Private Sub cmdEnd_Click()
    End
End Sub

Private Sub cmdLoad_Click()
    Form2.Show
End Sub

Private Sub cmdUnload_Click()
    Unload Me
End Sub

Private Sub Form_QueryUnload(Cancel As Integer, _
  UnloadMode As Integer)
Dim Frm As Form
    MsgBox "Unloading form1"
    For Each Frm In Forms
        Unload Frm
        Set Frm = Nothing
    Next Frm
End Sub
```

Now, add another form to the project. Place the following code in this form's code window:

```
Option Explicit
Private Sub Form_QueryUnload(Cancel As Integer, _
    UnloadMode As Integer)
    MsgBox "Unloading form 2"
End Sub
```

Run the project. Click the Load button so that Form2 will show. Click on Form1 so that it will stay on top. Click the End button. Do you see any message? The program terminates abruptly.

Run the project again. Repeat the preceding steps without clicking the End button. Instead, click the Unload button. Do you see any message? Run the project another time. This time, click the Close (x) button instead of the Unload button. Do you see any message?

Both forms' QueryUnload events are raised. You can place code in the form's QueryUnload or Unload event to take care of unfinished business for the form before it unloads. However, the code will be triggered only if your code uses the Unload (not the End) statement to quit.

11-7. What's the Difference: The Startup Form for MDI Applications. Work with a new project. Set the form's MDIChild property to True. Add an MDI form by following the steps explained in the text.

Run the project. What form(s) do you see? End the project.

Select the "Project 1 properties" option in the Project menu. Set the startup object to MDIForm1, instead of Form1. Run the project again. What form(s) do you see this time? This difference is mentioned in the text.

11-8. Are the Child Forms Really Unloaded When the MDI Form Unloads? You know that in an SDI application, when the startup form unloads, the other forms do not automatically unload. However, the text claims that the child forms will unload when the MDI (parent) form unloads. Design a code scheme to verify that. (*Hint:* Set up an MDI application that will allow you to create multiple copies of the child form; e.g., the New option of the File menu. Then place code to display some message in the child form's Unload event. Make sure that the message will allow you to identify which window [child form] is being unloaded. Test the project by clicking the MDI form's Close button while several child forms are open.)

11-9. Form Events and Methods. Some methods of the form cannot be used until the form is "ready." Draw a text box and a command button on a new form. Then enter the following code:

```
Private Sub Form_Load()
    Me.Print "Test"
    Text1.SetFocus
End Sub
```

Run the project. What results do you get?

Reverse the order of the two statements inside the procedure. Run again. Any difference?

Now, insert the following statement before both of the existing ones.

```
Me.Show
```

Run the project again. You should have no problem this time. In general, the form is not displayed until the Form Load event is complete. The Print method and controls' SetFocus method cannot be carried out until the form is shown. You can force the form to show in the Form Load event by using the form's Show method.

11-10. Sequence of Form Events and Availability of Data. This hands-on exercise is designed for you to inspect the life cycle of the form and the timing that controls properties and variables remain available. In a new project, add a new form so that you have two forms. In Form1, draw four command buttons and set their properties as follows:

Name	Caption
cmdShowForm2	Show Form 2
cmdUnloadForm2	Unload Form 2
cmdSetForm2ToNothing	Set Form 2 to Nothing
cmdShowData	Show Data

Then enter the following code (all in Form1):

```
Private Sub cmdShowForm2_Click()
    Form2.Show vbModal
End Sub

Private Sub cmdUnloadForm2_Click()
    Unload Form2
End Sub

Private Sub cmdSetForm2ToNothing_Click()
    Set Form2 = Nothing
End Sub
```

```
Private Sub cmdShowData_Click()
    Debug.Print "List1.Text =" & Form2.List1.Text
    Debug.Print "List1.listindex " & Form2.List1.ListIndex
    Debug.Print "Text =" & Form2.Text
End Sub

Private Sub Form_Initialize()
    Debug.Print "Form 1 is initialized"
End Sub

Private Sub Form_Load()
    Debug.Print "Form 1 is loaded"
End Sub

Private Sub Form_Activate()
    Debug.Print "Form 1 activated."
End Sub

Private Sub Form_Deactivate()
    Debug.Print "Form 1 deactivated."
End Sub

Private Sub Form_Terminate()
    Debug.Print "Form 1 is terminated"
End Sub

Private Sub Form_Unload(Cancel As Integer)
    Debug.Print "Form 1 is unloaded"
    Set Form1 = Nothing
End Sub
```

Note that the first four procedures pertain to the Command Click events, whereas the last six pertain to Form1's life cycle and activation.

In Form2, draw a list box and two command buttons. Set the two command button's properties as follows:

Name	Caption
cmdSetList	Set List
cmdHide	Hide Me

Then enter the following code (all in Form2):

```
Option Explicit
Public Text As String

Private Sub cmdSetList_Click()
Dim I As Integer
    For I = vbKeyA To vbKeyJ
        List1.AddItem Chr$(I)
    Next I
    List1.ListIndex = 0
End Sub

Private Sub List1_Click()
    Text = List1.Text
End Sub

Private Sub cmdHide_Click()
    Me.Hide
End Sub

Private Sub Form_Initialize()
    Debug.Print "Form2 initialized"
End Sub

Private Sub Form_Load()
    Debug.Print "Form 2 loaded"
End Sub

Private Sub Form_Activate()
    Debug.Print "Form 2 activated"
End Sub
```

```
Private Sub Form_Deactivate()
    Debug.Print "Form 2 deactivated"
End Sub
Private Sub Form_Unload(Cancel As Integer)
    Debug.Print "Form 2 unloaded"
End Sub
Private Sub Form_Terminate()
    Debug.Print "Form 2 terminated"
End Sub
```

Run the project. Perform the following and observe the messages displayed in the immediate window. You should be able to draw conclusions concerning when each of the form life cycle events occurs.

1. Click the "Show Form 2" button. What events occurred?
2. Click the "Set List" button on Form 2. Then click one of the items in the list.
3. Click the "Hide Me" button. What events occurred? Notice which form is activated and which is deactivated.
4. Click the "Show Data" button. What are the values for the List1 properties and the text? All data should be present.
5. Click the "Unload Form 2" button. What events are triggered?
6. Click the "Show Data" button again. What are the values for the List1 properties and the variable Text? Are they the same as before the form was unloaded? Does the variable Text still have the same value? Also, is there some event that gets triggered unexpectedly?
7. Click the "Set Form 2 to Nothing" button. What events are triggered?
8. Click the "Show Data" button again. What are the values of the List1 properties and the variable Text? Are there events that are triggered unexpectedly?
9. Click the Close button in Form1. What events do you observe?

When is Form2 actually terminated? It is terminated only after Form 1 is "ready" to unload and terminate, not when the statement to set it to Nothing is executed. We explore more about a form's life in Chapter 12.

Exercises

11-11. Creating Menus for a General Ledger Application. In a new project, create a menu system that has the following:

- On the menu bar, there are two items: File and Maintenance (with both items' first letter underlined.)
- In the File menu, there are four options: New, Open, Close, and Exit, with the N, O, C, and x underlined in each respective item. There should be a separator between Exit and Close.
- In the Maintenance menu, there are three options: Account Classification, Account Entry/Edit, and Statement Format. The letters underlined for the respective items are C, A, and S.
- Add the code so that the program will end when the user clicks the Exit option at runtime.

11-12. Creating a Menu for a Clinic. In a new project, create a menu system that has the following:

- On the menu bar, there are three items: Code Maintenance, Service, and Account/Patient. The first letter of each item is underlined.
- In the Code Maintenance menu, there are three items: Service Code, Diagnosis Code, and Billing Adjustment Code. The first letter of each item should be underlined.

- In the service menu, there are two items: Service and Reports (first letter of each is underlined). There is a line (separator) between the two items. The reports item has three options (third-level menu items): Daily Service by Patient Report (S in Service is underlined; shortcut key is Ctrl+S), Daily Service by Service Code Report (C in code is underlined), and Daily Patient Payment Report (P in payment is underlined; shortcut key is Ctrl+P).
- In the Account/Patient menu, there are two items: Account Entry/Edit and Patient Entry/Edit. The first letter of each item is underlined.

11-13. Creating a Pop-Up Menu for a Clinic. (continued from 11-12.) Add a pop-up menu to the preceding project. Name the menu mnuOther, which should have three options: Doctor, Hospital, and Lab. Follow the menu naming guide for these three items. Make sure that the menu does not show up in the menu bar. The menu should pop up when there is a right-click on the form.

11-14. Centering a Form Being Loaded. Provide the code to center the startup form on the screen as soon as the project starts. (*Hint:* Use the Move method. Both the Screen and Form objects have the Height and Width properties.) Note that the form has a StartUpPosition property that you can set to do the same. Pretend that the property does not exist.

11-15. A Sub Procedure to Center a Form. Write a Sub procedure in a standard module that will center a form that is passed as a parameter to this Sub. List different ways this Sub procedure can be used. (What event procedures can make use of this procedure?)

11-16. An Application with Two Forms. Design a project that does the following:

- As soon as the project starts, a login form appears to solicit a password from the user. The password is "master key." The text that the user enters into the password text box should be masked with "*." The password should not be case sensitive.
- If the password entered by the user is not correct, an error message to that effect should be displayed. Also, if the user fails three times, the program will terminate.
- If the password entered is correct, this password form is unloaded. Another form (the form designed for 11-11) is displayed until the user decides to quit.

11-17. When a Change Is Not Really a Change. Refer to the MDI example in the text. In handling the unloading of the child form, the Boolean variable TextChanged is checked in the form's QueryUnload event to decide whether to save the document. It was noted that the Boolean variable is set to True in the text box's Change event. However, the event is also raised when the code first loads an existing document in the text box. This should not really be considered a change to the text. Design a code scheme such that reading the file into the text box will not cause the Boolean variable to be set to True. (*Hint:* Use another Boolean variable. Set it to True at the point the file is being read. In the text box's Change event, check the value of this variable. If the value is True, set it to False and Exit Sub.)

11-18. An Application with a Sub Main Procedure. Modify Exercise 11-12 by adding the following:

1. Add Sub Main in a standard module that will become the startup object. The Sub Main will display a splash form for 3 seconds and then the menu form, which will serve as the main form from then on.
2. The splash form will display a logo with the title "Clinic Receivable Management System, Version 1." (Hint: Use a picture that will cover the entire form as its background. Select a font of your choice to make the title succinct and neat. Set the form's ControlBox property to False so that it cannot be resized or unloaded by the user.)

3. Add a File menu as the first menu in the menu bar. This menu should have New, Open, Close, and Exit as its menu options. There should be a separator between Exit and Close.
4. The program should terminate when the user clicks the Exit option.

11-19. Saving a Document for an MDI Application. Refer to Exercise 11-17. The SaveDoc Sub was not presented. Add the Sub to the standard module. (*Hint:* To obtain the filename to save, you may want to create a different function or modify the GetOpenFile function. Set the common dialog's flags such that it will warn the user of a potential write-over operation. Also, the ShowSave method, instead of the ShowOpen method, should be used to display the correct prompt.)

11-20. The Find and Replace Dialog Box. Refer to Exercise 11-19. Suppose the Find menu in the child form is revised to include Find and Find & Replace as it menu options. The Find (Search) dialog box has been presented in the example. Add the Find and Replace capability to the project.

Projects

11-21. A Form with a Custom Dialog Box (Sales Application). Refer to 8-18 for the product table of the inventory database. Create another table, Sales, with four columns: OrderID, Date, ProductID, and Quantity Sold. Then design a project for the sales order entry application. The form should have all the four fields (use a masked edit box for Date and text boxes for all other fields) and three command buttons (Save, Search, and Quit).

When the Save button is clicked, data will be saved. The Search button is placed by the ProductID. When it is clicked, a custom dialog box will appear to help the user find the ProductID given a product name. When the Quit button is clicked, the program quits.

The dialog box has a text box for the user to enter a portion of the product name. When the user clicks the Search button by the text box, all products matching the name will appear in a grid (use the HFG), which has two columns: Product Name and Product ID. When the user clicks a row in the grid, the corresponding data will show in the two labels above the grid. When the user clicks the OK button, this dialog box disappears.

The data-entry form should incorporate all error-checking routines necessary to ensure data validity before the record is saved into the Sales table.

11-22. An Application with a Menu Form and Two Additional Forms. (continued from 11-21.) Modify 11-21 in the following manner:

1. The project will start with a menu bar, which appears as follows:

File	Maintenance	Transaction
Open	Product	Sales
Exit	Customer	Purchase

2. The Open option of the File menu will invoke a common dialog box for the user to specify the location of the Inventory database. The Exit option will end the application.
3. The Product option of the Maintenance menu will invoke the form you created for 8-18.
4. The Sales option of the Transaction menu will invoke the form you created for 11-21.
5. When the Customer or Purchase options is clicked, display the message "Sorry! But the application is still under development."

11-23. A Generalized Find Dialog Box: Design for Code Reusability. The Find dialog box in the MDI example makes specific reference to the form and its text box. Such a design makes the dialog box difficult to use by other projects. One way to avoid referring to the calling form is to not call the dialog box directly. The mnuFind Click event procedure in the child form will instead call a Sub (call it FindText) in the dialog box form and pass the text box (the object, not the Text property) to be searched as a parameter. Its header should look like the following:

```
Public Sub FindText(TextBoxFromCaller As TextBox)
```

This Sub then sets this text box to yet another module-level text box variable (call it WorkingTextBox) so that other procedures in this form can refer to it. In addition, the FindText Sub should invoke the dialog box as a modal form. That is:

```
Set WorkingTextBox = TextBoxFromCaller
Me.Show vbModal
```

where WorkingTextBox is declared at the form level as follows:

```
Dim WorkingTextBox as TextBox
```

When the user clicks the "Find Next" button in the dialog box, the event procedure can then work with the variable WorkingTextbox in exactly the same manner as the text box in the MDI child form, performing search and highlighting. Neither the FindText Sub nor the cmdFindNext event procedure in the dialog box makes any direct reference to the MDI child form or the text box therein.

Notice that the FindText Sub does not really perform any "Find Text" but sets the text box to the working text box variable and invokes the form's Show method. However, this Sub is what another developer sees to provide the search text service. Because the dialog box form is named frmSearch and the text box to search on (in the calling form) is named txtDocument, this Sub can be invoked with the following statement:

```
frmSearch.FindText txtDocument
```

Modify the code for the text search functionality in the MDI project by implementing this design.

12 Object-Oriented Programming

You have been working with objects since the first day you worked with VB. Both forms and controls are recognized as objects. You can see them while you are designing your project. Still, there are objects such as Debug, Printer, and ADO that are not visible on your form. All these objects have been defined and provided by others (Microsoft and other software vendors).

In this chapter, we take a different angle. You will learn how to develop your own objects that you and other programmers can use. Before you can do so, you will need to learn terminology associated with objects. Section 12.1 discusses terms that are related to objects. The remaining sections deal with features that you can implement for the objects you develop.

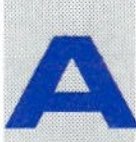

After completing this chapter, you should be able to:

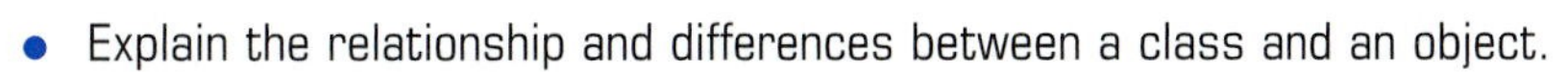

- Explain the relationship and differences between a class and an object.
- Appreciate the advantages of object-oriented programming.
- Develop code to create interfaces (properties, methods, and events) for a class.
- Implement additional features for a class, including enumerated constants, setting initial property values, raising events, and raising errors for improper uses of the object.
- Create and use an object from the class you have developed.
- Treat the form as an element of a class.
- Use the class builder utility to create a class template.

12.1 Classes and Objects

You have seen and worked with objects. An object consists of code and data that work together as a unit. As a programmer who uses objects, you can think of objects as black boxes because we do not know how they work internally. However, as you are aware, they do have defined behaviors. They provide properties and methods that you can use to perform desired activities. They also recognize events to which you can write code in response. These defined features and behaviors are the interfaces of the object and are exposed to its outside world (externally). All other code and data of the object are insulated from other programs (kept internally). This arrangement is recognized as ***encapsulation***.

Object and Class

Objects are derived (or more precisely, instantiated) from classes. A ***class*** is a code template or blueprint that defines the characteristics of an object. Thus, *an object is a special instance of a class*. To differentiate between a class and an object, consider the text box icon in the toolbox and a text box in your form. We know the general features that we can derive from the text box while it is in the toolbox. The appearances and behaviors of the text boxes we draw on a form can be quite different from each other. Each text box on the form is a special instance of the text box in the toolbox. The text box icon in the toolbox is a template and thus a class. On the other hand, a text box in the form is a special instance of the text box class and thus is an object.

In our daily language, we tend not to differentiate an object from a class. For example, we usually refer to an instance of the text box class as a text box, or just the text box, which in turn can really mean the text box class itself. Such references are harmless because a clear differentiation between the two is not really necessary in their context. However, in this chapter, we do need to understand the difference between the two. In Section 12.2, you will learn how to build a class, that is, a template (like the text box icon). You will then create special instances of that class (i.e., objects) that your program can use.

Advantages of Object-Oriented Programming

When you start to build your own classes and use your own objects, your thinking process and the resulting code can be quite different from the programs you write in the "traditional" way. In essence, you will be doing object-oriented programming. That is, instead of attacking the programming problem directly, you will be thinking in terms of building a class to solve a generic class of problems and creating an object from the class to handle the problem at hand. While you are developing the class, you are one step away from a particular programming problem.

Why build classes? Why use objects? Here are the advantages of this programming approach:

- *Encapsulation:* As already explained, each object keeps its own data, free from the interference of any part of the code in a project. Thus, the performance and accuracy of an object is independent of the other code in a project.
- *Code Reusability and Maintainability:* A class/object has well-defined interfaces (properties, methods, and events) and boundaries (encapsulation). You can easily incorporate a new object/class into your project. These interfaces are all you need to know about the class/object to use it properly. In addition, code update and maintenance can be much more convenient. For example, if there is a change in the class/object, the new version can replace the old one easily. When the class/object is provided through a Dynamic Link Library (DLL), replacing the old DLL with the new DLL is all it takes to "update" all the projects using that class. A project that is compiled using objects provided by a DLL does not embed (statically link) the code of these objects but rather just makes references to them. These objects are linked to the project dynamically at runtime. There is no need to tear down or recompile the project.
- *Uniform Data Validation Rules:* An interesting application of objects in business is their representation as a business entity. For example, an object can be used to represent a

student, an employee, or a product. (This appears to be a very different use compared with a text box as an object.) Then all the data associated with such a business object can be coded as the properties of the entity. You can then code all the data validation rules for each property in the object's property procedures (to be explained in Section 12.2). A company can require that all the programs dealing with the "business entity" (object) use that object instead of using their own definition. Imposing such a requirement on all programs will result in uniform data validation rules. The advantages should be obvious: (1) no unexpected exception will occur, and (2) any change of validation rules can be revised in only one location—where the class is defined. This point should become clearer after you complete Section 12.2.

- *Easier Project Management:* A big project can be more easily divided into smaller subprojects defined in terms of objects/classes that can be assigned to project team members. Each member can more easily focus on his or her own assignment because the interactions of his or her products are defined by the interfaces of the objects. These subprojects can then be assembled and tested by focusing on the behaviors of the interfaces.

12.2 Building and Using a Class

So, how do you build a class from which you can create objects? You build a class by writing code in a ***class module***. You can think of a class module as a form without its visual element; that is, a class module behaves like the code window of the form. Multiple copies of the same form can be loaded into the project (as can the class module), each being associated with a specific object.

Differences Between the Class Module and the Standard Module

The class module is also similar to the standard module in that they both can contain only code, with no visual element. However, they are different in several respects:

- Each standard module can have only one copy in a project, and it can contain unrelated data and code (Functions and Sub procedures). On the other hand, each class module can have multiple objects (copies) in the same project, but it should not contain unrelated code or data.
- A standard module exists for as long as the project runs. An object (instance of a class module) exists when it is created but is destroyed when it is out of scope. For example, if an object is created with an object variable in a procedure, the object is destroyed as soon as the procedure ends. In addition, an object can be destroyed by being set to Nothing (e.g., Set ObjVar = Nothing). There is no way to destroy a standard module in a project other than ending the project.
- Public Sub and Function procedures in standard modules are recognized as Subs and Functions accordingly. To invoke a procedure in a standard module, your code makes a reference to the procedure name. However, Public Sub and Function procedures in a class module are methods of the object. They can be accessible only when the object exists. To invoke a method in a class module, your code must qualify the name of the method with the object name (not the classname); that is, the code must have the following syntax:

  ```
  Object.Method
  ```

- Public variables in a standard module are accessible to all other modules in the duration of the project. There is only one copy of the variables in the project. Public variables of a class module are properties of the object; thus they are accessible only when the object exists and must be referenced with the object name as the qualifier. That is, you refer to the Public variables of a class module by the following syntax:

  ```
  Object.Variable
  ```

Note again that the qualifier of the variable is the object name, not the classname. Recall that you code the Text property of a text box named txtEmployee as follows:

txtEmployee.Text

Not

TextBox.Text

Because these public variables are properties of the object, there can be as many copies of these variables as the number of instances (objects) of the class in the project. These copies are independent of each other.

These differences are summarized in the following table.

Difference in	Class Module	Standard Module
Number of copies in a project	Multiple copies of the same module can be loaded.	Only one copy is loaded.
Data and code relationship	All data and code in one module should be related to the same class.	Unrelated code and data can exist in the same module.
Life duration	An object exists when it is created from the class module and disappears when it is destroyed.	A standard module exists throughout the life of the project.
Copies of Public procedures	As many as the number of the objects created from the same module.	Only one copy exists.
Reference to the Public procedures	Object.Method (A Public procedure is a method of an object and can be accessible only when the object exists.)	ProcedureName or ModuleName.ProcedureName.
Copies of Public variables	As many as the number of the objects created from the same module.	Only one copy per project.
Reference to the Public variables	Object.Variable (Public variables are properties of the object and can be accessible only when the object exists.)	VariableName or ModuleName.VariableName.

Adding a Class Module to a Project

To build a class, you need to add a class module to your project. To add a class module:

1. Click the Project menu.
2. Click the Add Class Module option. An Add Class Module dialog box will appear.
3. Make sure that the Class Module in the New tab is highlighted.
4. Click the Open button. A code window with the title "Project1-Class1 [Code]" should appear in place of the form. The Project Explorer window should also show Class1 as a part of its content (see Figure 12.1). (*Note:* In some systems, you may also see an Open Folder icon on top of each object [Class1 and Form1] under Project1.)

Once you have a class module in your project, you can use it to build a class. We show how a fixed asset class can be created and used next. For each class you want to build, you will need a class module. You can include as many class modules as you need in a project.

Figure 12.1
The Project Explorer Window with a Class Module

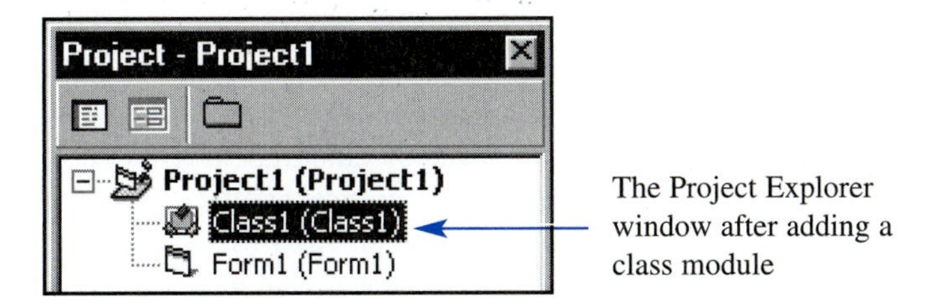

Creating the Fixed Asset Class

To illustrate how a class can be created and used, let's consider the creation of a FixedAsset class step by step. Suppose we would like to create this class with the following interfaces:

- Three properties:
  - Cost
  - Estimated life (in years)
  - The depreciation (accounting) method
- One method: net book value. This method will return the net book value of the fixed asset using the aforementioned three properties and a parameter to be discussed next.

How do you proceed? In general, the major steps are as follows:

1. Add a new class module to a new project. This has been explained in the preceding subsection.
2. Name the class module.
3. Add property procedures to create properties.
4. Add Public Sub and/or Function procedures for methods.

The following discussion assumes that you have added a class module to a new project.

Naming a Class. To create a class called FixedAsset, you will name the newly added class module FixedAsset. Follow these steps:

1. Double-click Class1 in the Project Explorer window (Figure 12.1); the class module code window will appear.
2. The Properties window will show Class1 as the object (Figure 12.2). You can then change the Name property in this window to FixedAsset. There is no difference between changing the name of a class module and that of a control or form.

Figure 12.2
Class1 Properties Window

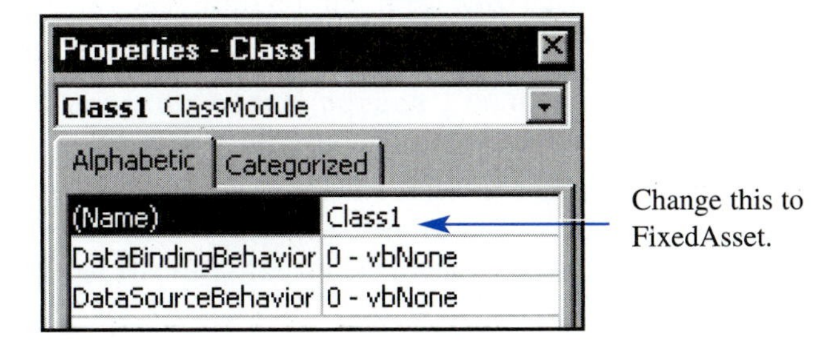

Creating a Property

In the class module, you use the ***Property Let*** and ***Property Get procedures*** to create properties. The Property Let procedure creates a property that allows the programmer to set the value (setting) for the property in another module and has the following syntax:

```
Public Property Let Name(ByVal Parameter As Type)
    'Statements
End Property
```

where *Name* is the name of the property and *Parameter* is the value passed from a calling procedure that sets the property value.

Notice that the Property Let procedure must be a Public (not a Private) procedure because a property must be Public to be recognized by other modules. Notice also that the parameter must be passed ByVal for scalar properties (properties that have only one value). Inside the Property Let procedure, you should assign the parameter to a variable that is private to the class module. You use a Private (instead of Public) variable so that the data passed to the class/object is insulated from other modules. In this way, data can be encapsulated.

In our example, you want the fixed asset class to have a "Cost" property. Thus, in the class module, you code the following:

```
Option Explicit
Private mCost As Double      ' this variable will keep the cost
                             ' property private in this class
    Public Property Let Cost(ByVal pCost As Double)
        mCost = pCost
    End Property
```

Notice the various names associated with "Cost." The name of the Property Let procedure is Cost, which is the name recognized by other modules as the property of any object created from this class module. The value that any other module sets for the object is passed as a parameter named pCost, which is then assigned to mCost, a module-level variable used to store the value of Cost internally for the object. The prefixes *p* and *m* are used to denote parameter and member variables. Notice also that the data type for both pCost and mCost should always be the same.

All Public variables in the class module will be set up as properties by the VB compiler. Thus, declaring Public variables in the class module is a shortcut to creating properties for the class. However, such a practice is not encouraged. In many cases, the property setting should be checked for validity before being accepted from other modules. The "natural" procedure to perform the checking is the Property Let procedure. The shortcut takes away this facility.

Using the Class and the Property. To see the effect of this property procedure, let's go back to the form. (Double-click Form1 in the Project Explorer window.) Draw a command button. Name it cmdCompute and set its Caption property to "Compute." In the button's Click event procedure, code the following:

```
Private Sub cmdCompute_Click()
Dim Land as Object 'Declare an object variable
' Create an instance of FixedAsset and refer to it as Land
    Set Land = New FixedAsset
    Land.Cost = 100000 'Assign value to the Cost property
End Sub
```

The Dim statement declares a variable (Land) of the Object type. The Set statement creates a new object of the FixedAsset class using the New keyword. This new object is referenced as Land. The creation of the Cost property in the FixedAsset class module now allows us to set the Cost property of Land to 100,000.

Notice that Land is declared to be a generic Object type so that you can see it as an object variable. In general, it is more efficient to declare an object variable as specific to the object type as possible; that is, if you know that the variable Land will be used exclusively as an instance of FixedAsset, you can make your code more efficient by declaring the following:

```
Dim Land as FixedAsset
```

Compare the preceding code with what you learned in Chapter 8, "Database and the ActiveX Data Objects," when working with the ADO objects. You should notice that there is no difference between the way you declare and use an object from a class you create for yourself and that from a class provided by others (as in the case of ADO).

Returning the Property Value. The Property Let procedure in the class module allows the code in other modules to set the property value of the object. What do you code to make the object return the value of the same property? For example, we would like in our form to inspect the value of the Cost property by coding the following:

```
MsgBox "Cost of the land is " & Land.Cost
```

What code/procedure do we need to add in the class module to enable this? (*Note:* Go back to the class module. All code from this point on should be placed in the class module.) It is the Property Get procedure. This procedure has the following syntax:

```
Public Property Get Name() As Type
    'Statements for the procedure
End Property
```

where *Name* is the property name. To enable the Cost property to return a value, we can code the following:

```
Public Property Get Cost() As Double
    Cost = mCost 'Return the property setting
End property
```

Note that the property name, Cost, is placed on the left side of the assignment statement so that the property will return a value. This is similar to the way we write code for a function to return a value. Also note that mCost is the Private variable that accepts the value of the same property in the Property Let procedure discussed previously. In addition, because a Property Get procedure returns a value, you will need to declare its data type with the As keyword (just like a Function procedure). The data type declared for the procedure is the same as that for mCost, which should also be of the same type as specified for the parameter in the Property Let procedure (pCost).

Read and Write Capabilities. In general, we say the Property Let procedure enables the code to "write" (set) the value for the property, whereas the Property Get procedure enables the code to "read" (return) the property. If you want to enable both the read and write capabilities for a property, you will need to provide both the Property Get and Property Let procedures. Whichever side of the property procedures you leave out will disable that particular capability; for example, a property without a Property Let procedure will disable its "write" capability and thus become read-only.

The Complete Property Procedures. Now you understand the relationship between the Property Let and Property Get Procedures in the class module and the properties of the class as previously illustrated. You can proceed in the same manner to code all other property procedures for the other properties (life and depreciation method) as initially planned. The complete code for the property procedures of the class module appears as follows:

```
Option Explicit
Private mCost As Double 'Local copy
Private mLife As Double 'Local copy
Private mDepreMethod As Integer 'Local copy
' The Cost property procedures
Public Property Let Cost(ByVal pCost As Double)
    mCost = pCost
End Property
Public Property Get Cost() As Double
    Cost = mCost
End Property
' The Life property procedures
Public Property Let Life(ByVal pLife As Double)
    mLife = pLife
End Property
Public Property Get Life() As Double
    Life = mLife
End Property
```

```
' The DepreMethod property procedures
Public Property Let DepreMethod(ByVal pDepreMethod As Integer)
    mDepreMethod = pDepreMethod
End Property
Public Property Get DepreMethod() As Integer
    DepreMethod = mDepreMethod
End Property
```

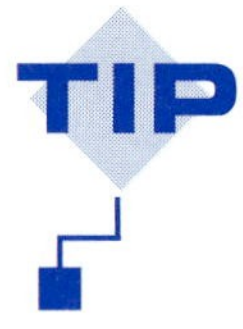

Notice that all the private copies of the Property variables have a prefix m, which is used to denote "member variable." (Some use mvar as the prefix.) The prefix makes it easy to recognize the nature of these variables and makes the code more readable. Follow this practice.

Creating a Method

How do we create a method for a class? The code for a method of an object is no different from a typical general Sub or Function procedure. In fact, you use exactly the same keywords: Sub and Function. To illustrate, we will create the NetBookValue method for the FixedAsset class to compute and return the net book value for the asset. In general, the net book value is computed by the following formula:

Net Book Value = Cost − Accumulated Depreciation

The amount of accumulated depreciation depends on the number of years the asset is in use and the depreciation method. For simplicity, assume the company uses only two accounting depreciation methods: no depreciation (0) and straight-line depreciation (1). The net book value of an asset can be computed as follows:

- If DepreMethod is 0, no depreciation needs to be taken for the asset (e.g., land). The asset's net book value should be the same as its cost.
- If the DepreMethod is 1, the straight-line depreciation is used. The annual depreciation can be computed by the following formula:

Annual Depreciation = (Cost − Salvage Value)/Life in Years

For simplicity again, we will assume a zero for the salvage value. Thus, the annual depreciation can be computed as follows:

Annual Depreciation = Cost/Life in Years

The accumulated depreciation will be computed as follows:

Accumulated Depreciation = Years in use x annual deprecation

Note that the maximum amount of accumulated depreciation is the cost of the asset. If the years the asset in use is greater than the asset's life, the net book value should be zero because the asset has been fully depreciated. Otherwise, the net book value should be equal to the cost minus the annual depreciation times the number of years in use. The years in use should be passed as a parameter to the NetBookValue procedure (method) so that it can perform the computation correctly.

The code for the NetBookValue method should be placed in the class module and should appear as follows:

```
Public Function NetBookValue(ByVal Years As Integer) As Double
    If mDepreMethod = 0 Then
    ' This deprecation method does not depreciate the asset.
        NetBookValue = mCost
    Else
```

```
    ' Straight line depreciation method
      If Years >= mLife Then
    'Asset has been fully depreciated; book value should be zero.
          NetBookValue = 0
      Else
      ' Compute net book value by subtracting accumulated
      ' depreciation from the cost
          NetBookValue = mCost - Years * (mCost / mLife)
      End If
    End If
End Function
```

Note that the parameter Years (representing years in use) has to be passed to the method (function) for the method to compute the net book value correctly. Also, very carefully examine the variables used in the formula to compute the net book value. Both the variables mCost and mLife are variables private to the FixedAsset class. Where are the sources of their values? They obtain their values when your code sets the values for the Cost and Life properties through their respective Property Let procedures. The flow of data can be depicted as in Figure 12.3.

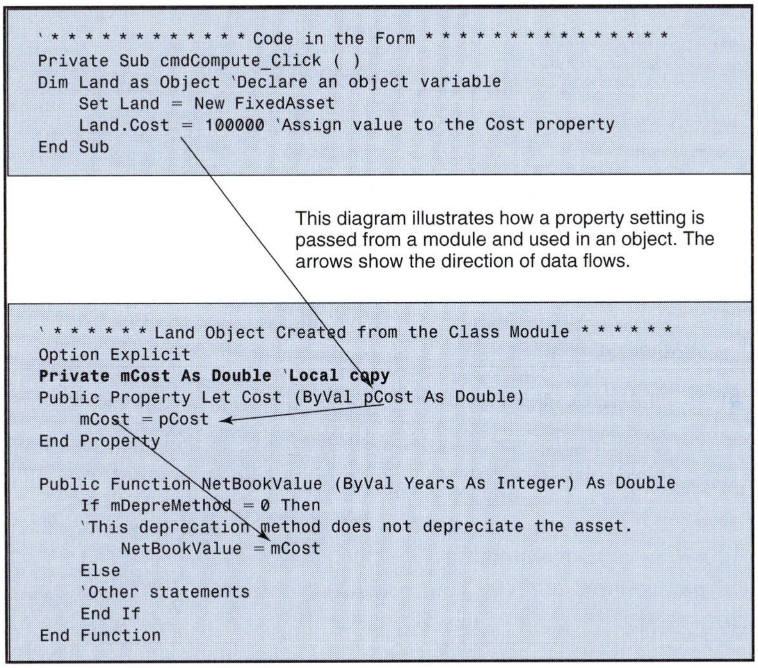

Figure 12.3
How a Property Setting Is Passed and Used

```
'************ Code in the Form **************
Private Sub cmdCompute_Click ( )
Dim Land as Object 'Declare an object variable
    Set Land = New FixedAsset
    Land.Cost = 100000 'Assign value to the Cost property
End Sub
```

This diagram illustrates how a property setting is passed from a module and used in an object. The arrows show the direction of data flows.

```
'****** Land Object Created from the Class Module ******
Option Explicit
Private mCost As Double 'Local copy
Public Property Let Cost (ByVal pCost As Double)
    mCost = pCost
End Property

Public Function NetBookValue (ByVal Years As Integer) As Double
    If mDepreMethod = 0 Then
    'This deprecation method does not depreciate the asset.
        NetBookValue = mCost
    Else
    'Other statements
    End If
End Function
```

Different Types of Methods. As you can see, when invoked, our NetBookValue method returns a value, the net book value. Therefore, we code it as a function. Not all methods need to return a value. If you need a method that only brings about a result, such as displaying data or moving an image, you should code it as a Sub.

Differences Between Methods and General Procedures. So, how are the methods in class modules different from those general procedures in standard modules? In logic and in syntax, there really is no difference. However, as we noted, the way the data are handled can and should be different. When designing your code, you always want to encapsulate the data as much as possible; that is, you will take care to eliminate contamination (unintentional interference) in the data you use in a procedure or a method. When dealing with the class/object, you accomplish this by encapsulating the properties. When working with procedures in the standard module, you will need to pass all required data elements as parameters. Thus, the number of parameters passed to a general procedure will tend to be more than that for a method, all other things being equal.

Another difference is the way that a method and the procedure are invoked. To invoke a method, you use the following syntax:

```
Object.Method(Parameter list)
```

whereas you usually invoke a procedure with the following syntax:

```
[ModuleName.]ProcedureName(Parameter List)
```

Note that to invoke a procedure, you refer to its name directly or qualify it with the module name, whereas you qualify the method with the object name (not the class name). Each object of the same class has its own data. Thus, you need not be concerned about data within a method being accidentally altered by another object. On the other hand, a procedure in a standard module deals with only one set of data. Therefore, you will need to be more careful about the possibility that some of its data can be a "leftover" from previous invocation or accidentally altered by other code.

These differences are summarized in the following table.

Difference in	Procedures in a Standard Module	Methods in a Class Module
Number of parameters	More	Less
Invocation (reference)	ProcName or Module.ProcName	Object.Method (not Module.Method)
Potential data contamination	Higher	Lower
Number of copies in a project	One	As many as objects created

Using the FixedAsset Class

Now that you have created a FixedAsset class, how do you use it in your project? As explained previously, the following is all you need to do:

1. Declare object variables of either the generic object class or the FixedAsset class.
2. Associate these variables with the instances of the class created using the New keyword.

From that point on, using the objects you have created will be exactly the same as using all the objects you have seen before.

For example, suppose you would like to create two fixed assets: Land and Factory. Each will be assigned different values of their properties. You will then use the NetBookValue method to determine their net book values after 10 years in use and use MsgBox to display the results.

You can rewrite the cmdCompute Click event procedure shown in the preceding subsection to satisfy these requirements. The code can appear as follows:

```
' Code in the form
Option Explicit

Private Sub cmdCompute_Click()
' Declare Land and Factory as variables of the FixedAsset class
Dim Land As FixedAsset
Dim Factory As FixedAsset
    Set Land = New FixedAsset 'Create a new Land object
    ' Set properties for Land
    Land.Cost = 100000
    Land.Life = 1000
    Land.DepreMethod = 0
    Set Factory = New FixedAsset 'Create a new Factory object
    ' Set properties for Factory
    Factory.Cost = 300000
    Factory.Life = 20
    Factory.DepreMethod = 1
```

```
    ' Display cost and net book value for Land
    MsgBox "Land cost is " & Land.Cost _
      & ". Net book value is  " & Land.NetBookValue(10) '10 years
    ' Display cost and net book value for Factory
    MsgBox "Factory cost is " & Factory.Cost _
      & ". Net book value is  " & Factory.NetBookValue(10)
    Set Land = Nothing 'Destroy the land object
    Set Factory = Nothing 'Destroy the Factory object
End Sub
```

In the preceding code, both Land and Factory are declared to be from the FixedAsset class (type). Recall that they can be declared "As Object." As noted, however, your code will be more efficient when you declare the object variable as specific as possible.

Notice in the preceding code that we use the NetBookValue method for both Land and Factory objects after their respective properties have been set. We do this intentionally for you to inspect the results. You should see each object retains its assigned cost and each object has a correct net book value: 100,000 and 150,000, respectively. The data for each object are encapsulated and isolated from each other's so that the property settings in one object will not affect the others. Imagine the net book value for each "object" is computed in a standard module. You will need to take special care to separate the data for the land from the factory, won't you?

Destroying Objects Explicitly. Note that the last two statements inside the procedure set the two objects to Nothing. This will explicitly destroy the objects, releasing the resources they use. In general, objects are destroyed when they go out of scope (similar to the way variables declared in a procedure are erased when the procedure ends). Thus, the two lines can be considered redundant. Most experienced programmers maintain that such a practice provides visual clues as to when the objects are actually destroyed and consider it good coding practice.

Building and Using a Class: A Recapitulation

The following table summarizes what you need to do to build a class and use an object created from thereof.

Objective	Action	Place Code in
To create a class	1. Add a class module to the project. 2. Set the class' Name property (e.g., from Class1 to FixedAsset).	Class module
To create a property	Add the Property Get procedure for the "read" capability. Add the Property Let procedure for the "write" capability.	
To create a method	Write a Function (that will return a value) or Sub (that does not return a value).	

To use an object	1. Declare an object variable of the class created; for example:
	`Dim Land As FixedAsset`
	2. Set the object variable to the object using the New keyword; for example:
	`Set Land = New FixedAsset`
		The module (form, standard module, or class module) that uses the object

To use a property or method of an object	Use the following syntax:
	`Object.Property or Object.Method`
	For example:
	`Land.Cost`	

12.3 Adding Features to the Class

Perhaps you have noticed some desirable improvements in the preceding example. This section considers several of these.

First, the depreciation (accounting) methods were coded with numbers: 0 for no depreciation and 1 for the straight-line depreciation method. We have advocated for the use of meaningful names for both constants and variables. Won't it be nice if we can do the same in this case? You can do the same for the property with the Enum statement.

Enumerated Constants

The Enum statement has the following syntax:

```
[Public ¦ Private] Enum name
    membername [= constant]
    membername [= constant]
    . . .
End Enum
```

where *name* represents a "generic" name for the data you are enumerating and *membername* is the name for the specific value you are designating.

For example, instead of using 0 and 1 to represent the depreciation (accounting) method in the previous example, you can place the following code *in the FixedAsset class module*:

```
Public Enum DepreType
    dprNoDepreciation = 0
    dprStraightLine = 1
End Enum
```

Note that the assignment of values to the enumerated names is optional. When you just list all names, the first one in the list will be assigned a value of zero. All subsequent names will be assigned a value of 1 greater than the preceding one. Also, you can assign any unique value to any name. Again, any subsequent names without being assigned a value will be assigned with one increment of its preceding one.

Revising the Property Procedures for the DepreMethod Property. Because you are going to use DepreType to enumerate the available settings with the depreciation (accounting) method property, the two property procedures for the DepreMethod should be revised as follows:

```
Public Property Let DepreMethod(ByVal pDepreMethod As DepreType)
    mDepreMethod = pDepreMethod
End Property

Public Property Get DepreMethod() As DepreType
    DepreMethod = mDepreMethod
End Property
```

Compare the headers of these procedures with the ones you had previously. The parameter pDepreMethod passed to the Property Let procedure now is declared to be the DepreType instead of the Integer type. The code informs the procedure to expect/accept only one of the two values (or names) declared in the Enum statement. Also, the Property Get procedure now is declared to be of the DepreType type. Again, this informs the procedure that it can return only one of the two values defined in the Enum statement. The declaration here must be consistent with that for the parameter in the Property Let procedure. Otherwise, the compiler will inform you of an error.

Effect of Enum on Code. How does this change affect your code? You can use the Enum data in both the class module and the form module. For example, in the class module, the NetBookValue method (function) contains a Select Case block that tests the value of the mDepreMethod. The block of code can be revised as follows:

```
If mDepreMethod = dprNoDepreciation Then
' This method does not depreciate the asset.
    NetBookValue = mCost
Else
' Straight line depreciation
    If Years >= mLife Then
        NetBookValue = 0
    Else
        NetBookValue = mCost - Years * (mCost / mLife)
    End If
End if
```

This revision should make the code more readable. In addition, in the form, you can now use the names in the Enum declaration to set the value for the DepreMethod in the Command Click event procedure. For example, you can now code the following:

```
Land.DepreMethod = dprNoDepreciation
```

Again, this change should make your code clearer and more readable. Indeed, while you are revising the code, you should see the IDE Intellisense displaying available choices as shown in Figure 12.4.

Figure 12.4
Effect of the Enum Declaration

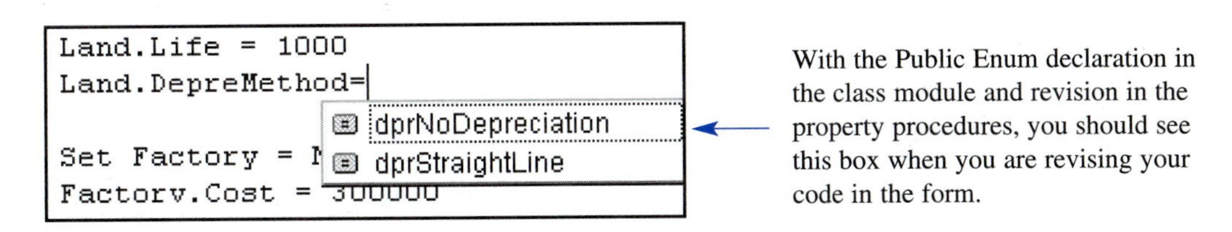

With the Public Enum declaration in the class module and revision in the property procedures, you should see this box when you are revising your code in the form.

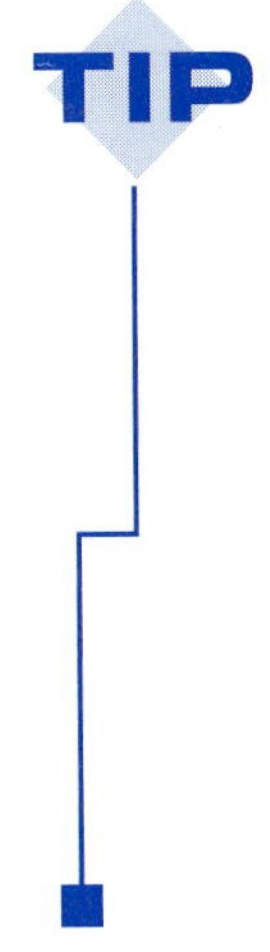

Enum data can also be used as a substitute for numeric indexes. Such a use can enhance the clarity of your code. For example, recall as discussed in Chapter 8 that the Authors table in the Biblio database has three fields: Au_ID, Author, and Year Born. Suppose you have constructed a recordset from the table and named it rsAuthors. For readability, the Author field is typically referenced as follows: rsAuthors!Author or rsAuthors("Author"). However, the use of numeric indexes executes much faster. That is, rsAuthors(1) is much more efficient. Unfortunately your code loses the readability. The solution? Use the Enum declaration for the numeric values. For example, you can declare the following:

```
Enum AuthorFld
    baAUID
    baAuthor
    baYearBorn
End Enum
```

Then refer to the author field as rsAuthors(baAuthor).

Default Property Setting

In the preceding fixed asset example, if you forget to set the property value for DepreMethod for a fixed asset object, its default value will be zero (i.e., no depreciation) because all numeric variables will be initialized to zero when a module (class, form, or standard) starts. However, most fixed assets are depreciable. Thus, the straight-line depreciation (accounting) method would be a better default. Is there a way to set the straight-line depreciation (accounting) method as the default for each fixed asset?

The class has two events: Initialize and Terminate. The class ***Terminate event*** is raised when the object is being destroyed. The class ***Initialize event*** is raised when a new object is being instantiated (created). You can use this latter event to set the initial value for various variables. Thus, if we want to set the value for DepreMethod to dprStraightLine for all fixed asset objects initially (as default), you can code the following:

```
Private Sub Class_Initialize()
    mDepreMethod = dprStraightLine
End Sub
```

After you add this code in the fixed asset class module, all fixed asset objects will have a default straight-line depreciation method.

To see the effect of the preceding code, let's go back to the form. Add a command button; name it cmdShow and give it the caption "Show." Then add the following code:

```
Private Sub cmdShow_Click()
Dim Furniture As FixedAsset
    Set Furniture = New FixedAsset
    MsgBox "DepreMethod for furniture is " & _
      Furniture.DepreMethod
End Sub
```

Keep in mind that in this event procedure, you have not yet set any value for any property of the Furniture object. However, if you run the project and click the button, you will see that the MsgBox displays the following message:

```
DepreMethod for furniture is 1
```

Raising Errors

In the preceding example, what if we accidentally set the value of the DepreMethod property to 2 for a fixed asset object? This value is apparently out of the valid range of the DepreType we declared for the property. The invalid setting will be ignored, and the object retains its default value. Although this provides some protection against errors in setting the value of the property, the result may not be exactly what you want. What if you meant to set the value to 0 (dprNoDepreciation)? The default setting (1) will be used, but we will not be alerted to the error.

Displaying Error Message in a Property Procedure. One alternative, of course, is to provide an error-checking routine in the Property Let procedure for the property of interest and to display an error message when the data is out of range. If you do so, when you test your program with an inappropriate property setting, you will encounter the message. However, the program continues to execute. You will have difficulty identifying the source of the code error.

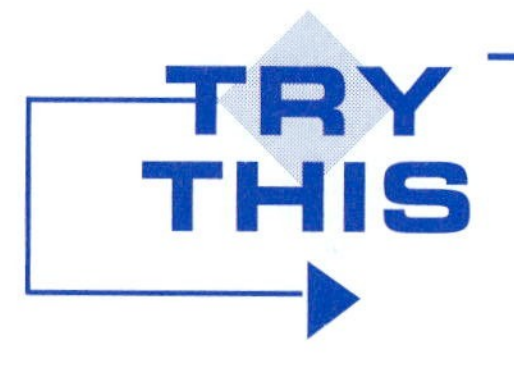

Modify your Property Let procedure for DepreMethod in the FixedAsset class as follows:

```
Public Property Let DepreMethod(ByVal pDepreMethod As _
    DepreType)
    If pDepreMethod > dprStraightLine Then
        MsgBox "Invalid property value."
        Exit Property
    Else
        mDepreMethod = pDepreMethod
    End If
End Property
```

Then in your cmdCompute Click event procedure, change the line to set DepreMethod for Land as follows:

```
Land.DepreMethod = 2
```

Run the project. Click the command button. You will see the error message "Invalid property value." However, your program continues to run after you click the OK button in the message box. After a few days of writing the code, will you still be able to figure out what goes wrong in your program when you see the message again?

Raising an Error. A better alternative is to raise an error condition in your class module, where you can specify the error number and the nature of the error. Raising an error emulates the error we encounter in our code. For example, when you fail to properly create an ADO recordset and proceed to use it, your program stops with the error "Object not set." When you raise an error in a class module, if an error occurs, the execution is halted at the point where your code attempts to set an invalid value. The error message will include your description of the error in the class module. This can be helpful to other programmers who are using the class you have developed. How do you raise an error? You use the ***Err object's Raise method***. The syntax appears as follows:

```
Err.Raise Number, Source, Description
```

where *Number* = the error number; it is recommended that you use a number at least 513 greater than the constant vbObjectError (e.g., vbObjectError + 513)

Source = the class from which the error is raised; optional; if omitted, the system provides a string representing the ID of the project and the class

Description = a text string you can use to articulate the error

Incorporating Error Raising in a Property Procedure. If you apply this alternative to treating the error for the depreciation (accounting) method, you can revise the code for its Property Let procedure as follows:

```
Public Property Let DepreMethod(ByVal pDepreMethod As DepreType)
     Select Case pDepreMethod
     Case dprNoDepreciation To dprStraightLine
          mDepreMethod = pDepreMethod 'Valid setting; accept
     Case Else
          Err.Raise vbObjectError + 513, , _
            "Property setting out of range."
     End Select
End Property
```

In this procedure, the Select Case block branches are based on whether the parameter value is within the valid range. If so, the property setting is assigned to the member variable mDepreMethod. Otherwise, the error number vbObjectError + 513 is raised. The description explains the nature of the error. You can explore the effect of this routine by using the following code in your cmdCompute_Click event procedure:

```
Land.DepreMethod = 2
```

When you test your program, execution will be halted on this line with the error message "Property setting out of range."

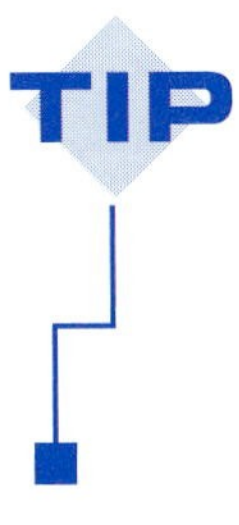

Be aware of the error-trapping setting in the VB IDE. The setting is specified in the General tab of the Options option of the Tools menu. Typically, it should be set to the "Break on unhandled errors." The previous description of error trapping by the IDE assumes this setting. If you are debugging the code in the class module, you may want to change the setting to "Break in class module." Under this setting, execution will stop on the line of the error in the class module, not on the line that calls a procedure in the class module.

Benefits of Raising Errors. When you work for a company, most of the programming projects are fairly large. They can be divided into smaller manageable subprojects, each assigned to different project team members. Most likely, you will be required to develop classes/objects to handle these subprojects. The classes/objects you have created will be used by your colleagues, while you will be using the classes/objects they have developed. You will appreciate your colleagues' classes/objects that raise errors to alert you to an error in your code. For the same reason, your colleagues will appreciate your objects that have similar implementations.

Additional Remarks. Admittedly, the fixed asset class we have created is very simple and can be enhanced in several ways. For example, you probably have noticed that various (accounting) depreciation methods exist. A "complete" fixed asset object should include all these methods for practical uses. Also, in reality, there are restrictive accounting rules governing the change of the depreciation method. You may want to incorporate an event (e.g., "DepreMethodChanged") in the class module when it detects an attempt to change the depreciation method. You can then place some code in that event to alert the user to the restriction when he or she attempts to change the depreciation method for an existing asset. In addition, you can also add methods for the class to compute the depreciation for the current year as well as the cumulative depreciation amount. These enhancements are left to you as exercises. The implementation of events in a class is discussed in the next subsection.

Implementing Events in a Class Module

Recall that objects have three types of interfaces: properties, methods, and events. You have seen how properties and methods are created in a class module. But how do you implement an event? In the class module, you use the event declaration statement to declare an event and the RaiseEvent statement to raise an event. The ***event declaration statement*** has the following syntax:

```
[Public] Event EventProcName(Parameter list)
```

where *EventProcName* is the name of the event procedure (e.g., Click) and *Parameter list* is the list of parameters to pass to the procedure.

Notice that the event must be declared at the module level as Public. All events must be recognized by other modules in order to be used. Therefore, an event declared as Private will not make any sense.

The following statement will declare an event, Insolvent, with two parameters, both of the Double type:

```
Public Event Insolvent(Cash As Double, PaymentsDue As Double)
```

The ***RaiseEvent statement*** has the following syntax:

```
RaiseEvent EventProcName[(Parameter List)]
```

where *EventProcName* and *Parameter list* have the same meaning as in the event declaration.

The RaiseEvent statement will fire (raise) the event and trigger the event procedure that is written to handle this event. The following code segment shows how the statement can be coded:

```
If Cash < PaymentsDue Then
    RaiseEvent Insolvent(Cash, PaymentsDue)
End If
```

Once an event is properly declared and raised in the class module, it can be used in other modules just like any typical event. The next subsection discusses additional details.

A Class with an Event: An Example

To illustrate how the two event statements are coded in a class module, let's consider a simple example. Suppose you want to create a SortEngine class, in which you will provide a BubbleSort method that can be used to sort any array of the Long type. Because you will be concerned about the amount of time that the method may take to sort the array, you would like to provide a means to inform the user of the progress in sorting. One way is to implement an event in the class module. The event (call it PercentChanged) can be raised at each percentage of completion (1%, 2%, and so on) and will give the percentage as well as an estimated remaining time.

Bubble Sort Without an Event. We will begin with coding the sorting routine in a new project. Because the procedure is a method in a class module, you will need to do the following:

1. Add a class module to the new project.
2. Change the class module name to SortEngine.
3. Enter the following code in the class module:

```
Option Explicit
Public Sub BubbleSort(X() As Long)
```

```
Dim I As Long
Dim J As Long
    For I = LBound(X) To UBound(X) - 1
        For J = LBound(X) To UBound(X) - I - 1
            If X(J) > X(J + 1) Then
            ' Out of order; swap
                X(J) = X(J) Xor X(J + 1)
                X(J + 1) = X(J) Xor X(J + 1)
                X(J) = X(J) Xor X(J + 1)
            End If
        Next J
    Next I
End Sub
```

The bubble sort algorithm was explained in Chapter 9, "Arrays and Their Uses." We use the Xor operator to perform the swap when the data in the array are out of order. The trick was explained in a Tip box in Chapter 6, "Input, Output, and Procedures."

Declaring the Event. The first step to implement an event is to declare the event using the Event statement. As described previously, the PercentChanged event will give two values: the percentage completed and the remaining time. The Event statement should be declared in the module-level declaration area as follows:

```
Public Event PercentChanged(Percent As Integer, TimeLeft As Single)
```

As you can see, the declaration looks very much like the header of a Sub procedure. The event must be declared as Public because you want it to be known to other modules in the projects. The Percent parameter is declared to be of the Integer type because we would like the number to be 1, 2, and 3 for 1%, 2%, and 3%, respectively. TimeLeft is declared to be a Single variable to show the estimated remaining time (in seconds). This statement should be placed in the general declaration area of the class module.

Raising the Event. The event should be raised each time the Percent variable increases by a percentile. The sorting time depends mainly on the number of comparisons to perform. As discussed in Chapter 9, for an array of N elements, the total number of comparisons for the bubble sort algorithm can be computed by the following formula:

$$\text{Comparisons} = (N - 1) + (N - 2) + \ldots + 2 + 1$$
$$= N * (N - 1)/2$$

The number of comparisons that has been performed can be computed in the inner loop with a variable (call it Counter) as follows:

```
Counter = Counter + 1
```

The percentage can then be computed by the following formula:

```
Percent = Int(100 * (Counter / Comparisons))
```

Assume the time at which the computation started (StartTime) has been obtained. Then the remaining time can be estimated as follows:

```
TimeLeft = (Timer - StartTime) / CSng(Percent) * _
    CSng(100 - Percent)
```

The preceding line explicitly converts Percent and (100 − Percent) to the Single type using the CSng function. Both TimeLeft and StartTime should be of the Single type to keep track of time in seconds. (Recall that the Timer function returns a Single value representing the number of seconds elapsed since midnight.) However, Percent should be declared as Integer (or Long) as implied in the preceding discussion. The use of CSng function makes the data type of all elements in the expression compatible and can help prevent unexpected results.

For efficiency, the event should not be raised until the value of Percent actually changes. To detect the change, another variable, OldPercent, can be used. When the procedure (method) is invoked, both Percent and OldPercent will initially be zero. Thus, the following If statement should detect the change:

```
If Percent > OldPercent Then
End If
```

Inside the If block, the RaiseEvent statement can be used to fire the event. In addition, OldPercent should be assigned with the value of Percent, ready to check for another change in Percent. Thus, you can code the following:

```
If Percent > OldPercent Then
    TimeLeft = (Timer - StartTime) / Percent * _
      CDbl(100 - Percent)
    RaiseEvent PercentChanged(Percent, TimeLeft)
' Revise OldPercent, so that this block will execute
' only when Percent has changed again.
    OldPercent = Percent
End If
```

Notice that the two arguments enclosed in the pair of parentheses correspond to the event declaration statement. The variable names do not have to be exactly the same as in the event declaration. The relationship of the argument list between RaiseEvent and Event declaration is the same as that between Call and Sub.

The Complete Class Module. The complete SortEngine class module appears as follows:

```
Option Explicit
Public Event PercentChanged(Percent As Integer, TimeLeft As Single)
Public Sub BubbleSort(X() As Long)
Dim I As Long, J As Long
Dim N As Long
Dim Counter As Long
Dim Comparisons As Long
Dim Percent As Integer
Dim OldPercent As Integer
Dim StartTime As Single
Dim TimeLeft As Single
    N = UBound(X) - LBound(X) + 1 'Number of elements in array
    Comparisons = N * (N - 1) / 2 'Number of comparisons
    StartTime = Timer 'starting time to sort
    For I = LBound(X) To UBound(X) - 1
        For J = LBound(X) To UBound(X) - I - 1
            ' Compare and order
            If X(J) > X(J + 1) Then
            ' Out of order; swap
                X(J) = X(J) Xor X(J + 1)
                X(J + 1) = X(J) Xor X(J + 1)
                X(J) = X(J) Xor X(J + 1)
            End If
            ' Code to handle event raising
            Counter = Counter + 1 'Count number of comparisons
            Percent = Int(100 * (Counter / Comparisons))
            If Percent > OldPercent Then
               TimeLeft = (Timer - StartTime) / CSng(Percent) * _
                  CSng(100 - Percent)
                RaiseEvent PercentChanged(Percent, TimeLeft)
                ' Revise OldPercent, so that this block will
                ' execute only when Percent has changed again.
                OldPercent = Percent
            End If
        Next J
    Next I
End Sub
```

Declaring and Using the Event. To use the event created in a class module, the object must be declared at the module (form) level with the WithEvents keyword. For example, assume an object, named Sorter, will be created from the preceding class module to sort arrays in a form. The Sorter object should be declared at the form level as follows:

```
' This code is placed in the form that will use
' the SortEngine class
Option Explicit
Dim WithEvents Sorter As SortEngine
```

Note that once the preceding line is placed in the code window of the form, you should be able to find the Sorter object in the code window's object box and the event in the procedure box as illustrated in Figure 12.5.

Figure 12.5
An Object Variable Declared With Events

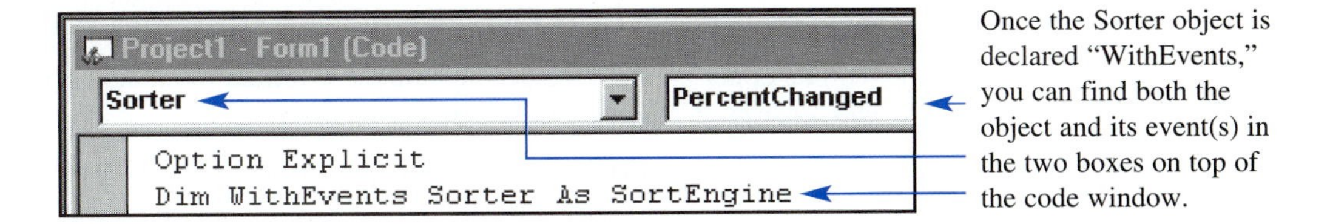
Project1 - Form1 (Code)
Sorter
PercentChanged
Option Explicit
Dim WithEvents Sorter As SortEngine
Once the Sorter object is declared "WithEvents," you can find both the object and its event(s) in the two boxes on top of the code window.

With this declaration, you can place code in the event in exactly the same manner as you can in all other events recognized by other objects.

Completing the Example. To continue and complete the example:

1. Go back to the form.
2. Draw a text box, two command buttons, and two labels.
3. Add a progress bar to the form.
   - 3.1 Click the Project menu and then select the Components option.
   - 3.2 Check "Microsoft Windows Common Controls 6.0" in the Components dialog box and click the OK button.
   - 3.3 Find the Progress Bar icon in the toolbox and draw it on the form.

The text box will be used to specify the upper bound for the array to sort. One command button will be used to generate random numbers, and the other will be used to call the BubbleSort method. One label will be used to display the percentage; the other will be used to show the time remaining. The progress bar will be used to indicate the percentage of progress in sorting. The following table indicates how the properties of these controls should be set.

Control	Property	Setting	Remarks
Text box	Name	txtNumber	To specify the upper limit for the array to hold numbers
	Text	(Cleared)	
Command button	Name	cmdGenerate	To generate the specified random numbers
	Caption	Generate	
Command button	Name	cmdSort	To call the bubble sort routine in the SortEngine class module
	Caption	Sort	
Label	Name	lblPercent	To display percentage of completion
	Caption	(Cleared)	
Label	Name	lblTimeLeft	To show remaining time to sort
	Caption	(Cleared)	
Progress bar	Name	prgPercent	To indicate percentage of completion

Figure 12.6 shows a sample visual interface in action.

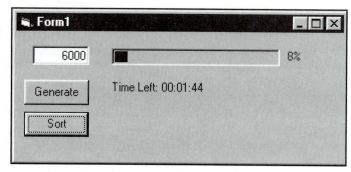

Figure 12.6
Sample Visual Interface in Action

When the user clicks the Generate button, the computer will generate an array of the Long type with its upper bound equal to the number specified in the text box txtNumber. The code in the ***cmdGenerate_Click procedure*** appears as follows:

```
Option Explicit
Dim WithEvents Sorter As SortEngine
Dim A() As Long

Private Sub cmdGenerate_Click()
Dim N As Long
Dim I As Long
    Randomize
    N = Val(txtNumber.Text)
    If N = 0 Then
        MsgBox "Please enter a number"
    End If
    ReDim A(N)
    For I = 0 To N
        A(I) = N * Rnd
    Next I
End Sub
```

When the user clicks the Sort button, your code will create a new Sorter object and use its BubbleSort method to sort the array generated in the cmdGenerate Click procedure. Thus, the ***cmdSort_Click procedure*** can appear as follows:

```
Private Sub cmdSort_Click()
    Set Sorter = New SortEngine
    Sorter.BubbleSort A()
    Set Sorter = Nothing
End Sub
```

Because the object variable Sorter has been declared in the general declaration area, it should not be declared again. This procedure simply creates a new SortEngine object and associates with Sorter. Sorter's BubbleSort method is then called to sort array A. As soon as this is done, the object is set to Nothing so that the object is destroyed. These three lines of code should be very familiar to you.

How do you code the PercentChanged event? This event is triggered when the percentage of comparisons changes by a full percent. You can use it to display the change in the labels and the progress bar. The code should appear as follows:

```
Private Sub Sorter_PercentChanged(Percent As Integer, _
  TimeLeft As Single)
Dim Remaining As Date
    lblPercent.Caption = Percent & "%"
    prgPercent.Value = Percent
    Remaining = DateAdd("s", TimeLeft, 0)
    lblTimeLeft.Caption = "Time Left: " & _
      Format$(Remaining, "hh:mm:ss")
    DoEvents
End Sub
```

Notice that you should obtain the event procedure template from the procedure box, not by writing your own. There is no difference between handling this event and handling any events generated by any VB objects. Notice that TimeLeft provided by the Sorter object is a Single value in seconds. We'd like to display the time in the hh:mm:ss format. Therefore, that value is converted to a Date/Time value using the DateAdd function. The result is assigned to the Date/Time variable, Remaining, which is declared at the beginning of this procedure and displayed with the Format$ function. Percent is used to set the progress bar and is also displayed in lblPercent. Notice also that the DoEvents statement is needed for the operating system to update the appearance (captions) of the labels.

Test this project with a different number for the upper bound of the array to get a feel. For a computer of 233 MHz, with an upper bound set to 10,000, you should see that it takes a few minutes to sort the array. Note that we use the bubble sort algorithm in this example to illustrate how the PercentChanged event can be implemented. Recall that this algorithm is the least efficient among all available sorting algorithms. You can think of its use here as a representation of a "process that takes a long time."

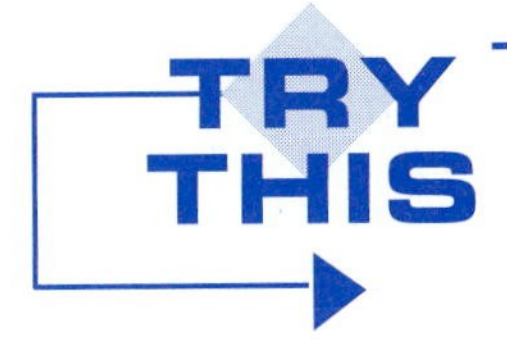

We mentioned that the code in the class module is more efficient if the event is raised only when the value of Percent is different from that of OldPercent. After you have obtained a feel of how the whole project works, go back to the class module. In the BubbleSort procedure, replace the following line:

```
If Percent > OldPercent Then
```

with

```
If Percent > 0 Then
```

Now run the project again. You should be able to observe a noticeable slowdown in performance. Raising events too often can make the program very slow.

Why Events? The sorting example illustrated thus far should give you a good appreciation of implementing events in class modules. Without the PercentChanged event, a programmer using the SortEngine class will have no way to implement code to inform the user of the progress in sorting. One possible alternative is to rewrite the method (BubbleSort) so that it will take two labels and a progress bar as it parameters. It can then display the progress in these controls. However, such a design is inflexible. The programmer who uses the method will be forced to provide these controls. In addition, these controls must be of the classes of the label and the progress bar.

On the other hand, when the PercentChanged event is implemented in the class module, the programmer who uses the class has complete flexibility in determining what to do with the object created from the class module. The programmer can ignore the event, or the programmer can code the event in any manner he or she sees fit. The combination of labels and the progress bar used in the preceding example is but one of the many possibilities.

12.4 Reusing Objects

Once a class is developed, you can use it not only in various modules in the current project but also in other projects. All the modules in the current project can use the class the same way as discussed previously. But how do you use the class in other projects?

Two Alternative Approaches to Reusing Objects

Basically, you can follow two different approaches in reusing a class:

1. *Add the class module to the project.* In the project that you want to use the class module, you can do the following:
   - Click the Project menu and select the Add Class Module option. The Add Class Module dialog box will appear.

- Click the Existing tab in the dialog box. The tab appears like an "Open File" common dialog box (see Figure 12.7).
- Browse the system and select the class module you want to include. Then click the Open button.

2. *Compile the class module as an ActiveX DLL.* The steps to create an ActiveX DLL are discussed in Chapter 14, "Beyond the Core." Once you have the class module compiled as an ActiveX DLL, you can use it like an object provided by others (e.g., the ADO objects).

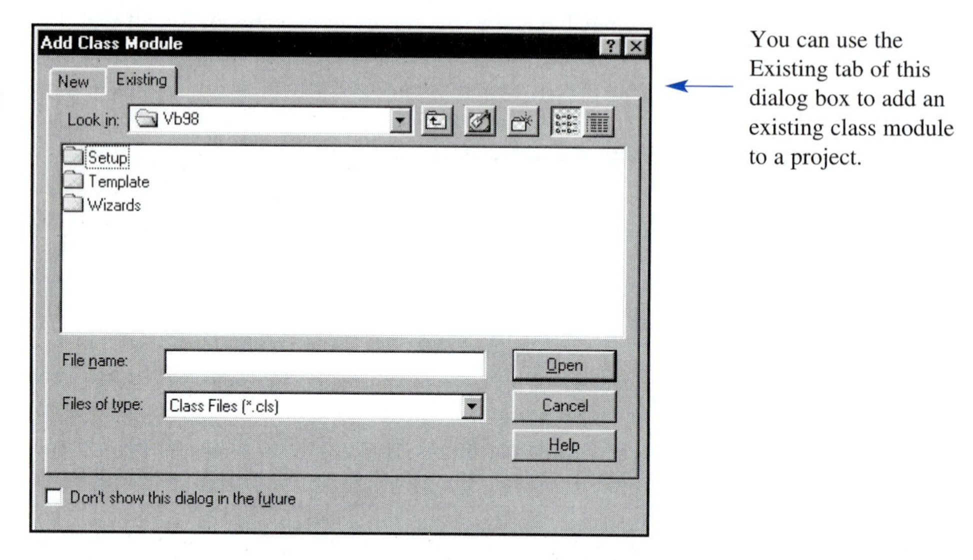

Figure 12.7
The Existing Tab of the Add Class Module Dialog Box

Relative Advantages and Disadvantages

The advantage of the first approach is its simplicity. Once you finish developing the class module, you need not to do anything more until you want to use it in another project.

The disadvantage is that it takes more effort to incorporate any subsequent changes you make to the class module. In general, your projects will be compiled into executable files for "production" once they are fully tested. If you subsequently revise the class module, all the projects using the class will need to be recompiled. This task calls for not only your time and effort to recompile the projects but also the additional effort of identifying the projects that have used the class. Furthermore, if your projects have been installed in many machines, you will need to reinstall/redistribute these projects onto those machines.

The advantage of the second approach is the elimination of the need to recompile the projects that have used the class if the class module is subsequently revised. All you need to do is to recompile the ActiveX DLL that contains the class module. If the projects using the class are installed in other machines, you need only to reinstall/redistribute the DLL. Nothing needs to be done with the projects that have used the class.

The disadvantage is that you will need to create the ActiveX DLL. However, the time and effort involved is relatively little. Thus, in general, *the way to reuse a class is to compile the class module as an ActiveX DLL.*

The following table summarizes the approaches to reusing objects.

Approach	Advantage	Disadvantage
Incorporate class module source code	No additional requirements after developing the module.	Revision of the class module calls for recompilation of all projects that have used the class. These projects need to be reinstalled in all machines that use the projects.

Approach	Advantage	Disadvantage
Compile class module as ActiveX DLL	Revision requires no need to recompile the projects that have used the class.	Compiling the class module into an ActiveX DLL takes time.

12.5 The Visual Element in an Object

In Chapter 11, "Menus and Multiple-Form Applications" we pointed out that the form has a visual element and a code module. At the beginning of this chapter, we stated that a class module is a form without the visual element. What if you need an object that requires the visual element?

Treating the Form as an Object

One possible alternative is to treat a form like a class module and code accordingly. Multiple copies of the same form can be created in exactly the same manner as the class module. For example, if you have created a form named frmEmployee, in another form, frmEmployee can be used in the following manner:

```
Dim Smith As frmEmployee
Dim Johnson As frmEmployee

' Create an employee object and name it Smith
Set Smith = New frmEmployee
' statements pertaining to Smith

' Create an employee object and name it Johnson
Set Johnson = New frmEmployee
' statements pertaining to Johnson
```

Of course, if you intend to treat the form as a class, you should code the form like a class module. That is, you should design the form such that it has properties, methods, and events that other modules (form, class, or standard modules) can use. Indeed, you have already worked with some of these elements. Public variables in the form are read-and-write properties, whereas Public procedures are methods.

The difference between a generic form and a form to be used as a class is that the latter is intended to be used for a broader applicability and should be written as a standalone unit. Thus, you should be careful in code design to avoid making specific references to objects in other forms and modules (unless these modules are intended to work together with that form as a unit).

The Disadvantage. Coding the form directly as an object has a potential disadvantage. A form in an ActiveX DLL is not visible to another project; that is, you cannot use a form in the ActiveX DLL directly from a project. Thus, if you want to use the form (as a class) in another project, you can only add it to the project. This will have the disadvantage of incorporating the source class module directly (the first approach) as discussed in the preceding section.

An Alternative Design. Alternatively, you can use a class module. From the class module, you can invoke the form that will provide the visual element for your class. This form is thus an integral part of the "object" and should not be exposed to (used directly by) other modules that are not a part of the object/class. You can then compile both the class module and the accompanied form into an ActiveX DLL. A project using the DLL will have no difficulty in accessing the class through which the visual element provided by the form can be invoked. Because it is easier to incorporate an object into a project using the ActiveX DLL approach (as discussed in the preceding section), you should use this design in creating a class with the visual element. Again, the steps to compile a class module (and with its form) are discussed in Chapter 14.

A Generalized "Search Engine"

To illustrate the inclusion of a form with a class module, imagine a data-entry form in which employee ID is required. To help the user search for the ID given an employee name, you can design a dialog box that shows the employee names and corresponding IDs based on the approximate name string entered by the user. When the user clicks a name, the corresponding ID is returned. There are actually many search problems of the same nature: to cite just two, searching for a customer ID given a customer name and searching for a product ID given a product name.

We can design a class with a form to work as a generalized "ID search engine." The "engine" will display the needed interface for the user to specify the text to search and allow the user to identify the record containing the ID. The details of the interface are discussed later. Here are the steps to set up the project:

1. Add a new form to the new project so that it contains two forms. Form1 will be used as the main form, and Form2 will be used as the visual element of the search engine. Name Form2 frmSearch, which will be called "the search form." (You can name Form1 any name you wish. Its name is not used in the code.)
2. Add a new class module to the project. Name this module clsSearch. This will be the module to code the class.
3. Add an MS HFG (Hierarchical FlexGrid) to the project. This grid is needed in the search form.

We begin with designing the visual interface for the search form. (Double-click frmSearch in the Project Explorer window so that the form will appear in the IDE.)

Visual Interface of the Search Form. The search form should have the following:

- A frame with the caption "Search Text." This frame will contain the following:
  - A text box for the user to enter the search text
  - A command button to initiate the search with the caption "Search"
- A command button to end the search with the caption "OK"
- An HFG to display the names (field to search on) and the IDs
- A label to display the value of the selected search-on field
- A label to display the ID of the selected record

This form (in action) should look like that in Figure 12.8. A list of selected property settings for these controls is shown in the following table.

Control	Property	Setting	Remark
Frame	Caption	Search Text	To contain the search text box and command button
Text box	Name	txtSearch	To specify search text
	Text	(Cleared)	
Command button	Name	cmdSearch	To initiate search in the database table
	Caption	Search	
Command button	Name	cmdOK	To go back to the class module
	Caption	OK	
HFG	Name	grdSearch	To display records found given the search text; this grid will be bound to the ADO recordset that gives the results of the search; setting FixedCols to 0 will allow data to be displayed in column 0
	FixedCols	0	

Control	Property	Setting	Remark
Label	Name	lblSearchOnField	To display the value of the SearchOnField of the selected record
	Caption	(Cleared)	
	BackColor	White	
	BorderStyle	1-Fixed Single	
Label	Name	lblID	To display the ID of the selected record
	Caption	(Cleared)	
	BackColor	White	
	BorderStyle	1-Fixed Single	

Expected Behavior of the Search Form. As you may infer from Figure 12.8, when the search form is in action:

- The user can enter the search text in the frame.
- When the user clicks the Search button, the program will search for the search text in the "search on" field and display in the HFG all the records that match the text.
- When the user clicks a row in the grid, the record is displayed in the labels above the grid.
- When the user clicks the OK button or the Close (x) button on the form, the form disappears.

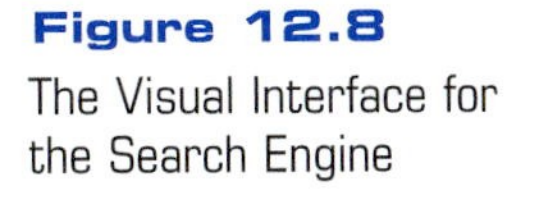

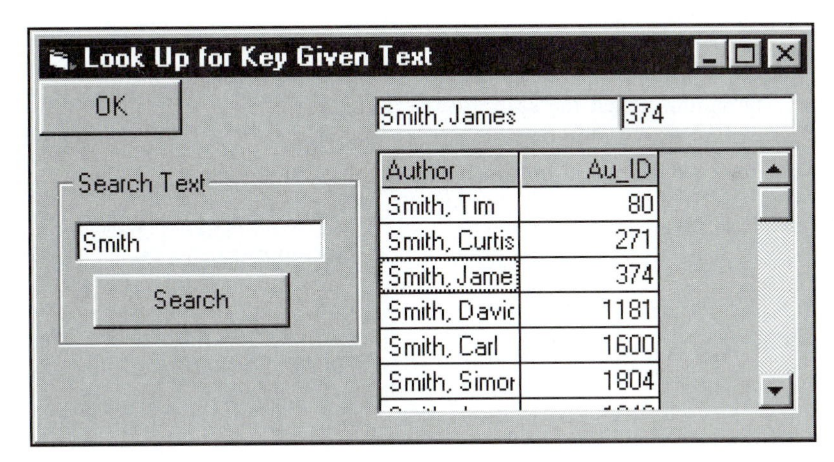

Figure 12.8
The Visual Interface for the Search Engine

Properties of the Class. Let's now turn our attention to the class module. The class should have the following properties:

- *DatabaseName:* a string to specify the database to search
- *TableName:* a string to specify the database table to search
- *SearchOnField:* a string to specify the field on which to search (e.g., Employee Name)
- *IDField:* a string to specify the ID field

This search engine should also have a Search method to initiate the search, which should return the ID of the selected record.

Coding the "Engine"

Let's consider the code in the search form. Before placing any code in the module, however, be sure that your project includes a reference to the ADO (2.1 or 2.0) Library.

Declarations in the General Area. The form will need to know the values of all four properties of the class. For simplicity, we can declare four Public variables of the same name in the form. The form will also need an ADO connection to connect to the database. The variable should be declared as a module-level variable because it will be used in more than one event procedure. Thus, the general declaration area should have the following statements:

```
Option Explicit
Public DatabaseName As String
Public TableName As String
Public SearchOnField As String
Public IDField As String
Private cnnSearch As ADODB.Connection
```

Setting Up the ADO Connection to the Database. The connection should be established as soon as the search form is called to action. Thus, the ADO connection object should be created in the Form Load event as follows:

```
Private Sub Form_Load()
Dim ConnStr As String
' Set up ADO connection
    ConnStr = "Provider=Microsoft.Jet.OLEDB.4.0;Data source=" & _
      DatabaseName
    Set cnnSearch = New ADODB.Connection
    cnnSearch.Open ConnStr
End Sub
```

The connection object should continue to exist until the form unloads. Thus, the object should be closed in the QueryUnload event. We consider this aspect later.

Searching for and Displaying the Matching Records. When the user clicks the Search button, the interface should display in the HFG all the records in the database table that match the search text. Thus, the code to perform the search should be placed in the command button's Click events as follows:

```
Private Sub cmdSearch_Click()
Dim rsSearch As ADODB.Recordset
Dim SQL As String
    SQL = "Select [" & SearchOnField & "], [" & IDField & _
      "] From " & TableName & " Where [" _
        & SearchOnField & "] Like '" & txtSearch.Text & "%';"
    ' Create a recordset object and associate it with rsSearch
    Set rsSearch = New ADODB.Recordset
    ' Open the recordset as static and read-only
    rsSearch.Open SQL, cnnSearch, adOpenStatic, adLockReadOnly, _
      adCmdText
    ' Bind the grid to the search results
    Set grdSearch.DataSource = rsSearch
    rsSearch.Close 'Close the recordset
    Set rsSearch = Nothing 'And destroy the object
End Sub
```

The procedure first constructs an SQL statement based on the entered search text. Both the values for SearchOnField and IDField are enclosed in a paired of brackets to avoid the problem with field names that may contain spaces. As required by the SQL syntax, the search text is attached with a wildcard "%" character and is enclosed with a pair of single quotes. After an ADO recordset object is created and associated with the variable rsSearch, the recordset is opened using the SQL as read-only because no update is required. Then, the Set statement binds the grid to the recordset so that the search results can be displayed in the grid with minimal code.

The recordset is immediately closed and set to Nothing because there is no further use of it. Recall that an object will be destroyed when the object variable goes out of scope. Thus, the statement that sets the recordset to Nothing is not really needed. However, it provides an explicit visual clue as to exactly when the object is destroyed. Including the statement is considered good programming practice.

Displaying the Selection. When the user clicks a cell in a row in the HFG, the record should be displayed in the two labels above the grid. Thus, the grid's Click event procedure can appear as follows:

```
Private Sub grdSearch_Click()
    With grdSearch
        lblSearchOnField.Caption = .TextMatrix(.Row, 0)
        lblID.Caption = .TextMatrix(.Row, 1)
    End With
End Sub
```

The HFG's TextMatrix property gives the grid's cell content in a tabular form. For example, the text content of the cell in row 0, column 0 can be accessed with the following syntax:

```
GridName.TextMatrix(0, 0)
```

When the user clicks a cell in the grid, the grid's Row and Col properties are set to point to this cell. Thus, the Row property can be used to retrieve the text in the cells of the row selected, as shown in the preceding code.

When the Search Is Complete. The user will click the OK button or the Close button when the record with the proper ID has been selected. The ID is stored in the label named lblID. As explained in Chapter 11, the data in a control will be lost if the form is unloaded. Thus, in either case, you should hide the form rather than unloading it. Thus, the Click event procedure for the OK button should appear as follows:

```
Private Sub cmdOK_Click()
    Me.Hide
End Sub
```

What happens when the user clicks the Close (X) button? Because you want to hide the form rather than unload it, your code should cancel the unloading operation and then use the form's Hide method. The QueryUnload event should be the most appropriate event to handle this.

Keep in mind the Unload command can also come from your code or the system at the end. You want to cancel the unloading operation only when the Close button is clicked. Recall also that the ADO connection object cnnSearch was open when the form was loaded and should be closed and destroyed when the form is unloaded. Thus, the code in the QueryUnload event procedure should appear as follows:

```
Private Sub Form_QueryUnload(Cancel As Integer, _
    UnloadMode As Integer)
    If UnloadMode = vbFormControlMenu Then
    ' Unload is initiated by clicking "X" button
    ' Hide instead of unload
        Cancel = True
        Me.Hide
    Else
    ' Unload is initiated by code.
        cnnSearch.Close  'Close the connection object
        Set cnnSearch = Nothing 'Destroy the object
    ' And proceed to unload (Do nothing with Cancel.)
    End If
End Sub
```

Recall that the second parameter, UnloadMode, allows your code to check for the source of the unload operation. The value vbFormControlMenu indicates that unload is initiated from the user's clicking the Close button. In that case, you will hide the form instead; otherwise, unload should proceed. The connection object should be closed and destroyed.

The preceding code completes the requirements in the search form. This form is invoked by the code in the class module, which provides the four properties and the Search method for other modules to use.

The following discussion pertains to the code in the class module named clsSearch.

When the Object Is Initialized and Terminated. When a search object is being created from the class module, the search form should also be loaded. In addition, when the object is being destroyed, the search form should also be unloaded and destroyed. In this way, the object and the form are "synchronized" as a unit. As explained previously, when an object is being created from the class, the Initialize event occurs; when the object is being destroyed, the Terminate event occurs. Thus, the code to synchronize the existence of the object and the search form can appear as follows:

```
Option Explicit
Private SearchForm As frmSearch 'Declare the search form object
Private Sub Class_Initialize()
    Set SearchForm = New frmSearch 'Create a new search form
End Sub
Private Sub Class_Terminate()
    Unload SearchForm 'unload the form
    Set SearchForm = Nothing 'Destroy the form module
End Sub
```

In the preceding code, notice that a module-level (object) variable, SearchForm is declared to be of the frmSearch type. In the Class Initialize event, a new object of this type is then created and associated with the variable SearchForm, making it possible to refer to the form by this variable in the duration of the object.

The Property Procedures. In the class module, each of the four properties can be implemented in a usual manner by using a module-level variable and the Property Let and Property Get procedures. For example, the DatabaseName property can be coded as follows:

```
Private mDatabaseName As String
Public Property Let DatabaseName(pDatabaseName As String)
    mDatabaseName = pDatabaseName
End Property
Public Property Get DatabaseName() As String
    DatabaseName = mDatabaseName
End Property
```

Without additional explanation, the property procedures for the other three properties are listed next. Note that these properties can simply be "declared" by using Public variables. However, such practice is not encouraged. In many cases, values assigned to the properties should be validated. The Property Let procedure is where the validation is carried out. Explicitly coding the property procedures facilitates the coding of validation rules.

```
Private mTableName As String
Private mSearchOnField As String
Private mIDField As String
' TableName Properties procedures
Public Property Let TableName(ByVal pTableName As String)
    mTableName = pTableName
End Property
Public Property Get TableName() As String
    TableName = mTableName
End Property
' SearchInField Property procedures
Public Property Let SearchOnField(ByVal pSearchOnField As String)
    mSearchOnField = pSearchOnField
End Property
Public Property Get SearchOnField() As String
    SearchOnField = mSearchOnField
End Property
' IDField Property procedures
Public Property Let IDField(ByVal pIDField As String)
    mIDField = pIDField
End Property
```

```
Public Property Get IDField() As String
     IDField = mIDField
End Property
```

The Search Method. The Search method will return an ID. Thus, it should be written as a Function procedure, not a Sub. In this function, the search form should be invoked to obtain the ID. Before the form is invoked, of course, all the settings for the properties required for the search must also be passed to the form. The value of the ID should come from the label lblID in the search form. Because the value will not be determined until the user signals an end of the search, the form should be invoked as modal. The procedure should appear as follows:

```
Public Function Search() As Variant
     With SearchForm
     ' Assign property settings to corresponding variables
     ' in search form
          .DatabaseName = mDatabaseName
          .TableName = mTableName
          .SearchOnField = mSearchOnField
          .IDField = mIDField
          .Show vbModal 'Display the search form as modal
          Search = .lblID.Caption 'Obtain and return ID
     End With
End Function
```

In this procedure, the first four assignment statements assign the settings of the four properties to the Public variables in the search form, which was created in the object's Initialize event. The search form is then invoked as modal by the Show method. After the form returns the execution control, the caption of the form's lblID is assigned to Search so that the method will return the ID to the caller.

Using the "Search Engine"

How can the preceding "search engine" be used? Consider the case of the familiar Biblio database. Suppose we are interested in finding an author's ID (AU_ID). We can use Form1 in our example as the startup form and test the "search engine." Here are the steps:

1. Draw a text box (name it txtAuID) with a command button (name it cmdBrowse) on its right. The text box will be used to display the Author ID.
2. Develop code so that when the command button is clicked, the program will do the following:
   2.1 Create a new clsSearch object.
   2.2 Set the object's properties required for the search.
   2.3 Invoke the Search method and place its returned value in the text box.

The code for the event procedure can appear as follows:

```
Private Sub cmdBrowse_Click()
Dim Biblio As clsSearch
     Set Biblio = New clsSearch
     With Biblio
          .DatabaseName = "C:\Program Files\" & _
            "Microsoft Visual Studio\Vb98\Biblio.mdb"
          .TableName = "Authors"
          .SearchOnField = "Author"
          .IDField = "Au_ID"
          txtAuID.Text = .Search
     End With
     Set Biblio = Nothing
End Sub
```

Run the project. You can verify whether it works properly with the following steps:

1. Click the Browse button. You should see the search form appear.
2. Enter a partial or complete name in the search text box (e.g., smi).

3. Click the Search button. If the search text has some matches in the Author field of the Authors table, you should see the authors' names with the corresponding author's ID displayed in the HFG.
4. Click a name. You should see the name and the ID displayed in the two labels above the grid.
5. Click the OK button or the Close (x) button on the search form. The form should disappear, and you should see that the Author ID you selected is now displayed in the Author ID text box in the main form (Form1).

Additional Remarks

Note that the Search class we just developed is a generalized ID search class. You can use it to identify a customer number for a customer, an account number for an account, or a product ID for a product, provided all the four required properties are set. You can also use it multiple times in a project for different "IDs."

However, the class can be improved in several respects. For example, it assumes that the "search on field" is of the String type. A truly generalized routine should allow different data types for that field. Also, the visual interface can also be improved. For example, the column widths of the grid can be adjusted to the widths of the data fields. Finally, no data validation is implemented for the required properties, making the source of error hard to trace when an error arises from setting one of these properties. All these desirable improvements are left to you as an exercise.

12.6 Using the Class Builder Utility

Some of the code needed to build a class is "routine." For example, the property procedures used to create the properties are similar. You can use the class builder utility that comes with VB6 as an add-in to handle this mechanical aspect. This utility program provides code templates for various object interfaces. This section shows you how to use this utility program.

Assume that you have just added a class module to your project. You would like to use the utility to add one method, one property, and one event. The major steps involved are as follows:

1. Add the class builder utility to the Add-In menu if the utility is not in the menu.
2. Start the class builder utility.
3. Specify the desired interfaces to add.
4. Quit the utility and "save" the results.

Now let's look at each step in more detail.

Adding the Class Builder Utility into the Add-Ins Menu

When you click the Add-Ins menu, if the class builder utility is not in the menu, you should be able to see a drop-down menu similar to that on the left in Figure 12.9. In this case, follow these steps to load the utility:

1. Click the Add-In Manager option. An Add-In Manager dialog box should appear.
2. Highlight VB 6 Class Builder Utility in the list box in the dialog box.
3. Check the Load/Unload check box at the lower portion of the dialog box.
4. Click the OK button.

The utility is now in the Add-Ins menu ready for use.

The following discussion assumes that you have already completed the preceding steps. In addition, you have added the class module Class1 to your project.

Figure 12.9
Add-In Menu Without and with the Class Builder Utility

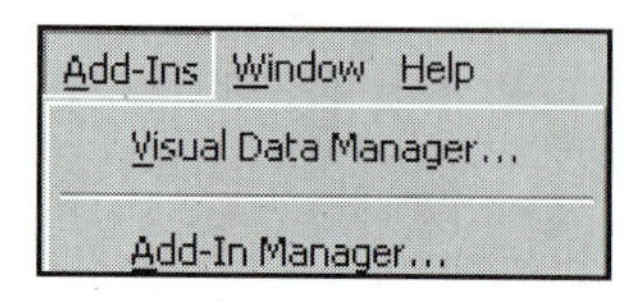

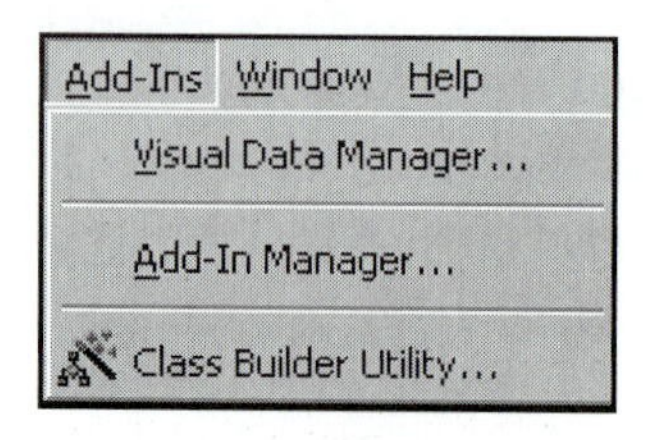

Working with the Class Builder Utility

To start the utility, click the Add-Ins menu and then select the "Class Builder Utility" option. The Class Builder dialog box should appear (see Figure 12.10). You can then use it to create a code template for a class with its features.

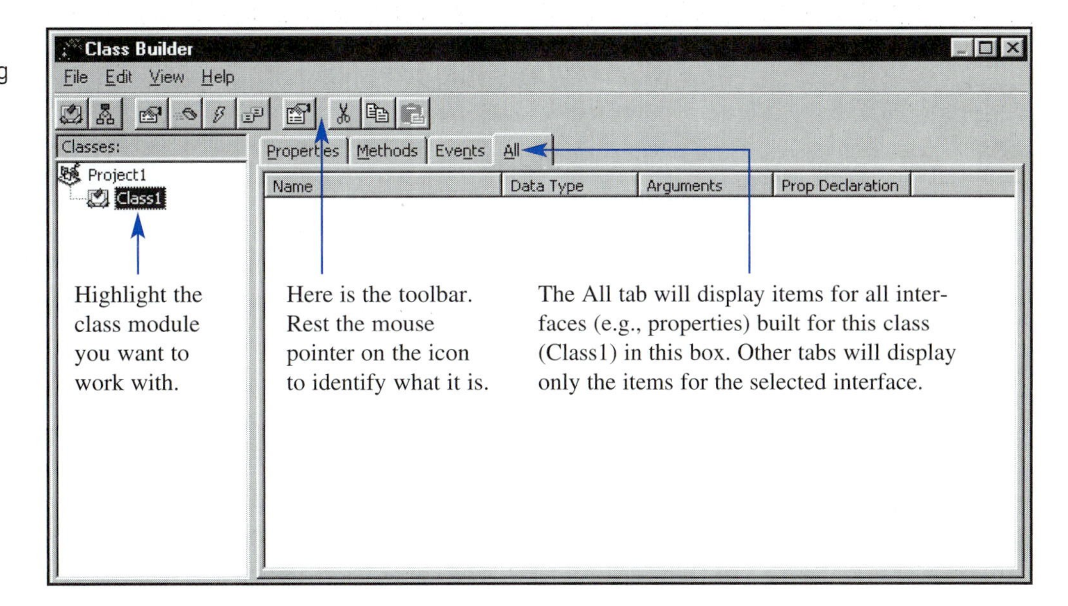
Class Builder
File Edit View Help
Classes:
Project1
Class1
Properties Methods Events All
Name Data Type Arguments Prop Declaration
Highlight the class module you want to work with.
Here is the toolbar. Rest the mouse pointer on the icon to identify what it is.
The All tab will display items for all interfaces (e.g., properties) built for this class (Class1) in this box. Other tabs will display only the items for the selected interface.

Figure 12.10 The Class Builder Dialog Box

Building the Interfaces for a Class. Suppose you would like to use this utility to build a fixed asset class with the Cost property, the NetBookValue method, and the CostChanged event. Here are the steps:

1. Change the name of class to clsFixedAsset. (Note that you can also use the Properties window to change the classname.)
   - 1.1 In the dialog box, you should see the name Class1 under Project1. Right-click on Class1. You should see a context pop-up menu.
   - 1.2 Select the Rename option. Class1 should now be highlighted and enclosed in a text box.
   - 1.3 Change Class1 to clsFixedAsset. Then press the Enter key.
2. Add the Cost property.
   - 2.1 Click the "Add New Property to Current Class" icon on the dialog box's toolbar. (If you are not sure which icon to click, rest the mouse pointer on each icon. The ToolTip text will appear to identify itself.) After you click the icon, the Property Builder dialog box will appear.
   - 2.2 Enter "Cost" in the Name box.
   - 2.3 Select Double as the data type from the Data Type combo box.
   - 2.4 Make sure that "Public Property" is the option chosen from the Declaration frame.
   - 2.5 Click the OK button.
3. Add the NetBookValue method. Note that this method takes the parameter Years (of the Integer type) and returns a value of the Double type representing the net book value of an asset.
   - 3.1 Click the "Add New Method to Current Class" icon. The Method Builder dialog box will appear.
   - 3.2 Enter NetBookValue in the Name box of the dialog box.
   - 3.3 Click the "+" sign by the Arguments box to add an argument. The Add Argument dialog box will appear.

3.3.1 Enter Years in the Name box of the dialog box.

3.3.2 Check the ByVal check box.

3.3.3 Select Integer from the Data Type combo box.

3.3.4 Make sure that the Optional check box is not checked.

3.3.5 Click the OK button.

3.4 Select Double from the Return Data Type combo box.

3.5 Make sure that neither the "Declare as Friend?" check box nor the "Default Method?" check box is checked.

3.6 Click the OK button.

4. Add the CostChanged event.

4.1 Click the "Add Event to Current Class" icon. The Event Builder dialog box will appear.

4.1.1 Enter OriginalCost in the Name box of the dialog box.

4.1.2 Click "+" on the right side of the Arguments box. The Add Argument dialog box will appear.

4.1.2.1 Enter OriginalCost in the Name box.

4.1.2.2 Check the ByVal check box.

4.1.2.3 Select Double from the Data Type combo box.

4.1.2.4 Click the OK button in the Add Argument dialog box.

4.2 Click the OK button in the Event Builder dialog box.

5. You have now completed the exercise of adding the three interfaces for the clsFixedAsset class. Click the close button of the Class Builder dialog box. You will be prompted whether to update project with changes. Click the Yes button.

The following code should appear in your clsFixedAsset class module:

```
Option Explicit
' local variable(s) to hold property value(s)
Private mvarCost As Double 'local copy
' To fire this event, use RaiseEvent with the following syntax:
' RaiseEvent CostChanged[(arg1, arg2, ... , argn)]
Public Event CostChanged(ByVal OriginalCost As Double)
Public Function NetBookValue(ByVal Years As Integer) As Double
End Function
Public Property Let Cost(ByVal vData As Double)
' used when assigning a value to the property, on the left side of
' an assignment.
' Syntax: X.Cost = 5
    mvarCost = vData
End Property
Public Property Get Cost() As Double
' used when retrieving value of a property, on the right side of
' an assignment.
' Syntax: Debug.Print X.Cost
    Cost = mvarCost
End Property
```

As you can see, the property procedures for the Cost property are fairly complete. The NetBookValue method has a function template for you to add necessary code. The CostChanged event is declared in the module-level declaration area. In addition, it provides a comment showing the syntax to raise the event.

Correcting Mistakes and Adding Additional Interfaces. Suppose that during the process of creating a property, you made a mistake in specifying its data type. Will you be able to correct it using the Class Builder Utility? It depends on whether you have "updated the project."

If you have not yet left the utility, you can do the following:

1. Find the property in either the Property tab or the All tab in the utility's dialog box and double-click the item. The Property Builder dialog box should appear.
2. Make the correct selection for the data type from the Data Type combo box. The step is the same as that previously described to create a new property. Note that you can no longer change the name of the property.

The steps to correct the parameters for a method or an event are similar.

If you have already left the utility, you will not be able to use it to make the correction. You can either correct the code in the class module manually or delete all the relevant code in the module and go back to the utility to add the property anew. To add additional interfaces, you can do the following:

1. Start the Class Builder Utility as described previously.
2. Click the target class module.
3. Add the desired interfaces using the steps described previously.
4. Click the Utility's File menu and select the "Update Project" option. Or, simply click the Close (x) button of the utility's dialog box and then click the Yes button when prompted whether to update the project.

You should be able to see all the newly added properties, methods, and/or events in the class module.

The class builder provides a convenient way to complete the mechanical aspect of the code. You will still need to know what you are doing to make the class work the way you want.

Summary

This chapter introduces you to object-oriented programming. The concepts of class and object are first clarified. Then the advantages of such a programming approach are explained. You have seen an example of developing a FixedAsset class with several properties and a method and using it to create different objects. You have also learned how to implement additional features such as raising errors and using the Enum declaration to enumerate all possible values for property settings. The use of error raising in class modules helps the programmer identify the source of errors. The use of Enum declaration enhances code readability.

In many cases, objects should also recognize events. The way to create events is explained. An example is also provided to show how an event is created in the class module and used in another (form) module. The implementation of events can be particularly useful for objects in which additional handling can best be done by code by the programmer who uses the objects.

We have also discussed treating the form as a class. Forms are indeed objects with visual elements. Thus, when you need an object with a visible window, you can treat the form as such. However, if you intend for the object to be reused by other projects, it is best that a class module be used to invoke the form. We have developed a generalized "search engine" as an example to illustrate how to implement the idea. Such a design makes it possible to compile the object (class) into an ActiveX DLL, a topic discussed in Chapter 14.

The focal point of object-oriented programming is encapsulation. Data and code within the module should be completely isolated from other modules. The only parts that can be exposed to the "outside world" are the object's properties, methods, and events. When you are developing a class, the importance of encapsulation cannot be overemphasized. Take care not to make direct reference to any objects outside the module.

Finally, we have also shown how the Class Builder Utility add-in program can be used to create a code template for a class module. The utility helps relieve you from having to handle the "mechanical" aspect of coding the property procedures and the declarations of methods and events. However, you are still the one to design and implement all the required features for the needed object.

Visual Basic Explorer

12-1. Timing of Creation and Destruction of an Object. Add a class module to a new form. Then place the following code in the class module:

```
Option Explicit

Private Sub Class_Initialize()
    Debug.Print "Object initialized"
End Sub

Private Sub Class_Terminate()
    Debug.Print "Object destroyed"
End Sub
```

And then place the following code in the code in the form:

```
Option Explicit

Private Sub Form_Click()
Dim MyObject As Class1
    Set MyObject = New Class1
End Sub
```

Run the project and click the form. Look for the messages in the immediate window. Are both "Object initialized" and "Object destroyed" messages displayed? Objects are destroyed when their associated variables are out of scope.

12-2. Timing of Creation and Destruction of an Object. (continued from 12-1). Revise the code in the form in the preceding exercise as follows:

```
Option Explicit
Dim MyObject As Class1
Private Sub Form_Click()
    Set MyObject = New Class1
End Sub
```

(Notice the location of the object variable declaration.)

Run the project and click the form. Look for the messages in the immediate window. Are both "Object initialized" and "Object destroyed" messages displayed? You should see only the "Object initialized" message.

Click the form's Close (x) button. Do you see the "Object destroyed" message? This reaffirms that objects are destroyed when their associated variables are out of scope.

12-3. Timing of Creation and Destruction of an Object. (continued from 12-2). Revise the code in the form in the preceding exercise as follows:

```
Option Explicit
Dim MyObject As Class1
Private Sub Form_Click()
    Set MyObject = New Class1
    Set MyObject = New Class1
End Sub
```

Run the project and click the form. Look for the messages in the immediate window. How many "Object initialized" and "Object destroyed" messages are displayed? You should see two "Object initialized" messages but only one "Object destroyed" message. What does this mean? The first object is destroyed when its associated object variable is associated with another object.

Click the form's Close (x) button. Do you see the "Object destroyed" message? The second object is destroyed. Again, objects are destroyed when their associated variables are out of scope.

12-4. Timing of Creation and Destruction of the Form Object. (continued from 12-3). Add a new form (Form2) to the preceding exercise. Place the following code in Form2:

```
Option Explicit
Private Sub Form_Initialize()
    Debug.Print "Form2 initialized"
End Sub
Private Sub Form_Terminate()
    Debug.Print "Form2 destroyed"
End Sub
```

Go back to Form1. Add a new command button in Form1. Name the control cmdShow and set its Caption property to "Show." Add the following code:

```
Private Sub cmdShow_Click()
Dim MyForm As Form2
    Set MyForm = New Form2
End Sub
```

Run the form and click the button. Look for the messages in the immediate window. Are both "Form initialized" and "Form destroyed" messages displayed? So far, objects are destroyed when they go out of scope.

12-5. Timing of Creation and Destruction of the Form Object. (continued from 12-4). Modify the code in Form1 as follows:

```
Private Sub cmdShow_Click()
Dim MyForm As Form2
    Set MyForm = New Form2
    MyForm.Show
End Sub
```

Run the form and click the button. Look for the messages in the immediate window. Are both "Form initialized" and "Form destroyed" messages displayed? You should see only the "Form initialized" message. The object variable MyForm goes out of scope, but the form object is not destroyed.

Click Form2's Close (x) button. Do you see the "Form destroyed" message? Once it is shown or loaded, the form object is destroyed only after it is unloaded.

12-6. Timing of Creation and Destruction of the Form Object. (continued from 12-5). Modify the code in the preceding exercise as follows:

```
Private Sub cmdShow_Click()
Dim MyForm As Form2
    Set MyForm = New Form2
    Load MyForm
End Sub
```

Run the form and click the button. Look for the messages in the immediate window. Are both "Form initialized" and "Form destroyed" messages displayed? You should see only the "Form initialized" message.

Click the Close (x) button on Form1. Although the form disappears, your program continues to run. (You can verify this by checking the toolbar. The Run icon is disabled, but the End icon is enabled.) Why? Form2 continues to run. Click the End icon to end the project. The user cannot unload or destroy an invisible form.

What are your conclusions after these six explorer exercises? Does it pay to explicitly unload a form and set an object to Nothing?

12-7. A Way to Inform What Happens in Another Form. Add a new form (Form2) to a new project. Draw a command button on this form (Form2). Name the button cmdClick and set its Caption property to "Click." Place the following code in this form:

```
Option Explicit
Event ActionOccurred()
```

```
Private Sub cmdClick_Click()
    RaiseEvent ActionOccurred
End Sub
```

Go back to Form1. Draw a command button on the form. Name the button cmdShow and set its Caption property to "Show Form2." Then place the following code in this form:

```
Option Explicit
Dim WithEvents ActionForm As Form2

Private Sub ActionForm_ActionOccurred()
    MsgBox "Someone has clicked the Click button"
End Sub

Private Sub cmdShow_Click()
    Set ActionForm = New Form2
    ActionForm.Show
End Sub
```

Run the project. Click the "Show Form2" button. Then click the "Click" button in Form2. Each time you do so, you should see the "Someone has clicked the Click button" message.

See the use of this code arrangement? One form (Form1) can be used to monitor the activities in another form (Form2), which can inform the other of what happens by raising an event.

12-8. Beware of the Difference. (continued from 12-7). Add the following code to Form1 in the preceding exercise:

```
Private Sub Form_Click()
    Form2.Show
End Sub
```

Run the project. Click on Form1 (the form itself, not the "Show Form2" button). When Form2 appears, click its "Click" button. Do you see any message displayed? Why?

Click Form1 to set focus on Form1. Then click the "Show Form2" button to display another Form2. Click the "Click" button on the newly displayed form. Do you see a message? Alternate the focus between the two Form2's and click the "Click" button to confirm that one sends messages and the other does not.

How do you explain the difference? ActionForm is an object variable declared "WithEvents." Thus, it is capable of recognizing the event(s) raised from the object (Form2). Form2 as referenced in the preceding code refers to the form template. Because this variable is not declared "WithEvents," it cannot recognize the event. You cannot even see Form2 in Form1's object box in the code window. The ActionForm_Click procedure is associated with the object variable ActionForm, not with Form2.

12-9. What Comes Next? Enter the following code in a new project:

```
Option Explicit
Enum TestType
    Test1
    Test2
    Test3
End Enum

Private Sub Form_Click()
    Debug.Print Test1; Test2; Test3
End Sub
```

Run the project and click the form. What numbers do you see in the immediate window?

Change Test1 in the Enum block as follows:

```
Test1 = 1
```

Run the project and click the form again. This time what do you see?

Change the Enum block so that it will appear as follows:

```
Enum TestType
     Test1
     Test2 = 2
     Test3
End Enum
```

Run the project and click the form again. This time what do you see? What is your conclusion concerning the items not being assigned with a value?

Exercises

12-10. An Employee Class. Create an employee class module named clsEmployee that has the following properties:

Field (Property)	Type
SSN	Long
Name	String
HourlyRate	Double

It has a GrossPay method that computes the gross pay of the employee. The method requires the number of hours worked (Double) as the parameter.

In the form, draw a command button. Set its Caption property to "Compute." When the user clicks the button, your program will create an employee object named objEmployee. Set its SSN, Name, and HourlyRate properties to 123456789, John Smith, and 70, respectively. Then use its GrossPay method to compute the gross pay for working 50 hours in a week (overtime pay is 1.5 times of the regular rate). Use a message box to display the following message:

John Smith (employee number 123-45-6789) worked 50 hours and is paid $x,xxx

(Replace x,xxx with proper amount.)

12-11. A Depositor Class. Create a depositor class module. Name it clsDepositor. The class should have the following properties:

Properties	Type
AccountNumber	Long
Name	String
Balance	Currency (read-only)

It has two methods: Deposit and Withdraw. Both methods require one parameter (Amount) of the Currency type. Deposit adds the value of the parameter to Balance, while Withdraw subtracts the value of the parameter from Balance. If the amount to be withdrawn is greater than the Balance, the object should deny the withdrawal. In addition, an error with a description "NSF" should be raised.

Test and use the class in a new project as follows:

1. Draw a text box, two option buttons, and two command buttons on the form. The text box will be used to enter the amount of deposit or withdrawal. The two option buttons will be used to indicate whether the amount is a deposit or withdrawal. One command button will have the caption "Process Transaction." When it is clicked, the

amount in the text box will be processed either by the Deposit method or Withdraw method, depending on the option button selected. The other command button will have the caption "Quit." When this button is clicked, your program quits.

2. The object's Account Number and Name properties should be set to 1111 and Jane Doe, respectively. The initial balance is zero.
3. When the program runs, the user can enter an amount in the text box, select the "proper" option button, and then click the Process command button. After the amount is processed, the balance is displayed in a message box and the text box is cleared. When the object raises the NSF error, your program should display an error message and deny the transaction. (Do not terminate the program. Handle the error with an error handler.)

12-12. A Student Class. Create a Student class that has the following properties:

Property	Type	Description
Number	Long	Student ID number
Name	String	Student name
CourseCount	Long	Returns the number of courses enrolled; read-only

The number and name properties can be set only once in the duration of the object. Attempts to set these properties more than once should cause a "Property already set" error.

The class has three methods:

- The Enroll method takes Course ID as a parameter and adds the Course ID to the Courses (array) property. (*Hint:* Use ReDim Preserve to increase the size of the array to accommodate the new course.) An attempt to enroll a course already in the course list will raise an error.
- The Drop method removes a course from the Courses list. An attempt to remove a course not already in the list will raise an error.
- The Courses method returns a string array that contains the courses in which the student has enrolled.

On the form, draw a text box and three command buttons. The text box (with proper label) will be used to enter the course ID. One command button has the caption "Enroll." When it is clicked, the course ID in the text box will be added to the student's course list. Another command button has the caption "Drop." When it is clicked, the course ID indicated in the text box will be removed from the course list. Finally, the third command button has the caption "Show." When it is clicked, the courses in which the student has enrolled will be displayed in a message box.

The Number and Name properties will be set to 123456789 and "John Doe," respectively, by code as soon as the project starts.

12-13. A Student Class with Database Tables. Modify the preceding exercise so that when the Number property is set for the Student object, the student name and the courses enrolled are retrieved from the Students database, which contains two tables: Students and StudentCourse Tables.

The Students table has the following fields:

Field	Description
RecordNo	Record number; auto number; primary key
Number	Student ID number (SSN), Long
Name	Student name, String

The StudentCourse table has the following fields:

Field	Description
Number	Student ID Number (SSN), Long
Course	Course ID (e.g., Acct5335-501)

The form that uses the Student object has the following:

- A text box (with a proper label) for the user to enter the student number
- A label to display the student name (with a proper label)
- A text box to enter/display a course ID
- A list box to display the courses enrolled
- A command button to enroll a new course
- A command button to drop a course
- A command button to quit the application

When your program runs, as soon as the user leaves the Student Number field (except for going to the list box or the Quit button), the program sets the Number property of the Student object, which then will proceed to set all other pertinent properties or internal member variable(s) (Courses and CourseCount). (*Hint:* Add a routine in the class module to retrieve the student enrollment data. Then use the resulting recordset to set mCourseCount and the mCourses array).

A student must already exist before he or she can enroll in or drop a course. The student name and courses enrolled in should be displayed in the controls described previously. Note that the Enroll and Drop methods should be modified to take care of adding records to and deleting records from the StudentCourse table when called.

12-14. **Revisiting the Fixed Asset Class.** Modify the FixedAsset class in the text as follows:

- Add an additional (accounting) depreciation method called the double declining balance method so that the DepreMethod will have three alternative settings (0, no depreciation; 1, straight line depreciation; and 2, double declining balance). This method is explained at the end of this exercise.
- Add the Depreciation (class) method and the CumulativeDepreciation method. Both methods will take Years as their parameter and return the current depreciation and the cumulative depreciation amount for the specified year(s).
- Add the DepreMethodChanged event. This event will be raised when the user tries to change the depreciation method for an existing asset; that is, the user is allowed to set the DepreMethod once. Any subsequent attempt to change the depreciation (accounting) method will cause this event to be raised. This event should have three parameters: OriginalMethod, NewMethod, and Cancel. The first two show the pertinent depreciation methods. The last parameter allows the user to cancel the change.

Use the following formula to compute the depreciation of the double declining balance method for a given year:

Depreciation = (2/N) * Current Net Book Value

Where N is the life of the asset in years and *Current Net Book Value* equals cost − cumulative depreciation

If the straight-line method on the current net book value results in a higher depreciation amount, the straight line method should be used. That is,

If Current net book value/Remaining life > Current net book value * (2/N), then Depreciation = Current net book value/Remaining life.

Test the class module by designing a user interface in the form that allows the user to enter/specify the asset's cost, life, years in use and the deprecation method. Use option buttons for depreciation methods. Each time an option button is clicked, the DepreMethod property is set. Clicking these buttons more than once should raise the DepreMethodChanged event. Your program should then warn the user of the change and ask if the user means to change. A No answer should cancel the change. When the user clicks the Compute command button, your program should show the current depreciation, cumulative deprecation, and book value in three textboxes, respectively.

12-15. Revisiting the Search Engine. Modify the Search Engine example in the text so that it will ensure that all properties must have been set before the Search method will attempt to search; that is, if any of these required properties has not been set, an error should be raised.

Then in the main form, design a visual interface for the user to specify the database name, the table name, the search field name, and the ID field name. This should involve one text box and three (3) combo boxes (with proper labels). The user can either enter the database name in the textbox (check for the Enter key in your program) or by clicking a command button with a caption, "Browse . . ." Once the database name is available, your program should populate the first combo box with the table names in the database. As soon as the user selects a table name, your program should populate the other two combo boxes with field names in the table. (*Hint:* Use the ADO connection's OpenSchema method to handle all of these. The form will look much neater if all these controls are placed within a frame.)

Then in a separate area of the same form, place another text box for ID (with a proper label). Place a command button by the text box. Set the button's caption to "Search." When the user clicks this command button, the SearchEngine should be created and properly set with the specified properties. The Search method should then be invoked, and its search result should be placed in the ID text box. The errors caused by not specifying all properties should be properly handled. (Test the program by not selecting data from some of the combo boxes.)

12-16. A Simulation Engine. Refer to Exercise 7-34. Modify the project so that the simulation process is done in an object. The visual interface in the form can then be used to accept input from the user and call the object.

12-17. A Sort Class with an Event. Create a Sort class module with two of your favorite sorting algorithms. The SortAlgorithm property allows the user (or programmer) to specify the sorting algorithm to use. The programmer should be able to specify the sorting algorithm by a named constant, such as sortBubble or sortQuick. One of these algorithms should be set as the default. The class has an Exec method that will carry out the sorting. This method takes an array as its parameter, which will be sorted. In both sorting routines, implement an event, called PercentChanged, which will be fired as the percentile of sort completion changes. The event should provide the following header template:

```
Private Sub Object_PercentChanged(Percent As Integer)
```

In a new form, draw two option buttons, two command buttons, a list box, and a label. The option buttons will be used to specify the sorting algorithm to use. One command button will have the caption "Generate." When it is clicked, 10,000 random numbers of the Long type will be generated. Another command button will have the caption "Sort." When it is clicked, it will invoke the sort object's Exec method to perform the sorting. The result will be displayed in the list box. As the sorting is in progress, the label should display the (estimated) percentage of completion.

12-18. A Data-Entry Server. Refer to Exercise 10-20, whose resulting project includes various Sub procedures to check for valid keys. Create a class module (call it EntryServer) that will include all these Subs at its Private procedures. The class module will provide a method,

VerifyKey, which takes ActiveControl and KeyAscii as its parameters and returns a Boolean value to indicate whether there is a problem with the key. A True value will indicate that the key is wrong. The wrong key will be suppressed in the method. All controls should have their Tag properties set according to the specifications in those exercises in Chapter 10.

Also include a ClearScreen method in this class module. The method should take a form as its parameter. All the text boxes, masked edit boxes, check boxes, and option buttons in the form should be cleared. All list boxes and combo boxes in the form should have their ListIndex properties set to −1. Also clear all selections if a list box allows multiselections because of its MultiSelect or Style setting.

Test the class module using a form with a visual interface that includes all text boxes and masked edit boxes needed to test each type of key. In addition, add a check box, two option buttons, a list box, and a combo box to test the ClearScreen method.

12-19. A Tic-Tac-Toe Game Object. Modify the Tic-Tac-Toe example in Chapter 9 so that the game board is an object (to be triggered from a class module). The object should allow the user to specify the back color, font size, and board size (a number for both the width and height). Also, provide the "Play" method to start the game.

Test the module by creating a Tic-Tac-Toe object and call its Play method from the main form.

12-20. A Progress Meter. Create a progress meter object that has two properties: Total and CurrentValue. Both are of the Long type. The Total property represents the total expected iterations of a process, whereas CurrentValue gives the current iteration number. The object will display the percentage of completion in a progress bar and in a label. It will also display the estimated time remaining. This object should also have a Cancel button, which will raise the CancelByUser event when clicked. Test the use of this object with Exercise 12-16. (*Hint:* Use a class module to work with the properties. Use a form to handle the required visual element.)

Projects

12-21. The Inventory Valuation Object. Develop a generalized inventory valuation class. The class will provide three different inventory valuation methods to compute the dollar value of the ending inventory for a product. The transactions of this product are kept in a database table described later.

The inventory valuation methods should be coded as methods of the object. These methods are as follows:

1. The *weighted average method,* which determines the ending inventory by using the following formulas:

   Weighted average cost = Total purchase costs/Total units purchased

   Ending inventory = Weighted average cost x units on hand

   where *Units on hand* represents total purchased units − total sold units.

2. The *FIFO (First-In First-Out) method,* which retains the unit costs of the most recent purchases. For example, if 1,000 units are on hand and the most recent purchases (in reverse chronological order) consist of 400 units @ $5 and 800 units @ $6, the ending inventory can be computed as follows:

   Ending inventory = 400 × 5 + 600 × 6 = 5,600

   Notice that only 600 units of the 800 units are used in the computation because there are only 1,000 units of inventory, which should include 400 of the most current purchase plus a quantity from the next most recent purchase to make the total equal to 1,000.

3. The *LIFO (Last-In First-Out) method,* which retains the unit costs of the oldest purchases. For example, if 1,000 units are on hand, the oldest purchases consist of (oldest first) 700 units @ $4 and 800 units @ $5. The ending inventory will be computed as follows:

   Ending inventory = $700 \times 4 + 300 \times 5 = 4{,}300$

The class will have five properties (set by the caller) that provide information on the product's transactions:

1. *DatabaseName:* the database name of the inventory file
2. *TableName:* the data table that contains the inventory information
3. *DateOfTrans:* the field name for the dates on which a purchase or sale is made
4. *Quantity:* the field name for the quantities of the inventory purchased or sold; a positive number represents a purchase; a negative number, a sale
5. *UnitCost:* the field name for the cost per unit if the transaction is a purchase; there should be no cost if the transaction is a sale

Note that items 3 through 5 must be field (column) names for item 2. Your class should include data validation code to verify that the settings for all properties are made before any of the methods can be called.

12-22. The Inventory Acquisition–Handling System. An inventory acquisition–handling system contains three classes: Vendor, Product, and Purchase.

The Vendor class has properties that correspond to data fields in the Vendors table of the Inventory database. These fields are as follows:

Field/Property	Type	Length
VendorID	Long	5 digits
Name	String	32 characters
Address	String	32 characters
State	String	2 characters
Zip	Long	5 or 9 digits
ContactName	String	24 characters
ContactPhone	Currency	10 digits

The primary key of the table is VendorID.

The Vendor class has two methods: GetVendor and SaveVendor. Both methods take VendorID as the parameter. The GetVendor method will retrieve the vendor using the VendorID parameter to look for the record. If the record is found, the method will return a recordset containing the record. In addition, it will set the properties of the object to the value of the fields. If the record is not found, it will return an empty recordset and clear the property setting.

The SaveVendor method will check whether VendorID exists in the Vendors table. If so, the corresponding record is updated; otherwise, a new record is added to the table.

The Product class has properties that correspond to data fields in the Products table of the Inventory database. These fields are as follows:

Field/Property	Type	Length
ProductID	String	5 characters
ProductName	String	25 characters
Description	String	32 characters
VendorID	Long	5 digits

The primary key of the Products table is ProductID.

The product class has two methods: GetProduct and SaveProduct. Both methods take ProductID as the parameter and work in exactly the same manner as the two methods for the Vendor class.

Finally, the Purchase class has properties that correspond to data fields in the Transactions table in the Inventory database. These data fields are as follows:

Field/Property	Type	Length
Date	Date/Time	MM/DD/YYYY
ProductID	String	5 characters
Quantity	Long	Up to 6 digits
UnitCost	Currency	6 digits (including two decimal places)
VendorID	Long	5 digits

The Purchase class has a SavePurchase method that can be used to save a purchase transaction.

Required: Design a project as follows:

- Have a data-entry screen to enter, edit, and save vendors. The form will use the Vendor object but is not a visual part of the object.
- Have a data-entry screen to enter, edit, and save products. The form will use the Product object but is not a visual part of the object.
- Have a data-entry screen to enter and save the purchase transaction. This form will use the Purchase class to save the entry but is not a part of the Purchase object.
- Include and use the generalized Search Engine as illustrated in the text to help identify/look up the VendorID and ProductID in the data-entry screens where the need is present.
- Implement all necessary checking for data-entry errors.

13 Selected Topics in Input and Output

This chapter considers a few selected topics in input and output. Output media can be classified into those that are invisible to human eyes (e.g., disks or tapes, which are termed secondary storage) and those that are visible (e.g., the screen or printer). This chapter focuses on the visible output. Most visible output is in the form of tables and reports, which also tend to contain large amount of information structured around a few (or quite a few) attributes of various entities or activities. A control with grid capabilities is most suitable for displaying this type of output on screen. More specifically, we discuss the use of Microsoft Hierarchical FlexGrid (HFG) for such purposes.

Often, tables and reports are also printed on paper. In VB, there are several ways to print output on the printer. Among these, the most flexible approach is to use the Printer object, which can even conveniently be used to print pictures. We begin this chapter with a look into this object.

For input, many data-entry applications call for multiple lines of input of the same type. For example, a sales order may require scores of different products. A journal entry may contain several debit and/or credit accounts and amounts. Again, the HFG control appears ideal for this type of data-entry application. However, this control is limited in its capability in accepting keyboard input. Therefore, you will need to add code to handle the keyboard for it to work properly. This chapter shows how the HFG can be programmed to accept input from the keyboard.

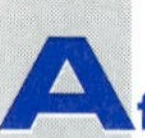

After completing this chapter, you should be able to:

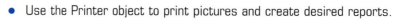

- Use the Printer object to print pictures and create desired reports.
- Use the MS HFG to display tables and reports.
- Program the HFG to accept keyboard input for data entry purposes.

13.1 Using the Printer Object

VB provides the Printer object to handle output to the printer. In Chapter 5, "Decision," you learned how to use the Print method to print text onto a printer. You can think of the Printer object as a sheet of paper on which you can draw graphs, print pictures, and print texts. You can go anywhere back and forth on the sheet to perform whatever output you desire until you use the ***EndDoc method*** to eject the page or the ***NewPage method*** to move to another sheet of paper.

Drawing a graph on the Printer object is no different than drawing a graph on a form or picture box. Drawing graphics is discussed in Appendix B, "Graphics, Animation, Drag and Drop." Here, we focus our discussion on printing pictures and texts. In this section, we use several examples to show how to use the object. We begin with a look at a few selected properties.

Selected Printer Properties

The Printer object has many properties. Before we show the examples, let's briefly look at a few selected properties, which are listed in the following table.

Property	Use
CurrentX	Sets or returns horizontal position
CurrentY	Sets or returns vertical position
Orientation	Sets or returns how output will be oriented: portrait or landscape
Page	Returns current page number
Font	Sets or returns the font; font also can be an object, which contains several properties

You have seen how CurrentX and CurrentY can be used to set the coordinate for the starting print position. In one of the examples here, we further illustrate their uses. The ***Orientation property*** can be used to set the orientation of the output. The Portrait orientation orients output vertically with the longer side of the sheet, whereas the landscape orientation orients output horizontally, as illustrated here:

The Portrait orientation prints a sheet this way.	The Landscape orientation prints the sheet this way.

The ***Page property*** keeps track of the page count of the "current document." As you start printing a document, the page property begins with one. Each time you advance the page by the NewPage method, the page count is increased by one until the EndDoc method is used. Afterward, the page count begins with one again.

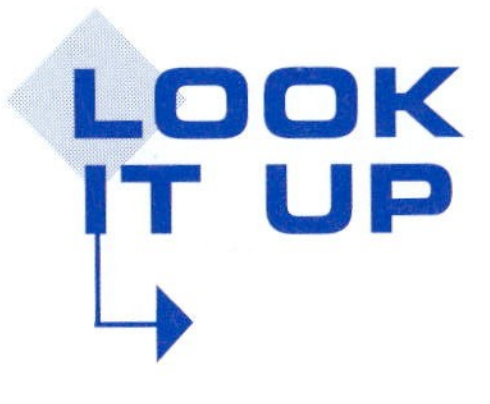

Use the keyword "Printer Object" (Visual Basic Reference) to search the Index tab of the online Help file. Its Properties link shows many properties that can be of interest to you. Some of them are discussed later in this chapter. The following properties should interest you: Copies, Count, Fonts, FontCount, and FontSize. Many additional properties pertain to drawing graphics. Browse those properties when you study Appendix B.

Setting the Printer Font

The Printer object has the Font object (property) that contains several properties, including Name, Size, Underline, and Bold. These are summarized in the following table.

Property	Type	Description
Name	String	A string giving the name of the font (e.g., Courier)
Size	Integer	A value giving the size of the font (e.g., 10)
UnderLine	Boolean	A value indicating whether a string is underlined
Bold	Boolean	A value indicating whether a string is boldfaced

All these properties are both read and write; that is, their settings can be set or returned. For example, the following code will display the current font in use and replace it with the Courier font:

```
MsgBox "The current font is " & Printer.Font.Name
Printer.Font.Name = "Courier"
```

The Printer object also has the Fonts property, which contains the names of all available fonts. The FontCount property gives the number of available fonts. All these properties together can be used to allow the user to set the desired font.

Using Printer Fonts: An Illustration. To illustrate, consider the user interface in Figure 13.1.

FIGURE 13.1
A User Interface for Printer Font Selection

Here is a user interface that will allow the user to set the Printer font and experiment with the output.

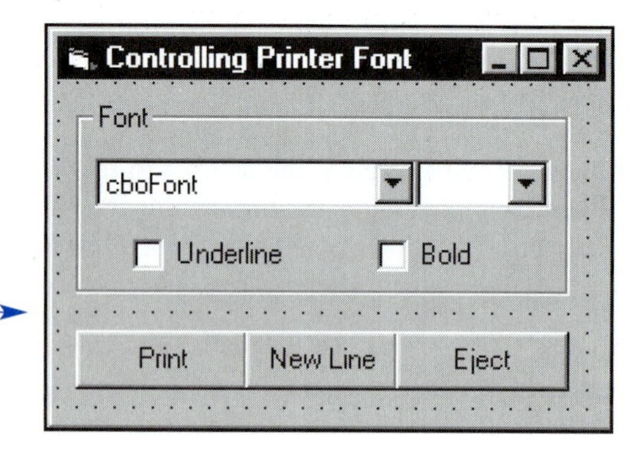

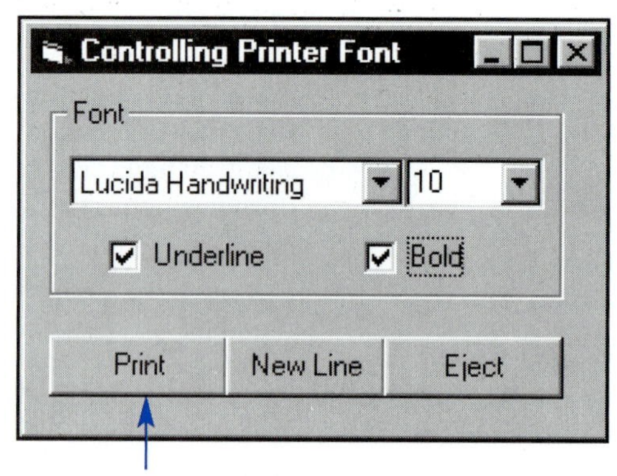

If you make the selection as shown above and click the Print button, the Printer will print the following:

Lucida Handwriting 10 Underlined Bold

The following table provides a list of selected properties of the controls involved in coding the project.

Control	Property	Setting	Remark
Combo box	Name	cboFont	To display available fonts and for the user to
	Style	2-Dropdown List	specify the font to use
Combo box	Name	cboSize	For the user to specify font size
Check box	Name	chkUnderLine	For the user to specify whether to underline
	Caption	UnderLine	
Check box	Name	chkBold	For the user to specify whether to use
	Caption	Bold	Bold font
Command button	Name	cmdPrint	To print the current font
	Caption	Print	
Command button	Name	cmdNewLine	To move to a new line
	Caption	New Line	

Control	Property	Setting	Remark
Command button	Name	cmdEject	To finish the document
	Caption	Eject	

We would like the combo box (on the left for font) to be populated with all the available printer fonts as soon as the program starts. The user can then select various combinations of font name, size, underline, and bold settings. When he or she clicks the Print button, the program will print the selected property settings with the same settings. The output will continue on the same line until the user clicks the New Line button. Finally, when the user clicks the Eject button, the sheet is actually printed. Ready?

Populating the Font Combo Box. The following code will populate the combo box cboFont with all the available printer fonts:

```
Dim I As Integer
    For I = 0 To Printer.FontCount - 1
        cboFont.AddItem Printer.Fonts(I)
    Next I
```

As you can see, the available fonts are enumerated with a For loop whose counter parameter is set from 0 to FontCount - 1. The ***Fonts property*** gives the names of the available fonts and is indexed for that range. Note that the printer can only print a font that is available in the driver. You should not allow the user to enter a font not listed in the combo box. Thus, you should set the combo box's Style property to 2 (Dropdown List) as shown in the preceding table.

You can set the font to any "reasonable" size. So, we will populate the combo box for size (cboSize) in the range of 8 to 24 (even numbers only) as follows:

```
For I = 8 To 24 Step 2
    cboSize.AddItem I
Next I
```

The user may rather use a different size than the ones given in the combo box. Thus, you should set the combo box's Style property to its default setting, 0 (Dropdown Combo).

These two combo boxes should be populated as soon as the program starts. In addition, to prevent errors, you may want to set default selections for both the name and size. The complete code to populate the font combo boxes is shown as follows:

```
Private Sub Form_Load()
Dim I As Integer
    'Populate cboFont with available fonts
    For I = 0 To Printer.FontCount - 1
        cboFont.AddItem Printer.Fonts(I)
    Next I
    cboFont.ListIndex = 0 'Set default font to the first
    For I = 8 To 24 Step 2
        cboSize.AddItem I
    Next I
    cboSize.ListIndex = 1 'Set size to 10
End Sub
```

Setting the Printer Font. As shown previously, to set the font for the printer, assign the printer's font name with the desired font. Thus, the following code will set the printer's font and size to those in the combo boxes cboFont and cboSize:

```
Printer.Print "";
Printer.Font.Name = cboFont.Text
Printer.Font.Size = cboSize.Text
```

Notice there is a Printer.Print " " statement, which actually prints nothing. The statement is needed for the first time for the font change to take effect. (Think of the first Print statement as one that opens the object.)

Printing Font Settings. When the Print button is clicked, your program should first set the font (using the code shown above) and proceed to print the settings. The procedure can appear as follows:

```
Private Sub cmdPrint_Click()
    With Printer
        Printer.Print "";
        .Font.Name = cboFont.Text 'set font name
        .Font.Size = cboSize.Text 'Set font size
        'Print font name and size
        Printer.Print cboFont.Text; cboSize.Text;
        If chkBold.Value = vbChecked Then
        'If "Bond" is checked, then print "Bond" in Bold
            .Font.Bold = True
            Printer.Print "Bold";
        Else
             .Font.Bold = False
        End If
        If chkUnderline = vbChecked Then
            'If "Underline" is checked, then print "Underline"
            underlined
            .Font.Underline = True
            Printer.Print "Underlined";
        Else
            .Font.Underline = False
        End If
        Printer.Print "  "; 'leave a few spaces between settings
    End With
End Sub
```

The preceding procedure first sets the font's name and size based on the values given in the proper combo boxes. Then it proceeds to print the settings using the Print method. Note how the Bold and Underline properties are set. Both are of the Boolean type and are turned on and off by the values True and False.

Notice also that all Print statements end with a semicolon (;). Recall that a semicolon informs the object (Printer) to stay at the same position after printing so that the next printing operation will continue on the same line, instead of on a new line.

You may have noticed that even within the "With Printer" block, the Print method is qualified by the Printer object (i.e., Printer.Print). This is necessary; otherwise, you will encounter a syntax error. Some methods must be qualified by the object even within the With block. The Print method belongs to this group.

New Line and Eject. As you may recall, to conclude a print line so that the next printing operation will start with a new line, the Print statement should conclude with the data to be printed and without a semicolon. Thus, the code to handle the New Line click button appears as follows:

```
Private Sub cmdNewLine_Click()
    Printer.Print ""
End Sub
```

When the user clicks the Eject button (named cmdEject), the printing operation logically ends. Thus, you will use the EndDoc method to force the actual printing:

```
Private Sub cmdEject_Click()
    Printer.EndDoc 'Eject
End Sub
```

Printing a Picture

You can use the ***PaintPicture method*** to print a picture in an object such as the Printer or a picture box. The PaintPicture method has the following syntax:

```
object.PaintPicture picture, x1, y1, width1, height1, _
    x2, y2, width2, height2
```

where *object* = an object such as the Printer object

Picture = the picture to be printed (e.g., picCheck.Picture)

x1, y1 = the coordinate to start printing the picture (e.g., 0, 0 will print the picture starting from the upper-left corner of the object [sheet])

width1, height1 = the width and height of the region in the sheet to print the picture

x2, y2 = the upper-left corner of the picture to "clip" and print (e.g., 0, 0 [default] will print the picture starting from its upper-left corner)

width2, height2 = the width and height of the picture region to "clip" and print

For example, the following code will print the upper-left quarter of the picture in picCheck on the upper-left corner of the sheet:

```
Printer.PaintPicture picCheck.Picture, 0, 0,,, _
  0, 0, picCheck.Width / 2, picCheck.Height / 2
```

Printing a Picture Step by Step. To illustrate, let's work with an example step by step. This example project will print a check (whose width and height will be twice that of the check that appears on the screen) with the landscape orientation at the center of the sheet. Here are the steps:

1. Start a new project.
2. Draw a picture box on the form. So that the shape of the picture box will look like a check, make sure it is drawn such that its width is at least twice as long as its height. Name the control picCheck.
3. Set the Picture property of picCheck to Check.wmf, which is located in the following folder: Microsoft Visual Studio\Common\Graphics\Metafile\Business.
4. Draw a command button on the form. Name it cmdPrint and set its Caption property to "Print." The completed visual interface should look like the graph shown in Figure 13.2.
5. Enter the following code:

```
Option Explicit
Private Sub cmdPrint_Click()
    With Printer
        .Orientation = vbPRORLandscape
        .PaintPicture picCheck.Picture, _
          (.ScaleWidth - 2 * picCheck.Width) / 2, _
          (.ScaleHeight - 2 * picCheck.Height) / 2, _
          2 * picCheck.Width, 2 * picCheck.Height
        .EndDoc
    End With
End Sub
```

Run the program and click the Print button. You should see a check picture on the sheet printed in Landscape orientation.

Notice that the last four parameters of the PaintPicture method are omitted. This will result in the entire source picture being printed on the sheet. Notice also that the Printer's Orientation property is assigned a value vbPRORLandscape (2) to effect the Landscape orientation. The default setting is vbPRORPortrait (1).

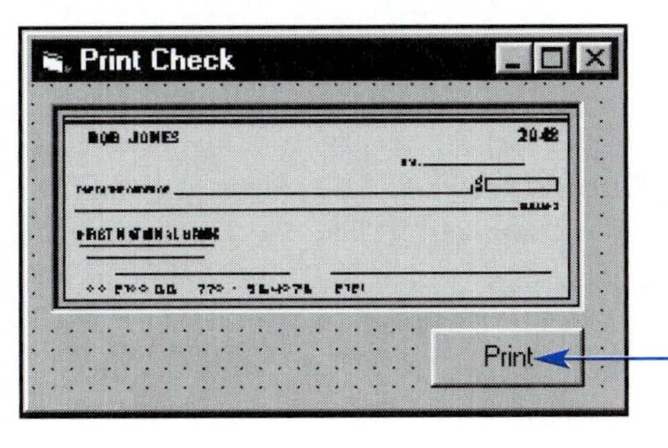

FIGURE 13.2
The Check Picture to Be Printed

When the user clicks the Print button, the code in the cmdPrint event procedure will print a hard copy of this check. Both the width and height will be twice in measurement as shown here.

Printing Mailing Labels

Writing code to print hard copies takes a lot of detailed design and computation. To illustrate, let's design a project to print mailing labels using the Avery 5160 Laser labels. The "form" contains 30 mailing labels per sheet (10 labels per column; 3 per row). Each label is 1" × 2 ⅝" in dimension. There is a ⅛" horizontal gap but no vertical gap between the labels. The first row starts ½" from the top and the last row is ½" from the bottom of the sheet. (See the layout in Figure 13.3.)

The names and addresses for the mailing labels are contained in a recordset. Each record in the recordset includes name, address, city, state, and zip code. A sample label appears in Figure 13.3.

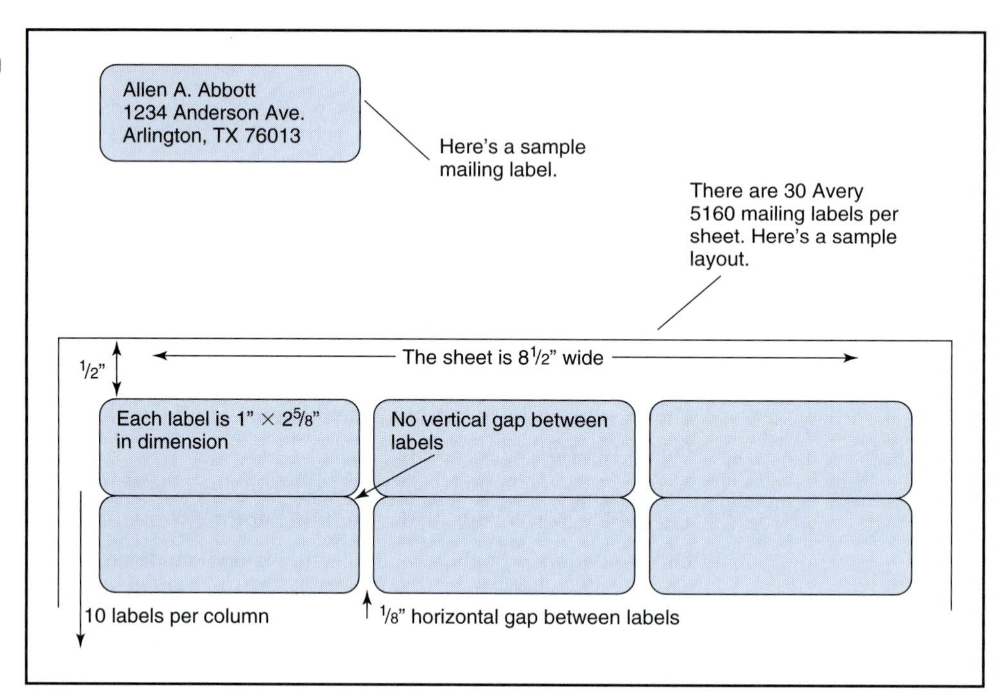

FIGURE 13.3
Layout of the Avery 5160 Laser Labels

Printing One Label. Let's consider how one label can be printed. Assume the upper-left corner of the label has been computed to be at a coordinate (x, y). Also assume the name of the recordset containing the address is rsContact. Then, the first line (name) of the mailing label can be printed with the following code:

```
With rsContact
    Printer.CurrentY = Y
    Printer.CurrentX = X
    Printer.Print !Name
End With
```

What about the second and third lines? Each will need to start at the same X horizontal position but one line below. Thus, the next two lines can be printed as follows:

```
Printer.CurrentX = X 'Left margin of current column
Printer.Print !Address
Printer.CurrentX = X 'Left margin of current column
Printer.Print Trim$(!City) & ", " & !State & " " & !ZipCode
```

These statements should be placed above the End With statement in the preceding "With rsContact" block.

Determining the Coordinate for the Label to Print. The question, then, is "How can X and Y be computed?" The coordinate depends on the label count in the sheet. For example, the first label will start at (0,0), assuming no position adjustment is needed. Now, suppose that we would like to print labels columnwise; that is, we will print the first 10 addresses on the first column, then the next 10 on the second column, and so on. The second label will start at one label lower; that is, (1,0) label position. The eleventh label will start at the top of the second column; that is, ((0,1) label position).

Let *LabelNo* = the label count in a sheet (zero based, i.e., 0 for the first label)

LabelHeight, LabelWidth = the dimension of the label

Then X and Y can be computed as follows:

```
Col = Int(LabelNo / 10) 'Col of the label
Row = LabelNo Mod 10  'Row of the label
'Compute current label horizontal position
X = Col * LabelWidth + XAdj
'Compute current label vertical position
Y = Row * LabelHeight + YAdj
```

This routine first computes the column and row of the current label based on the label count in the sheet. Each column has 10 labels. Thus, the formula Int(LabelNo/10) should give the column position of the label (again, zero based). In addition, the formula LabelNo Mod 10 should give the row position (zero based). Then, X (Y) is computed by multiplying the Col (Row) by LabelWidth (LabelHeight) value plus an adjustment value, XAdj (YAd;).

If you prefer to print mailing labels row by row, use the following formulas to compute Row and Column:

```
Row = Int(LabelNo / 3)
Col = LabelNo Mod 3
```

Setting Values for Some Variables. In the preceding computation, we take the variables LabelNo, LabelWidth, and LabelHeight as given. How are these values obtained?

In the original description, we stated that each label is 1" × $2\frac{5}{8}$". However, there is a $\frac{1}{8}$" horizontal gap. Thus, the width for each label is in effect $2\frac{3}{4}$". The default scale of the printer is twips. There are 1440 twips in 1 inch. Thus, LabelWidth and LabelHeight can be computed as follows:

```
LabelHeight = 1440
LabelWidth = 2.75 * 1440
```

Handling Multiple Pages. Recall that in the previous discussion, LabelNo is defined as "the label count *in a sheet.*" Each sheet has 30 labels. What if the number of labels exceeds 30? We can use another variable to perform the overall count and take the remainder of this variable divided by 30. That is, if we let Count represent the overall label count (again, zero based), then LabelNo can be computed by the following formula:

```
LabelNo = Count Mod 30
```

If the count exceeds 30, each time it reaches the multiple of 30, a new sheet will need to be used. We can use the NewPage method to effect this:

```
Count = Count + 1
If (Count Mod 30) = 0 Then
    Printer.NewPage 'Print on a new sheet
End If
```

Computing the Position for the First Mailing Label. In the preceding formulas, both X and Y are adjusted by an adjustment value. Why is there the need for the adjustment, and how should each be computed?

The adjustment is needed because of the difference in the physical margin of the sheet and printable margin of the printer. Consider the vertical margin. The first label margin starts ½" from the top of the sheet. However, the printable area of the printer starts much closer to the top. The height of the entire sheet is measured by the Printer object's Height property, whereas the printable height is represented by the ScaleHeight property.

Keep in mind that the CurrentX and CurrentY properties that are used to set the starting print position are associated with the printable area. That is, setting the two properties at (0,0) will start the printing at beginning of the printable area, not the sheet's upper-left corner of the first mailing label. The relation among the sheet, the first label, and CurrentY at 0 is depicted in Figure 13.4.

FIGURE 13.4
A Sketch of Various Vertical Positions from the Sheet Top

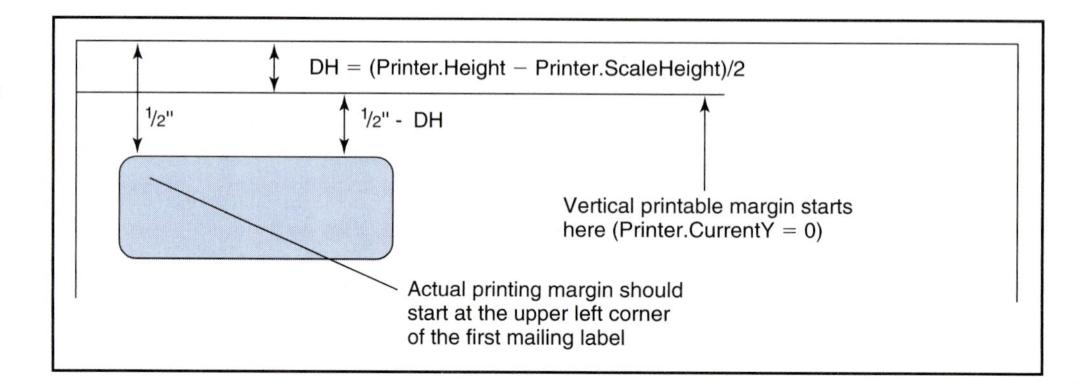

As you can see from the figure, the distance between the sheet top and the printable area is measured by the following formula:

DH = (Printer.Height – Printer.ScaleHeight)/2

The formula is derived from the fact that the difference between the sheet and printable area is equally divided between the top and bottom of the sheet. The actual printing margin, however, should start ½" from the top. Thus, the CurrentY property at 0 is not the proper starting position. The first label actually is located vertically at ½" – DH from the printable margin (see Figure 13.4). Recall that 1 inch equals 1440 twips. Thus, the proper expression for the starting vertical label margin should be as follows:

720 - (Printer.Height - Printer.ScaleHeight)/2

However, you will not start to print the address at this position because it is too close to the label margin. Assume that you would rather start one print line from the label margin. You can compute YAdj as follows:

```
YAdj= 720 - (Printer.Height - Printer.ScaleHeight) / 2 + _
    Printer.TextHeight("H")
```

As explained in Chapter 6, "Input, Output, and Procedures," the TextHeight method returns the Height of the text string.

With the same reasoning, you can develop the formula for XAdj. The left column labels are $3/16$" from the sheet's left margin. Thus, the formula for XAdj can be written as follows:

```
XAdj = 270 - (Printer.Width - Printer.ScaleWidth) / 2 + _
    Printer.TextWidth("H")
```

You may be tempted to adjust the printable area of the Printer object by setting the ScaleWidth and ScaleHeight property. For example, if the first label is ½" from the top, can we set the ScaleHeight property using the following formula?

```
Printer.ScaleHeight = Printer.Height / 2 - 720
```

No. The physical printable area remains the same. The preceding statement tells the computer to change the measuring scale so that the printable area has the number of units as computed. That is, if you assign 1,000 to the ScaleHeight property, the entire printable area will have 1,000 units. Assigning 500 to the CurrentY property will start the printing half way from the top.

Putting Everything Together. Now, we have considered all the important details. Let's put everything together. The routine to print one mailing label can be written as a Sub procedure. As indicated, the source data come from a recordset. Thus, the header of the Sub procedure can appear as follows:

```
Sub Print1Label(rsContact As ADODB.Recordset)
```

We need to preserve the value for Count even after the procedure finishes printing a mailing label. In addition, the label's dimension as well as the adjustment values to X and Y should be computed only once. Thus, we should declare these variables as Static:

```
Static Count As Long
Static LabelHeight As Single
Static LabelWidth As Single
Static XAdj As Single
Static YAdj As Single
```

Other variables can be declared as follows:

```
Dim LabelNo As Integer
Dim Row As Integer
Dim Col As Integer
Dim X As Single
```

When this procedure is called the first time, the label's dimension and the adjustment values should be computed. We should also set the font for the printer. The code for this preparatory activity appears as follows:

```
If Count = 0 Then
   'If this is the first label, then
   'SetFont
   Printer.Print "";
   Printer.Font.Name = "Times New Roman"
   Printer.Font.Size = "10"
   ' Compute Label height and width
   LabelHeight = 1440
   LabelWidth = 2.75 * 1440 'Set to 2 3/4"
   'Compute the horizontal and vertical margin for labels
     XAdj = 270 - (Printer.Width - Printer.ScaleWidth) / 2 + _
       Printer.TextWidth("H")
     YAdj= 720 - (Printer.Height - Printer.ScaleHeight) / 2 + _
       Printer.TextHeight("H")
End If
```

The complete Print1Label procedure appears as follows:

```
Sub Print1Label(rsContact As ADODB.Recordset)
Static Count As Long
Static LabelHeight As Single
Static LabelWidth As Single
Static XAdj As Single
Static YAdj As Single
Dim LabelNo As Integer
Dim Row As Integer
Dim Col As Integer
Dim X As Single
    If Count = 0 Then
    'If this the first label, then
        'SetFont
        Printer.Print "";
```

```
            Printer.Font.Name = "Times New Roman"
            Printer.Font.Size = "10"
            ' Set the desired font and compute Label height and width
            LabelHeight = 1440
            LabelWidth = 2.75 * 1440 'Set to 2 3/4"
            XAdj = 270 - (Printer.Width - Printer.ScaleWidth) / 2 + _
              Printer.TextWidth("H")
            YAdj= 720 - (Printer.Height - Printer.ScaleHeight) / 2 + _
            Printer.TextHeight("H")
        End If
        'Find the (row, col) position for the current label
        LabelNo = Count Mod 30
        Col = Int(LabelNo / 10)
        Row = LabelNo Mod 10
        'Compute current label vertical position
        Printer.CurrentY = Row * LabelHeight + YAdj 'This is Y
        'Compute current label horizontal position
        X = Col * LabelWidth + Xadj
        With rsContact
            Printer.CurrentX = X
            Printer.Print !Name
            Printer.CurrentX = X 'Left margin of current column
            Printer.Print !Address
            Printer.CurrentX = X 'Left margin of current column
            Printer.Print Trim$(!City) & ", " & !State & " " & !ZipCode
        End With
        Count = Count + 1 'Update label count
        If (Count Mod 30) = 0 Then
            Printer.NewPage 'start a new sheet
        End If
    End Sub
```

Using the Procedure. To use the preceding procedure, you can open an ADO recordset. Make sure that the recordset contains the fields Name, Address, City, State, and ZipCode. Then the following loop can be used to call the procedure and print the content of the recordset:

```
rsContact.MoveFirst
Do Until rsContact.EOF
    Print1Label rsContact
    rsContact.MoveNext
Loop
Printer.EndDoc
```

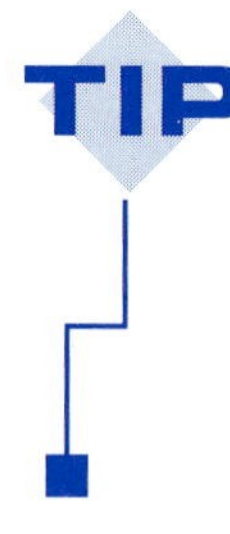

If your database table does not contain the exact field names as expected by the Print1Label Sub procedure, you can still construct a recordset with those names by using the As keyword in the SQL as long as the table has the fields. For example, assume you have an Employee table that has these fields: EmpName, Addr, City, State, and ZipCode. The following SQL should produce the expected field names:

```
SQL = "Select EmpName As Name, Addr As Address, City, State," & _
"ZipCode From Employee"
```

Additional Remarks. The mailing label printing procedure can be improved in several respects:

- The routine will print mailing labels column by column. A Tip box shows the formula to compute the label positions to print row by row. Actually, the routine can be written to allow the user to choose between the two ways of printing.
- For simplicity, we use Times New Roman 10 to print the mailing labels. The routine can be modified to allow the user to make his or her own choice of font.

- In computing the starting printing position for the first mailing label (XAdj and YAdj), we arbitrarily set it one line below the top margin and one character to the right. A more generalized program should allow the user to decide these adjustment values and perhaps even provide an option to print the address centered.

These desired refinements are left to you as an exercise.

Headings, Multiple-Page Reports, and Right-Alignment

In nearly all cases, the report generated from your program will need to show the title. In addition, columns in the report will require headings. Numeric fields need to be right-aligned. How can these be handled?

Print a Column Right-Aligned. The Printer object does not have a property to print a selected column right-aligned. In fact, there is no property that explicitly handles columns. You will need to compute the column boundaries by code, as you may have inferred from the preceding examples. Handling right-alignment for a column would have been fairly easy if all fonts were of fixed width; that is, each printed character was of the same width. However, many available fonts on the printer are proportional fonts, which have varying widths for different characters. An easy way to handle the right-alignment problem regardless of the font involved is to define the column's right margin instead of the left margin. For example, let RightMargin be the right margin of a particular column. Then, to print the text string Text right-aligned, you can code the following:

```
Printer.CurrentX = RightMargin - Printer.TextWidth(Text) + 1
Printer.Print Text
```

That is, from the right margin, you can compute the starting point to print. Notice that one is added to the difference between RightMargin and the text width to arrive at the beginning position so that the ending position will be right on the margin. Because the default measurement unit is twips, which is so small, whether or not one is added will not result in any noticeable difference.

Page Title and Column Headers. Many reports can span over multiple pages. However, each page will need to show the same title with a page number and column headings. Therefore, it is a good idea to write a separate Sub procedure to print the title and headings. The procedure can also print the page number each time it is called. A sketch of the top portion of a report appears in Figure 13.5.

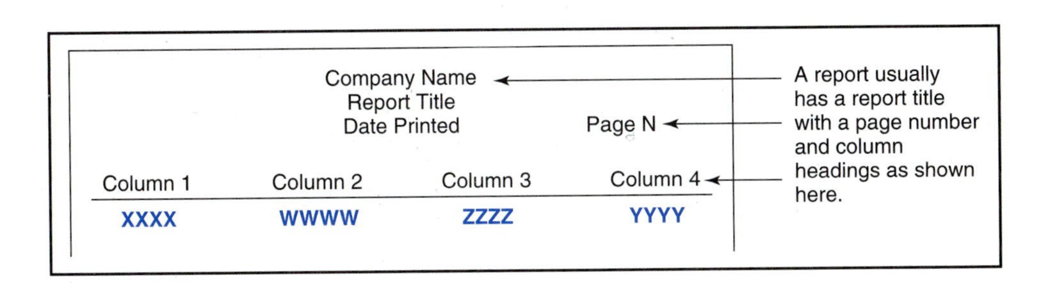

FIGURE 13.5 Typical Page Top of a Report

To print the page title, this procedure needs to know the title to print. A title can have several lines, each with a different length. This parameter (Title) can be passed as a string array. To print column headings, this procedure needs to know not only the headings but also the starting point of each column. For simplicity, we will assume that each column header has only one line. The procedure can then expect a string array for the headings (ColHeader) and another array for the column starting position (ColStart) . Thus, the procedure header can appear as follows:

```
Sub PrintTitle(Title() As String, ColHeader() As String, _
    ColStart() As Single)
```

As discussed, some columns can be right-aligned. How can this alignment be specified in the ColStart parameter? One way is to specify a right-aligned column with a negative value. Then in the Sub, each element of ColStart can be checked to see whether it is negative. If so, the routine will change the value back to positive and use the formula shown previously to compute the starting point to print the text. For an element I in the ColStart array, the following routine should compute the starting position properly:

```
If ColStart(I) > 0 Then
        .CurrentX = ColStart(I)
    Else
        .CurrentX = -ColStart(I) - _
          .TextWidth(ColHeader(I)) + 1
    End If
```

The PrintTitle Procedure. The following procedure (named PrintTitle) should print a page title with the page number (beginning ½" below the page top) and the column headings underlined all in bold.

```
Sub PrintTitle(Title() As String, ColHeader() As String, _
     ColStart() As Single)
'This Sub prints a centered page title given in the title
'parameter (starting at 1/2'' below the page top)
'It also prints column headers given in ColHeader at the position
'Specified in the ColStart parameter
'A negative value of an element in ColStart indicates that the
'column is right-aligned at that position
Dim I As Integer
Dim PageNo As String
    With Printer
        'Start at 1/2'' from the top
        .CurrentY = 720 - _
          (Printer.Height - Printer.ScaleHeight) / 2
        .Font.Bold = True
        ' Print page title
        For I = 0 To UBound(Title)
            'Center the title line
            .CurrentX = (.ScaleWidth - .TextWidth(Title(I))) / 2
            Printer.Print Title(I)
        Next I
        ' Print page number
        PageNo = "Page " & .Page
        ' Go back to the preceding line
        .CurrentY = .CurrentY - .TextHeight("H")
        ' Right-align "Page n" at 95% of the printable line
        .CurrentX = 0.95 * .ScaleWidth - .TextWidth(PageNo)
        Printer.Print PageNo
        Printer.Print 'Skip a line
        .Font.Underline = True 'Underline Column header
        ' Print column headers
        For I = 0 To UBound(ColHeader)
            If ColStart(I) > 0 Then
            .CurrentX = ColStart(I)
            Else
                .CurrentX = -ColStart(I) - _
                  .TextWidth(ColHeader(I)) + 1
            End If
            Printer.Print ColHeader(I);
        Next I
        .Font.Underline = False 'No more underline
        .Font.Bold = False
        Printer.Print 'Next line
    End With
End Sub
```

Notice the difference between the statement to print the page title and that to print the column headers. The former ends without a semicolon because each title line should be printed on a separate line. The latter ends with a semicolon because all these fields for column headers should be on the same line.

Notice also how the page number is printed. The routine first constructs the text for PageNo by concatenating "Page" with the Printer object's Page property. The CurrentY property is then subtracted by the TextHeight to go back to the previous line, the last title line. Then, the following formula:

```
.CurrentX = 0.95 * .ScaleWidth - .TextWidth(PageNo)
```

will align on the right at 95% of the ScaleWidth when the variable PageNo is printed.

The ***Page property*** starts with a value one when the printing starts. Each time the NewPage method is executed, the property increases the value by one. When the EndDoc method is executed, this property resets to one again.

Using the PrintTitle Sub Procedure. To illustrate how the preceding Sub procedure can be used, let's consider an example. Suppose we would like to print a customer contact list that will show the company name, contact name, contact title, and phone number. A sample recordset can be extracted from the NWInd database that comes with VB. The Customers table has all these data fields and has 91 records. The printout will require more than a page. The recordset can be obtained with the following statements using the ADO:

```
Dim SQL As String, ConnStr As String
Dim rsContact As ADODB.Recordset
    'Construct recordset
    ConnStr = "Provider=Microsoft.Jet.OLEDB.4.0;" & _
      "Data Source=C:\Program Files\" & _
      "Microsoft Visual Studio\VB98\NWIND.mdb"
    SQL = "select CompanyName, ContactName, ContactTitle," & _
      " Phone From customers"
    Set rsContact = New ADODB.Recordset
    rsContact.Open SQL, ConnStr, adOpenForwardOnly, _
      adLockReadOnly, adCmdText
```

The recordset is opened as forward and read-only because all we need is to read and print. Now, suppose we would like for the page title to look as follows:

```
North Wind Traders
Customer Contact Listing
(Date Printed)
```

We will need to set up a *title array*, which can appear as follows:

```
Dim Title(2) As String
    ' Set up Report Title
    Title(0) = "North Wind Traders"
    Title(1) = "Customer Contact Listing"
    Title(2) = Format$(Date, "mm/dd/yyyy")
```

Similarly, the *column headers* can be set up as follows (note that the extra spaces are added to draw wider underlines to properly cover the respective columns):

```
'set up column headers
ColHeader(0) = "Company Name" & Space(30)
ColHeader(1) = "Contact Name" & Space(20)
ColHeader(2) = "Contact Title" & Space(16)
ColHeader(3) = Space(16) & "Phone"
```

The first three columns will be left-aligned, but assume we would like the last column (phone) to be right-aligned. Also assume that we would like both left and right margins to be 5% of the printable area. Then the ***column "start" positions*** can be computed as follows:

```
'Set up column start position
With Printer
    ColStart(0) = 0.05 * .ScaleWidth
    ColStart(1) = 0.35 * .ScaleWidth
    ColStart(2) = 0.6 * .ScaleWidth
    ColStart(3) = -0.95 * .ScaleWidth 'Right-aligned
```

Recall that the ScaleWidth property gives the measurement units of the width of the printable area. Using the approach explained previously, the positive percentage multiplied by the ScaleWidth will give the starting position of the column. The negative value, –95% of the ScaleWidth, indicates that the column will be right-aligned with its right margin at 95% of the printable width. (Notice that we leave the "With Printer" block open from here on.)

To ensure that all fields can be printed within the specified column widths, we can set the font to Times New Roman 10 as follows:

```
'Set up printer font
Printer.Print "";
.Font = "Times New Roman"
.Font.Size = 10
```

How many lines should we print on a page? Rather than thinking in terms of lines, we could set the margin for the bottom. For example, because the page starts $\frac{1}{2}$" below the top, we can also set the bottom margin $\frac{1}{2}$" above the bottom of the page. Recall that the entire printable height is measured by the ScaleHeight property. As explained previously, the distance from the printable area to the top (or bottom) of the sheet is (Height –ScaleHeight)/2. Adding the two values should give (Height + ScaleHeight)/2. Thus, the value of the CurrentY property that is $\frac{1}{2}$" from the bottom can be computed as follows:

```
Dim PageBottom As Single
'Set page bottom at half inch above sheet margin
  PageBottom = (.Height + .ScaleHeight) / 2 - 720
```

When the next line to print goes below PageBottom, we can start a new page and print the title and column headings then print the line.

Now, we are ready to print the customer contact list. Each customer will be printed on one line. We can set up a typical loop to retrieve and print a record in each iteration. Each column will start at the same position as its column header. The routine should appear as follows:

```
Dim I As Integer
'Ready; print Title
PrintTitle Title(), ColHeader(), ColStart()
rsContact.MoveFirst
Do Until rsContact.EOF
     If .CurrentY >= PageBottom Then
          .NewPage
          PrintTitle Title(), ColHeader(), ColStart()
     End If
     ' Print recordset fields
     For I = 0 To rsContact.Fields.Count - 1
          If ColStart(I) > 0 Then
               .CurrentX = ColStart(I)
          Else
               .CurrentX = -ColStart(I) - .TextWidth(rsContact(I))
          End If
          Printer.Print rsContact(I);
     Next I <br>
     'Move down by 1.2 lines
     .CurrentY = .CurrentY + .TextHeight("H") * 1.2
     rsContact.MoveNext
Loop
```

Before the loop, the routine calls the PrintTitle Sub procedure to print the page title and column headers. Within the Do loop, the first If statement checks whether the Printer's CurrentY property is beyond the page bottom computed previously. If so, the NewPage method is executed to start a new page and the PrintTitle Sub is called to print the page title and column headers.

For each record in the recordset, the For I loop is executed. In the loop, each field, referenced using the syntax rsContact(I), is printed. Its starting position, the printer's CurrentX is computed with a different expression, depending on whether the ColStart(I) value is positive or negative (left- or right-aligned). If ColStart(I) is positive, the value is assigned to the printer's CurrentX; otherwise, it is converted to a positive value and the TextWidth of the text to be printed is subtracted from that positive value. This will give the starting value for a right-aligned column. Notice that the statement to print the recordset field ends with a semicolon so that all fields are printed on the same line.

After all the fields in a record are printed (below the For loop), it is time to move to the next print line. In most cases, you would use the Printer.Print " " statement to accomplish this. However, if you do so in this case, you may find that the output lines are too close to each other, making the list hard to read. You can use the same Printer.Print " " statement again to effect double space between lines. However, there then appears to be too much space between lines. To illustrate that the next line does not have to be exactly on a "fixed" line position, we compute the printer's CurrentY position 1.2 of the text height as follows:

```
'Move down by 1.2 lines
.CurrentY = .CurrentY + .TextHeight("H") * 1.2
```

After all these, the loop is ready to print another record; therefore, the last statement in the loop is the execution of the recordset's MoveNext method.

What do we do after the Do loop (i.e., after all records have been printed)? The printed document should be released with the EndDoc method, and the "With" block should be closed:

```
    .EndDoc
End With
```

Finally, the recordset should be closed and set to Nothing:

```
rsContact.Close
Set rsContact = Nothing
```

The Complete Code. Suppose you have a new project with a command button named cmdPrint. You can put all the preceding code to print the customer contact list in the command button's Click event procedure. By rearranging all the Dim statements at the beginning of the procedure, the complete print procedure should appear as follows:

```
Private Sub cmdPrint_Click()
Dim Title(2) As String
Dim ColHeader(3) As String
Dim ColStart(3) As Single
Dim PageBottom As Single
Dim I As Integer
Dim SQL As String
Dim ConnStr As String
Dim rsContact As ADODB.Recordset
    'Construct recordset
    ConnStr = "Provider=Microsoft.Jet.OLEDB.4.0;" & _
      "Data Source=C:\Program Files\" & _
        "Microsoft Visual Studio\VB98\NWIND.mdb"
    SQL = "select CompanyName, ContactName, " & _
      "ContactTitle,Phone From customers"
    Set rsContact = New ADODB.Recordset
    rsContact.Open SQL, ConnStr, adOpenForwardOnly, _
      adLockReadOnly, adCmdText
    ' Set up Report Title
    Title(0) = "North Wind Traders"
    Title(1) = "Customer Contact Listing"
    Title(2) = Format$(Date, "mm/dd/yyyy")
    'set up column headers
    ColHeader(0) = "Company Name" & Space(30)
    ColHeader(1) = "Contact Name" & Space(20)
    ColHeader(2) = "Contact Title" & Space(16)
    ColHeader(3) = Space(16) & "Phone"
    'Set up column start position
    With Printer
        ColStart(0) = 0.05 * .ScaleWidth
        ColStart(1) = 0.35 * .ScaleWidth
        ColStart(2) = 0.6 * .ScaleWidth
        ColStart(3) = -0.95 * .ScaleWidth 'Right-aligned
```

```
                ' Set up printer font
                Printer.Print "";
                .Font = "Times New Roman"
                .Font.Size = 10 <br>
                ' set Page bottom at half inch from bottom margin
                PageBottom = (.Height + .ScaleHeight) / 2 - 720
                ' Ready; print Title
                PrintTitle Title(), ColHeader(), ColStart()
                Do Until rsContact.EOF
                    If .CurrentY > PageBottom Then
                        .NewPage
                        PrintTitle Title(), ColHeader(), ColStart()
                    End If
                    ' Print recordset fields
                    For I = 0 To rsContact.Fields.Count - 1
                    If ColStart(I) > 0 Then
                        .CurrentX = ColStart(I)
                    Else
                        .CurrentX = -ColStart(I) -.TextWidth(rsContact(I))
                    End If
                    Printer.Print rsContact(I);
                Next I
                ' Move down by 1.2 lines
                .CurrentY = .CurrentY + .TextHeight("H") * 1.2
                rsContact.MoveNext
            Loop
            .EndDoc
            End With
            rsContact.Close
            Set rsContact = Nothing
        End Sub
```

Notice that this event procedure uses the PrintTitle Sub procedure presented previously. To test this project, you will also need to include that Sub procedure.

Setting the Printer Object

If your system has several printers, one of them is set as the default by the Windows system. This will be the printer that the Printer object is initially associated with. The Printers collection contains the information on all the printers available in the system. The ***DeviceName property*** of the Printer object gives the model name of the printer. The following code will populate a combo box named cboPrinter with all the printer's names:

```
Dim Pr As Printer
    For Each Pr In Printers
    cboPrinter.AddItem Pr.DeviceName
    Next Pr
```

You will be able to allow the user to select a printer from the available device by setting the Printer object to the printer selected. For example, the following code will set the Printer object to the printer selected from the combo box cboPrinter:

```
Private Sub cboPrinter_Click()
    Set Printer = Printers(cboPrinter.ListIndex)
End Sub
```

13.2 Using the MS HFG for Reports

In Chapter 8, "Database and the ActiveX Data Objects," we introduced the MS HFG as a control bound to the ADODC and to the hierarchical recordset. There we mentioned that this control has many more features. It can be used to display various kinds of reports or tables either being bound or without being bound to a recordset. Let's now take a closer look at this control.

Selected Features of the MS HFG

The HFG has several properties that allow you to present data in a very flexible manner. To cite a few, the RowHeight and ColWidth properties allow you to set different heights and widths for different rows and columns. The ***WordWrap property*** allows texts to be wrapped and displayed in multiple lines in the grid's cells. The ***Sort*** and ***Merge properties*** allow the data to be sorted and/or merged. There are also cell-specific properties that allow individual cells to behave differently from each other.

This section demonstrates a few of these features that can be used for reporting purposes. We begin with an example to display the present value factor of $1 with different interest rates and time periods.

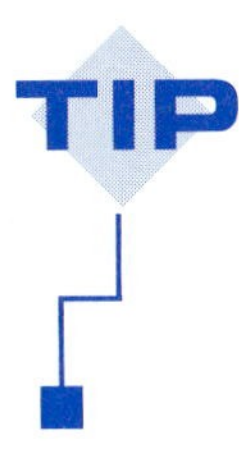

Actually, there is another grid control that has features very similar to the MS HFG. That control is named MS FlexGrid (FG) and was introduced in VB5. The HFG can be bound only to ADO recordsets, whereas the FG can be bound only to VB's intrinsic data control. If you plan to use the grid without binding it to any recordset, you should consider the FG as a substitute for the HFG. The FG uses fewer system resources than the HFG. We discuss only HFG in the text so that some of their minor differences will not sidetrack our attention.

Presenting a Table of Present Values with the HFG

The present value factor of $1 can be computed with the following formula:

$$PV = (1 + r)^{-n}$$

where r is the rate of interest per period (usually year) and n is the number of periods (years).

Suppose we would like to display the present value at various rates and time periods in a table. The HFG with its multiple rows and columns lends itself as a good candidate to serve as a display table for such a purpose. Assume we would like the rates to vary from 4% to 12% and the periods to vary from 1 to 20 years (see Figure 13.6). How do we proceed?

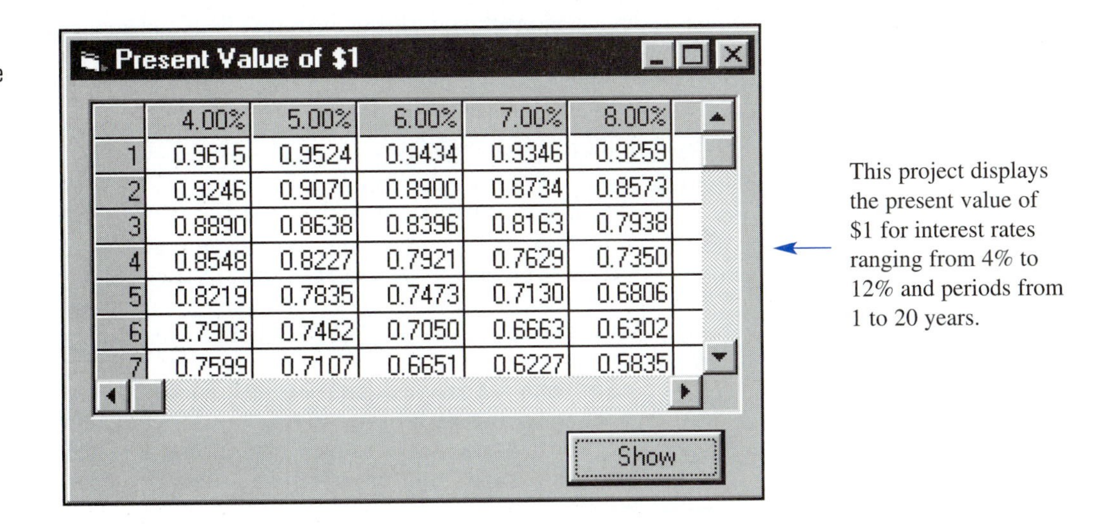

FIGURE 13.6
Table of Present Value of $1

This project displays the present value of $1 for interest rates ranging from 4% to 12% and periods from 1 to 20 years.

We can solve this problem by answering the following questions:

1. How can the grid be set up to contain the desired number of rows and columns?
2. How can the various present value factors be computed?
3. How can these present value factors be populated into the grid?
4. How can the column and row headings be added?

Setting Up the Grid. The desired number of rows and columns for a grid can be set at design time or at runtime. To set the rows and columns at design time, you can do the following:

1. Double click the Custom property in the Properties window of the grid. A Property Pages dialog box will appear.
2. Enter the desired number of rows and columns in the proper boxes.

To set the number of rows and columns at runtime, assign the proper values to the Rows and Cols properties. In this example, we will use this approach. Because there are 20 periods and 9 different interest rates, we will set the Rows and Cols properties to 21 and 10, respectively. (This will take care of the need for the extra row and column for headings.)

In addition, the width of each column also should be set properly. The grid's ColWidth property allows the column widths to be set at runtime. This property is indexed by a number, with 0 representing the first column. That is, grdTable.ColWidth(0) refers to the width of the first column (column zero). Incidentally, the index –1 refers to all columns.

The following code should set the grid's Rows and Cols properties as well as the widths for all columns:

```
With grdTable
     .Rows = 21
     .Cols = 10
     W = Me.TextWidth("H")
     .ColWidth(-1) = 6 * W 'Set width for all columns
     .ColWidth(0) = 3 * W 'Set width for Column 0
End With
```

Notice that we use the form's TextWidth method to compute the width of the letter "H" for the grid. The grid does not have the TextWidth method. However, it usually has the same font as the form. All columns are then assigned with a value equal to the width of six "H"'s. Because column 0 displays the number of periods, its width is set to three widths of "H."

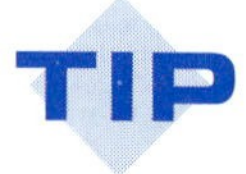

If you are unsure that the form has the same font and font size as the grid but the precise column width is important, you can set the form's Font and Font.Size properties to those of the grid's before using the form's TextWidth method. Of course, you should take care to restore the two properties for the form after the column width is obtained. The following code demonstrates how this can be done:

```
Dim FormFont As String
Dim FormFontSize As Long
     FormFont = Me.Font.Name 'Save the form's original font
     FormFontSize = Me.Font.Size 'Save the form's font size
     Me.Font.Name = grdTable.Font.Name 'Set the font to
                                       'that of the grid
     Me.Font.Size = grdTable.Font.Size 'Set to the grid's
                                       'font size
     'Set the width of col. 0 to three 0s wide
     grdTable.ColWidth(0) = Me.TextWidth("000")
     Me.Font.Name = FormFont 'Restore the form's font
     Me.Font.Size = FormFontSize 'Restore the form's font size
```

Computing the Present Value Factor. Let the variable PVFactor be the present value factor of $1. Then, the following routine should produce the results for the specified rates and time periods.

```
Rate = 0.04
For Col = 1 To 9
     Factor1 = 1 / (1 + Rate)
     PVFactor = 1
```

```
        For Period = 1 To 20
            PVFactor = PVFactor * Factor1 'This will get (1 + R)
                                          '^ -N
        Next Period
        Rate = Rate + 0.01
    Next Col
```

This routine involves two loops. The outer loop varies Col from 1 to 9 (there are 9 rates from 4% to 12%), and the inner loop varies the periods from 1 to 20. Rather than using the original formula as shown previously, we optimize the code by computing the discount factor for one period first (as represented by Factor1). Then in the inner loop, this value is used to multiply the present value factor of the previous period to produce the factor for the current period. This technique avoids the use of "raising a number to certain power" and was discussed in Chapter 7, "Repetition."

Why use Col as the loop counter for the outer loop instead of the rate directly? Usually, floating point variables are not very good as loop counters. The results of adding the increment parameter (the value after the keyword "Step") may not be exactly accurate. A minor error can cause the loop to iterate one more (or less) time than we would expect.

Populating the Results in the Grid. Each of the resulting PVFactor should be displayed in the grid. How? The grid has a property, ***TextMatrix,*** that can be used to set the text directly in each cell. This property allows you to refer to the cell content directly in a matrix style by a pair of indexes as follows:

```
Object.TextMatrix(Row, Col)
```

where *Object* is an expression that refers to the grid and *Row, Col* represents a pair of values that point to the cell's row and column position; (0, 0) refers to the first cell in the grid.

Assuming the grid is named grdTable, you can populate the grid by assigning the resulting present value factor to its cells with the following statement:

```
grdTable.TextMatrix(Period, Col) = Format$(PVFactor, "0.0000")
```

This statement uses the Format$ function to format the output so that the results will align neatly. (The "0" format character forces all trailing zeros to be shown as "0"'s instead of blank spaces.) This statement can be added right after PVFactor is computed.

Notice that the PVFactor is computed and populated into the cell, varying the number of periods for the same interest rate (column). This suggests that the results are populated into the grid column by column, not row by row.

Setting the Column Headings and Showing Periods. The column headings (for the interest rates) should be shown in the first row immediately following the computation for Col. The following statement should accomplish this:

```
grdTable.TextMatrix(0, Col) = Format$(Rate, "Percent")
```

Notice that we use the named format string "Percent" so that the rate will be displayed in percentage instead of a fractional number.

A separate loop will be needed to display the number of periods in column 0 for all rows. The code fragment appears as follows:

```
' Show time periods in the first column
For Period = 1 To 20
    grdTable.TextMatrix(Period, 0) = Period
Next Period
```

The Complete Code. Assume the present value factors are to be displayed when the user clicks a command button named cmdShow. The complete code can be put together as follows:

```
Option Explicit

Private Sub cmdShow_Click()
Dim Rate As Single
Dim Period As Integer
Dim Factor1 As Single
Dim PVFactor As Single
```

```
Dim Col As Integer
Dim W As Integer
    'Set up the grid rows and columns
    With grdTable
        .Rows = 21
        .Cols = 10
        W = Me.TextWidth("H")
        .ColWidth(-1) = 6 * W
        .ColWidth(0) = 3 * W
    End With
    ' Show time periods in the first column
    For Period = 1 To 20
        grdTable.TextMatrix(Period, 0) = Period
    Next Period
    Rate = 0.04
    For Col = 1 To 9
        'Show rate as the column title
        grdTable.TextMatrix(0, Col) = Format$(Rate, "Percent")
        Factor1 = 1 / (1 + Rate)
        PVFactor = 1
        For Period = 1 To 20
            PVFactor = PVFactor * Factor1
            grdTable.TextMatrix(Period, Col) = _
              Format$(PVFactor, "0.0000")
        Next Period
        Rate = Rate + 0.01
    Next Col
End Sub
```

Of course, this procedure can easily be modified to allow the user to specify the number of periods and the range of rates to show the present value factors. Such a refinement is left to you as an exercise.

The Sort and Merge Capabilities of the HFG

Often, the user needs to inspect a report by different sort orders. Imagine a sales report that shows detailed sales by salesperson, customer, and product. The user (manager) may first wish to inspect sales sorted by product. Later, he or she may wish to inspect sales by sales person or customer. The HFG has the ***Sort property*** that can perform sorting with minimum code. This property, available only at runtime, enables you to specify the type of sorting to perform on the selected columns. For example, setting this property to 1 (flexSortGenericAscending) will make the grid guess the type of data (numeric or string) and sort the selected columns in ascending order accordingly.

To specify the columns to sort, you can do the following:

1. Set the grid's Col (column) and ColSel (column selected) properties. The Col property specifies the starting column, and ColSel specifies the ending column.
2. Specify the type of sorting to perform by setting the Sort property.

For example, the following code fragment will sort grdTable, treating Columns 1 and 2 as the sort key of the String type.

```
With grdTable
    .Col = 1 'Define beginning col to sort
    .ColSel = 2 'Define ending col to sort
    .Sort = flexSortStringAscending 'Tell how to sort the grid
End With
```

Note that when assigning the values to the Col and ColSel properties, you must assign the value for the Col property first. Otherwise, the ColSel property will take on the same value as the Col property.

In addition, the HFG can perform merge. The ***MergeCells property*** lets you specify how the cells should be merged when the neighboring cells have the same value. For example, setting this property to 1 (flexMergeFree) will enable you to specify columns as well as rows to merge.

You should also set the ***MergeCol()*** and ***MergeRow() properties*** to True for the columns and rows to merge. For example, the following code fragment will merge the neighboring cells of the same value in Column 1.

```
.MergeCells = flexMergeFree 'Allow cell merge for col & row
.MergeCol(1) = True 'Merge cells of same value for Col(1)
```

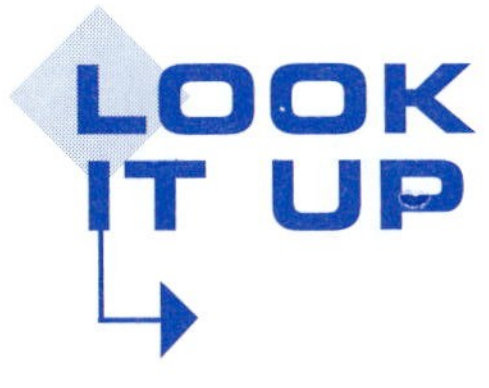

Use "MSHFlexGrid constant" as the keyword to search in the Index tab of the online Help file for the various constant values (and named constants) you can set for the Sort and MergeCells properties.

To illustrate how these properties work together, let's consider a simple example. Suppose we would like to show the Authors table in the Biblio database in a HFG. When the user clicks a column, the data will be displayed in ascending order by that column. Start a new project and follow these steps:

1. Add the HFG to the toolbox. The steps are similar to adding a masked edit box and other nonstandard controls.
2. Draw an HFG control on the form.
3. Set properties for the HFG. Name the HFG grdAuthors. To allow the user to adjust the column size, set the AllowUserResize to 1 (flexResizeColumns).
4. Add a reference of the ADO 2.1 (or 2.0 if 2.1 is not available) library to the project. The steps are explained in Chapter 8. (Use the References option instead of the Components option in the Project menu.)
5. Open the connection and recordset for the Authors table and bind the grid (by code) to the recordset. The code appears as follows:

```
Private Sub Form_Load()
Dim cnnBiblio As ADODB.Connection
Dim rsAuthors As ADODB.Recordset
Dim cnnStr As String
    cnnStr = "Provider=Microsoft.Jet.OLEDB.4.0;" & _
      "Data Source=" & _
      "C:\Program Files\Microsoft Visual Studio\Vb98\Biblio.mdb"
    Set cnnBiblio = New ADODB.Connection
    cnnBiblio.Open cnnStr
    Set rsAuthors = New ADODB.Recordset
    rsAuthors.Open "Authors", cnnBiblio, adOpenStatic, _
      adLockReadOnly
    Set grdAuthors.DataSource = rsAuthors
End Sub
```

   Notice that the grid's DataSource property is associated with the recordset rsAuthors by a Set statement. The recordset is an object and cannot be assigned to the property using an assignment statement (without the Set keyword).

6. Enable the HFG's sort and merge capabilities. Enter the following code. Notice that we place the code in the grid's Click event procedure.

```
Private Sub grdAuthors_Click()
Dim N As Integer
    ' Allow the grid to merge cell
    grdAuthors.MergeCells = flexMergeFree
    N = grdAuthors.Col 'this is the column selected
    ' Merge cells on the sorted column
    grdAuthors.MergeCol(N) = True
    'Specify type of sort to perform
```

```
    grdAuthors.Sort = flexSortGenericAscending
End Sub
```

Run the project and click on different columns in the grid. You should be able to verify that whichever column you click, the data are sorted and merged (for cells with the same data values) by that column.

How the Code Works. When the user clicks a cell in the HFG (named grdAuthors), the grid's Col, Row, and Text properties are set to this cell. For example, if the user clicks on the cell located at column 2 and row 3, the grid's Col and Row properties will be set to 2 and 3, respectively. In addition, the grid's Text property also will be set to the content of this cell. In the preceding code, the MergeCells property is assigned a value, flexMergeFree, indicating that cell merge can be for both row and column. The value of the Col property (the column that the user clicks) is assigned to the variable N, which is then used to specify the column to merge. (This is done just for code clarity. The Col property setting could have been used as the index in the MergeCol property for the assignment statement.) Finally, the last statement before End Sub specifies the type of sorting to perform. A sample result is shown in Figure 13.7.

FIGURE 13.7
Sample Results of Using the HFG's Sort and Merge Features

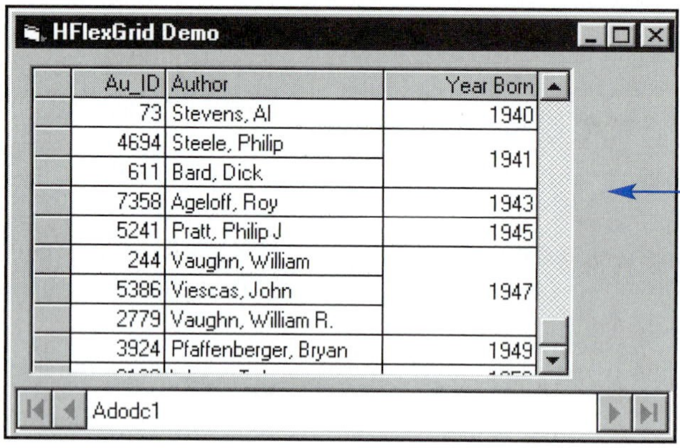

HFlexGrid Demo

Au_ID	Author	Year Born
73	Stevens, Al	1940
4694	Steele, Philip	1941
611	Bard, Dick	
7358	Ageloff, Roy	1943
5241	Pratt, Philip J	1945
244	Vaughn, William	1947
5386	Viescas, John	
2779	Vaughn, William R.	
3924	Pfaffenberger, Bryan	1949

Adodc1

The sort/merge feature of the HFG in action; with the code provided in the text in place, when the user clicks a column, the grid sorts by that column. This one shows the results of clicking the "Year Born" column. Cells of the same year are merged. Note that sorts performed by the grid are faster than by the SQL because data are already in memory.

Displaying a Recordset Without Binding

The preceding example shows how the HFG can display, sort, and merge data when bound to a recordset. The HFG also can be used to display a recordset without binding. Why not just bind the grid to the recordset? There are at least two possible reasons for not binding:

1. You may want to have complete control over the display format. For example, a field containing the Social Security number may be internally stored as a Long integer. However, you would rather present the field with proper dashes (-).
2. You may also recall that bound grids (DataGrid and HFG) cannot properly display a recordset opened with the cursor type adOpenForwardOnly (the only type from the connection's Execute method). Thus, if you open a recordset of this cursor type, you must provide your own code to display the content in the grid.

The AddItem Method. One convenient way to display the content of a recordset in the HFG without binding is to use the control's AddItem method, which works similarly to the list box's. The AddItem method adds one row of data at a time and has the following syntax:

```
Object.AddItem String[, Row]
```

where *Object* = the name of the HFG

String = a string containing the data for the row to be added

Row = the row number to insert the current string; if omitted, the new row is appended as the last row

Fields in the string to be added are separated by the tab character vbTab. The grid's Cols property determines the maximum number of cells in each row to add. If the number of elements in the string exceeds Cols, the extra elements are dropped. If the number is smaller, the remaining columns of the grid are left blank. The following code will add a row with its first three cells containing 1, 2, and 3 to the HFG named grdTest:

```
grdTest.AddItem 1 & vbTab & 2 vbTab & 3
```

To illustrate how to populate the grid without binding it to a recordset, let's consider an example. This project involves displaying selected titles from the Biblio database. There is a text box (named txtSearch) for the user to enter a portion of the title to search for. When the user clicks a command button captioned "Search" (named cmdSearch), the program will display the titles that matches the search string, along with the publisher's names. A sample result appears in Figure 13.8.

FIGURE 13.8
Sample Output on an HFG

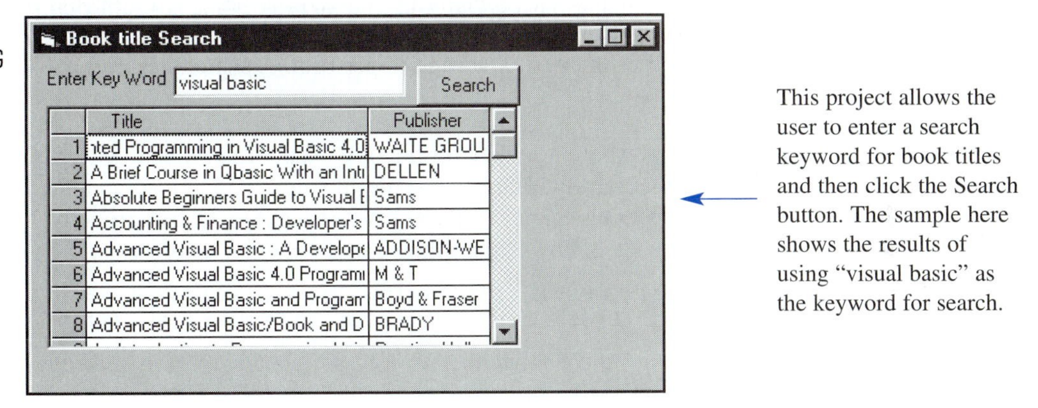

This project involves three major steps:

1. Set up the connection and create the recordset with the proper SQL statement. We will name the recordset rsTitles.
2. Prepare the HFG. Adjust its size and position. Set up its rows, columns, and column titles. We will name this grid grdTitles.
3. Populate the grid with the records.

The connection can be opened as soon as the program starts. The code to open the connection cnnBiblio appears as follows:

```
Option Explicit
Dim cnnBiblio As ADODB.Connection
Private Sub Form_Load()
Dim ConnStr As String
' Open the connection
    ConnStr = "Provider=Microsoft.Jet.OLEDB.4.0;" & _
      "Data Source=" & _
      "c:\program files\Microsoft Visual Studio\vb98\Biblio.mdb"
    Set cnnBiblio = New ADODB.Connection
    cnnBiblio.Open ConnStr
End Sub
```

You will also need to construct an SQL statement to obtain the book titles and publisher names. If you inspect the Biblio database, you should see that the Title field is in the Titles table and the Name field of the publishers is in the Publishers table. Both tables have the PubID field, which can be "inner joined" to obtain the desired results. The SQL statement should appear as follows:

```
Select Titles.Title, Publishers.Name From Titles _
    Inner Join Publishers On Titles.PubID = Publishers.PubID _
```

```
        Where Titles.Title Like '%<text from the text box>%' _
          Order By Titles.Title
```

Notice that we place the wildcard search character "%" before and after the entered search text. This will allow a match for the text in any part of the title, not just the beginning of the title. We can use this statement as a parameter in the connection's Execute method to return a recordset:

```
SearchStr = "Select Titles.Title, Publishers.Name" & _
     " From Titles Inner join Publishers" & _
     " on Titles.PubId = publishers.pubId " & _
     " where titles.Title Like '%" & Trim$(txtSearch.Text) & _
     "%' Order by Title"
Set rsTitles = cnnBiblio.Execute(SearchStr, , adCmdText)
```

Setting Up the HFG. As discussed previously, the HFG has the Cols and Rows properties that can be used to set the number of columns and rows for the grid. As implied, we will add data to the grid using the AddItem method. Thus, we will start the grid with one row to display the column titles. The grid should have three columns. Thus:

```
grdTitles.Cols = 3
grdTitles.Rows = 1
```

The first column will be for the row count. The remaining two columns will be for Title and Name, respectively. Thus, we would like to assign "Title" and "Name" to the second and third cells in this row. Recall that you can use the TextMatrix property to identify the cells to set to any texts. The following two lines should assign the proper column titles:

```
grdTitles.TextMatrix(0, 1) = "Title"
grdTitles.TextMatrix(0,2) = "Publisher Name"
```

However, there is another way to set up the column headings. It involves the use of the FormatString property.

The FormatString Property. This property allows you to set up the column and row headings, the column widths, and the column alignment all at one time for the grid. The headings are separated by the special character "|." The first group of headings are assigned to columns. The semicolon (;) is used to separate the column headings from the row headings. For example, consider the following statement:

```
grdTest.FormatString = "¦A¦B¦C;¦1¦2¦3"
```

The first three elements before the semicolon will be the column headings, and the last three elements will be the row titles, as show in Figure 13.9.

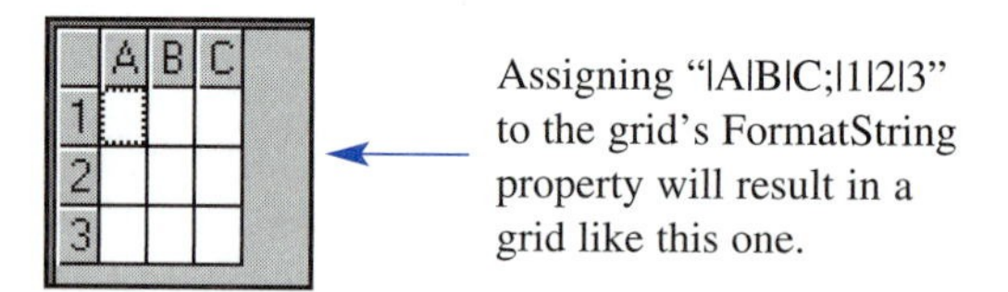
A
B
C
1
2
3
Assigning "|A|B|C;|1|2|3" to the grid's FormatString property will result in a grid like this one.

FIGURE 13.9
Effect of Assigning a Format String

Notice that the first "|" in either group is not preceded by anything, suggesting that the first column (row) is left blank. This string also implicitly sets the grid to four columns and four rows. (See the resulting grid in Figure 13.9 again.) However, if you have previously set the grid to more than four columns or rows, the additional columns or rows will not be deleted. Notice also that each column will be only one character wide because there is only one character in each column heading. If you wish to have a wider column, add additional spaces to the heading. You can also precede the column headings with the characters ">" (right-aligned), "<" (left-aligned), and "^" (centered) to effect the column alignment.

Back to our example project, the column headings can also be set up using the FormatString property as follows:

```
grdTitles.FormatString = "¦Title ¦Publisher Name "
```

Notice that this statement should precede the statement that assigns the Rows property to 1 (i.e., .Rows = 1). The FormatString property will not work properly when there is only one row in the grid.

Populating the HFG. Now, how do you populate the grid by code? As mentioned, we can use the grid's AddItem method. Because this method works similarly to that for the list box, the code to populate an HFG should be familiar. The following code should populate the HFG with the data in the recordset.

```
With rsTitles
     If .BOF And .EOF Then Exit Sub 'no data; return to caller
     .MoveFirst
     Do Until .EOF
          Row = Row + 1
          Text = Row & vbTab & !Title & vbTab & !Name
          grdTitles.AddItem Text
          .MoveNext
     Loop
End With
```

If the recordset contains many records, populating the HFG can take a long time. One way to speed up the operation is to set the grid's Redraw property to False before the loop and set it to True after the loop. This will save the grid from attempting to redraw its appearance after each row of data is added. Its appearance will be "updated" only after the Redraw property is set to True again.

Populating the FlexGrid: The "Complete" Code. The settings for the grid appearance and the creation of the connection should be done only once (e.g., in the Form Load event), whereas populating the grid should be done whenever the user clicks the Search button. The "complete" code appears as follows:

```
Option Explicit
Dim cnnBiblio As ADODB.Connection
Private Sub Form_Load()
Dim ConnStr As String
     ' Set up the HFG with column headings
     With grdTitles
          grdTitles.FormatString = "¦Title ¦Name "
          .Cols = 3
          .Rows = 1
     End With
     ' Open the connection with the file path for Biblio.mdb
     ConnStr = "Provider=Microsoft.Jet.OLEDB.4.0;" & _
       "Data Source=" & _
       "C:\Program Files\Microsoft Visual Studio\Vb98\Biblio.mdb"
     Set cnnBiblio = New ADODB.Connection
     cnnBiblio.Open ConnStr
End Sub
Private Sub cmdSearch_Click()
Dim rsTitles As ADODB.Recordset
Dim SearchStr As String
Dim Text As String
Dim Row As Integer
     SearchStr = "Select Titles.Title, Publishers.Name" & _
       " From Titles Inner join Publishers" & _
       " on Titles.PubId = Publishers.PubId " & _
       " where Titles.Title Like '%" & Trim$(txtSearch.Text) _
       & "%' Order by Title"
     Set rsTitles = cnnBiblio.Execute(SearchStr, , adCmdText)
```

```
        grdTitles.Rows = 1 'Clear the grid except the column titles
        With rsTitles
        If .BOF And .EOF Then Exit Sub 'no record to populate
            .MoveFirst
            Do Until .EOF
                Row = Row + 1
                Text = Row & vbTab & !Title & vbTab & !Name
                grdTitles.AddItem Text
                .MoveNext
            Loop
        End With
        grdTitles.FixedRows = 1
    End Sub
```

Notice that we have also included the following statement:

```
grdTitles.FixedRows = 1
```

The statement sets the number of fixed rows to 1, which was the original default. However, when we assigned the Rows property to 1, VB automatically set the number of fixed rows to 0 because there must be at least one nonfixed row in the grid. After additional rows are added by the AddItem method, we can reset the number of fixed rows to 1 so that the headings will appear "properly."

The preceding example shows how to work with some of the HFG's properties (e.g., Cols, Rows, TextMatrix, FormatString) and how to populate the HFG by code. As you can see, you have complete control on what data to include (e.g., the row number is included as the first column).

A Finishing Touch. The preceding code will work; however, when you run the project, you might find it takes "a few seconds" to show the results. The SQL query takes time. Populating the grid also takes time. You can speed up the latter by setting the grid's Redraw property to False before the loop to add items and setting the same property to True after the loop. That is, to speed up execution, the code structure can be modified as follows:

```
With rsTitles
If .BOF And .EOF Then Exit Sub 'no record to populate
    grdTitles.Redraw = False
    .MoveFirst
    Do Until .EOF
        Row = Row + 1
        Text = Row & vbTab & !Title & vbTab & !Name
        grdTitles.AddItem Text
        .MoveNext
    Loop
    grdTitles.Redraw = True
End With
```

Setting the Redraw property to False will prevent the grid from attempting to update its appearance as each item is added to the grid. After all the data have been added, you can reset it to True so that the grid will update its appearance. The effect of these two statements can be "dramatic" when your recordset is huge.

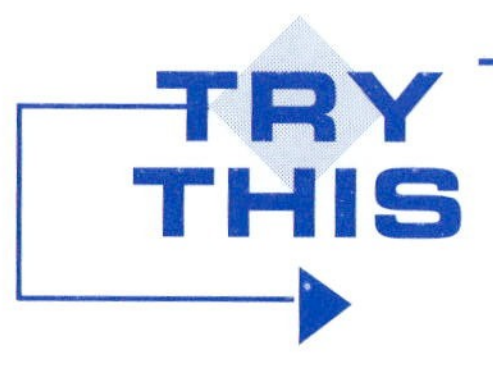

Add a label at the bottom of the form in the unbound HFG project. Name it lblTime. Then do the following:

1. Add the two "Redraw" statements as shown in the text.
2. Add the following statements to the cmdSearch_Click event procedure as suggested in the comments:

```
Dim T As Single ' Place this at the beginning of the procedure
T = Timer 'Place this immediately before
          ' grdTitles.Redraw = False
lblTime.Caption = Timer - T      'Place this after
                                 ' grdTitles.Redraw = True
```

3. Run the project. Enter "Visual" in the text box and click the Search button. Observe the time shown in the label.
4. Comment out the Redraw statements and repeat the same query. Observe the time again.

See any difference in performance? The difference will be even greater if the recordset is larger.

13.3 Programming the MS HFG for Data Entry

The preceding section discusses the uses of the MS HFG for the purposes of presenting tables and reports. This section focuses on programming it for data entry purposes.

Implementation Strategy

In many business applications, data are entered in a tabular form. For example, an order from a customer may request a long list of product items. Each item can be entered in a row, containing details such as item number, quantity ordered, and price. The HFG appears to be a good choice to handle this. However, this control is not versatile in accepting keys. To make the grid appear to accept keys, we can do the following:

1. Place a floating text box on the cell in the grid to accept the key input. The user is then led to perceive that data are actually entered into the grid.
2. Program the text box to float onto the cell to which the user moves the focus. So that the text box is fully utilized to handle the keys, this control must get the focus even when the grid is meant to be the one receiving the focus.
3. Ensure that as the text box moves away from a cell, the content of the text box is left in that cell. In addition, the text box should pick up the content of the cell into which the text box moves, making the content ready for editing.

Setting Up the Project

To illustrate how this design strategy can be implemented, we will set up a visual interface as shown in Figure 13.10.

Some selected properties of the controls in the interface are set as indicated in the following table:

Object	Property	Setting	Remarks
Form	Name	frmGridDemo	
	Caption	Grid for Data Entry	
Text box	Name	txtAboveGrid	To serve as a control above the grid
	TabIndex	0	
HFlexGrid	Name	grdInput	Used to illustrate how a text box can
	Cols	5	float around its cells
	Rows	11	
	FixedCols	1	
	FixedRows	1	
	TabIndex	1	
Text box	Name	txtEdit	A floating text box to accept
	BackColor	vbDeskTop	keyboard input on behalf of the grid
	BorderStyle	0-None	
	Visible	False	
	TabStop	False	

Object	Property	Setting	Remarks
Command button	Name	cmdSave	To serve as a control below the grid
	Caption	Save	
	TabIndex	2	

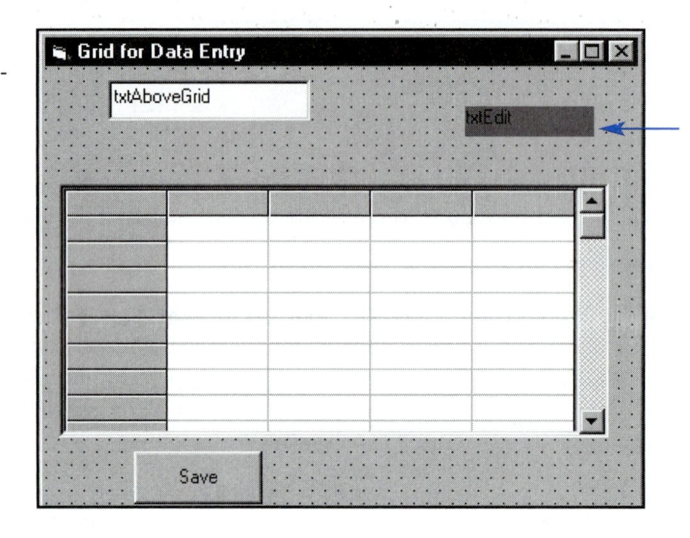

FIGURE 13.10
Visual Interface for Data-Entry Illustration

This project illustrates how a floating text box (txtEdit) can be programmed to navigate around cells in a grid control and to accept keyboard input. The two additional controls (txtAboveGrid and cmdSave) serve to play the roles of "other controls" on the same form.

Showing the Text Box on the Grid

Fixed rows and fixed columns of a grid cannot receive focus. When the user clicks on a particular nonfixed cell on the grid, that cell receives the focus and becomes the active cell. The grid's Col, Row, and Text properties all refer to this cell. For example, if the user clicks on grdInput at cell(1,3), which contains the text "Here," grdInput.Row, grdInput.Col, and grdInput.Text will have the values, 1, 3, and "Here," respectively.

Presetting the Row and Col Properties. When the user uses the Tab key to move focus to the grid, the grid's previous settings for the Col and Row properties remain the same. Therefore, it is a good idea to explicitly set the Col and Row properties when the program starts to ensure that the proper cell gets the focus. The following code can be placed in the Form Load event procedure for this purpose.

```
Private Sub Form_Load()
' To ensure that focus will be set at cell(1,1) when the grid
'receives the focus
' Be sure to place these two lines AFTER all statements to
' setup the appearance of the grid
   grdInput.Row = 1
   grdInput.Col = 1
End Sub
```

Showing the Text Box in the Grid. When the grid receives the focus, the text box should be placed on top of the active cell. This involves several steps:

1. Compute the location at which to place the text box.
2. Move the text box to the computed location, adjusting its size to the cell's.
3. Place the cell content in the text box.
4. Display the text box and ensure that the text box stays on top of the screen (not behind the grid).
5. Highlight the content of the text box.

Computing the Location of Cell Position. To calculate the position where the text box should appear, we will need to use the ***CellLeft*** and ***CellTop properties*** of the active cell. These properties give the upper-left corner position of the cell, similar to the ***Left*** and ***Top properties*** of most VB controls. However, the values are set relative to the grid; that is, the upper-left corner of the grid is considered (0, 0). The text box's Left and Top properties, on the other hand, are relative to the form. To place the text box at the correct location in the form, the cell's Left and Top property values should be adjusted by the Left and Top property values of the grid. Let (X, Y) be the coordinate of the upper-left corner of the active cell on the form. Then the pair can be computed as follows:

```
With grdInput
     X = .Left + .CellLeft
     Y = .Top + .CellTop
```

Note that the With block is left open without the End With statement. The following discussion will be included in this With block.

Placing the Floating Text Box on the Cell. The resulting X and Y values can then be used to locate the text box using its Move method, which can also adjust the text box's width and height to the width and height of the active cell. Thus, the following line can be added:

```
txtEdit.Move X, Y, .CellWidth, .CellHeight
```

The third and fourth parameters of the Move method set the Width and Height of the text box, which should fit in the cell that the text box overlays. The CellWidth and CellHeight properties of the HFG give the width and height of the active cell. These property settings are exactly what are called for by the Move method.

Showing the Content of the Cell. The content of the cell can be moved to the text box with the following statement:

```
     txtEdit.Text = .Text 'Place cell content in text box
End With
```

Notice the End With statement is added to close the With block for the grid.

To display the text box, the text box's Visible property can be set to True. In addition, we need to ensure that the text box will be placed on top of (not behind) the grid. This can be done with the text box's ZOrder method. Also, as soon as it appears, the text box should be ready to accept input on behalf of the grid. Thus, it should receive the focus. The code appears as follows:

```
With txtEdit
     .Visible = True 'make the text box show
     .ZOrder 'ensure the text box stays on top
     .SetFocus 'Set the focus on the text box to accept data
End With
```

The ZOrder Method. The ***ZOrder method*** places a control either at the top or bottom of the screen where two or more controls overlap. The general syntax for the ZOrder method is as follows:

```
Object.ZOrder Position
```

If the position value is either 0 or omitted, the object is placed on top (front) of the screen. A position value of one will place the object in the bottom (behind).

Highlighting the Content. Finally, we can highlight the content of the text box by setting its SelStart and SelLength properties (add these lines within the With block for the text box):

```
.SelStart = 0
.SelLength = Len(.Text)
```

The "Complete" Procedure. We will put all the steps discussed in a Sub procedure and name it ShowEditBox. The complete code appears as follows:

```
Sub ShowEditBox()
'The Proc moves the floating text box onto the Grid's cell which
' has the focus
Dim X As Long
Dim Y As Long
Dim Adj As Long
    With grdInput
    'Calculate text pos & size
        X = .Left + .CellLeft
        Y = .Top + .CellTop
    'place the floating text box at (x, y)
    ' and fit its size to the cell
        txtEdit.Move X, Y, .CellWidth, .CellHeight
    'Display cell text using the edit box
        txtEdit.Text = .Text
    End With
    With txtEdit
        .Visible = True 'Make the text box visible
        .ZOrder 'ensure the text box stays on top
        .SetFocus 'So that the text box is ready for edit/key entry
        ' Highlight the content
        .SelStart = 0
        .SelLength = Len(.Text)
    End With
End Sub
```

Using the ShowEditBox Procedure. As soon as the grid receives the focus, the floating text box should be displayed at its active cell. In effect, the focus is shifted to the text box. The code appears as follows:

```
Private Sub grdInput_GotFocus()
    ShowEditBox
End Sub
```

Handling Mouse Clicks

What should happen when the user clicks another part of the grid or another control in the form? The text box will lose its focus. The content of the text box should be assigned to the cell where the text box is. However, notice that this cell may no longer be the cell with the current grdInput.Col and grdInput.Row. Why? Because as soon as the user clicks on another cell, this new cell immediately becomes the active cell that the grdInput.Col and grdInput.Row are pointing to, leaving the text box behind.

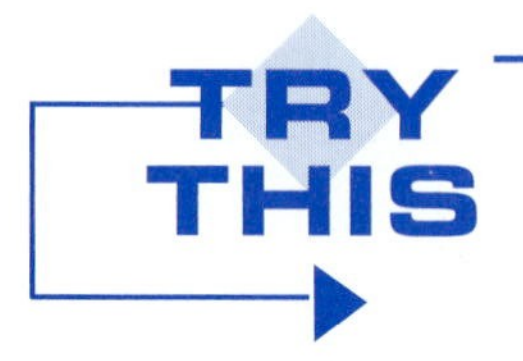

Add the following event procedure to your current project:

```
Private Sub grdInput_Click
    Debug.Print grdInput.Row; grdInput.Col
End Sub
```

Run the program and click on the grid a few times. You should see that each time you click on the grid, the Row and Col properties of the active cell appear in the Debug window. This means that as soon as the user clicks a cell, it immediately becomes the active cell. The cell that the edit box resides in is no longer the active cell to which grdInput.Row and grdInput.Col are pointing.

Recall that when the grid received its focus, the text box was moved to the then active cell, whose Col and Row property values pointed to the cell where the text box was (and still is).

Thus, the following code scheme should be able to keep track of this cell position. In the general declaration section, add the following lines:

```
Dim CurRow As Integer
Dim CurCol As Integer
```

Now insert the following lines immediately below the "With grdInput" line in the ShowEditBox Sub Procedure.

```
' keep the col and row values for future use
    CurRow = .Row
    CurCol = .Col
```

Once this is done, the following event procedure will leave the content of the text box in the cell that is "losing focus."

```
Private Sub txtEdit_LostFocus()
     'drop the content in the cell where the text box is
     grdInput.TextMatrix(CurRow, CurCol) = txtEdit.Text
     txtEdit.Visible = False 'and disappear
End Sub
```

Notice that the LostFocus event procedure is associated with the text box, not with the grid. As explained, once the grid receives the focus, the ShowEditBox procedure is called and the focus is immediately shifted to the text box so that the latter can accept keys on behalf of the grid. Once losing the focus, the text box's Visible property is set to False so that it will disappear from the grid in case the control receiving the focus is no longer the grid.

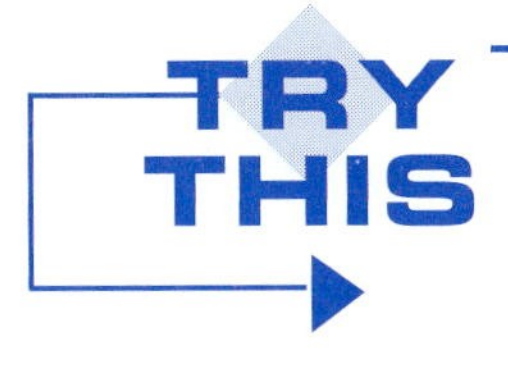

Enter all the code just provided with proper settings of controls listed at the beginning. Start the project. You should be able to see the text box moving around the grid as you click on different cells. In addition, whatever you enter into the text box should appear in the cell after you click on another cell as well as the Save command. In the latter case, the text box should disappear. If you click on a cell in which you have entered data previously, the text should appear in the text box highlighted.

Handling the Scrollbars on the Grid. Before we leave this subsection, there is a fine detail that needs to be taken care: The user may use the grid's scrollbar to change the cell positions in the grid. Because the relative position of the active cell will have been changed in this situation, the text box's position will have to be adjusted as well. The MS HFG has a Scroll event, which is raised when the user moves the scrollbar. The code to adjust the text box's position in the grid can be coded in this event procedure:

```
Private Sub grdInput_Scroll()
     ShowEditBox 'Reposition the text box
End Sub
```

Handling Navigation Keys

Instead of using the mouse to move around the grid, most likely the user will use the navigation keys, such the Enter key or the arrow keys. Let's consider the Enter key first. In a typical spreadsheet application, the Enter key either moves the focus to the cell on the right or below. We will assume that this key will move the focus to the right because in most data-entry applications, data in a table are entered row by row.

Coding the Enter Key. When the Enter key is pressed, before the cursor is moved, the content of the text box should be assigned to the active cell. The program should then move the focus (the text box) to the cell on the right. The event procedure to handle this is txtEdit_KeyPress, as shown in the following code. In the procedure, the value of the key pressed is checked against the named constant vbKeyReturn (13). After assigning the content of the text box to the active cell, the procedure calls another procedure, MoveToCellRight. In addition, the key's ASCII value is replaced with a zero so that no further processing is performed on the key. Notice that the circumstance of this event is quite different from that of the mouse click as described previously. The text box still has the focus and is still sitting on top of the active cell. Thus, there is no need to consider where the active cell was.

```
Private Sub txtEdit_KeyPress(KeyAscii As Integer)
    If KeyAscii = vbKeyReturn Then
        grdInput.Text = txtEdit.Text 'Drop content in the cell
        MoveToCellRight 'Move focus to the right
        KeyAscii = 0 'Suppress the Return key
    End If
End Sub
```

Coding the MoveToCellRight Sub. Let's consider the code for the MoveToCellRight Sub procedure. This procedure should handle the movement of the text box when the user presses the Enter key. We need to take into account three possible situations of the cell location:

1. The active cell is not at the rightmost position of the grid. The next active cell should be set to the right. All we need to do is to increase the Col property by 1 (Note that .Col and CurCol have the same value at this point):

   ```
   .Col = CurCol + 1
   ```

2. The active cell is at the rightmost position of the grid, but the current row is not the last row of the grid. The next active cell should be set to the leftmost nonfixed cell (column 1) of the row below. That is, the Row property should be increased by 1, and Col property should be assigned a value of 1:

   ```
   .Row = CurRow + 1
   .Col = 1
   ```

3. The active cell is the rightmost cell of the grid's bottom row. In this case, the focus should be moved to the next control. The text box should be invisible. No additional code in the current procedure should be executed (Exit Sub). The code should appear as follows:

   ```
   cmdSave.SetFocus 'set focus on next control
   txtEdit.Visible = False 'disappear once lost focus
   Exit Sub
   ```

In cases 1 and 2, the ShowEditBox Sub procedure should be called to move and display the text box in the new active cell. The complete procedure appears as follows:

```
Sub MoveToCellRight()
    With grdInput
        If CurCol < .Cols - 1 Then
            ' typical move to next cell
            .Col = CurCol + 1
        ElseIf CurRow < .Rows - 1 Then
            ' cursor at the rightmost col,
            'move to first cell of next row
            .Row = CurRow + 1
            .Col = 1
        Else
           ' at rightmost cell of bottom row; move to next control
            cmdSave.SetFocus 'set focus on next control
            txtEdit.Visible = False 'disappear
            Exit Sub
        End If
    End with
    ShowEditBox
End Sub
```

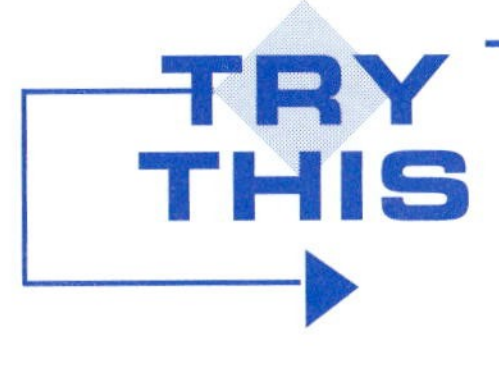

Add the preceding code to the project and run the project. Press the Enter key repetitively when the grid has the focus. The text box should move from left to right until it reaches the end of a row. Then it will move to the beginning (first nonfixed column) of the next row. When the text box reaches the end of the grid, pressing the Enter key again will move the focus to the next control.

Coding the Arrow Keys. How should the arrow keys behave? The left- and right-arrow keys are used inside the text box to move the cursor left or right. If we program these keys such that they will move between cells, we in effect take away the ability for the user to use these keys to move the cursor to edit the text in the text box. Inconsistent behaviors of the keys can make it confusing for the user.

One possible solution is to have these keys behave as they normally do when no Shift key is pressed. Only when one of the Shift keys (including Ctrl and Alt keys) is pressed simultaneously with the arrow keys should the cell focus be moved. The arrow keys and the Shift keys can be captured in the KeyDown event. The code to implement this design is shown here:

```
Private Sub txtEdit_KeyDown(KeyCode As Integer, Shift As Integer)
    If Shift = 0 Then Exit Sub    'handle arrow keys only if a shift
                                  ' key is pressed
    If KeyCode < vbKeyLeft Then Exit Sub 'Not an arrow key
    If KeyCode > vbKeyDown Then Exit Sub 'Not an arrow key
    grdInput.Text = txtEdit.Text 'Leave the content in cell
    Select Case KeyCode
    Case vbKeyLeft ' Arrow key left (37)
        MoveToCellLeft
    Case vbKeyUp ' Arrow key up (38)
        MoveToCellAbove
    Case vbKeyRight ' Arrow key right (39)
        MoveToCellRight
    Case vbKeyDown ' Arrow key down (40)
        MoveToCellBelow
    End Select
    KeyCode = 0
End Sub
```

The code first checks whether a Shift key has been pressed. If not (i.e., Shift = 0), the key will not be processed. In addition, if the key is not an arrow key, there is no need to handle it. The next two statements ensure that only arrow keys will be handled in this procedure. The key code values for the left-, up-, right-, and down-arrow keys are 37, 38, 39, and 40, respectively. These keys have predefined system constant names: vbKeyLeft, vbKeyUp, vbKeyRight, and vbKeyDown.

Notice that when an arrow key is pressed, the current content of the text box is assigned to the active cell first. Then in the Select Case block, a separate Sub procedure is used to handle the key movement. Note also that the right-arrow key uses the same procedure as the Enter key because both are to behave the same way (move to the right).

The code for the three additional Sub procedures is shown next. The logic for each of these procedures is similar to that for MoveToCellRight explained previously.

```
Sub MoveToCellLeft()
    With grdInput
        If CurCol > .FixedCols Then
            ' typical move to cell to the left
             .Col = CurCol - 1
            ElseIf CurRow > .FixedRows Then
            ' at the leftmost col; move to last cell of the row
            above
            .Row = CurRow - 1
            .Col = .Cols - 1
```

```
            Else
            ' at first cell of the grid; move to the control above
                txtAboveGrid.SetFocus
                txtEdit.Visible = False
                Exit Sub
            End If
        End With
        ShowEditBox
    End Sub

    Sub MoveToCellBelow()
        With grdInput
            If CurRow < .Rows - 1 Then
            ' typical move to row below
                .Row = CurRow + 1
            Else
            ' at bottom row; move to the control below the grid
                cmdSave.SetFocus
                txtEdit.Visible = False
                Exit Sub
            End If
        End With
        ShowEditBox
    End Sub

    Sub MoveToCellAbove()
        With grdInput
            If CurRow > .FixedRows Then
            ' typical move to row above
                .Row = CurRow - 1
            Else
            ' grid boundary; move to the control above
                txtAboveGrid.SetFocus
                txtEdit.Visible = False
                Exit Sub
            End If
        End With
        ShowEditBox
    End Sub
```

Additional Remarks

The data entered onto the grid should be further processed and/or saved. As discussed previously, its TextMatrix property makes it easy to access the text in all cells. For example, the following code fragment will accumulate the total for column 1 of the grid named grdInput:

```
Dim R As Integer
Dim Total As Double
 'Assuming that Row 0 is fixed (used for column titles)
With grdInput
    For R = 1 to .Rows - 1
        Total = total + Val(.TextMatrix(R, 1))
    Next R
End With
```

Error Checking. Data-entry programs typically require that all data entered be checked for possible errors. Using the preceding approach, keys pressed into the text box should all be checked for correct data type (key press level check). In addition, when the text box is being moved from a cell, its content should be checked for field validity (field level check).

The key press level check (as explained in Chapter 10, "Special Topics in Data Entry") can be coded in the text box's KeyPress event procedure (not in the form's KeyPress event). *The key pressed can be checked for the correct data type by the column of the grid.* For example, assume that CheckNumeric and CheckAlphabet Sub procedures are available (as illustrated in Chapter

10), columns 1 and 4 of grdInput call for numeric data, and columns 2 and 3 require alphabetic data. The following event procedure can be used:

```
Private Sub txtEdit_KeyPress(KeyAscii as Integer)
    Select Case grdInput.Col
        Case 1,4
            ' Column 1 and 4 require numeric data
            CheckNumeric KeyAscii
        Case 2,3
            ' Column 2 and 3 require alphabetic data
            CheckAlpha KeyAscii
        End Select
End Sub
```

You should perform the field-level data validation when the user leaves a cell. If the user leaves a cell by clicking another part of the grid or form, the text box will lose focus. If the user leaves a cell by using a navigation key, the move is recognized by the KeyDown event. In each of these event procedures, you can insert code at the beginning to check for field-level errors. For example, the following fragments of code should prevent the focus from being moved when the cell is empty:

```
Function Missing(T as String) as Boolean
    Missing = Len(Trim$(T)) = 0
End Function
Private Sub txtEdit_LostFocus(Cancel As Boolean)
'***the following lines are inserted for data validation
    If Missing(txtEdit.Text) then
        MsgBox "Must have data"
        grdInput.Col = CurCol 'set focus to the previous
        grdInput.Row = CurRow 'cell
        ShowEditBox 'go back to that previous cell
        Exit Sub
    End If
'*** the preceding lines are inserted for data validation
    grdInput.TextMatrix(CurRow, CurCol) = txtEdit.Text
    txtEdit.Visible = False
End Sub
```

Notice in the preceding code, the active cell is reset to the previous one because the mouse click may have changed the current active cell if a part of the grid has been clicked. It is not necessary to reset the focus if the attempted move is done by a navigation key (the active cell is still the same) as shown here:

```
Private Sub txtEdit_KeyDown(KeyCode As Integer, Shift As Integer)
    If Shift = 0 Then Exit Sub    'handle arrow keys only if
                                  'a shift key is pressed
    '****the following lines are inserted for data validation
    If KeyCode >= vbKeyLeft and KeyCode <= vbKeyDown then
        If Missing(txtEdit) then
            MsgBox "Must have data"
            Exit Sub
        End If
    Else
        Exit Sub 'Not an arrow key; ignore.
    End If
    '******the preceding lines are inserted for data validation
    ' Typical handling for the arrow keys
    Select Case KeyCode
    Case vbKeyLeft ' Arrow key left (37)
        grdInput.Text = txtEdit.Text
        MoveToCellLeft
  .
  .
  .
End Sub
```

The preceding illustration does not take into account the possibility of allowing the user to move back (up) without checking, which can be desirable in most cases. Neither does it show how to check for errors when the user presses the Enter key. However, it should be similar to handling the right-arrow key. The needed code is left to you as an exercise.

Clearing the Grid

After the data entered on the grid are handled (e.g., saved), it may be desirable to clear the grid for the next entry. The MS HFG has a Clear method that can be used to clear all cells. However, this may not be exactly what you want to do because your grid probably has column headings and row numbers that you have set and would rather keep. You can use its FillStyle property to handle the clearing elegantly in this case.

The ***FillStyle property*** can be set to either flexFillSingle (0; default) or flexFillRepeat (1). When this property is set to flexFillSingle, a change to the text and formatting properties applies only to the active cell. When this property is set to flexFillRepeat, a change to the text applies to all the selected cells. Thus, you can clear all the nonfixed cells by doing the following:

1. Setting the FillStyle property to flexFillRepeat
2. Selecting all nonfixed cells
3. Assigning a zero-length string to the Text property

To ensure that changing the FillStyle property in a procedure will not accidentally affect the grid's FillStyle behavior in any part of your project, you should restore the property to its original setting. The following sample code takes this into account by keeping the original setting before the property is changed and reassigning the original value before the procedure ends.

```
Private Sub ClearGrid()
Dim DefaultSetting As Integer
    With grdInput
        DefaultSetting = .FillStyle 'Keep the original setting
        .FillStyle = flexFillRepeat 'Change FillStyle to "Repeat"
        ' Select all non-fixed cells
        .Col = 1
        .Row = 1
        .ColSel = .Cols - 1
        .RowSel = .Rows - 1
        .Text = "" ' Clear all selected cells
        .FillStyle = DefaultSetting 'Restore the original setting
        .ColSel = 1 ' Set the selection to (1, 1)
        .RowSel = 1 ' So that the grid will not show highlight
    End With
End Sub
```

Summary

We took a closer look at two VB objects in this chapter: the Printer object and the MS HFG. Our goals were to explore the capabilities of the two objects for reporting (and possibly other output) purposes as well as the use of the grid for tabular input (data entry). Both the Printer object and the HFG provide a lot of flexibility in handling output.

Although the Printer object is limited to one sheet in *active* operations, you can produce complex reports with careful analysis and design. We illustrated how the fonts (and their sizes) can be set. We also showed how the object can be used to print pictures and how to compute the coordinates to print any output at the desired locations. These illustrations should provide you with sufficient foundation to design your own reports or any other kind of output.

The HFG has many interesting features. We showed how it can be used to display tables and any tabular reports, whether bound to an ADO recordset or not. The HFG's sort and merge capabilities are worth noting. Reports can be designed so that the user can select columns to sort. Your imagination can be the only limit to exploit the potential of this feature to present useful and flexible reports for management.

Although our focus was on displaying texts, the grid can also be used to show pictures. This capability is illustrated in one of the Visual Basic Explorer exercises.

We noted that although many business applications call for data to be entered in a tabular form, none of the existing VB controls can handle this type of operation conveniently. Section 13.3 shows an approach to overlay a text box in the HFG for such purposes. Hopefully, the illustration provides you not only with a solution to a problem but also with an example as to how you can enhance the capability of an existing control.

Visual Basic Explorer

13-1. The NewPage and EndDoc Method and the Page Property. Draw two command buttons on a new form. Name the first one cmdNewPage and set its Caption property to "New Page." Name the second one cmdEnddoc and set its Caption property to "End Doc." Enter the following code:

```
Option Explicit

Private Sub cmdNewPage_Click()
Static Count
    With Printer
        .CurrentX = 72
        .CurrentY = 720
        Count = Count + 1
        Printer.Print "Page " & Printer.Page; _
          " Count = " & Count
        Printer.NewPage
    End With
End Sub

Private Sub cmdEnddoc_Click()
    Printer.EndDoc
End Sub
```

Run the project and click the New Page button two times. Then click the End Doc button. Repeat the same clicks. Inspect the printout. You should see Count continues to go up on each additional output sheet. However, the page number starts over from 1 after you click the End Doc button. What have you learned?

13-2. Text Height and Line Height. Run the following code in a new project and click the form.

```
Private Sub Form_Click()
Dim Y As Single
    Y = Printer.CurrentY
    Printer.Print
    Me.Print Printer.CurrentY - Y
    Me.Print Printer.TextHeight("H")
End Sub
```

What numbers do you see on the form? The expression "Printer.CurrentY – Y" gives the printer current line height. So, is it the same as the printer's text height? Can you use the text height to approximate the line height?

13-3. What if the Font Size Changes? Modify the preceding code so that it appears as follows. Run the project and click the form.

```
Private Sub Form_Click()
Dim Y As Single
    Printer.Print "";
    Printer.Font.Size = 14
    Y = Printer.CurrentY
    Printer.Print
    Me.Print Printer.CurrentY - Y
```

```
    Me.Print Printer.TextHeight("H")
End Sub
```

What numbers do you see on the form this time? Are the two numbers still the same? Are they the same as the two in 13-2? What conclusion can you draw?

13-4. The ScaleMode Property of the Printer Object. Enter the following code in a new project.

```
Private Sub Form_Click()
    Printer.ScaleMode = vbInches
    Print Printer.TextHeight("H"); Printer.TextWidth("H")
    Printer.CurrentX = 6
    Printer.Print "H"

    Printer.ScaleMode = vbPixels
    Print Printer.TextHeight("H"); Printer.TextWidth("H")
    Printer.CurrentX = 6
    Printer.Print "H"

    Printer.ScaleMode = vbPoints
    Print Printer.TextHeight("H"); Printer.TextWidth("H")
    Printer.CurrentX = 6
    Printer.Print "H"

    Printer.ScaleMode = vbTwips
    Print Printer.TextHeight("H"); Printer.TextWidth("H")
    Printer.CurrentX = 6
    Printer.Print "H"
End Sub
```

Run the project, click the form, and study the four pairs of numbers. What do the numbers tell you? They give you the size of "H" under different measurement units. (Under the scale mode of vbInches, "H" should be only a fractional number because it size is only a fraction of an inch.)

Notice that when the program ends, the printer prints all four "H"'s in the same size but at a different horizontal position. The setting of ScaleMode property affects how CurrentX and CurrentY are measured but does not affect the font size.

13-5. Setting the ScaleHeight Property. Start a new project. Enter the following code:

```
Option Explicit

Private Sub Form_Click()
    Debug.Print Printer.ScaleMode
    Printer.ScaleHeight = 100
    Debug.Print Printer.ScaleMode
    Printer.CurrentY = 50
    Printer.Print "CurrentY at 50"
End Sub
```

Run the project. Click the form. What do you see in the Debug window? The ScaleMode changed from 1 (vbTwips) to 0 (vbUser) after the ScaleHeight property was assigned a value (100).

Examine the printout. Where is the line printed? It should be about half way from the top of the page. Assigning a value to the ScaleHeight (or ScaleWidth) property does not change the physical printable area. Rather, it changes how the area is measured. After executing the preceding code, the entire printable height is 100 units. Setting CurrentY to 100 will start the printing at the bottom of the printable area.

13-6. The PrintForm Method. Start a new project. Draw a command button on the form. Name it cmdPrintForm and set its Caption property to "Print Form." Then enter the following code:

```
Private Sub cmdPrintForm_Click()
    Me.PrintForm
End Sub
```

Run the project and click the button. Do you see a form printed? Notice that the method is provided by the form, not by the Printer object.

13-7. The FormatString Property of the HFG. Draw an HFG on a new form. Name it grdTest. In the Form Load event procedure, type in the following code:

```
grdTest.FormatString = _
      " ¦^S-S-N ¦<Name ¦<Home Address ¦>Zip Code "
```

Run the project. How does the grid appear? How many columns are there in the grid? Do you see any field headings? How are they aligned? What do you think the character “|” is for? How about “^,”“<,” and “>”? They do not appear in the headings, but do they serve some purposes?

13-8. More on the FormatString Property. Modify the preceding code to the following:

```
grdTest.FormatString = _
      " ¦^S-S-N ¦<Name ¦<Home Address ¦>Zip Code " & _
         ";¦1¦2¦3"
```

Run the project. What do you see this time? What do you think the semicolon (;) in the format string is for?

13-9. The CellPicture Property of the HFG. Add the following code to the preceding project.

```
With grdTest
     .ColWidth(0) = .ColWidth(0) * 2
     .RowHeight(0) = .RowHeight(0) * 2
     .Col = 0
     .Row = 0
     Set .CellPicture = LoadPicture _
        ("C:\Program Files\Microsoft Visual Studio\Common" & _
           "\Graphics\Icons\Traffic\Trffc10a.ico")
End With
```

Run the project. Do you see a picture in the grid? The CellPicture property of the HFG can be used to display a picture in a cell.

13-10. The ColAlignment and CellAlignment Properties of the HFG. Draw an HFG on a new form. Name the grid grdTest. Set it Rows property to 3. Enter the following code:

```
Private Sub Form_Click()
     With grdTest
          .ColAlignment(1) = flexAlignRightCenter
          .TextMatrix(0, 1) = "ABC"
          .TextMatrix(1, 1) = "ABC"
          .TextMatrix(2, 1) = "ABC"
     End With
End Sub
```

Run the project and click the form. How are the texts aligned in the grid? The ColAlignment property affects only the nonfixed cells.

Insert the following code within the With block.

```
     .Col = 1
     .Row = 0
     .CellAlignment = flexAlignRightCenter
     .Row = 1
     .CellAlignment = flexAlignLeftCenter
```

Test the program again. What do you see this time? The CellAlignment property can be used to specify the alignment for any cell. However, notice how the property setting is assigned. You must first specify the current (active) cell (by assigning numbers to Row and Col properties) before specifying the alignment. For the list of alignment constants, search the Index tab of the online Help file for the keyword "ColAlignment property." (*Note:* You can also use the ColAlignmentFixed property to set alignment for the fixed cells. This property has syntax similar to that for the ColAlignment property.)

13-11. The TextArray Property of the HFG. (continued from 13-10). Insert the following statement immediately before the End With statement in the preceding project:

```
.TextArray(1) = "CDE"
```

Run the project and click the form. Where does "CDE" appear? You know another way to make the same text appear in the same cell. So, how are the TextArray and TextMatrix properties related to each other?

13-12. The MouseRow and MouseCol Property. (continued from 13-11). Add the following code to the preceding project. (Note that the event is grdTest_Click, not Form_Click.)

```
Private Sub grdTest_Click()
    With grdTest
        Debug.Print .Row; .Col
        Debug.Print .MouseRow; .MouseCol
    End With
End Sub
```

Run the project. Click a nonfixed cell. What do you see in the immediate window? The two pairs of numbers should be the same.

Click a fixed cell. Now, what do you see? The pair (MouseRow, MouseCol) gives the correct cell clicked. However, the pair (Row, Col) gives the nearest nonfixed cell. Beware of how you use the Row and Col properties in response to the Click event.

13-13. The Clip Property of the HFG. Draw an HFG on a new form. Name it grdTest. Enter the following code:

```
Option Explicit

Private Sub Form_Click()
Dim Text As String
Dim I As Integer
    With grdTest
        .Rows = 3
        For I = 0 To 5
            .TextArray(I) = Chr$(65 + I)
        Next I
        .Row = 0
        .Col = 0
        .RowSel = 2
        .ColSel = 1
        Text = grdTest.Clip
        Debug.Print Text; Len(Text)
    End With
End Sub
```

Run the project and click the form. What do you see in the grid? (For an explanation of the TextArray property, see 13-11.) What do you see in the immediate window? The Clip property returns data in the cells selected in the pairs of (Row, Col) and (RowSel, and ColSel). Data between cells in the same row are separated by vbTab characters. Data between rows are separated by vbCr characters. (*Note:* If you see nothing but the number 0 in the Debug window, you need to download Visual Studio SP3 [Service pack 3] from Microsoft and install the patches to correct the bugs in the original package.)

13-14. The TopRow and LeftCol Property. Draw an HFG on a new form. Name the grid grdTester. Set its Cols and Rows properties to 20 and 200, respectively (use the Property

Pages dialog box by double-clicking the Custom property in the Properties window). Then type in the following code:

```
Private Sub grdTester_Scroll()
    MsgBox "Top Row = " & grdTester.TopRow & _
      ".LeftCol = " & grdTester.LeftCol
End Sub
```

Run the project. Use the grid's scrollbar to make the grid to show different cells in the grid. Also you can use the arrow keys to move the focus between cells when the grid has the focus. You should see the message box display a message each time the visible area of the grid changes. When is the Scroll event fired? What do the TopRow and LeftCol properties tell you?

Exercises

13-15. Printing a Picture. Draw an image control and a command button on a new form. Name the image control imgLapTop. Set its Stretch property to True and its Picture property to LapTop1.wmf, which is located in the following folder: Common\Graphics\MetaFile\Business (under the Microsoft Visual Studio).

Name the command button cmdPrint and set its Caption property to "Print." Provide the code to print the laptop computer with the Landscape orientation in the image control when the user clicks the Print button. The computer should be printed at the center of the sheet and should be 50% wider and taller than the picture in the image control. (*Note:* Use the EndDoc method to effect the printing instead of waiting for the program to end.)

13-16. Adding Text to a Picture. (continued from 13-15). Add code to the preceding project so that "My Favorite Computer" will be printed on the screen of the laptop computer. Use the Lucida Handwriting font (size 10). If your printer does not have the specified font, use your favorite font as a substitute. (*Hint:* The text should start approximately at the middle of the sheet horizontally and three lines above the center vertically.)

13-17. Right-Alignment on a Column for the Printer. Write a Sub with the following header:

```
Sub PrintRightAligned(Text As String, ColEnd As Single)
```

The Sub procedure will print the Text parameter right-aligned; that is, the text will end at the position as specified by the ColEnd parameter. Test the Sub with 10 random numbers that are generated by the following code:

```
Format$(1000000 * Rnd, "Currency")
```

In addition, specify that the column ends at half of the printer width (use the ScaleWdith property).

13-18. Printing the Present Value Factors. Develop a project to print a hard copy of the present value factors for interest rates from 4% to 12% (increment by 1%) and periods from 1 to 20 years (increment by 1 year). The text provides a sample program to compute the same but display in a grid.

Print the results with the Landscape orientation. Also notice that the columns should be right-aligned. Thus, the Sub you developed for 13-17 can come in handy.

13-19. Allowing the User to Specify Fonts for the Table for the Present Value Factors. (continued from 13-18). Modify the project in the preceding exercise so that the user can specify the following:

- Font and font size
- Range of interest rates (assume an increment of 1%)
- Range of periods (assume an increment of one period).

(*Hint:* Use combo boxes and populate each with pertinent data so that the user can select without having to enter the required data. Be sure to set the Style property for the combo box for fonts to 2-Dropdown List.)

13-20. Allowing the User to Specify Fonts, Mailing Labels. Develop a project to printing mailing labels. The user should be able to specify the following:

- Font and font size
- Horizontal and vertical space to shift (adjust) in $1/10$ of an inch (i.e., 0.1, 0.2, and so on) (*Hint:* There are 1440 twips per inch.)
- Database and the table containing the address information

You can use the Sub procedure Print1Label illustrated in the text to handle the actual printing.

13-21. Multipage Report with Page Numbers. Modify the Title-Publisher project presented in this chapter in the following manner:

- The data will be sorted on the column that the user clicks.
- Add a command button. Name it cmdPrint and set its Caption property to "Print."
- When the user clicks the Print button, the data in the grid will be printed on the printer. Note that the "report" can be several pages long. Make sure that each page has the report title, column headings, and page number.

13-22. Present Value Table Specified by the User. Modify the present value project in this chapter so that the user can specify the lower rate, upper rate, and increment rate for the table. In addition, the user can also specify the maximum number of years, instead of 20 years as in the example.

13-23. A Loan Payment Table. Develop a project to display a loan (monthly) payment table assuming a principal amount of $100,000. The interest rates should vary from 5% to 12%. The payment periods should vary from 5 to 15 years. (Note that the periods are by year but the payments are monthly.) The output should have a format as follows:

Year/Rate	5%	6%	7%	...
5	(amount)	(amount)	...	
6	(amount)	...		
7	...			

Use the HFG to display the table. (*Hint:* Use the Pmt function to obtain the monthly payment amounts. Search the Index tab of the online Help file using the keyword "Pmt function" for additional information on how to use this function.)

13-24. A Mortgage Amortization Table. A mortgage amortization table shows how fixed monthly payments are allocated between interest and principal over the life of the mortgage. For example, a mortgage of $100,000 for 5 years (60 months) at a rate of 9% requires a monthly payment of $2,075.84. An amortization table for the mortgage can be prepared as follows:

	Beginning Balance	Payment	Interest	Principal Reduced
1	100,000	2,075.84	750.00	1,325.84
2	98,674.16	2,075.84	740.06	1,335.78
3	.	.	.	.

Develop a project that will do the following:

- Allow the user to enter the amount of mortgage, interest rate (annual percentage rate), and loan life (in months).
- Compute the monthly payment.
- Display an amortization table for the mortgage using the HFG.

(*Hint:* The amount of interest is computed with the following formula:
Interest = Beginning Balance × Annual Percentage Rate/12.)

13-25. A Depreciation Schedule: The Sum-of-Years-Digit Method. In accounting, fixed assets are depreciated based on the depreciable base and life (in years). Under the sum-of-years-digit method, the depreciation amount for each year is computed by multiplying the base by a factor derived as follows:

Let B = Depreciable base (Cost – Salvage value)
L = Life in years

The sum-of-years-digit can be computed as follows:

$$S = 1 + 2 + 3 + \ldots + L = L\,(L + 1)/2$$

Then the depreciation amount for each year is computed as follows:

Year	Depreciation
1	B (L/S)
2	B ((L –1))/S)
3	B ((L –2))/S)
4	. . .

For example, a fixed asset with a depreciable base of $100,000 and 4 years of useful life will have a depreciation schedule as follows:

Year	Depreciation	Accumulated Depreciation
1	4,000	4,000
2	3,000	7,000
3	2,000	9,000
4	1,000	10,000

Where the accumulated depreciation is total depreciation from the beginning up to (inclusive) the year of computation.

Develop a VB project that will do the following:

- Allow the user to enter the depreciable base and the useful life.
- Compute and display the depreciation schedule in an HFG when the user clicks a command button with the caption "Compute."

13-26. Present Value of Annuity Table. The present value of an annuity of $1 is computed using the following formula:

$$P = (1 + r)^{-1} + (1 + r)^{-2} + \ldots + (1 + r)^{-n}$$

where r is the rate of interest and n is the number of periods (years).

Develop a VB project that will do the following:

- Allow the user to enter the range of interest rates (assume an increment of 1%) and the maximum number of periods.
- Compute the present values of the annuity under different rates and time periods when the user clicks a command button with the caption "Compute." The results should be displayed in an HFG in a format similar to the following:

	5%	6%	7%	...
1	0.9524	0.9434	0.9346	
2	1.8594	...		
3	...			

13-27. Query and Sort and Merge. Develop a project to search the Biblio database by year of publication. When the user enters the year in a text box and clicks a command button captioned "Search," the program will display in an HFG all the book titles published in that year along with the publisher, the author, and the ISBN. Also, the first column should give the count (row number).

Use the ADO connection's Execute method to obtain the recordset. Also provide the code so that when the user clicks a column, the data are sorted by that column. Cells in the publisher column and the author column (respectively) should be merged if the neighboring cells have the same data.

13-28. Sort and Merge with the HFG. The NWInd database has a Customers table. Use ADO by code to display all customers in an HFG (use the connection object's Execute method to obtain the recordset). Then when the user clicks on a particular column, the data will sort in ascending order by that column. Also, all cells with the same value in that column should be merged.

13-29. Browsing Database Tables with the MS HFG Control (SQL). Develop a project that will perform the following:

1. Prompt the user for the file location for the NWInd database, which will be concatenated to the connection string to be used for a query.
2. Retrieve the data from the database based on the range of required dates (in the Orders table) specified by the user. These dates are entered in two masked edit boxes. When the user clicks the Search button, the following fields should be retrieved and displayed in an HFG:

Field	Field Name	In Table
Date Required	RequiredDate	Orders
Date Shipped	ShippedDate	Orders
Order ID	OrderID	Orders
Contact Name	ContactName	Customers
Phone	Phone	Customers
Product Name	ProductName	Products

Requirement 1 should be done as soon as the program starts. Requirement 2 should be carried out when the user clicks the Browse command button. The results should be sorted by date required (first level), then by date shipped (second level). Use the grid's sort capability. Cells in the HFG with the same date required should be merged. Also, set the "Allow User Resize" property of the HFG to flexResizeColumns (1). (*Hint:* Enclose the date in a pair of "#" signs, e.g., #01/31/1998# for SQL statements. To facilitate sorting, format dates with "yyyy/mm/dd" as the format string.)

Projects

13-30. Importing Comma-Delimited Files. Develop a project that will import comma-delimited files to a database table. The form should have a tab control, which will be used so that the program will behave in the following manner:

1. In Tab 0, there should be a text box for the user to specify the text file to be imported. By the text box, there should be a command button to allow the user to browse the system and select the file. (The file must exist. This file should be opened in Tab 1, not here. See Figure 13.11.)
2. In Tab 1 (Figure 13.11), there should be a text box for the user to specify the number of fields per record. By this text box, there should be a command button to click when the user is ready to import. Your program will then read the text file and display the data in an MS HFG, which should have one more column than the number of fields per record. The first column is used to display record number; the other columns are used to display the fields of each record.
3. In Tab 2 (Figure 13.11), there should be a text box for the user to specify the database name to import the text file. By the text box, there should be a command button to allow the user to browse the system and select the database. (The database must exist.) Below the text box there should be a combo box, which will be filled with the table names found in the database specified. The user is expected to enter a new table name. Existing table names are not allowed.
4. In Tab 3 (Figure 13.11), there should be a text box to enter the field name. The field is selected from an HFG, which has two rows. The first row is a fixed row and is initially blank. The second row contains the first record copied from the HFG in Tab 1. When the user clicks on a column of the HFG, the data in that column will be displayed in a label below the text box. After the user enters the field name in the text box, the name will be placed in the first row of the selected (clicked) column and in the second column of another grid, which is used tp keep track of the fields selected. Thus, each field selected with the name specified becomes a row in this second grid, whose first column shows the field number, second column shows the field name, and third column gives the data of the field selected from the first HFG. If the user double-clicks a field name in the second grid, the row is removed. When the user clicks the Save button in this tab, all the selected fields of all records in the imported grid (in Tab 1) will be saved in the database table specified in Tab 2.

Your program should ensure that the proper sequence of actions is followed (Tab 0 is completed before proceeding to Tab 1, and so on). It should have additional labels to provide necessary instructions in each step. It should also check for all potential errors. Figure 13.11 provides a sample visual interface for each tab.

FIGURE 13.11
Sample Visual Interface for the Text File Importer

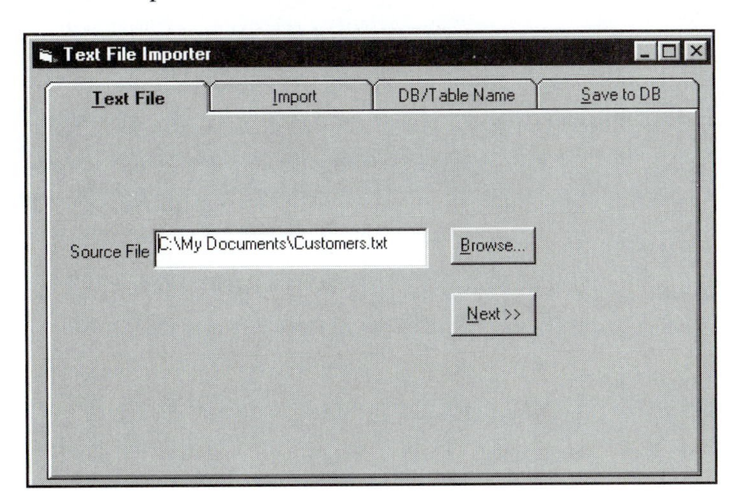

Tab0 should allow the user to specify the source file.

continues

FIGURE 13.11
Sample Visual Interface for the Text File Importer

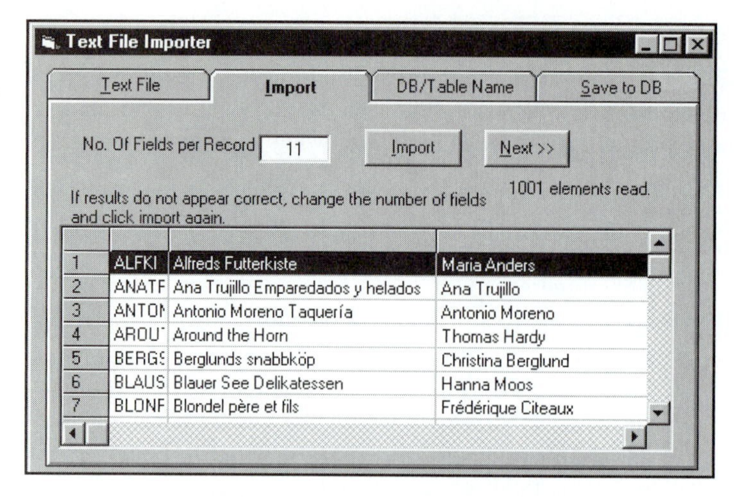

Tab1 should allow the user to specify the number of fields per record. When the user clicks the Import button, the program will read the text file and display the records.

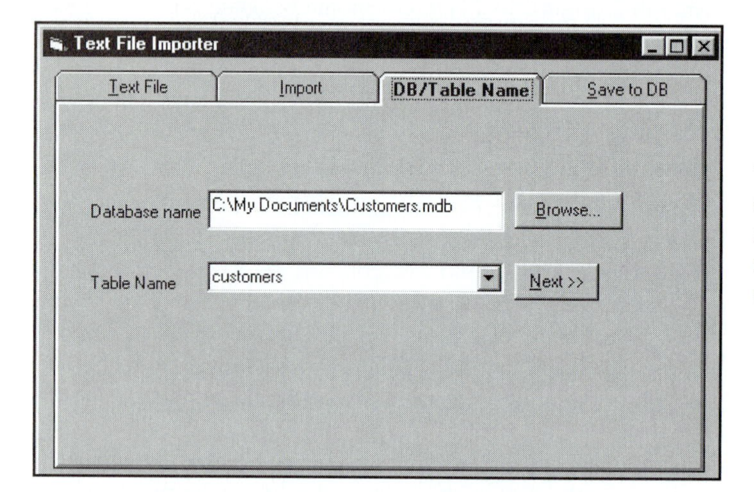

Tab2 should allow the user to specify the database name and table name. The database must exist, and the table name must be new.

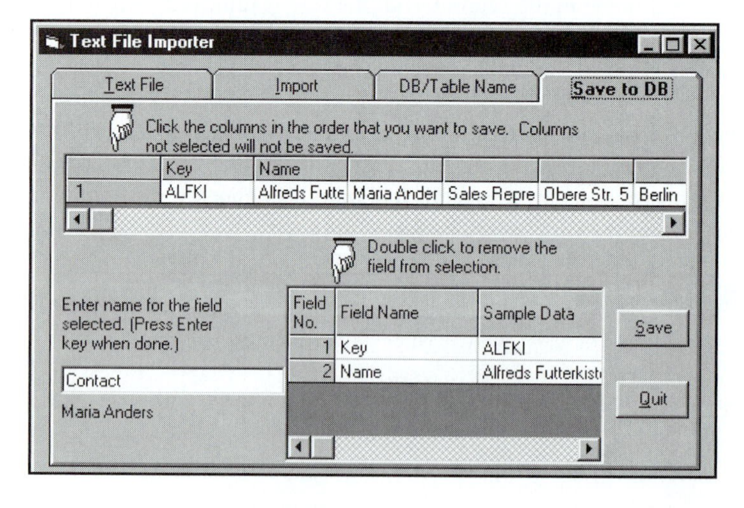

Tab3 will display the first imported record in the first HFG and allow the user to select a field and specify the field name. When the user presses the Enter key after entering the field name, the field name and the sample data will appear in the second HFG. Selected fields of the imported records will be saved in the database table specified in Tab2 when the user clicks the Save button.

13-31. Sales Order Entry Screen. You are engaged in developing a sales order entry project. The program should have a visual interface as in Figure 13.12:

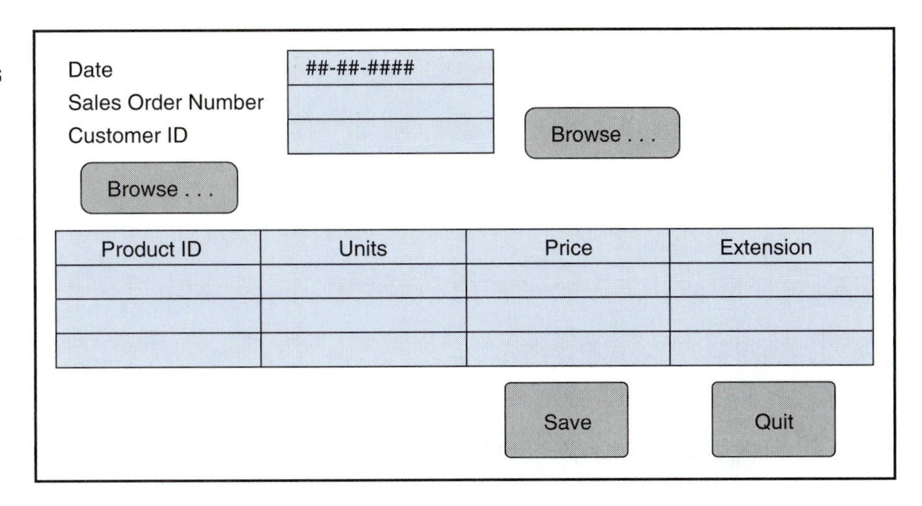

FIGURE 13.12
Visual Interface for Sales Order Entry

Required: Develop a project so that the user can enter required data. Additional specification/requirements:

1. Use the MS HFG to handle the order detail lines (which can go as many as 30 lines, of which 5 lines should be visible).
2. The user can leave a cell either by using the mouse or by using the Enter key or Shift+<arrow key>. The extension column should be computed when the user leaves the Price field. This column should be "protected" from the user; that is, the column should not be accessible to the user by any key or mouse click.
3. Data validation should be done as follows:
   A. Key-level checking: Date, Sales Order Number, Product ID, Units, and Prices must be numeric. Customer ID must be alphabetic.
   B. Field-level checking: Date must be valid. Customer ID and Product ID must exist. (Use the Customers and Products tables in the NWInd.mdb that comes with VB6 to verify Customer ID and Product ID.)
   C. Screen-level checking: All header fields (those data fields above the grid) must have data. A line must be either complete or blank. There should not be blank lines between entered items.
4. When the user clicks the Quit button, if there are unsaved data, the program should verify with the user that he or she means to quit.
5. When the user clicks the Save button, your program should clear the screen and display a "Data saved" message (after successfully completing screen-level error checking).
6. When the user clicks the "Browse..." button by the Customer ID box, a dialog box will appear to allow the user to select a proper Customer ID (using the Customer ID in the Customers table of the NWInd.mdb).
7. When the user clicks the "Browse..." button by the Product ID box, a dialog box will appear to allow the user to select a proper Product ID (using the Product ID in the Products table of the NWInd.mdb).

14 Beyond the Core

This chapter presents topics that are "beyond the core" of VB. However, these topics are very important. They deal with the extensibility of VB. A good knowledge of this chapter will enable you to extend VB's power beyond the level you can currently imagine.

We begin with introducing the Windows API (acronym for Application Program Interface), which is a set of functions provided by the Windows operating systems to perform lower-level services. You can use these functions either to implement capabilities that are not available in VB or to perform certain operations more efficiently.

In Section 14.2, you will be introduced to the Windows registry, a database maintained by the Windows operating system to facilitate its own and other application program's operations. We limit our discussion to how the registry can be used to maintain data needed for the proper operation of your application.

The subsequent sections introduce you to ActiveX components, which are based on an open, extensible standard recognized as the Component Object Model (COM). We first explain concepts and terms. We then illustrate how to use some of the components. Finally, we discuss how to create one type of component, the ActiveX DLL (Dynamic Link Library).

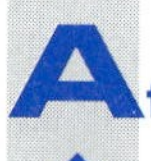

After completing this chapter, you should be able to:

- Understand how to make an API call and appreciate the power of API.
- Have a good working knowledge of how to save and retrieve data from the Windows registry.
- Understand the terms and concepts associated with the component object model.
- Set up the environment and/or create the code to use components.
- Create and use the ActiveX DLL.

14.1 Using the Windows API

API is a set of functions (commands) in the Windows operating system that provide lower-level services to application programs. The Windows API comes with the Windows operating system and is available to all languages (programs), not just VB. Many of the services provided by the operating system for VB have been encapsulated into the language so that we rarely need to make direct API calls.

Why API?

There are cases in which your VB program needs to perform a function that either is not provided by the language or can be much more efficiently performed by an API call. In these cases, using the API will be either the only or the better solution. We introduce API so that you are equipped to find a solution through this route when you encounter this type of situation. However, what we introduce here is merely a very small portion of the available API. To have a complete reference, you will need to consult a book specialized in this area, such as Dan Appleman's *Visual Basic Programmer's Guide to the Win32 API* (Sams, 1999).

Using API

How does a VB program make an API call? Calling an API function is almost the same as calling a VB Sub or function. However, you need to be aware of at least the following issues:

- The program libraries (DLLs) that contain the API functions are not a part of the VB itself. Therefore, you will first need to provide information to the VB compiler on the name of the function that you are calling and in which library the function is located. You use the Declare statement to perform the declaration of the API function. (Note that this is not the same as the familiar Dim statement we use to declare variables.)
- There is a scope restriction on the Declare statement and the Const statement (often used to declare constants used in an API call). If you place these statements in a form or class module, they must be preceded with the keyword Private. That is, you cannot declare API functions as Public in a form or class module.
- API functions have been developed in the C programming language. Parameters expected in C functions are passed by value by default. In contrast, by default, parameters expected in VB functions are passed by reference. Thus, in most cases, API functions expect that parameters are passed by value. When declaring an API function in your VB program, you should take special care to ensure that the keyword ByVal is used for each parameter when called for.
- Internally, VB and C handle strings quite differently. Strings in VB are structured as BSTRs. Under this structure, each string variable contains a header, which includes information on its length and the address of the string itself. Thus, the actual address of the string is different from its "apparent" address. C strings are so called lpSTRs. The pointer to a lpSTR points to the beginning address of the string itself. The null character (Chr$(0)) is used to terminate lpSTRs. Thus, a string's length is "calculated" by searching for the null character from the beginning address. This difference between the two languages requires extra care and code when strings are involved in an API call.
- Some parameters in some API functions can be of any data type. In such a case, the parameter is declared as Any in the parameter list. Such a declaration suppresses data type checking by the VB compiler. You must be extra careful in ensuring that the data passed in a given situation is exactly the data type expected in that particular operation. Otherwise, errors will result. Worse yet, the program may hang. In addition, a parameter declared as Any is passed by reference, not by value. Thus, if "by value" is what is expected for a given operation, you must explicitly state such when calling the function. We will show how to handle this in one of our examples.

The API Text Viewer

Although VB provides a way for you to call API functions, its documentation support is limited to an API viewer, which provides all the necessary texts for the declaration of functions, constants, and user-defined types used in the API. The API Text Viewer comes with the VB software package. You can find and use the Viewer in a computer that has VB installed by the following steps:

1. Click the Windows Start icon at the lower-left corner of the screen.
2. Highlight the Programs menu.
3. Highlight Microsoft Visual Basic 6.0 in the Programs menu.
4. Highlight Microsoft Visual Basic 6.0 Tools.
5. Click the API Text Viewer.

Note that if you have the Microsoft Visual Studio installed, the steps may vary slightly.

When started, the viewer's dialog box appears as in Figure 14.1.

FIGURE 14.1
The API Viewer

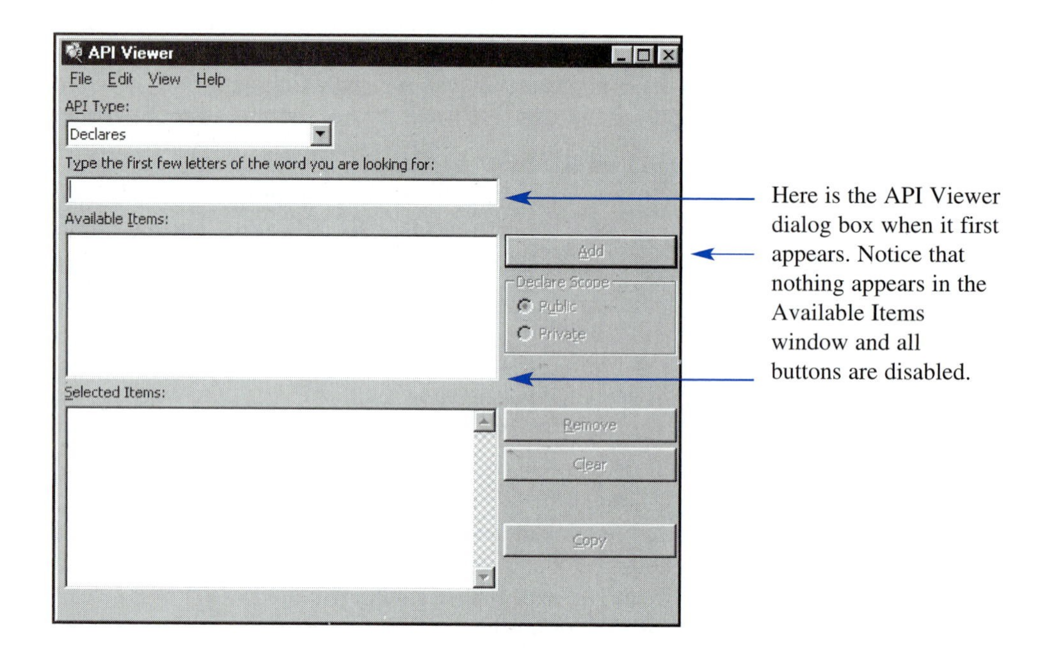

When you start the API viewer, nothing will appear in the Available Items window until you load the API text file or the database file. If you are using the viewer for the first time, only the text file will be readily available.

To load the text file:

1. Click the File drop-down menu in the API viewer.
2. Click the Load Text File option. You should see a Select an API Text file dialog box.
3. Select Win32api.txt in the dialog box and click the Open button.

Three Kinds of "Declarations." Once the API text file is open, you should see items appearing in the Available Items window (list box). Depending on the API type you choose, the list will be different. If you click the API type combo box, you should see that three different types are available:

- The ***Constant*** type provides a list of Constants used in the API.
- The ***Declare*** type gives a list of API functions.
- The ***Type*** type supplies a list of the user-defined types used in the API.

Once you click an item in the Available Items list box, the Add button is enabled. If you click that button, the item you have selected along with the proper VB declaration required for that item will appear in the Selected Items list box. The Clear and Copy buttons are then enabled. If you click an item in this list box, the Remove button will also be enabled. Clicking this button will remove the item you have selected from the list box. You can use the Clear button to clear all items selected in the list box. The Copy button copies all selected items into the Clipboard, which can then be pasted into your code window in the VB IDE.

Also notice that the Declare Scope frame contains two options for the scope of your declaration. If you are declaring the API functions in a form or class module, be sure to select the Private option button before selecting any item in the list box.

Converting to and Using the API Database File. If you use the API viewer often, you should find that loading the database file makes the search faster. You can make the database file available to load by following these steps:

1. Load the text file from the File menu as explained previously.
2. Click the "Convert text to database" option in the File menu. (This option is enabled only after the text file is loaded.) A dialog box will appear to prompt for the database name. (The default is Win32api.mdb.)
3. Click the Save button and the conversion will proceed.

The database file will be available to load from then on.

Sample Uses of API

The following examples illustrate how an API function can be used. They also suggest solutions to application situations in which equivalent capability is either not provided by VB or an API function can perform more efficiently.

Example 1. Trapping the Tab Key. If you have more than one control in a form and some controls have their ***TabStop property*** set to True, there is no VB event procedure in which you can detect that the Tab key has been pressed. (If a control's TabStop property is set to False, the control will not receive the focus when the user uses the Tab key to tab through the controls in the form. The property's default setting is True.) The API function GetKeyState has this capability. This function requires the following declaration statement (the steps to obtain this declaration using the API viewer are presented later):

```
Private Declare Function GetKeyState Lib "user32" _
    (ByVal nVirtKey As Long) As Integer
```

The statement starts with the keywords Private Declare, followed by the keyword Function and the name of the function. The Lib keyword gives the name of the DLL ("user32" in this case). The remainder of the statement is the parameter list (enclosed in a pair of parentheses) and the data type (Integer) that the function is expected to return.

The GetKeyState function requires a Long type parameter that represents the key whose state you are interested to know. The function returns an integer that represents the state of the key at the time the function is invoked. To test whether the Tab key is pressed, you can code the following:

```
KeyTabState = GetKeyState(vbKeyTab)
```

The named constant vbKeyTab is the key code value for the Tab key. Thus, this API call requests the function to return the state of the Tab key. A negative returned value indicates that the Tab key has been pressed.

In what event procedure can this call be placed? You may recall that the Tab key does not trigger the KeyDown, KeyPress, or KeyUp event. Thus, placing the statement in any of these events will not result in the detection of the Tab key. However, the Tab key will trigger the LostFocus event. Therefore, you can test for the Tab key in this event. Suppose that you want to know if the Tab key is pressed in a text box named txtEdit, you can code the following:

```
Private Declare Function GetKeyState Lib "user32" _
    (ByVal nVirtKey As Long) As Integer
Private Sub txtEdit_LostFocus()
Dim KeyTabState As Integer
        KeyTabState = GetKeyState(vbKeyTab)
        If KeyTabState < 0 Then
            MsgBox "Tab Key has been pressed."
        End If
End Sub
```

You may wonder why you would attempt to detect the Tab key in the LostFocus event. After all, pressing the Tab key will result in the control's losing the focus. Recall, however, that the user can also click another control to cause the current active control to lose the focus. The preceding code enables you to differentiate between the two situations.

In Chapter 10, "Special Topics in Data Entry," we used the Validate event to perform data validation when the user leaves a field. You may be tempted to use the same event to trap the Tab key. This is not advisable. Why? If the control receiving the focus after the Tab key has its CausesValidation property set to False, the Validate event will not be raised. You will then not be able to trap the Tab key.

Getting Help from the API Viewer. You may also wonder how to know what to declare for a function. As implied in the previous discussion, once you know the name of the function, the easiest way to declare the function is to use the API Text Viewer. To use the viewer for this purpose, follow these steps:

1. Start the API viewer and load either the text file or the database (see Figure 14.2). The steps have been already outlined.
2. Ensure that "Declares" is selected in the API Type combo box.
3. Select the Private option button in the Declare Scope frame.
4. Type the function name GetKeyState into the text box below the instruction "Type the first few letters of the word you are looking for:" (In version 5, there is no such text box. You type the keyword in the Items Available list box instead. Also, your typing must be continuous; otherwise, the search starts over from the point you pause.)
5. You should see the function name highlighted in the Available Items list box.
6. Double-click the item or click the Add button after you make a selection. You should see a line of code (declaration) in the Selected Items list box. The result should appear as in Figure 14.2.
7. Click the Copy button.
8. Go back to the code window of your VB IDE.
9. Select the Paste option in the Edit drop-down menu in your VB IDE to paste the declaration into your code window.

Example 2. Locating the System Directory. Occasionally, when your program is installed in a user's computer, you may need to place some specific files in the Windows system directory. However, each computer may have a different disk drive/folder where this directory is located. There is no specific VB function to find such directory. However, an API function is available that can perform this service. The name of the function is

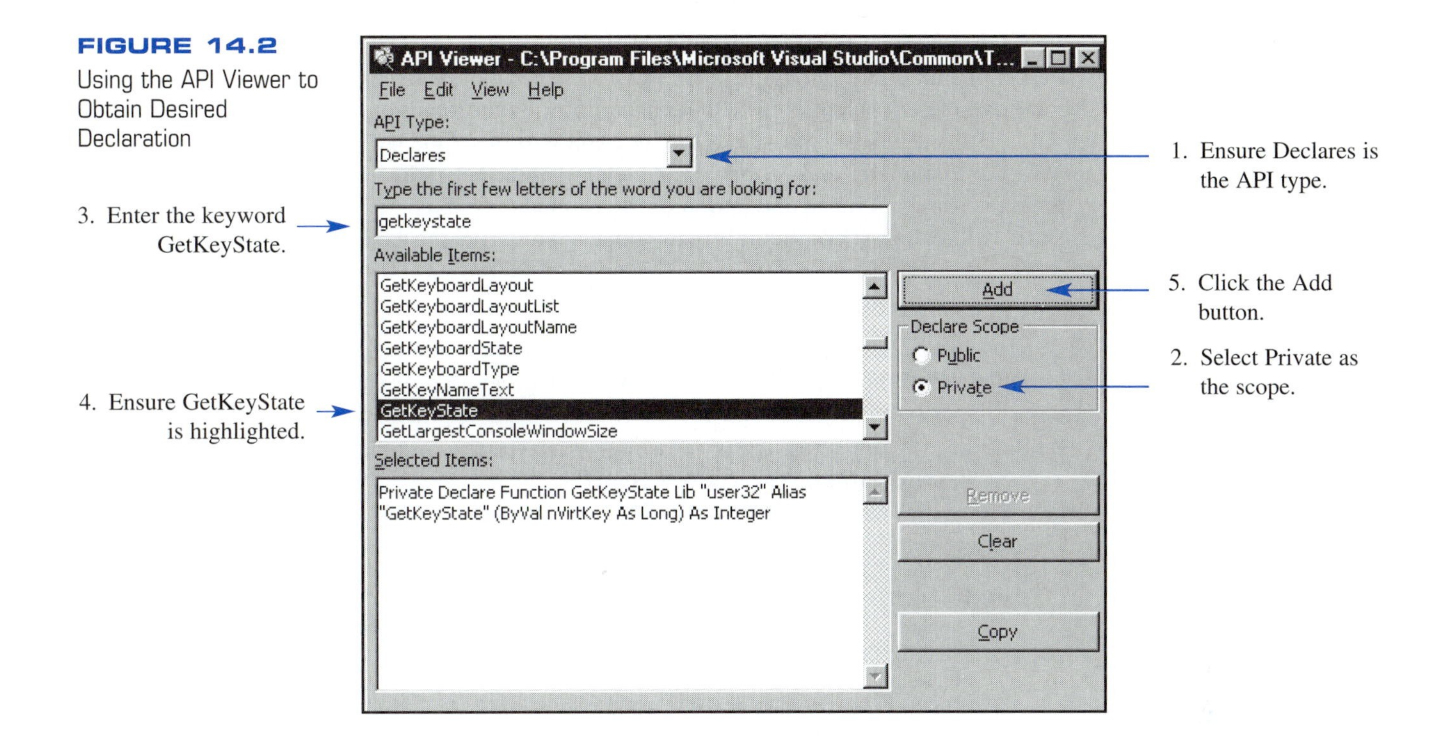

FIGURE 14.2
Using the API Viewer to Obtain Desired Declaration

GetSystemDirectory. The required declaration appears as follows (follow the steps outlined previously to obtain the declaration from the API viewer):

```
Private Declare Function GetSystemDirectory Lib "kernel32" _
    Alias "GetSystemDirectoryA" _
      (ByVal lpBuffer As String, ByVal nSize As Long) As Long
```

As you can see in the statement, the DLL in which this function is located is kernel32, not the same as user32 for the GetKeyState function. This statement also contains the Alias keyword, which indicates that the name given first (GetSystemDirectory) is an alias of the function name GetSystemDirectoryA, which is the actual name in the DLL kernel32.

Again, the remainder of the statement is the familiar parameter list required for the function (enclosed in the pair of parentheses) and the type of the function, Long. VB6 operates under the 32-bit operating system and uses 32-bit API functions (as the name of the DLL "kernel32" also implies). In most cases, when numeric values are involved, these functions use and return the Long type.

The GetSystemDirectory function takes two parameters. The first is a string variable used as an area for the function to place the path of the system directory, and the second informs the API of the size (number of bytes) of the string.

As indicated in the preceding discussion, API functions, being developed in C, handle strings differently from a typical VB procedure. Specifically, *any string variable to be used by an API function must have its size set ready*; for example, if the API function needs a string variable 32 characters long, you must make sure that the string is of a length at least 32 characters before calling the function. Otherwise, your program can crash.

Thus, to call GetSystemDirectory, you will need to set up a string long enough to hold the pathname of the system directory. Not knowing how long the path can go, we'd better be on the safe side by creating one longer than is actually needed, for example, 128. So, the code to call this function can appear as follows:

```
Dim PathOfDir As String
Dim LengthOfDir As Long
PathOfDir = String$(128, 0)
LengthOfDir = GetSystemDirectory(PathOfDir, 128)
```

The String$ function returns a string with 128 characters of Chr$(0), which is assigned to the variable PathOfDir, which is in turn passed to the GetSystemDirectory API function. The second parameter (128) of the API function informs the function of the length of the string variable PathOfDir. Once invoked, the function will place the pathname of the system directory in this parameter and return a Long type value that indicates the actual length of the pathname. That is, if the actual length of the pathname is 35 characters long, the function will return a value of 35. Thus, the following code should give the exact path of the system directory:

```
Left$(PathOfDir, LengthOfDir)
```

Suppose that you have a form with a command button named cmdGetSysDir and a text box txtDirPath. When the user clicks the button, your program will show the path of the system directory. The complete code to perform this task should appear as follows:

```
Private Declare Function GetSystemDirectory Lib "kernel32" _
     Alias "GetSystemDirectoryA" _
       (ByVal lpBuffer As String, ByVal nSize As Long) As Long
Private Sub cmdGetSysDir_Click()
Dim LengthOfDir As Long
Dim PathOfDir As String
     ' Set up the string buffer for the pathname
     PathOfDir = String$(128, 0)
     ' Call the API function
     LengthOfDir = GetSystemDirectory(PathOfDir, 128)
     ' Place the pathname of system directory in the text box
     txtDirPath.Text = Left$(PathOfDir, LengthOfDir)
End Sub
```

Example 3. Horizontal Scrollbar for the List Box. The list box will automatically add a vertical scrollbar when its physical size is not sufficient to present all data items in the list. However, it does not automatically provide a horizontal scrollbar when its width is not sufficient to show the entire length of the items in the list. What can you do?

You can use the ***SendMessage API function*** to make the list box add the horizontal scrollbar. Again, you can use the API viewer to obtain the appropriate declaration for the function, which should appear as follows:

```
Private Declare Function SendMessage Lib "user32" Alias _
   "SendMessageA" (ByVal hwnd As Long, ByVal wMsg As Long, _
   ByVal wParam As Long, lParam As Any) As Long
```

This function takes four parameters. The first one is the "handle" of the "window" (hwnd). In this context, the ***handle*** is a numeric value that represents the ID of a window, which is a visual object such as a form, a text box, or a list box. All "windows" have their unique IDs. The second parameter is a Long type value that represents the "message" that you wish to send to the window. The message tells the window what to perform. Depending on the message, the third and fourth parameters vary and, in some cases, only one is used.

The function returns a Long type value. Depending on the message used, the returned value can mean different things. You will see some of them in the following discussion.

As you can imagine, there are countless messages that your program can send to various windows. It will be difficult to remember all the constants needed to send the proper messages. The API viewer can help you in this regard. Recall that you can specify three different API types in the viewer. One you have seen is "Declare." Another one is "Constant." You can search this type for the proper message value. For example, our current objective is to send a message to a list box to set a horizontal scrollbar. The name of the constant is LB_SETHORIZONTALEXTENT. (Note that *LB* = list box; and the second part reads: Set Horizontal Extent.) The declaration appears as follows:

```
Private Const LB_SETHORIZONTALEXTENT = &H194
```

Notice that these messages are not a part of the VB language. The constant names are not recognized by VB. Thus, the constant declaration must be included in the code. Once you have the function and the constant properly declared, you can use the function to set the horizontal scrollbar for a list box. For example, the following statement will set a horizontal scrollbar to 300 pixels wide for a list box named lstName. A sample output is given in Figure 14.3.

```
Dim M As Long
M = SendMessage(lstName.hwnd, LB_SETHORIZONTALEXTENT, 300, 0)
```

Note that the fourth parameter is not used in this case. However, because it is required in the syntax, a zero is inserted as a "dummy" value. The returned value in this case represents an error code.

FIGURE 14.3

A List Box with the Horizontal Scrollbar

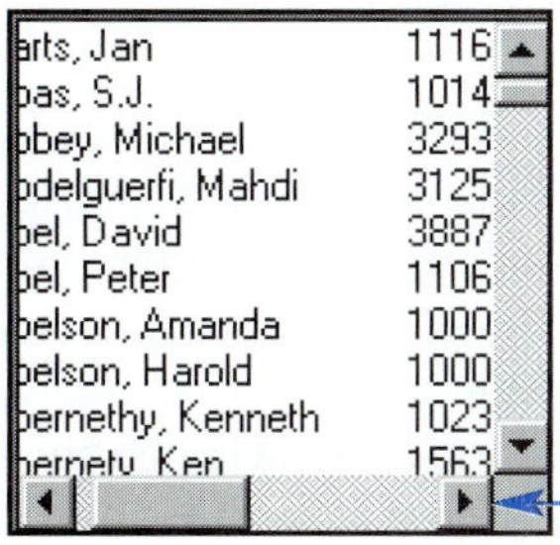

Here is a list box with the horizontal scrollbar created with the SendMessage API call. Now you are able to scroll both vertically and horizontally.

The preceding code can be placed in any event procedure. Because the list box needs to set its horizontal scrollbar only once, it is appropriate to place the code in the Form Load event. The complete code can then appear as follows:

```
Option Explicit
Private Declare Function SendMessage Lib "user32" Alias _
  "SendMessageA" (ByVal hwnd As Long, ByVal wMsg As Long, _
  ByVal wParam As Long, lParam As Any) As Long
Private Const LB_SETHORIZONTALEXTENT = &H194

Private Sub Form_Load()
    Dim M As Long
    M = SendMessage(lstName.hwnd, _
      LB_SETHORIZONTALEXTENT, 300, 0)
End Sub
```

The SendMessage function is indeed very versatile. Example 4 presents another use.

Example 4. Searching for a String in a List Box. Suppose you would like to search a list box (lstNames) for a string that partially matches a search string specified by the user in a text box (txtName) when the user clicks the Search button. What can you do? You can set up a loop and compare each item in the list with the search string until a match is found or until the list runs out.

However, there is another way that should be more efficient. You can use the FindString (for exact match, use the FINDSTRINGEXACT) message via the SendMessage API. For the list box, the declaration for the message constant appears as follows:

```
Private Const LB_FINDSTRING = &H18F
```

Again, once both the functions and the constant are declared, you can call the function as follows:

```
Private Sub cmdSearch_Click()
Dim Pos as Long
Dim TheName as String
    TheName = txtName.Text
    'Find the position of the name in the list box
    Pos = SendMessage(lstNames.hwnd, LB_FINDSTRING, 0, _
      ByVal TheName)
    'Highlight the item found
    lstNames.ListIndex = Pos
End Sub
```

Notice that in this case, the third parameter is not used. Thus, a zero is inserted. Also notice that the *ByVal keyword is needed for the fourth parameter* (TheName) for the API function to perform correctly.

Example 5. Disabling the Shift Key and Sending the Tab Key. In Chapter 10, we presented a way to auto tab a text field when the cursor reaches its maximum length. The procedure is reproduced here:

```
Private Sub Form_KeyUp(KeyCode As Integer, Shift As Integer)
    If TypeName(ActiveControl) = "TextBox" Then
        If ActiveControl.SelStart >= ActiveControl.MaxLength Then
            SendKeys vbTab
        End If
    End If
End Sub
```

This procedure will work fine under "normal" conditions. However, when the user is entering the last key in the text box, if he or she also presses the Shift key to capitalize a letter, the focus will go to the control above the current text box, not the one below. Why? Because the Shift key plus the Tab key sent by the SendKeys statement in the procedure results in a Shift+Tab key combination. Thus, if there is a possibility that the user will press the Shift key when entering data, the routine may cause unexpected results from time to time.

Is there a way to suppress the Shift key? There is an API function, keybd_event, that emulates the keyboard event, much like the SendKeys statement. It can handle situations that SendKeys cannot. Suppressing the Shift key is an example. The keybd_event API should be declared as follows:

```
Private Declare Sub keybd_event Lib "user32" (ByVal bVk As Byte, _
  ByVal bScan As Byte, ByVal dwFlags As Long, _
  ByVal dwExtraInfo As Long)
```

where *bVk* = the key code to emulate

bScan = the scan code for the key

dwFlags = a Long integer that can have a value of zero or one of the two constants: (1) *KEYEVENTF_EXTENDEDKEY* = the key is an extended key (two bytes) and (2) *KEYEVENTF_KEYUP* = emulates a key release

dwExtrInfo = seldom used

As you can see, the dwFlags parameter provides a way to release (suppress) a key. This is exactly what we need to suppress the Shift key. The following statement should suppress the Shift key:

```
keybd_event vbKeyShift, 0, KEYEVENTF_KEYUP, 0
```

In the code, we provide 0 for both the second and last parameters because they are not needed. Similarly, we can use this API to send a Tab key as follows:

```
keybd_event vbKeyTab, 0, 0, 0
```

Thus, a better routine to handle the auto tabbing of text boxes can be written as follows:

```
Option Explicit
Private Declare Sub keybd_event Lib "user32" (ByVal bVk As Byte, _
  ByVal bScan As Byte, ByVal dwFlags As Long, _
  ByVal dwExtraInfo As Long)
Private Const KEYEVENTF_KEYUP = &H2

Private Sub Form_KeyUp(KeyCode As Integer, Shift As Integer)
    If TypeName(ActiveControl) = "TextBox" Then
        If ActiveControl.SelStart >= ActiveControl.MaxLength Then
            If Shift And vbShiftMask Then
                'Suppress the Shift key
                keybd_event vbKeyShift, 0, KEYEVENTF_KEYUP, 0
            End If
            'Send the Tab key using the keybd_event API
            keybd_event vbKeyTab, 0, 0, 0
        End If
    End If
End Sub
```

In the preceding code, the keybd_event API is used both to release the Shift key and to send the Tab key (in place of the SendKeys statement). This makes internal working of the code more compatible with each other, reducing the need to consider the timing (sequencing) that the keys are handled.

If you use the API viewer to declare the keybd_event function, you may find that there is additional "Alias" text after "user32." Sometimes, the Alias declaration appears to be exactly the same as the original function name. In such a case, the extra text is not needed.

Additional Remarks

If used properly, API functions can be very powerful and can add a lot of additional capabilities to VB. However, because API functions are not "native" to VB, their uses involve additional effort and care in coding. In incorporating the API functions into your programs, you should always think about the reusability of the code. One practice that experienced VB programmers follow is to encapsulate the frequently used API calls in VB functions. That is, rather than calling the API functions directly, you create VB functions that "wrap" the API calls in them. All subsequent uses of the API functions will then be handled through the VB functions you have created, saving you the effort to look for the details needed for the API calls. These VB functions are recognized as API "wrappers."

For example, to set the horizontal scrollbar, you can create a generalized VB function that takes two parameters: the list box handle and the width. This function will in turn use these two parameters to call the SendMessage API to perform the LB_SETHORIZONTALEXTENT message. This function can be placed in a standard module (or a class module) available to all projects. All subsequent needs to set the horizontal scrollbar can be performed by calling this function. Wrapping the API calls in VB functions is left to you as an exercise.

14.2 Using the Windows Registry

Often, you will encounter a situation in which you would like your program to have some VB control properties set to certain values but you are hesitant to hard-code the values simply because you want to allow your user to choose these values. Sometimes, it is also because the values can be properly set only when your program runs in a particular computer.

One possible solution to this problem is to create a special file that keeps track of these special settings. However, this solution has several shortcomings. The code to handle the file can take quite a few lines. Determining the proper file path can also be an issue. Finally, you will need to secure the file from the user's accidental alteration or destruction.

A better alternative is to use the Windows registry, which is a database that the operating system maintains to support the system's and applications' operations. This section illustrates how you can use the Windows registry in your program to handle some of its operational needs.

A Simple Text Browser Project

Consider the simple text browser application whose visual interface is shown in Figure 14.4. The form has a command button that allows your user to specify the text file he or she wants to read. Once the filename is specified, your program proceeds to load the file content into a text box on the form. You also want to allow your user to view the text with any font available in the system. The available fonts are listed in a combo box. When the user makes a selection from this box, the font in the text box changes accordingly. *The challenge is this: You want your program to use this same font when it starts next time.* This means your program must find some way to save this font before it quits and to retrieve the same next time.

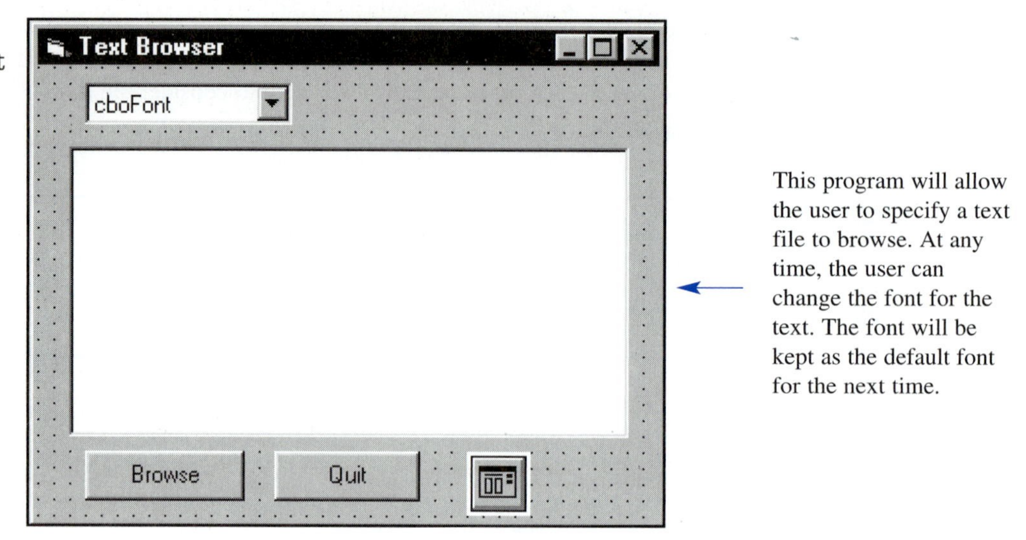
Text Browser
cboFont
Browse
Quit
This program will allow the user to specify a text file to browse. At any time, the user can change the font for the text. The font will be kept as the default font for the next time.

FIGURE 14.4
Visual Interface for a Text Browser

Selected settings of the controls used in the form are listed in the following table.

Control	Property	Setting	Remarks
Text box	Name	txtTextBrowser	To display text file for read only
	MultiLine	True	
	Locked	True	
Combo box	Name	cboFont	To display available fonts for selection
	Style	2 (Dropdown List)	
Command button	Name	cmdBrowse	To initiate browsing for a file
	Caption	Browse	
Command button	Name	cmdQuit	To quit the application
	Caption	Quit	
Common dialog	Name	cdlFile	

The code to populate the combo box with the available fonts appears as follows:

```
Private Sub Form_Load()
Dim I As Integer
     ' Populate combo box with font names
     For I = 0 To Screen.FontCount - 1
          cboFont.AddItem Screen.Fonts(I)
     Next I
End Sub
```

The Screen Object. In the preceding code, the available fonts are obtained from the ***Screen object***, which represents the "screen" that contains several properties common to all forms used in an application. These properties include the Fonts and FontCount properties. The Fonts property is an array that contains the names of all the fonts available for display, and FontCount gives the number of these fonts.

Setting the Font. The combo box now contains the available fonts. The user can select any font from this combo box. The code to set the font for the text box to reflect the selection should appear as follows:

```
Private Sub cboFont_Click()
'Set the text box's font to the one selected
     txtTextBrowser.Font.Name = cboFont.Text
End Sub
```

"Remembering" the "Default" Font

Now, suppose you want your program to "remember" the font that the user has selected so that next time the program can use the same font as the default. How would you do this? One possibility is to create a file and use it to keep the font name. This approach requires your program to handle several details, including the file path and opening and closing the file. In addition, your program will need to check to ensure the file exists before it attempts to open the file. What initially appears to be a fairly simple problem seems to require some effort.

Accessing the Registry from VB. A better alternative is to use the Windows registry, which is a database maintained by the Windows operating system and available to all applications to keep track of information for their own uses. (Of course, the Windows operating system also uses the registry for various purposes. However, a discussion of these uses is beyond the scope of this book.) VB provides several procedures that you can use to access the registry easily. The following table lists three selected procedures.

Procedure	Type	Uses
GetSetting	Function	To retrieve data from the registry
SaveSetting	Statement	To save data in the registry
DeleteSetting	Statement	To delete data from the registry

In our example, we can use the registry to save the font name by using the SaveSetting statement, which has the following syntax:

```
SaveSetting AppName, SectionName, Key, Setting
```

where *AppName* = a string representing your application name

SectionName = a string representing the section name

Key = a string representing the key for your data (setting).

For example, to save the font in the registry selected from the combo box by the user, you can code the following:

```
SaveSetting "TextBrowser", "TextFont", "FontName", cboFont.Text
```

If the font selected by the user is Courier, the preceding statement will save "Courier" in the location that represents an application named TextBrowser with the Section name TextFont and Key name FontName.

Where should the preceding statement be placed? Recall that the purpose of saving the font is to allow the same font to be used as the default for the next time. Thus, the most appropriate time to save it is before the program quits. We can place the code either in the Unload or the QueryUnload event:

```
Private Sub Form_QueryUnload(Cancel As Integer, UnloadMode As _
      Integer)
      ' Save font for next time
     SaveSetting "TextBrowser", "TextFont", "FontName", cboFont.Text
End Sub
```

Retrieving the Setting. So, how can the setting be retrieved from the registry? You can use the GetSetting function, which has the following syntax:

```
Setting = GetSetting(AppName, SectionName, Key[, DefaultSetting])
```

where the *AppName, SectionName,* and *Key* parameters must match those provided when the setting was saved. You can also provide a value for the default setting, which will be the returned value if there is no previous setting in the registry. For our example problem, we can code the following:

```
' Retrieve Font name and size from registry
TextFontName = GetSetting("TextBrowser", "TextFont", _
   "FontName", txtTextBrowser.Font.Name)
```

Note that we use the text box's font name as the default setting in the preceding statement. This works well because when there is no previous setting, the "safest" to do is to use the same font as the current font of the text box. If you omit the default setting and nothing is found in the registry, the function will return a zero-length string.

Showing the Font in the Combo Box. Once you retrieve the font from the registry, you also want the combo box to reflect the current setting. Recall that the combo box has its Style property set to 2- Dropdown List. Under this setting, its Text property cannot be assigned directly. However, you can set its ListIndex property to show its text. To set the proper value for the ListIndex property, the combo box's list must be searched for the item that matches the font retrieved from the registry. Of course, you can set up a loop and compare the retrieved font with the items in the list. However, a more elegant way will be to take advantage of the SendMessage API discussed in the preceding section. The constant to find a match in a combo box is CB_FINDSTRING. Assume proper declarations have been made. Then the statements to find a match and set the ListIndex property appear as follows:

```
' Find a match in the combo box
P = SendMessage(cboFont.hwnd, CB_FINDSTRING, 0, _
    ByVal  TextFontName)
cboFont.ListIndex = P 'Note this will also trigger the Click event
```

All the statements related to retrieving the font and setting the ListIndex property should be coded in the Form Load event. The revised event procedure, including the proper declarations, appears as follows:

```
' In the general declaration area
Option Explicit
Private Declare Function SendMessage Lib "user32" Alias _
   "SendMessageA" (ByVal hwnd As Long, ByVal wMsg As Long, _
  ByVal wParam As Long, lParam As Any) As Long
Private Const CB_FINDSTRING = &H14C
Dim TextFontName As String

Private Sub Form_Load()
Dim I As Integer
Dim P As Integer
    ' Populate combo box with font names
    For I = 0 To Screen.FontCount - 1
        cboFont.AddItem Screen.Fonts(I)
    Next I
    ' Retrieve Font name and size from registry
    TextFontName = GetSetting("TextBrowser", "TextFont", _
      "FontName", txtTextBrowser.Font.Name)
    ' Find a match in the cmbo box
    P = SendMessage(cboFont.hwnd, CB_FINDSTRING, 0, _
      ByVal TextFontName)
    ' Display the font in the combo box
    cboFont.ListIndex = P 'Note this will also trigger the Click
                          ' event
End Sub
```

Note that the assignment of the ListIndex Property of the combo box will also trigger its Click event, which has the code that sets the font for the text box. This will work exactly the way we want: Whatever appears in the combo box is the font used in the text box.

Deleting the Setting. If for any reason, the setting should be removed from the registry, the DeleteSetting statement can be used. The statement has the following syntax:

DeleteSetting *AppName, SectionName[, Key]*

To remove the font from the registry, you will code the following:

```
DeleteSetting "TextBrowser", "TextFont", "FontName"
```

Assume you have a command button named cmdDeleteSetting for the user to initiate the deletion. Your code will appear as follows:

```
Private Sub cmdDeleteSetting_Click()
    DeleteSetting "TextBrowser", "TextFont", "FontName"
End Sub
```

Completing the Example. Our example actually requires more code than the preceding code. We should also provide the code for the user to specify the file to browse, open the file, and read the content into the text box. By now you should be familiar enough with the code to handle this. The following code is provided without further explanation.

```
Private Sub cmdBrowse_Click()
Dim FileName As String
Dim FileNo As Integer
    FileName = GetFileName
    If Len(FileName) = 0 Then Exit Sub
    FileNo = FreeFile
    Open FileName For Input As #FileNo
    txtTextBrowser.Text = Input(LOF(FileNo), FileNo)
    Close #FileNo
End Sub

Function GetFileName() As String
    On Error GoTo DoNothing
    With cdlFile
        .DialogTitle = "Please specify text filename to open"
        .Filter = "text File (*.txt)¦*.txt¦All Files (*.*)¦*.*"
        .Flags = cdlOFNFileMustExist
        .CancelError = True
        .ShowOpen
        GetFileName = .FileName
        Exit Function
    End With
DoNothing:
End Function
```

Additional Remarks

As you can see from the preceding example, you can use the Windows registry to keep information that your program needs from one run to the next. Other examples of using the registry for this purpose include saving the user password, keeping a file path as the default, and saving various settings of the visual interface (e.g., foreground and back ground colors) as the default.

Using the registry for such purposes has several advantages:

- It makes your program more flexible. Your program does not have to start with a setting that is hard-coded. The user can set the default and stay with it for as long as he or she wishes. Also, some specific systems may not have the hard-coded setting. This can cause problems. Thus, avoiding hard-coding settings also enhances your program's applicability to different systems.
- Compared with using a file to save settings, it is much more convenient for the following reasons:
  - You don't have to worry about in which folder this file should be kept.
  - You don't have to check to ensure that the file exists before opening it.
  - The registry is less susceptible to user errors, such as mistakenly erasing the file or altering the file content.

Proper Use of the Registry. Because of the convenience, you may be tempted to use the registry to save anything that your program needs to read back in the future. Keep in mind, however, that the registry is used by the operating system to keep information for many other purposes. Overloading the registry will slow down the performance of the computer system.

You should use the registry only to maintain information that is pertinent to the operation of your program itself, not the type of data that the user needs to maintain his or her application. For example, suppose your payroll program allows the user to set background colors for various controls. It would be appropriate to keep this type of information in the registry. On the other hand, the data that pertain to the payroll operations (e.g., employees' earnings records) should be kept in files or database, rather than in the registry.

14.3 Automation

This section and the next discuss ActiveX components. An ActiveX component is a unit of executable code that is compliant with the ActiveX specification for providing objects. You have been introduced to several ActiveX components in this book. For example, in Chapter 8, "Database and the ActiveX Data Objects," you worked with the ADO (ActiveX Data Objects). In other chapters, you have also worked with controls that are not intrinsic to VB, including the masked edit control, the common dialog control, and the Microsoft Hierarchical FlexGrid. These are ActiveX controls.

All these objects and controls are created following the ActiveX specification based on the Component Object Model (COM). Components created under the COM model can be easily incorporated into VB programs. (Recall that all you have to do to use an ActiveX control is to add the control to the toolbox from the Components option of the Project menu.) The ActiveX technology makes VB easily extensible into any application. For example, if you acquire a bar code control, you can quickly develop an application performing bar coding operations. If you obtain a numerical analysis DLL, you can easily turn your VB program into a computing engine.

Types of ActiveX Components

There are four types of ActiveX components:

1. Code component—***ActiveX DLL***: Unlike VB controls, this type of component does not provide visible elements at design time. (Therefore, you can manipulate its properties only at runtime.) The component is used as objects in the VB program. For example, the ADO objects belong to this type. This type of component runs "in process," using the same thread of execution as the VB program.
2. Code component—***ActiveX EXE***: Like the ActiveX DLL, this type of component does not provide visible elements at design time for you to set its properties. It is also used as objects in the VB program. This type of component runs "out of process," executing in a different thread of execution from your VB program; that is, once it is invoked, it runs as a separate application. Because initiating actions requires communication across the process boundary, using this type of component executes more slowly. A feature of this type of component is that it can run by itself as an application. Programs in the Microsoft Office suite are of this type. Later in this section, we show how they can be used from within the VB program.
3. ***ActiveX Control***: This type of component has an OCX extension. For example, the filename for the MS HFG is "MSHFLXGD.OCX." It provides a visual interface that you can use to design its appearance and set its properties. ActiveX controls run "in process," like the ActiveX DLL.
4. ***ActiveX Document:*** Active documents are forms that can appear within the Internet browser windows. They are mainly developed for Internet applications. They can run either in process or out of process and have an EXE extension for their filenames.

The classification of these components are summarized in the following table.

Type	File Extension	Process	Recognized in VB Program as
Code component	DLL	In process	Object
	EXE	Out of process	Object
ActiveX control	OCX	In process	Control
ActiveX document	EXE	In or out of process	Form

VB allows you *not only to use but also to create* all four types of components. The remainder of this chapter discusses the first three types of components. In this section, we pay particular attention to using the components. Because you have already learned how to work with objects in the ActiveX DLL (e.g., the ADO) and ActiveX controls (e.g., the masked edit control), we limit our discussion on how to use objects provided by the ActiveX EXE.

Using a Code Component EXE

Using a code component EXE is not much different from using a code component DLL. Both are recognized in VB as objects. To use the component, you should do the following:

1. Set up an object variable and associate it with the object that you create from the component.
2. Manipulate the object by setting the object's properties or using its methods.
3. Terminate the object and set the object variable to nothing.

Creating an Object from the Component. Your method to create an object depends on whether the component provides an object library and registers with VB. If the component does, you can create an object by doing the following:

1. Setting the reference to the component library
2. Declaring directly in your program the object using the names provided by the library

These steps are exactly the same as using the ADO. For example, MS Word 97 provides the object library and registers with VB (assuming your system has the software installed). Thus, you can set a reference to the component by following these steps:

1. Click the Project menu and select the References option. The References dialog box will appear.
2. Locate Microsoft Word Object 8.0 Object Library in the Available References list box and check it on.

Once you have the reference to the component, you can declare an object to refer to it. The declaration can appear as follows:

```
Dim MSWord As Word.Application
```

You can then create an object using the New keyword and associate it with the variable:

```
Set MSWord = New Word.Application
```

Using the Word Objects

To use the Word application, you will need to know the properties and methods that Word provides. The following code will create a Word application object, use it to open a document (i.e., Chapter 14.doc) for read-only, and print pages 3 and 4 in the background.

```
Option Explicit
Dim MSWord As Word.Application
Private Sub cmdPrint_Click()
    Set MSWord = New Word.Application
    With MSWord
        .ChangeFileOpenDirectory "C:\My Documents\VBBook\"
        .Documents.Open FileName:="Chapter 14.doc", _
          ReadOnly:=True
        .PrintOut Range:=wdPrintRangeOfPages, Item:= _
          wdPrintDocumentContent, Copies:=1, Pages:="3-4", _
```

```
                PageType:= wdPrintAllPages, Background:=True
              .ActiveDocument.Close
          End With
      End Sub
```

The preceding code uses named parameters instead of positional parameters to specify arguments to pass to the methods of the MSWord object. You can specify parameters by name if you know the names of the parameters. Chapter 6, "Input, Output, and Procedures," has a brief discussion of named parameters. Not all methods or procedures allow named parameters.

You can, of course, make the program more general by replacing the file path and the value assigned to the Pages parameter of the PrintOut method with proper variables. Notice that the document is closed at the end of the procedure using the Close method of the active document. If you intend to use the procedure to open different documents and print different pages, this should be a good idea. The Word application object will then be working with only one document as you continue to open new ones.

Before Your Program Quits. Recall that in Chapter 8 and Chapter 12, "Object-Oriented Programming," you were urged to set the object to Nothing to clear out the reference so that the object will not be orphaned and continue to stay in memory. The same thing is true with the component EXE. In addition, because the component gets started as a separate application, you should terminate the application even before you set the object variable to Nothing. Assume you will continue to use the object until the form unloads. Your code to close the Word application will appear as follows:

```
Private Sub Form_Unload(Cancel As Integer)
    MSWord.Quit 'Tell Word to quit
    Set MSWord = Nothing 'Set the object variable to nothing
End Sub
```

If you fail to terminate the component, even if you set the object variable to Nothing, the application will continue to stay in memory doing nothing.

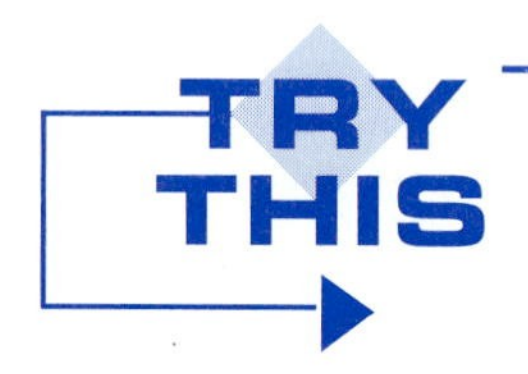

Modify the preceding code so that you can print a few pages of a document in your system using Word. Comment out the line:

```
MsWord.Quit
```

Run the project. After your program quits, press Ctrl+Alt+Delete so that the Windows system will show a list of active tasks in the Close Program window. You should see WinWord among the list. This means the application continues to stay in memory. Highlight it and select the End Task button to terminate the application.

Using Excel in Your VB Program

You can use Excel in your VB program in almost the same way as you use Word. In a similar manner, you can make a reference to the Excel object library by following these steps:

1. Click the Project menu and select the References option. The References dialog box should appear.
2. Look for the Microsoft Excel 8.0 Object Library in the dialog box's list box and check the item.

Now you will be able to use code to use the objects in the library. As an illustration, suppose you have a command button named cmdCreate in your form. When the user clicks the button, the following code in the event procedure will do the following:

1. Create a new Excel workbook.
2. Change the name of the sheet to "Annuity Table."
3. Copy the content of a grid (named grdAnnTable) to the active sheet.

4. Create in Cell E3 the title "Present Value of Annuity Table" with the proper font.
5. Align Cell A3 to the right.
6. Double underline the first row (for interest rates).
7. Save the workbook in "C:\Temp\Annuity.xls."
8. Quit the Excel application.

```
Option Explicit
Private Sub cmdCreate_Click()
Dim MsExcel As Excel.Application
Dim Col As Integer
Dim Row As Integer
    Set MsExcel = New Excel.Application
    With MsExcel
        .Workbooks.Add 'Start with 1 workbook
        .Sheets("Sheet1").Select 'Use sheet1
        .Sheets("Sheet1").Name = "Annuity Table" 'Change name
        'Copy data from grid to worksheet
        For Col = 0 To grdAnnTable.Cols - 1
            For Row = 0 To grdAnnTable.Rows - 1
            'Copy content of grid Cell to Excel Cell
                .ActiveSheet.Cells(Row + 3, Col + 1) = _
                  grdAnnTable.TextMatrix(Row, Col)
            Next Row
        Next Col
        'set up table title in Cell E1
        .Range("E1").Select
        .ActiveCell.FormulaR1C1 = "Present Value of Annuity Table"
        'Use Aerial bold 14 for the title
        With Selection.Font
            .Name = "Arial"
            .FontStyle = "Bold"
            .Size = 14
        End With
        'Align right for "Years"
        .Range("A3").HorizontalAlignment = xlRight
        .Range("A3").VerticalAlignment = xlBottom
        'Double underline the rates
        .Range("B3:K3").Select
        With Selection.Borders(xlEdgeBottom)
            .LineStyle = xlDouble
            .Weight = xlThick
            .ColorIndex = xlAutomatic
        End With
        'Save the workbook
        .ActiveWorkbook.SaveAs FileName:="c:\temp\annuity.xls"
        .Workbooks.Close 'Close the workbook
        .Quit 'Terminate the application
    End With
    Set MsExcel = Nothing 'Clear the object
End Sub
```

Notice that at the end, the workbook should be closed with the Close method and the Excel application should be terminated with its Quit method. Without these statements, the workbook and Excel will continue to stay in memory, doing nothing.

The grid that the preceding procedure uses is a present value of annuity table created with the following code:

```
Private Sub cmdAnnuity_Click()
Dim Rate As Double
Dim Disc As Double
Dim Factor As Double
Dim PVAnnuity As Double
Dim Col As Integer, Row As Integer
'Create a PV of annuity table on grid
```

```
        With grdAnnTable
            .Rows = 21
            .Cols = 11
            'Show Number of years in col 1
            .TextMatrix(0, 0) = "Years"
            For Row = 1 To 20
                .TextMatrix(Row, 0) = Row
            Next Row
            Rate = 0.05 'Create annuity table starting with 5%
            For Col = 1 To 10
                .TextMatrix(0, Col) = Format$(Rate, "Percent")
                Disc = 1 / (1 + Rate)
                Factor = 1
                PVAnnuity = 0
                For Row = 1 To 20
                    Factor = Factor * Disc
                    PVAnnuity = PVAnnuity + Factor
                    .TextMatrix(Row, Col) = _
                      Format$(PVAnnuity, "###.###00")
                Next Row
                Rate = Rate + 0.01
            Next Col
        End With
    End Sub
```

To test the code, you will need to do the following:

1. Draw a command button on the form and name it cmdCreate.
2. Add the HFG component to your project.
3. Draw an HFG on your form and name the HFG grdAnnTable.

Admittedly, the results of the computations could have been assigned directly to the cells in the Excel worksheet without involving the grid. However, you may find the use of a grid in your project "handy" because in many cases, you would probably want to inspect the results in your program before deciding to save them in an Excel worksheet. You can also imagine that the grid contains the results of a database query of sales or other transaction summary. Once the results are transferred to the Excel worksheet, you can perform many additional analyses and further processing.

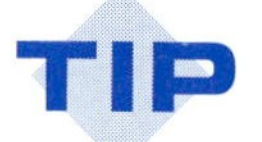

If you are not familiar with the objects, properties, and methods available in the Word or Excel application, there is one way you can learn about them fairly easily. Each application provides a mechanism to record your commands while working with the application. For example, in the Word application, you can create a Macro with the following steps:

1. Click the Tools menu and highlight the Macro option. A submenu will appear.
2. Select Record Macro and enter a name for the Macro.
3. Start your activities that you want to record in the Macro (e.g., retrieve a document and print).
4. Click the Stop recording button in the small form that appears after step 2 to stop recording. If you do not see the small form, click the Tools menu and highlight the Macro option. Then click the "Stop Recording" option in the submenu.

To view the macro you have recorded:

1. Click the Tools menu and highlight the Macro option.
2. Select Macro from the submenu. A Macro dialog box will appear.
3. Highlight the macro of interest. Then Click the Edit button. You should see the code in a code window. From there you can study or modify the code.

The Contents and Index option in the Help menu provides you with all the needed information to learn about the language of the application, VBA (Visual Basic for Applications). You can do the same in Excel.

Creating an Object Without the Object Library

The previous examples show how to create and use a component when it provides the VB IDE with an object library and registers with VB. What if it does not register with VB? You will then need to use the CreateObject or GetObject function to create or get the object and associate it with an object variable. Indeed, even if a component provides an object library and registers with VB, if you choose to ignore it, you can also use these two functions to create or obtain the appropriate object.

The ***CreateObject function*** has the following syntax:

```
Set ObjectName = CreateObject(Class)
```

where *ObjectName* is the name of the object variable and *Class* is a string that gives the application and class name in the following format:

```
AppName.ObjectType
```

where *AppName* is the application name (e.g., Word or Excel) and *ObjectType* is the class name of the object (e.g., Application or Workbook).

As the name implies, the function is used to create an object from a code component (either DLL or EXE). You can use the following code to create a Word application object:

```
Dim MsWord As Object
Set MsWord = CreateObject("Word.Application")
```

Note that *the argument is a string*, not an object type as in the previous case where a reference has been made in VB. Once the object is created and associated with the object variable, the latter can be used in exactly the same manner as we did previously. For example, using the CreateObject function, the cmdPrint Click event procedure our previous Word example can be modified as follows:

```
Option Explicit
Dim MSWord As Object
Private Sub cmdPrint_Click()
    Set MSWord = CreateObject("Word.Application")
    With MSWord
        .ChangeFileOpenDirectory "C:\My Documents\VBBook\"
        .Documents.Open FileName:="Chapter 14.doc", _
          ReadOnly:=True
        .PrintOut Range:=wdPrintRangeOfPages, Item:= _
           wdPrintDocumentContent, Copies:=1, Pages:="3-4", _
           PageType:=wdPrintAllPages, Background:=True
        .ActiveDocument.Close
    End With
End Sub
```

The ***GetObject function*** is used when a component has already been created and you do not need (want) another instance of the same. It has the following syntax:

```
Set ObjectName = GetObject([FilePath],[Class])
```

where *ObjectName* = name of the object variable

FilePath = the filename for the component

Class = a string that gives the application and class name as explained for the CreateObject function

For example, after the Word application object is already activated, you can refer to the same object by coding:

```
Set MsWord = GetObject("", "Word.Application")
```

Notice that the first parameter is coded as a zero-length string, which ensures that GetObject returns the active object. (Note also, if there are several instances of the object, there is no way to predict which instance will be returned.) If the first parameter is omitted, the function will return a new instance of the object. There are additional fine points and restrictions on the use of GetObject function. Search the Index tab of the online Help file using the keyword "GetObject function" for additional information.

If you wish to minimize the number of instances of the same object in the system, you can create a function similar to the following:

```
Function GetOneObject(Class As string) As Object
    On Error Resume Next
    ' Get the object if it exists.
    Set GetOneObject = GetObject("", Class)
    If Err.Number Then
    ' GetObject failed. Create the object.
        Set GetOneObject = CreateObject(Class)
    End If
    If Err.Number Then
    ' CreateObject failed. Out of magic. Give the error.
        MsgBox "Can't create the specified object; " & _
          Err.Description
    End If
End Function
```

The preceding function will first attempt to get and return an object of the specified class using the GetObject function. If it is unsuccessful, an error will be raised, causing the Err.Number to be nonzero and the statement in the If block to execute. The CreateObject function will then attempt to create and return a new object. If it is still unsuccessful, another error will be raised, causing the error message to be displayed.

To Reference or Not. As you can see from this code, the only difference between making a reference to the object library and not making it is in the declaration of the object variable and the creation of the object. So, why bother with setting a reference to the object library as we did previously? Once you try both ways, you should immediately notice the difference in the "assistance" you get from the IDE.

When you set the reference to the component, the object library is available when you are coding. Thus, after you type the object's name with a dot (.), you will immediately see all the available properties and methods of the object displayed in the code window, making your coding job much easier (see Figure 14.5). On the other hand, when you use the CreateObject method directly, you will not be able to see the same. Not only must you remember the exact names of all the properties and methods, but you also must type out every keystroke of them while coding. Your choice of which way to go should be obvious. You will always want to make a reference to the object library when it is provided.

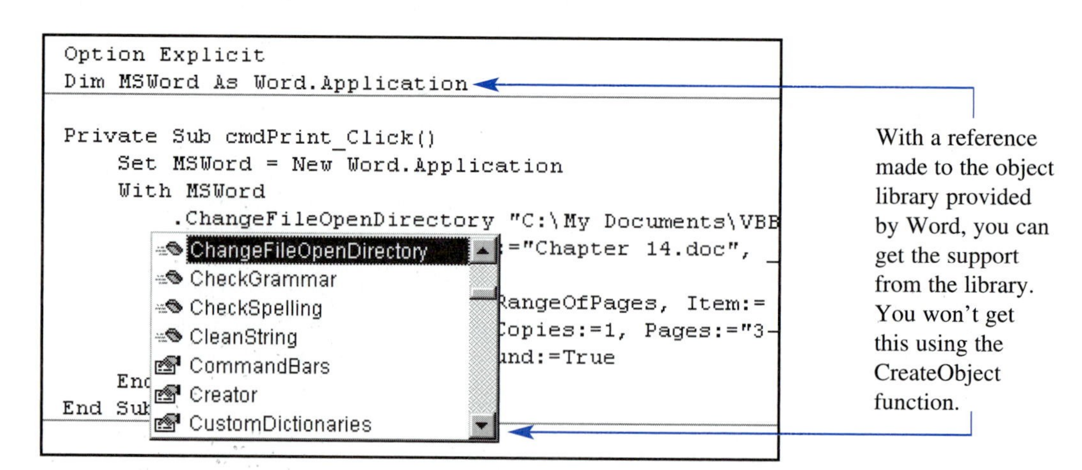

FIGURE 14.5
Coding the Word Application with the Inclusion of the Component

Automation and Extensibility

The examples in this section illustrate that VB can easily extend its capability with its ability to use ActiveX code components. For example, using VB code, you can make your program perform tasks that Word or Excel specializes, without having to reinvent the wheels. The possibility is there for you to explore and take advantage.

Incidentally, the ActiveX code components used to be termed as OLE automation, where *OLE* is the acronym for object linking and embedding. The ActiveX components were termed OLE servers but now are referred to as ActiveX servers. The term *servers* is used because these components provide services. Your VB program is termed a *client* because it uses the services of the components.

In the next section, we turn our attention to creating ActiveX components. More specifically, we discuss how to create ActiveX DLL. The process will lay a foundation for you to create other kinds of components.

14.4 Creating an ActiveX DLL

To create an ActiveX DLL, you can do the following:

1. Start with a new ActiveX DLL project.
2. Use the class module to create a class.
3. Get the project compiled as an ActiveX DLL.

To illustrate, let's consider a project. In this project, we will create a Financial DLL, in which we will create a class that can be used to show a present value table in an MS HFG for a specified range of interest rates for years from 1 to the number specified. The algorithm to show the table was explained in Chapter 13, "Selected Topics in Input and Output," although not in a class module but in a form module. We use the same problem so that you can focus more on the creation of the DLL than on the details in creating the class module itself.

More specifically, in this project, you will create a class module, which will allow the user to specify three properties: the LowerRate, the HigherRate, and the Years. These properties will then be used to compute and display the present value of $1 in a HFG in a form. The rates will vary from the specified lower rate to the higher rate by an increment of 1 percent. The years will vary from 1 to the number of years specified. A sample result is given in Figure 14.6.

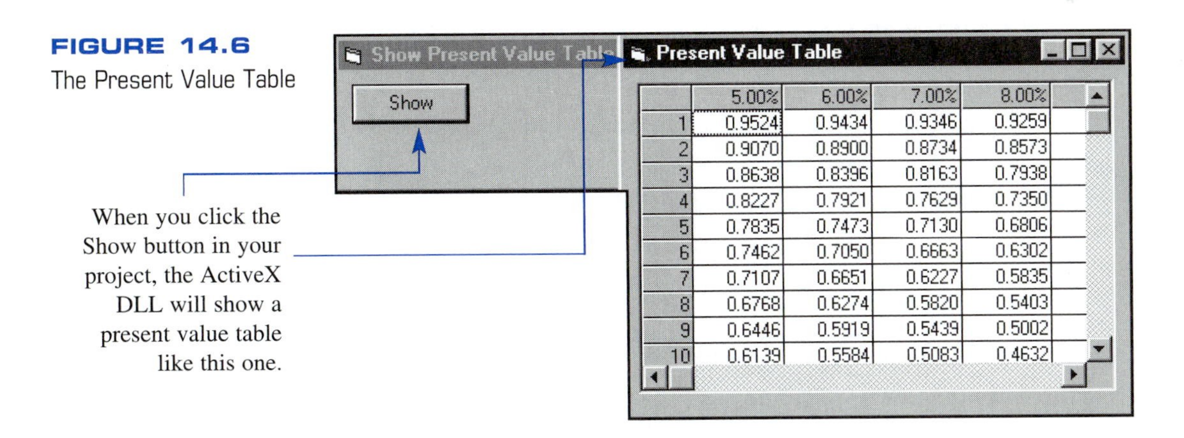
Show Present Value Table
Show
Present Value Table
When you click the Show button in your project, the ActiveX DLL will show a present value table like this one.

	5.00%	6.00%	7.00%	8.00%
1	0.9524	0.9434	0.9346	0.9259
2	0.9070	0.8900	0.8734	0.8573
3	0.8638	0.8396	0.8163	0.7938
4	0.8227	0.7921	0.7629	0.7350
5	0.7835	0.7473	0.7130	0.6806
6	0.7462	0.7050	0.6663	0.6302
7	0.7107	0.6651	0.6227	0.5835
8	0.6768	0.6274	0.5820	0.5403
9	0.6446	0.5919	0.5439	0.5002
10	0.6139	0.5584	0.5083	0.4632

FIGURE 14.6
The Present Value Table

Recall that although a form is an object (or class), it cannot be created directly by another project and thus has to be created from another module (standard module or class module) in the same project. *This project thus involves a class module as well as a form module.* The main difference between this project and any of the previous projects is that we will create an ActiveX DLL as the result.

Setting Up the Project

Follow these steps to set up the ActiveX DLL project:

1. From the VB IDE, click the File menu and select the New Project option.

2. Select the ActiveX DLL icon (instead of the familiar Standard EXE) from the New Project dialog box. Then click the OK button. A new project with a new class module should appear.
3. Click the Project menu and select the Project1 Properties option. The Project Properties dialog box will appear.
4. Change the Project Name from Project1 to Financial, which will become the name of the DLL you will create. Enter "Personal Financial Library" in the Description box. Leave all other boxes the same. The result should appear as in Figure 14.7.
5. Use the Properties window to change the name of the class module to PVTable from Class1.
6. Enter the following code in the class module:

```
Option Explicit
Private frmFinTable As frmFinTable 'Declare a form object variable
'local variable(s) to hold property value(s)
Private mLowerRate As Double 'local copy
Private mHigherRate As Double 'local copy
Private mYears As Integer 'local copy

Public Property Let Years(ByVal pYears As Integer)
    mYears = pYears
End Property
Public Property Get Years() As Integer
    Years = mYears
End Property

Public Property Let HigherRate(ByVal pvHigherRate As Double)
    mHigherRate = pHigherRate
End Property
Public Property Get HigherRate() As Double
    HigherRate = mHigherRate
End Property

Public Property Let LowerRate(ByVal vData As Double)
    mLowerRate = pLowerRate
End Property
Public Property Get LowerRate() As Double
    LowerRate = mLowerRate
End Property
```

This code sets up the three properties (Years, HigherRate, and LowerRate) for the PVTable class.

7. Enter the following code for the class events:

```
Private Sub Class_Initialize()
    Set frmFinTable = New frmFinTable
    Load frmFinTable
End Sub
Private Sub Class_Terminate()
    Unload frmFinTable
    Set frmFinTable = Nothing
End Sub
```

This code will create and load the form to display the present value table when the class is initialized and will unload the form and destroy the form module when the class is terminated.

8. Enter the following code for the ShowTable method:

```
Public Sub ShowPVTable()
Dim Rate As Double
Dim Period As Integer
Dim Factor1 As Double
Dim PVFactor As Double
Dim Col As Integer
Dim W As Integer
```

```
    With frmFinTable.grdTable
        .Rows = mYears + 1
        .Cols = (mHigherRate - mLowerRate) * 100 + 2
        W = frmFinTable.TextWidth("H")
        .ColWidth(-1) = 7 * W
        .ColWidth(0) = 4 * W
        ' show periods in the first column
        For Period = 1 To mYears
            .TextMatrix(Period, 0) = Period
        Next Period
        Rate = mLowerRate
        For Col = 1 To .Cols - 1
            'Show rate as the column title
            .TextMatrix(0, Col) = Format$(Rate, "Percent")
            'Compute PV for the rate for different years
            Factor1 = 1 / (1 + Rate)
            PVFactor = 1
            For Period = 1 To mvYears
                PVFactor = PVFactor * Factor1
                .TextMatrix(Period, Col) = _
                  Format$(PVFactor, "0.0000")
            Next Period
            Rate = Rate + 0.01
        Next Col
    End With
    'Display the result
    frmFinTable.Show
End Sub
```

The code here is basically the same as that presented in Chapter 13. Notice, however, that the HFG cannot be placed on the class module directly. It has to be placed in a form. The HFG is still named grdTable, but it has to be referenced by qualifying it with the form variable name frmFinTable. Notice also that "Years" is now a property. Thus, the name of the local copy mvYears (instead of Years) is used in the procedure.

9. Add a new form and change its name to frmFinTable. The required steps should be exactly the same as those in a standard EXE project.
10. Add an HFG to the form and change its name to grdTable. Notice that you must add the HFG component to your project first.

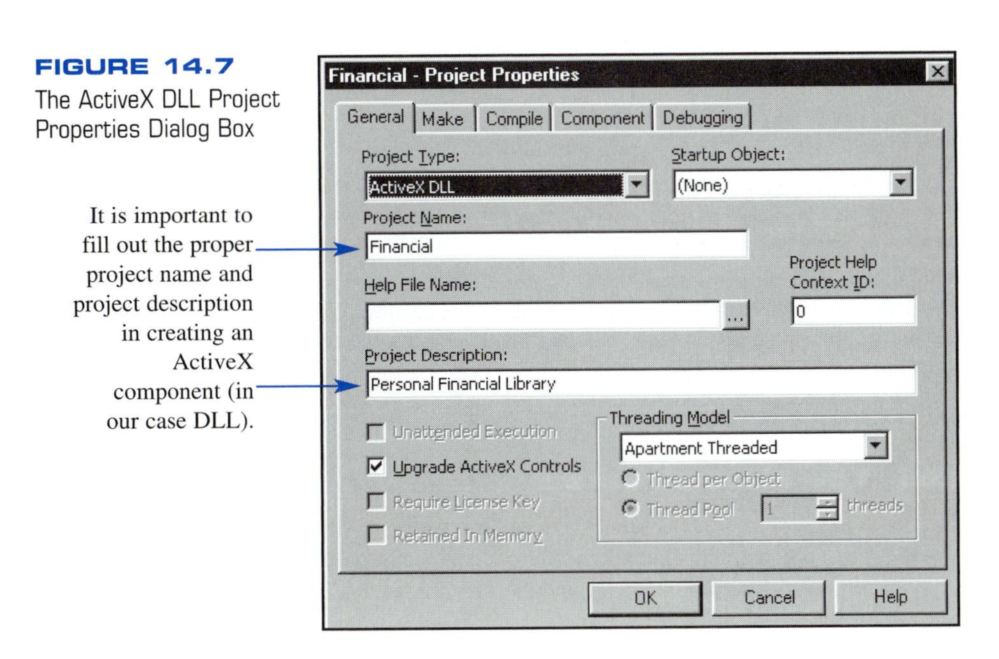

FIGURE 14.7
The ActiveX DLL Project Properties Dialog Box

Compiling the ActiveX DLL Project

If everything is done correctly, you are ready to compile the project and make it an ActiveX DLL for future uses. Follow these steps:

1. Click the PVTable icon in the Project Explorer window so that the PVTable class module will appear in the Properties Window.
2. Make sure the Instancing property is MultiUse (5), not Private (1). (See Figure 14.8.) This will make the PVTable class exposed as a Public class, instead of being Private, which can be recognized only inside a project. Only the Public class can be used by other projects.
3. Click the File menu. Locate and select the "Make Financial.dll" option. You will be prompted for the folder to save the DLL. Select a folder of your choice and click the OK button.
4. When the VB IDE finishes compiling without any error message, the ActiveX DLL is successfully created. You are now able to use the object in the DLL.

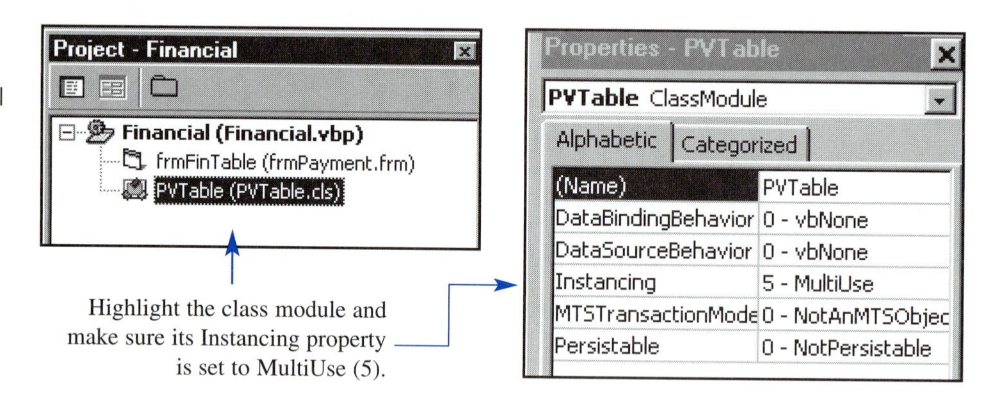

FIGURE 14.8 Setting the Instancing Property of the Financial Class Module

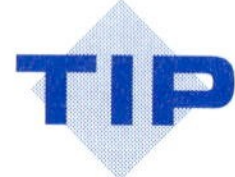

TIP

Suppose you have developed a class module through a standard EXE project and you would like to create an ActiveX DLL with the class module. Is there an easy way? Yes. You can do the following:

1. Start a new ActiveX DLL project.
2. Add the class module you have created to the current project. Click the Project menu and select the Add Class Module option to add the existing class module to the project.
3. Set the Instancing property of the class module to MultiUse.
4. Remove the empty (Class1) class module from the project. Highlight Class1 in the Project Explorer window. Then click the Project menu and select the Remove Class1 option.
5. Set the appropriate properties for the project. Click the Project menu and select the Project1 Properties option. In the General tab of the Project Properties dialog box, enter the project name and project description in the proper boxes.
6. Compile the ActiveX DLL project.

Using the ActiveX DLL You Have Created

Using the object(s) in an ActiveX DLL you have created is no different than using other ActiveX DLL such as the ADO objects. You can add a reference of the DLL to your project (like the way you added ADO to your project) or you can use the GetObject and/or CreateObject function to create the object. To get a feel, let's continue our example by incorporating the PVTable in a new standard EXE project. Here are the steps:

1. Start a new standard EXE project.
2. Click the Project menu and select the References option. The References dialog box will appear.
3. Look for "Personal Financial Library" (this string is what you entered in the project description box in the Project1 Properties dialog box described previously) in the Available References list box. Check the item and click the OK button. (See Figure 14.9.)
4. Draw a command button in the form. Set its Caption property to "Show PV Table" and name it cmdShow.
5. Add the following code:

```
Option Explicit
Dim PresentValueTable As Financial.PVTable
Private Sub cmdShow_Click()
    Set PresentValueTable = New Financial.PVTable
    With PresentValueTable
        .HigherRate = 0.2
        .LowerRate = 0.05
        .Years = 30
        .ShowPVTable
    End With
End Sub
Private Sub Form_QueryUnload(Cancel As Integer, _
    UnloadMode As Integer)
    Set PresentValueTable = Nothing
End Sub
```

The code declares an object, PresentValueTable, as the Financial.PVTable class. Recall that Financial is the project we created for the DLL and PVTable is the name of the class module. The cmdShow Click event procedure creates a new Financial PVTable object and associates it with the object variable PresentValueTable. It then sets the properties for the object and calls the object's ShowPVTable method to display the present value table. When you click the command button, you should see the form with an HFG display the table as shown in Figure 14.6.

Notice that we have declared the PresentValueTable object variable in the general declaration area rather than in the event procedure. The object is destroyed (set to Nothing) in the form's QueryUnload event. The object should remain alive even after the Click event procedure is executed. If the object is declared within the event procedure, the present value table will be displayed and destroyed as soon as the event procedure finishes because the object will go "out of scope."

FIGURE 14.9
The References Dialog Box After Compiling the Financial ActiveX DLL

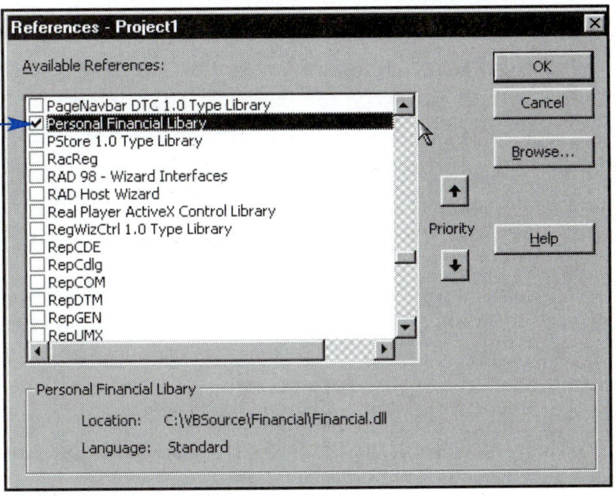

When you compile your ActiveX DLL with the proper project description entered, the description shows here as an item in the Available References list box of the References dialog box.

This illustration shows that not only the steps but also the way to declare and use the PVTable object in the Financial DLL are exactly the same as it took to use those objects in the ADO library. With this capability to create an ActiveX DLL, you can make your code truly reusable. Any collection of routines of similar nature that you want to use in other projects can be created as a class or classes and compiled as an ActiveX DLL (or other types of components).

In addition, the objects in the ActiveX DLL are not statically linked into the compiled standard EXE programs. Instead, they are dynamically linked to the programs at runtime. That is, rather than incorporating the objects in your ActiveX DLL when a client program is compiled, it makes a reference to only the object in the DLL. Thus, if you need to revise any class in the DLL, you can do so and update the DLL without having to recompile the programs that use the objects.

You may wonder how VB becomes aware of your Financial project. When your ActiveX DLL project was compiled successfully, VB also automatically registered (placed a reference in the Windows registry) for the DLL, saving you all the extra trouble to tell VB where to look for it.

Developing and Debugging an ActiveX DLL Project

When you are developing an ActiveX DLL project, you will need to test the code you have developed. Because your DLL project will be an object to be created and used by other standard projects, you should use a standard project to test it.

Suppose you want to debug the preceding Financial project while you are developing the code. You can add a standard EXE project to the IDE to form a ***project group*** and then test the two projects as a group. The steps are as follows:

1. Load your Financial ActiveX DLL project into the IDE. If this is your new project, you will need to create the project by following all the steps for setting up the project as outlined previously.
2. Add a new standard EXE project.
   - 2.1 Click the File menu and select the Add Project option. (Note: Do not select the New Project option.) The Add Project dialog box will appear.
   - 2.2 Select standard EXE project in the dialog box and click the Open button. You should now see two projects in the Project Explorer window.
3. Make Project1 (instead of the Financial project) the startup project.
   - 3.1 Right-click Project1 in the Project Explorer window to invoke the context menu.
   - 3.2 Select the "Set as Start Up" option. The startup project should be displayed in bold (see Figure 14.10).
4. Set a reference to the Financial project. Click the Project menu and select the References option. Locate and check "Financial" in the Available References list box. Note that this item is placed near the beginning of the list and does not appear in alphabetical order. Note also, here the project name, not the project description, is used.
5. Set up the visual interface and enter code in Project 1 to test the Financial project. For example, you can draw a command button on the new form. Name it cmdShow and set its Caption property to "Show." Then enter the code from step 5 (the cmdShow click event procedure) of the preceding subsection.
6. Press Ctrl+F5 (Start with Full Compile) to test your project. Although you can start the project by pressing the F5 key, pressing Ctrl+F5 will force a full compile so that the Financial ActiveX DLL project is truly ready for a test.

From there on, you can test, identify, and correct the problem(s) in both of the projects in the group. Of course, you should save all your work for both projects as you progress. You should also save the project group so that you can load the two projects as a group in the future. These steps are similar to those for a single project.

You should be aware of the error-trapping setting during your testing process. By default, error trapping is set to "Break on Unhandled Errors." Under this setting, an error that occurs in the class module will be trapped in the module that uses an interface (method or property) in that class module, making it diffculty to locate the error. To pinpoint the root of any errors in the

FIGURE 14.10
The Project Explorer Window After Setting Project1 as the Startup Project

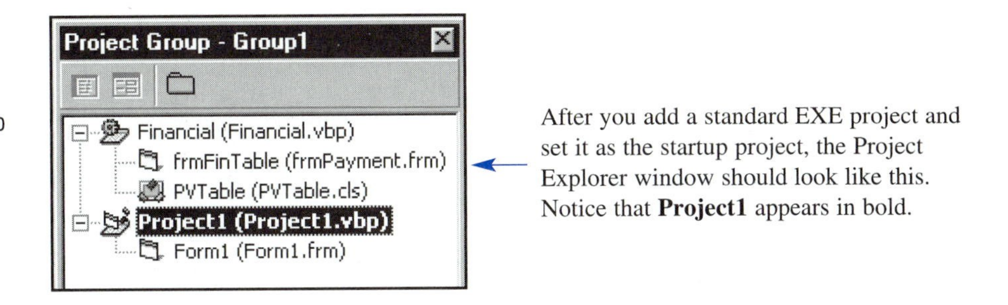
Project Group - Group1
Financial (Financial.vbp)
frmFinTable (frmPayment.frm)
PVTable (PVTable.cls)
Project1 (Project1.vbp)
Form1 (Form1.frm)
After you add a standard EXE project and set it as the startup project, the Project Explorer window should look like this. Notice that **Project1** appears in bold.

class module, make sure that the error trapping is set to "Break in Class Module." To change the setting:

1. Click the Tools menu and then click the Options option. The Options dialog box will appear.
2. Click the General tab.
3. In the Error Trapping frame, select the "Break in Class Module" option.
4. Click the OK button in the dialog box.

After your ActiveX DLL project is fully tested, you will be ready to compile it into a DLL:

1. Remove the test project (Project1) from the project group. Right-click Project1 in the Project Explorer window to invoke the context menu. Select the Remove Project option.
2. Compile the remaining ActiveX DLL project. The steps have been given previously.

Summary

In this chapter, you have learned three topics that extend the capabilities of VB: the API functions, the Windows registry, and the ActiveX components. API functions can be used to perform services that are not built into the VB language. In some cases, API functions also can be used to perform tasks more efficiently than VB code. You have seen several examples that illustrate the case. Because API functions are not native to the VB language, coding with API takes additional care and effort. It is suggested that each function used be "wrapped" by a VB procedure. Once the procedure is created, you can call the procedure in the future without having to deal with the technical details in the API and constant declarations.

The Windows registry is a neat facility that your program can use to maintain data peculiar to the operations of your program. These types of data typically involve various settings that your program allows the user to customize the application. These can include user passwords; the file paths or databases that the user maintains; and the fonts, form position, and/or background color of a particular form when it is loaded.

Once one becomes well acquainted with the registry, there might be a tendency to overuse it because of the convenience. Overusing the registry, however, is not advisable because it can slow down the operation of the entire computer system. Again, the data to be saved in the registry should be limited to the internal operation of the application. Data pertaining to the user's business operations (e.g., sales orders) should be kept in a database or file.

You have also been introduced to the ActiveX component technology. We listed four types of ActiveX components but limited the discussion to only three types. In the discussion, it was pointed out that you have used two types of ActiveX components before reaching this chapter. These are the ActiveX DLL (e.g., the ADO) and the ActiveX OCX (e.g., the masked edit box). We then discussed how to use the ActiveX EXE such as those objects provided by Excel and Word. We presented one example of each. We also showed an alternative way to use these objects by using the CreateObject and GetObject functions when the code component's object library is not referenced in VB. Finally, you learned how to create and debug an ActiveX DLL. This experience should provide you with the foundation to create other types of components.

The theme of this chapter is "extensibility." You have been exposed to the various ways to extend the functionality of VB. With a solid knowledge of VB that you have learned from the previous chapters and a peek into the extensibility arena, the rest is all yours. Happy VBing!

Visual Basic Explorer

14-1. Trapping the Tab Key. Now You See Me. Now You Don't. It is generally understood that the Tab key is not trappable in any of the keyboard events. Let's explore this "truth." Draw a text box on a new form. Set the form's KeyPreview property to True. Place the following code in the code window:

```
Private Sub Form_KeyDown(KeyCode As Integer, Shift As Integer)
     If KeyCode = vbKeyTab Then
          MsgBox "Got the Tab key!"
     End If
End Sub
```

Run the project and press the Tab key. Do you see the Tab key trapped? So, why does the text say the Tab key is not trappable in VB?

Draw another text box on the form. Run the project and press the Tab key again. This time, do you see any message displayed? So, the Tab key is not really trappable?

Wait. Try another thing. Set the TabStop property of both text boxes to False. Run the project and press the Tab key again. Now, do you see the message displayed?

The Tab key is trappable only if at most one control's TabStop property is set to True. In this case, you will have to manage the Tab key by your own code; that is, the Tab key can no longer be relied on to move focus. Still want to trap the Tab key using the KeyUp and KeyDown events?

14-2. Shell and SendKeys: A Way to Communicate with Other Applications. You can use the Shell function to start another application and then use the Clipboard object and SendKeys statements to communicate with another application. Draw a command button on a new form. Name it cmdToNotePad and set its Caption property to "To Notepad." Then try the following code:

```
Option Explicit

Private Sub cmdToNotepad_Click()
Dim D As Double
     'Set up the Clipboard
     Clipboard.Clear
     'Place text in the clipboard
     Clipboard.SetText "This comes from my VB program."

     D = Shell("Notepad", vbNormalFocus) 'Start notepad
     DoEvents
     AppActivate D 'Activate Notepad (set focus)
     DoEvents
     'Send Alt+E key & P key (Edit, paste)
     'This will paste the text in Clipboard in Notepad
     SendKeys "%ep", True
End Sub
```

Run the program and click the command button. What do you see?

The procedure first places a text string in the Clipboard object. Then it starts the Notepad application and sets the focus on it with the AppActivate statement. The SendKeys statement sends Alt+E (for the Edit menu) and P (for Paste) keys to the active window (Notepad), causing the text in the Clipboard to show in Notepad. Note that the DoEvents statements in the procedure are necessary for the system to start the application and set focus.

14-3. Common Dialog Box Without a Form. Recall that before you can use the common dialog box control, you have to add it to your project from the Components option of the Project menu and draw it on a form. What if you want to use it in a general procedure in a standard or class module so that the procedure can be used in various projects? Place the following code in a standard module and call the procedure from your Form Click event.

```
'In the standard module
Function GetFileName()
Dim cdlFile As Object
    Set cdlFile = CreateObject("msComDlg.CommonDialog")
    With cdlFile
        .CancelError = True
        .ShowOpen
        GetFileName = .FileName
    End With
    Set cdlFile = Nothing
End Function
'In the form
Private Sub Form_Click()
Dim FileName As String
    FileName = GetFileName
    MsgBox "FileName = " & FileName
End Sub
```

Run the project and click the form. What result do you obtain? What are the advantages and disadvantages of using this approach?

14-4. What Is Exposed? In Chapter 12, we stated that a form in an ActiveX DLL is not visible to another project. Here is a way to verify:

1. Start a new standard project. This should be shown as Project1.
2. Add (not Open) an ActiveX DLL project. This should be shown as Project2.
3. Add a new form to Project2.
4. Click the Project menu and select the Project2 Properties option. (Make sure Project2 has the focus in the Project Explorer window before you start.)
5. Change the project name in the Project2 Project Properties dialog box from Project2 to Testing and click the OK button.
6. Click Project1 to highlight the project.
7. Click the Project menu and select the References option. The References – Project1 dialog box should appear.
8. Look for Testing in the list box and check this item. Then click the OK button.
9. Double-click Form1 under Project1 in the Project Explorer window. The form will appear in the IDE.
10. Double-click the form so that its code window will appear.
11. Enter the following code:

```
Dim MyObject As Testing
```

At this point you should see only Class1 (no form1) appears in the object browser box. Conclusion? A class module but not a form as an object in an ActiveX DLL module can be exposed to another project.

14-5. The Dictionary Object. This project will create a dictionary object that you can use to index phone numbers by name. Draw a text box, a masked edit box, and two command buttons on a new form. Name the text box txtName. Name the masked edit box mskPhone and set its Mask property to "(###)-###-####" (you can also add proper labels for these two controls). Name the first command button cmdIndex and set its Caption property to "Index." Name the second command button cmdRetrieve and set its Caption property to "Retrieve." Then enter the following code:

```
Option Explicit
Dim dicPhone As Object
Private Sub Form_Load()
    Set dicPhone = CreateObject("scripting.Dictionary")
End Sub

Private Sub cmdIndex_Click()
    'Build the index
    dicPhone.Add txtName.Text, mskPhone.ClipText
    'Clear the fields
    txtName.Text = ""
    mskPhone.Mask = ""
    mskPhone.Text = ""
    mskPhone.Mask = "(###)-###-####"
End Sub

Private Sub cmdRetrieve_Click()
    On Error GoTo errhand
    'Retrieve phone number by name; If fail, display error msg
    mskPhone.Text = Format$(dicPhone(txtName.Text), _
      "(000)-000-0000")
    Exit Sub
errhand:
    MsgBox "Name not found."
End Sub
```

Run the project. Enter the following names and phone numbers into the text box and mask edit control, one set at a time. When complete, click the Index button.

Name	Phone Number
Jerry	972-225-3838
Jesse	817-999-1234
Jody	214-333-5555

Then enter any name in the text box and click the Retrieve button. If the name you enter is one of those you have previously entered, you should be able to get the phone number. Otherwise, you should see an error message displayed. Can you see how the Dictionary object works and how it can facilitate building an index?

14-6. Dictionary Object Again. When you entered the code in 14-5, it should have felt quite different from your "typical" experience in coding. The IDE did not show much support in providing hints about the methods or properties of the dictionary object.

Try to code the same project with the following modification:

A. Set a reference to the scripting library. Its name is "Microsoft Scripting Runtime."

B. Change the declaration of the variable, dicPhone as follows:

```
Dim dicPhone As New Scripting.Dictionary
```

C. Change the Form Load procedure as follows:

```
Private Sub Form_Load()
    Set dicPhone = Scripting.Dictionary
End Sub
```

Feel any different when entering the Set statement? Try the program again. Does it work the same way? Which way do you prefer to code?

14-7. The FileSystemObject. (continued from 14-6). The Scripting library has another object called the FileSystemObject; this library provides a host of file services. Enter the following code:

```
Private Sub Form_Click()
Dim myFileObj As Scripting.FileSystemObject
        Set myFileObj = New Scripting.FileSystemObject
        If myFileObj.DriveExists("C") Then
            MsgBox "Drive C exists"
        Else
            MsgBox "There's no drive C"
    End If
End Sub
```

Run the project and click the form. What message do you see? What do you think the DriveExists method can be used for?

Exercises

14-8. Trapping the Shift Key in the LostFocus Event. The text demonstrates how the Tab key can be trapped in the LostFocus Event. It would be desirable to also check whether the Shift key has been pressed in that same event. Provide the code to perform the check. (*Hint:* You can use the GetKeyState API in the same event several times to check for the state of different keys. Find the key code constant value of the Shift key from the VB online Help file. Have your routine print the returned value from the API function so that you can see what value to check for when the Shift key is pressed.)

14-9. The GetComputerName API. Want to know the name of the computer you are working with? The GetComputerName API answers your wish. It works similarly to the GetSystemDirectory API except that the length of the computer name is set in the second parameter, rather than as a returned function value. Develop a project to get the name of your computer using this API. You should be able to obtain proper declaration information from the API text viewer.

14-10. A "Wrapper" for the List Box Horizontal Scrollbar. Write a VB function with the following header:

```
Public Function SetLbHScrollBar(HWnd As Long, Width As Long) _
  As Long
```

where *HWnd* is the handle for the list box and *Width* is the width of the horizontal scrollbar in pixels.

The function will set the horizontal scrollbar of the list box referenced by the HWnd to the width parameter. It will return whatever the value returned by the SendMessage API function.

14-11. Doubling the Width of the List Box. Write a function that will double the width of the horizontal scrollbar of the list box. The name of the message to obtain the width of the list box is LB_GETHORIZONTALEXTENT. The header of the function should be as follows:

```
Public Function SetLbDblHsb(TheLB As ListBox) As Long
```

The function will return whatever the value the SendMessage API returns. (*Hint:* The return value [not the third parameter] of the SendMessage API will give the horizontal extent when the message is LB_GETHORIZONTALEXTENT. It will return a value of zero before the LB_SETHORIZONTALEXTENT message is used. In such a case, use the following formula to compute the original width before sending the "set" message: Width = TheLB.Width/Screen.TwipsPerPixelX.)

14-12. A Wrapper for Finding a String in the List Box. Write a function that will return the position of the string in the list box that matches the search string. The function should have the following header:

```
Function FindLbString(Hwnd As Long, Text As String)
```

where *HWnd* is the handle for the list box and *Text* is the search string.

The message named constant has been used in the text as an illustration for the SendMessage API.

14-13. Searching the Combo Box for a String. Using the example to search a list box for a string, write a routine to search the combo box for a string. Note that messages having something to do with the combo box start with the two letters CB, instead of LB. (The key purpose of this exercise is for you to look for a constant in the API viewer.)

14-14. Searching the Combo Box for an Exact Match. Write a function that will return the position of the item in a combo box that matches exactly the search string. This function should be based on the SendMessage API. Note that the name of the constant is CB_FINDSTRINGEXACT. The function header should appear as follows:

```
Function FindCBExactMatch(HWnd As Long, Text As string) As Long
```

where *HWnd* is the handle of the combo box and *Text* is the search string.

The function should return the position of the search string in the combo box.

14-15. Finding Free Disk Space. The name of the API function to find the free space in a disk is GetDiskFreeSpace, which returns a Long Integer indicating whether the call is successful (nonzero = success; zero = failure). The first parameter in its parameter list is a string parameter specifying the drive to check for space. All other parameters are "loaded" (set) by the function and are self-explanatory (provided you obtain the declaration from the API viewer). Write a "wrapper" function (call it FindFreeSpace) that will (1) take a disk drive name as the parameter, (2) call the GetDiskFreeSpace function, and (3) compute and return the free disk space in bytes. Note that the drive should be specified with proper trailing characters. For example, Drive C should be specified as "C:\" (without quotes).

14-16. Saving the Biblio.mdb File Path. In many of your projects that involve using the Biblio.mdb file, you have either hard-coded its file path or used the common dialog box to prompt for the file path. Add code to one of these projects so that when the project starts, it will do the following:

- Prompt for the file path (using the common dialog box) if the program cannot find the setting from the registry.
- Save the file path in the registry when the program quits.
- Retrieve the file path when the program restarts. Your program should not prompt for the file path again, if the program can open the database without any problem.

14-17. Saving the Form Location and WindowState. Develop a project so that when the program restarts, it will appear at the previous location with the same previous WindowState; that is, if the form was previously maximized when it quit, it will be maximized when it runs again. (*Hint:* Save the form's Left, Top, and WindowState properties with three different keys in the QueryUnload event and retrieve these settings in the Form Load event.)

14-18. A Login Form. Design a login form that will be the first form to greet the user when he or she starts an application. The form should have two option buttons: Login and New User.

If the New User option button is clicked, the form displays three boxes: Username, Password, and Confirm. It also displays an OK command button. The user is expected to enter the username and the password twice: once in the password box and once in the confirm box. He or she then clicks the OK button. If the two passwords match, the username and the encrypted password should be saved in the registry. Each character of the password should be encrypted then the OK button clicked. If the two passwords match, the username and the encrypted password shuold be saved in the registry. Each character of the password should be encrypted with the value 15, which should also be used to decrypt the password when the latter is retrieved. (*Hint:* Use the Xor operator to encrypt the ASCII value of each letter with 15.) If the passwords in the password and confirm boxes do not match, the form continues to prompt for the same.

If the user clicks the Login option button, the form should ask the user for the username and password. When the user finishes the entry, he or she clicks a Login command button. If the username exists, your program will compare the password with the one saved in the registry and proceed to the "application" if they match; otherwise, the login form will continue to prompt for the username and password.

14-19. Printing a Word Document. Modify the MS Word project presented in this chapter so that the user can specify the document, the page numbers, and the number of copies to print. Use three text boxes to take input from the user. There should be a command button by the text box for document (file path). When the user clicks this button, it will trigger a common dialog box for the user to browse the system to find the file. The user will specify the page numbers to print by entering two numbers with a dash in between. For example, "12-34" means page 12 through page 34.

14-20. Showing a Pie Chart. Create a VB project for the user to enter the sales amounts for four regions (east, west, north, and south). When the user clicks the command button with the caption "Show Pie Chart," your program creates an Excel object, inserts the four sales amounts in a worksheet, and uses Excel's chart object to draw and display a pie chart based on those amounts. (*Hint:* To make Excel appear, set the application's Visible property to True.)

14-21. Building a Copy File Class. You have seen how to use the common dialog box without a form. You have also been introduced to the FileSystemObject in the MS Scripting library (Visual Basic Explorer exercise 14-7). This object has a CopyFile method that can be used to copy a file.

Create a method (call it CopyAFile) in class module (call it FileObject) that can be used to copy a file. When the method is invoked, it uses the common dialog box to prompt for the source file (file to be copy from) and then prompts for the target file path. Note that the source file must exist. In addition, if the target file exists, the user should be warned and should confirm the write-over to proceed.

14-22. Creating an ActiveX DLL for FileObject. (continued from 14-21). Create a component DLL for the FileObject class you created in 14-21. Name the project FileService and use "My File Service Library" as the project description. After you have the project compiled successfully, test to ensure that the method works properly. (*Hint:* Start a new ActiveX DLL project. Add the class module FileObject to the project. Make sure its Instancing property is set properly before getting the project compiled.)

Projects

14-23. An ActiveX DLL for Log in. Modify the project you created in 14-18 so that it is suitable to be compiled as an ActiveX DLL. Note that you will need to use a class module to activate the form. Then add a standard EXE project to form a project group. Write code to use the component. Test and debug the project group. When the project group performs properly, compile the ActiveX DLL project. Test the compiled version again, using the same Standard EXE project.

14-24. Sales Order Entry Screen and Its Configuration. Refer to project 13-31, the sales order entry project. Modify the project as follows:

A. Add a form that serves as the startup object. The form should contain the following menu structure:

File	Transactions	Customers	Products	Utilities
Open . . .	Sales	Add/Edit	Add/Edit	Configure
Exit	Purchase	Query	Query	Clear Registry

B. Add another form that will be used as a custom dialog box for "entry forms" configuration. The form is invoked when the user clicks the Configure option in the Utilities menu and will allow the user to specify foreground and background colors for boxes (text boxes, combo boxes, and masked edit boxes as a group), label captions, and command buttons, respectively. (Hint: Use text boxes for the user to enter values. However, provide a way for the user to use the common dialog box to make the color choices.) These values should be saved in the Windows registry. When the Sales Order Entry form is invoked (see E), these values are retrieved and applied to the controls on the form. (Use their default colors if the registry contains no applicable values.)

C. When the program starts, it checks the Windows registry to determine whether it contains the file path for the Products database, which contains Sales Order table. If the registry has no such entry, your program invokes a common dialog box to prompt the user for the file path. For simplicity, use NWInd.mdb as the surrogate for this purpose. After obtaining the file path (either from the user or from the registry), your program should make an ADO connection. (Do not actually perform any input or output.) If the attempt to open the database is unsuccessful, your program should ask the user whether to specify another path or quit. The file path should be saved in the Windows registry before the program quits.

D. The Open option in the File menu will invoke a common dialog box for the user to specify the file path for the Products database. Follow the same instructions as in C to handle making an ADO connection. This option allows the user to specify another file path in case the database has been moved.

E. When the user clicks the Sales option in the Transactions menu, the sale order entry form will be invoked. (This was the original form created in 13-31.) Modify this form as follows:

   1. Replace all SendKeys statements in the module with proper API calls to avoid the potential problems with the Shift key as discussed in this chapter.
   2. Add a list box. Each time a sale order is entered (after the user clicks the Save button and pretends to have the order saved), the order number is added to the list box if it is not found in the list box. Use the proper API call to verify whether the order number exists.

F. When the user clicks the Clear Registry option in the Utilities menu, all registry entries should be removed after confirming with the user.

G. When the user clicks the Exit option in the File menu, the program quits.

H. When the user clicks on an option in any menu that is not defined already, display the message "Under Development."

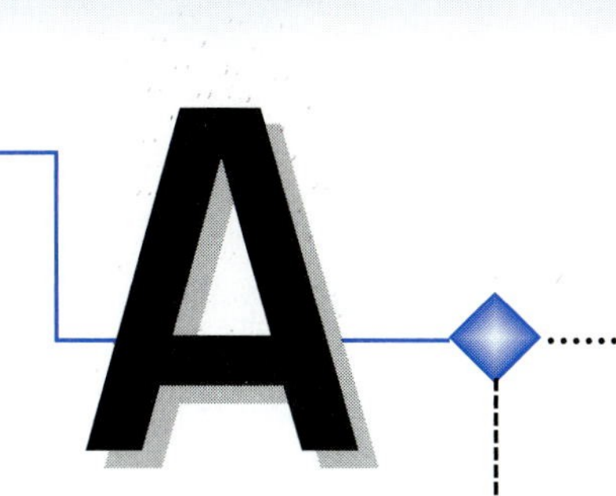

Data Management Using Files

In Chapter 8, "Database and the ActiveX Data Objects," we discussed the use of relational database for data management. In business applications, the database approach to data management was introduced long after the file-oriented approach. Under the file-oriented approach, all data that need to be kept for uses by the computer are stored in the secondary storage as files. VB provides three different file types to handle data:

1. Sequential files
2. Binary files
3. Random files

Sequential files were discussed in Chapter 6, "Input, Output, and Procedures." This appendix focuses mainly on binary files and random files.

A.1. Opening and Closing a File

As explained in Chapter 6, regardless of the file type you will be dealing with, the first step to work with a file is to open it. The syntax is as follows:

```
Open FileName For Mode As [#]FileNumber [Len = Length]
```

The mode determines how a file is to behave. The following table provides a summary.

File Mode	File Behavior	Applicable Statements
Input	Sequential input	Input statement; Input function; Line Input statement
Output	Sequential output (previous content will be erased)	Print statement; Write statement
Append	Sequential output (new data are added at end of previous content)	Print statement; Write statement
Binary	Any byte position in the file can be read or written	Get statement; Put statement
Random	Any record position in the file can be read or written	Get statement; Put statement

For example, to open a file with a path "C:\Temp\TempFile.txt" for sequential input, you will code the following:

```
Dim TempFile As Integer
TempFile = FreeFile
Open "C:\Temp\TempFile.txt" For Input As #TempFile
```

In the preceding code, the variable TempFile is assigned with a file number provided by the FreeFile function, which is explained in Chapter 6.

To close the same file, you code the following:

```
Close #TempFile
```

File Mode and File Type

Note that given an existing file, you can open it with any mode you wish. However, it is more logical that a file is opened with a mode that is consistent with the file type when it is created. That is, if a file is initially created as a sequential file, you will encounter far fewer technical problems if you open it with one of the three modes for the sequential files. By the same token, if you create a file with the binary mode, it will be much easier to work with the same file with the same binary mode. This point should become apparent as we proceed through the following sections, which explain in more detail the uses of the binary file and random file.

A.2. Working with Binary Files

How Does a Binary File Work?

Perhaps it is easier to understand how a binary file works by comparing it with a sequential file.

Input and Output Allowed. You can perform input from a sequential file only if it is opened with the Input mode and perform output only if it is opened in Output or Append mode. However, you can perform both input and output at the same time on a file opened with the binary mode.

Data Access. You can access data in a sequential file only "sequentially"; that is, you read or write one data element at a time. Once you pass that element, you cannot go back until you close the file and reopen for another round. (*Note:* Technically, this is not exactly true with the case of the Input function. However, it is still advisable to observe this general rule.) In contrast, you can have access to any position of a binary file in any order any time. Thus, you have complete "freedom of movement" around a binary file.

Data Conversion for Output. All output to a sequential file is converted to text strings before actual output is carried out. However, no data conversion is performed on output to a binary file. Thus, a 9-digit number of the Long type will be written onto a sequential file as a 9-digit character string (plus any delimiters) but on a binary file as a 4-byte field. (Recall that a Long type variable requires 4 bytes of storage.) This difference in I/O operation can be tricky to a beginner and is further illustrated later.

Data Conversion for Input. All numeric input from a sequential file is converted to the data type of the variable specified. In contrast, the data read from a binary file is taken "at face value." The data obtained is assigned directly to the variable used in the Get statement (for binary input) without any data conversion.

Delimiters. In the sequential file output operation, delimiters are inserted automatically. Recall that if you use a Write statement to output a string, it adds a pair of double quotes to enclose the string and a comma before it if it is not the first item in the output list. Each line in the sequential file (whether done by the Write or Print statement) is delimited by the character pair vbCrLf (Chr$(13)Chr$(10)). However, no delimiter characters are automatically inserted to any output in a binary file. (Thus, if you create a file with the binary mode and reopen the file with the Input mode, you will most likely see only one long line of data.)

These differences are summarized in the following table.

Difference in	Sequential File	Binary File
Mode and I/O	Either Input for input; or Append or Output for output	Binary
Access	Sequential; either input or output	Direct; input and output at any byte position
Data conversion in output	Numeric data are converted to string before output	No conversion; each byte in memory is output as a byte in file
Data conversion in input	Strings read in for numeric variables will be converted to numbers	No conversion; each byte in file is read in as a byte into memory
Delimiters	Added automatically	No delimiter added

Opening a File with the Binary Mode

To open a file (with a path "C:\Payroll\Special.dat") for the Binary mode, you code the following:

```
Dim SpecialFile As Integer
SpecialFile = FreeFile
Open "C:\Payroll\Special.dat" for Binary As #SpecialFile
```

As you can see, the difference between opening a sequential file and a binary file is the keyword for the file mode. You use the keyword "for Binary" to open a binary file.

Output and Input with a Binary File

Once open, a binary file can be used to perform any input or output. To perform output, you use the Put statement, which has the following syntax:

```
Put #FileNumber, [Position], VariableName
```

For example, to output a value 65 to the preceding file, you can code the following:

```
Dim SixtyFive As Integer
SixtyFive = 65
Put #SpecialFile, 1, SixtyFive
```

The Position Value in the Binary File. The Put statement in the preceding code instructs the computer to output the variable SixtyFive to the binary file, SpecialFile, starting at position 1 (first position). The position is expressed in byte (e.g., position 1 is the first byte position). As explained, you can place the output in any position of the file. This holds even for the first output operation. Thus, if you change the position to 1,000,001 in the preceding statement, it will still work. However, you will leave the first 1,000,000 bytes unused. Unless you have something planned for that storage area, it is just not advisable to skip that many bytes in a file.

Retrieving Data from the Binary file. To retrieve the data from a binary file, you use the Get statement, which has the following syntax:

```
Get #FileNumber, [Position], VariableName
```

For example, to read the data stored in the preceding example, you can code the following:

```
Dim RetrievedData As Integer
Get #SpecialFile, 1, RetrievedData
```

Notice that to retrieve the stored data correctly, *the position and the data type of the variable must match that specified in the original Put statement.* The binary file is very precise in this respect. Count on an unexpected result if you fail to observe this rule.

To ensure correct results, match the exact position and data type of the data you are retrieving with what were originally stored in a binary file.

Data Type and Binary I/O. Why is it so important to match the data type between input and output in a binary file? After all, you may recall that in working with the sequential file, any data can be read as a string or variant without any errors in the results. This is certainly not the case for the binary file. Recall that data saved in the binary file are done without any conversion. Thus, the preceding Put statement will result in a 2-byte integer image being placed in the first 2 bytes of the file. Once the data are left in the file, the computer no longer remembers the format of the data. It relies on your code to provide the correct format (data type) to retrieve the same data. A different data type will make the computer interpret the data differently and therefore incorrectly.

For example, consider the following code to retrieve the same data saved previously:

```
Dim Tester As String * 2
Get #SpecialFile, 1, Tester
```

The result will be quite different. The 2-byte Integer image will be retrieved from the file. No conversion is performed. Thus, you should expect to see the character representation of the numeric value; that is, Chr$(Value of first byte) & Chr$(Value of second byte).

To illustrate, let's put all the preceding code together (with some minor modifications) in a command Click event procedure (draw a command button on a new form and name it cmdTest before coding) as follows:

```
Private Sub cmdTest_Click()
Dim SpecialFile As Integer
Dim SixtyFive As Integer
Dim RetrievedData As Integer
Dim Tester As String * 2
```

```
        SpecialFile = FreeFile
        Open "C:\Temp\Special.dat" For Binary As #SpecialFile
        SixtyFive = 65
        Put #SpecialFile, 1, SixtyFive
        Get #SpecialFile, 1, RetrievedData
        Print RetrievedData
        Get #SpecialFile, 1, Tester
        Print Tester
    End Sub
```

When you run the program and click the command button, you should see two values on the form:

65

A

The variable RetrievedData gives the correct result because its data type matches that of SixtyFive. However, Tester shows "A" because the first byte in the file has a code value of 65, the ASCII value for "A." Incidentally, when the computer saves a numeric field, the lowest byte is saved first, as you might have inferred from these results.

Omitting the Position Parameter? As implied in the preceding syntax, the position parameter in both Put and Get statements can be omitted. If left unspecified, the position that VB actually uses is the value that is determined by the Seek function, which returns a value representing a position in the file. In general, when you leave the position parameter unspecified, you leave the control at the mercy of the computer. Always specify the position parameter to ensure the accuracy of the results.

Handling String Data. Writing string data to the binary file is fairly simple and presents no problem. For example, the following statement will write the name "John Smith" to SpecialFile starting from byte position 3.

```
Put #SpecialFile, 3, "John Smith"
```

But how do you read it back? The following fragment of code will *not* work properly. (Test it in an event procedure such as Form Click. You will see nothing printed.)

```
Dim TheName As String
Get #SpecialFile, 3, TheName
Print TheName
```

Why? Recall that the Get statement relies on your code to provide the data type (and its implicit length) to retrieve the data. Although the code declares TheName as a string variable, it has yet to indicate the length of the string. The default length of the string variable is zero. Thus, nothing is read. To read the name back, you will need to specify the length for the string variable first. The following code fragment should work properly:

```
Dim TheName As String
'Generate a string of 10 null characters
TheName = String$(10, 0)
Get #SpecialFile, 3, TheName
Print TheName
```

Using Fixed Length String for I/O. To repeat, the position and data type (and its length) to be read must match the data that was originally created for the Get statement to retrieve the data accurately. For this reason, string I/O in the binary file is usually done with fixed-length string variables. This eliminates the need to set the length for the variable before the Get statement. Assume 24 characters are appropriate to store any names. You can revise the preceding code as follows:

```
' In the general declaration area
Dim TheName As String * 24
    ' To output
    TheName = "John Smith"
    Put #SpecialFile, 3, TheName
```

```
' To Input
Get #SpecialFile, 3, TheName
Print TheName
```

Note, however, the effect of this fragment of code will be a bit different from the previous example where the constant "John Smith" is "put" in the file. In the current example, the field is 24 characters long. The fixed-length variable TheName ensures that the remaining field after the name is filled with blank spaces. In the previous example, the content beyond "John Smith" is unknown.

Saving and Retrieving an Array. You can also save into and retrieve from a binary file an array of data. For example, the following code fragment will save 100 random numbers in a binary file called RandNumFile:

```
Dim RandNumFile As Integer
Dim I As Integer
Dim MyArray(99) As Long
    For I = 0 To 99
        MyArray(I) = 1000 * Rnd
    Next I
    RandNumFile = FreeFile
    Open "RandNum.dat" For Binary As #RandNumFile
    Put #RandNumFile, 1, MyArray
    Close RandNumFile
```

To retrieve the same data from the file into another array, you can code the following:

```
Dim RandNumFile As Integer
Dim I As Integer
Dim YourArray(99) As Long
    RandNumFile = FreeFile
    Open "RandNum.dat" For Binary As #RandNumFile
    Get #RandNumFile, 1, YourArray
    Close RandNumFile
```

Note that you do not have to read the entire array at one time. Once the data are saved, you can retrieve only the part that you need. For example, if you need to read only the last 50 elements of the number back, you can code the following:

```
Dim RandNumFile As Integer
Dim I As Integer
Dim HisArray(49) As Long
    RandNumFile = FreeFile
    Open "RandNum.dat" For Binary As #RandNumFile
    Get #RandNumFile, 201, HisArray
    Close RandNumFile
```

Notice that HisArray has only 50 elements. Also, the byte position in the Get statement is 201 because each element of the Long type is 4 bytes long. Finally, if HisArray is a scalar variable (not an array), the Get statement in the preceding code will read the fifty-first element from the file.

A.3. Working with Random Files

How Does a Random File Work?

In many ways, the random file works similarly to the binary file. Indeed, once a file is created using the Random file mode, you can reopen the same file in the Binary mode and access the same data without any problem, provided that "you know what you are doing." Here are the similarity and differences between the binary file and the random file:

- Both file modes/types use the Get and Put statements for input and output. However, the second parameter (the number) in these statements has quite a different meaning. In the binary file, the number refers to the byte position, whereas in the random file, it refers to the record position. For example, consider the following statement:

  ```
  Get #SpecialFile, 3, TheName
  ```

If SpecialFile is open with the Binary mode, 3 will refer to the third byte position of the file. If the file is open with the Random mode, 3 will refer to the third record. The actual byte position will depend on the specified record length. This also means that in the Binary mode, you can access data starting at any position in the file. However, in the Random mode, you can access data only at the beginning of a record position. You have much more flexibility in the Binary mode than in the Random mode.

- In the Open statement, the Len parameter refers to the buffer size if the file mode is Binary. However, it refers to the record length if the file mode is Random. Thus, omitting this parameter for the binary file will not cause any problem but can have serious unexpected consequence for the random file. In the Random file mode, the Get and Put statements rely on the specified record length to compute the byte position to store or retrieve a record. A wrong record length will result in accessing the wrong data.
- Because data in a random file can be accessed only at a record position (rather than at a byte position), it is only logical that the I/O operation involves an entire record instead of only a field (data element). The technique to structure a record is discussed in the next subsection.
- In Binary mode, the data type and length of data can vary from field to field. In Random mode, the maximum length of the record is defined in the Open statement. Varying the record size in Random mode will result in waste of storage space.

These differences are summarized in the following table.

Differences in	Binary File	Random File
Get and Put statements	The second parameter of Get and Put statements refers to byte position	The second parameter refers to record position
Len parameter in Open statement	Refers to buffer size	Refers to the record size for address computation. Subsequent access to the file cannot specify any record size that exceeds this limit
Access	By field	By record
Variability in data	Extremely flexible	Limited

An Example

To illustrate how the random file can be used, let's consider the familiar phone book application. Suppose you would like to keep your friends' phone numbers, addresses, and email addresses in a random file. You have designed the visual interface as shown in Figure A.1.

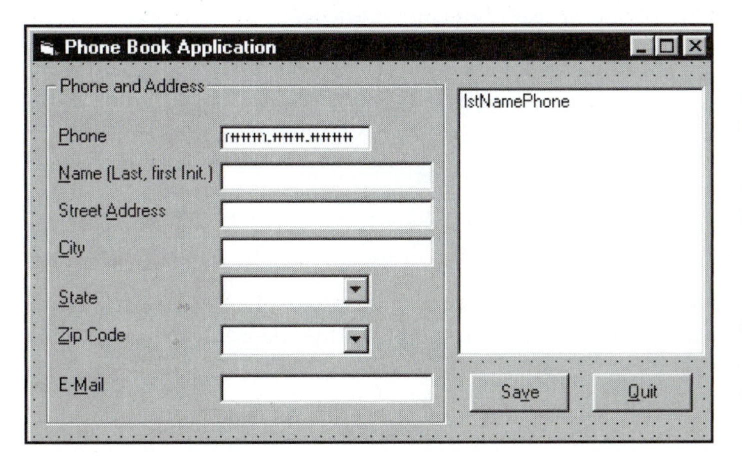

FIGURE A.1
Visual Interface for the Phone Book Application

This project will allow you to keep records in a random file. When the program starts, the list box will show phone numbers and names of existing records. Double-clicking an item in the list box will retrieve the corresponding record. The Save button will add the record if it is new; otherwise, it will update the record.

The list box (named lstNamePhone) will be used to display names and phone numbers. So that your user can easily find the name of interest, the list box's Sorted property is set to True. (Thus, the list box will display names in alphabetical order when populated.) When the user clicks a name, the record will be retrieved from the file and displayed on the form. When the user clicks the Save button, your program will determine whether it is a new record. If so, it will be added to the file; otherwise, the existing record will be updated.

The following table shows the layout of each record and the name of the control for each field.

Field	Data Type	Field Length	Description	Control Name/Remark
Phone	String	10	Phone number	mskPhone; set Mask to "(###)-###-####"
Name	String	24	Last, First Init.	txtName; set MaxLength to 24
Address	String	32		txtAddress; set MaxLength to 32
City	String	28		txtCity; set MaxLength to 28
State Code	String	2		cboStateCode
Zip Code	Long	4		cboZipCode
Email	String	48		txtEMail

Notice the length of the Zip Code field. Although "externally" we see the zip code to be a five-digit number, its data type is Long and will be saved as such, which takes 4 bytes of storage. Also, the Mask property of mskPhone should be set to "(###)-###-####" for proper entry in the field.

Recall from the previous discussion that each record in the file will have to be saved or retrieved in one Put or Get operation. How do we then group all these data elements into a "record"? The next subsection answers this question.

The User-Defined Type

The data types we have learned in Chapter 4, "Data, Operations, and Built-In Functions," such as Boolean, Integer, Long, Single, and so on, are recognized as intrinsic data types. You can combine any of these data types together to form a new type, which is recognized as the "user-defined type" (UDT, which sometimes is also called a "structure"). Once defined, it can be used as a data type to declare a variable, just like the keyword "Integer" can be used to declare an Integer variable.

Defining the User-Defined Type. To define a UDT, you use the Type structure that appears as follows:

```
[Private¦Public] Type TypeName
     Name1 As Type [* Length]
     Name2 As Type [* Length]
          :
          :
End Type
```

where *TypeName* = a name for the UDT you are defining

Name1, Name2 = field (variable) names

Type = data type; can be an intrinsic type or another UDT

Length = number of bytes to define a fixed-length string

Notice that a UDT defined in a form must be the Private type. For the phone book application, we can first define a data type for the record structure as follows:

```
Option Explicit
Private Type PhoneRecType
```

```
        Phone As String * 10
        Name As String * 24
        Address As String * 32
        City As String * 28
        StateCode As String * 2
        ZipCode As Long
        EMail As String * 48
    End Type
```

Notice that all string elements are declared with a length and are thus fixed-length strings. Although variable-length strings are allowed in the UDT, for those UDTs that are to be used as records (to save in random files), variable-length strings can cause many problems. You will be far better off using fixed-length strings in defining your records.

Declaring and Using a UDT Variable. We can then use the preceding UDT to declare a variable that can be used as the record for input and output with the random file. The familiar Dim statement can be used for such purposes:

```
Dim PhoneRecord As PhoneRecType
```

Note that you can declare as many variables of the same UDT as you want (just like you can declare as many Integer variables as you wish). However, all we need for this example is one variable, PhoneRecord.

How do you refer to an element in the record? You qualify the data element with the UDT variable. For example, the following expression refers to the name in the PhoneRecord record.

```
PhoneRecord.Name
```

Once we declare the record, we are ready to open a random file to perform I/O operations.

Opening a File for Random Mode

To open the preceding PhoneBook file with the Random mode, you would code the following:

```
Dim PhoneFile As Integer
PhoneFile = FreeFile
Open "PhoneBook.dat" For Random As #PhoneFile _
    Len = 148
```

The Open statement "declares" that each of the record is 148 bytes long. As explained, under the Random mode, each record is expected to be of the same length. In general, however, it is not a good idea to hard-code the record length while your program is still "under development." You may find a need to change the record structure and thus its length. Each change will necessitate changing this number. An alternative is to use the Len function (explained in Chapter 4) to perform the length computation. The Open statement can be revised as follows:

```
Open "PhoneBook.dat" For Random As #PhoneFile _
    Len = Len(PhoneRecord)
```

Performing Input and Output with a Random File

Once the file is open and the record is defined, you can use the Get and Put statement to perform the I/O operation. For example, to read the first record from the Phone Book File, you can code the following:

```
Get #PhoneFile, 1, PhoneRecord
```

Similarly, to save a phone record in the third record position, you can code as follows:

```
Put #PhoneFile, 3, PhoneRecord
```

For our example, the record retrieved should be displayed in the visual interface, whereas the data source for the record to save comes from the visual interface. It is a good idea to write generalized Sub procedures to perform these operations. These procedures can then be called from wherever such activities need to be carried out. The two procedures are presented as follows:

```
Sub ShowRecord(RecNum As Long)
' This Procedure displays a record in the visual interface
```

```
        Get #PhoneFile, RecNum, PhoneRecord
        With PhoneRecord
            mskPhone.Text = Format$Val(.Phone, "(000)-000-0000")
            txtName.Text = .Name
            txtAddress.Text = .Address
            txtCity.Text = .City
            cboStateCode.Text = .StateCode
            cboZipCode.Text = .ZipCode
            txtEMail.Text = .EMail
        End With
    End Sub
```

Notice that the phone number is formatted with the format string "(000)-000-0000." The masked edit box's Mask property has been set to "(###)-###-####." The data stored in the file, however, is a 10-digit string with no embedded parentheses or dashes. Thus, it is converted to a number using the Val function first. The 0's in the format string ensure that a phone number shorter than 10 digits will be filled with leading zeros. The format string also added the parentheses and the dashes so that the resulting string will fit the mask.

```
    Sub SaveRecord(RecNum As Long)
    ' This procedure saves a record from the visual interface
        With PhoneRecord
            .Phone = mskPhone.ClipText
            .Name = txtName.Text
            .Address = txtAddress.Text
            .City = txtCity.Text
            .StateCode = cboStateCode.Text
            .ZipCode = cboZipCode.Text
            .EMail = txtEMail.Text
        End With
        Put #PhoneFile, RecNum, PhoneRecord
    End Sub
```

Notice that the mskPhone's ClipText property (not the Text property) is moved to the Phone field in the record to save. Recall that the ClipText property extracts only those characters that are actually input by the user, not those literal constants added by the Mask property. The resulting string should be a 10-digit number without parentheses or dashes.

In both procedures, the RecNum parameter gives the record position, which is used in the Get or Put statement to perform the necessary input or output operation.

Completing the Example

With the two I/O procedures in place, let's recapitulate the requirements of the project and complete the code. The program should do the following:

1. Open the file and populate the list box with names and phone numbers of the existing records in the file as soon as the program starts.
2. Display the record that the user selects from the list box by clicking the item.
3. Save the record in the visual interface when the user clicks the Save button. The program should determine whether the record exists by searching for the entered phone number (in the masked edit box) in the list box. If it is found, the data on the visual interface should be used to update the record in the file. Otherwise, the record should be added as a new one.

General Declaration. The following code should be placed in the general declaration area:

```
    Option Explicit
    Private Type PhoneRecType
        Phone As String * 10
        Name As String * 24
        Address As String * 32
        City As String * 28
        StateCode As String * 2
        ZipCode As Long
        EMail As String * 48
    End Type
```

```
Dim PhoneRecord As PhoneRecType
Dim PhoneFile As Integer
```

As explained previously, the Type block is used to declare a user-defined type. We use the block to declare a structure for the phone record. The Dim statement following the Type block creates a variable, PhoneRecord, of the PhoneRecType type. This variable is used in the SaveRecord and ShowRecord Sub procedures. Also, the variable PhoneFile is declared as a form-level (module-level) variable so that the file can be referenced in various procedures.

Populating the List Box. As soon as the program starts, it should open the phone book file and populate the list box with the existing data. The following procedure should accomplish this:

```
Private Sub Form_Load()
Dim R As Long
Dim Records As Long
     PhoneFile = FreeFile
     Open "PhoneBook.dat" For Random As PhoneFile _
       Len = Len(PhoneRecord)
     Records = LOF(PhoneFile) / Len(PhoneRecord)
     'Populate the list box
     For R = 1 To Records
          Get #PhoneFile, R, PhoneRecord
          lstNamePhone.AddItem Trim$(PhoneRecord.Name) & vbTab & _
            Format$(PhoneRecord.Phone, "(000)-000-0000")
          'Keep record position for ease of record retrieval
          lstNamePhone.ItemData(lstNamePhone.NewIndex) = R
     Next R
End Sub
```

The procedure first opens the phone file for random with a record length equal to that of the variable PhoneRecord. It then proceeds to compute the number of records in the file in preparation of populating the list box. The number of records in the file is computed with the following formula:

```
Records = LOF(PhoneFile) / Len(PhoneRecord)
```

Recall that the LOF function gives the number of bytes of the file and the Len function returns the length of the string (record). Once the number of records is determined, the list box can be populated with a For loop, in which the records are read from the file and the names and the phone numbers are added to the list with the AddItem method. Note that Name in the record has been declared as a fixed string field of 24 characters. Its extra spaces are stripped with the Trim$ function before the content is placed in the list box.

The ItemData and NewIndex Properties. Notice that names in the list box will be sorted in order (because the Sorted property is set to True). Thus, the position of the name in the list box will not be the same as the position of the record in the file. To keep track of the latter so that the record can be retrieved from the file conveniently, the list box's ***ItemData property*** is used. Similar to the List and Selected properties, this property is an array with the same index. When a new item is added to the list in whichever position, all these three properties are pointed to by the ***NewIndex property***. The ItemData property is of the Long type and can be used to hold any integer data. Here we use it the keep the record position that corresponds to the position of the new item in the list box.

Retrieving Selected Record. When the user clicks an item in the list box, the program is expected to retrieve the data from the file and display the result in the visual interface. Because the ItemData property holds the record position, this property provides the needed information to retrieve the record. The code appears as follows:

```
Private Sub lstNamePhone_Click()
Dim R As Long
'ListIndex points to the item selected
```

```
' Use it to retrieve the record number stored in ItemData
    R = lstNamePhone.ItemData(lstNamePhone.ListIndex)
    ShowRecord R 'Show record R, using the ShowRecord Sub
End Sub
```

Saving a Record. When the user clicks the Save button, the program should check whether the current record (in the visual interface) exists in the file. Each record is identified by the phone number (i.e., phone number is the record key). Thus, the phone number as given in mskPhone is passed to the function FindPhone, which searches through the list box to find a match of the phone number. If found, the function returns the record position. Otherwise, -1 is returned.

If the FindPhone function returns −1, the record does not exist. The program should do the following:

- Provide a record position for the new record. This value can be calculated by using the following formula:

  ```
  Records = LOF(PhoneFile) / Len(PhoneRecord) + 1
  ```

- Add the name and phone number to the list box. The record position of the new record should also be kept in the ItemData property for future retrieval.

All records, new or existing, can be saved with the same procedure, SaveRecord, which has been shown previously. The Save button's Click event procedure appears as follows:

```
Private Sub cmdSave_Click()
Dim R As Long
    'Note: Data validation should be performed here
    R = FindPhone(mskPhone.Text)
    If R < 0 Then
    ' New record; add to the end of file
        R = LOF(PhoneFile) / Len(PhoneRecord) + 1
    ' Add phone & name to the list box
        With lstNamePhone
            .AddItem txtName.Text & vbTab & _
              mskPhone.Text
    ' Also keep the record number in ItemData
            .ItemData(.NewIndex) = R
        End With
    End If
    SaveRecord R
End Sub
```

The function to search for the phone number in the list box is given next:

```
Function FindPhone(Phone As String) As Long
' This function returns the record position for a given phone number.
' If the phone number is not found, -1 is returned.
Dim I As Long
    With lstNamePhone
        FindPhone = -1 'Assume Not found; return -1
        For I = 0 To .ListIndex - 1
            If Phone = Right$(.List(I), 14) Then
                'Found; return the record position
                FindPhone = .ItemData(I)
                Exit For
            End If
        Next I
    End With
End Function
```

As you can see, in the function, the return value is first set to −1. If the ensuing search for the phone number is unsuccessful, this will be the value returned. Then in the For loop, the phone number being searched for is compared with the phone number in the list box (extracted with the Right$ function) one by one. When a match is found, the corresponding value in the ItemData property (which holds the record position) is returned and the search terminates.

Additional Remarks

You may have noticed that the visual interface includes two combo boxes: one for state code and another for zip code. The style property of both boxes is set to its default, Dropdown Combo (0) so that the user can enter the data like in a text box. In a real application, you can populate the combo boxes with known data so that the user can select from the list instead of actually keying the data. These data can come from a separate file, or they can be obtained from the existing phone records. Also, for real applications, error-checking routines should be added and the screen should be cleared after the data are saved. These refinements are left to you as an exercise.

Because of its simplicity, the phone book problem is used to illustrate the basic I/O operations not only here but also in Chapter 6 (sequential I/O) and in Chapter 8 (database). You may want to compare these solutions to gain a good assessment of the relative advantages of different data management approaches in terms of design and code complexity. In terms of speed, using the random file should be the fastest, and the sequential file should be the slowest.

Although the random file approach is the fastest, the current trend in data management is toward the use of the database approach. The latter approach has the advantages of developing new applications and handling complex queries much more easily and therefore more rapidly. All the complexities associated with data management are "absorbed" by the database management system (software), which offers the SQL capability.

If you use the random file approach for complex applications, you will need to develop all the capabilities to handle the queries and other data management requirements. This can be a tremendous undertaking. In addition, it may not be very easy to modify the code to deal with a new application. The development efforts and lead time for each application are typically much longer than the database approach. Thus, unless the application's requirements are fairly simple, the database approach is usually the way to go.

A Technical Note

Notice that the preceding random file can also be opened with the Binary mode. For example, the following code fragment will open the same file in Binary mode:

```
PhoneFile = FreeFile
Open "PhoneBook.dat" For Binary As PhoneFile
```

Then to read the Ith record, you will code the following:

```
Get #PhoneFile, (I - 1) * Len(PhoneRecord) + 1, PhoneRecord
```

Indeed, you can even just access an individual byte (or field) in the file. However, as you can see, the computation of the byte position can become cumbersome. So, in general, *the binary file has the most flexibility but can become pretty tricky for your program to keep track of the location of data.*

A.4. Design Considerations

Despite of the relative advantages of the database approach to data management, there will always be cases where the file-oriented approach is more suitable, especially when the application problem setting is fairly simple. The file-oriented approach has the advantage of requiring far fewer systems resources. This section provides a summary of the situations in which each of the three file structures (sequential, binary, and random) is most suitable.

File Characteristics and Suitable Applications

Based on the discussion in this appendix and in Chapter 6, the characteristics of the three file types are summarized in the following table.

Factor	Sequential	Binary	Random
Access	Data can be accessed only in one direction. A file must be opened for output and input separately.	Data can be accessed at the byte level. Any position in the file can be read or written.	Data can be accessed at the record level. Record size must be defined in the Open statement.
Speed	Slow	Fast	Fast
Remarks	Data in the file can be inspected easily or changed by use of other word processing applications such as Notepad or Word.	Numeric (binary) data are kept "as is." The file is extremely flexible in handling any possible data structures. However, the programmer has to devise a systematic way of keeping track of the location of the data. A minor error can cause chaos.	Numeric (binary) data are kept "as is." Each record should have the same length. The file type is not as flexible as the binary file in handling varying data structures in the same file but is capable of handling records of the same type in huge number.
Potentially suitable applications	Text files for word processing applications; data for one-time processing only (import/export files); small system configuration files.	System configuration files; small tables (tax rate table); numeric arrays (statistic data); files requiring speed and/or complex structures (e.g., index files.)	Files for fairly large volume data processing applications (e.g., master files and transaction files for various business applications, when the database approach is not used.)

Summary

This appendix discusses the use of binary and random files. The differences among sequential, binary, and random files are explained. They mainly differ in the way data are handled and accessed. Numeric data are converted to strings before being saved onto a sequential file, and strings are converted to numeric data type when they are read from a sequential file (if the variable involved is a numeric variable). On the other hand, data are saved or retrieved from the file without any conversion when the file mode is either Binary or Random. Data in a sequential file can be accessed only sequentially, whereas data in a binary file and random file can be accessed randomly. In Binary mode, the file can be accessed at any byte position, whereas in random mode, the file can be accessed only by the record position. Understanding these differences can help you select the right file type given a set of requirements for a file in a particular application. The preceding section provides a summary in this respect.

Because a random file can be accessed only by the record position, it is only logical that each I/O operation involves a record (not just a field). Section A.3 shows how the UDT can be used to construct a record for such purposes. UDTs can also be used to build very complex data structures. Their introduction in this appendix gives you a preview to such possibilities.

Visual Basic Explorer

A-1. Mismatching Data Types Between Input and Output. Enter the following code:

```
Option Explicit

Private Sub Form_Click()
Dim TestFile As Integer
Dim TheData As Long
    TestFile = FreeFile
    Open "C:\Temp\TestFile.dat" For Output As #TestFile
    Print #TestFile, "ABCD"
```

```
        Close #TestFile
        Open "C:\Temp\TestFile.dat" For Binary As #TestFile
        Print LOF(TestFile)
        Get #TestFile, 1, TheData
        Print TheData; Hex$(TheData)
        Print &H44434241
    End Sub
```

Run the program and click the form. You should see the following three lines of output on the form:

```
6
1145258561 44434241
1145258561
```

The print statement should print "ABCD" in the file. Why does the LOF function return 6? (*Hint:* The vbCrLf characters have been added at the end.)

Why does TheData have a value 1145258561? The Get statement reads a 4-byte image "ABCD," which has that corresponding numeric value. When you use the Hex$ function to show the Hex decimal representation of TheData, it gives 44434241. This means internally, TheData contains &H44434241. This is confirmed by the output of the last print statement. Note that &H41, &H42, &H43, and &H44 are the ASCII values for A, B, C, and D, respectively. Recall again, when numeric data are output, the lowest byte is written first. Conversely, when a numeric field is read, the first byte is read as the lowest byte in the value.

A-2. Binary File and File Size. Draw a command button on a new form. Name it cmdTest and set its Caption property to "Test." Enter the following code:

```
Option Explicit
Private Sub cmdTest_Click()
Dim BinaryFile As Integer
    BinaryFile = FreeFile
    Open "C:\Temp\Binary.dat" For Binary As #BinaryFile
    Put #BinaryFile, 2001, 0&
    Print LOF(BinaryFile)
End Sub
```

Start the project and click the button. What value do you see? You have just put the Long integer value 0 onto the file. Why does the LOF function return 2004?

A-3. Variable-Length String and Length of UDT. Draw a command button on a new form. Name it cmdShow and set its Caption property to "Show Length." Enter the following code:

```
Option Explicit
Private Type MyDataType
    TheString As String
    TheLong As Long
End Type
Dim MyData As MyDataType
Private Sub cmdShow_Click()
    Print Len(MyData)
End Sub
```

Run the project and click the button. What value do you see on the form? The Long integer is 4 bytes long. However, you have not assigned any value to the string yet. Why is the length of the UDT variable 8? A variable-length string in VB is structured as a BSTR, which consists of a "header" and the string itself. The header contains information on the location and length of the string. What is included in the length count of the UDT is the length of the header, not the length of the string.

A-4. Variable-Length Strings, UDT, and Input/Output. (continued from A-3). Add one more command button to your preceding project. Name it cmdPut and set its Caption property to "Put." Add the following code:

```
Dim UDTFile As Integer 'place this line in general declaration

Private Sub cmdPut_Click()
    UDTFile = FreeFile
    MsgBox "Length of MyData is " & Len(MyData)
    Open "C:\Temp\UDTFile.dat" For Random As #UDTFile _
      Len = Len(MyData)
    MyData.TheString = "ABC"
    MyData.TheLong = 100
    Put #UDTFile, 1, MyData
End Sub
```

Run the project and click the button. What do you see? Why is there a bad record length error? Change the Len line to the following:

```
Len = Len(MyData) + 3
```

Run the project again. Does it work this time? Why? (See next exercise.)

A-5. Variable-Length Strings, UDT, and Input/Output. (continued from A-4). To be sure the data can be retrieved, add another command button to your preceding project. Name it cmdGet and set its Caption property to "Get." Add the following code:

```
Private Sub cmdGet_Click()
    Get #UDTFile, 1, MyData
    Print MyData.TheString
    Print MyData.TheLong
End Sub
```

Run the project. Click the Put command and then click the Get command. Is everything working properly? The reason 3 has to be added to the record length is that both the string and the string header are included in the output. The record length declared in the Open statement must be at least the same as the record size used in the I/O operation. Keep in mind that the record lengths for all records in the file are assumed to be the same by the system. Thus, variable-length strings are not really suitable for random file I/O.

Exercises

A-6. FICA Tax Brackets. The current (1999) FICA taxes for each employee per year are as follows:

Medicare tax: 1.45% for all amount of payroll

Social Security tax: 6.2% for the first $72,600 of pay, 0% beyond $72,600

Design a file structure to save the data for later use of determining withholdings for employees during payroll calculation. There should be a user interface to display and update the saved data.

A-7. Income Tax Rate Brackets. Two of the four 1997 Income Tax Rate schedules are as follow:

SCHEDULE X (FOR HEAD OF HOUSEHOLD)

Taxable Income Between	Applicable Rate (on the Indicate Range)
0–24,650	15%
24,650–59,750	28%
59,750–124,650	31%
124,650–271,050	36%
271,050–. . .	39.6%

SCHEDULE Z (FOR SINGLE)

Taxable Income Between	Applicable Rate (on the Indicate Range)
0–33,050	15%
33,050–85,350	28%
85,350–138,200	31%
138,200–271,050	36%
271,050–. . .	39.6%

Develop a project to save and retrieve these tables. There should be a user interface to display and update the retrieved/saved data. (*Hint:* You can save these data as arrays in a binary file. Notice that although the tax income brackets are shown in two columns, a one-dimensional array should be able to take care of each schedule. The tax rates can be saved in another array. If you are concerned about the possibility that the number of brackets can change in the future, store that number as the first element in the file. Because you are working with multiple tables, you should find the SSTab useful in your interface design.)

A-8. General Ledger Account File. Each of the general ledger accounts in a file is structured as follows:

Field Name	Data Type	Internal Length	External Length
Account Number	Long	4	5
Account Name	String	24	24
Beginning Balance	Currency	8	12
Y-T-D Debit Amount	Currency	8	12
Y-T-D Credit Amount	Currency	8	12

Develop a project with a visual interface to enter, edit, and save the account records. In real applications, the three amounts should be updated by transactions. However, for the purposes of practice, include them in your interface. (*Hint:* Use a visual interface design similar to the phone book example in this appendix.)

A-9. Clinic Account Holder Basic Info File. Each of the account holders of a clinic is structured as follows:

Field Name	Data Type	Internal Length	External Length
Account Number	Long	4	5
Account Holder Name (Last, First Init.)	String	32	32
Date of Birth	Date/Time	8	10 (with "-")
Sex	String	1	1
S-S-N	Long	4	11(with "-")
Street Address	String	32	32
City	String	24	24
State	String	2	2
Zip Code	Long	4	5 or 9
Home Phone	Currency	8	14; for example, (817)-222-3333
Work Phone	Currency	8	14 (see above)
Employer	String	32	32

Develop a project that will allow the user to enter and update account holder information. (*Hint:* You can still design a user interface similar to the phone book application in this appendix. The actual number of accounts can be much more than that of a phone book. This means for a real application, your routine for looking up an account can be much more complex using the file-oriented approach than using the database approach.)

A-10. Clinic Patient Basic ID Info File. (continued from A-9). The Clinic Patient Basic Info file has the following fields:

Field Name	Data Type	Internal Length	External Length
Account Number	Long	5	5
Sequence Number	Integer	2	2
Patient Name (Last, First Init.)	String	24	24
Date of Birth	Date/Time	8	10
Sex	String	1	1

Develop a project that will allow the user to enter and update patient information records using the random file structure. Keep in mind that a patient record cannot exist without an account holder record. The sequence number 0 should be reserved for the account holder; 1 for spouse; and 2 and on for other dependents. Note also that not all records pertaining to a family will be entered in consecutive order. (*Hint:* Use two list boxes: one to hold account holders and another to hold patients. The former can be used to verify the existence of an account. The latter can be used to determine whether to add or to update a patient record. Of course, this approach assumes that the number of records for both files is relatively small. For large files, a more complex algorithm will have to be used. Identify the patient by combining the account number and sequence number.) (*Question:* If both the account holder and patient info data had been presented to you as one problem, will your design for the files be different? Notice that some fields in the account holder info record have to be repeated in the patient info file.)

A-11. Clinic Patient Visit File. Each time a patient visits the clinic, a transaction record should be created. A simplified layout is given as follows:

Field Name	Data Type	Internal Length	External Length
Date	Date/Time	8	10
Account Number	Long	4	5
Sequence Number	Integer	2	2
Diagnostic Code	String	7	3 to 7
Service Code	Currency	8	5 to 8
Total Service Fee	Currency	8	8
Insurance Company Code	String	12	12

Develop a project to allow the user to enter patient visit/service records. Keep in mind that the patient record must exist before any patient visit record can be entered. Again, identify the patient by combining the account number with the sequence number.

B Graphics, Animation, Drag and Drop

This appendix discusses topics related to graphics. When we introduced the picture box and the image control in Chapter 3, "Some Visual Basic Controls and Events," we briefly discussed how to load pictures into these controls. In Chapter 13, "Selected Topics in Input and Output," we also discussed the use of the Printer object's PaintPicture method to print pictures. The first section here discusses how to draw graphs in the picture box or the form. Most of the techniques discussed should also apply to the Printer object. Once we have an understanding of graphic techniques, we will be able to consider topics in animation, which is discussed in Section B.2. Another interesting application of graphics is the drag-and-drop operation, which can provide the user a very convenient way to specify operations that can otherwise be fairly complex to describe. This type of application can be exciting and dynamic. We discuss drag and drop in Section B.3.

B.1. Drawing Graphs

Drawing graphs involves using one of the object's graphic methods: the ***Pset method***, the ***Circle method***, or the ***Line method***. Before discussing these methods in detail, let's first take a look at a few concepts that are fundamental to graphs.

Basic Concepts

When you are drawing a graph, you will always need to decide the position to begin or end your drawing. The coordinate and the measurement units jointly determine the numeric value of the position. In addition, the attractiveness of a graph is significantly affected by the color you use. This subsection introduces you to the basics of coordinates, measurement units, and colors.

Coordinates. The object (form, picture box, or the Printer object) on which you draw a graph has a coordinate system that is different than the familiar Cartesian coordinate system. In the latter system, the horizontal coordinate, x, increases from left to right and the vertical coordinate, y, increases from bottom to top. With an object, the horizontal coordinate, x, also increases from left to right, with the leftmost margin being 0. The vertical coordinate, y, however, starts from top to bottom, with the topmost margin being 0. This system is depicted in Figure B.1.

FIGURE B.1
VB Object's Coordinate

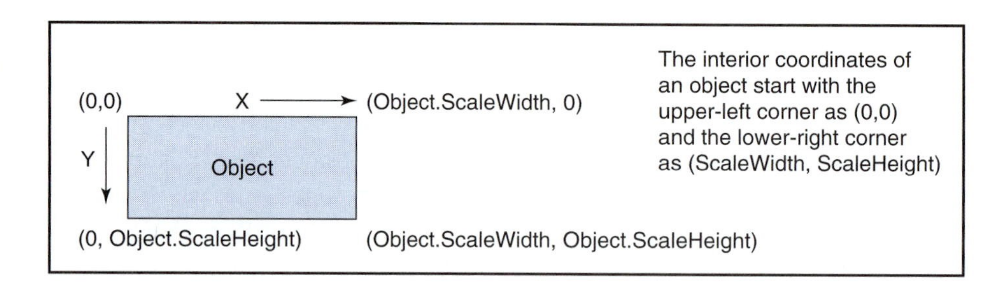

You need to be aware of this difference so that you can draw on an object correctly. Notice that the available interior area is measured by the object's ScaleWidth and ScaleHeight properties.

Measurement Units. The ***units of measurement*** used in the graphics methods are determined by the ScaleMode property. A change of this property will change the object's measurement units for the ScaleWidth, ScaleHeight, CurrentX, and CurrentY properties. A selected list of ScaleMode settings is presented in the following table.

ScaleMode Setting	Value	Measurement Units
vbTwips	1 (Default)	Twip; 1440 twips per logical inch
vbPoints	2	Point; 72 points per logical inch
vbPixels	3	Pixel; smallest unit of monitor or printer resolution
vbInches	5	Inch

As the table indicates, the default measurement units are twips. The examples in this appendix assume the default ScaleMode setting (twips).

Colors. A color is represented by a Long integer value that represents the relative intensity of the red, green, and blue (RGB) color composition. The intensity is represented by a value ranging from &HO to &HFF (0 to 255). The following table provides a sample of the colors of different RGB intensities.

R Value	G value	B value	Color Name
0	0	0	vbBlack
0	0	&HFF	vbBlue

R Value	G value	B value	Color Name
0	&HFF	0	vbGreen
0	&HFF	&HFF	vbCyan
&HFF	0	0	vbRed
&HFF	0	&HFF	vbMagenta
&HFF	&HFF	0	vbYellow
&HFF	&HFF	&HFF	vbWhite

VB provides a function named RGB that you can use to construct any color combination. The function has the following syntax:

```
Color = RGB(Red, Green, Blue)
```

where *Color* is a Long variable to represent a color and *Red, Green, Blue* are Integers representing the intensity of respective colors.

With an understanding of the coordinate system, the measurement units, and colors, you are now ready to take a look at two of the graphics methods: the Pset method and the Circle method.

The Pset Method

The Pset method draws a point at a specified position and has the following syntax:

```
object.PSet [Step] (x, y), [color]
```

where *object* = a picture box, the form, or the Printer object

Step = this optional keyword, if specified, indicates that the (x, y) parameter is relative to the current position as given by the object's CurrentX and CurrentY properties

(x, y) = the coordinate to draw the point; notice that the pair of parentheses are required

Color = a Long value that specifies the color to use

For example, the following will draw a red point at (100, 100) on a form when you click it:

```
Private Sub Form_Click()
    Me.PSet (100, 100), vbRed
End Sub
```

How big is the point? It depends on the setting of the ***DrawWidth property*** of the object. For example, if the DrawWidth property has a value of 1, the point will be 1 pixel. You can set the DrawWidth at runtime to dynamically change the sizes of points drawn. If you wish to have a point that is 5 pixels big, you can code the following instead:

```
Private Sub Form_Click()
    Me.DrawWidth = 5
    Me.PSet (100, 100), vbRed
End Sub
```

You may not be able to see any red point with the following code:

```
Private Sub Form_Load()
    Me.DrawWidth = 5
    Me.PSet (100, 100), vbRed
End Sub
```

Why? When the point is being drawn on the form, the form has not yet appeared. Thus, nothing is drawn on the screen. Either place the statement Me.Show before the drawing or set the form's AutoRedraw property to True to obtain the desired result.

Free-Hand Drawing. The Pset method can conveniently be used to provide the user the free-hand drawing capability with the mouse. For example, the MouseMove event is triggered when the user moves the mouse. You can track the mouse movement and draw a point where the mouse moves. The MouseMove event has the following header:

```
Private Sub object_MouseMove([index As Integer,] _
    Button As Integer, Shift As Integer, x As Single, y As Single)
```

where *object* = form or a picture box

Index = specified if the object is an element of a control array

Button = an integer representing the flags for the mouse button(s) pressed; bit 0 (the lowest bit), 1, and 2 correspond to left, right, and middle buttons, respectively; if a button is pressed, the corresponding bit is set on (e.g., if the right button is pressed, Button will have a value 2 [bit 1 is on])

Shift = an integer representing the flags for the Shift key(s) pressed; bit 0, 1, and 2 correspond to Shift, Ctrl, and Alt keys, respectively; if a key is pressed, the corresponding bit is turned on (e.g., if the Alt key is pressed, Shift will have a value of 4)

x, y = represents the coordinate of the current mouse location; as you move the mouse, x and y will change

To draw points on a form as the mouse moves, you can code the following:

```
Private Sub Form_MouseMove(Button As Integer, Shift As Integer, _
    X As Single, Y As Single)
        Me.DrawWidth = 1 'Or set it to a value you like
        Me.PSet (X, Y), vbRed
End Sub
```

This procedure will draw red points (1 pixel each as specified by the DrawWidth property) on the form wherever the mouse goes.

Usually, however, this is not exactly what you want. For example, you will probably want to draw only when you drag the mouse, not just anytime you move it. You can accomplish this by doing the following:

1. Introducing a module-level Boolean variable (e.g., DrawingOn)
2. Setting it on when the mouse is down (in the MouseDown event) and turning it off when the mouse is up (in the MouseUp event)
3. Drawing the point(s) in the MouseMove event only when this variable is on

The following procedures will implement this:

```
Option Explicit
Dim DrawingOn As Boolean 'Declare a module level variable

Private Sub Form_MouseDown(Button As Integer, Shift As Integer, X
As Single, Y As Single)
        'Signal it's ok to draw
        DrawingOn = True
End Sub

Private Sub Form_MouseUp(Button As Integer, Shift As Integer, _
    X As Single, Y As Single)
        'Turn off drawing
        DrawingOn = False
End Sub

Private Sub Form_MouseMove(Button As Integer, Shift As Integer, _
    X As Single, Y As Single)
        If DrawingOn Then
        'Draw only if DrawingOn is true
            Me.DrawWidth = 1
            Me.PSet (X, Y), vbRed
        End If
End Sub
```

The Circle Method

The Circle method draws a circle, ellipse, or arc on the object. It has the following syntax:

```
object.Circle [Step] (x, y), radius _
    [,color][, start][, end][, aspect]
```

where *object* = form, picture box, or the Printer object

Step = this optional keyword, if present, indicates that the coordinate (x, y) is relative to the current position as given by the object's CurrentX and CurrentY; otherwise, the coordinate (x, y) specifies the absolute position in the object

X, Y = the coordinate of the center of the circle

Radius = radius of the circle

Color = color to draw the circle; if not specified, the object's ForeColor property setting is used

Start, End = the starting and ending angles (in radians) to draw the arc; if omitted, 0 and 2 π (for the complete circle) will be the default

Aspect = the aspect ratio for the circle; a value of 1 (default) will give a perfect circle; a value different from 1 will result in a different shape of ellipse

The following code examples produce the graphs given in Figure B.2.

```
Option Explicit
Const Pi As Single = 3.14159
Private Sub Form_Click()
    Me.DrawWidth = 1
    ' Circle with a radius 200
    Me.Circle (400, 400), 200, vbRed ' (1)
    ' (2) an ellipse with a radius 200 and
    ' aspect ratio .6
    Me.Circle (1200, 400), 200, vbBlue, , , 0.6 ' (2)
    ' (3) An arc in the first quadrant
    Me.Circle (2000, 400), 200, vbGreen , 0, Pi / 2 ' (3)
End Sub
```

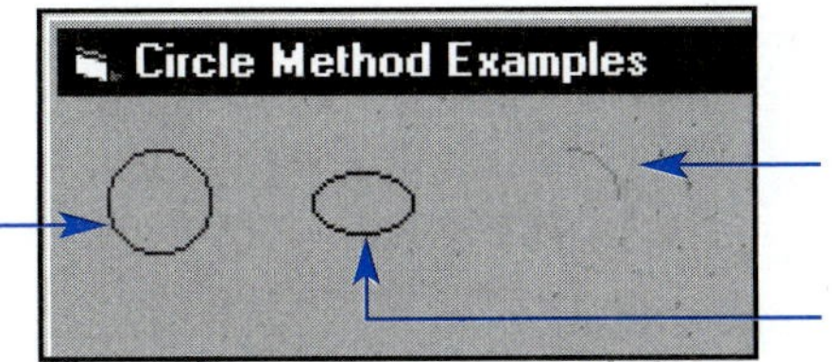

FIGURE B.2
Results of the Circle Method

The statement marked as (1) produces this circle.

The statement marked as (3) produces this arc.

The statement marked as (2) produces this ellipse.

Let's take a look at each statement that involves the Circle method:

```
Me.Circle (400, 400), 200, vbRed
```

This statement draws a circle with the center at 400 twips from the left margin and 400 twips from the top. (Note that the coordinate values are enclosed with a pair of parentheses, which are required.) The radius is 200 twips long, and the color to draw the circle is red (vbRed).

```
Me.Circle (1200, 400), 200, vbBlue, , , 0.6
```

This statement draws an ellipse with its center at (1200, 400) and a radius of 200 twips long. The Start and End parameters are not specified, indicating the drawing should be encircled. If the last (aspect) parameter were not specified, the result would have been a circle. However, the last parameter specifies an aspect ratio of 60%, resulting in an ellipse that looks like an egg.

Finally:

```
Me.Circle (2000, 400), 200, vbGreen , 0, Pi / 2
```

This statement specifies the Start and End values without the aspect parameter. The two values (representing angles in radians) are used to compute the x and y value relative to the center. For a given angle, θ, and with the center at the point of origin, the coordinate (x, y) is determined as shown in Figure B.3. When the angle is zero, the point will be at (Radius, 0). When the angle is π/2 (90 degrees because a complete circle is 2π), the point will be at (0, Radius). Thus, the preceding statement will draw an arc that covers the first quadrant.

FIGURE B.3
Arc of an Angle y

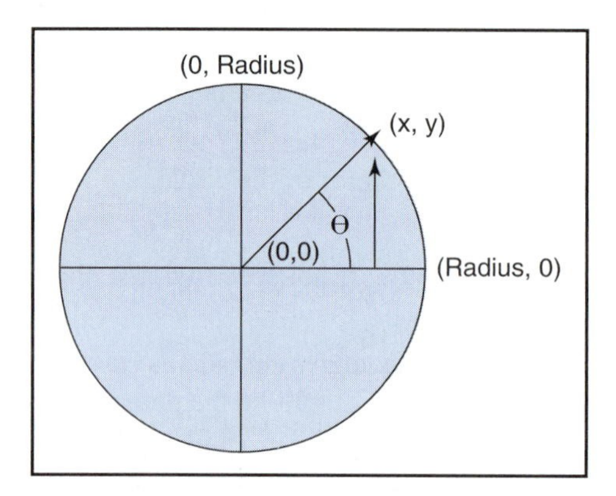

Combined with colors, the different shapes produced by the Circle method can produce an interesting presentation. For example, you can draw ellipses on the sides of a picture box with assorted colors. These ellipses can look like Christmas lights.

An Example: Christmas Lights

Let's develop a project that will draw Christmas lights on the sides of a picture box. When the picture is complete, it will look like Figure B.4.

FIGURE B.4
Christmas Lights

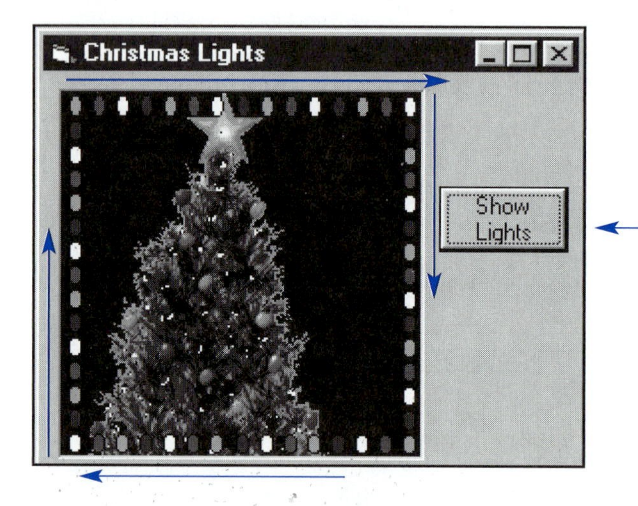

This project draws the Christmas lights around the sides of the picture box starting at the upper-left corner. Lights are drawn clockwise as the arrows show. The Christmas tree is loaded to the Picture property at design time. You can download a similar picture from various Web sites on the Internet, although you do not have to have the tree to work on this project.

To create the picture, follow these steps:

1. Draw a picture box on a new form, adjusting its size and location.
2. Name the picture box picLights and set its BackColor property to black.
3. Set the picture box's Picture property to a Christmas tree picture. The Graphics folder that comes with VB6 does not have one. However, you can download one from Web sites on the Internet that feature clip art. You do not have to have a tree picture to do this project, although the result will look nicer.
4. Draw a command button on the form. Name it cmdShow and set its Caption property to "Show Lights."
5. Develop the code to draw the lights.

To draw the lights we need to answer the following questions:

1. How do we compute the size of the lights and the distance between them?
2. How do we compute the position of each light and draw it?
3. How do we alternate the colors for the lights?

Computing the Distance and Size of the Lights. As soon as the program starts, the distance and size of the lights can be computed. These parameters can then be used to determine the position of each light. To make our job easier, we will force the picture box to be square, using the longer of the width and height. We will draw 14 lights on each side.

Let *Distance* = the distance between the lights

Radius = the radius of each light

Then, we can compute the two variables as follows:

```
Distance = Scale Width / 15
Radius = 75% of (Distance / 2)
```

Although we state that we will draw 14 lights on each side, each side will "appear" to have 15 lights because the first light of each side will start at a corner, which will overlap two sides. Consider a simple case of drawing two lights on each side. The graph will end up with three lights (two plus one extra) on each side as depicted in Figure B.5.

FIGURE B.5
Drawing Two Lights on Each Side

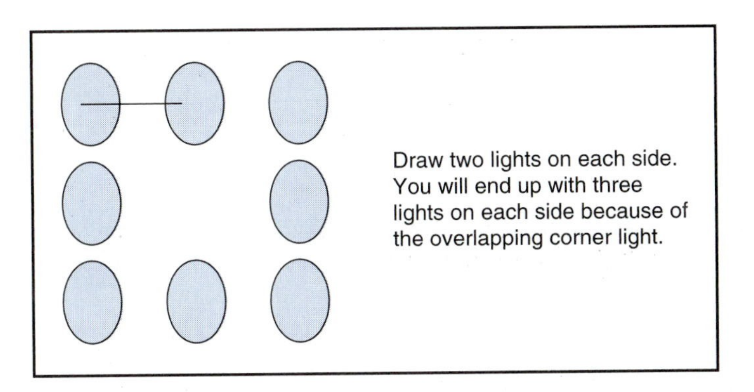

Draw two lights on each side.
You will end up with three
lights on each side because of
the overlapping corner light.

Note also that the distance is measured from the center of each light. Thus, the maximum value that the radius can take is half the distance. However, such a value will cause the lights to overlap each other. A 75% of that maximum value appears to keep a "proper distance" between lights. This is how the preceding formula for the radius is derived.

The following Form Load Sub procedure will carry out the computations.

```
Option Explicit
Dim Distance As Single
Dim Radius As Single

Private Sub Form_Load()
    'Set the picture box squared
    With picLights
        If .Height > .Width Then
            .Width = .Height
        Else
            .Height = .Width
        End If

        'Compute distance between each light bulb
        Distance = .ScaleWidth / 15
        ' Radius is a bit shorter than half distance
        Radius = 0.75 * Distance / 2
    End With
End Sub
```

Notice that both Distance and Radius will be used by other procedures. Therefore, they are declared as the module-level variables right after the Option Explicit statement.

In the procedure, the If block compares the picture box's height with its width and changes the shorter one to the longer to make the picture box square. Then the variable Distance is computed by dividing the ScaleWidth property by 15. Recall that the ScaleHeight and ScaleWidth properties represent the available space inside the box. These two properties also reflect the proper values for the units of measurement, given any scale mode.

Computing the Position for Each Light. Recall that there are 56 lights. For computation, we will identify each light by its position counting clockwise from the upper-left corner starting with number 0. With this scheme, the first 14 lights will be drawn on the top from left to right; the next 14, on the right side, top down; the next 14, at the bottom from right to left; and finally, the last 14 on the left side, bottom up. We can then compute the position of a light based on its number. (There are simpler ways to draw the lights. The reason to draw the lights our way is explained later.)

For example, consider the first light bulb (position 0). Its center should be placed at the half distance from the left and the top of the picture box. The second light bulb (position 1) should be *a full distance from the first one*; and the third will be another full distance from the second light. This means the x coordinate will increase by a full distance for each next light, whereas the y coordinate remains the same. Thus:

Let X = the x coordinate of the light bulb

Y = the y coordinate of the light bulb

P = the position number of the light (0 = first position)

Then the positions of the *first 14 light bulbs* can be computed as follows:

```
X = Distance / 2 + P * Distance
Y = Distance / 2
```

The next 14 light bulbs will go on the right side and down vertically. The x coordinate for these light bulbs will remain the same, whereas y will increase by a full distance for each subsequent light. Their positions can be computed as follows:

```
X = Distance / 2 + 14 * Distance; that is,
X = 14.5 * Distance
Y = Distance / 2 + (P - 14) * Distance; that is,
Y = (P – 13.5) * Distance
```

Notice that in computing Y, 14 is subtracted from P so that light number 14 (the first light for this side) is on the corner (half distance from the top); and light number 15 is one position below light number 14.

For the bottom side, the lights will go from the right to the left. As the position value increases, the X value decreases. This first light for this side (number 28) should be 14.5 times the distance from the left, same as all lights on the right side.

Let P = position of a light on this side

Then, the X value of the light position can be computed as follows:

```
X = (28 – P) * Distance + 14.5 * Distance; that is,
Y = (42.5 – P) * Distance
```

In a similar fashion, the formula for the light positions on the left side can be developed.

Drawing the Light Bulb. Once the position is computed, it is fairly easy to draw the light bulb using the Circle method. One thing to consider is the aspect ratio. *An aspect ratio greater than 1 will produce an ellipse whose vertical height is greater than its width.* For our purpose, 1.5 appears to be a good choice. Thus, the statement to draw a light bulb can be as follows:

```
picLights.Circle (X, Y), Radius, , , , 1.5
```

This statement alone, however, does not draw an ellipse that is filled with a color as shown in Figure B.4. To fill a color inside an enclosed area (e.g., in an ellipse or a circle), we need to set the FillStyle and FillColor properties. The ***FillColor property*** specifies the color to fill in the area, and the ***FillStyle property*** specifies how the area should be filled. There are eight different styles, including solid (vbFSSolid), transparent (vbFSTransparent), and diagonal cross (vbDiagonalCross). For our purpose, the area should be filled solid. The following statements will draw a red light bulb:

```
picLights.FillStyle = vbFSSolid
picLights.FillColor = vbRed
picLights.Circle (X, Y), Radius, , , , 1.5
```

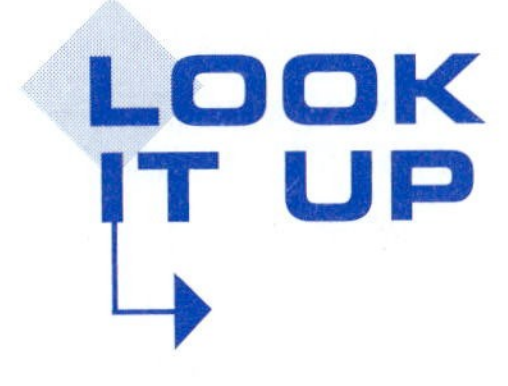

Use the keyword "FillStyle" to search the Index tab of the online Help file. The page explains how the FillStyle property works. It also lists all the eight styles that you can use to fill an area.

The DrawBulb Procedure. Now, we are ready to write the procedure that computes the position and draws a light bulb. We will make it a Sub procedure, named DrawBulb. This procedure requires two parameters: P, the position number of the light bulb; and Color, the color for the light bulb. The complete procedure appears as follows:

```
Sub DrawBulb(ByVal P As Integer, ByVal Color As Long)
Dim R As Single
Dim C As Single
Dim X As Single
Dim Y As Single
'Step 1: Compute the position (x, y) of the light bulb
     Select Case P
     Case 0 To 13
     ' on the top
          X = Distance / 2 + P * Distance
          Y = Distance / 2 'Y is fixed for the top row
     Case 14 To 27
     ' on the right margin
          X = 14.5 * Distance 'X is fixed on the right
          Y = (P - 13.5) * Distance
     Case 28 To 41
     ' at the bottom
          X = (42.5 - P) * Distance
          Y = 14.5 * Distance 'Y is fixed
     Case 42 To 55
     'on the left
          X = Distance / 2 'X is fixed
          Y = (56.5 - P) * Distance
     End Select
' Step 2: Draw the light bulb
     'Set the fill style so that each drawing
     ' is filled with solid color
     picLights.FillStyle = vbFSSolid
     ' Fill the light bulb with the color specified
     picLights.FillColor = Color
     'Draw a light bulb
     picLights.Circle (X, Y), Radius, , , , 1.5
End Sub
```

Calling the Procedure. The preceding procedure can be called to draw all the 56 light bulbs. It should be called when the user clicks the "Draw Lights" button. We would like to alternate the light colors among green, red, white, and blue. For simplicity, we will use four lines of code, using different colors for each call. The complete procedure appears as follows:

```
Private Sub cmdShow_Click()
Dim I As Integer
    ' This loop draws 56 light bulbs starting with position 0
    ' The colors are: green, red, white, and blue
    For I = 0 To 52 Step 4
        DrawBulb I, vbGreen
        DrawBulb I + 1, vbRed
        DrawBulb I + 2, vbWhite
        DrawBulb I + 3, vbBlue
    Next I
End Sub
```

The procedure uses a For loop to call the DrawBulb Sub. Because each iteration calls DrawBulb four times using different color parameters, the loop counter is incremented by 4. Notice that the fourth call sets the bulb position to I + 3. Thus, when I reaches 52, the last light bulb (number 55) will be drawn. I should not go beyond 52.

Why Compute the Bulb Positions That Way? Our DrawBulb procedure appears to be a bit complex. You may have figured out a simpler way to compute the positions for the light bulbs given the program requirements. Thus, you may wonder why such a "complex" procedure. There is a reason. The procedure can easily be modified to perform animation, which is discussed in the next section. We will revisit this project to illustrate how one type of animation can be implemented.

Saving the Picture You Draw

Often, you may want to save what you draw in a file for future use. The ***SavePicture*** statement allows you to do so. The SavePicture statement has the following syntax:

```
SavePicture Picture, FilePath
```

where *Picture* is the Picture or Image property of an object and *FilePath* is the filename to save the picture.

You must understand, however, that what you draw on the screen (a form or a picture box) is not reflected in the Picture property of the object. *The picture you draw is kept in the object's Image property if you set the object's AutoRedraw property to True.* In such a case, the picture on the screen is kept in the ***Image property*** so that if the picture is erased (e.g., you minimize the form), it can be redrawn when the object is restored on the screen. Thus, to save the preceding picture, you will need to do the following:

1. Set the AutoRedraw property to True either at design time or at runtime.
2. Use the SavePicture statement to save the image as follows:

```
SavePicture picLights.Image,"C:\Temp\ChristmasLights.bmp"
```

Notice that the picture in the Image property will always be saved in the bmp format.

B.2. Animation

Animations take different forms. For example, you can show different pictures at a fixed time intervals in the same or different positions. While one picture is displayed, all other pictures of the same objects are made invisible. Usually, a timer is used to regulate the timing to display. This creates an illusion that the object is moving. You can also create animations by drawing instead of using existing pictures. For example, you can draw different colors on the same graph, again at a fixed time interval. This can create an impression that the object is blinking or the lights are moving. Also, you can create a rotating object (or an object with different motions) by drawing some part of the object at a different relative position while the object moves. In this section, we use three examples to illustrate how each of these ideas can be done.

The Flying Butterfly

In this project, we show a butterfly flying at a random height and distance (width) from the lower-left corner toward the upper-right corner of the form. Follow these steps to set up the project:

1. Draw two image controls and a timer on a new form. (*Note:* Always use the image control instead of the picture box when all you need is to display a picture. The image control uses fewer system resources.)
2. Name the image controls imgFly1 and imgFly2. Then set the Picture properties to Bfly1.bmp and Bfly2.bmp for the two controls, respectively. These two bmp files are located in the following folder:

Microsoft Visual Studio\MSDN98\98VS\1033\SAMPLES\VB98\Vcr

3. Name the timer control tmrFly. Set its Interval property to 350. (You can change this setting depending on how fast you want the butterfly to flip and fly.)
4. Develop the code to perform the animation. The following discussion focuses on this aspect.

The initial form setup appears as in Figure B.6.

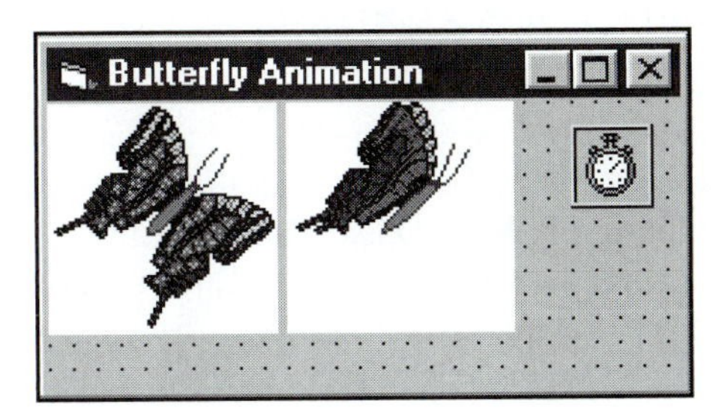

FIGURE B.6
Initial Setup for the Flying Butterfly Project

The Form Load Event Procedure. As soon the project starts, the program should perform a few preparatory steps:

- Set the WindowState property to vbMaximized so that we can view the butterfly flying over the entire screen.
- Set the form's BackColor property to white so that it will correspond with that of the pictures.
- Move the pictures to the lower-left corner so that they cannot be seen; that is, each picture is placed an entire width of itself to the left and entire height of itself below the form. (See the sketch in Figure B.7.)
- Randomize the seed for the Rnd function because this function will be used.

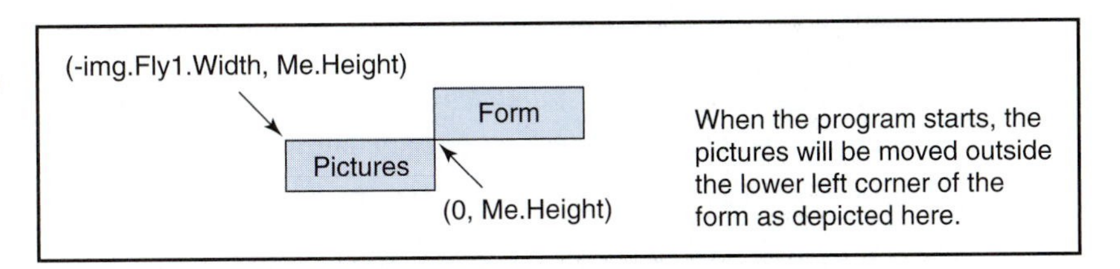

FIGURE B.7
Initial Position of the Two Images

The following procedure should accomplish these requirements.

```
Option Explicit
Private Sub Form_Load()
    Me.WindowState = vbMaximized 'maximize the form
    Me.BackColor = vbWhite 'set background to white
    Me.Show 'So that the form's height and width reflect the size
```

```
        imgFly1.Move -imgFly1.Width, Me.Height 'Start images at the
        imgFly2.Move -imgFly2.Width, Me.Height ' lower left corner
        Randomize 'Randomize the seed
    End Sub
```

Notice that we have inserted a statement that uses the form's Show method to make the form appear after the WindowState property is set to vbMaximized. This is needed because the form's Width and Height properties will not change until the form actually appears. The form's height is used to set the positions for the two pictures.

Toggling the Images. This animation involves only two pictures, so we can use a Static Boolean variable (FlyWingsOpen) to determine which picture should appear. The code structure can appear as follows:

```
    Static FlyWingsOpen As Boolean
        FlyWingsOpen = Not FlyWingsOpen 'Toggle wings open state
        If FlyWingsOpen Then
        'Compute the Wings-open picture position
        Else
        'Compute the wings-closed picture position
        End If
        imgFly1.Visble = FlyWingsOpen
        imgFly2.Visible = Not FlyWingsOpen
```

The first "Not" statement will toggle the value of FlyWingsOpen. The Visible property of the first picture is set to the value of FlyWingsOpen. Thus, if the variable is True, that picture will appear; otherwise, it will disappear. On the other hand, the second picture's Visible property is set to the opposite (Not) value of FlyWingsOpen. Thus, when the variable is True, the second picture will not be visible; otherwise, it will be visible. Thus, the last two statements in the preceding code will make one picture appear and the other disappear depending on the value of FlyWingsOpen, which is toggled (with the Not statement) between procedure calls.

Computing the Picture Position. The current picture will move on average half its own width and a quarter of its own height from the position of the previous picture. That is, imgFly1's position (x, y) can be computed as follows:

```
    X = imgFly2.Left + Rnd * imgFly1.Width
    Y = imgFly2.Top - Rnd * 0.5 * imgFly1.Height
```

Notice that the previous position of imgFly1 is based on that of imgFly2 because the two images take turns to appear. Notice also that Rnd * imgFly1.Width will result in a horizontal move on average by half of the first picture's width because Rnd generates a random number between 0 and 1, whose expected (average) value is 0.5. Multiplying this expected value by 0.5 should obtain an expected value of $\frac{1}{4}$. Thus, the second formula should result in a vertical move up by $\frac{1}{4}$ of the image's height. Similar formulas can be used to compute the new position for imgFly2.

When the Butterfly Disappears from the Form. As soon as the butterfly disappears from the form, we can start the two image controls from the lower-right corner again. The butterfly disappears when either of the image control's Left property is greater than or equal to the form's width or when its Top property plus its Height is less than zero. For code simplicity we will test only the first image control. The code structure will appear as follows:

```
    If imgFly1.Left >  Me.Width Or _
      imgFly1.Top + imgFly1.Height < 0 Then
    ' the butterfly has completely disappeared, start at
    ' the lower left corner again
        imgFly1.Move -imgFly1.Width, Me.Height
        imgFly2.Move -imgFly2.Width, Me.Height
    End If
```

The test for the image control's position should be done before any computation of the control's new position. Therefore, this block of code should appear at the top of the procedure.

The Complete Timer Procedure. The placement and appearance of the butterfly should be regulated by the timer's interval. Thus, the code to perform the animation should be placed in the timer's Timer event. The complete timer procedure appears as follows:

```
Private Sub tmrFly_Timer()
Static FlyWingsOpen As Boolean 'Declare a static variable
    If imgFly1.Left >  Me.Width Or _
      imgFly1.Top + imgFly1.Height < 0 Then
    ' the fly has completely disappeared, start at
    ' the lower left corner again
        imgFly1.Move -imgFly1.Width, Me.Height
        imgFly2.Move -imgFly2.Width, Me.Height
     End If
    FlyWingsOpen = Not FlyWingsOpen 'Toggle the state
    If FlyWingsOpen Then
    'Move the wings-open image
        imgFly1.Move imgFly2.Left + Rnd * imgFly1.Width, _
        imgFly2.Top - Rnd * 0.5 * imgFly1.Height
    Else
    ' Move the wings-closed image
         imgFly2.Move imgFly1.Left + Rnd * imgFly2.Width, _
         imgFly1.Top - Rnd * 0.5 * imgFly2.Height
    End If
    'Show wings-open picture if FlyWingsOpen is True
    imgFly1.Visible = FlyWingsOpen
    'Make wings-closed image appear if FlyWingsOpen is False
    imgFly2.Visible = Not FlyWingsOpen
End Sub
```

Rotating Light Colors

By rotating the colors for the "light bulbs," you can create an impression that the lights are moving. Our previous Christmas lights project can easily be modified to show this effect. Reload the project and then follow these steps:

1. Save the form and the project as a different project (e.g., Christmas2 for both the form and the project files) in a new folder.
2. Draw a timer control on the form. Name it tmrLights. Set its Interval property to 250.
3. Add code in the Timer event. The following discussion focuses on this aspect.

Actually, the code in the Timer event should be pretty much like the one in the previous cmdShow_Click event. Consider the For loop in that procedure:

```
For I = 0 To 52 Step 4
  ' Statements to display green, red, white and blue lights
Next I
```

The loop begins with drawing a green light at position 0 and rotates among the four colors as it proceeds. After the loop is complete, 56 lights are drawn. Suppose the next time the procedure is called, the loop will begin with drawing a green light at position 1 and proceed from there to draw 56 lights. Then this 56th light will be drawn at position 56, one position more than the last (55). Notice, however, position 0 has not yet been drawn. Thus, if we subtract 56 from the position number when it exceeds 55, we make the drawing starting from position 0 again. The loop can then be made to draw a complete rotation from whichever position it begins to draw the lights. That is, if we let BegPos be the position the loop starts, we can modify the loop parameters as follows:

```
For I = BegPos To 52 + BegPos Step 4
' statements to draw the lights
Next I
```

We can increase the value of BegPos by 1 each time the procedure is called. There are four colors. Thus, there is no need to have this variable take on more than 4 values (from 0 to 3). Thus, we can code the following:

```
BegPos = BegPos + 1
If BegPos > 3 Then BegPos = 0
```

The complete Timer event procedure can appear as follows:

```
Private Sub tmrLights_Timer()
Dim I As Integer
Static BegPos As Integer
    'Draw 56 lights in rotation
    ' The colors are: green, red, white, and blue
    For I = BegPos To 52 + BegPos Step 4
        DrawBulb I, vbGreen
        DrawBulb I + 1, vbRed
        DrawBulb I + 2, vbWhite
        DrawBulb I + 3, vbBlue
    Next I
    BegPos = BegPos + 1
    If BegPos > 3 Then BegPos = 0
End Sub
```

Notice that BegPos is declared as a Static variable so that its value can be preserved between the Timer event procedure calls.

The Timer event procedure does not really take care of the situation in which the light position exceeds 55. This can easily be handled in the DrawBulb procedure as follows:

```
Sub DrawBulb(ByVal P As Integer, ByVal Color As Long)
Dim R As Single
Dim C As Single
Dim X As Single
Dim Y As Single
'Step 0: Adjust value for P
    If P > 55 Then P = P - 56
'Step 1: Compute the position of the light bulb
' Other statements (remain the same)
End Sub
```

After you modify the project as shown, you are ready to see the effect. Run the program. You should be able to see lights rotating around the picture frame. Incidentally, you no longer need the command button (captioned Show Lights) or its Click event procedure. You can delete both from the project without affecting the results.

The Rolling Wheel

This example project will emulate a rolling wheel on the form. The rolling wheel will appear from the right side and roll across the form. As soon as it disappears, it will appear from the right side again. To set up this project, bring a timer on a new form. Name the timer tmrWheel and set its interval to 100.

This project presents two issues. First, to "move" the wheel, you need not only to draw the wheel at the new position but also to erase the wheel at its previous location. Second, you need to show that the wheel not only moves forward but also rolls. To show the wheel is rolling, we can draw a line similar to the clock hand in the wheel and make it appear at different angles. A glimpse of the resulting form appears in Figure B.8

FIGURE B.8
The Rolling Wheel

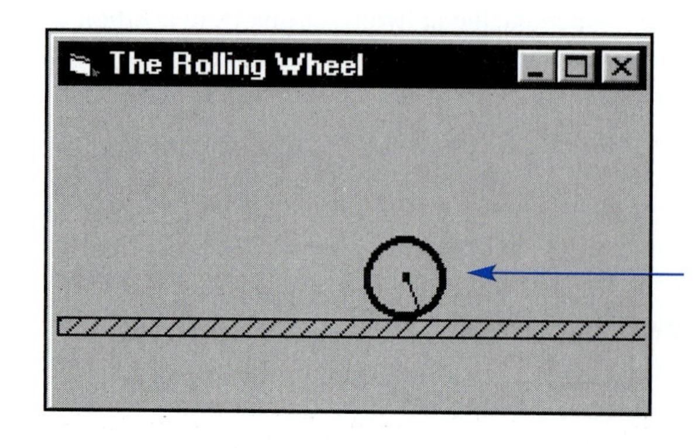

This project draws a wheel rolling across the form. As the wheel moves from right to left, its hand rotates, making the wheel appear to roll.

As the wheel "turns," the hand will rotate. The distance that the wheel travels and the angle that the hand rotates should be consistent.

Let *WheelRadius* = the wheel radius

AngleTurned = the angle (in radians) that the hand rotates

Then the distance the wheel travels can be computed as follows:

```
Distance = WheelRadius * AngleTurned
```

Here is a roundabout way of explaining how the preceding formula works:

The length of the whole circle is 2 π WheelRadius.

The ratio of the distance traveled to the circle for an angle, AngleTurned (in radians), is AngledTurned/2 π. Thus,

Distance = Circle × Ratio

= (2 π WheelRadius) (AngelTurned/2 π)

= WheelRadius × AngleTurned

Assume that we will move the wheel 16 times to complete a full rotation (whole circle). Then AngleTurned can be computed as follows:

```
AngleTurned = 2 Pi / 16; that is,
AngleTurned = Pi / 8
```

There should also be a "road" below the wheel. To show the road, we will draw a box at 60% of the form's height. We can use the ***Line method*** to draw the box. The Line method has the following syntax:

```
object.Line [Step] (x1, y1) [Step] - (x2, y2), [color], [B][F]
```

where *Object* = form, picture box, or the Printer object

X1, Y1 = the coordinate of the beginning point to draw the line

Step = the optional keyword to indicate the coordinate is relative to the object's CurrentX, CurrentY coordinate

X2, Y2 = the coordinate of the ending point for the line

Color = the color of the line; if omitted, the object's ForeColor is used

B = the optional keyword to indicate the coordinates are to be used to draw a box instead of a line

F = the optional keyword to indicate the box should be filled with a color specified by the FillColor property; the B optional keyword must be used if F is to be specified

For our purpose, to draw the road, we can code the following:

```
Y = Me.ScaleHeight * 0.6
Me.FillStyle = vbDownwardDiagonal
Me.Line (0, Y)-(Me.ScaleWidth, Y + 100), , B
```

The code specifies that the FillStyle will be downward diagonal. The Line method is then used to draw a box from left of the form at 60% of the form height (as computed for Y) across the entire width. The box has a height of 100 twips (Y versus Y + 100) as depicted in Figure B.9.

FIGURE B.9
Drawing a Box with the Line Method

(0, Y)
(Me.ScaleWidth, Y + 100)
The "line" starts at (0, Y) and ends at (Me.ScaleWidth, Y + 100). With "B" specified, it is drawn as a box.

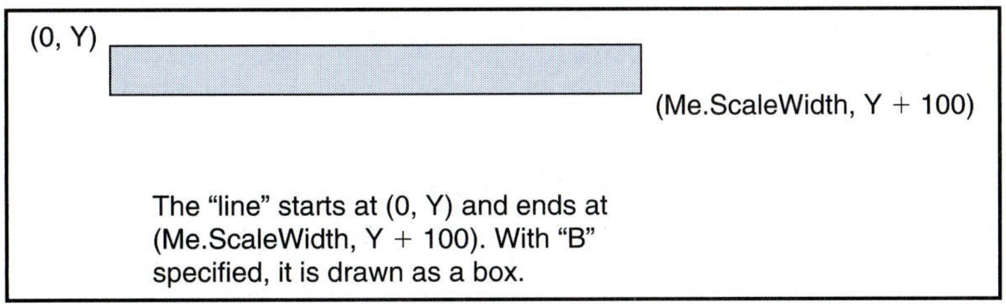

Setting the Initial Position of the Wheel. The wheel will go from right to left on the form. Initially, it will not be seen. So, the center of its X coordinate should be the form's width plus it radius. The center of its Y coordinate should be immediately above the road. The wheel itself should not be drawn on the road to avoid drawing over. Let WheelX and WheelY be the coordinate for the wheel's center. Then, they can be computed as follows:

```
WheelX = Me.ScaleWidth + WheelRadius 'On the form's right margin
'Place the bottom of the wheel two pixels above the road
WheelY = 0.6 * Me.ScaleHeight - _
    WheelRadius - 2 * Screen.TwipsPerPixelY
```

The formula for WheelY indicates that the lowest portion of the wheel will be drawn 2 pixels above the road. Because all other variables and properties are measured in twips, the pixels are converted to twips with the conversion rate, ***Screen.TwipsPerPixelY,*** a property of the Screen object. The Screen object provides several properties that your application can use to handle forms on the desktop (screen). The TwipsPerPixelY property gives the number of vertical twips per pixel, as the name suggests.

The Form Load Procedure. All the preceding discussion pertains to the computations required as soon as the program starts. The code can be placed in the Form Load event as follows:

```
Option Explicit
Private Const Pi As Single = 3.14159
Dim Distance As Single
Dim WheelRadius As Single
Dim AngleTurned As Single 'angle turned in each period
Dim WheelX As Single
Dim WheelY As Single

Private Sub Form_Load()
Dim Y As Single
    ' Compute parameter values
    WheelRadius = Me.ScaleHeight * 0.1
    AngleTurned = Pi / 8
    Distance = WheelRadius * AngleTurned
    'Draw the wheel path
    Me.DrawWidth = 1 'Use 1 pixel to draw
    Y = Me.ScaleHeight * 0.6
    Me.FillStyle = vbDownwardDiagonal
    'Note: To make this road show,
    'set Form's AutoRedraw property to True at design time.
    Me.Line (0, Y)-(Me.ScaleWidth, Y + 100), , B
    Me.FillStyle = vbFSTransparent 'Restore FillStyle
    ' Initialize wheel center
    WheelX = Me.ScaleWidth + WheelRadius 'On the form's right margin
    'Place the bottom of the wheel two pixels above the road
    WheelY = 0.6 * Me.ScaleHeight - _
      WheelRadius - 2 * Screen.TwipsPerPixelY
End Sub
```

Notice that we have declared all five variables as module-level variables because they will be used in other procedures. Notice also that we have inserted a statement to set the FillStyle property to vbFSTransparent after it was initially set to vbDownwardDiagonal to draw the box. This is needed because all the subsequent drawing will be done without filling anything in the enclosed drawing area.

Drawing the Wheel. The wheel has three parts: the circle, the center point, and the hand. Given the wheel center at (Xc,Yc) with a Radius and a Color, the circle for the wheel can be drawn on the form with the following code:

```
Me.Circle (Xc, Yc), Radius, Color 'Draw the wheel
```

We would also like to draw a point at the center. This can be done with the following code:

```
Me.PSet (Xc, Yc), Color 'Draw the center point
```

The hand will connect the center point to the circle with a line. The hand's position on the circle depends on the angle. Given an angle, Theta (in radians), its coordinate can be computed with the following formula:

```
X = Xc + Cos(Theta) * Radius
Y = Yc - Sin(Theta) * Radius
```

Recall that by definition, at the point of origin (0, 0), Sin(Theta) = Y/Radius. (Refer to Figure B.3 for a visual hint.) Thus, at that point, Y = Sin(Theta) × Radius. Notice, however, that the Y value computed in this formula is based on the Cartesian coordinate. The Y coordinate of an object in VB goes the other way: the closer a position is to the top, the smaller the value is. Thus, the Y value should be subtracted from (rather than added to) Yc. Thus, Y can be computed with the preceding formula.

Similarly, at the point of origin, Cos(Theta) = X/Radius. Thus, X = Cos(Theta) × Radius. The X coordinate under the Cartesian system is consistent with that for the object in VB. Thus, this value is added to Xc, the X coordinate of the wheel center. The hand then can be drawn with the following statement:

```
Me.Line (Xc, Yc)-(Xc + Cos(Theta) * Radius, _
    Yc - Sin(Theta) * Radius), Color
```

The Sub procedure to draw a wheel (DrawWheel) can then appear as follows:

```
Sub DrawWheel(Xc As Single, Yc As Single, Radius As Single, _
  Theta As Single, Color As Long)
    Me.DrawWidth = 3 'Use 3 pixels to draw the wheel
    Me.Circle (Xc, Yc), Radius, Color 'Draw the wheel
    Me.PSet (Xc, Yc), Color 'Draw the center
    Me.DrawWidth = 1 'Use 1 pixel to draw the "hand"
    'Draw the hand from the center
    Me.Line (Xc, Yc)-(Xc + Cos(Theta) * Radius, _
      Yc - Sin(Theta) * Radius), Color
End Sub
```

Notice that we have inserted the statements to set the DrawWidth property. The circle and the point are drawn with a width of 3 pixels. However, the line (hand) is drawn with 1 pixel.

Rolling the Wheel. The DrawWheel Sub procedure can be used to roll the wheel across the form. This should be done in the Timer event procedure. In each event call, the original wheel should be erased. Then another wheel should be drawn at a new location.

To erase the wheel, you can draw it at the same location with the BackColor. This will restore every part of the wheel to the BackColor, making it disappear.

To draw another wheel at a new location, we will need to know the wheel's current coordinate. Recall that we have calculated the original coordinate for the wheel in the Form Load procedure. There, we also calculated the distance the wheel would travel each time. The module-level variables for the coordinate are WheelX and WheelY, and the variable for the distance traveled is named Distance. WheelY should remain the same. However, WheelX should be decreased (because the wheel is going from right to left) by Distance for the distance the wheel will travel; that is:

```
WheelX = WheelX – Distance
```

When the wheel completely disappears from the form, it will reappear from the right. If the wheel has disappeared from the left side, the WheelX value should be less than the negative value of the radius. Thus, we can code the following:

```
If WheelX < -WheelRadius Then
    ' wheel has disappeared; start from right again
    WheelX = Me.ScaleWidth + WheelRadius
End If
```

The wheel rolls counter-clockwise. This means, as the wheel rolls, the angle Theta is increased by the angle turned, which is represented by the variable AngleTurned and was also computed in the form load procedure. Thus:

```
Theta = Theta + AngleTurned
```

We can start the value for Theta at zero, and then check whether the value is greater than or equal to 2π. If so, the wheel has turned a complete round and Theta can be reset to 0. Thus, the code will appear as follows:

```
If Theta >= 2 * Pi Then
    ' Set theta to 0
    Theta = 0
End If
```

To put everything together, the complete Timer event procedure should appear as follows:

```
Private Sub tmrWheel_Timer()
Static Theta As Single
    ' Erase wheel drawn previously
    DrawWheel WheelX, WheelY, WheelRadius, Theta, Me.BackColor
    If WheelX < -WheelRadius Then
    ' wheel has disappeared; start from right again
        WheelX = Me.Width + WheelRadius
    End If
    'Change the angle (turn)
    Theta = Theta + AngleTurned
    If Theta >= 2 * Pi Then
    ' Set theta to 0 to start over
        Theta = 0
    End If
    ' Move the wheel by a fixed distance
    WheelX = WheelX - Distance
    DrawWheel WheelX, WheelY, WheelRadius, Theta, Me.ForeColor
End Sub
```

Notice that Theta is declared to be a Static variable in the procedure so that its value between event calls can be preserved. Notice also the DrawWheel Sub is called twice. The first time, the form's BackColor is used as the color parameter so that the previous wheel can be erased. The second time, the new wheel position, the new angle, and the ForeColor are passed to draw the wheel.

This rolling wheel project includes the Form Load event procedure, the DrawWheel Sub procedure, and the tmrWheel Timer event procedure. Try the project and get a feel for how the wheel turns. You can change the timer interval and the denominator for the AngleTurned formula to get a different speed for the wheel.

The following table summarizes the methods, properties, and a statement (SavePicture) pertinent to graphic operations discussed in these two sections.

Type	Name	Applicable Object	Description	Example
Method	Pset	Form, picture box, Printer object	To draw a point	`picLights.Pset (x,y), _ vbGreen`
	Circle		To draw circle, ellipse, or arc	`Me.Circle (x, y), _ Radius, Color, _ 0, Pi, Aspect`
	Line		To draw line or box	`Printer.Line _ (X1, Y1)- (X2, Y2), _ Color, B, F`
Property	AutoRedraw	Form, picture box	Set AutoRedraw to True to save drawn image in memory	`Me.AutoRedraw = True`
	FillStyle	Form, picture box, Printer object	To specify style to fill a drawing area	`picLights.FillStyle = _ vbFSSolid`
	FillColor		To specify the color to fill in the drawing area	`Me.FillColor = vbBlue`

Type	Name	Applicable Object	Description	Example
	DrawWidth		To specify the width to draw	`Printer.DrawWidth = 2`
	ScaleMode		To specify the units of measurement for graphics methods	`picLight.ScaleMode = _ vbPixels`
Statement	SavePicture	Form, picture box, image control	To save picture in the Picture or image property	`SavePicture picLights.Image, _ "Lights.bmp"`

B.3. Drag and Drop

Drag and drop provides an interesting and easy way for the user to specify operations that can be too complex to express by some other means. A typical drag-and-drop operation involves dragging an icon to another icon at another location to initiate certain activities. For example, a file can be dragged into a trash can to delete the file. Typically, in this type of operation, three icons are involved. In the case of dumping a file, one icon will represent the file, another will represent an empty trash can (before the file is dragged), and the other will represent the trash can containing the dumped file (after the file is dropped). Only one of the two trash cans will be visible at a given time.

Playing with Drag and Drop

To illustrate how the drag-and-drop operation is done in VB, let's do some hands-on experiments with a new project:

1. Draw an image control on the new form. Name the control imgDisk. Set its Picture property to Disk03.ico, which is located in the following folder:

   Microsoft Visual Studio\Common\Graphics\Icons\Computer

2. Run the project and try to drag the icon around the form. Nothing will happen. End the program.
3. Set the control's ***DragMode property*** to 1 – Automatic. Run the program and try to drag the icon again. This time, you should see a square image moving (while the icon itself remains still) as you drag. When you release the mouse button, the icon stays at its original location. Terminate the program.
4. Set the image control's ***DragIcon property*** to Disk01.ico, which can be found in the same folder mentioned in number 1. Run the project and drag the icon again. As you drag, you should see the Disk01 icon moving. However, Disk03 remains at the same location when you release the mouse button, whereas Disk01 disappears. End the program.
5. Enter the following in the code window:

```
Private Sub Form_DragDrop(Source As Control, X As Single, _
    Y As Single)
    Source.Move X, Y
End Sub
```

6. Run the program again. Drag the icon around the form. This time, you should see the Disk03 icon moves to the location where you release the mouse button.

You have learned several things about drag and drop from this experiment:

- To allow a control to be dragged, you can set its DragMode property to automatic (1), although this is not the only way.
- To show an icon different from a square image while a control is being dragged, you can set the control's DragIcon property to an icon of your choice.

- The control being dragged is the Source control. The control or form that will handle the drag-and-drop result is the ***target object***, whose DragDrop event is the procedure in which to place the code to perform the operations.

In the preceding example, we leave the control at the location of the drag and drop. In other cases, we may perform different operations.

Keeping a Disk in the Holder: An Example

To illustrate, let's expand our example. We will allow the user to drag the disk and drop it in a disk holder. When the operation is complete, the disk will disappear as if it had been placed in the holder. The disk holder will change colors to indicate that it is holding the disk.

Follow these steps to perform additional setup for the project:

1. Draw two more image controls onto the form. Name the first one imgDiskHolder1. Name the second one imgDiskHolder2 and set its Visible property to False.
2. Set imgDiskHolder1's Picture property to Disks03.ico and imgDiskHolder2's Picture property to Disks04.ico. (Note the names of both files. They start with "Disks," not just "Disk.")
3. Position the icons so that they will appear in the form as in Figure B.10.

FIGURE B.10
Initial Setup for Disk Drag and Drop

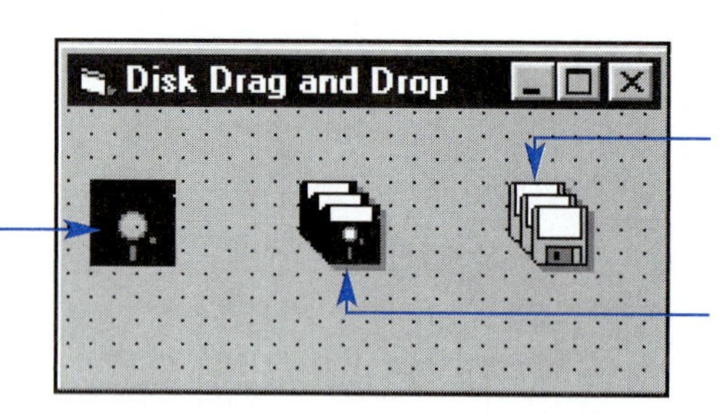

Place imgDisk here. Once this disk is dragged to the "empty holder" and dropped, it will disappear.

Place imgDiskHolder1 here. When the program starts, this holder appears. After the disk is dragged and dropped here, the other holder will appear here in its place.

Place imgDiskHolder2 here. When your program starts, this holder will not be visible.

When the project starts, the disk on the left can be dragged to the disk holder on the right. Thus, imgDiskHolder1 is the target control. Our code should be placed in its DragDrop event to handle the operation. The code should make imgDisk disappear. In addition, imgDiskHolder2 should take the place of imgDiskHolder1; that is, imgDiskHolder2 should appear at the location of imgDiskHolder1, which should then disappear. This description yields the following code:

```
Private Sub imgDiskHolder1_DragDrop(Source As Control, _
    X As Single, Y As Single)
        Source.Visible = False 'Make the disk disappear
        With imgDiskHolder1
            imgDiskHolder2.Move .Left, .Top 'Move holder2 to holder1
            .Visible = False 'Make holder1 disappear
        End With
        imgDiskHolder2.Visible = True 'Make holder2 appear
End Sub
```

You can now test the program. When you drag the disk on the form, you can leave it anywhere (from the code in our previous experiment). However, when you drop the disk on the disk holder, the disk should disappear. In addition, the disk holder changes color (disk holder 1 is replaced by disk holder 2).

The drag-and-drop operation is not limited to icons. In addition, the operation need not involve more than one control. For example, an item in a list box can be dragged to a different position. In this way, the user can rearrange the order of the items in the list box. You can also allow the user to drag and drop a column or a row to a different position in an MS Hierarchical FlexGrid (HFG). The following example shows how this can be done.

Dragging and Dropping a Column in an MS HFG

In this example, we show how a column in an MS HFG can be dragged to another column position. When the program starts, it will populate the HFG with 100 numbers ranging from 1 to 100 in four columns. (This is done for simplicity of illustration. You can bind it to a recordset from a database query as an alternative.) The routine uses the TextArray property to populate the grid. The property maps the grid's cells as a linear array, beginning with Cell(0, 0) as TextArray(0), Cell(0, 1) as TextArray(1), and so on. We assume you are familiar with the HFG (discussed in Chapter 8, "Database and the ActiveX Data Objects," and Chapter 13) and will therefore provide the code for setting up the grid without explanation. Follow these steps to set up the project:

1. Add the HFG to the toolbox of a new project using the Components option of the Project menu.
2. Draw an HFG on the new form. Adjust its size so that it can accommodate about four columns and eight rows. Name the HFG grdNumbers. Set its DragIcon property to Drag1pg.ico, which is located in the subfolder DragDrop of the aforementioned Icons folder.
3. Type in the following code:

```
Private Sub Form_Load()
Dim I As Integer
    With grdNumbers
        .Cols = 4
        .Rows = 25
        .FixedCols = 0
        For I = 1 To 100
            .TextArray(I - 1) = I
        Next I
    End With
End Sub
```

When the project starts, you should be able to see the grid displaying the data as shown in Figure B.11.

FIGURE B.11
HFG for Drag-and-Drop Demo

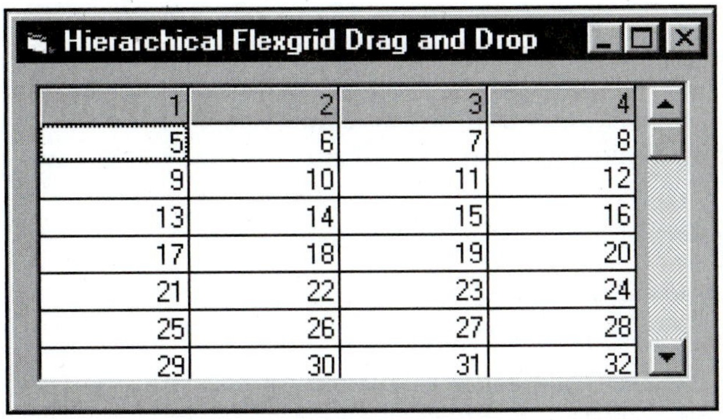

Hierarchical Flexgrid Drag and Drop

1	2	3	4
5	6	7	8
9	10	11	12
13	14	15	16
17	18	19	20
21	22	23	24
25	26	27	28
29	30	31	32

Let's now consider the drag-and-drop aspect of the program. We would like the user to start the dragging operation only when he or she presses the mouse on a column title; that is, if the mouse pointer is on the nonfixed portion of the grid, we will ignore the drag and drop. In which event should we place the code?

When the user presses the mouse button, the MouseDown event is triggered. This is the event we can use to check whether the mouse pointer is on a column title. The cell that the mouse is at is reflected by the MouseRow and MouseCol properties. If the mouse pointer is on a column title, the MouseRow property should be zero. Thus, in the MouseDown event, we can code the following:

```
 'Not on the column header. Ignore.
If grdNumbers.MouseRow > 0 Then Exit Sub
```

Recall that in this project, we did not set the DragMode property to automatic. The default is 0 - Manual, meaning that we will need to use the code to initiate the drag. Most VB controls have the Drag method that allows us to specify how to handle the drag and drop operation. For example, the following code will start the HFG's drag operation:

```
grdNumbers.Drag vbBeginDrag
```

Because we will be dragging the column to a different position, we will need to keep track of the current column number. Thus, we will also need to code the following:

```
ColDragged = grdNumbers.MouseCol
```

In sum, the MouseDown event procedure should appear as follows:

```
Option Explicit
Dim ColDragged As Integer
Private Sub grdNumbers_MouseDown(Button As Integer, _
  Shift As Integer, x As Single, y As Single)
    'Ignore dragging, if mouse is not on a column title
    If grdNumbers.MouseRow > 0 Then Exit Sub
    grdNumbers.Drag vbBeginDrag 'Start dragging
    ColDragged = grdNumbers.MouseCol 'Keep the Col. No. to drag
End Sub
```

Notice that we have declared ColDragged as a module-level variable so that its value can be used in other procedures.

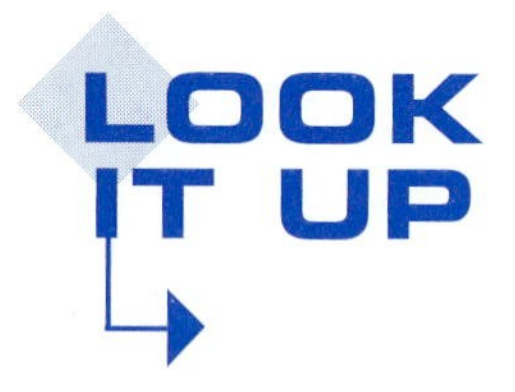

Search the keyword "Drag Method" in the Index tab of the online Help file. The page explains additional uses of the Drag method. It also gives other named constants that can be used to specify how a drag should be handled.

Moving the Dragged Column. When the drag and drop is complete, we will need to move the dragged column to the dropped position. The HFG has the ***ColPosition property*** that can be used to specify the new column position for any column. For example, the following code will move column 2 to column 1. (Read it: the new column position for column 2 is 1.)

```
grdNumbers.ColPosition(2) = 1
```

The event to handle the drag and drop is the DragDrop event procedure. Thus, the code to perform the move is as follows:

```
Private Sub grdNumbers_DragDrop(Source As Control, _
  x As Single, y As Single)
    'Move Column dragged to the current column
    grdNumbers.ColPosition(ColDragged) = grdNumbers.MouseCol
End Sub
```

Notice that the MouseCol property in this procedure has the current cell position, not the position when the mouse was down. As a side note, the HFG also has the ***RowPosition property***, which works similarly to its ColPosition property.

Run the project and try to drag any column to another. As long as your drag-and-drop operation is performed on a column title, you should be successful. However, you will not even be able to see the drag icon if you attempt to start the drag in a nonfixed cell. Thus, this example also shows the flexibility you can have when you set the DragMode property to Manual instead of Automatic.

The following table provides a summary of our discussion of the object's interfaces pertinent to the drag-and-drop operation.

Type of Interface	Name	Object Involved	Explanation	Example
Property	DragMode	Source control	Specifies whether the control is to be dragged automatically or only initiated by its Drag method	Set to 1 (automatic) at design time
	DragIcon	Source control	Specifies the icon to display when the control is being dragged	Set to an icon of your choice
Method	Drag	Source control	Specifies how the drag is to be handled	`ImgDisk.Drag vbBeginDrag`
Event	DragDrop	Target control	You provide the code to handle the drag and drop	`Source.Visible = False`
Property	ColPosition RowPosition	MS HFG	Specifies new column position or row position	`grdNumbers.ColPosition(Old) _ = Mouse.Col`

Summary

This appendix presents topics related to graphics. You have learned how to draw graphs using the Pset, Circle, and Line methods, combining several properties pertaining to drawing. A summary of these methods and properties are presented at the end of Section B.2. You have also been introduced to several animation techniques. They should provide you with a good peek into the exciting world of animation.

You have also learned how to code the drag-and-drop operation. As stated in the introduction, drag and drop provides a means for the user to specify an operation that can otherwise be very complex to express. Consider the last example that allows the user to drag and drop an HFG column to another location. How else can you design a way for the user to specify the same operation? Now you have learned the "trick." Take advantage of the technique to its fullest extent in your design of the user interface for your applications.

Visual Basic Explorer

B-1. The ScaleMode Property. Enter the following code in a new form:

```
Private Sub Form_Click()
Dim I As Integer
    For I = 1 To 7
        Me.ScaleMode = I
        Print I; Me.ScaleWidth; Me.ScaleHeight; Me.CurrentX; _
          Me.CurrentY
    Next I
End Sub
```

Run the project and click the form. You should see five numbers in each line of output on the form. The first number gives the ScaleMode. The next two numbers give the available interior width and height given the ScaleMode. The last two numbers give the current location of the "cursor"; that is, the current value of x and y to print data. Note that the form's available interior width and height are the same. However, its ScaleWidth and ScaleHeight properties are changed to reflect the same size under different measurement units.

B-2. The AutoRedraw Property. Enter the following code:

```
Private Sub Form_Click()
    Me.Circle (300, 300), 100, vbRed
End Sub
```

Run the project and click the form. What do you see?

Minimize the form then restore it from the taskbar. Now, do you see the circle?

Set the AutoRedraw property to True and repeat the experiment. Do you always see the circle now?

B-3. The Cls Method and AutoRedraw Property. Add a command button to the form in the preceding project (B-2). Set its Caption property to "Clear" and name it cmdClear. Add the following code:

```
Private Sub cmdClear_Click()
    Me.Cls
End Sub
```

Run the project again. Click the form then click the button. Does the red circle disappear? Anything you draw on an object can be erased with the Cls method.

B-4. Box, the FillStyle and the FillColor Properties. Enter the following code into a new project:

```
Private Sub Form_Click()
    Me.FillColor = vbGreen
    Me.Line (100, 300)-(1000, 400), vbRed, B
End Sub
```

Run the project and click the form. Do you see any green?

Add the following line as the first statement in the preceding event procedure.

```
    Me.FillStyle = vbDiagonalCross
```

Run the project and click the form again. Do you see the green? The default for the FillStyle property is vbFSTransparent. The FillColor is ignored with this setting. Be sure to set the FillStyle property so that the FillColor property has an effect.

Exercises

B-5. Free-Hand Drawing on the Right Button. Modify the free-hand drawing project in this appendix so that the computer will draw only when the right mouse button is being pressed.

B-6. Draw a Sector. Draw a sector that is one-quarter of a circle. The sector should be enclosed by an arc and two lines joining at the arc center. The radius of the arc is 250 twips.

B-7. Rotating Christmas Lights. Modify the first Christmas lights project in this appendix so that every fourth light will go out in rotation every quarter of a second. That is, the first quarter of a second, lights 0, 4, 8, and so on will go out; the second quarter of a second, lights 1, 5, 9, and so on will go out, whereas lights 0, 4, 8, and so on will come back on. (*Hint:* Fill the light bulb with the black color to make it "go out." Fill the light bulb with its original color to make it "come back on." Note that all lights to be restored are the same color.)

B-8. Add Color to the Rolling Wheel. Modify the rolling wheel project in this appendix so that the wheel's color is white. Make sure when the wheel is "erased," the white color also "disappears."

B-9. Emulating the Clock. Draw a clock with a second hand. The hand will tick every second and complete a full rotation on the clock every minute.

B-10. Take the Sad Face to the Happy Home. Draw two image controls and a frame on a new form. Name the two image controls imgSad and imgHappy. Set the Picture properties of the two image controls to Sad.bmp and Happy.bmp. These two files are located in the Assorted subfolder of the Bitmaps folder under the Graphics folder. Set the frame's caption to "Happy Home" and name it fraHappyHome.

Provide the code so that at runtime the sad face will show but the happy face is not visible. When it is dragged into the "Happy Home" frame, it turns into the happy face. (*Hint:* Use the following statement to make fraHappyHome the logical container of imgHappy.

```
Set imgHappy.Container = fraHappyHome
```

Then, use imgHappy's Move method to move it into the frame.)

B-11. Drag and Drop in a List Box. Draw a list box on a new form. Set its List property to contain 10 of your friends' names. Provide the code so that at runtime you can drag and drop the names to rearrange the list in any order. (*Hint:* Use the AddItem and RemoveItem methods to add and delete an item in a particular position. Be aware that the ListIndex can change after either of the two methods. Thus, it is easier to handle [add or delete] the higher position first. Also, use the MouseDown and MouseUp events, not the DragDrop event.)

B-12. Drag and Drop Between Two List Boxes. Draw two list boxes onto a form. Populate both boxes with your friends' names. Provide the code so that at runtime, you can drag any name from one control and drop it into another control. Be aware that the user may drop a name on the same list box from which the name is dragged. (*Hint:* In the DragDrop event, check the Source name against the name of the other list box.)

B-13. Drag and Drop for Two List Boxes. Modify the code in Exercise B-12 so that the user can drag and drop either within the same list box or between two list boxes. (*Hint:* You will still need to check the name of the Source to perform the correct operations. Once drag and drop is started, the ListIndex does not change. You will need to use Y to compute the new position when the drag and drop is within the same list box.)

B-14. Drag and Drop the Row for the HFG. Modify the HFG project in this appendix so that the user can also drag and drop a row in the HFG. Allow the operation only when the user drags on column zero.

Index

Symbols

A

B

D

E

F

G

H

I

J

K

L

M

P

Q

R

S

T